Perioperative Assessment of the Maxillofacial Surgery Patient

AF831509

Elie M. Ferneini
Jeffrey D. Bennett
Editors

Perioperative Assessment of the Maxillofacial Surgery Patient

Problem-based Patient Management

Springer

Editors
Elie M. Ferneini
University of Connecticut
Farmington, CT
USA

Jeffrey D. Bennett
Indianapolis, IN
USA

ISBN 978-3-030-09636-6 ISBN 978-3-319-58868-1 (eBook)
https://doi.org/10.1007/978-3-319-58868-1

© Springer International Publishing AG 2018
Softcover re-print of the Hardcover 1st edition 2018
This work is subject to copyright. All rights are reserved by the Publisher, whether the whole or part of the material is concerned, specifically the rights of translation, reprinting, reuse of illustrations, recitation, broadcasting, reproduction on microfilms or in any other physical way, and transmission or information storage and retrieval, electronic adaptation, computer software, or by similar or dissimilar methodology now known or hereafter developed.
The use of general descriptive names, registered names, trademarks, service marks, etc. in this publication does not imply, even in the absence of a specific statement, that such names are exempt from the relevant protective laws and regulations and therefore free for general use.
The publisher, the authors and the editors are safe to assume that the advice and information in this book are believed to be true and accurate at the date of publication. Neither the publisher nor the authors or the editors give a warranty, express or implied, with respect to the material contained herein or for any errors or omissions that may have been made. The publisher remains neutral with regard to jurisdictional claims in published maps and institutional affiliations.

Printed on acid-free paper

This Springer imprint is published by Springer Nature
The registered company is Springer International Publishing AG
The registered company address is: Gewerbestrasse 11, 6330 Cham, Switzerland

Foreword

The preoperative management and assessment of the maxillofacial surgery patient has become more complex in recent years. The aging of our population, increased chronic disease, and increased medical treatments of illness make preoperative assessment critical to a successful surgical outcome. This book blends the art and science to enhance the clinical wisdom of the surgeon. Francis W. Peabody said in 1927 "the secret of the care of the patient is in caring for the patient." Surgical technique must have an abundant amount of personal caring in the doctor-patient relationship, but it also must be based on the latest and best medical information. The text accomplishes its goals well.

The scope of the material covered in this text is wide but relevant. The advances in surgery such as navigation and importance of behavioral issues are covered for the first time in the same surgical text. Issues of drug interactions, medical management of the surgical patients, and complications are detailed in a readable and useful manner. The chapters emphasize interprofessional management in providing the best surgical treatment and the best outcome.

Boston, MA, USA R. Bruce Donoff

Contents

Contributors

Marconi Abreu, M.D. Division of Endocrinology, Department of Internal Medicine, University of Texas Southwestern Medical Center, Dallas, TX, USA

Odette M. Aguirre, D.D.S., M.S., M.P.H. Department of Biomedical and Applied Sciences, Indiana University School of Dentistry, Indianapolis, IN, USA

Mahmood Ahmad, M.D. Shaheed Zulfiqar Ali Bhutto Medical University, Islamabad, Pakistan

Rishal Ambaram, D.D.S. Division of Oral and Maxillofacial Surgery, School of Dental Medicine, University of Connecticut, Farmington, CT, USA

Joelle El Amm, M.D. Division of Hematology and Oncology, School of Medicine, Lebanese American University, Beirut, Lebanon

Sarah T. Araji, M.D. PGY3 Obstetrics and Gynecology, Saint Joseph's Regional Medical Center, Paterson, NJ, USA

Chakib M. Ayoub, M.D., M.B.A. Department of Anesthsiology, Duke University School of Medicine, Durham, NC, USA

Roger S. Badwal, D.M.D., M.D. Division of Oral and Maxillofacial Surgery, Danbury Hospital, Danbury, CT, USA

Mohammad Banki, M.D., D.M.D., F.A.C.S. Artistic Contours, Warwick, RI, USA

Department of Surgery, Warren Alpert Medical School of Brown University, Providence, RI, USA

Division of Oral and Maxillofacial Surgery, University of Connecticut, Farmington, CT, USA

Lydia Aoun Barakat, M.D. Section of Infectious Disease, Yale University School of Medicine, New Haven, CT, USA

Jeffrey D. Bennett, D.M.D. Indianapolis, IN, USA

Michael S. Block, D.M.D. Private Practice, Metairie, LA, USA

Gary F. Bouloux, M.D., D.D.S., M.D.Sc. Division of Oral and Maxillofacial Surgery, Department of Surgery, Emory University School of Medicine, Atlanta, GA, USA

Yulanka Castro-Dominguez, M.D. Division of Cardiology, Department of Internal Medicine, Yale University School of Medicine, New Haven, CT, USA

Victor A. Chang, M.D. Yale University School of Medicine, New Haven, CT, USA

Marc Ciampi, M.D., F.A.C.P., F.A.S.N. Quinnipiac University Netter School of Medicine, North Haven, CT, USA

Yale University School of Medicine, New Haven, CT, USA

Joseph E. Cillo Jr, D.M.D., M.P.H., Ph.D., F.A.C.S. Division of Oral and Maxillofacial Surgery, Drexel University College of Medicine, Allegheny General Hospital, Allegheny Health Network, Pittsburgh, PA, USA

Jeremy D. Clark, M.D. Oculofacial Plastic and Orbital Surgery, Indianapolis, IN, USA

Department of Ophthalmology and Visual Sciences, University of Louisville, Louisville, KY, USA

Bernard J. Costello, D.M.D., M.D., F.A.C.S. Faculty Affairs, University of Pittsburgh School of Dental Medicine, Pittsburgh, PA, USA

Department of Oral and Maxillofacial Surgery, University of Pittsburgh, Pittsburgh, PA, USA

Department of Otolaryngology, University of Pittsburgh, Pittsburgh, PA, USA

H. Alexander Crisp, D.M.D. Department of Oral and Maxillofacial Surgery, Medical University of South Carolina College of Dental Medicine, Charleston, SC, USA

Roselle E. Crombie, M.D. General Surgery, Hyperbaric Medicine, Surgical Critical Care, Bridgeport Hospital, Bridgeport, CT, USA

Jasjit Dillon, D.D.S., M.B.B.S., F.D.S.R.C.S. Department of Oral and Maxillofacial Surgery, Harborview Medical Center, University of Washington, Seattle, WA, USA

Deena Elkafrawi, B.A. St. George's University School of Medicine, True Blue, Grenada

Annibal Faddoul, M.D. Department of Anesthesiology, American University of Beirut Medical Center, Beirut, Lebanon

Pooia Fattahi, M.D. Department of Neurology and Internal Medicine, Yale University, New Haven, CT, USA

Brendan Faulkner, Esq. RisCassi & Davis P.C., Hartford, CT, USA

Elie M. Ferneini, M.D., D.M.D., M.H.S., F.A.C.S. Division of Oral and Maxillofacial Surgery, University of Connecticut, Farmington, CT, USA

Beau Visage Med Spa/Greater Waterbury OMS, Cheshire, CT, USA

Antoine Ferneini, M.D., F.A.C.S. Division of Vascular Surgery, Yale-New Haven Hospital/St. Raphael Campus, North Haven, CT, USA

Connecticut Vascular Center, PC, North Haven, CT, USA

Lawrence P. Garetto, Ph.D. Department of Oral Pathology, Medicine and Radiology, Indiana University School of Dentistry, Indianapolis, IN, USA

Charles Warren Fairbanks Center for Medical Ethics, IU Health Methodist Hospital, Indianapolis, IN, USA

Marwan Ghabril, M.D. Division of Gastroenterology and Hepatology, Indiana University School of Medicine, Indianapolis, IN, USA

G.E. Ghali, D.D.S., M.D., F.A.C.S. Louisiana State University Health Sciences Center-Shreveport, Shreveport, LA, USA

Hady Ghanem, M.D. Division of Hematology and Oncology, Lebanese American University, School of Medicine, Beirut, Lebanon

Andre Ghantous, M.D., F.A.C.C. Division of Cardiology, Department of Internal Medicine, Yale University School of Medicine, New Haven, CT, USA

William Gossett, M.S.H.C.M., B.S.N., R.N., N.R.P. Department of Emergency Medicine, Indiana University Health—Ball Memorial Hospital, Muncie, IN, USA

Avni Gupta, M.D. Department of Psychiatry & Behavioral Medicine, University of Illinois-Peoria, Peoria, IL, USA

Millennium Pain Center, Unity Point Health-Methodist Hospital, Peoria, IL, USA

Thomas M. Halaszynski, D.M.D., M.D., M.B.A. Department of Anesthesiology, Yale University School of Medicine, New Haven, CT, USA

Hui Bae Harold Lee, M.D., F.A.C.S. Oculofacial Plastic and Orbital Surgery, Indianapolis, IN, USA

Jennifer Hartwell, M.D., F.A.C.S. Department of Surgery, IU Health/Methodist Hospital, Indianapolis, IN, USA

Jagdev S. Heir, M.D., D.M.D., F.A.C.S. Sacramento Surgical Arts, PC, Sacramento, CA, USA

Andrew Herlich, D.M.D., M.D., F.A.A.P. Department of Anesthesiology, University of Pittsburgh School of Medicine, Pittsburgh, PA, USA

Thomas Hickey, M.D. Yale School of Medicine, New Haven, CT, USA

VA Connecticut Healthcare System, West Haven, CT, USA

Steven Hugenberg, M.D. Rheumatology Division, Department of Medicine, Indiana University School of Medicine, Indianapolis, IN, USA

James R. Hupp, D.M.D., M.D., J.D., M.B.A. Journal of Oral Maxillofacial Surgery, Fairfield Glade, TN, USA

Emeritus of Oral-Maxillofacial Surgery, School of Dental Medicine, East Carolina University, Greenville, NC, USA

Michael P. Johnson, D.M.D., F.A.C.S Oral and Maxillofacial Surgery, Yale New Haven Hospital, Yale University, New Haven, CT, USA

Douglas Johnson, D.M.D. Oral and Facial Surgical Center, St. Augustine, FL, USA

Jayesh Kamath, M.D., Ph.D. Psychiatry and Immunology, Mood and Anxiety Program, University of Connecticut Health Center, Farmington, CT, USA

Katherine Kedzierski, M.D. Department of Neurology, Yale University, New Haven, CT, USA

Waterbury Neurology, Waterbury, CT, USA

Patrick J. Kennedy, Esq. RisCassi & Davis P.C., Hartford, CT, USA

Hassan Khalid, M.D. Division of Endocrinology, Department of Internal Medicine, University of Texas Southwestern Medical Center, Dallas, TX, USA

Shakaib Khan, M.D. Department of Psychiatry, University of Connecticut Health Center, Farmington, CT, USA

Roderick Youngdo Kim University of Michigan Oral and Maxillofacial Surgery, Ann Arbor, MI, USA

Head and Neck Oncologic and Microvascular Reconstructive Surgery, John Peter Smith Hospital, Baylor Scott & White, Fort Worth, TX, USA

Jan R. Kornilow, M.D., F.A.C.E.P., F.A.A.E.M. Department of Emergency Medicine, Indiana University Health—Ball Memorial Hospital, Muncie, IN, USA

Kyle J. Kramer, D.D.S., M.S. Department of Oral Surgery and Hospital Dentistry, Indiana University School of Dentistry, Indianapolis, IN, USA

Deepak G. Krishnan, D.D.S., F.A.C.S. Oral Maxillofacial Surgery, University of Cincinnati, Cincinnati, OH, USA

Michael Kwakye, M.D. Yale New Haven Hospital, New Haven, CT, USA

Carolyn McDonald, C.R.N.A. Department of Anesthesiology, Richard L. Roudebush VA Medical Center, Indianapolis, IN, USA

Daniel McNally, M.D. Division of Pulmonary, Critical Care and Sleep Medicine, Department of Medicine, University of Connecticut School of Medicine, Farmington, CT, USA

Julie McNeish, D.M.D., M.D. Division of Oral and Maxillofacial Surgery, School of Dental Medicine, University of Connecticut, Farmington, CT, USA

Jacques Emile Mokhbat, M.D. Division of Infectious Diseases, Department of Medicine, Lebanese American University School of Medicine, Beirut, Lebanon,

Christian A. Moore, D.M.D. Department of Oral and Maxillofacial Surgery, University of Pittsburgh, Pittsburgh, PA, USA

Kristine Mosier, D.M.D., Ph.D. Department of Radiology, Indiana University School of Medicine, Indianapolis, IN, USA

Elie Tony Nader, M.D. Division of Pulmonary and Critical Care Medicine, Norton Community Physicians Group, Norton, VA, USA

Michele Obeid, M.D. Division of Hematology and Oncology, Lebanese American University, School of Medicine, Beirut, Lebanon

James Omlie, D.D.S., M.D. Department of Oral and Maxillofacial Surgery, University of Pittsburgh Medical Center, Pittsburgh, PA, USA

Adriana D. Oprea, M.D. Department of Anesthesiology, Yale School of Medicine, New Haven, CT, USA

Frank Paletta, M.D., D.M.D., F.A.C.S. MSL Facial and Oral Surgery, Warwick, RI, USA

Warren Alpert Medical School, Brown University, Providence, RI, USA

LisaMarie Di Pasquale, D.D.S., M.D. Division of Oral and Maxillofacial Surgery, School of Dental Medicine, University of Connecticut, Farmington, CT, USA

George Sunny Pazhayattil, M.D., F.A.C.P. Quinnipiac University Netter School of Medicine, North Haven, CT, USA

Yale University School of Medicine, New Haven, CT, USA

Dmitry Peysakhov, D.M.D. Bothell Oral, Maxillofacial and Implant Surgery, Bothell, WA, USA

Timothy H. Pohlman, M.D., F.A.C.S. Department of Surgery, Section of Acute Care Surgery, Indiana University Health—Methodist Hospital, Indianapolis, IN, USA

Issa Rezek, M.D. Department of Surgery, Yale University School of Medicine, New Haven, CT, USA

Laura Romito, D.D.S., M.S., M.B.A. Nicotine Dependence Program, Indiana University School of Dentistry, Indianapolis, IN, USA

Sashidhar Sagi, M.D. Division of Gastroenterology and Hepatology, Indiana University School of Medicine, Indianapolis, IN, USA

David S. Shapiro, M.D., F.A.C.S., F.C.C.M. Department of Surgery, Saint Francis Hospital & Medical Center, Hartfort, CT, USA

Julie Ann Smith, D.D.S., M.D., M.C.R., F.I.C.D. Willamette Dental Group, Portland, OR, USA

Department of Oral and Maxillofacial Surgery, Oregon Health and Science University, Portland, OR, USA

Amit Sood, D.M.D., M.D. Division of Oral and Maxillofacial Surgery, School of Dental Medicine, University of Connecticut, Farmington, CT, USA

Martin B. Steed, D.D.S., F.A.C.S. Department of Oral and Maxillofacial Surgery, Medical University of South Carolina College of Dental Medicine, Charleston, SC, USA

Sean M. Stokes, Esq. RisCassi & Davis P.C., Hartford, CT, USA

Elisabeth M. Swanson, Esq. RisCassi & Davis P.C., Hartford, CT, USA

Pavan Tankha, D.O. Department of Anesthesiology, Yale School of Medicine, New Haven, CT, USA

Pain Management Section, VA Connecticut Healthcare System, West Haven, CT, USA

Youssef Tfaili, M.D. Department of Anesthesiology, American University of Beirut Medical Center, Beirut, Lebanon

Akashdeep Villing, D.M.D. Department of Oral and Maxillofacial Surgery, University of Washington, Seattle, WA, USA

Brent Benson Ward, M.D., D.D.S. Department of Surgery, Section of Oral and Maxillofacial Surgery, University of Michigan, Ann Arbor, MI, USA

Jennifer E. Woerner, D.M.D., M.D., F.A.C.S. Louisiana State University Health Sciences Center-Shreveport, Shreveport, LA, USA

Virginia Workman, M.D. Division of Cardiology, Department of Internal Medicine, Yale University School of Medicine, New Haven, CT, USA

Georges Yared, M.D. Department of OB/GYN, Lebanese American University School of Medicine, Beirut, Lebanon

Masoud Yeganegi, M.D., M.A.Sc. Waterbury Neurology, Waterbury, CT, USA

Jagiellonian University Medical College, Kraków, Poland

Tian Ran Zhu, M.D. Warren Alpert Medical School, Brown University, Providence, RI, USA

Tony G. Zreik, M.D., M.B.A. Department of OB/GYN, Lebanese American University School of Medicine, Beirut, Lebanon

Part 1

General Concepts in Assessment and Management of the Surgical Patient

1 Patient Safety

Jeffrey D. Bennett

Abstract

Excellent patient care is dependent upon attention to patient safety. There are many elements of patient safety that the practitioner must attend to; first and foremost is obtaining a complete medical and medication history. The more medically compromised the patient, the more time will be required to develop a thorough understanding of the patient's medical status and its implication in risk assessment. Ensuring that the correct treatment is provided is absolute. In a busy office, errors can occur. Steps, such as "time-out," to verify name and identify information, procedure, specific medical conditions, and allergies, can minimize medical errors and optimize care. Patient care extends beyond the actual time in treatment, and appropriate planning is required for continuance of care once the patient leaves the office. Despite the best of intentions and care, adverse events occur and the office must be prepared to manage these situations appropriately. Patient safety is an evolving process, and operating under the philosophy of "we have always done it this way" is no longer adequate or appropriate. This chapter will address several of these issues and others that are critical to patient safety.

1.1 Introduction

The goal of each patient encounter is to provide optimal care. A fundamental principle in medicine is "primum non nocere," translated as "first, do no harm." Patient safety is the basis for good patient care. In this chapter we will address various aspects that impact patient safety: patient selection; medical history and physical examination; management of a patient's pre-, intra-, and postoperative medications; checklists/time-out; monitoring; discharge, transference, and continuity of care; inter-professional communication; and staff and office preparation and training.

J.D. Bennett, D.M.D.
Indianapolis, IN, USA
e-mail: jb2omfs@gmail.com

© Springer International Publishing AG 2018

E.M. Ferneini, J.D. Bennett (eds.), *Perioperative Assessment of the Maxillofacial Surgery Patient*,
https://doi.org/10.1007/978-3-319-58868-1_1

1.2 The Basis for Patient Safety

Healthcare is potentially hazardous. A 2016 publication estimates that medical error is the third greatest cause of death in the United States [1]. Surgical care accounts for two-thirds of the in-hospital deaths [2]. Medical errors permeate through all aspects of patient care. These medical errors can be categorized as diagnostic errors, medication errors, anesthetic errors, surgical errors, instrument errors, and procedural errors (which may include infection control, discharge/continuity/transference of care, and communication errors).

A medical error may be *the act of neglecting or doing something wrong*, which is an "act of commission," or the *act of failing to do the correct thing* that may be secondary to a lack of knowledge or understanding, which is an "act of omission" [3].

Healthcare is complex. Care may involve that of a medically complex patient. The surgical procedure may be one that the practitioner performs routinely, but every patient is unique and the unexpected may present itself at any time. Alternatively, the procedure may be one that the surgeon rarely performs and thus presents its own challenges. While oral and maxillofacial surgeons have traditionally safely administered anesthesia to their surgical patients, such a practice is not mundane but requires a well-trained, attentive, and cohesive anesthetic team. With the changing environment of healthcare, there has been a growth in office-based ambulatory anesthesia and surgery among other specialties both in medicine and dentistry. Each of the above, the patient, the procedure, the anesthetic, and the postoperative care following a procedure, is potentially fraught with error and provides the opportunity for the occurrence of an adverse event. It is inherent for each practitioner, as well as their offices, to be observant and learn from other organizations (such as the aviation and/nuclear industry) where high-risk acts are performed and accomplished with excellent safety records on how to minimize risk.

Processes, such as medication reconciliation, medication preparation and medication dispensation, time-outs, checklists, routine and emergency care manuals, and simulated patient care, have all been shown to reduce adverse events. Patient safety is a dynamic and developing activity. Hospitals have implemented these and various systems to reduce patient risk. The challenge to the outpatient office is to implement a comparable plan, most likely without the assistance of a staff consisting of risk officers, quality control officers, and compliance officers.

1.3 Medical History

The care of every patient begins with a good history. A good medical history requires that the practitioner listen and observe the patient. It begins with listing the patient's medical ailments/illnesses, surgeries, medications, and allergies. Many offices may use a form with a checklist of medical conditions, which may be completed by the patient, staff member, or practitioner. A checklist form completed and signed by the patient endorses that this is their understanding of their medical history. However, for a patient with a low health literacy, confusion with the items may contribute to an inaccurate response; and for the patient who anticipates difficulty in receiving treatment, the form may be intentionally falsely completed.

It is clear, therefore, that the checklist form by itself is insufficient and inadequate in providing a complete medical history. The checklist, however, provides information to guide and tailor further questioning as the practitioner next completes a review of systems. The review of systems confirms the diagnosis, defines the severity of a known illness, and/or identifies signs and symptoms suggestive of a previously unrecognized or defined illness.

1.4 Medication Management

A list of a patient's medications provides further insight into the patient's medical ailments. A medication for which a medical illness was not listed may identify a need for further exploration into the medical history. Multiple medications or specific medications for a medical ailment may provide insight into the severity of that condition. Knowing the patient's medications is an essential element to providing optimal care.

Many patients take over-the-counter medications, herbal or dietary supplements, and/or prescription medications. Herbal or dietary supplements may go unreported, as many patients do not consider these to be medications; yet approximately 20% of the population may be taking such supplements [4]. This is further compounded by the inability of many patients to provide an accurate and complete list of their medications.

Medication reconciliation, which is the process of ensuring a complete and accurate list of medications that the patient is taking, is a critical safety matter.

The practitioner is responsible for continuance or discontinuance of medications during the perioperative period. The decision to continue or discontinue a medication cannot solely be deferred to a medical consultant, as they may not have a full comprehension of the planned treatment and the effect of continuance or discontinuance of the medication on patient treatment [5]. An example of this is the ability to maintain hemostatic-altering medications (e.g., warfarin, antiplatelet medications) for most dentoalveolar surgery through the perioperative period; yet if the practitioner inquires about management of these medications during the perioperative period, the consultant response will frequently suggest their discontinuance.

An adverse drug event (ADE) is an injury, which results secondary to medication use. Adverse drug events are one of the most common contributing factors to morbidity and mortality. The ADE may be anticipatable as a known side effect or toxic reaction, which may be potentially avoidable. This entails being fully knowledgeable with the medications and either using an alternative medication if such is available or employing appropriate monitoring to recognize an unwanted effect and minimizing the adverse consequences. Alternatively, the ADE may be unforeseeable as an idiosyncratic or allergic reaction. Adverse drug events are not all the result of medication error; but it is critical to implement safety steps that can minimize medication error that can contribute to adverse drug events.

Many patients take multiple medications with the prevalence higher as the patient ages. The potential for drug interactions increases with polypharmacy. Drug–drug interactions have been reported to be responsible for an adverse drug interaction or altered drug efficacy in approximately 25% of the patients in an outpatient population [6, 7]. In the patient who presents taking multiple medications, drug–drug interactions may already exist being on the threshold to manifest their effect. An example of this may be the alteration in the homeostatic balance (e.g., acid–base change) as a result of patient treatment, which affects available drug concentrations.

The delivery of anesthesia entails its unique challenges. Anesthesia-related medication errors for both general anesthesia and sedation were reported to occur at a rate of one for every 20 medication administrations with one-third of the occurrences resulting in patient harm [8]. There are multiple factors that may contribute to anesthesia-related medication errors. The medical community has experienced various drug shortages over the past several years necessitating practitioners to use drugs with which that they may be less familiar. Drug shortages have also resulted in the lack of availability of the regularly used drug concentration. The use of infusion pumps, which require the input of medication, medication concentration, bolus, and infusion rate, may contribute to an increased level of complexity and incidence of error. One study in which anesthesiologist's ability to calculate drug concentrations demonstrated that approximately 60% of the participants made significant miscalculations resulting in drug concentrations which ranged between 50 times too low and 50 times too high [9]. This may be evident when formulating drug mixtures, such as propofol–remifentanil, or diluting emergency medications such as phenylephrine to the correct concentration for intravenous administration.

The potential for error with preparation of emergency medications is compounded when the medication preparation is urgently required.

Medication errors and/or adverse drug events may be minimized by:

1. Familiarity and knowledge of medications
2. Labeling all syringes with drug name and concentration after it is drawn up into the syringe
3. Avoidance of maintaining the same drug at different concentrations
4. Verifying that the vial contains the correct drug concentration
5. Avoidance of look-alike vials
6. Avoidance of using soundalike drug names
7. Medications (e.g., phenylephrine) in ready-to-use concentrations
8. Storage of medications in a temperature-controlled environment
9. Limiting the use of a multidose vial to a single patient
10. The use of sterile technique when preparing all medications (as not swabbing with alcohol before opening a multidose vial was associated with an incidence of contamination up to 18%)
11. Connecting a medication infusion (e.g., propofol–remifentanil) to the most proximal intravenous port
12. Ensuring a patent continuous running intravenous line (which will prevent an inadvertent medication bolus when patency of an obstructed line is reestablished)
13. Appropriate (closed-loop) communication
14. Utilizing readily available manuals/aids to determine dosing for both adult and pediatric patients
15. Preventing distraction

The greater the number of perioperative medications administered during an anesthetic, the more likely for a medical error or an adverse drug event to occur. The relatively limited number of anesthetic medications administered during an office-based anesthetic is associated with a decreased incidence of medication errors and adverse drug events.

1.5 Patient Selection

Based on the medical history and physical examination of the patient, the practitioner can determine what is the appropriate anesthetic depth and where the surgery should be performed. The following criteria may dictate the anesthetic depth: ASA classification, patient age, comorbidities, and/or treatment location. The practitioner must be cognizant of anatomic and physiologic developmental stages in the pediatric patient as they impact anesthetic care.

1.6 Tracking Patient Information

The management of a diverse and complex patient population entails the use of diagnostic testing, such as laboratory tests, imaging, and/or anatomic pathology.

Failure to track these diagnostic tests may result in misdiagnosis or failure or delay to diagnose [10, 11]. The office must ensure that the patient understands the purpose for and is aware of scheduled tests. The office must subsequently follow through if the patient does not obtain such testing and either reschedule or appropriately document if the failure is secondary to noncompliance with care. The office must maintain a logbook to safeguard that it tracks all ordered tests such that all specimens are received, no abnormal results are missed, and all test results are communicated to the patient.

1.7 Checklists and Time-Outs

Healthcare is a complex process that has many steps and tasks that make risk inevitable. Several industries, such as aviation, nuclear energy, and construction, as described by Atul Gawande in his book *The Checklist Manifesto: How To Get Things Right*, have implemented processes to optimize both safety and outcome quality while minimizing risk that have only begun to be adopted within healthcare [12].

An ideal checklist is a simple standardized process. It is designed to anticipate errors, intercept them, and prevent harm from occurring. A checklist establishes protection by developing redundancy and multiple layers or steps that need to be cross-checked. At times it may force a task to be performed.

A time-out is a period of interdisciplinary discussion. It ensures communication between the team members, minimizes misunderstandings, and ensures that everybody comprehends the intended procedure.

The World Health Organization (WHO) checklist/time-out process for surgery consists of three stages: sign in, time-out, sign out [13, 14]. The process has to be simple and flexible to incorporate different approaches, such that it will be used by practitioners in various types of facilities (e.g., hospital and office), yet exacting to achieve its goal. A primary principle goal of the Joint Commission is to prevent wrong patient and wrong site surgery, which is achieved by having that the entire surgical and anesthetic teams along with the patient verify correct patient, correct procedure, correct site, and patient allergies [15]. This is not a problem that occurs solely with hospital-based surgery but is a problem in the oral and maxillofacial surgery office. As recently as 2007, wrong site surgery in oral and maxillofacial surgery accounted for 14% of the malpractice claims compared to only 2% of the claims in orthopedic surgery [16].

It facilitates that all team members are introduced and know each other as when the team is familiar with each other, it functions best. It directs those caring for the patient to discuss any anticipated critical events prior to surgery as well those involved with postoperative care to discuss recovery management. The checklist ensures critical events that optimize outcomes are completed and confirmed by the team such as antibiotic prophylaxis administration, appropriate imaging is displayed, instrument and material counts both at commencement and completion of surgery are correct, implantable biologics/devices are appropriately documented, and specimens are appropriately logged.

Anesthesia is a critical aspect of care both in the hospital and office. An anesthesia checklist confirms working instrumentation, readiness of routine and emergency medications, accessibility of emergency manuals and protocols, and system functionality.

Combined, a checklist and time-out optimize communication, team cohesiveness, and consistency of care. The introduction of a surgical checklist to patient care has resulted in a decrease in both death rate and complication rate [17]. What is achieved by the checklist and time-out goes beyond the basic concept as it results in a modification in behavior fostering a culture of safety [18]. Office-based ambulatory surgery is susceptible to the same risks that occur within the hospital. Is it not time to incorporate these concepts into the office?

1.8 Training, Guidelines, and Aids

There is significant truth to the old adage that "you are only as good as your staff." Good care is dependent on a well-organized and quality staff. Creating and maintaining a quality team entails several components: staff and team training, office guidelines, and cognitive aids.

Staff and team training consists of two components. The first aspect of staff training focuses on knowledge and skill acquisition. Each office based on the scope of surgery that is performed will require individualized and precise instruction to attain the expertise specific to that office; however, a common core among most oral and maxillofacial surgery practices is the provision of deep sedation and general anesthesia. Knowledge base must be acquired and maintained in airway management, interpretation of monitoring information and data (e.g., ECG rhythm recognition), anesthetic pharmacology and techniques, recovery and discharge assessment, and anesthetic and emergency preparation and management. The second component of staff training focuses on team functionality or *crew resource management*. Teamwork training focuses on leadership, decision-making, information management, knowledge sharing, staff member empowerment, role delegation, individual responsibility, (closed-loop) communication, collaboration, workload distribution, and situational awareness.

Task simulators provide the opportunity to acquire specific skills. Airway management is a critical aspect of anesthesia care, with adverse airway events being the highest contributor to anesthetic morbidity and mortality [19–21]. Simple airway mannequins have been shown to teach airway skills that transfer well to clinical care. These simulators allow the individual to develop skill with bag-valve-mask ventilation, oral and nasal airway placement, supraglottic airway placement, and endotracheal intubation. However, most airway instruction, which is provided in conjunction with BLS and ACLS courses, employs simple airway simulators, which unfortunately do not replicate the difficult and complex airway that may be encountered in a real emergency. The importance of the staff acquiring and maintaining airway management skill within the ambulatory office relates to the incidence in which it contributes to morbidity and the limited personnel available within the ambulatory facility who can respond to a situation.

In the hospital, the practitioner team leader sole responsibility is observing, assessing, interpreting, and directing the team, which frequently consists of nursing, respiratory, and pharmacy staff in addition to other practitioners. In the ambulatory office, the personnel is more limited with a typical solely practitioner office having in addition to the surgeon, an anesthetic assistant, a surgical assistant, and a front desk staff member. The difference in staff support is obvious and is further compounded if the staff is not adequately skilled to provide assistance to the surgeon such that the surgeon is also tasked with providing most aspects of care in addition to directing such care. While there is a lack of literature pertaining to the OMS model, the emergency and simulation literature would support staff training to optimize patient care. Practitioners must appreciate that emergency management entails a level of skill and team training above what is required for routine anesthetic delivery.

Team functionality is achieved with simulation-based training. Simulation-based training replicates the "real" event. It provides an environment in which the entire office team can repetitively immerse themselves into both routine and emergent situations. It provides the opportunity to analytically assess the operation and functionality of the individuals, team, resource allocation, and office environment without placing a patient at risk of an adverse outcome. Because knowledge and skill diminish with time, simulation-based training must be regularly scheduled as "one does best what one does often." Repetitive training reinforces knowledge and skills [22].

While all of the points listed above in regard to teamwork training are critical to a functional team, I would like to emphasize the significance and importance of staff empowerment and leveling the hierarchy of command, especially in the office environment. In most OMS offices, the incidence of emergent events is few, making the event rare for not only the staff but also the practitioner. With significant responsibility placed on the practitioner, the practitioner's focus may be misdirected. A knowledgeable staff that is empowered and understands their role and responsibility in "speaking up" may make a contribution that could critically impact the outcome of events.

"Best practice" is achieved through the establishment of a structured protocol, which may be documented in critical care pathways. Much of routine practice adheres to a specific care pathway which when used to direct care both optimizes patient outcome and minimizes adverse events. The availability of critical care pathways is even more important when confronting an emergent situation. The stress associated with an emergent situation may impair the team's ability to retrieve knowledge that is rarely used, even if the office routinely is involved in simulation exercises. Cognitive aids and manuals, which are readily available and possibly posted on the operatory wall, have the ability to provide relevant information and facilitate emergency intervention.

1.9 Discharge and Transference of Care

Continuity of patient care is critical to optimizing patient outcome. Factors contributing to a lack of continuity occur in areas of transition. Transition of care can occur when a patient is shifted from an area of acute monitoring, such as the operating room or ambulatory office operatory, to an area less supervised, such as the recovery area (especially in the ambulatory office), and finally discharged home. Transition of care may also occur secondary to the changing dynamics of medical/dental care in which several different practitioners may care for one patient. Transition of care may occur between the consultation and surgery, surgery and postoperative care, outpatient and inpatient, and/or day and night. Transition of care is a potential weakness in patient care because it provides the opportunity for miscommunication among healthcare professionals. Patient care is complex, and clinical disagreements among doctors regarding patient care in addition to miscommunication have both contributed to adverse outcomes [23, 24].

It is precisely for these reasons that the utmost diligence must be taken when transitioning a patient from one area to another area or from one practitioner to another practitioner. There are protocols that may optimize patient care. For example, continuance of respiratory monitoring (oxygen saturation and respiratory rate) and intravenous access up to discharge in the ambulatory environment after an anesthetic observes for respiratory depression which is the greatest contributor to adverse events in the sedated patient while maintaining intravenous access simplifies the ability to provide necessary intervention.

For the sedated patient, there are established criteria and parameters to guide patient assessment. A systematic approach with checklists is as advantageous for discharge as they are to prior to the surgical procedure. It is prudent that the practitioner empower their staff. The staff that has been monitoring the patient may have observed concerns that may require assessment by the practitioner prior to discharge. Ultimately, it is the practitioner's responsibility to make the final decision to discharge the patient.

1.9.1 Postoperative Analgesia

Surgery inflicts pain, and appropriate pain management is a vital component of continuity of care. Short-acting opioids are frequently administered intraoperatively. These medications smoothen the anesthetic and reduce the requirement for anesthetic agents. However, short-acting opioids, such as fentanyl, do not provide significant postoperative analgesia. The practitioner may consider the intraoperative use of long-acting local anesthetic nerve blocks, infiltration of liposomal local anesthetics, intravenous NSAIDS, and/or intravenous acetaminophen to provide initial postoperative analgesia.

Enteral postoperative medications will usually be indicated for the initial home recovery period. NSAIDs, acetaminophen, opioids, or combinations of the above may be prescribed. NSAIDs have been shown to provide comparable if not superior analgesia to the opioid/acetaminophen combination [25]. A recommended regimen for postoperative analgesia is to take a NSAID (if not contraindicated) preemptively which is initiated either just prior to, intraoperatively, or immediately after surgery at a regular interval for the first 48 h. This has been demonstrated to reduce the severity of surgical pain. An opioid/acetaminophen combination can be used to supplement the NSAID medication; however, the preemptive NSAID administration should reduce and potentially negate the need for the opioid requirement and the adverse effects associated with opioid administration. It is not inappropriate to prescribe opioids as opioids or opioid combinations may be indicated, but the medical profession must understand that there is an opioid epidemic for which overprescribing postoperative opioid analgesia is contributing to.

1.10 Equipment Safety

Equipment safety is critical to patient and staff safety. It pertains to radiation safety, anesthetic gas scavenging, sterilization efficacy, monitoring device accuracy, correctness of anesthetic gas plumbing, as well as "backup" power and lighting.

Assembly or dysfunction of any component of equipment critical to patient care can contribute to an adverse outcome. This may be illustrated by the following examples. A failure to monitor autoclave function can result in ineffective instrument sterilization with transmission of disease. An inaccuracy in anesthetic plumbing may result in the administration of the wrong anesthetic gas (e.g., a gas other than oxygen coming from the oxygen outlet). This has resulted in resuscitation of patients with anoxic gas mixtures. This can only be avoided by having an oxygen sensor within the oxygen line. Inadequate reserve power and lighting can leave the practitioner "blind" (without monitoring, without suction, without emergency equipment) and unable to provide proper care. Maintaining a checklist will force task completion to ensure a functional environment.

Regulations differ based on medical or dental licensure, whether you participate in the AAOMS office anesthesia evaluation (OAE) program or have an accredited or non-accredited office, and/or state regulations. As dental and medical professionals, it is important to ensure standards that will optimize patient and staff safety.

Conclusion

It is important that we learn from others and that we recognize our mistakes and do not repeat them. We must understand that just because we managed a situation and avoided a catastraphe does not indicate that the overall management (planned and emergent) for the patient was correct. We must understand that not all "near misses" may have been recognized and that we were simply lucky. This chapter simply introduces the reader to concepts that are being implemented in all accredited hospitals. Is it not appropriate that a facility in which surgery and anesthesia are provided adopts these same standards to optimize patient care and minimize adverse events?

References

1. Makary MA, Daniel M. Medical error—the third leading cause of death in the United States. BMJ. 2016;353:i2139.
2. de Vries EN, Ramrattan MA, SM S, et al. The incidence and nature of in-hospital adverse events: a systematic review. Qual Saf Health Care. 2008;17(3):216–23.
3. Wachter RM. The nature and frequency of medical errors and adverse events. In: Wachter RM, editor. Understanding patient safety. New York: McGraw-Hill; 2012. p. 3–9.
4. Qato DM, Wilder J, Schumm LP, et al. Changes in prescription and over-the-counter medication and dietary supplement use among older adults in the United States, 2005 vs 2011. JAMA Intern Med. 2016;176:473.
5. Gary CJ, Glick M. Medical clearance. An issue of professional autonomy, not a crutch. JADA. 2014;143:1180–1.
6. Tulner LR, Frankfort SV, Gijsen GJ, et al. Drug-drug interactions in a geriatric outpatient cohort: prevalence and relevance. Drugs Aging. 2008;25(4):343–55.
7. Gandhi TK, Weingart SN, Borus J, et al. Adverse drug events in ambulatory care. N Engl J Med. 2003;348:1556–64.
8. Nanji KC, Patel A, Shaikh S, et al. Evaluation of perioperative medication errors and adverse drug events. Anesthesiology. 2016;124:24–34.
9. Avidan A, Levin PD, Weissman C, et al. Anesthesiologists' ability in calculating weight-based concentrations for pediatric drug infusion: an observational study. J Clin Anesth. 2014;26:276–80.
10. Graber ML, Franklin N, Gordon R. Diagnostic error in internal medicine. Arch Intern Med. 2005;165:1493.
11. West DR, James KA, Fernald DH, et al. Laboratory medicine handoff gaps experienced by primary care practices: a report from the shared networks of collaborative ambulatory practices and partners (SNOCAP). J Am Board Fam Med. 2017;27:796.
12. Gawande A. The checklist manifesto: how to get things right. Basingstoke: Picador; 2009.
13. Haynes AB, Weiser TG, Berry WR, et al. Safe Surgery Saves Lives Study Group A surgical safety checklist to reduce morbidity and mortality in a global population. NEJM. 2009;360:491–9.
14. The WHO surgical safety checklist and implementation manual. Geneva: World Health Organization Press; 2016.
15. The Joint Commission Ambulatory Care Patient Safety Goals. http://www.jointcommission.org/assets/1/6/2016_NPSG_AHC_ER.pdf. Viewed on January 5, 2017.
16. Lee JS, Curley JD, Smith RA. Prevention of wrong site tooth extraction: clinical guidelines. Br J Oral Maxillofac Surg. 2009;65:1793–9.
17. ABM H, Weiser TG, Berry WR, et al. A surgical safety checklist to reduce morbidity and mortality in a global population. N Engl J Med. 2009;360:491–9.
18. Hill MR, Roberts MJ, Alderson ML, Gale TCE. Safety culture and the 5 steps to safer surgery: an intervention study. Br J Anaesth. 2015;114(6):958–62. https://doi.org/10.1093/bja/aev063. Epub 2015 Mar 16.

19. Metzner J, Posner KL, Domino KB. The risk and safety of anesthesia at remote locations: the US closed claims analysis. Curr Opin Anaesthesiol. 2009;22:502–8.
20. Bhananker SM, Posner KL, Cheney FW, et al. Injury and liability associated with monitored anesthesia care: a closed claims analysis. Anesthesiology. 2006;1045:228–34.
21. Cheney FW, Posner KL, Cheney FW. Trends in anesthesia-related death and brain damage: a closed claims analysis. Anesthesiology. 2006;105:1081–6.
22. Neily J, Mills PD, Young-Xu Y, et al. Association between implementation of a medical team training program and surgical mortality. JAMA. 2010;304:1693–700.
23. Greenberg C, Regenbogen S, Studder D, et al. Patterns of communication breakdowns resulting in injury to surgical patients. J Am Coll Surg. 2007;204:533–40.
24. Hilsden R, Molfat B, Knowles S, et al. Surgeon agreement at the time of handover, a prospective cohort study. World J Emerg Surg. 2016;11:11. https://doi.org/10.1186/s13017-016-0065-6.
25. Moore PA, WIffen PJ, Derry S, et al. Non-prescription (OTC) oral analgesics for acute pain: an overview of Cochrane reviews. Cochrane Database Syst Rev. 2015;11:CD010794.

2 Preoperative Assessment and Evaluation for Maxillofacial Surgery

Thomas M. Halaszynski

Abstract

Maxillofacial patient's surgical condition(s), medical problems, and additional healthcare comorbidities should be preoperatively identified and managed appropriately to minimize postoperative complications or reduce the likelihood of admission to a critical care setting for convalescence. Appropriate judgment and effective medical management of the maxillofacial surgery patient can be achieved by incorporating insightful actions ranging from routine preoperative assessment to extensive evaluation, therapeutic interventions, and subspecialty consultation when needed. Optimal perioperative management for the maxillofacial surgery patient reveals its greatest impact is by preparing patients for surgery and ensuring their safe and effective transition to home. Maxillofacial surgery patient preoperative care should focus on improving outcomes, implementing the discovery from innovative preoperative practice models, improving information technology, and contributing to the evolution of evidenced-based practice principles through physician leadership and redesign of pre- and perioperative processes.

2.1 Introduction

Appropriate judgment and effective medical management of the uncomplicated maxillofacial surgery patient through to and including those with significant and complex medical comorbidities can be achieved by incorporating insightful actions ranging from routine preoperative assessment to more extensive evaluation, therapeutic interventions, and subspecialty consultation. A multimodal team consisting of the maxillofacial surgeon, anesthesiologist, patient primary care provider(s), and/or medical specialty consultants often conducts the evaluation and assessment which may, in selected cases, include admission to a specialty care unit for preoperative optimization [1].

T.M. Halaszynski, D.M.D., M.D., M.B.A.
Department of Anesthesiology, Yale University School of Medicine, New Haven, CT, USA
e-mail: thomas.halaszynski@yale.edu

© Springer International Publishing AG 2018

E.M. Ferneini, J.D. Bennett (eds.), *Perioperative Assessment of the Maxillofacial Surgery Patient*,
https://doi.org/10.1007/978-3-319-58868-1_2

Optimizing preoperative preparation has a twofold benefit toward curtailing the need for extensive postoperative care and/or ICU admission. First, it is in the best interest of the patient, medical institution, and healthcare system providers to minimize the need for intensive postoperative care management and to maximize patient surgical outcome(s). As an analogy, it has been shown that high-risk elderly patients who undergo medical optimization prior to high-risk surgical interventions have decreased mortality rates [2–4]. Second, less costly healthcare resources are consumed by preoperatively addressing significant comorbid diseases in order to curtail adverse perioperative incidents without the need for postoperative admission to a more intensive care or critical care setting. In addition, the era of managed care and cost containment places increasingly more stringent guidelines as to what constitutes "appropriate" (i.e., reimbursable) utilization of hospital inpatient resources.

It is important for healthcare personnel involved in maxillofacial preoperative assessment and preparation to comprehend all the patient needs and then to coordinate perioperative care efforts, especially in those patients who are likely to require more extensive perioperative evaluation, management, and care. This remains necessary as in some situations, a patient's medical problems may extend beyond the expertise of a single practitioner. However, it still remains optimal to have one individual coordinate the several preoperative assessment and management modalities should they become necessary to perform. Prior to implementation of the managed care era, even healthy patients were being admitted to the hospital at least 1 day prior to their scheduled surgery date so that routine testing (and often times conducting excessive testing) could be performed and reviewed.

However, in the past few decades, the aforementioned preoperative preparation protocol models have been modified, and these once traditional processes have become increasingly difficult to arrange. Instead, it is the responsibility of the maxillofacial surgical practitioner to ensure adequate, and when necessary, more comprehensive preoperative patient preparation(s). Therefore, it is important for the oral surgeon to establish a working framework of perioperative management, including appropriate and comprehensive preoperative assessment(s) as needed, that will minimize preoperative inefficiencies and maximize patient surgical preparedness to yield more optimal maxillofacial surgery outcomes. The preoperative interview is also a great opportunity to discuss options for postoperative analgesia, including multimodal analgesia in order to minimize postoperative pain and morbidity.

2.2 Preadmission Testing Centers

Well-established preadmission testing (PAT) centers, structured to address the needs of performing thorough and coordinated preoperative assessment of surgical patients, have become common in medical centers throughout the United States. These centers perform anesthesia, surgical, and nursing assessments of surgical patients days prior to scheduled surgery. The centers are staffed with healthcare providers capable of performing all the necessary presurgery workups and competencies for patient optimization protocols in anticipation of elective surgical intervention(s). These centers can improve perioperative care of patients as well as augment the satisfaction of surgeons and patients alike.

The PAT center has typically been staffed and coordinated by an anesthesiologist capable of performing and supervising activities related to the preoperative assessment and management of the maxillofacial surgical patient. These responsibilities include the preoperative anesthesia history and physical (H&P) examination, the requisite general H&P, attainment and review of laboratory data, decisions as to the need for further consultation, and patient instructions regarding which medications should be discontinued, continued, or initiated prior to surgery.

The time and resources invested in scheduling maxillofacial patients for a PAT visit can result in significant direct and indirect savings related to several other aspects of a patient's perioperative care [5, 6]. For example, healthcare dollars can be saved by elimination of unnecessary or excessive "routine" laboratory testing [5–9]. Evidence has shown that another important and impactful aspect of scheduling a preoperative PAT visit is improved perioperative efficiency along with decreases in last-minute delays (i.e., obtaining old medical/surgical records, requirements for additional medical testing, or need for further specialty consultation), reduced surgical cancelations, and a decrease in length of hospital stay [10]/[11]/[12]. Additional indirect influences and positive impact from effective preoperative preparation are related to the postoperative well-being of those patients with complicated medical comorbidities.

2.3 Preoperative Assessment

Components of the maxillofacial preoperative history and physical examination along with an anesthesiology preoperative assessment can overlap as they both include a review of systems and physical examination, history of present illness, review of allergies and adverse reactions, listing of medications, prior surgeries, and family history review for evidence of any genetic or inherited healthcare issues/complications. Additionally, the preoperative portion of an anesthesiology assessment/interview will examine a patient's history for any specific anesthesia-related issues or problems (i.e., adverse medication reactions, difficult airway, need for postoperative mechanical ventilation, unanticipated ICU admission, poorly controlled pain, persistent nausea, and/or vomiting) as well as any evidence for a family history of anesthesia-related issues (e.g., pseudocholinesterase deficiency, malignant hyperthermia). An anesthesia preoperative history and physical examination also focuses on the airway, heart, and lungs, seeking to identify evidence of any disorders or abnormalities of these organ systems that could compromise intraoperative anesthesia management and postoperative surgical care.

More extensive and in-depth examination, optimization, and management of specific medical disorders or organ system compromise (neurologic, cardiac, vascular, pulmonary, hepatic, electrolytes, bariatric, psychiatric, and hematologic) are sometimes necessary that would constitute medical subspecialty consultation separate from the more "routine" preoperative surgical assessment described above. For example, preoperative preparation of the high-risk maxillofacial surgical patient may benefit from consultation by those who will be subsequently collaborating with the surgeon during the postoperative period if critical care management of high-risk surgical patients should become necessary. This consultation process can be coordinated between the surgeons in conjunction with the protocols established by the practitioners from the preadmission testing center. A similar concept, known as the "Perioperative Surgical Home" (PSH, further described below), permits for a more seamless transition for the patient should any need for postoperative critical care management become necessary. However, decisions regarding specialty consultation, how and when such requests should be made, may not always be obvious. Therefore, several subspecialty organizations have developed protocols and guidelines for the practitioner to implement such as those provided by the American College of Cardiology and American Heart Association (ACC/AHA) [13]. These guidelines can provide a level of consistency when concerns related to the high-risk maxillofacial surgical patient (i.e., symptomatic or new-onset cardiovascular disease) are presented to the surgeon.

Summations from a host of aspects of the maxillofacial patient's preoperative assessment, based on their medical condition(s) and any necessary input from consultants, will permit the anesthesiologist to grade each patient according to a I-to-V (along with modifier E and optional VI) rating scale. Table 2.1 describes such a system that has become a well-established terminology grading mechanism and identified as the American Society of Anesthesiologists (ASA) physical status classification [14, 15]. These patient physical status classification categories have proven efficacious for assessing the fitness of patients prior to surgery, as well as predict perioperative morbidity and mortality [8, 16, 17].

Table 2.1 ASA physical status classification

Modified from American Society of Anesthesiologists physical status classification*		
Class	*Description*	*Examples*
I	• There are no organic, physiologic, biochemical, or psychiatric disturbances • Surgical etiology does not entail a systemic disturbance • Surgical problem is localized	Otherwise healthy patient [Patient for "routine" (nonimpacted) dental extraction(s), bunion repair, hernia repair, lumpectomy, asymptomatic fibroids]
II	• Mild to moderate systemic disturbance(s) • Systemic disturbance may or may not be related to the reason for surgery	Well-controlled hypertension, h/o asthma, anemia, tobacco use, controlled diabetes, mild obesity, age < 1 year or >70 years, malignancy without evidence of significant spread or physiological disturbance, controlled seizure disorder, moderate hyperparathyroidism, treated hyper- or hypothyroidism, localized colitis, localized Crohn's or diverticulitis, renal stones, asymptomatic pituitary tumor, painful or moderately bleeding fibroids
III	• Severe (but not incapacitating or acutely life-threatening) systemic disturbance that may or may not be related to the reason for surgery	Angina, poorly controlled hypertension, poorly controlled diabetes, symptomatic COPD or asthma, massive obesity, renal failure on dialysis, poorly controlled thyroid dysfunction, widespread inflammatory bowel disease, S/P chemotherapy, pituitary tumor with systemic effects, brain tumor with focal signs, sleep apnea, O_2 sat 90–93%, atrial fibrillation with controlled heart rate, h/o cerebrovascular accident, fibroids causing significant anemia (leading to hypotension and/or need for transfusion)
IV	• Severe systemic disturbance that is life-threatening with or without surgery • Systemic disturbance where invasive monitoring likely required to manage the patient prior to induction of anesthesia	"Unstable" angina, CHF, debilitating respiratory disease, hepatorenal failure, brain tumor with significant neurological dysfunction or increased ICP, severe sleep apnea with pulmonary hypertension, O_2 sat < 90 at rest, recurrent V-tach/V-fib, significant compromise from atrial fibrillation, recent CVA (≤ 1 month) or recurrent TIAs, symptomatic cerebral aneurysm or arteriovenous malformation, fibroids causing dangerous deep vein thrombosis requiring current anticoagulation (h/o significant threat of pulmonary embolus)
V	• Moribund patient who has little chance of survival • Patient submitted to surgery as a last resort • Desperation measure and/or resuscitation effort	Patient with acutely deteriorating brain function due to bleeding cerebral aneurysm, "crash" in cardiac catheterization laboratory
VI	• Brain-dead patient for organ harvesting	
E	• Modifier for any patient in whom an emergency operation is required	Patient with acute trauma, recent food ingestion, postoperative problem requiring emergency surgery

COPD chronic obstructive pulmonary disease, *S/P* status-post, *h/o* history of, *CHF* congestive heart failure, *ICP* intracranial pressure, *V* ventricular, *CVA* cardiovascular accident, *TIA* transient ischemic attack

There remain three important components of the anesthesiologist's preoperative assessment process that the ASA physical status classification system does not directly address including, but not limited to:

1. Reports or history of airway problems (e.g., difficult mask ventilation/intubation, sleep apnea) and examination of the difficult airway (seek additional references for more detailed information)
2. Risk(s) and/or complexity associated with the maxillofacial surgical procedure
3. Potential for any adverse reaction(s) to administration of anesthesia secondary to an anesthesia-specific patient disorder (unless the etiology itself would be a cause for a higher ASA physical status score)

However, these concerns must always be incorporated into perioperative perspectives when managing a maxillofacial patients' surgical care. Even though influences and effects of a maxillofacial patient's surgical condition on systemic well-being is incorporated into the ASA physical status scoring system, the nature and complexity of the actual planned surgical procedure(s) is not part of and should not influence the score.

A possible negative impact upon patients from proposed maxillofacial surgery and influence on the focus of the preoperative assessment has been emphasized by the ACC/AHA in the guidelines for cardiac evaluation prior to noncardiac surgery [13]. This impact is related to the nature of the planned surgery and its capacity to have any effect upon parameters of the preoperative assessment that has also been addressed in the literature [8, 18]. Several investigators, authors, and other practitioners have classified surgery into three (or more subdivisions) categories by risk stratification in order to assess for potential patient-specific compromise associated with planned maxillofacial surgery:

- Low risk—minimal physiologic stress potential or risk toward the patient (independent of a patient's medical condition), rarely requires the need for blood transfusion, invasive monitoring, or ICU care, e.g., office-based surgery and minor surgery (routine dental extraction).
- Moderate risk—increased physiologic stress and risk (such as fluid shifts), typically with minimal blood loss, but the potential must be appreciated, e.g., full-mouth extractions secondary to the teeth that have been affected by extensive caries and/or periodontal disease.
- High risk—significant perioperative stress and potential for added postoperative physiologic stress, increased likelihood to require a blood transfusion and/or larger amounts of fluids or body fluid shifts, invasive monitoring, and postoperative management in ICU setting, e.g., extensive maxillofacial surgery linked to short-term stroke and heart attack risk or maxillofacial surgery that deals with high-risk medically compromising patients.

There are patients presenting for maxillofacial surgery where the potential for an associated disorder can be inferred. For example, patients with a medical history of aortic and/or peripheral vascular disease have a higher likelihood of significant coronary artery disease, or when a patient's diabetes is associated with an autonomic neuropathy, they are also predisposed to an increased likelihood of coronary artery disease [18]. It has been suggested that structuring preoperative interventions, especially in the medically compromised patient, be designed to lessen the probability of adverse perioperative outcomes. This is possible when preoperative assessments on those with significant comorbidities are structured in accordance with what has been termed "precaution protocols" (i.e., cardiac ischemia precautions (grades 1–3) and hypertension precautions). Degree(s) of precaution incorporated should be made dependent on both the severity of underlying disease and possible ramifications toward the surgical risk(s) involved [19].

2.3.1 Assessment of Anesthesia-Related and Anesthesia-Specific Disorders

Systemic disorders, as well as a history of an adverse perioperative reaction/interaction to medications, can have an impact on perioperative care of the surgical patient and predispose patients to the need for unanticipated perioperative events. Preoperative assessment of the maxillofacial patient should involve identification of disorders, adverse reactions to, or allergy from use of any of the anticipated intraoperative anesthetic agent(s) or antibiotics used during surgery [20–26]. For example, use of inhalational agents (anesthetic agent possessing general anesthetic properties delivered by inhalation) should be avoided in the patient with a history of or immediate family member with a history of malignant hyperthermia.

Patients describing a history (or family history) of prolonged intubation hours following minor surgery could have a likely diagnosis of atypical pseudocholinesterase that causes an inability to metabolize succinylcholine (depolarizing neuromuscular blocking drug). Such a diagnosis can be confirmed with a blood test identifying decreased pseudocholinesterase activity that should be further explored and then caution expressed to perioperative team members to avoid use of succinylcholine [21]. Patients with a diagnosis of myasthenia gravis can also present with perioperative prolonged muscle paralysis precipitated by anesthesia. Myasthenia gravis is characterized as autoimmune destruction of acetylcholine receptors capable of resulting in progressive weakness (neuromuscular "fade") following repeated muscle stimulation or persistent muscle activity [22]. Damage to the acetylcholine receptors will predispose the muscular system neuromuscular junction complex to exaggerated responses caused by non-depolarizing neuromuscular blocking medications (i.e., curare, pancuronium, vecuronium, atracurium, and rocuronium). Management of the maxillofacial surgery patient with a history of myasthenia gravis during preoperative planning is to determine if it is appropriate to discontinue anticholinesterase medications the day prior to scheduled surgery (cessation of anticholinesterase drugs facilitates anesthesia management since such agents can influence effects of neuromuscular blocking agents). However, making such a decision should not be attempted in those with a history of severe muscle weakness or for patients who are anticholinesterase-dependent.

Malignant hyperthermia is a true life-threatening systemic response. It is caused by increased intracellular concentrations of calcium that can be precipitated by inhalational anesthetic agents (alter muscle cell membrane integrity) and depolarizing muscle relaxants like succinylcholine (leading to simultaneous contractions of skeletal muscles) [23]. Clinical signs/symptoms include hypercarbia, hyperthermia, arrhythmias, acidosis, muscle rigidity, increased creatinine kinase, and myoglobinuria. Safe anesthesia management of the susceptible MH patient is first to recognize the condition (by patient report or history of diagnosis in an immediate family member) and to then plan accordingly by avoiding known triggering agents during the perioperative period. Without a prior history of MH, it cannot be diagnosed until a crisis develops in a susceptible patient. However, there is an increased possibility of MH in some patients with particular diagnosis such as muscular dystrophy, those with strabismus, and patients with neurofibromatosis. Confirmation of MH can be made with muscle biopsy testing showing a positive caffeine-halothane contracture test.

Historically, mortality was high from MH prior to the introduction of dantrolene (an antidote medication that can stabilize muscle cell membranes and limits intracellular calcium levels). There was a time when anesthesiologists would electively administer dantrolene (prophylactic dantrolene can cause muscle weakness and gastrointestinal upset) and pretreat the MH-susceptible patient. However, it is now believed that dantrolene pretreatment is not necessary, provided non-triggering anesthetics are administered. Therefore, total intravenous anesthesia (TIVA) can be employed using an oxygen-flushed anesthesia machine, monitoring end-expired carbon dioxide, and having dantrolene along with MH protocol supplies readily available. Table 2.2 summarizes the treatment regimen/protocol to be used if a potential diagnosis of MH is suspected and/or confirmed. In addition, MH may first become recognized during the postoperative period, further necessitating an understanding of the potential signs and symptoms along with knowledge of diagnostic and therapeutic interventions.

Adverse reactions and life-threatening responses to neuromuscular blocking agents may occur in patients with denervating disorders/diseases including amyotrophic lateral sclerosis, history of massive tissue trauma, denervating injuries (stroke or major nerve injury), and muscle disorders (muscular dystrophy) [21–23]. Patients with serious denervation disorders can experience proliferation of extra-junctional acetylcholine receptors such that when these receptors are exposed to succinylcholine an exaggerated efflux of potassium can occur along with life-threatening hyperkalemia and profound muscle contractions. Burn injury patients and those who have suffered from major soft tissue trauma are also predisposed to succinylcholine-induced hyperkalemia [27]. Muscle integrity can also be compromised by myopathies such that fasciculations (brief and spontaneous uncoordinated muscle contractions) caused by succinylcholine could result in a massive efflux of potassium or precipitate rhabdomyolysis [24–26].

Table 2.2 Treatment protocol for malignant hyperthermia

1.	Call for *help*
2.	Remove all possible *triggering agents*. Discontinue the anesthesia and stop surgery as soon as possible. Change the airway tubing and/or anesthesia machine if possible
3.	*Hyperventilate* with 100% oxygen in order to decrease $PaCO_2$ and increase oxygenation
4.	Administer *dantrolene* (≥2.5 mg Kg^{-1} IV, repeated as needed (i.e., titrate to heart rate, temperature, pCO_2 or followed by a rapid infusion of an additional 7.5 mg Kg^{-1}). Most cases will respond to 3–5 mg Kg^{-1}. Alternatively, infuse 1 mg kg^{-1} min^{-1} until relief of adverse signs is detected, and then repeat half the initial dose at 4-hour intervals until all signs and symptoms have resolved. If the episode does not resolve within several minutes, then an additional 10 mg Kg^{-1} (possibly much higher doses) should be used, or a rapid infusion may be titrated to effect
5.	Place an arterial line, CVP catheter, urinary catheter, and core temperature monitor
6.	*If severe hyperthermia is present*, cool the patient by packing in ice, infusing cooled saline, and possibly lavaging the stomach, rectum, and peritoneum (cooling measures should be stopped when the body temperature reaches approximately 38 °C to avoid hypothermia)
7.	*If acidosis is severe and unresolving*, consider administering sodium bicarbonate. Otherwise, it may be best to avoid the Na^+ and bicarbonate load that is also provided by the dantrolene solution
8.	*Maintain urine output* with fluids and diuretics, BUT NOT with lactated Ringer's solution as it contains K^+ and Ca^{2+}. An output of ≥0.2 mL kg^{-1} hr^{-1} should prevent myoglobin cast formation
9.	Administer *procainamide* (≤1 gm/70 kg/30 min) if arrhythmias persist following dantrolene administration. In addition to procainamide being an antiarrhythmic, it inhibits drug-induced contractures in MH-susceptible muscle in vitro (not as effectively as dantrolene). Procainamide may be infused until the arrhythmias have resolved, unless the QT interval is prolonged by 50% or more. Such prolongation indicates significant cardiac depression, which may be treated with isoproterenol. The safety of other antiarrhythmics has not been proven; lidocaine and other amide local anesthetics have been used safely; calcium channel blockers are less helpful and may be contraindicated
10.	*Maintain cardiac output*, which may be compromised in the context of acidosis, hyperkalemia, hemoconcentration, arrhythmias, and their treatment
11.	Treat *hyperkalemia* (using insulin at 0.1–0.2 units kg^{-1} and dextrose at 0.5–1.0 mg Kg^{-1}), *hypoglycemia* (which may result from the hypermetabolic state), *hypovolemia, coagulopathy,* and other related abnormalities. If hypokalemia develops, treat it slowly because of potentially decreased renal function and the possibility that a marked increase in K^+ may retrigger an MH episode

Monitor patients for a minimum of 24–48 h. An MH crisis can recrudesce following successful resolution of the initial episode. Recrudescence is especially likely if all parameters have not fully returned too normal (e.g., heart rate). *Dantrolene should be continued for* several doses (possibly for 24 h), and the dosing interval should be titrated to symptoms (taking into account that the $t_{1/2}$ of dantrolene given IV is 12 h and that therapeutic plasma levels (>2.5 μg mL^{-1}) typically persist for 4–6 h following 2.5 mg kg^{-1} IV)

Note: The Malignant Hyperthermia Association of the United States (MHAUS) is an organization with 24-hour numbers:
209-634-4917 for emergency calls as well as public information
607-674-7901 for patients and families
800-644-9737 (800-MH HYPER) for immediate expert consultation
website: http://www.mhaus.org

2.3.2 Preoperative Laboratory Testing of the Maxillofacial Patient

Across the board, ordering of preoperative screening tests, as opposed to a more coordinated and directed testing approach, has been reviewed in the literature [7, 8, 28–33]. Directed testing has proven to be more cost-effective and efficient [34–36].

There is evidence that routine testing and indiscriminate blood screenings are of little-to-no direct patient benefit. For example, even for the older patient, it has been found that "routine" laboratory testing protocols were less predictive of perioperative morbidity than ASA physical status classification or surgical risk stratification [37]. It is also identified that the more tests that are ordered, there is a greater likelihood that an abnormal testing result will be found ("…for every 20 tests ordered, the chance that all results will be in the normal range is only 36%.") [16]. Arbitrarily, performing preoperative screening tests that have a low specificity for a significant disorder and/or low prevalence in a given patient population can result in false-positive findings that could further lead to costly, time-consuming, and even hazardous patient workups.

It has been shown to be more preferable and cost-effective to establish preoperative testing guidelines wherein strategic testing parameters are based upon information obtained during the preoperative assessment such as:

1. Presence of a medical condition determined from the preoperative history and physical examination (as reflected by overall ASA physical status or specific disease/disorder);
2. Patient categorized in a "high-risk" group based on epidemiology data (i.e., EKG for male patient ≥70 years of age);
3. Legitimate benefit from obtaining an otherwise nonselective baseline testing parameter secondary to the real potential of intra- and/or postoperative change(s) (i.e., high-risk surgical intervention); and
4. Anticipated need for more intensive postoperative care (ICU admission) that would have an impact upon preoperative tested indices.

Consistent with the above criteria [7], the ASA has also proposed general guidelines for preoperative testing [38]; however, *total* evidence to identify explicit decision parameters or rules for ordering preoperative tests based on specific patient factors is lacking.

A proposed preoperative laboratory testing guideline for the maxillofacial surgery patient is identified in Fig. 2.1. It has been developed by selecting specific guideline data from several national organizations and tailored to the maxillofacial surgery patient in order to facilitate preoperative assessment and preparation (providing consistency while maintaining practitioner flexibility). Indications toward determining testing parameters are based on patient age (i.e., no testing required in a healthy patient <45 years old who is undergoing minor surgery), surgical risk stratification (i.e., minor-, moderate-, or high-risk surgery), and medical disease or comorbidities. The columns of the figure include suggestions for additional testing that may be required prior to different surgical procedures (based on overall surgical complexity as well as specific medical comorbidity aspects) and/or recommended testing due to varied medical conditions in order to assess for readiness of surgery as well as provide baseline information for those patients where perioperative problems may be suspected intra- or postoperatively. Some testing selections should be performed within 30 days of planned surgery (shaded areas) as the results of these tests may prove vital to the assessment of the given disease/disorder. Additional testing (including repeat testing on the day of surgery) may be indicated if new or worsening of existing medical issues should surface or with exacerbation of preexisting disease(s) and/or surgical signs and symptoms. As per a recent ASA Practice Advisory, "More recent test results may be desirable if the medical history has changed, or when test results may play a role in the selection of a specific anesthetic" [38].

2.3.2.1 Instructions for Optimization of Patient Medications

On the day of scheduled surgery (despite the desire to minimize oral intake several hours prior to surgery), patients are typically directed to take some of their morning prescription medications with just enough water to swallow the medication. The prescription agents routinely taken/continued on the day of surgery include cardiac (digitalis and beta-blockers), respiratory/asthma (e.g., metered-dose inhalers), antiseizure, endocrine, steroid, and gastrointestinal medications (for treatment of gastroesophageal reflux disease). Other groups of medications that should be continued on the day of surgery if scheduled to be taken in the morning, with few exceptions, include analgesics and chronic pain agents (possible exception, aspirin-containing medications and nonsteroidal anti-inflammatory drugs), antianxiety drugs (possible exception, monoamine oxidase inhibitors (MAOIs) and tricyclic antidepressants), and antihypertensive

TEST	MINOR SURG. IN HEALTHY PATIENT (w/in 90 days)				Additive Medical Factors for Moderate & High Risk Maxillo facial Surgery: HIGHRisk Surgical Procedures (within 90days)			Additive Medical Factors for Moderate & High Risk Maxillo facial Surgery: ClinicallySignificantandChanging Medical Disorders and/or Medication (white-w/in 90 days; gray-given test for given disorder likely should be w/in 30 days)																			
	HealthyAdult <45	45-54 y/o	55-69 y/o	≥70 y/o			Anticipate > 2u	Hypertension	Smoking	Morbid Obesity	h/o Stroke	Cancer (?metastatic)	Seizure Meds	Cardiovascular	Respiratory	Daibetes	Hepatic	Renal	Fluid or Lyte Loss	Autoimmune/Lupus	EtoH/DrugAbuse	Steroids/Cushings	HIV	Parathyroid	Unstable Thyroid	Anticoag/Bleeding	Suspected Pregnan.
ECG		M	Y	Y	Y		Y	Y	Y	Y	Y	Y		Y	Y	Y	Y	Y	±	Y	Y	Y	Y	Y	Y		
CBC+plates			Y	Y	Y		Y			Y	Y	Y	Y	Y	Y	Y	Y	Y	Y	Y	Y	Y	Y	Y	Y	Y	
Lytes				Y	Y		Y	Y		Y	Y	Y		Y	Y	Y	Y	Y	Y	Y	Y	Y	Y	Y	Y		
BUN/Creat				Y	Y		Y	Y			Y	Y		Y	Y	Y	Y	Y		Y	Y	Y	Y	Y	Y		
Glucose				Y	Y		Y			Y	Y	Y		Y		Y	Y	Y			Y	Y	Y	Y	Y		
LFTs					±							Y	Y				Y				Y		Y				
Calcium																								Y			
PT/PTT					S		Y										Y	Y		Y	Y					Y	
U/A (?culture)					S																						
CXR					±							S			Y								S				
Hormone Levels					±																				Y		
Bleed Time																										±	
Pregnancy					Y																						Y
DrugLevels													S								±						
TumorMarkers												S															
Clot	**Depends primarily on extensiveness of proposed surgery andper Institutional Blood Bank guidelines.**																										

Fig. 2.1 General suggestions for adult maxillofacial surgery preoperative testing. *Y* usually indicated, *M* usually indicated for male, *S* may be requested and reviewed by surgeon as part of surgical w/u,; ± if situation acute/severe. *Comments*: (1) Testing for a given disorder depends on severity of the disorder in the context of planned surgery, i.e., are the tests likely to generate potentially clinically significant information and provide information that would be an important component of the H&P (e.g., a brief course of steroids or a h/o asymptomatic mitral valve prolapse does not warrant testing). (2) Times and test listings are suggestions: they are not absolute and should not preclude other testings in given settings nor should they prevent a case from proceeding if the anesthesiologist and surgeon deem that to be appropriate. (3) An anesthesiologist would not routinely order a chest X-ray unless there is suspected airway compromise or an acute pulmonary problem; if the surgeon or PCP wants a CXR for another reason (e.g., metastatic workup), then it is the responsibility of that individual to follow up on the report

medications (possible exception, angiotensin converting enzyme (ACE) inhibitors and angiotensin II receptor blockers). There are also differences among certain classes of medications that could prove critical to patient perioperative management and must be appreciated. For example, to decrease the risk of intraoperative acid aspiration, it is a routine to continue H2-blockers and proton pump antagonists. However, over-the-counter particulate antacids such as Tums should be withheld (and substituted with an alternative medication if deemed necessary) on the day of surgery due to potential adverse deleterious effects (i.e., aspiration of the drug particulate matter).

2.3.3 Antihyperglycemic Medications

On the morning of a patient's maxillofacial surgery, oral hypoglycemic agents should be withheld in addition to consideration that some of these medications (i.e., the long-acting agents) be discontinued on the evening prior to surgery, especially if a patient is prone to morning hypoglycemia.

Patient instructions on insulin (short-acting versus long-acting) administration on the day of scheduled surgery can be complex and are handled differently for inpatients compared to outpatient surgery candidates. On the morning of surgery for an inpatient, a portion of the morning insulin dose is commonly provided (to facilitate "tight" blood sugar control) with an ability to administer intravenous glucose if required. However, for the outpatient coming in from home on the day of surgery, they should be instructed not to take any of their morning insulin (concerns of inducing hypoglycemia while patients are en route or waiting in the hospital). Further challenges arise when instructing an insulin-dependent patient's evening prior to surgery insulin administration. For example, depending upon the likelihood of hypoglycemia if a patient does not eat breakfast upon awakening, consideration toward the amount of long-acting insulin taken the night before surgery may need to be reduced. For all insulin-dependent patients upon arrival to the hospital on the day of their scheduled surgery, dosing of insulin for outpatients can be titrated according to blood sugar concentration testing.

2.3.4 Antihypertensive Medications

Preoperative assessment of the maxillofacial surgery patient must include queries about hemodynamic status, presence of hypo- or hypertension, use and duration of antihypertensive medications, and duration and evidence of any changes in the diagnosis of the disorder or prescription medications used for treating the disease. Hypertension can be associated with an increased surgical risk ranging from benign perioperative blood pressure fluctuations (stage I (mild) and stage II (moderate) hypertension with systolic <180 mmHg and diastolic <110 mmHg) to a more escalated concern of hyper- and/or hypotension with the potential for progression to myocardial ischemia and stroke in more extreme circumstances [13, 39–42]. However, moderate hypertension could also be associated with pathophysiology of organ injury and predispose patients to dangerously high pressures during the intraoperative period. Such patients would benefit from enhanced at-home therapy, and these individuals may also require intervention and treatment on the morning of surgery. Medical intervention/treatment and possibility of delaying elective maxillofacial surgery should be seriously considered for the patient presenting with stage III hypertension (severe, systolic >180 mmHg or diastolic >110 mmHg) in order to permit medical therapy [13, 40, 43, 44] as the ACC/AHA guidelines recommend that such blood pressure be "controlled" before surgery [13].

Hypertensive patients can also present with left ventricular hypertrophy (associated with increased afterload from persistent vasoconstriction), coronary artery disease, poor exercise tolerance, chronic renal insufficiency and hypovolemia, and/or history of cerebrovascular disease (i.e., transient ischemic attaches). When end-organ disease/damage is suspected, an electrocardiogram and serum creatinine measurement should be obtained [38]. History of difficult and/or poorly controlled hypertension should alert the practitioner to look for evidence of other treatable causes such as: pheochromocytoma, hyperthyroidism, increased intracranial pressure, coarctation, hyperadrenalism, renal disease, renal artery stenosis, acromegaly, hypercalcemia, and extreme anxiety.

Maxillofacial surgery patients should be maintained on most of their antihypertensive medications, especially beta-blockers, up to and including the morning of surgery [13, 38]. Withdrawal of beta-blocker antihypertensive medications, like many other antihypertensive agents, could result in a perioperative situation associated with "rebound" hypertension and tachycardia [41]. However, there are certain classes of hypertensive medication that should be routinely withheld unless preoperative consultant recommendations indicate that such agents should be continued to avoid patient compromise or harm. These classes of antihypertensive drugs that should be withheld on the day of surgery include:

1. Diuretic medications (unless they are vital to the management of congestive heart failure or continued treatment is necessary due to fluid and electrolyte disturbances) to avoid hemodynamic compromise, intravascular volume depletion, and excessive bladder filling during surgery
2. Angiotensin converting enzyme (ACE) inhibitors
3. Angiotensin receptor blockers (ARBs) unless continuation is vital to the prevention of severe hypertension or administration is necessary to reduce afterload in a failing heart [44]

Therefore, it is recommended to withhold these antihypertensive medications on the day of surgery since continuing them can result in significant intraoperative hypotension and hypovolemia that can become even more pronounced with perioperative blood or fluid losses and general anesthesia [44, 45].

2.3.5 Antithrombotic Medications

Tables 2.3 and 2.4 provide information related to both the classes (Table 2.3) in addition to preoperative guidelines (Table 2.4) for the surgical patient who is taking coagulation-altering medications. There are several other sources and data-based protocols that can be used to help instruct and guide the surgeon when dealing with those patients taking coagulation-altering medications [46–52]. The perioperative care team needs to have a general understanding of information within these guidelines in order to more properly instruct the maxillofacial surgery patient related to how to best manage these agents preoperatively and to determine if, and when, to withhold medications with antiplatelet and anticoagulant effects.

Table 2.3 Classes of hemostasis-altering medications

Herbal medications [53] • Garlic • Ginkgo • Ginseng
Antiplatelet medications • Aspirin (ASA) • Nonsteroidal anti-inflammatory drugs (NSAIDs) • Thienopyridine derivatives (ticlopidine, clopidogrel) • Platelet glycoprotein IIb/IIIa inhibitors (GPIIb/IIIa receptor antagonists)
Unfractionated heparin (UFH) intravenous and subcutaneous
Low-molecular-weight heparin (LMWH)
Vitamin K antagonists: warfarin
Thrombin (factor IIa) inhibitors • Desirudin • Lepirudin • Bivalirudin • Argatroban
Factor Xa inhibitors • Fondaparinux • Rivaroxaban • Apixaban • Edoxaban
Thrombolytic and fibrinolysis medications • Tissue plasminogen activator (tPA) • Streptokinase • Urokinase • Anistreplase

Table 2.4 General guidelines for drugs that influence platelet function and coagulation

Drugs	Typical guidelines for withholding	Comments
• Aspirin or aspirin-containing products (effect lasts 7–10 days, duration of the platelet)	• Up to 10 days prior to surgery	• Aspirin as an analgesic or other nonspecific reasons • Decision by surgeon, anesthesiologist, primary care physician, and/or cardiologist based on risks/benefits [54] • At times, continued for those with cardiac (CABG), carotid, and pacemaker surgery (unless otherwise indicated)
• Nonsteroidal anti-inflammatory drugs (NSAIDs)	• Up to 5 days prior to surgery	• PCP or surgeon should determine if patient can tolerate discontinuance (e.g., may lead to flare-up of arthritis?)
• Cyclooxygenase inhibitors (COX-2 inhibitors)	• Up to 5 days prior to surgery	• Many surgeons elect to maintain patients on cyclooxygenase type 2 inhibitors, in that they do not appear to affect platelet function [55–57]
Clopidogrel (Plavix) Ticlopidine (Ticlid)	• Up to 7–10 days prior to surgery • Up to 10–14 days prior to surgery (the actual risk of spinal hematoma with ticlopidine and clopidogrel is unknown)	• Often discontinued even if aspirin continued • Patients who have had recent percutaneous coronary intervention may require antiplatelet therapy with clopidogrel or ticlopidine for several weeks [58–62] • Consult and follow instructions provided by internist, cardiologist, or cardiac surgeon in context of perioperative risk with respect to surgical bleeding or stent thrombosis • Platelet transfusion (possibly methylprednisolone) may reverse effects of thienopyridines
Dipyridamole (Persantine)	• Discontinue use 1 day prior to surgery	• Consult and follow instructions provided by internist, cardiologist, or cardiac surgeon in context of perioperative risk with respect to surgical bleeding or thrombotic event [63, 64]
GPIIb/IIIa inhibitors (profound effect on platelet aggregation)	• GP IIb/IIIa antagonists are discontinued within 4 weeks of surgery (the actual risk of spinal hematoma with the GP IIb/IIIa antagonists is unknown)	• Time to normal platelet aggregation is 24–48 h for abciximab and 4–8 h for eptifibatide and tirofiban • Patients of recent percutaneous coronary intervention may require antiplatelet therapy for several weeks
Anticoagulants		
Coumadin [65–70]	• Up to 4–5 days prior to surgery	• If surgery is minimally invasive, may not need to return prothrombin time to baseline • If anticoagulation is critical, add low-molecular-weight heparin or IV/SQ heparin after Coumadin stopped • Check INR or prothrombin time to confirm return of normal coagulation
Low-molecular-weight heparin (e.g., enoxaparin (Lovenox)) [71–73]	• Discontinue use 12 h prior to surgery	• May replace Coumadin preoperatively because of its short half-life • Increased risk of bleeding if given in combination with other agents

Table 2.4 (continued)

Drugs	Typical guidelines for withholding	Comments
IV/SQ heparin (therapeutic and full- or low-dose and prophylactic standard heparin)	• Discontinue use 2–4 h (IV) and 4–6 h (SQ) prior to surgery	• Increased risk of bleeding if given in combination with other agents
Thrombotic agents (e.g., streptokinase, tPA)	• Discontinue use 1–2 days prior to surgery	
Fondaparinux 2.5 mg SC QD	4 days	With a shared assessment, a 2 half-life interval discontinuation may be considered in low-risk maxillofacial surgery
Dabigatran	4–5 days (normal renal function) 6 days (impaired renal function)	With a shared assessment, a 2 half-life interval discontinuation may be considered in low-risk maxillofacial surgery
Rivaroxaban	3 days	With a shared assessment, a 2 half-life interval discontinuations may be considered in low-risk maxillofacial surgery
Apixaban	3–5 days	With a shared assessment, a 2 half-life interval discontinuations may be considered in low-risk maxillofacial surgery

2.4 Perioperative Surgical Home as a Model for Preoperative Assessment of the Maxillofacial Surgery Patient

Healthcare in the United States has been a subject of national debate and is facing continued concerns toward the quality, scope, quantity, and cost of delivering care. Solutions for the most optimal answers are complex and multifactorial, but perioperative care, especially providing an ideal means of preoperative surgical assessment, is one dilemma to improve upon and to provide added value toward healthcare in the United States. An ideal preoperative surgical assessment, structured as a component of the current perioperative system, is one way to better (1) manage the increasing costs of delivery of surgical care, (2) focus on reducing perioperative complications, (3) minimize longer than necessary lengths of hospital stays, and (4) eliminate or reduce excess readmission rates [74–76].

The Perioperative Surgical Home (PSH) is a practice model being proposed as a potential solution to the current fragmented perioperative system. The PSH is defined as "a patient-centered and physician-led multidisciplinary and team-based system of coordinated care that guides the patient throughout the entire surgical experience" (as stated by the American Society of Anesthesiologists) [76, 77]. Goals of the PSH is to provide improved clinical outcomes with better perioperative service (inclusive of optimal preoperative assessment) with the purpose to achieve these goals and establish benefits for all users of the service (patients, surgeons, hospital administrators, etc.) from this practice model.

Concept of the PSH model and context of the preoperative surgical assessment aim to reduce the variability in perioperative care given that variability increases the likelihood for errors and/or complications. Variability could be reduced through assuring continuity of care and treating the entire perioperative episode of care as a "continuum" rather than discrete episodes (i.e., preoperative, intraoperative, postoperative, and post-discharge). Such an endeavor can be accomplished by having one team responsible for managing all aspects of the continuum from the time that the patient and the surgeon make the decision for surgery until a predetermined number of days post-discharge. During the surgical encounter, goals of the PSH are to ensure that the best evidence and best practices are applied and utilized in a consistent and standardized way for all patients scheduled for surgery. If such a paradigm does not exist or is not clear, then the PSH team should develop an agreement to establish standardization for that particular practice model that can then be applied to all patients. Localized systems and policies remain important in decision-making; for example, at each step of the continuum from the decision to undergo maxillofacial surgery until a predetermined number of days after surgery, patients will be informed, educated, and involved in decision-making and treatment planning. By applying these types of concepts, a unique opportunity exists to improve outcomes and decrease the length of stay and other metrics to improve surgical experiences and patient satisfaction.

There are major differences between the current structure of perioperative care and the future patient-focused system under a PSH model. Briefly, patient-centered care and shared decision-making would replace the present physician-centered care under the PSH model. PSH model considers preferences and values of the patient in all healthcare decisions that are often found to be associated with better outcomes, decreased utilization of expensive preoperative tests and procedures, and decreased "routine" use of preoperative specialty consultation [78]. Patient expectation management, including standardized protocol-driven preoperative health and risk assessment, preoperative optimization of underlying medical conditions, perioperative standardized anesthesia/nursing/surgical protocols, strategies for fluid management, and discharge planning (enhanced recovery after surgery), is determined in advance through the PSH pathway. Multimodal analgesia, a targeted postoperative recovery plan, early ambulation, nutrition management, rescue protocols from perioperative complications, and smooth transition of care to an appropriate discharge setting are all part of a PSH pathway. An important aspect and aim of the PSH is not to replace the surgeon's role in the perioperative period, but rather to assure adherence to mutually agreed upon pre-, peri-, and post-recovery protocols and to better manage any medical issues that arise during each episode of surgical care.

2.5 Preoperative Optimization of the Maxillofacial Surgery Patient

Preoperative consultation with critical care team consultants is sometimes necessary for the care of selected high-risk maxillofacial surgery patients [35, 74]. Such preoperative planning provides an opportunity to optimize a high-risk patient's preoperative condition, obtain necessary baseline presurgical laboratory screening values, and improve planning for any potential postoperative medical requirements [79]. However, such preoperative interventions can be costly and are not always effective, and any mild improvement in physiological indices does not necessarily translate into improved clinical outcomes. Therefore, for those maxillofacial surgery patients whose preoperative physiologic parameters are not severely deranged, routine preoperative optimization in the critical care setting is not well established and frequently adds nothing that could not otherwise be achieved with careful preoperative screening and management performed in a PAT center along with the patient's primary care physician preoperative evaluation and adequate perioperative preparation and instruction by the maxillofacial surgeon. As an example, it has been suggested that postoperative morbidity in the patient with ischemic heart disease is reduced with preoperative optimization (i.e., guided by a pulmonary artery catheter) [80]. This may be important for the patient with significant left ventricular dysfunction or enable one to increase cardiac performance in the compromised patient, but according to the classification of evidence used by the ACC/AHA guidelines (2002 and 2008), there is no conclusive evidence that it is useful or effective in noncardiac surgery [81].

Goals for an optimal preoperative assessment would be to decrease the number of unnecessary tests and screening procedures, reduce the need for intraoperative blood transfusions, avoid extending the length of time in the hospital following surgery, improve upon a patient's pain management experience, enhance communication with consulting physicians (when necessary) and surgeon, and optimize surgical outcomes with heightened patient satisfaction. There is an evolving concept of more rigorously coordinating and integrating preoperative assessment during perioperative management, referred to as the PSH, that has parallels to the advantageous concept of a patient-centered medical home. This model shares a vision of improved clinical outcomes, reductions in cost of care, patient engagement throughout the surgical care plan, and improved surgical care coordination between all players of the healthcare team. The literature reports consistent and significant positive findings related to the PSH initiatives and guidelines.

Conclusion

An optimal perioperative management plan for the maxillofacial surgery patient may have the greatest impact on preparing patients for surgery and ensuring their safe and effective transition to home or other designated facilities (i.e., postoperative rehabilitation). Optimization and enhancement of care should continue to focus on comparison of improved outcomes from changing policies and practices to research focused on the discovery of innovative preoperative practice models, improving information technology, and contributing to the implementation and evolution of evidenced-based practice principles through physician leadership and redesign of pre- and perioperative processes.

References

1. Kehlet H. Multimodal strategies to improve surgical outcome. Am J Surg. 2002;183(6):630–41.
2. Williams FM, Bergin JD. Cardiac screening before noncardiac surgery. Surg Clin North Am. 2009;89(4):747–62.
3. Cecconi M, Corredor C, Arulkumaran N, et al. Clinical review: goal-directed therapy-what is the evidence in surgical patients? The effect on different risk groups. Crit Care. 2013;17(2):209.
4. Kern JW, Shoemaker WC. Meta-analysis of hemodynamic optimization in high-risk patients. Crit Care Med. 2002;30:1686–92.
5. Fisher SP. Cost-effective preoperative evaluation and testing. Chest. 1999;115(suppl):96–100.
6. Katz RI, Dexter F, Rosenfeld K, et al. Survey study of anesthesiologists' and surgeons' ordering of unnecessary preoperative laboratory tests. Anesth Analg. 2011;112(1):207–12.
7. Czoski-Murray C, Lloyd Jones M, McCabe C, et al. What is the value of routinely testing full blood count, electrolytes and urea, and pulmonary function tests before elective surgery in patients with no apparent clinical indication and in subgroups of patients with common comorbidities: a systematic review of the clinical and cost-effective literature. Health Technol Assess. 2012;16(50):i–xvi, 1–159.
8. Main C, Moxham T, Wyatt JC, Kay J, Anderson R, Stein K. Computerised decision support systems in order communication for diagnostic, screening or monitoring test ordering: systematic reviews of the effects and cost-effectiveness of systems. Health Technol Assess. 2010;14(48):1–227.
9. Michota FA Jr. The preoperative evaluation and use of laboratory testing. Cleve Clin J Med. 2006;73(Suppl 1):S4–7.
10. Dexter F, Maxbauer T, Stout C, et al. Relative influence on total cancelled operating room time from patients who are inpatients or outpatients preoperatively. Anesth Analg. 2014;118(5):1072–80.
11. Lemmens LC, Kerkkamp HE, van Klei WA, et al. Implementation of outpatient preoperative evaluation clinics: facilitating and limiting factors. Br J Anaesth. 2008;100(5):645–51.
12. van Klei WA, Moons KG, Rutten CL, et al. The effect of outpatient preoperative evaluation of hospital inpatients on cancellation of surgery and length of hospital stay. Anesth Analg. 2002;94(3):644–9.
13. Fleisher LA, Beckman JA, et al. ACC/AHA 2007 guidelines on perioperative cardiovascular evaluation and care for noncardiac surgery: executive summary: a report of the American College of Cardiology/American Heart Association Task Force on Practice Guidelines (Writing Committee to Revise the 2002 Guidelines on Perioperative Cardiovascular Evaluation for Noncardiac Surgery). American College of Cardiology/American Heart Association Task Force on Practice Guidelines (Writing Committee to Revise the 2002 Guidelines on Perioperative Cardiovascular Evaluation for Noncardiac Surgery)., American Society of Echocardiography., American Society of Nuclear Cardiology., Heart Rhythm Society., Society of Cardiovascular Anesthesiologists., Society for Cardiovascular Angiography and Interventions., Society for Vascular Medicine and Biology., Society for Vascular Surgery. Anesth Analg. 2008;106(3):685–712.
14. Hopkins TJ, Raghunathan K, Barbeito A, et al. Associations between ASA physical status and postoperative mortality at 48 h: a contemporary dataset analysis compared to a historical cohort. Perioper Med (Lond). 2016;5:29.
15. Owens WD. American Society of Anesthesiologist physical classification system is not a risk classification system. Anesthesiology. 2001;94(2):378.

16. Maddox TM. Preoperative cardiovascular evaluation for noncardiac surgery. Mt Sinai J Med. 2005;72(3):185–92.
17. Holt NF. Perioperative cardiac risk reduction. Am Fam Physician. 2012;85(3):239–46.
18. Roizen MF. Preoperative testing. In: Schweitzer BJ, editor. Chapter 3: handbook of preoperative assessment and management. Philadelphia: Lippincott Williams and Wilkins; 2000.
19. Beattie C, Chung OY, Pierce DF Jr. Risk assessment and risk modification. In: Schweitzer BJ, editor. Chapter 1: handbook of preoperative assessment and management. Philadelphia: Lippincott Williams and Wilkins; 2000.
20. Jones CM, Quinn MS, Minisi AJ. Reflex control of sympathetic outflow and depressed baroreflex sensitivity following myocardial infarction. Auton Neurosci. 2008;141(1–2):46–53.
21. Silverman DG, Donati F. Factors affecting pseudocholinesterase and the pharmacokinetics and pharmacodynamics of succinylcholine. In: Silverman DG, editor. Chapter 17: neuromuscular block in anesthesia and intensive care. Philadelphia: J.B. Lippincott; 1995.
22. Morrison BM. Neuromuscular diseases. Semin Neurol. 2016;36(5):409–18.
23. Robinson R, Carpenter D, Shaw MA, et al. Mutations in RYR1 in malignant hyperthermia and central core disease. Hum Mutat. 2006;27(10):977–89.
24. Silverman DG, Donati F. Undesirable effects of succinylcholine. In: Silverman DG, editor. Chapter 18: neuromuscular block in anesthesia and intensive care. Philadelphia: J.B. Lippincott; 1995.
25. Al-Takrouri H, Martin TW, Mayhew JF. Hyperkalemic cardiac arrest following succinylcholine administration: the use of extracorporeal membrane oxygenation in an emergency situation. J Clin Anesth. 2004;16(6):449–51.
26. Gronert J. Cardiac arrest after succinylcholine: mortality greater with rhabdomyolysis than receptor upregulation. Anesthesiology. 2001;94(3):523–9.
27. Cox SG, Martinez R, Glick A, et al. A review of community management of paediatric burns. Burns. 2015;41(8):1805–10.
28. Benarroch-Gampel J, Riall TS. What laboratory tests are required for ambulatory surgery? Adv Surg. 2013;47:81–98.
29. Smetana GW, Macpherson DS. The case against routine preoperative laboratory testing. Med Clin North Am. 2003;87(1):7–40.
30. White PF, White LM, Monk T, et al. Perioperative care for the older outpatient undergoing ambulatory surgery. Anesth Analg. 2012;114(6):1190–215.
31. Ajimura FY, Maia AS, Hachiya A, et al. Preoperative laboratory evaluation of patients aged over 40 years undergoing elective non-cardiac surgery. Sao Paulo Med J. 2005;123(2):50–3.
32. Feely MA, Collins CS, Daniels PR, Kebede EB, Jatoi A, Mauck KF. Preoperative testing before noncardiac surgery: guidelines and recommendations. Am Fam Physician. 2013;87(6):414–8.
33. Bryson GL, Wyand A, Bragg PR. Preoperative testing is inconsistent with published guidelines and rarely changes management. Can J Anaesth. 2006;53(3):236–41.
34. Cecconi M, Corredor C, Arulkumaran N, et al. Clinical review: goal-directed therapy-what is the evidence in surgical patients? The effect on different risk groups. Crit Care. 2013;17(2):209.
35. de Vos M, Graafmans W, Keesman E, et al. Quality measurement at intensive care units: which indicators should we use? J Crit Care. 2007;22(4):267–74.
36. Schouten O, Bax JJ, Poldermans D. Coronary risk assessment in the management of patients undergoing noncardiac vascular surgery. Rev Esp Cardiol. 2007;60(10):1083–91.
37. Fritsch G, Flamm M, Hepner DL, et al. Abnormal preoperative tests, pathologic findings of medical history, and their predictive value for perioperative complications. Acta Anaesthesiol Scand. 2012;56(3):339–50.
38. Apfelbaum JL, Connis RT, Nickinovich DG, American Society of Anesthesiologists Task Force on Preanesthesia Evaluation, Pasternak LR, Arens JF, Caplan RA, Connis RT, Fleisher LA, et al. Practice advisory for preanesthesia evaluation: an updated report by the American Society of Anesthesiologists Task Force on Preanesthesia evaluation. Committee on standards and practice parameters. Anesthesiology. 2012;116(3):522–38.
39. Stokes GS. Treatment of isolated systolic hypertension. Curr Hypertens Rep. 2006;8(5):377–83.
40. Ong HT. Are angiotensin-converting enzyme inhibitors and angiotensin receptor blockers especially useful for cardiovascular protection? J Am Board Fam Med. 2009;22(6):686–97.
41. Davis C, Tait G, Carroll J, et al. The revised cardiac risk index in the new millennium: a single-centre prospective cohort re-evaluation of the original variables in 9,519 consecutive elective surgical patients. Can J Anaesth. 2013;60(9):855–63.
42. Radovanović D, Kolak R, Stokić A, et al. Cardiac perioperative complications in noncardiac surgery. Med Pregl. 2008;61(7-8):375–82.
43. HY W, Huang JW, Lin HJ, et al. Comparative effectiveness of renin-angiotensin system blockers and other antihypertensive drugs in patients with diabetes: systematic review and bayesian network meta-analysis. BMJ. 2013;347:f6008.
44. Tandon P, Abraldes JG, Berzigotti A, et al. Renin-angiotensin-aldosterone inhibitors in the reduction of portal pressure: a systematic review and meta-analysis. J Hepatol. 2010;53(2):273–82.
45. Xie X, Liu Y, Perkovic V, et al. Renin-angiotensin system inhibitors and kidney and cardiovascular outcomes in patients with CKD: a bayesian network meta-analysis of randomized clinical trials. Am J Kidney Dis. 2016;67(5):728–41.
46. Horlocker TT, Wedel DJ, Rowlingson JC, Enneking FK, Kopp SL, Benzon HT, et al. Regional anesthesia in the patient receiving antithrombotic or thrombolytic therapy: American Society of Regional Anesthesia

and Pain Medicine evidence-based guidelines (third edition). Reg Anesth Pain Med. 2010;35:64–101.
47. Daniels PR. Peri-procedural management of patients taking oral anticoagulants. BMJ. 2015;351:h2391.
48. Levy JH, Faraoni D, Spring JL, Douketis JD, Samama CM. Managing new oral anticoagulants in the perioperative and intensive care unit setting. Anesthesiology. 2013;118:1466–74.
49. American Society of Regional Anesthesia and Pain Medicine. Regional anesthesia in the patient receiving antithrombotic or thrombolytic therapy: American Society of Regional Anesthesia and Pain Medicine Evidence-Based Guidelines (interim update 2015). 2015. https://http://www.asra.com/advisory-guidelines/article/1/anticoagulation-3rd-edition. Accessed 09 May 2016.
50. Halaszynski T. Administration of coagulation-altering therapy in the patient presenting for oral health and maxillofacial surgery. Oral Maxillofac Surg Clin North Am. 2016;28(4):443–60.
51. Veen i v, JJ MM. Management of peri-operative antithrombotic therapy. Anaesthesia. 2015;70(Suppl 1):58–67, e21–3.
52. Eisele R, Melzer N, Bramlage P. Perioperative management of anticoagulation. Chirurg. 2014;85:513–9.
53. McEwen BJ. The influence of herbal medicine on platelet function and coagulation: a narrative review. Semin Thromb Hemost. 2015;41(3):300–14.
54. Guthrie R. Review and management of side effects associated with antiplatelet therapy for prevention of recurrent cerebrovascular events. Adv Ther. 2011;28(6):473–82.
55. Silverman DG, Halaszynski T, Sinatra R, Luther M, Rinder CS. Rofecoxib does not compromise platelet aggregation during anesthesia and surgery: [le rofecoxib n'altere pas l'agregation plaquettaire pendant l'anesthesie et la chirurgie]. Can J Anaesth. 2003;50(10):1004–8.
56. FitzGerald GA, Patrono C. Drug therapy: the coxibs, selective inhibitors of cyclooxygenase-2. N Engl J Med. 2001;345:433–42.
57. Sinatra RS, Shen QJ, Halaszynski T, Luther MA, Shaheen Y. Preoperative rofecoxib oral suspension as an analgesic adjunct after lower abdominal surgery: the effects on effort-dependent pain and pulmonary function. Anesth Analg. 2004;98(1):135–40.
58. Serebruany VL, Malinin AI, Pokov AN, Hanley DF. Antiplatelet profiles of the fixed-dose combination of extended-release dipyridamole and low-dose aspirin compared with clopidogrel with or without aspirin in patients with type 2 diabetes and a history of transient ischemic attack: a randomized, single-blind, 30-day trial. Clin Ther. 2008;30(2):249–59.
59. Cornett O, Ocava LC, Singh M, Malhotra S, Rosenbaum DM. Antithrombotic and thrombolytic therapy for ischemic stroke. Cardiol Clin. 2008;26(2):251–65.
60. Vande Griend JP, Saseen JJ. Combination antiplatelet agents for secondary prevention of ischemic stroke. Pharmacotherapy. 2008;28(10):1233–42.
61. Bath PM, Cotton D, Martin RH, PRoFESS Study Group, et al. Effect of combined aspirin and extended-release dipyridamole versus clopidogrel on functional outcome and recurrence in acute, mild ischemic stroke: PRoFESS subgroup analysis. Stroke. 2010;41(4):732–8.
62. Arora RR, Rai F. Antiplatelet intervention in acute coronary syndrome. Am J Ther. 2009;16(5):e29–40.
63. Lievens D, von Hundelshausen P. Platelets in atherosclerosis. Thromb Haemost. 2011;106(5):827–38.
64. De Luca G, Biondi-Zoccai G, Marino P. Transferring patients with ST-segment elevation myocardial infarction for mechanical reperfusion: a meta-regression analysis of randomized trials. Ann Emerg Med. 2008;52(6):665–76.
65. You JJ, Singer DE, Howard PA, et al. Antithrombotic therapy for atrial fibrillation: antithrombotic therapy and prevention of thrombosis, 9th ed: American College of Chest Physicians Evidence-Based Clinical Practice Guidelines. Chest. 2012;141(2 Suppl):e531S–75S.
66. Adam SS, McDuffie JR, Ortel TL, Williams JW Jr. Comparative effectiveness of warfarin and new oral anticoagulants for the management of atrial fibrillation and venous thromboembolism: a systematic review. Ann Intern Med. 2012;157(11):796–807.
67. Salazar CA, del Aguila D, Cordova EG. Direct thrombin inhibitors versus vitamin K antagonists for preventing cerebral or systemic embolism in people with non-valvular atrial fibrillation. Cochrane Database Syst Rev. 2014;3:CD009893.
68. Chandra D, Gupta A, Grover V, Kumar Gupta V. When should you restart anticoagulation in patients who suffer an intracranial bleed who also have a prosthetic valve? Interact Cardiovasc Thorac Surg. 2013;16(4):520–3.
69. Abildgaard U, Sandset PM, Hammerstrøm J, et al. Management of pregnant women with mechanical heart valve prosthesis: thromboprophylaxis with low molecular weight heparin. Thromb Res. 2009;124(3):262–7.
70. Watson L, Broderick C, Armon MP. Thrombolysis for acute deep vein thrombosis. Cochrane Database Syst Rev. 2014;1:CD002783.
71. Caldeira D, Rodrigues FB, Barra M, et al. Non-vitamin K antagonist oral anticoagulants and major bleeding-related fatality in patients with atrial fibrillation and venous thromboembolism: a systematic review and meta-analysis. Heart. 2015;101(15):1204–11.
72. Lip GY, Mitchell SA, Liu X, et al. Relative efficacy and safety of non-vitamin K oral anticoagulants for non-valvular atrial fibrillation: network meta-analysis comparing apixaban, dabigatran, rivaroxaban and edoxaban in three patient subgroups. Int J Cardiol. 2016;204:88–94.
73. Sharma M, Cornelius VR, Patel JP, Davies JG, Molokhia M. Efficacy and harms of direct oral anticoagulants in the elderly for stroke prevention in atrial fibrillation and secondary prevention of venous thromboembolism: systematic review and meta-analysis. Circulation. 2015;132(3):194–204.

74. Barry MJ, Edgman-Levitan S. Shared decision making–pinnacle of patient-centered care. N Engl J Med. 2012;366:780–1.
75. Ghaferi AA, Birkmeyer JD, Dimick JB. Variation in hospital mortality associated with inpatient surgery. N Engl J Med. 2009;361:1368–75.
76. Ravikumar TS, Sharma C, Marini C, Steele GD Jr, Ritter G, Barrera R, Kim M, Safyer SM, Vandervoort K, De Geronimo M, Baker L, Levi P, Pierdon S, Horgan M, Maynor K, Maloney G, Wojtowicz M, Nelson K. A validated value-based model to improve hospital-wide perioperative outcomes: adaptability to combined medical/surgical inpatient cohorts. Ann Surg. 2010;252:486–96.
77. Vetter TR, Goeddel LA, Boudreaux AM, Hunt TR, Jones KA, Pittet JF. The perioperative surgical home: how can it make the case so everyone wins? BMC Anesthesiol. 2013;13:6.
78. Adamina M, Kehlet H, Tomlinson GA, et al. Enhanced recovery pathways optimize health outcomes and resource utilization: a meta-analysis of randomized con- trolled trials in colorectal surgery. Surgery. 2011;149:830–40.
79. Cecconi M, Corredor C, Arulkumaran N, et al. Clinical review: goal-directed therapy-what is the evidence in surgical patients? The effect on different risk groups. Crit Care. 2013;17(2):209.
80. Dalfino L, Giglio MT, Puntillo F, et al. Haemodynamic goal-directed therapy and postoperative infections: earlier is better. A systematic review and meta-analysis. Crit Care. 2011;15(3):R154.
81. Tracy CM, Epstein AE, Darbar D, , et al. 2012 ACCF/AHA/HRS focused update of the 2008 guidelines for device-based therapy of cardiac rhythm abnormalities: a report of the American College of Cardiology Foundation/American Heart Association Task Force on Practice Guidelines and the Heart Rhythm Society. [corrected]. Circulation 2012; 126(14):1784–1800.

3 Anesthesia Care in Maxillofacial Surgery

Annibal Faddoul, Youssef Tfaili,
and Chakib M. Ayoub

Abstract

Maxillofacial surgery requires specifically tailored anesthetic care. Working in close proximity to the airway warrants continuous communication between the teams. The advent of the videolaryngoscope and many other modalities for airway management over the recent years reflects an important evolution in the field and broadens the anesthesiologist's armament in managing difficult cases. The intraoperative management includes interventions that would optimize the surgical conditions and improve the patient's recovery, as well as minimize the potential for complications. The emergence phase remains one of the more dangerous phases of the anesthetic management and demands heightened presence and critical decision-making on the anesthesiologist's behalf. Naturally, managing pediatric or geriatric populations also poses challenges of their own and requires specific care and different techniques.

3.1 Introduction

The purpose of this chapter is to present a point of view from the other side of the drapes, in order for surgeons to have a closer look at how anesthesiologists perceive this area of surgery.

In light of the considerable advances in maxillofacial surgery techniques in the last decades, anesthesia management has substantially evolved with the advent of new airway management techniques, specifically the evolution of fiberoptic scopes and video-assisted laryngoscopes. Because surgical sites in this kind of procedures may be in the vicinity or even involving parts of the airway, anesthesiologists have developed skills that could preserve oxygen delivery throughout the procedure and deal with any unanticipated complications.

Whether the surgery in question is a simple skin lesion excision or a major maxillary tumor excision, an extensive training is required before an anesthesiologist can manage various maxillofacial procedures.

This chapter will tackle the multidisciplinary approach to the management of all kinds of surgi-

A. Faddoul, M.D. • Y. Tfaili, M.D.
Department of Anesthesiology, American University of Beirut Medical Center, Beirut, Lebanon

C.M. Ayoub, M.D., M.B.A. (✉)
Department of Anesthsiology, Duke University School of Medicine, Durham, NC, USA
e-mail: chakib.ayoub@duke.edu

© Springer International Publishing AG 2018

E.M. Ferneini, J.D. Bennett (eds.), *Perioperative Assessment of the Maxillofacial Surgery Patient*,
https://doi.org/10.1007/978-3-319-58868-1_3

cal procedures in this field, how to choose surgical candidates after careful preoperative assessment, how to secure an airway, how to maintain hemodynamic stability throughout the case, and how to guarantee a smooth and safe emergence from anesthesia.

3.2 Airway Management and Induction

Maxillofacial surgery poses a unique challenge to the anesthesiologist in the matter of airway management. Indeed, when the surgical field involves proximity to the airway, cooperation between the surgical and anesthesia teams is of paramount importance. As such, the modalities for securing the airway should be thoroughly reviewed and discussed in the preoperative phase. The need for intubation will vary among the different types of surgery, as short procedures may sometimes be carried out on awake patients with the use of local anesthetic infiltration combined with monitored anesthesia care (MAC).

A thorough physical examination of the airway is always warranted in any kind of surgery, more so in the maxillofacial cases. An attempt to determine whether invasive airway management may be difficult is of utmost importance, although not always reliable using the available means. Some anatomical features have been shown to be associated with difficult airways, but the level of evidence is low. The ASA task force on management of the difficult airway has published practice guidelines for difficult airway management, in which it stresses on the importance of the physical examination of the airway [1]. Some of the components of the physical examination of the airway include but are not limited to the visualization of the uvula (better known as the Mallampati score), the thyromental or sternomental distances, the interincisor distance, the presence of retrognathia, and temporomandibular joint mobility. Reviewing the patient's anesthetic history is also helpful in determining the best course of action. In some cases, additional testing may be warranted but needs to be clinically decided on a per-case basis, such as radiography or CT scans.

3.3 Intraoperative Management and Maintenance

3.3.1 Induced Hypotension

By definition, induced hypotension is the reduction of the systolic blood pressure to 80–90 mmHg, a reduction of mean arterial pressure (MAP) to 50–65 mmHg, or a 30% reduction of baseline MAP. It is a technique that helps in providing a bloodless surgical field for better visibility, reducing hemodynamic changes and decreasing the need for blood transfusion. Blood loss is linked to MAP rather than cardiac output and can be reduced to 40% when MAP is maintained at 50 instead of 60 mmHg.

Hypotensive anesthesia, while indicated in many surgical specialties, is better avoided in patients who are at high risk of myocardial ischemia, strokes, or end-organ damage due to hypoperfusion.

This can be achieved by a wide variety of pharmacological agents; as inhalational anesthetics naturally cause vasodilation in a dose-dependent manner, increasing the depth of anesthesia can assist to reach the desired BP [2]. Opioids are also a good choice to decrease the BP and may be a better option than inhaled agents alone especially when using ultrashort-acting drugs like remifentanil. In case where the balanced anesthesia technique will be disrupted, vasodilators like sodium nitroprusside or nitroglycerin can be used safely as continuous infusions to decrease the BP. Some patients have uncontrolled hypotension, and decreasing their BP may require short-acting beta-blockers like esmolol or labetalol.

3.3.2 Blood and Fluid Requirements

Maxillofacial surgeries are classified into minor, intermediate, major, and supra-major surgeries depending on the site and duration. For example, mandibular tumor resections are long procedures involving dissection of soft tissues and bones over a long period of time. These surgeries are accompanied by increased blood loss, while minor procedures like a simple nose lesion excision may have minimal tissue injury.

Factors that increase the risk of bleeding include hard tissue lesions, the use of anticoagulant or antiplatelet drugs, and lesions invading nearby vessels.

The correlation between expected blood loss and specific maxillofacial surgeries has been demonstrated [3], which requires a thorough preoperative assessment of the patient's medical status. The availability of several blood units prior to the start of the procedure is very important along with preoperative baseline hematocrit values.

Intraoperative thromboelastography can guide the anesthesiologist in maintaining a stable blood volume throughout the case. The isovolemic hemodilution technique can decrease the need for allogenic transfusion to avoid undesirable side effects.

In parallel, fluid maintenance in maxillofacial surgery follows the same rules as other types of surgery. In cases where the anesthesiologist expects large fluid and blood loss, one or two large bore IV lines are inserted, and the volume to be infused is calculated according to the patient's age, weight, extent of tissue exposure, duration of the surgery, and preoperative NPO status.

3.3.3 Monitoring

Standard monitoring is required for all maxillofacial surgeries, with the exception of cases with major fluid shifts where an arterial line is needed for real-time BP monitoring.

3.3.4 Positioning

Patient positioning during these cases is similar to other disciplines. Head-up and supine positions are routinely used, with the demonstrated benefit of the head-up position in decreasing desaturations and improving the rib cage expansion. Special attention should be given to avoid any compression to the neck that may compromise venous return. Soft rolls and silicone pads can be used under the head and shoulders to decrease the risk of cervical and brachial plexus injuries, while eye pads and other eye protection precautions are used to decrease the risk of ocular ischemia and corneal abrasions.

3.3.5 Complications

A wide range of possible complications can occur during maxillofacial procedures, but airway problems can be fatal. Prevention should start by securing the ET tube and fixing it to avoid any dislodgment during manipulation of the head or neck. Compression of the neck or chest by the surgeon may decrease the ventilation and cause high airway pressures. It is also very important to make sure that the cuff is well inflated when using cuffed tubes to prevent blood and secretions from leaking into the trachea and lungs which may compromise intraoperative ventilation and emergence.

Manipulation of the neck vessels can cause either decreased venous drainage or decreased blood perfusion to the brain.

As mentioned earlier, the use of vasopressor infiltration to decrease bleeding may cause tachyarrhythmia and require the use of antiarrhythmic agents.

Another issue that may cause devastating complications is airway fires, when inflammable anesthetics or high FiO_2 levels are used while the surgeon is operating with electrocautery.

3.4 Emergence and Extubation

As the surgical procedure comes to a close, the emergence phase of anesthesia begins. Often likened to the landing of a plane, emergence is one of the most critical parts of the anesthetic plan. During this phase, anesthetics are weaned, and the patient needs to recover his vital functions to tolerate extubation and become autonomous. The goals to achieve during emergence are to recover airway protective reflexes, regain consciousness, and be free of pain, all while maintaining normal hemodynamics.

Some amount of time prior to placing the last stitches, the maintenance anesthetics are switched off, with the longer-acting ones to be discontinued first. A reversal agent for the neuromuscular blockade is administered as needed and documented with the return of a TOF ratio of 0.9 on a quantitative neuromuscular monitor (such as an NMT or a TOF watch) when available. It has been determined that most clinical signs of return to normal function are unreliable, and the use of a quantitative monitor, rather than the detection of twitch fade by the clinician, should become the standard of care [4]. The goal of this practice is the prevention of residual weakness in the postoperative phase, which could cause weakness in the laryngeal airway protection muscles and therefore increase the risk of pulmonary complications. The reversal agent, typically an acetylcholinesterase inhibitor combined with an anticholinergic agent, should be injected ideally at a TOF count of 4 and 15–20 min prior to tracheal extubation, to maximize recovery of neuromuscular function.

Inhaled anesthetics should be switched off and washed out of the circuit with the use of higher fresh gas flows. It is important to avoid extubation when the patient is still in light planes of anesthesia, as the risk of laryngospasm is increased, especially in the pediatric population. Opioids should be titrated ideally to a respiratory rate of 8–12 breaths per minute, to promote adequate analgesia.

3.4.1 Criteria for Extubation

For a patient to be extubated, certain criteria need to be fulfilled to ensure the patient would tolerate an unassisted airway. In a controlled environment such as the operating room, with patients undergoing non-emergent uncomplicated surgeries, the following should be observed prior to the removal of the endotracheal tube:

- Adequate oxygenation (as measured by pulse oximetry or blood gas analysis)
- Adequate ventilation (tidal volume higher than 5 mL/kg, end-tidal CO_2 below 50 mmHg)
- Stable hemodynamics
- Full reversal of muscle relaxation with a TOF ratio of 0.9
- Neurological status (obeying verbal commands, intact cough reflex)
- Appropriate acid-base status
- Normal metabolic status (adequate hydration and electrolyte balance)
- Normothermia

3.4.2 Awake vs. Deep Extubation

It is common knowledge with anesthesiologists that while a light plane of anesthesia (defined as patients whose cough reflexes have recovered but are unresponsive to verbal commands) increases laryngospasm risk after extubation, a deep plane of anesthesia may allow for a deep extubation. It should be noted that patients at high risk of aspiration, upper airway obstruction, or difficult airways are poor candidates for this technique. However, deep extubation isn't without its benefits, especially in the field of ENT or maxillofacial surgery.

To achieve a successful deep extubation, the patient should be weaned from mechanical ventilation and spontaneous ventilation should be elicited. This can be achieved by decreasing the minute ventilation to allow the blood CO_2 level to rise, thus triggering a central response for spontaneous ventilation. Neuromuscular paralysis should be reversed while keeping the maintenance anesthetics running. The respiratory rate will then be a useful tool to ensure analgesia, as we titrate the opioid analgesics to a respiratory rate ranging from 8 to 12 breaths per minute, after which good supralaryngeal and gastric suctioning would be performed, and the tube removed. Typically, an oropharyngeal or nasopharyngeal (with the benefit of causing no gag reflex) is inserted to relieve upper airway obstruction, and an oxygen face mask would be applied.

The major benefits of a deep extubation come with the avoidance of coughing on the tube seen in awake extubations (colloquially known as bucking), which increases the intrathoracic pressure, in turn increasing central venous pressure and arterial blood pressure. This technique is commonly used in the setting of intraocular surgery, to avoid a sudden increase in intraocular pressure. In maxillofacial surgery, specifically after intricate dissection which leaves room for hematoma formation, a deep extubation might be beneficial. It should also be considered in patients with cardiovascular instability and hyperactive airways.

On the other hand, care should be taken in patients who underwent surgery on the upper airway, as bleeding into the pharynx may increase risk of aspiration or airway irritation, which may cause a laryngospasm as the patient is recovering from the anesthetics.

An LMA would be beneficial here too, as it typically minimizes laryngeal stimulation and does not require very deep levels of anesthesia to allow the patients to breathe spontaneously. Some clinicians suggest the switching from an ETT to an LMA prior to emergence to render the extubation process smoother.

It has also been relatively common practice to administer IV lidocaine (1–2 mg/kg) prior to weaning as an attempt to decrease tracheal irritation on emergence.

3.4.3 Emergence Complications

As mentioned earlier, emergence is a critical step in the anesthetic management, and its complications should be anticipated and treated accordingly by the clinician.

- Airway edema: a significant postoperative complication, particularly in the pediatric population, where the airway may become edematous and would cause symptoms ranging from stridor to airway obstruction after extubation. A strong predictor for edema is the leak test, where the tracheal tube cuff would be deflated and an airway pressure of 30 cm of water would be applied to elicit a leak around the tube. When the leak cannot be achieved, an edematous airway should be anticipated, and treatment administered as needed, in the form of intravenous steroids, racemic nebulized epinephrine, or both. Their effectiveness has however yet to be determined.
- Laryngospasm: regarded as a common post extubation complication, it may be avoided by deep extubation, removal of the tube during the inspiratory phase, injection of lidocaine (usage described in many modalities including intravenous, intratracheal, within the tube cuff), or replacing the tube with an LMA prior to discontinuing anesthetics. It may be treated by positive pressure ventilation with face mask, low dose of succinylcholine, or deepening of the anesthetics and reintubation. In certain cases, negative pressure pulmonary edema may appear after a laryngospasm, due to attempts of breathing against a closed airway.
- Laryngeal dysfunction: defined as the inability of a patient to protect his airway from aspiration, laryngeal dysfunction may occur after prolonged intubation of an oversized tube. It may also be due to residual paralysis due to an incomplete neuromuscular block reversal. It puts the patient at an increased risk for aspiration.
- Sore throat: sometimes reported in as high as 90% of the postoperative intubated patients. It may be due to mechanical damage to the airway as in overinflated cuffs or airway irritation due to the use of lubricant [5].

3.5 Pediatric Considerations

Anesthesiologists deal with diverse patient population and surgical subspecialties, but the pediatric population warrants a special attention because of specific anatomical and physiological differences from adult patient. In the maxillofacial discipline, anesthesiologists should have deep knowledge of the pediatric response to pharmacological agents, including inhaled and intravenous medications, while considering the dosages and routes of administration.

Because corrective and reconstructive maxillofacial surgery is often indicated since the first weeks of life, pediatric anesthesiologist should be trained to manage pediatric critical newborn surgeries such as palatoplasties in patients having serious comorbidities and syndromes. The most important skill is pediatric airway management, including pediatric fiberoptic scope usage, which would prevent disastrous outcomes in patients with severe maxillofacial malformations like Treacher Collins, Klippel-Feil, Goldenhar, Pierre Robin, and Apert syndromes. For some anesthesiologists, elective cases would be postponed until hemodynamic conditions are favorable. A large portion of patients presenting for palatoplasties may have chronic aspirations, recurrent otitis media, and upper respiratory tract infections with cough and fever; starting a preoperative antibiotics course would be a wise decision. This should be decided in coordination with the surgery team in order to provide the best care for high-risk pediatric patients.

Congenital cardiovascular malformations are frequently associated with many facial malformations, which require a thorough preoperative assessment (EKG, echocardiogram, etc.) and the use of cardiac medications intraoperatively; this is best planned with a pediatric cardiologist on board.

For example, patients with facial deformities causing chronic aspiration necessitating enteral feeding are at a high risk for intraoperative and postoperative complications. The decision to proceed should be made after weighing risk/benefit ratio, taking into consideration that anesthesia management can have a critical impact on the patient's outcome [6]. Most of these surgeries are done under GA in an operating room fully equipped with advanced airway and supraglottic devices, not to mention different ET tubes (preformed, reinforced, etc.) and laryngeal masks.

For the induction process of pediatric patients, inhaled anesthetic induction is widely used to put the patients to sleep before inserting an IV line and then proceed to give muscle relaxation and analgesics then securing the airway. In some exceptions, an awake fiberoptic intubation (oral/nasal) is indicated if the child is cooperative, with the help and consent of the parents who play a major role in facilitating the procedure [7].

Maintenance of these patients under anesthesia follows the same guidelines as other pediatric surgeries, regarding TIVA or inhaled anesthetics, depending on the type of the surgery and the modes of ventilation. Sevoflurane is the most common gas used because it causes the least hemodynamic side effects, while propofol and short-acting opioids are the gold standard for intravenous anesthetics. Ketamine also plays a role in both premedication and sedation for pediatric patients; although it might cause severe hallucinations in children, it is used in parallel with benzodiazepines to induce amnesia.

Some centers only use muscle relaxants for induction and abstain to use it during maintenance; this technique requires keeping the patient deeply anesthetized providing immobility. Other centers do not use muscle relaxants at all especially in younger patients, despite the recent literature endorsing their usage routinely.

The use of laryngeal masks in the pediatric population has been widely described in the last decade, with many authors advocating for their benefit intra- and postoperatively, especially describing removing LMAs in the lateral decubitus position rather than the supine position [8].

As with adult maxillofacial surgery, pediatric patients are under the risk of arrhythmias when adrenaline is used to decrease surgical bleeding. In addition, the mixture to be injected contains lidocaine and adrenaline, which raises the issue of local anesthetic toxicity in pediatric patients.

Fluid and blood resuscitation follows the same rules as other pediatric surgeries, with the goal of preserving the intravascular volume and oxygen carrying capacity without excessive fluid replenishment to decrease the risk of pulmonary edema in patients with congenital heart diseases undergoing long procedures.

Standard monitors are used in pediatric cases with rare need for invasive arterial BP monitoring. Special attention to ventilation and $EtCO_2$ monitors should be warranted because of the risk of losing the airway during manipulation and repositioning. Other complications include airway edema because of overinflated ETT cuffs, which may compromise extubation, and blood aspiration, which is usually avoided by using throat packs.

The role of warming is crucial in pediatric patients, where behavioral modification and thermoregulatory mechanisms are abolished by anesthesia; unintended hypothermia could easily happen which can lead to increased risk of wound infections, prolonged drug effects, bleeding diatheses, delayed emergence, and prolonged hospital stay [9].

When the surgery is done, the decision to extubate is made according to the duration of the surgery, the severity of the fluid shift, and the possibility of airway edema in pediatric patients. Some patients may be kept intubated overnight or sent to the pediatric ICU for close monitoring. As for patients who will be extubated, a smooth emergence should be planned in order to decrease the risk of aspiration and severe coughing that may compromise the surgical work and cause bleeding.

3.6 Geriatric Considerations

As the median population age is advancing in most developed nations, it is important for the practitioner to acknowledge the significance of becoming familiar with treating elderly patients. While aging should not be considered a disease in itself, the occurrence of chronic illnesses increases exponentially with advanced age. This puts the geriatric population at an increased risk of perioperative morbidity and mortality and makes the cases more difficult to manage. However, generalizations are difficult to make since discrepancies between the stated age and the biological or physiological age are common. A 70-year-old man who has been taking good care of his health and is active daily might respond to anesthetics like a healthy 50-year-old would.

On the cardiovascular aspect, aging usually entails a loss of elasticity in the circulatory system, which often grows into left ventricular hypertrophy and hypertension. This in turn makes the feedback baroreceptor reflex dysfunctional, and the patient becomes more prone to wide fluctuations in blood pressure and cardiovascular status. Incidence of coronary artery disease is also prevalent in the geriatric population.

The nervous system is greatly affected by age, even when no symptoms are present. Degeneration of neurons happens at an increased rate in the elderly and places the patients at risk for cognitive dysfunction, including dementia, delirium, and depression, which may be exacerbated in the acute postoperative phase.

Respiratory changes are closely tied with advanced age, with gradual degeneration of tissues causing decreased efficiency of oxygen delivery and removal of carbon dioxide. This is due to the increase in instances of ventilation perfusion mismatch and even more so in the increase in dead space.

As a patient ages, the hepatic and renal metabolism and clearance of drugs in the systemic circulation slow down, and organ damage is difficult to quantify in the preoperative phase. This causes an increased sensitivity to intravenous anesthetics, especially for the drugs which have active metabolites.

The abovementioned physiological changes necessitate tailoring of the anesthetic plan and careful titration of the dosage of many of the drugs used in cases of general anesthesia. Close monitoring is paramount, and per the type of the surgery and preoperative status of the patient, the clinician may opt to use more invasive monitoring methods such as intra-arterial blood pressure, among others.

Airway management may also become a challenge as degenerative conditions of the musculoskeletal system may limit neck mobility [10].

Conclusion

Through this chapter, we hope we have managed to give a brief but enlightening view from an anesthesiologist's perspective when it comes to dealing with the challenging field of maxillofacial surgery. Here, more than most types of surgery, cross-disciplinary communication is key. The team effort expressed through good practice and safety would culminate with the painless and successful transit of the patient through the operating theater.

References

1. American Society of Anesthesiologists. Practice guidelines for management of the difficult airway. Anesthesiology. 2013;118(2):251–70.

2. Degoute C. Controlled hypotension: a guide to drug choice. Drugs. 2007;67(7):1053–76.
3. Akinbami BO, Onajin-Obembe B. Assessment of intraoperative blood loss during oral and maxillofacial surgical procedures in a Nigerian tertiary health care center. J Blood Transfus. 2014;2014:301467.
4. Brull SJ, Murphy GS. Residual neuromuscular block: lessons unlearned. Part ii: methods to reduce the risk of residual weakness. Anesth Analg. 2010;111(1):129–40.
5. Karmarkar S, Varshney S. Tracheal extubation. Contin Educ Anaesth Crit Care Pain. 2008;8(6):214–20.
6. Nguyen T, Freilich MM, Macpherson BA. Complications of oral and maxillofacial surgery under general anesthesia in tube-fed children: a retrospective analysis. J Can Dent Assoc. 2016;82:g16.
7. Blanco G, Melman E, Cuairan V, Moyao D, Ortiz-Monasterio F. Fiberoptic nasal intubation in children with anticipated and unanticipated difficult intubation. Paediatr Anaesth. 2001;11(1):49–53.
8. Thomas-Kattappurathu G, Kasisomayajula A, Short J. Best position and depth of anaesthesia for laryngeal mask airway removal in children: a prospective randomised controlled trial. Eur J Anaesthesiol. 2015;32(9):624–30.
9. Hart SR, Bordes B, Hart J, Corsino D, Harmon D. Unintended perioperative hypothermia. Ochsner J. 2011;11(3):259–70.
10. Hevesi ZG, Hammel LL. Geriatric disorders. In: Hines RL, Marschall KE, editors. Stoelting's anesthesia and co-existing disease. Philadelphia: Elsevier Saunders; 2014. p. 642–54.

4 Initial Management of the Trauma Patient in Maxillofacial Surgery

Timothy H. Pohlman, William Gossett, and Jan R. Kornilow

"Shock is a rude unhinging of the machinery of life."

—*Samuel Gross. 1871*

Abstract

Oral maxillofacial surgeons must be integral members of the trauma team. With the unique skill sets of this specialty, OMFS is a certain critical participant in the initial evaluation and management of patients with multiple injuries, particularly with critical issues such as a difficult airway due to injuries involving the head and neck, massive hemorrhage from these areas, and threatened vision loss. Although definitive repair of injuries within the area of OMFS generally does not occur until several days past the resuscitation of the critically injured, early participation of the oral and maxillofacial surgeon in optimal care of trauma victims promotes a more thorough understanding of the complex pathophysiology that may adversely affect perioperative preparation for these cases. Moreover, familiarity with recent advances in resuscitation of shock following trauma prepares the surgeon for catastrophic bleeding that may occasionally complicate OMFS. Fundamental knowledge of cardiovascular physiology, a detailed understanding of the coagulation system, and appreciation for the intricate pathways and delicate balance of homeostasis provide an arguably necessary scientific foundation for safe and effective surgical practice of any specialty.

4.1 Introduction

Trauma is the most common cause of death in individuals at the age of 44, and unintentional injury is the fourth most common cause of death for anyone throughout life. From 2000 to 2010, the population in the USA increased approximately 10% yet violent death increased 23% [1]. In 2014, the age-adjusted death rate for all types of traumatic injury, in both males and females,

T.H. Pohlman, M.D., F.A.C.S. (✉)
Department of Surgery, Section of Acute Care Surgery, Indiana University Health—Methodist Hospital, Indianapolis, IN, USA
e-mail: tpohlman@iuhealth.org

W. Gossett, M.S.H.C.M., B.S.N., R.N., N.R.P.
J.R. Kornilow, MD, FACEP, FAAEM, BCEMSP
Department of Emergency Medicine, Indiana University Health—Ball Memorial Hospital, Muncie, IN, USA

© Springer International Publishing AG 2018
E.M. Ferneini, J.D. Bennett (eds.), *Perioperative Assessment of the Maxillofacial Surgery Patient*,
https://doi.org/10.1007/978-3-319-58868-1_4

Table 4.1 Characteristics of different stages in the optimal care of trauma victims with severe and/or multiple injuries

	Rescue	Resuscitation	Repair	Rehabilitation
Location	Scene	Emergency department Shock room/trauma bay	Acute care hosp OR Radiology ICU	LTAC Rehabilitation hosp
Personnel involved	EMR EMT AEMT Paramedic	EM physician Trauma surgeon TCRN/TNCC Support personnel	Trauma surgeon Orthopedic surgeon OMF surgeon Other specialists RN Case manager	Physiatrist Physical therapist Occupation therapist Vocational therapist Social worker
Applicable educational modules	BLS ALS PHTLS	ATLS ACLS PALS	–	–
Time frame	Minutes	Hours	Days	Weeks

BLS basic life support, *ALS* advanced life support, *PHTLS* prehospital trauma life support, *ATLS* advanced trauma life support, *ACLS* advanced cardiac life support, *LTAC* long-term acute care
In every case, the rescue, resuscitation, repair (or reconstruction), and rehabilitation of victims should and do seemlessly overlap. Moreover, the success of one particular stage of care profoundly influences the outcome of the one to follow. Effective state trauma systems in part assure the effective coordination of these different stages of care

was 58.2 per 100,000 [2]. Or, at a more personal level, the chance that an individual born in 2013 will die from injury is 1 in 20. In the USA, trauma accounts for 30% of all life-years lost [2], compared to 16% and 12% life-years lost due to cancer and heart disease, respectively, which translates into an annual economic burden of trauma-related death and disability estimated at $671 billion. Moreover, approximately one-quarter of all trauma deaths are potentially survivable and therefore preventable with optimal care of the injured [3].

The optimal care of the multiply injured patient can be divided into four arbitrary overlapping clinical areas (Table 4.1). An initial rescue involves management of immediate life-threatening conditions by first responders, generally in accordance with NAEMT[1] Prehospital Trauma Life Support (PHTLS) guidelines. Patients are then triaged and transported expeditiously to the most appropriate level of care based on guidelines developed by the centers for disease control and prevention and adopted by most state trauma systems. Resuscitation continues in the emergency department (ED), with immediate responses to conditions identified in the primary survey that affect airway, breathing, and circulation. Nothing else happens until the patient has an open, protected airway; satisfactory, symmetrical ventilation; and convincing evidence of sufficient and stable perfusion of vital organs. This is followed by systematic identification of injuries revealed in the secondary survey and confirmed by findings from relevant imaging. In the days that follow, the patient then begins definitive reconstruction of specific injuries and reconstitution of normal physiology. Lastly the patient moves on to rehabilitation, sometimes lasting weeks that may be required to maximize recovery from injuries, whether that recovery is partial or complete.

Extensive injuries to the head, face, and neck are frequently found in patients who have sustained either penetrating or blunt force trauma [4], and such injuries typically are considered for non-emergent repair days after a substantial amount of trauma care has been completed. Nonetheless, the initial care of the trauma patient can be enhanced, when oral and maxillofacial surgeons are included with other principal members of the trauma team. For this, working knowledge of the often extensive hemodynamic, hemostatic, and homeostatic derangements that develop in the multiple trauma patient is required. This complex pathophysiology evolves rapidly in the severely injured during the early phases of care. A bears on preparation of the patient for surgical

[1]National Association of Emergency Medical Technicians

procedures later in the hospital course. A synergistic interaction between oral and maxillofacial surgery (OMFS) and other surgical specialties is critical to effective management of specific issues such as difficult airways complicating maxillofacial trauma, massive hemorrhage from facial fractures or arterial injuries of the face and neck, or injuries that threaten vision [5, 6]. In addition, for Level 1 or Level 2 trauma center verification, the American College of Surgeons Committee on Trauma (ACSCOT) requires a multidisciplinary approach to complex craniofacial trauma.

Initial management of the multiply injured patient centers mainly on restoring adequate oxygen transport. Oxygen transport encompasses several biophysical and biochemical processes that mediate the transfer of oxygen from the atmosphere (partial pressure = 150 mmHg) to tissue (partial pressure = 40 mmHg). Fundamentally, the pathophysiology of shock relates to disruption of one or more of these processes. Oxygen must be continually supplied to generate sufficient amounts of adenosine triphosphate (ATP) for normal cellular metabolism. Furthermore, the total quantity of ATP maintained in the human body at any given moment is approximately 0.1 mole, although the cellular energy needed daily by an adult requires hydrolysis of 200–300 moles of ATP. Therefore, ATP must be continuously replenished 2000–3000 times during a 24-h period with essentially no interruption to maintain satisfactory cellular metabolism, preserve normal organ system function, and thereby assure survival of the critically injured patient. Consequently, the foremost objective of the initial care of the trauma patient is expeditious identification and correction of abnormalities of oxygen transport.

Here, we examine the initial care, essentially the perioperative care, of the trauma patient based on a detailed understanding of the complex pathophysiology that complicates multiple injuries. We also discuss management strategies, particularly for resuscitation, that have evolved in the last decade from the war-time experience of surgeons deployed to Iraq and Afghanistan. Definitive surgical management of specific injuries to the head face and neck are beyond the scope of this chapter. The reader is referred to recent comprehensive reviews and book chapters for specific discussions on these topics [7–22].

4.2 Pathophysiology

4.2.1 Shock

4.2.1.1 Etiology of Shock in the Trauma Patient

Fundamentally, shock can be defined as disruption of normal oxygen transport to peripheral tissue, which requires rapid correction before a physiologic oxygen reserve is exhausted. This can occur by airway obstruction, inadequate ventilation, or circulatory failure. Circulatory failure falls into two major categories: (1) decreased cardiac output, but mechanisms of flow distribution and oxygen extraction are unaffected, and (2) disruption of microvascular flow or extraction of oxygen, although cardiac output is either normal or elevated. Shock due to a decrease in cardiac output can be subdivided into conditions that reduce preload, diminish contractility, or increase afterload.

Loss of airway is the most obvious of these pathological processes, and an airway may be compromised by the process itself of establishing an airway. Immediate and severe arterial oxygen desaturation can occur with right mainstem intubation due to absent hypoxic pulmonary vasoconstriction (von Euler-Liljestrand mechanism) in multiply injured trauma patients. Potentially, 50% of cardiac output continues to the unventilated left lung after right mainstem intubation, whereas in a normal individual with a right mainstem intubation, saturation does not fall. Other problems with airways once they are established include unrecognized extubation; obstruction of the tube with mucus plugs, blood clots, or both; and the patient biting down on the tube as emergence from sedation used for intubation occurs.

Life-threatening conditions in the chest that must be recognized initially during the primary survey include open pneumothorax (sucking chest wound), flail chest, tension pneumothorax, massive hemothorax, and pericardial tamponade. A traumatic tear of the thoracic aorta will result in immediate exsanguination at the scene or will be contained by a hematoma that will never be large enough to produce shock. Indeed, if a patient with a known injury to the thoracic aorta exhibits signs of hypovolemic shock, another injury with ongoing hemorrhage should be assumed to be present until ruled out.

Because the right ventricle (RV) operates normally under low pressure, conditions that lower the pulmonary artery compliance or increase pulmonary vascular resistance to only a minor extent may significantly increase afterload on the RV, reduce output from the RV, and consequently reduce preload to the left ventricle [23]. Massive hemothorax can produce profound shock due to a combination of profound hypovolemia (decreased preload) and so-called tension physiology (increased afterload). These may be further compounded by a decrease in contractility secondary to extensive myocardial contusion. Therefore, massive hemothorax is often fatal because of simultaneous negative impact on all the three determinants of cardiac output.

Multiple derangements in oxygen transport also characterize the pathophysiology of smoke inhalation injuries. First, contained fires consume oxygen and can reduce the partial pressure of oxygen below ambient levels. Second, carbon monoxide can be generated in large quantities in fires and will raise levels of carboxyhemoglobin in victims of smoke inhalation to very high percentages. Carboxyhemoglobin has an affinity for oxygen 20 times that of normal hemoglobin and fails to offload oxygen in the periphery. Third, older combustible items give off cyanide that poisons oxidative phosphorylation (cytopathic hypoxia). Thus, victims of fires in an oxygen-poor environment tend not to offload what oxygen they do obtain, and what little is offloaded cannot be used effectively by mitochondria.

4.2.1.2 Hemorrhagic Shock

Hemorrhage induces a characteristic adaptive response, mediated by an increase in sympathetic autonomic activity in conjunction with secretion of several hormones that sustains vital organ function despite an acute reduction in circulating blood volume. Under this intense neurohormonal stimulation, an initial clinical state of *compensated shock* develops characterized by the activities of several physiological mechanisms that tend to mitigate the reduction in perfusion to peripheral tissue. In a previously healthy patient, these early compensatory processes can be highly effective and can create a deceptive clinical state that may suggest stability when, in fact, a substantial oxygen debt may be accruing and significant cellular dysfunction may be increasing. In the absence of intervention, ongoing hemorrhage may then progress to *decompensated shock*, characterized by hemodynamic instability and insufficient blood flow to sustain vital organ function [24], and finally to *refractory shock* (also referred to as irreversible shock), associated with catastrophic hemodynamic collapse and organ failure [25, 26]. For a patient in compensated hemorrhagic shock (HS), a resuscitation begun early and guided by accepted standards of care generally is effective. However, resuscitation becomes progressively less effective during the decompensated phase of HS as physiological reserves are exhausted and essentially is ineffective during the refractory phase as accumulating cell death prevents recovery of organ function. A patient can tolerate loss of 30% of his or her blood volume[2] and appear on superficial inspection to not be injured [27], but a blood loss of only 55–65% of blood volume is almost always fatal.

Because acceleration in heart rate (chronotropy) tends to produce a substantial increase in CO, tachycardia is observed as a primary compensatory response to hemorrhage, although this response can be limited by a reduction in SV due to a tachycardia-associated decrease in diastolic filling time. However, SV is preserved or even expanded secondary to several other compensatory mechanisms involving the heart operating in concert with an increase in heart rate. In addition to an increase in ventricular inotropy, these mechanisms include atrial contraction, accelerated ventricular relaxation during diastole (lusitropy), and reduced right ventricular afterload secondary to pulmonary artery vasodilatation [28]. Awareness of possible disruptions of these various physiological adaptations can be helpful to the trauma team attempting to discern unusual clinical presentations. For example, in trauma patients with ventricular diastolic dysfunction secondary to preexisting heart disease or as a consequence of certain cardiopulmonary injuries, diminished RV relaxation results in lower RV end-diastolic volume at a higher RV end-diastolic pressure [29]. Loss of this component of

[2]Blood volume for males is 75 mL/kg, for females 65 mL/kg.

compensation for acute blood loss may lead unexpectedly to a further fall in stroke volume as the chronotropic and inotropic components become active. In addition, similar neurohumoral mechanisms that mediate a compensatory response to acute blood loss are activated chronically in heart failure patients to compensate for deteriorating myocardial performance. A chronic increase in sympathetic tone due to heart failure downregulates heart adrenergic receptors, which would attenuate the chronotropic and inotropic effects of these agents where they expressed acutely to compensate for acute hemorrhage [28].

The blood a patient loses in severe traumatic injury can usually be found in one of four places: (1) blood left at the scene, (2) massive hemothorax, (3) hemoperitoneum, and (4) pelvis/retroperitoneum. Mortality for patients in shock with pelvic fracture remains high despite advances in the diagnosis and management of pelvic hemorrhage [30]. Pelvic fractures often occur in the setting of multisystem trauma and are associated with significant injuries and hemorrhage in other anatomic areas [31]. Pelvic fractures are classified according to Young-Burgess as lateral compression I–III, anterior-posterior compression I–III, and vertical shear (Fig. 4.1). There

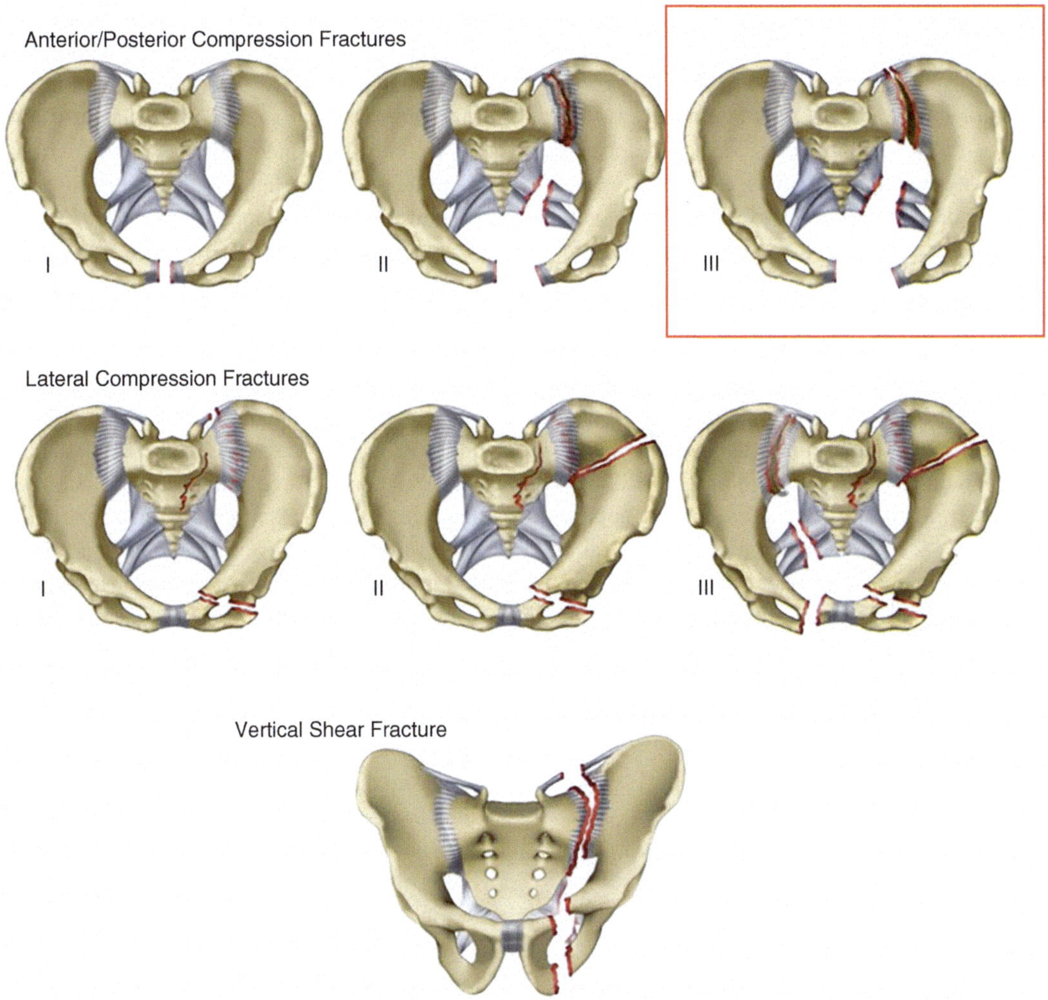

Fig. 4.1 Patterns of force cause distinct, recognizable, radiographic appearances of the fractured pelvis, described by Young, J.W., Burgess, A.R., et al.{Young, 1986 #2280}. These patterns are {Alton, 2014 #2278}

are also open pelvic fracture patterns that complement the Young-Burgess classification system. From the American Association for the Surgery of Trauma Multi-Institutional Trials Committee database, the most common pelvic fracture pattern is lateral compression I. The fracture pattern most likely to require a hemorrhage control intervention was anterior-posterior compression III.

4.2.2 Trauma-Induced Coagulopathies

4.2.2.1 Bleeding in the Trauma Patient

Predictably, disorders of hemostasis contribute to hemorrhage following severe injury and significantly complicate resuscitation. Dilution of platelets and coagulation factors during resuscitation was previously considered to be the principal cause of injury-associated coagulopathy (technically, resuscitation-associated coagulopathy). With the exception of transfusion events exceeding one blood volume (approximately 12 units), however, and in the absence of hypothermia and acidosis, hemodilution during resuscitation is now considered to have an inconsequential effect on coagulation [32]. Several other distinct hemostatic abnormalities have now been identified that are induced specifically by injury, collectively referred to as trauma-induced coagulopathy [33–37]. Trauma-induced coagulopathy (TIC) is detectable at the time of admission in approximately 25–56% of seriously injured trauma patients [38, 39], and once present, TIC is an independent predictor of adverse outcomes such as prolongation of ICU and hospital lengths of stay, as well as a fourfold increase in mortality [40]. The recognition of coagulopathy at admission is crucial in that this abnormality predicts a subsequent transfusion requirement [41].

4.2.2.2 Etiology of Trauma-Induced Coagulopathy

TIC is attributed to one of four basic mechanisms including (1) a qualitative platelet defect (particularly after traumatic brain injury [TBI]) [42–45], (2) diffuse endothelial cell injury (shock-induced endotheliopathy) [46], (3) depletion of coagulation factors and platelets through hemorrhage and deposition into injuries, or (4) consumption of platelets and coagulation factors secondary to disseminated intravascular coagulation (DIC) or hyperfibrinolysis [35, 47–49]. It must be recognized that trauma patients may have multiple or overlapping causes of coagulopathy and that the etiology or etiologies of a trauma-related bleeding diathesis will shift frequently, unpredictably, and without warning through the course of resuscitation. Therefore, frequent reassessment of the coagulation system by any means is an essential diagnostic objective. Furthermore, TIC by whatever mechanism or combination of mechanisms is intensified and perpetuated by acidosis and hypothermia. Indeed, the close association of these three abnormalities in critically injured patients is underscored by the colloquialism, "lethal triad of trauma." Complicating matters still further, patients may manifest a bleeding diathesis initially but subsequently convert within hours to a hypercoagulable state acquiring a risk for thromboembolic complications [50].

A qualitative platelet defect related to injury may develop in trauma patients [43, 51], and this specific acquired disorder occurs characteristically in patients with traumatic brain injury [42]. Early impairment in platelet aggregation after severe TBI is due in part to downregulation of platelet $P2Y_{12}$ receptor. $P2Y_{12}$ binds platelet agonist ADP and is the site of action of a frequently prescribed anticoagulant, clopidogrel (Plavix™). $P2Y_{12}$ inhibition correlates strongly with severity of TBI and TBI-related mortality, although AA receptor inhibition does not. The mechanism responsible for TBI-induced $P2Y_{12}$ downregulation is not clearly defined, and this type of platelet dysfunction is often overlooked in the TBI patient who is bleeding, particularly when the platelet count is normal.

Shock-mediated injury of the vascular endothelium has been examined as a mechanism of TIC. This injury also involves disruption of the covering glycocalyx, a 50–100 nm extracellular layer on the luminal side of blood vessels throughout the vascular space [52–54]. Shedding of the endothelial glycocalyx is suggested by detection of circulating levels of a somewhat nonspecific heparin sulfate proteoglycan, syndecan-1, and is associated with autoheparinization, which contributes to TIC in a small percentage of patients [55, 56]. High levels of syndecan-1 are independently associated with increased mortality after trauma [55].

Detached endothelial cells circulating in blood, and detection of specific biomarkers indicating endothelial cell injury, including angiopoietin-2, von Willebrand factor antigen, ristocetin cofactor activity, and soluble thrombomodulin, suggest some form of disruption of vascular endothelium [52] as part of a dysfunctional hemostatic response to injury. Although the exact cellular and molecular manifestations of endothelial cell perturbation in patients after significant trauma have not been clarified, enhanced expression both of the protein C receptor (EPCR) and of TM are thought to occur, which results in a substantial accumulation of aPC. Following activation of protein C (PC) by thrombin on this endothelial cell receptor platform, inactivation of FVa and FVIIIa is accelerated resulting in endogenous anticoagulation. Evidence also suggests that endothelial cell injury results in the release of substantial amounts of stored tissue-type plasminogen activator (tPA) from specific endothelial cell intracellular granules [57]. Furthermore, the concurrent activation of PC activation will also result in an increase in aPC-mediated degradation of plasminogen activator inhibitor-1 (PAI-1), which contributes to accumulation of tPA [58, 59]. Thus by more than one mechanism, overexpression of endothelial anticoagulation properties in the trauma patient destabilizes the balance between coagulation and fibrinolysis leading to a disproportionate amount of clot lysis over clot formation.

Coagulation factor depletion after injury and specifically hypofibrinogenemia are increasingly recognized as a frequent cause of TIC. Acquired hypofibrinogenemia also occurs as a result of reduced synthesis in patients with advance liver disease. Fibrinogen may be rapidly consumed in patients with DIC and secondary hyperfibrinolysis occurring in response to the diffuse prothrombotic state that characterizes DIC. Upregulation of tPA for any reason can generate plasmin in sufficient quantities to proteolytically degrade fibrinogen.

Fibrinogen circulates in plasma at a concentration of 200–400 mg/dL (substantially more than other coagulation factors) and has a half-life of approximately 3.75 days [60], second only in coagulation factor stability to FXIII (plasma half-life, 8 days). In response to systemic inflammatory processes, fibrinogen concentrations increase substantially as an acute-phase reactant, whereas, fibrinogen levels fall rapidly after trauma. Clot strength and the resistance of clot to sheer stress are attributed to the interaction between platelets and fibrinogen. Although recent viscoelastic data confirm that both platelets and fibrinogen are indeed important to clot strength following trauma, these data suggest, in fact, that platelets have a measurably greater impact at every time point after injury assessed out to 72 h [61].

DIC as a cause of TIC has recently been reexamined [49, 62], although DIC developing after trauma has been disputed [58, 63, 64]. In fact, most textbook descriptions of DIC consistently include trauma along with sepsis, obstetric crises, and severe immunologic responses as the clinical conditions most often complicated by DIC [65]. DIC is not a disease process as such, but rather the result of a distinct underlying pathology. DIC involves both the thrombin-generating and plasmin-generating pathways of hemostasis, and, as such, any clinical manifestation of DIC will be determined by the degree of activity of one pathway relative to the other. Generally, DIC is regarded as a hypercoagulable state characterized by nonspecific and diffuse deposition of microthrombi in smaller vessels causing a thrombotic microangiopathy. A deficiency of TFPI increases susceptibility to the development of DIC initiated by TF [66]. Ultimately the microangiopathy results in inadequate flow and disruption of oxygen delivery leading to organ dysfunction. Depletion of platelets and coagulation factors frequently occur as these are consumed in microvascular thrombi which manifests secondarily as coagulopathy. Because fibrinolytic activity, albeit reduced, may compensate somewhat for intravascular microthrombosis, antifibrinolytic therapy for DIC is not therefore recommended, except in rare cases when fibrinolysis dominates the clinical course (hyperfibrinolysis) [67]. An important exception to this pathologic course is a fulminate form of DIC that may occur after trauma during pregnancy complicated by injury to the gravid uterus as, for example, uterine laceration, amniotic fluid embolism, or placenta abruption [68]. A profound coagulopathy characterizes this clinical course due to a very rapid and almost complete consumption of platelets and coagulation factors [69]. An obstetrical hemorrhagic crisis combined with any of the other coagulopathies induced by trauma may cause catastrophic bleeding that is difficult, if not impossible, to control.

Severe injury (ISS > 25) may lead to the onset of uncontrolled lysis of fibrin and fibrinogen (fibrinogenolysis) as a primary process causing a bleeding diathesis (referred to as hyperfibrinolysis [HF]). HF develops in 2–20% of trauma patients, increasing to 53% in a subgroup who progress to massive transfusion [70–72] and who suffer worse outcomes [73]. However, TEG assessment of coagulation demonstrates that clinically significant hyperfibrinolysis may actually occur less frequently, developing in less than 3% of trauma patients [74]. Progressive hemodilution during resuscitation can decrease endogenous antifibrinolytic proteins including PAI-1, α_2-antiplasmin, and thrombin-activatable fibrinolysis inhibitor (TAFI) and contribute to the hyperfibrinolytic propensity associated with severe injury [75]. HF is characterized by viscoelastic assay as fulminant, intermediate, or late, resulting in 100%, 91%, or 73% mortality, respectively [76].

Both fibrin and fibrinogen degradation products in excess contribute to the coagulopathy by interfering with fibrin covalent polymerization and clot stability [77] and by blocking ADP-induced platelet aggregation [78]. Also this bleeding diathesis is potentiated by preexisting liver disease, severe liver injury, and hypoxic injury to the liver (shock liver) that tend to compromise hepatic clearance of these degradation products. A decrease in α_2-plasmin, an inhibitor that functions similar to PAI-1, is suggested as an additional mechanism of unopposed plasmin formation that characterizes hyperfibrinolysis complicating TBI [79].

4.2.3 Homeostatic Imbalances

4.2.3.1 Acid-Base Disturbances

A normal H+ concentration ([H+]) in blood and extracellular fluid is 40 nmol/L. A rise in [H+] secondary to hypoperfusion is relatively very small. In addition to detection of acidemia, an acidosis can be characterized by the amount of base that is required to return intravascular fluid and all other extracellular fluid pH to 7.4. This quantity is usually referred to by convention as base excess (BE) and is proceeded by a negative sign if base must be added to neutralize an excess [H+] and achieve a pH of 7.4; or BE is expressed without a negative sign if base would need to be removed as would be the case for an alkalosis. Thus, a BE of −3.0 mmol/L in a hemorrhaging patient would signify an acidemia likely secondary to lactic acidosis, while progression of the BE to −6.0 mmol/L in the same patient indicates a more severe lactic acidosis and progression of shock [79]. A negative BE is suggested to be the most accurate indicator of hypovolemic shock, and a worsening BE is a sensitive indicator of transfusion a requirement [80, 81]. Exogenously administered bicarbonate affects determination of BE and prevents the utilization of sequential determinations of this important parameter for decisions during resuscitation. Ethanol intoxication deepens a negative BE in trauma patients, but in general this should not confound identification of patients who are severely injured. Acidemia associated with a very high anion gap (AG) out of proportion to the fall in serum bicarbonate (i.e., the presence of excess unmeasured anions; $\Delta AG/\Delta HCO3 >> 1$) may suggest rhabdomyolysis complicating a lactic acidosis due to hypoperfusion [82] or severe hypophosphatemia [83].

4.2.3.2 Hypothermia

A decrease in core body temperature increases mortality of patients in hemorrhagic shock. Coagulation processes are profoundly altered by even mild hypothermia. Specifically, the enzymatic specificity constants of coagulation factors in hemostatic pathways and platelet activity are negatively affected to a significant degree by hypothermia. Coagulation factor activity is reduced approximately 10–15% for each 1 °C drop in temperature. However, the activity of endogenous anticoagulants, TFPIβ, antithrombin, and protein C, are also modified by hypothermia [84]. Hypothermia has a more important clinical effect on coagulation by inhibiting von Willebrand factor-platelet glycoprotein Ib-IX-V interactions [85]. Hyperfibrinolysis has been suggested as a potential mechanism of hypothermia-mediated coagulopathy [86], but accelerated clot lysis does not appear to be involved in this process when interrogated by viscoelastography [87].

In the hypovolemic patient, mild hypothermia may increase cardiac output and oxygen demand, whereas moderate or severe hypothermia can depress myocardial contractility and reduce cardiac output [88]. Hypothermia decreases compliance of the pulmonary artery, which imposes an increase in afterload on the RV. Metabolism is significantly diminished in hemorrhaging patients, and consequently heat production is reduced limiting passive rewarming [89]. Although external rewarming methods help to prevent heat loss, these transfer no heat to the patient.

Hypothermia is made worse by infusion of room-temperature fluids or cold blood components. Infusion of room-temperature fluids is equivalent to a 16 kcal/L heat loss, which will decrease the body temperature of a mildly hypothermic patient approximately 0.3 °C for every 2 L of infused crystalloid. For example, a patient will need to generate an additional 16 kcal to warm 1 L of room temperature (21 °C) crystalloid to 37 °C. However, patients cannot generate this additional heat because of diminished oxygen consumption due to shock [90]. Countercurrent rapid transfusion devices enable the infusion of up to 800 mL of saline, or 1 unit of blood, per minute at a temperature of 37–40 °C, equivalent to transfusing 5–8 kcal of heat per liter or 18–28 kcal of heat/12 units transfused [89, 91].

4.2.3.3 Electrolyte Imbalance

Reduced circulating ionized calcium and magnesium levels develop less from trauma and more from resuscitation-induced citrate toxicity. High transfusion rates of citrate-containing blood components often exceed the liver's capacity to clear the infused citrate. Furthermore, citrate metabolism may be reduced secondary to preexisting liver disease or impaired hepatic function from hypothermia. Citrate accumulation during resuscitation and citrate-mediated hypocalcemia are often made worse by dilution of calcium. Hypocalcemia reduces myocardial contractility and impairs maintenance of vasomotor tone. Hypomagnesemia also develops due to citrate accumulation and dilution. Hypomagnesemia and hypocalcemia are associated with disruption of myocardial repolarization characterized by a prolonged QT interval and a risk for development of torsades de pointes. Intravenous calcium gluconate or calcium chloride may be administered [92–94].

4.3 Hospital Evaluation and Management

4.3.1 Assessment for Shock

4.3.1.1 Physical Findings

Airway stridor is generally obvious, although the possibility of an impending loss of the airway should always be considered. For example, bilateral mandibular rami fractures may free the base of the tongue allowing the tongue to potentially slide posteriorly, obstructing the airway, which may occur suddenly, without warning if the patient's level of consciousness alters or his position on the gurney changes. An imminent loss of airway should be considered in patients with maxillofacial trauma who struggle to sit forward despite verbal or physical restraints. An expanding hematoma in the neck of an awake and alert patient from either blunt force or penetrating mechanisms mandates immediate intubation.

After intubation, a sudden increase in airway pressure (or the respiratory therapist reports that the patient has become "more difficult to bag") associated with a rapid fall in arterial oxygen saturation may suggest migration of the endotracheal tube into the right mainstem, a mucus plug, or an awake patient and no bite block. Asymmetry of chest wall excursions after intubation may suggest developing pneumo-, tension pneumo-, or hemopneumothorax. Paradoxical movement of a portion of the chest wall (inward movement during inspiration, outward movement during expiration) indicates flail chest (defined as an incompetent segment of the chest wall large enough to impair respiration [95]). An important pathological component of flail chest is the underlying severe pulmonary contusion that is invariably observed. A high-energy force vectored into the chest wall that damages the chest wall so extensively often does not dissipate completely before reaching the lung. A large V/Q mismatch from pulmonary contusion in concert with marked destabilization of chest wall mechanics precipitates deep respiratory failure, which will be suggested by an evident increase in work of breathing.

Inspection of the neck under a rigid collar should occur frequently during the resuscitation phase. Tracheal deviation is difficult to appreciate on inspection of the neck. Tracheal deviation is much easier to discern on the portable chest radiograph that is obtained as an adjunct to the primary survey. However, tracheal deviation usually indicates tension pneumothorax that requires immediate decompression, and therefore detection of tracheal deviation implies an error (delay) in management. Neck veins may be found in four conditions, including pericardial tamponade, tension pneumothorax, massive hemothorax, and congestive heart failure. For the last two conditions, distension will not generally be seen until fluid resuscitation is begun, and the last condition will be suggested by the appearance of pink, frothy sputum after initiation of resuscitation (as seen, e.g., in patient brought from a crash caused by a loss of control of the vehicle precipitated by sudden massive loss of consciousness after a sudden massive myocardial infarction).

Physical findings of hypoperfusion may be subtle or absent in the early phases of shock. Also there is substantial variability in the relationship of blood loss and clinical signs, making it difficult to establish clinical triggers to initiate interventions [96]. Capillary refill is simple and highly suggestive of hypoperfusion if a blanched fingernail bed does not return to normal in under 2 s. Traditional signs of hypoperfusion due to hemorrhagic shock, including cold, pale, and mottled skin (livedo reticularis), rapid and shallow breathing, weak to absent peripheral pulses, and confusion, are late signs reflecting decompensated shock and implying a delay in diagnosis if the patient presents before these signs develop.

Hypotension (systolic blood pressure [SBP] 90 mmHg) is inaccurate as a clinical indicator of shock, particularly hemorrhagic shock [97, 98]. A change in heart rate (HR) assessed out of context with other parameters is also an insensitive as well as a nonspecific sign of hemorrhage. However, the ratio of heart rate (HR) to SBP, or shock index (SI),[3] may identify hypoperfusion before decompensated shock develops [99, 100]. When healthy blood donors were subjected to a defined blood loss of 450 mL, the SI substantially increased, whereas the HR and SBP, taken as separate values, still remained within normal ranges [101]. A classification of shock based on SI was recently published (Table 4.2) [102]. Because age reduces physiological reserve, the product of SI and age is suggested as a more accurate clinical sign of hypoperfusion compared to SI alone [103]. A more sensitive indication of occult hemorrhage is obtained by dividing HR by pulse pressure (PP; equal to SBP minus DBP) ((HR/PP), referred to as the pulse rate over pressure evaluation (ROPE) index. Based on results in an animal model of acute blood loss, the inverse of the ROPE index (PP/HR) has been suggested as an even more sensitive reflection of changes in stroke volume during hemorrhagic shock [104, 105].

[3] Expression of clinical data in canonical forms tends to substantially expand the informational content of the raw data, and consequently data in this form are utilized whenever possible during assessment and management of a multiple trauma patient. For example, any one PaO_2 value expressed in relation to the fractional amount of oxygen in the gas the patient is inspiring when the PaO_2 is drawn, referred to as the P/F ratio, may now indicate one of several different clinical conditions. Thus, a P/F ratio = 100 for a ventilated, critically injured patient with a PaO_2 of 100 mmHg on a FiO_2 of 1.0 implies severe respiratory failure. This is, of course, a substantially different scenario compared to a healthy individual breathing room air who also has a PaO_2 of 100 mmHg (P/F = 100/0.2 = 500).

Table 4.2 Different conditions associated with a decrease or an increase in oxygen saturation of blood sampled from the central venous circulation ($ScvO_2$) $ScvO_2$ can be used as a close approximation of SvO_2 in the absence of a pulmonary artery catheter

↓$ScvO_2$ (<65% → ↑O_2ER)	↑$ScvO_2$ (>80% → ↓O_2ER)
A. ↓O_2 delivery • ↓*CaO_2* ↓[Hgb] (anemia) ↓SaO_2 (hypoxia) • ↓*Cardiac output* ↓Preload ↓Contractility ↑Afterload ↓Venous return	**A. ↑O_2 delivery** • ↑*Cardiac output* SIRS/sepsis Liver failure Shunt
B. ↑O_2 consumption • Adrenergic stimulation • Stress/inflammation • Pain/delirium • Hyperthermia/shivering	**B. ↓O_2 consumption** • Analgesia/sedation • Hypothermia • Mechanical ventilation • Hypothyroidism • Starvation • Paralysis
C. ↑P_{50} • ↑Temp • ↑[2,3-DPG] • ↑[H^+] (acidosis)	**C. ↓P_{50}** • ↓Temp • ↓[2,3-DPG] • ↓[H^+] (alkalosis)

PP will change as SV changes. A PP less than 25% of SBP is considered abnormally low (also referred to as narrowed) and is typically discernable before a fall in MAP (that is to say, before the patient enters a state of decompensated shock). PP narrowing reflects a downward trend in SBP due to diminished SV in concert with an upward trend in DBP secondary to an increase in vascular resistance, a compensatory circulatory response for an acute reduction in SV.

4.3.1.2 CVP

The measurement of central venous pressure (CVP) has been used extensively for several decades to guide fluid therapy in critical ill patients, including patients undergoing fluid resuscitation for hemorrhagic shock secondary to blunt force or penetrating trauma. The use of CVP measurements in this manner is based on, arguably, an incorrect assumption that CVP accurately reflects right ventricular end-diastolic volume (RVEDV) and therefore correctly predicts whether or not an increase CO can be achieved by increasing preload (i.e., whether or not the patient is fluid responsive) (Fig. 4.2). However, two extensive meta-analyses of several published

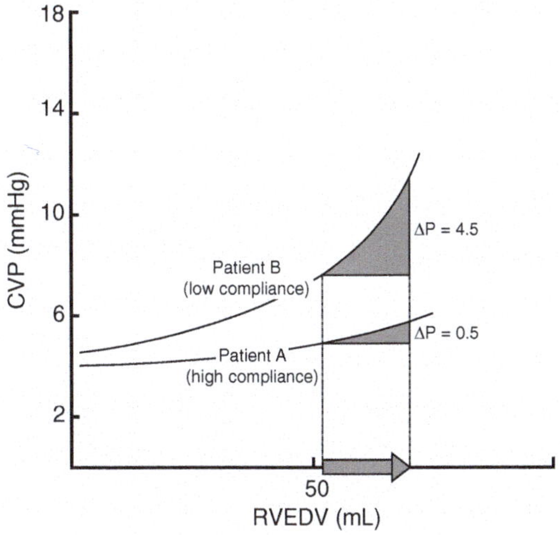

Fig. 4.2 Central venous pressure (CVP) is dependent on compliance. Two hypothetical patients, one (**a**) exhibiting low, and the other (**b**) high, elastance of the ventricular wall (high compliance and low compliance, respectively). Although both ventricles are filled to the same volume, and have the same preload, CVP readings suggest different preloads leading possibly to excess fluid being given to patient A and an insufficient resuscitation of patient B

studies that examine the utility of this hemodynamic parameter used in this manner indicate that CVP monitoring, in fact, neither predicts fluid responsiveness nor correlates with fluid administration [106–108]. Because of highly variable right ventricular compliance, there is an inconsistent relationship between right atrial pressure (CVP) and RVEDV, and hence one does not reflect the other. This is particularly the case in trauma patients in whom significant reductions in ventricular compliance may occur secondary to myocardial contusion. Also, during elevations in intrathoracic pressure induced by mechanical ventilation, CVP increases although there is generally a decrease in RVEDV. Moreover, the normal response of the right ventricle to fluid resuscitation characteristically results in little change or even a small drop in CVP as cardiac output increases. This response is essential for maintenance of a pressure gradient between P_{ms} and right atrial pressure that promotes sufficient venous return. Consequently, CVP measurements used to guide fluid therapy may lead to clinical decisions that are potentially harmful.

4.3.1.3 Oximetry

The saturation of Hgb with oxygen is the most accurately measured ex vivo in a sample of blood by a CO-oximeter (designated SaO_2 or SvO_2 for arterial or venous blood samples, respectively). Modern CO-oximeters also detect certain acquired dyshemoglobins such as methemoglobin and carboxyhemoglobin [109]. Pulse oximetry (SpO_2) is used to routinely assess arterial oxygen saturation indirectly by absorbance of light of specific wavelengths [109]. Conventional SpO_2 sensors are placed on a finger, toe, or earlobe, which permit adequate transmission and measurement of light absorbance at opposing surfaces of the tissue bed. Finger probes are more accurate than toe or earlobe probes [110].Low-flow states degrade absorbance-based SpO_2 accuracy significantly, at a time when an accurate signal is most needed. Forehead SpO_2 sensors use reflectance technology rather than absorbance, which improves accuracy of data in critically ill trauma patients [111] and patients on flow-restricting high-dose vasopressors [112].

Mixed venous oxygen saturation (SvO_2) reflects the balance between delivery (DO_2) and oxygen utilization (VO_2), (also referred to as oxygen uptake), which is maintained by the fraction of oxygen extracted from DO_2 (O_2ER) required to hold VO_2 at a level that exactly matches oxygen consumption. Shock is defined as a reduction in DO_2 to a level (DO_2crit) below which VO_2 cannot be sustained, irrespective of the pathological process that disrupts oxygen transport balance. Specific correlations between DO_2 and VO_2 differentiate stages of circulatory shock such as compensated decompensated or refractory shock; *and SvO_2 can effectively serve as a meaningful endpoint of resuscitation.* In addition, SvO_2 may be utilized to estimate cardiac output or to trend a cardiac output response to a specific intervention. Furthermore, SvO_2 may unmask unexpected microvascular dysfunction, illuminate plausible etiologies for a hypoxia that elude diagnosis, and provide data to rapidly calculate useful approximations of venous admixture[4] [113].

SvO_2 is obtained on blood sampled from the pulmonary artery, usually through the most distal port of a balloon-tipped, flow-directed pulmonary artery catheter (Swan-Ganz® catheter). In the early phases of resuscitation, these catheters are not inserted. However, an acceptable approximation of SvO_2 ($ScvO_2$) can be obtained from blood drawn from a central venous catheter (Table 4.2). The best approximation is obtained with the tip of the catheter in the right atrium. However, in the acute setting introducer-type catheters which are of large bore and short length are occasionally put into the central circulation for rapid fluid administration. Even if the tip of these catheters resides in an innominate vein, $ScvO_2$ can be used to approximate SvO_2. Typically, blood returning from the upper part of the body is lower in saturation than mixed venous SvO_2. Blood returning from the lower part of the body is more highly saturated with oxygen than normal SvO_2 due to a large amount of blood flow to the kidneys, which extract proportionally less oxygen. Blood from the inferior vena cava obtained from a femoral catheter is probably not useful.

When blood is aspirated through a central venous catheter for determination of $ScvO_2$, it is

[4]During subsequent phases of management, determination of $ScvO_2$ may be used to uncover risk for reintubation in patients who successfully have met all other criteria for extubation.

important to bring back the plunger in the syringe smoothly but also to not draw with excessive force, to avoid high negative pressure in a relatively long, narrow triple lumen catheter channel. Blood in the catheter lumen under substantial negative pressure may cause cavitation inception which theoretically could distort the oxygen saturation of the sample. Also, allowing the blood sample to equilibrate with an air bubble above the plunger in the syringe may also distort $ScvO_2$.

Near-infrared spectroscopy (NIRS) of peripheral nonpulsatile blood also may be utilized to assess peripheral perfusion. In determining hemoglobin saturation (denoted as StO_2), NIRS does not sample transmitted pulsatile arterial signals and nonpulsatile venous signals (as in SpO_2 determinations), but instead assesses nonpulsatile reflective absorbance of blood in capillaries and venules [114]. As such, changes in StO_2 in peripheral muscle (usually a probe is placed over the thenar prominence or deltoid muscles) reflect changes in oxygen demand, oxygen delivery, or both; oxygen delivery, in turn, is a function of cardiac output and total systemic resistance. In the setting of hemorrhagic shock, with diminished flow to the periphery, one may assume that oxygen demand is constant and therefore plausibly infer that a fall in StO_2 is indicative of an increase in oxygen extraction occurring in response to a reduction in flow, reduced hemoglobin concentration, or microvascular dysfunction. StO_2 measurements indicate inadequate perfusion with a sensitivity similar to a negative base excess sensitivity for hemorrhagic shock, but in contrast to repetitive blood draws for repeat determination of base excess, StO_2 is a noninvasive continuous signal [115]. A low StO_2 may precede hemodynamic deterioration and provide an early warning of imminent decompensation.

In addition to baseline measurements of StO_2, a vascular occlusion test (VOT) is performed with a rapid inflation of a pneumatic cuff to a pressure well above the SBP for a brief period of time. The vascular VOT assesses the response of the microvascular blood flow to a defined local hypoxic stimulus, by determining the slope of StO_2 desaturation during the ischemic period and the rate of change of StO_2 during a reactive hyperemia after the cuff is deflated [116].

4.3.1.4 Metabolic Markers of Shock

Hemorrhagic shock produces a type A lactic acidosis due to hypoperfusion. A serum lactate in a trauma patient >2.5 mg/dL on admission is an independent marker of increased mortality [117], even though an elevated lactate in shock is generally considered an adaptive protective mechanism by providing an alternate energy source to glucose for the brain and heart. Lactic acidosis is associated with a negative base excess, and resolution of this value is considered the most reliable endpoint of resuscitation. A lactate to pyruvate ratio in extracellular fluid of >25–30 indicates a type A lactic acidosis consistent with hypoperfusion and may be a more sensitive marker of impaired oxygen delivery than a negative base excess [118]. However, determination of a lactate to pyruvate ratio requires specialized point-of-care monitoring technology presently not applicable in acute settings. There is no detectable difference in lactate level between arterial, central venous, and peripheral venous blood samples, although a peripheral venous sample for lactate determination should not be drawn below a tourniquet [119]. Failure to normalize blood lactate levels (<2.5 mmol/L) also is associated with increased morbidity and mortality [120].

Although $ScvO_2$ detects perfusion failure at a macrocirculatory level with acceptable sensitivity, $ScvO_2$ is somewhat insensitive to the presence of tissue hypoperfusion due to dysfunction in microcirculatory beds, which ultimately may be the major determination of patient outcomes. As a consequence of deficiencies in the regional distribution of blood flow through arterioles or secondary to reduced diffusion of oxygen from capillary erythrocytes to peripheral cells, tissue hypoxia may be present even though a normal $ScvO_2$ value is measured. CO_2 is an end product of metabolism, and therefore the content of CO_2 in effluent venous blood from tissue is higher than the content of CO_2 in afferent arterial blood transported to tissue. Also, due to its high plasma solubility, CO_2 lacks diffusion limitations compared to O_2. For these reasons, an increase in the difference between the partial pressure of CO_2 (pCO_2) in central venous blood ($pcvCO_2$) and arterial blood ($paCO_2$), referred to as the central venous-to-arterial CO_2gap

(ΔpCO_2gap; normal <6 mmHg), can be used to identify shock in patients for whom $ScvO_2$ is normal [121, 122]. $\Delta pCO_2gap/(CaO_2\text{-}CvO_2)$ may predict whether or not an increase in DO_2 induced by infusion of fluids will result in an increase in VO_2 [123] (Table 4.3).

4.3.1.5 Ultrasound

Bedside ultrasound directed by specific protocols is an essential diagnostic tool for assessment of hypovolemic shock, although this technique provides information at one moment in time. These imaging algorithms include focused cardiac ultrasound (FOCUSED), focused assessed transthoracic echo (FATE), rapid ultrasound for shock and hypotension (RUSH), focused assessment with sonography in trauma (FAST), extended FAST (e-FAST), and bedside organ assessment with sonography after trauma (BOAST). Evaluation of the inferior vena cava (IVC) by ultrasound contributes important information to the diagnosis of hypovolemia. Sonographic views in different axes of the IVC may be obtained with either a subxiphoid or lateral abdominal wall window. For spontaneously breathing patients, an inspiratory decrease in IVC diameter relative to expiratory diameter correlates with right atrial pressure (Fig. 4.3). Conversely, in patients supported by positive pressure ventilation, the IVC distends during the inspiratory phase relative to the expiratory phase, and increasing distension suggests fluid responsiveness.

Table 4.3 Causes of circulatory shock in trauma

1) ↓CO, ↓$ScvO_2$, ↓ΔpCO_2gap, ↓RPAP
- ↓Preload (e.g., hemorrhagic shock)
- ↓Contractility (e.g., post-MI; cardiogenic)
- ↑Afterload (e.g., tension pneumothorax)

2) ↑CO, ↑$ScvO_2$, ↑ΔpCO_2gap, ↓RPAP
- Sepsis
- Neurogenic

3) ↑CO, ↑$ScvO_2$, ↑ΔpCO_2gap, ↑RPAP
- Liver failure

4.3.2 Assessment of Coagulation

4.3.2.1 Conventional Laboratory Tests of Coagulation

The coagulation system is routinely screened by measuring the activated partial thromboplastin time (aPTT) and prothrombin time (PT, also expressed as an international normalized ratio, or INR). A platelet count is usually obtained, but although qualitative platelet defects are as common as quantitative defects, platelet function is not routinely assessed. Fibrinogen concentration

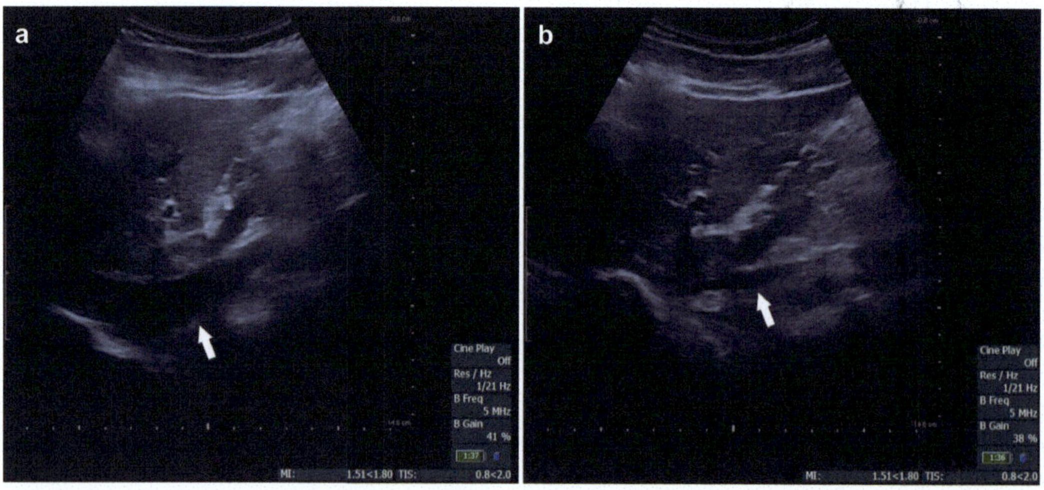

Fig. 4.3 Shock room focused assessment with sonography for trauma (FAST) examination demonstrating the inferior vena cava in sagittal projection (white arrows) during (**a**) expiration and (**b**) inspiration (Images courtesy of Dr. Grace Rozycki, Indiana University School of Medicine)

may form part of a coagulation screen. The presence or absence of products of fibrinolysis or the proteolytic digestion of fibrinogen may be determined. Data from these tests performed in most clinical laboratories often are not available within a time frame that is useful for assessment of an actively bleeding trauma patient [124].

Assays available for determination of fibrinogen used most often in hospitals are Clauss and PT-derived fibrinogen. Reduced fibrinogen by Clauss assay does not differentiate whether the decreased fibrinogen activity is caused by hypofibrinogenemia, a dysfunctional protein present in normal amounts (dysfibrinogenemia), or the combination of a dysfunctional protein circulating in plasma at an abnormal concentration. Also, the presence of heparin reduces the amount of fibrinogen detectable by Clauss due to inhibition of thrombin as a reagent in the assay, which may incorrectly suggest hypofibrinogenemia. The presence of direct thrombin inhibitors (e.g., bivalirudin or argatroban) also causes inaccurate fibrinogen determinations by Clauss [125]. Currently available methods for determination of fibrinogen also include enzyme immunoassays, as well as immunoturbidimetric assays, radial immunodiffusion, and electroimmunoassays [126].

Conventional clinical laboratory assays do not completely describe the various coagulation abnormalities associated with trauma [127–130]. PT and aPTT, for example, only assay the function of a discrete number of procoagulant proteins, are insensitive to plasma levels of the endogenous anticoagulants, and, more importantly, do not include the contribution of cellular elements to coagulation [131]. Indeed, neither PT, initially developed for titration of warfarin therapy, nor aPTT, developed to monitor certain inherited bleeding disorders, has been validated for the evaluation of coagulation system in trauma [132]. One other assay, the clot formation and lysis (CloFAL) assay, does measure the net hemostatic balance between coagulation and fibrinolytic capacities, but this particular laboratory test is not performed routinely. Moreover, customary coagulation assays are not capable of detecting hypercoagulable disorders [133], which complicate severe injury as frequently as bleeding disorders.

4.3.2.2 Viscoelastic Assay

A blood clot is a viscoelastic polymer with the elastic properties of a spring combined with the properties of a viscous fluid. Together these physical properties maintain clot integrity and reversible deformation despite the shear force of flowing blood. Measures of coagulation more relevant in trauma patients may include assessment of the rate of clot formation, clot strength, and the resistance of the newly formed clot to lysis. Three systems, SONOCLOT™, thromboelastography (TEG™, Haemonetics Corp., Niles, IL, USA), and rotational thromboelastometry (ROTEM™, Tem International GmbH, Munich, Germany), are used clinically to determine the viscoelastic properties of a blood clot. TEG and ROTEM are similar in that they interrogate essentially the same viscoelastic properties of a fibrin clot under low shear stress conditions (simulating rheologic conditions in veins), including rates of clot formation, clot elasticity, and overall stability of clot. They are also somewhat distinct due to certain technical differences and different nomenclatures for the same measured parameters (Fig. 4.4). A viscoelastic hemostatic assay is in essence an integrated assessment of the several components involved in clot formation and is comprised of five basic measurements, which have been correlated with different phases of coagulation [134–136] and different disorders of coagulation. Both TEG and ROTEM provide results earlier than are usually available with conventional tests of coagulation [137]. Basic viscoelastic hemostatic assays are limited in that these do not specifically evaluate endothelial cell function in coagulation and therefore cannot detect the various forms of von Willebrand disease, expression of thrombomodulin, or release of various molecules stored in endothelial cell Weibel-Palade bodies.

The strength of a formed clot is dependent in large part upon an interaction between platelets and fibrinogen [138, 139]. Both are critical for clot resistance to disruption by intravascular hydrodynamic forces. Clot strength is measured in both viscoelastic systems and is designated maximal amplitude (MA) in the TEG system, whereas it is designated maximal clot firmness

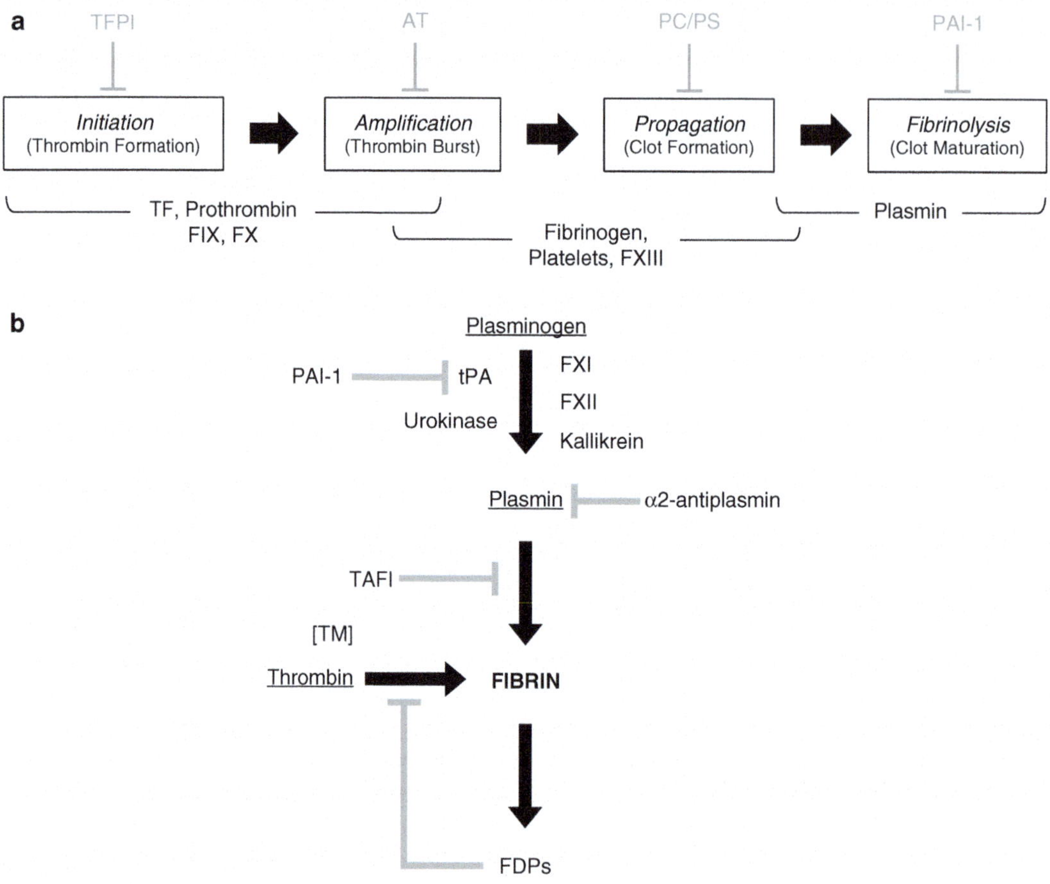

Fig. 4.4 Coagulation and fibrinolysis. Fundamentally, coagulation is the generation of two key enzymes, *thrombin* and *plasmin*, that act on two key substrates, *fibrinogen* and *fibrin*, respectively. In (**a**), a cell-based model of coagulation is shown, consisting of formation of a small amount of thrombin that leads to thrombin-mediated activation of many other supporting components. This initiates rapid acceleration of reactions leading to a so-called thrombin burst and the initiation of fibrinogen conversion to fibrin strands, which are ultimately cross-linked by FXIII. Although endogenous inhibitors, tissue factor pathway inhibitor (TFPI), antithrombin (AT), and protein C | thrombomodulin are shown in fairly specific interactions, more cross-reactivity exists. In (**b**), the generation of plasmin from plasminogen is shown. Also depicted are the regulatory pathways of fibrinolysis, including the major endogenous inhibitor of fibrinolysis, plasminogen activator inhibitor-1 (PAI-1). Fibrinolysis (referred to as secondary fibrinolysis) is required as part of normal hemostasis. A physiological release of endogenous tPA in response to trauma is thought to be essential to prevent propagation of the clotting process beyond sites of injury. In particular, control of coagulation by fibrinolysis averts intravascular thrombosis in microvascular circuits. Disruption of microvascular perfusion, if extensive, may precipitate organ failure. The exact physiological function of fibrinolysis in clot formation is made less clear, however, by the observation that neither congenital plasminogen deficiency nor congenital dysplasminogenemia is causally linked to any thromboembolic phenomena [190]. An inherited hypofibrinolytic phenotype due to excessive PAI-1 expression associated with an increased thrombotic risk occurs in patients with 4G/5G polymorphism of the PAI-1 gene [191]. Tranexamic acid (TXA; Cyklokapron™) is a synthetic lysine that occupies plasminogen and plasmin lysine binding sites and blocks binding of plasminogen and plasmin to lysine sites on fibrin. Tranexamic acid has eight times the antifibrinolytic activity of a second lysine analogue, ε-aminocaproic acid (aminocaproic acid; Amacar™)

(MCF) in the ROTEM system. Traditional viscoelastic parameters reflecting fibrinogen function, k-time (TEG), clot formation time (ROTEM), and α-angle (TEG and ROTEM) correlate to some degree with fibrinogen concentration. However the agreement between these parameters and fibrinogen levels determined by standard von Clauss assay is not sufficiently strong to be useful clinically [140, 141]. To overcome this limitation in TEG assays, the specific contributions of fibrinogen and platelets to clot strength ($MA_{fibrinogen}$ and $MA_{platelets}$, respectively) are determined by measurement of MA before and after the addition of an inhibitor of the platelet glycoprotein IIb/IIIa receptor for fibrinogen (abciximab; ReoPro™) [140]. In ROTEM assays, cytochalasin D, which inhibits platelet function by blocking platelet actin contractile elements, is added to assess the relative contributions of fibrinogen and platelets to MCF [142]. Recent observations indicate that the viscoelastic evaluation of fibrinogen by platelet GPIIb/IIIa receptor inhibition is less effective compared to the reduction of a platelet contribution to clot strength with cytochalasin D. The combination of a GPIIb/IIIa receptor blockade and cytochalasin D added in viscoelastic assays may improve agreement with a fibrinogen level by von Clauss determination [142]. In that there is growing recognition that trauma-induced hypofibrinogenemia develops frequently and that improvement in survival is realized with infusion of fibrinogen [143], accurate determination of fibrinogen by viscoelastic hemostatic assay is an important consideration.

In the TEG system, additional measures of clot strength can be computed. Coagulation index (CI) is derived from r, k-time, α-angle, and MA, with a normal CI −3.0 to +3.0; > +3.0 suggests hypercoagulable state and <−3.0 suggests coagulopathy. CI can be used to differentiate a trauma-associated consumptive process caused by either DIC or primary hyperfibrinolysis and whether to administer heparin or an antifibrinolytic. The shear elastic module strength, designated, G, is a computer-generated quantity that reflects an integrated measure of clot strength incorporating TEG parameters determined by the initial thrombin burst, amplification, propagation, and fibrinolysis ($G = [5000 \times \text{amplitude}/ [100 - \text{amplitude}]$; $G = 5.3–12.4$ dynes/cm^2 is considered normal, $G < 5.3$ dynes/cm^2 is indicative of coagulopathy, and $G > 12.4$ dynes/cm^2 is indicative of a hypercoagulable state). Conceptually G is the best measure of clot strength because it reflects the contributions of the enzymatic and platelet components of hemostasis [144, 145]. Speed of clot propagation is given by maximum rate of thrombus generation (MRTG; dynes/cm^2 s^{-1}) [146].

4.3.3 Management of Shock

4.3.3.1 Airway

Airway problems characteristically complicate maxillofacial trauma, whether caused by a penetrating or a blunt force mechanism, and these readily justify inclusion of the most experienced airway experts among principal members of the trauma team. Anatomic distortion of the pharynx because of restricted mouth opening, tongue base prolapse, pharyngeal edema, pharyngeal hematomas, or uncontrolled hemorrhage prevents the correct seating of supraglottic airway devices (so-called airway rescue devices) or obscures the glottic opening challenging the placement of an endotracheal tube [147]. Maxillofacial trauma is often associated with a cervical spine fracture [148], and, in fact, for every patient in the process of airway evaluation and management, the cervical spine is assumed to be fractured and the fracture is assumed to be unstable until proven otherwise [15].

Other factors also considered in recognition of a difficult airway include, but are not limited to, the experience of the surgeon, whether or not airway protection is the sole indication, and the amount of time available for preoxygenation. Although advanced airway management in the setting of maxillofacial trauma is, predictably, often indicated to assure airway patency, airway management is critical to the goals of restoring and maintaining oxygen transport. Therefore, the risk of cardiovascular collapse that is possible with any airway intervention must be factored into identification of the difficult airway. Specifically, risks of airway interventions include the development of hypoxemia, systemic arterial hypotension, metabolic acidosis, and acute right ventricular failure. The process of oral endotracheal intubation may precipitate rapid desaturation, which may result in hemodynamic instability, hypoxic brain injury, and potentially cardiopulmonary arrest [149]. Conversion of a low transpleural pressure in the spontaneous breathing patient, inadequate though the patient's ventilation may be, to a markedly increased transpleural pressure with intubation and positive pressure ventilation potentially reduces the pressure gradient ((P_{MS} – [R] atrial pressure), from Eq. (1)) responsible for venous return to the right heart. In this scenario, systemic hypotension is managed by infusion of isotonic (or hypertonic) crystalloid, colloid, or a blood component; α- and β-adrenergic stimulation with norepinephrine (Levophed™) or α_1-adrenergic stimulation with phenylephrine (Neo-Synephrine™) would most likely further reduce perfusion of tissue close to an anaerobic threshold.

Emergent percutaneous cricothyrotomy using a narrow-bore cannula (with either Seldinger or trocar methods) may prove ineffective, and the use of jet ventilation is associated with a higher incidence of serious complications (e.g., device failure or barotrauma). Repeated attempts at endotracheal intubation may compromise maintaining oxygenation and increase the risk of aspiration. Therefore, to secure the airway before a "cannot intubate/cannot oxygenate" crisis develops, surgical cricothyrotomy may be considered early. An open cricothyrotomy performed by an experienced operator is associated with the highest success rate and carries the lowest incidence of complications. Factors associated with unsuccessful cricothyrotomy are failure to localize the cricothyroid membrane and an incision (whether transverse or horizontal) that fails to accommodate the size of the patient, the experience of the operator, or both. We place a cuffed size 6 endotracheal through the tracheotomy directly or over a boogie tube exchanger. Care should be taken not to perforate either the left or right mainstem bronchus by a rigid end of any airway exchange device.

4.3.3.2 Ventilation

Management of chest trauma in the initial period of evaluation involves decompression of air, blood, or both that have accumulated in one or the other hemithorax for a variety of reasons. For this, treatment modalities consist of needle decompression chest tube placement or ED thoracotomy in escalating degrees of invasiveness. During the primary survey, it is paramount to determine symmetrical ventilation to the right and left hemithoraces. Commonly, an emergent placement of a chest tube is incorrectly passed off as a minor procedure. However, a chest tube placed without proper indication, utilizing imperfect technique, or not managed appropriately after placement may result in substantial morbidity [150]. A chest tube is indicated whenever fluid, air, or both must be drained from the chest. Patients at risk for tension pneumothorax (e.g., patients with chest injuries requiring air transport or patients who cannot be monitored) should have prophylactic chest tubes placed. We prefer placement through the fifth intercostal space (or the inframammary crease) between anterior and midaxillary lines. Placement of a chest tube in the fifth intercostal space on the right side runs the risk of placement into the horizontal fissure separating the upper and middle lobes of the right lung, and, in this location, a chest tube may not function properly. This may be avoided by using a tube exchanger as an introducer, which can be directed away from the fissure with the tip of the tube positioned in the apex of the thoracic cavity.

Confirmation of entry into pleural space by inserting a finger through the thoracostomy incision while placing a chest tube in a trauma patient carries considerable risk of puncture injury and transmission of blood-borne pathogens. Rib fracture ends may be sharply splintered and displaced and capable of harm in this way. The authors prefer to complete the dissection with a large curved Kelly clamp run along the superior surface of the rib below the interspace chosen to enter. Once it is ascertained that the rib is smooth, we place a finger on the rib and then over the superior aspect of the rib to confirm the pleural space and pleural space contents. The lung can be identified by its spongy feel, and the diaphragm identified by a tactile sense similar to uncooked skinned chicken breast. We prefer a 36 Fr straight chest tube to ensure complete evacuation of any blood in the pleural space.

Exploratory thoracotomy for traumatic hemothorax is mandated if more than 1200 mL of blood is evacuated immediately. If the initial amount drained is less than 1200 mL, then the rate of bleeding from the chest becomes the determining parameter in deciding whether to explore the chest. This rate is somewhat variable, from 500 mL/h to 150 mL/4 h. Often the decision to perform exploratory thoracotomy for bleeding must be made within a shorter time frame. We explore the chest if output is >100 mL/15 mins at any time in the first hour, greater than 1500 mL for 24 h after that, or if after placement of the chest tube, bleeding from the chest continues at a rate of 150–200 mL/2 h. A third consideration is ongoing blood transfusion requirement or the institution of massive transfusion with a suggested source in the chest.

4.3.3.3 Perfusion

Hemodynamic Resuscitation

The volume of blood a severely injured patient may have lost prior to arrival to the hospital can be difficult to quantify, and the rate of ongoing hemorrhage in the trauma bay often cannot be measured. Up to 35% of blood volume may be lost acutely before hemodynamic decompensation occurs, and tachycardia or systemic hypotension becomes evident [27]. Therefore, development of hypotension during initial assessment of the trauma patient implies a delayed diagnosis of shock.

Under physiologic and pathophysiological conditions, regulation of blood flow is determined by metabolic demand. Autoregulatory mechanisms involving cerebral and coronary artery circulations maintain adequate blood flow over a wide range of mean arterial blood pressures (MAPs). Consequently, a MAP of 45 to 50 mmHg is sufficient to maintain adequate perfusion of the heart and brain in acute situations [97]. Under certain circumstances, however, when the capacity to compensate for a change in perfusion pressure is compromised, a higher MAP may be indicated. For example, a MAP of 65 to 70 mmHg may be required if the patient has a significant traumatic brain injury, which tends to disable cerebral autoregulatory mechanisms, or for the patient who harbors a comorbidity that renders autoregulation inoperative such as atherosclerotic coronary artery disease or aortic stenosis.

Red blood cell transfusion is the critical component of hemodynamic resuscitation but may be adversely affected by rapid deterioration of many biophysical and biochemical properties of erythrocytes stored at 4 °C (for up to 42 days). These abnormalities are collectively referred to as a red cell storage lesion [151]. For example, exhaustion of energy stores during storage leads to depletion of erythrocyte 2,3-diphosphoglycerate (2,3-DPG). Binding of 2,3-DPG to hemoglobin decreases the affinity of hemoglobin for oxygen (rightward shift of the oxyhemoglobin dissociation curve), which facilitates offloading of oxygen from hemoglobin in tissue despite a relatively low partial pressure of oxygen in this environment. Depending on length of time in storage, packed RBCs transfused during resuscitation may not offload oxygen in sufficient amounts to meet cellular demand due to low levels of erythrocyte 2,3-DPG. Methemoglobin (hemoglobin containing iron in an oxidized ferric state), which increases hemoglobin affinity for oxygen, accumulates in erythrocytes during storage and could potentially exacerbate a leftward shift of the oxyhemoglobin dissociation curve (higher hemoglobin affinity for oxygen, lower P_{50}) induced by low levels of 2,3-DPG [152]. Furthermore, the oxygen affinity of hemoglobin in transfused RBCs may be driven even higher by hypophosphatemia or hypothermia in the recipient [153, 154]. A leftward shift in the oxyhemoglobin dissociation curve may be offset by a rightward shift due to an elevated plasma H^+ concentration (Bohr Effect). The relative contributions of hypothermia and acidosis to the final P_{50} can be determined by calculation of this parameter with the sigaard- andersen oxygen status algorithm, or the Hill Equation [155] (Table 4.4). Thus an ostensibly resuscitated patient could potentially remain acidotic despite every indication of adequate perfusion and transport of oxygen to the periphery. This complex abnormality in oxygen transport would be suggested by an elevated $ScvO_2$ and/or elevated ΔpCO_2gap if these two parameters are included as resuscitation endpoints.

Table 4.4 Calculation of P_{50} at various temperatures and at different levels of pH

	7.4 $[H^+]$ = 40 nm/L	7.3 $[H^+]$ = 50 nm/L	7.2 $[H^+]$ = 63 nm/L	7.5 $[H^+]$ = 31 nm/L
37°	26.6	29.4	32.3	24.5
36°	25.4	27.8	30.5	23.5
35°	24.0	26.3	28.9	21.9
34°	22.7	24.9	27.3	20.7
33°	21.5	23.6	25.9	19.6
32°	20.3	22.3	24.5	18.6
31°	19.3	21.1	23.1	17.6
30°	18.2	20.0	21.9	16.6
28°	16.3	17.9	19.6	14.8

In addition to these metabolic abnormalities, morphologic transformation in stored erythrocytes from flexible biconcave discs to rigid echinocytes (burr cells) and then to sphero-echinocytes decreases microvascular flow due to obstruction of capillaries. RBC-mediated regulation of microvascular blood flow mediated by release of nitric oxide (NO) and adenosine triphosphate (ATP) is abolished by storage [156]. This indirectly promotes a systemic proinflammatory state by triggering innate immune activation and by generating procoagulant bioactive phospholipids that are associated with an increased risk of acute lung injury [157].

Whether transfusion of RBCs stored for shorter periods of time (<21 days) conveys an additional benefit by limiting adverse effects in the recipient remains controversial. However, storage of red blood cell may be improved by cryopreservation at −80 °C in a glycerol buffer solution to prevent membrane damage from ice crystal formation. Cryopreserved RBC transfusions are associated with improved transport of oxygen and an attenuated propensity for proinflammatory complications including surgical site infection, transfusion-related acute lung injury, multiple organ dysfunction syndrome, and multiple organ system failure [158].

4.3.3.4 Reperfusion Injury

Reperfusion injury is caused by a rapid restoration of normal blood flow to hypoperfused tissue and may appear early during the resuscitation phase [159]. Nonspecific activation of coagulation/fibrinolysis system and diffuse activation of innate immune and contact activation processes characterize and constitute the basic pathological mechanisms. The dissemination of constitutive intracellular molecules released from disrupted cells in areas of ischemia and damaged tissue underlies the trigger of activation. These molecules bear specific molecular structures referred to as damage-associated molecular patterns (DAMP) [160–162]. DAMPs are recognized by pattern recognition receptors (PRRs). High mobility group box 1 protein (HMGB1), the prototype host molecule with a DAMP motif that is recognized by Toll-like receptor 4 (TLR4), expressed on several cell types of inflammatory cells, as well as endothelial cells and platelets. HMGB1-TLR4 interactions activate a broad range of procoagulant and proinflammatory activities, which mediate an autoinflammatory response expressed clinically as a systemic inflammatory response syndrome (SIRS) [163]. Diffuse interstitial edema and cellular swelling are the most significant consequences of systemic autoinflammatory syndrome. RBCs stored for long periods release free hemoglobin containing DAMP structures, which exacerbates reperfusion injury [164].

Greatly diminished perfusion of the gut is a characteristic feature of the compensatory mechanisms that operate in response to massive blood loss. Subsequent mesenteric reperfusion produces significant bowel wall edema leading to intra-abdominal hypertension (IAH)143, 144. IAH produces a reduction in inferior vena cava blood flow leading to a reduction in RV preload and decreased CO. Bowel edema during reperfusion occurs early, and IAH may progress to intra-abdominal compartment syndrome and organ failure [165].

Hemostatic Resuscitation

Hemostatic resuscitation is achieved by transfusion of equivalent numbers of units of plasma and platelets relative to packed RBC transfusion to, in effect, transfuse whole blood during resuscitation. Hemostatic resuscitation also can be goal-directed by applying point-of-care viscoelastic coagulation testing. In practical terms, resuscitation may begin with transfusion of empiric amounts of components in a ratio of 1:1:1 (i.e., transfusion of "whole blood") and be followed by specific component transfusions, with the quantity and timing of transfusion adapted to the patient's coagulation profile.

Stored thawed plasma, which contains acceptable coagulation factor activity for up to 5 days [166], is the chief plasma product in most centers. Unless blood type of the recipient is known, technically group AB plasma is used as a "universal donor" plasma type (because group AB plasma lacks antibodies against either group A or group B antigen). AB plasma is generally in limited supply, and never maintained thawed, which slows delivery to the shock room at the initiation of resuscitation. A reduction in the time to first plasma transfusion during resuscitation significantly reduces mortality [167]. To minimize these problems, group A plasma can be used before a blood type of the recipient is known [168–170]. The risk of a blood group mismatch transfusion reaction is decreased by the fact that the most common encountered blood group in a recipient will be group A, and anti-B antibodies in group A donated plasma, which can be screened for (but typically are not) and generally are low, especially if the donor is a North American male and >50 years old.

Bleeding-associated coagulopathy may occur secondary to the rapid development of fibrinogen depletion, aggravated by consumption of fibrinogen (hyperfibrinogenolysis). The proteolytic breakdown of fibrinogen occurs secondary to overexpression of endogenous plasminogen activator, downregulation of PAI-1, upregulation of C4b-binding protein expression [171–174] (a complement activation regulatory protein), or a combination of these activities that are normally restricted to fibrin cross-reacting with fibrinogen. Acidosis, which frequently complicates resuscitation, accelerates plasmin-mediated hyperfibrinogenolysis, as well as hyperfibrinolysis. Diminished synthesis secondary to preexisting liver disease and hypothermia compounds depletion and consumption of fibrinogen [79, 175]. Transfusion of four units of plasma provides approximately 2.5 g of fibrinogen (600 mg fibrinogen/unit), which should be a sufficient amount of fibrinogen (expected to raise plasma fibrinogen concentration in a 70-kg man by 70 mg/dL) to obviate cryoprecipitate transfusion (the usual source of fibrinogen in the USA). FXIII that crosslinks thrombin-generated fibrin strands and stabilizes forming clot is enriched in cryoprecipitate, but not in transfused plasma, and therefore a substantial increase in FXIII will likely not be seen if cryoprecipitate is not infused.

Reconstituted lyophilized plasma (RLP) is another source of this blood component that may be used immediately for a recipient of any blood type because of dilution and neutralization of anti-A and anti-B hemagglutinins. RLP, which contains coagulation factor levels equivalent to FFP, has been used by different military forces, including the French Army, Israeli Defense Forces, and US Special Operations Forces.

Standardized solvent/detergent-treated pooled (S/D-P) plasma has been developed as a safer alternative to untreated plasma for transfusion for several indications [176]. In addition to a lower rate of pathogen transmission, there is lower risk of transfusion-related acute lung injury (TRALI) with S/D-P plasma due to dilution of anti-HLA and anti-HNA antibodies. Coagulation factor activity in S/D-P plasma is comparable to factor activity in fresh-frozen plasma (FFP), although S/D-P plasma is more procoagulant than FFP due to degradation of protein S activity by S/D treatment. Consequently S/D-P plasma is suggested as a more efficacious component than thawed plasma for hemostatic resuscitation [177]. However, α2-antiplasmin is also degraded by S/D treatment and is reduced 35–76% in S/D-P plasma (depending on the specific product). Consequently, fibrinolysis may be potentiated if S/D-P plasma is used in place of thawed plasma during resuscitation. An antifibrinolytic agent should be considered for patients with TIC undergoing resuscitation with S/D-treated plasma [177].

The admission platelet count in trauma patients is inversely correlated with 24-hour mortality [178]. A normal platelet count may be insufficient after severe trauma, and as a result, these patients may benefit from a lower platelet transfusion threshold. One unit of platelets obtained by apheresis contains approximately the same number of platelets as a 6-random donor unit pooled concentrate, or approximately 6×10^{11} platelets. A 6-unit pooled random donor platelet concentrate or 1 unit of apheresis platelets can be expected to increase the platelet count by approximately 30,000–60,000/μL (30×10^3 to $60 \times 10^3/mm^3$) in a 70 kg nonhemorrhaging patient; 1-h and 24-h increments are consistently higher with apheresis platelets when compared to pooled platelets [179]. Platelets are suspended in plasma and therefore harbor risk of plasma-mediated febrile nonhemolytic transfusion and allergic reactions. One apheresis platelet unit contains approximately 200–400 mL of plasma and therefore provides 500 mg of fibrinogen as well as other coagulation factors. Also, bacterial contamination as a consequence of platelet storage at room temperature (24 °C) occurs at equivalent rates for both random donor pools and apheresis platelets [180]. Platelet transfusion-associated sepsis is the third leading cause of transfusion-related mortality.

Plasma-derived and recombinant coagulation factor concentrates are considered as an alternative to blood components for hemostatic resuscitation. These agents effectively and rapidly control hemorrhage-associated coagulopathy, reduce total blood use during resuscitation, and preclude component transfusion-related complications [181]. In Europe, fibrinogen concentrate is now used in place of allogeneic blood products as a first-line treatment for hypofibrinogenemia [182]. Fibrinogen concentrate is commercially available in the USA and approved by the FDA to treat hereditary fibrinogen disorders, but correction of acquired fibrinogen deficiency complicating hemorrhagic shock is not FDA-approved [140]. Administration of FXIII concentrate with fibrinogen concentrate has been considered in the management of massive hemorrhage [183, 184]. In some patients undergoing massive transfusion, an acquired FXIII deficiency is suggested by persistent coagulopathy and diminished clot strength despite adequate fibrinogen levels and platelets, and administration of FXIII concentrate may prove effective for this clinical state [181].

Prothrombin complex concentrates (PCCs) include vitamin K-dependent factors, FII, FVII, FIX, and FX. PCC products are considered either three-factor PCCs (containing a negligible concentration of FVII) or four-factor PCCs (with a higher concentration of FVII). Most newer PCC products should be considered 6-factor PCCs because these contain two additional vitamin K covalently modified proteins, PC and protein S (a cofactor for aPC). Thrombotic complications associated with PCCs include venous thromboembolism, disseminated DIC, microvascular thrombosis, and myocardial infarction [185]. Although these agents have specific indications for reversal of pharmacological anticoagulation in trauma patients, the use and timing of PCCs for management of TIC remains to be defined.

A large manufacturer-sponsored trial involving 150 international sites that was designed to assess the potential for mortality and morbidity benefits associated with use of rFVIIa in blunt and penetrating trauma was terminated when a preplanned interim data analysis predicted a low likelihood of observing a significant difference in the primary mortality endpoint [186]. From a further analysis of a large and comprehensive cohort involved in placebo-controlled trials of rFVIIa, it was reported that treatment with high doses of rFVIIa on an off-label basis significantly increased the risk of arterial thromboembolic events (e.g., coronary artery thrombosis), especially among the elderly.

Cryoprecipitate (cryo) is transfused during resuscitation for suspected hypofibrinogenemia (or possibly acquired fibrinogen dysfunction) in the exsanguinating trauma patient. In addition to fibrinogen, the precipitated proteins in cryo include von Willebrand factor, FVIII, and FXIII. Each unit of cryo (20 mL) contains approximately 250 mg of fibrinogen, and therefore, a 200 mL-10 unit dose of cryo will deliver 2.5g of fibrinogen. A unit of plasma (~250 mL) contains approximately 600 mg of fibrinogen. Thus, 4 units of plasma provide 2.4 g fibrinogen, equivalent to a 10-unit dose of cryoprecipitate, although at 5 times the volume [187]. One apheresis platelet unit contains approximately 200–400 mL of plasma and therefore provides 500 mg of fibrinogen as well as other coagulation factors. Hence, provided that resuscitation with plasma and platelets is initiated early, and transfusion of these components is continued using high ratios of plasma and platelets in relation to RBCs, a quantity of fibrinogen will be provided that approaches the amount delivered by a standard dose of cryo [188]. However, a relative deficiency of FXIII may develop as a result of hemorrhage or secondary to dilution by massive transfusion, and depletion of this specific coagulation factor may be associated with an increased risk for bleeding [189]. Empiric treatment of TIC with cryo can reverse this specific hemostatic abnormality, whereas plasma will not be as effective.

Acknowledgments The authors gratefully acknowledge many helpful discussions with Jill Castor, R.N., T.C.R.N., and Tracy Spitzer, M.S.N., R.N., C.C.R.N., T.C.R.N., during preparation of this manuscript.

References

1. Rhee P, Joseph B, Pandit V, Aziz H, Vercruysse G, Kulvatunyou N, Friese RS. Increasing trauma deaths in the United States. Ann Surg. 2014;260(1):13–21. https://doi.org/10.1097/SLA.0000000000000600.
2. Center for Disease Control. 2017. https://wisqars.cdc.gov:8443/cdcMapFramework/mapModuleInterface.jsp. Accessed 29 Mar 2017.
3. Kwon AM, Garbett NC, Kloecker GH. Pooled preventable death rates in trauma patients: meta analysis and systematic review since 1990. Eur J Trauma Emerg Surg. 2014;40(3):279–85. https://doi.org/10.1007/s00068-013-0364-5.
4. Lynham AJ, Hirst JP, Cosson JA, Chapman PJ, McEniery P. Emergency department management of maxillofacial trauma. EMA. 2004;16(1):7–12.
5. Choonthar MM, Raghothaman A, Prasad R, Pradeep S, Pandya K. Head injury- a maxillofacial surgeon's perspective. J Clin Diagn Res. 2016;10(1):ZE01–6. https://doi.org/10.7860/JCDR/2016/16112.7122.
6. Krausz AA, Krausz MM, Picetti E. Maxillofacial and neck trauma: a damage control approach. World J Emerg Surg. 2015;10:31. https://doi.org/10.1186/s13017-015-0022-9.
7. O'Connor RC, Shakib K, Brennan PA. Recent advances in the management of oral and maxillofacial trauma. Br J Oral Maxillofac Surg. 2015;53(10):913–21. https://doi.org/10.1016/j.bjoms.2015.08.261.
8. Mast G, Ehrenfeld M, Cornelius CP, Litschel R, Tasman AJ. Maxillofacial fractures: midface and internal orbit-part I: classification and assessment. Facial Plast Surg. 2015;31(4):351–6. https://doi.org/10.1055/s-0035-1563692.
9. Mast G, Ehrenfeld M, Cornelius CP, Tasman AJ, Litschel R. Maxillofacial fractures: midface and internal orbit-part II: principles and surgical treatment. Facial Plast Surg. 2015;31(4):357–67. https://doi.org/10.1055/s-0035-1563693.
10. Coppola S, Froio S, Merli G, Chiumello D. Maxillofacial trauma in the emergency department: pearls and pitfalls in airway management. Minerva Anestesiol. 2015;81(12):1346–58.
11. Tong DC, Breeze J. Damage control surgery and combat-related maxillofacial and cervical injuries: a systematic review. Br J Oral Maxillofac Surg. 2016;54(1):8–12. https://doi.org/10.1016/j.bjoms.2015.10.013.
12. Kuhnel TS, Reichert TE. Trauma of the midface. GMS Curr Top Otorhinolaryngol Head Neck Surg. 2015;14:Doc06. https://doi.org/10.3205/cto000121.
13. Kieliszak CR, Larson SR, Keller CR, Selinsky CR, Joshi AS. Interrelationship of structure and function in maxillofacial fractures. J Am Osteopath Assoc. 2016;116(2):e8–e12. https://doi.org/10.7556/jaoa.2016.026.
14. Sahni V. Maxillofacial trauma scoring systems. Injury. 2016;47(7):1388–92. https://doi.org/10.1016/j.injury.2016.02.001.
15. Jose A, Nagori SA, Agarwal B, Bhutia O, Roychoudhury A. Management of maxillofacial trauma in emergency: an update of challenges and controversies. J Emerg Trauma Shock. 2016;9(2):73–80. https://doi.org/10.4103/0974-2700.179456.
16. Powers DB. Classification of mandibular condylar fractures. Atlas Oral Maxillofac Surg Clin North Am. 2017;25(1):1–10. https://doi.org/10.1016/j.cxom.2016.11.001.
17. Azarmehr I, Stokbro K, Bell RB, Thygesen T. Surgical navigation: a systematic review of indications, treatments, and outcomes in oral and maxillofacial surgery. J Oral Maxillofac Surg. 2017;75(9):1987–2005. https://doi.org/10.1016/j.joms.2017.01.004.

18. Noy D, Rachmiel A, Emodi O, Amsalem Y, Israel Y, Nagler RM. Transarterial embolization in maxillofacial intractable potentially life-threatening hemorrhage. J Oral Maxillofac Surg. 2017;75(6):1223–31. https://doi.org/10.1016/j.joms.2017.01.033.
19. Mitchener TA, Chan R, Simecek JW. Oral-maxillofacial injury surveillance of U.S. military personnel in Iraq and Afghanistan, 2001 to 2014. Mil Med. 2017;182(3):e1767–73. https://doi.org/10.7205/MILMED-D-16-00117.
20. Manodh P, Prabhu Shankar D, Pradeep D, Santhosh R, Murugan A. Incidence and patterns of maxillofacial trauma-a retrospective analysis of 3611 patients-an update. Oral Maxillofac Surg. 2016;20(4):377–83. https://doi.org/10.1007/s10006-016-0576-z.
21. Haq J, Gately F, Bentley R. Implementation of an oral and maxillofacial surgery trauma team in a major trauma centre. Br J Oral Maxillofac Surg. 2017;55(4):396–9. https://doi.org/10.1016/j.bjoms.2016.12.016.
22. Fonseca RJ, Barber HD, Walker VW, Powers MP, Frost DE. Oral and maxillofacial trauma 2013.
23. Leigh-Smith S, Harris T. Tension pneumothorax-DOUBLEHYPHENtime for a re-think? Emerg Med J. 2005;22(1):8–16. https://doi.org/10.1136/emj.2003.010421.
24. Orlinsky M, Shoemaker W, Reis ED, Kerstein MD. Current controversies in shock and resuscitation. Surg Clin North Am. 2001;81(6):1217–62.
25. Cowley RA, Mergner WJ, Fisher RS, Jones RT, Trump BF. The subcellular pathology of shock in trauma patients: studies using the immediate autopsy. Am Surg. 1979;45(4):255–69.
26. Guan J, Jin DD, Jin LJ, Lu Q. Apoptosis in organs of rats in early stage after polytrauma combined with shock. J Trauma. 2002;52(1):104–11.
27. Mackersie RC. Pitfalls in the evaluation and resuscitation of the trauma patient. Emerg Med Clin North Am. 2010;28(1):1–27. https://doi.org/10.1016/j.emc.2009.10.001.
28. Klabunde RE. Cardiovascular physiology concepts. 2nd ed. Philadelphia: Lippincott Williams & Wilkins; 2012.
29. Kitzman DW, Little WC, Brubaker PH, Anderson RT, Hundley WG, Marburger CT, Brosnihan B, Morgan TM, Stewart KP. Pathophysiological characterization of isolated diastolic heart failure in comparison to systolic heart failure. JAMA. 2002;288(17):2144–50.
30. Costantini TW, Coimbra R, Holcomb JB, Podbielski JM, Catalano R, Blackburn A, Scalea TM, Stein DM, Williams L, Conflitti J, Keeney S, Suleiman G, Zhou T, Sperry J, Skiada D, Inaba K, Williams BH, Minei JP, Privette A, Mackersie RC, Robinson BR, Moore FO, Group APFS. Current management of hemorrhage from severe pelvic fractures: results of an American Association for the Surgery of Trauma multi-institutional trial. J Trauma Acute Care Surg. 2016;80(5):717–723; discussion 723-715. https://doi.org/10.1097/TA.0000000000001034.
31. Costantini TW, Coimbra R, Holcomb JB, Podbielski JM, Catalano R, Blackburn A, Scalea TM, Stein DM, Williams L, Conflitti J, Keeney S, Hoey C, Zhou T, Sperry J, Skiada D, Inaba K, Williams BH, Minei JP, Privette A, Mackersie RC, Robinson BR, Moore FO, Group APFS. Pelvic fracture pattern predicts the need for hemorrhage control intervention DOUBLEHYPHEN results of a AAST multi-institutional study. J Trauma Acute Care Surg. 2017. https://doi.org/10.1097/TA.0000000000001465.
32. Wohlauer MV, Moore EE, Droz NM, Harr J, Gonzalez E, Fragoso M, Silliman CC. Hemodilution is not critical in the pathogenesis of the acute coagulopathy of trauma. J Surg Res. 2012;173(1):26–30. https://doi.org/10.1016/j.jss.2011.04.047.
33. Cohen MJ, Christie SA. Coagulopathy of trauma. Crit Care Clin. 2017;33(1):101–18. https://doi.org/10.1016/j.ccc.2016.08.003.
34. Davenport RA, Brohi K. Cause of trauma-induced coagulopathy. Curr Opin Anaesthesiol. 2016;29(2):212–9. https://doi.org/10.1097/ACO.0000000000000295.
35. Gando S, Wada H, Kim HK, Kurosawa S, Nielsen JD, Thachil J, Toh CH, Scientific, Standardization Committee on DICotI. Comparison of disseminated intravascular coagulation in trauma with coagulopathy of trauma/acute coagulopathy of trauma-shock. J Thromb Haemost. 2012;10(12):2593–5.
36. Grottke O, Fries D, Nascimento B. Perioperatively acquired disorders of coagulation. Curr Opin Anaesthesiol. 2015;28(2):113–22. https://doi.org/10.1097/ACO.0000000000000176.
37. Hayakawa M. Pathophysiology of trauma-induced coagulopathy: disseminated intravascular coagulation with the fibrinolytic phenotype. J Intensive Care. 2017;5:14. https://doi.org/10.1186/s40560-016-0200-1.
38. Brohi K, Singh J, Heron M, Coats T. Acute traumatic coagulopathy. J Trauma. 2003;54(6):1127–30. https://doi.org/10.1097/01.TA.0000069184.82147.06.
39. Floccard B, Rugeri L, Faure A, Denis MS, Boyle EM, Peguet O, Levrat A, Guillaume C, Marcotte G, Vulliez A, Hautin E, David JS, Négrier C, Allaouchiche B. Early coagulopathy in trauma patients: an on-scene and hospital admission study. Injury. 2012;43(1):26–32. https://doi.org/10.1016/j.injury.2010.11.003.
40. MacLeod JB. Trauma and coagulopathy: a new paradigm to consider. Arch Surg. 2008;143(8):797–801. https://doi.org/10.1001/archsurg.143.8.797.
41. Brohi K. Prediction of acute traumatic coagulopathy and massive transfusion - is this the best we can do? Resuscitation. 2011;82(9):1128–1129. S0300-9572(11)00398-4. https://doi.org/10.1016/j.resuscitation.2011.06.022.
42. Davis PK, Musunuru H, Walsh M, Cassady R, Yount R, Losiniecki A, Moore EE, Wohlauer MV, Howard J, Ploplis VA, Castellino FJ, Thomas SG. Platelet dysfunction is an early marker for traumatic brain injury-induced coagulopathy. Neurocrit Care. 2013;18(2):201–8. https://doi.org/10.1007/s12028-012-9745-6.

43. Kutcher ME, Redick BJ, McCreery RC, Crane IM, Greenberg MD, Cachola LM, Nelson MF, Cohen MJ. Characterization of platelet dysfunction after trauma. J Trauma Acute Care Surg. 2012;73(1):13–9. https://doi.org/10.1097/TA.0b013e318256deab.
44. Solomon C, Traintinger S, Ziegler B, Hanke A, Rahe-Meyer N, Voelckel W, Schochl H. Platelet function following trauma. A multiple electrode aggregometry study. Thromb Haemost. 2011;106(2):322–30. https://doi.org/10.1160/TH11-03-0175.
45. Windelov NA, Sorensen AM, Perner A, Wanscher M, Larsen CF, Ostrowski SR, Johansson PI, Rasmussen LS. Platelet aggregation following trauma: a prospective study. Blood Coagul Fibrinolysis. 2014;25(1):67–73. https://doi.org/10.1097/MBC.0b013e328364c2da.
46. Johansson P, Stensballe J, Ostrowski S. Shock induced endotheliopathy (SHINE) in acute critical illness - a unifying pathophysiologic mechanism. Crit Care. 2017;21(1):25. https://doi.org/10.1186/s13054-017-1605-5.
47. Frith D, Brohi K. The pathophysiology of trauma-induced coagulopathy. Curr Opin Crit Care. 2012;18(6):631–6. https://doi.org/10.1097/MCC.0b013e3283599ab9.
48. Frith D, Davenport R, Brohi K. Acute traumatic coagulopathy. Curr Opin Anaesthesiol. 2012;25(2):229–34. https://doi.org/10.1097/ACO.0b013e3283509675.
49. Gando S, Sawamura A, Hayakawa M. Trauma, shock, and disseminated intravascular coagulation: lessons from the classical literature. Ann Surg. 2011;254(1):10–9. https://doi.org/10.1097/SLA.0b013e31821221b1.
50. Selby R, Geerts W, Ofosu FA, Craven S, Dewar L, Phillips A, Szalai JP. Hypercoagulability after trauma: hemostatic changes and relationship to venous thromboembolism. Thromb Res. 2009; 124(3):281–7. https://doi.org/10.1016/j.thromres.2008.10.002.
51. Wohlauer MV, Moore EE, Thomas S, Sauaia A, Evans E, Harr J, Silliman CC, Ploplis V, Castellino FJ, Walsh M. Early platelet dysfunction: an unrecognized role in the acute coagulopathy of trauma. J Am Coll Surg. 2012;214(5):739–46. https://doi.org/10.1016/j.jamcollsurg.2012.01.050.
52. Johansson PI, SØRensen AM, Perner A, Welling KL, Wanscher M, Larsen CF, Ostrowski SR. High sCD40L levels early after trauma are associated with enhanced shock, sympathoadrenal activation, tissue and endothelial damage, coagulopathy and mortality. J Thromb Haemost. 2012;10(2):207–16. https://doi.org/10.1111/j.1538-7836.2011.04589.x.
53. Johansson PI, Stensballe J, Rasmussen LS, Ostrowski SR. A high admission syndecan-1 level, a marker of endothelial glycocalyx degradation, is associated with inflammation, protein C depletion, fibrinolysis, and increased mortality in trauma patients. Ann Surg. 2011;254(2):194–200. https://doi.org/10.1097/SLA.0b013e318226113d.
54. Johansson PI, Stensballe J, Rasmussen LS, Ostrowski SR. High circulating adrenaline levels at admission predict increased mortality after trauma. J Trauma Acute Care Surg. 2012;72(2):428–36.
55. Ostrowski SR, Johansson PI. Endothelial glycocalyx degradation induces endogenous heparinization in patients with severe injury and early traumatic coagulopathy. J Trauma Acute Care Surg. 2012;73(1):60–6. https://doi.org/10.1097/TA.0b013e31825b5c10.
56. Senzolo M, Coppell J, Cholongitas E, Riddell A, Triantos CK, Perry D, Burroughs AK. The effects of glycosaminoglycans on coagulation: a thromboelastographic study. Blood Coagul Fibrinolysis. 2007;18(3):227–36. https://doi.org/10.1097/MBC.0b013e328010bd3d.
57. Johansson PI, Stensballe J, Oliveri R, Wade CE, Ostrowski SR, Holcomb JB. How I treat patients with massive hemorrhage. Blood. 2014. https://doi.org/10.1182/blood-2014-05-575340.
58. Johansson PI, Sorensen AM, Perner A, Welling KL, Wanscher M, Larsen CF, Ostrowski SR. Disseminated intravascular coagulation or acute coagulopathy of trauma shock early after trauma? An observational study. Crit Care. 2011;15(6):R272. https://doi.org/10.1186/cc10553.
59. Johansson PI, Stensballe J, Ostrowski SR. Current management of massive hemorrhage in trauma. Scand J Trauma Resusc Emerg Med. 2012;20:47. https://doi.org/10.1186/1757-7241-20-47.
60. Tennent GA, Brennan SO, Stangou AJ, O'Grady J, Hawkins PN, Pepys MB. Human plasma fibrinogen is synthesized in the liver. Blood. 2007;109(5):1971–4. https://doi.org/10.1182/blood-2006-08-040956.
61. Kornblith LZ, Kutcher ME, Redick BJ, Calfee CS, Vilardi RF, Cohen MJ. Fibrinogen and platelet contributions to clot formation: implications for trauma resuscitation and thromboprophylaxis. J Trauma Acute Care Surg. 2014;76(2):255–63. https://doi.org/10.1097/TA.0000000000000108.
62. Gando S, Otomo Y. Local hemostasis, immunothrombosis, and systemic disseminated intravascular coagulation in trauma and traumatic shock. Crit Care. 2015;19:72. https://doi.org/10.1186/s13054-015-0735-x.
63. Hess JR, Brohi K, Dutton RP, Hauser CJ, Holcomb JB, Kluger Y, Mackway-Jones K, Parr MJ, Rizoli SB, Yukioka T, Hoyt DB, Bouillon B. The coagulopathy of trauma: a review of mechanisms. J Trauma. 2008;65(4):748–54. https://doi.org/10.1097/TA.0b013e3181877a9c.
64. Hess JR, Lawson JH. The coagulopathy of trauma versus disseminated intravascular coagulation. J Trauma. 2006;60(6 Suppl):S12–9. https://doi.org/10.1097/01.ta.0000199545.06536.22.
65. Levi M. Disseminated intravascular coagulation. In: Hoffman R, Benz EJ, Silberstein LE, Heslop HE, Weitz JI, Anastasi J, editors. Hematology: basic principles and practice. 6th ed. Philadelphia: Saunders; 2013. p. 2001–12.

66. Wood JP, Ellery PE, Maroney SA, Mast AE. Biology of tissue factor pathway inhibitor. Blood. 2014;123(19):2934–43. https://doi.org/10.1182/blood-2013-11-512764.
67. Levi M, Toh CH, Thachil J, Watson HG. Guidelines for the diagnosis and management of disseminated intravascular coagulation. Br J Haematol. 2009;145(1):24–33. https://doi.org/10.1111/j.1365-2141.2009.07600.x.
68. Muench MV, Canterino JC. Trauma in pregnancy. Obstet Gynecol Clin N Am. 2007;34(3):555–83. https://doi.org/10.1016/j.ogc.2007.06.001.
69. McLintock C, James AH. Obstetric hemorrhage. J Thromb Haemost. 2011;9(8):1441–51. https://doi.org/10.1111/j.1538-7836.2011.04398.x.
70. Davenport R. Pathogenesis of acute traumatic coagulopathy. Transfusion. 2013;53(Suppl 1):23S–7S. https://doi.org/10.1111/trf.12032.
71. Raza I, Davenport R, Rourke C, Platton S, Manson J, Spoors C, Khan S, De'ath HD, Allard S, Hart DP, Pasi KJ, Hunt BJ, Stanworth S, MacCallum PK, Brohi K. The incidence and magnitude of fibrinolytic activation in trauma patients. J Thromb Haemost. 2013;11(2):307–14. https://doi.org/10.1111/jth.12078.
72. Schochl H, Voelckel W, Maegele M, Solomon C. Trauma-associated hyperfibrinolysis. Hamostaseologie. 2012;32(1):22–7. https://doi.org/10.5482/ha-1178.
73. Cardenas JC, Wade CE, Holcomb JB. Mechanisms of trauma-induced coagulopathy. Curr Opin Hematol. 2014;21(5):404–9. https://doi.org/10.1097/MOH.0000000000000063.
74. Cotton BA, Harvin JA, Kostousouv V, Minei KM, Radwan ZA, Schochl H, Wade CE, Holcomb JB, Matijevic N. Hyperfibrinolysis at admission is an uncommon but highly lethal event associated with shock and prehospital fluid administration. J Trauma Acute Care Surg. 2012;73(2):365–70. https://doi.org/10.1097/TA.0b013e31825c1234.
75. Bolliger D, Szlam F, Levy JH, Molinaro RJ, Tanaka KA. Haemodilution-induced profibrinolytic state is mitigated by fresh-frozen plasma: implications for early haemostatic intervention in massive haemorrhage. Br J Anaesth. 2010;104(3):318–25. https://doi.org/10.1093/bja/aeq001.
76. Schochl H, Frietsch T, Pavelka M, Jambor C. Hyperfibrinolysis after major trauma: differential diagnosis of lysis patterns and prognostic value of thrombelastometry. J Trauma. 2009;67(1):125–31. https://doi.org/10.1097/TA.0b013e31818b2483. 00005373-200907000-00022 [pii]
77. Hunt BJ, Segal H. Hyperfibrinolysis. J Clin Pathol. 1996;49(12):958.
78. Stachurska J, Latallo Z, Kopec M. Inhibition of platelet aggregation by dialysable fibrinogen degradation products (FDP). Thromb Diath Haemorrh. 1970;23(1):91–8.
79. Kushimoto S, Shibata Y, Yamamoto Y. Implications of fibrinogenolysis in patients with closed head injury. J Neurotrauma. 2003;20(4):357–63. https://doi.org/10.1089/089771503765172318.
80. Riskin DJ, Tsai TC, Riskin L, Hernandez-Boussard T, Purtill M, Maggio PM, Spain DA, Brundage SI. Massive transfusion protocols: the role of aggressive resuscitation versus product ratio in mortality reduction. J Am Coll Surg. 2009;209(2):198–205. https://doi.org/10.1016/j.jamcollsurg.2009.04.016.
81. Spinella PC, Perkins JG, Grathwohl KW, Beekley AC, Holcomb JB. Warm fresh whole blood is independently associated with improved survival for patients with combat-related traumatic injuries. J Trauma. 2009;66(4 Suppl):S69–76. https://doi.org/10.1097/TA.0b013e31819d85fb.
82. McCarron DA, Elliott WC, Rose JS, Bennett WM. Severe mixed metabolic acidosis secondary to rhabdomyolysis. Am J Med. 1979;67(5):905–8.
83. Kraut JA, Madias NE. Serum anion gap: its uses and limitations in clinical medicine. CJASN. 2007;2(1):162–74. https://doi.org/10.2215/CJN.03020906.
84. Murthi SB, Stansbury LG, Dutton RP, Edelman BB, Scalea TM, Hess JR. Transfusion medicine in trauma patients: an update. Expert Rev Hematol. 2011;4(5):527–37. https://doi.org/10.1586/ehm.11.49.
85. Kermode JC, Zheng Q, Milner EP. Marked temperature dependence of the platelet calcium signal induced by human von Willebrand factor. Blood. 1999;94(1):199–207.
86. Hardy JF, de Moerloose P, Samama CM. The coagulopathy of massive transfusion. Vox Sang. 2005;89(3):123–7. https://doi.org/10.1111/j.1423-0410.2005.00678.x.
87. Watts DD, Trask A, Soeken K, Perdue P, Dols S, Kaufmann C. Hypothermic coagulopathy in trauma: effect of varying levels of hypothermia on enzyme speed, platelet function, and fibrinolytic activity. J Trauma. 1998;44(5):846–54.
88. Peng RY, Bongard FS. Hypothermia in trauma patients. J Am Coll Surg. 1999;188(6):685–96.
89. Gentilello LM, Moujaes S. Treatment of hypothermia in trauma victims: thermodynamic considerations. J Intensive Care Med. 1995;10(1):5–14.
90. Barthel ER, Pierce JR. Steady-state and time-dependent thermodynamic modeling of the effect of intravenous infusion of warm and cold fluids. J Trauma Acute Care Surg. 2012;72(6):1590–600. https://doi.org/10.1097/TA.0b013e31824a7943.
91. Gentilello LM, Pierson DJ. Trauma critical care. Am J Respir Crit Care Med. 2001;163(3 Pt 1):604–7.
92. Davis TM, Singh B, Choo KE, Ibrahim J, Spencer JL, St John A. Dynamic assessment of the electrocardiographic QT interval during citrate infusion in healthy volunteers. Br Heart J. 1995;73(6):523–6.
93. Kramer L, Bauer E, Joukhadar C, Strobl W, Gendo A, Madl C, Gangl A. Citrate pharmacokinetics and metabolism in cirrhotic and noncirrhotic critically ill patients. Crit Care Med. 2003;31(10):2450–5. https://doi.org/10.1097/01.CCM.0000084871.76568.E6.
94. Passman R, Kadish A. Polymorphic ventricular tachycardia, long Q-T syndrome, and torsades de pointes. Med Clin North Am. 2001;85(2):321–41.

95. Mayberry JC, Trunkey DD. The fractured rib in chest wall trauma. Chest Surg Clin N Am. 1997;7(2):239–61.
96. Pacagnella RC, Souza JP, Durocher J, Perel P, Blum J, Winikoff B, Gulmezoglu AM. A systematic review of the relationship between blood loss and clinical signs. PLoS One. 2013;8(3):e57594. https://doi.org/10.1371/journal.pone.0057594.
97. Dunser MW, Takala J, Brunauer A, Bakker J. Re-thinking resuscitation: leaving blood pressure cosmetics behind and moving forward to permissive hypotension and a tissue perfusion-based approach. Crit Care. 2013;17(5):326. https://doi.org/10.1186/cc12727.
98. Wilson M, Davis DP, Coimbra R. Diagnosis and monitoring of hemorrhagic shock during the initial resuscitation of multiple trauma patients: a review. J Emerg Med. 2003;24(4):413–22.
99. Cannon CM, Braxton CC, Kling-Smith M, Mahnken JD, Carlton E, Moncure M. Utility of the shock index in predicting mortality in traumatically injured patients. J Trauma. 2009;67(6):1426–30. https://doi.org/10.1097/TA.0b013e3181bbf728.
100. Vandromme MJ, Griffin RL, Kerby JD, McGwin G Jr, Rue LW 3rd, Weinberg JA. Identifying risk for massive transfusion in the relatively normotensive patient: utility of the prehospital shock index. J Trauma. 2011;70(2):384–8. https://doi.org/10.1097/TA.0b013e3182095a0a. 00005373-201102000-00020 [pii]
101. Birkhahn RH, Gaeta TJ, Terry D, Bove JJ, Tloczkowski J. Shock index in diagnosing early acute hypovolemia. Am J Emerg Med. 2005;23(3):323–6.
102. Mutschler M, Nienaber U, Munzberg M, Wolfl C, Schoechl H, Paffrath T, Bouillon B, Maegele M, The TraumaRegister DGU. The shock index revisited - a fast guide to transfusion requirement? A retrospective analysis on 21,853 patients derived from the TraumaRegister DGU(R). Crit Care. 2013;17(4):R172. https://doi.org/10.1186/cc12851.
103. Zarzaur BL, Croce MA, Magnotti LJ, Fabian TC. Identifying life-threatening shock in the older injured patient: an analysis of the National Trauma Data Bank. J Trauma. 2010;68(5):1134–8. https://doi.org/10.1097/TA.0b013e3181d87488.
104. Ardagh MW, Hodgson T, Shaw L, Turner D. Pulse rate over pressure evaluation (ROPE) is useful in the assessment of compensated haemorrhagic shock. Emerg Med (Fremantle). 2001;13(1):43–6.
105. Campbell R, Ardagh MW, Than M. Validation of the pulse rate over pressure evaluation index as a detector of early occult hemorrhage: a prospective observational study. J Trauma Acute Care Surg. 2012;73(1):286–8. https://doi.org/10.1097/TA.0b013e318253b52e.
106. Funk DJ, Kumar A. If the central venous pressure is [x], call me ... Maybe. Crit Care Med. 2013;41(7):1823–4. https://doi.org/10.1097/CCM.0b013e3182913685.
107. Marik PE, Baram M, Vahid B. Does central venous pressure predict fluid responsiveness? A systematic review of the literature and the tale of seven mares. Chest. 2008;134(1):172–8. https://doi.org/10.1378/chest.07-2331.
108. Marik PE, Cavallazzi R. Does the central venous pressure predict fluid responsiveness? An updated meta-analysis and a plea for some common sense. Crit Care Med. 2013;41(7):1774–81. https://doi.org/10.1097/CCM.0b013e31828a25fd.
109. Jubran A. Pulse oximetry. Crit Care. 2015;19:272. https://doi.org/10.1186/s13054-015-0984-8.
110. Clayton DG, Webb RK, Ralston AC, Duthie D, Runciman WB. Pulse oximeter probes. A comparison between finger, nose, ear and forehead probes under conditions of poor perfusion. Anaesthesia. 1991;46(4):260–5.
111. Schallom L, Sona C, McSweeney M, Mazuski J. Comparison of forehead and digit oximetry in surgical/trauma patients at risk for decreased peripheral perfusion. Heart Lung. 2007;36(3):188–94. https://doi.org/10.1016/j.hrtlng.2006.07.007.
112. Nesseler N, Frenel JV, Launey Y, Morcet J, Malledant Y, Seguin P. Pulse oximetry and high-dose vasopressors: a comparison between forehead reflectance and finger transmission sensors. Intensive Care Med. 2012;38(10):1718–22. https://doi.org/10.1007/s00134-012-2659-0.
113. Walley KR. Use of central venous oxygen saturation to guide therapy. Am J Respir Crit Care Med. 2011;184(5):514–20. https://doi.org/10.1164/rccm.201010-1584CI.
114. Hampton DA, Schreiber MA. Near infrared spectroscopy: clinical and research uses. Transfusion. 2013;53(Suppl 1):52S–8S. https://doi.org/10.1111/trf.12036.
115. Cohn SM, Nathens AB, Moore FA, Rhee P, Puyana JC, Moore EE, Beilman GJ, St OTPTI. Tissue oxygen saturation predicts the development of organ dysfunction during traumatic shock resuscitation. J Trauma. 2007;62(1):44–54. https://doi.org/10.1097/TA.0b013e31802eb817.
116. Gomez H, Torres A, Polanco P, Kim HK, Zenker S, Puyana JC, Pinsky MR. Use of non-invasive NIRS during a vascular occlusion test to assess dynamic tissue O(2) saturation response. Intensive Care Med. 2008;34(9):1600–7. https://doi.org/10.1007/s00134-008-1145-1.
117. Odom SR, Howell MD, Silva GS, Nielsen VM, Gupta A, Shapiro NI, Talmor D. Lactate clearance as a predictor of mortality in trauma patients. J Trauma Acute Care Surg. 2013;74(4):999–1004. https://doi.org/10.1097/TA.0b013e3182858a3e.
118. Bursa F, Pleva L. Anaerobic metabolism associated with traumatic hemorrhagic shock monitored by microdialysis of muscle tissue is dependent on the levels of hemoglobin and central venous oxygen saturation: a prospective, observational study. Scand J Trauma Resusc Emerg Med. 2014;22:11. https://doi.org/10.1186/1757-7241-22-11.
119. Lavery RF, Livingston DH, Tortella BJ, Sambol JT, Slomovitz BM, Siegel JH. The utility of venous lactate to triage injured patients in the trauma center. J Am Coll Surg. 2000;190(6):656–64.

120. Vincent JL, Quintairos ESA, Couto L Jr, Taccone FS. The value of blood lactate kinetics in critically ill patients: a systematic review. Crit Care. 2016;20(1):257. https://doi.org/10.1186/s13054-016-1403-5.
121. Futier E, Robin E, Jabaudon M, Guerin R, Petit A, Bazin JE, Constantin JM, Vallet B. Central venous O(2) saturation and venous-to-arterial CO(2) difference as complementary tools for goal-directed therapy during high-risk surgery. Crit Care. 2010;14(5):R193. https://doi.org/10.1186/cc9310.
122. Mallat J, Lazkani A, Lemyze M, Pepy F, Meddour M, Gasan G, Temime J, Vangrunderbeeck N, Tronchon L, Thevenin D. Repeatability of blood gas parameters, PCO2 gap, and PCO2 gap to arterial-to-venous oxygen content difference in critically ill adult patients. Medicine. 2015;94(3):e415. https://doi.org/10.1097/MD.0000000000000415.
123. Monnet X, Julien F, Ait-Hamou N, Lequoy M, Gosset C, Jozwiak M, Persichini R, Anguel N, Richard C, Teboul JL. Lactate and venoarterial carbon dioxide difference/arterial-venous oxygen difference ratio, but not central venous oxygen saturation, predict increase in oxygen consumption in fluid responders. Crit Care Med. 2013;41(6):1412–20. https://doi.org/10.1097/CCM.0b013e318275cece.
124. Maani CV, DeSocio PA, Holcomb JB. Coagulopathy in trauma patients: what are the main influence factors? Curr Opin Anaesthesiol. 2009;22(2):255–60. https://doi.org/10.1097/ACO.0b013e32832922be.
125. Besser MW, MacDonald SG. Acquired hypofibrinogenemia: current perspectives. J Blood Med. 2016;7:217–25. https://doi.org/10.2147/JBM.S90693.
126. Miesbach W, Schenk J, Alesci S, Lindhoff-Last E. Comparison of the fibrinogen Clauss assay and the fibrinogen PT derived method in patients with dysfibrinogenemia. Thromb Res. 2010;126(6):e428–33. https://doi.org/10.1016/j.thromres.2010.09.004.
127. Chowdary P, Saayman AG, Paulus U, Findlay GP, Collins PW. Efficacy of standard dose and 30 ml/kg fresh frozen plasma in correcting laboratory parameters of haemostasis in critically ill patients. Br J Haematol. 2004;125(1):69–73.
128. Martini WZ, Cortez DS, Dubick MA, Park MS, Holcomb JB. Thrombelastography is better than PT, aPTT, and activated clotting time in detecting clinically relevant clotting abnormalities after hypothermia, hemorrhagic shock and resuscitation in pigs. J Trauma. 2008;65(3):535–43. https://doi.org/10.1097/TA.0b013e31818379a6. 00005373-200809000-00005 [pii]
129. Meyer AS, Meyer MA, Sorensen AM, Rasmussen LS, Hansen MB, Holcomb JB, Cotton BA, Wade CE, Ostrowski SR, Johansson PI. Thrombelastography and rotational thromboelastometry early amplitudes in 182 trauma patients with clinical suspicion of severe injury. J Trauma Acute Care Surg. 2014;76(3):682–90. https://doi.org/10.1097/TA.0000000000000134.
130. Park MS, Martini WZ, Dubick MA, Salinas J, Butenas S, Kheirabadi BS, Pusateri AE, Vos JA, Guymon CH, Wolf SE, Mann KG, Holcomb JB. Thromboelastography as a better indicator of hypercoagulable state after injury than prothrombin time or activated partial thromboplastin time. J Trauma. 2009;67(2):266–275; discussion 275-266. https://doi.org/10.1097/TA.0b013e3181ae6f1c.
131. Weeder PD, Porte RJ, Lisman T. Hemostasis in liver disease: implications of new concepts for peri-operative management. Transfus Med Rev. 2014;28(3):107–13.
132. Johansson PI. Coagulation monitoring of the bleeding traumatized patient. Curr Opin Anaesthesiol. 2012;25(2):235–41. https://doi.org/10.1097/ACO.0b013e32834fab76.
133. Curnow JL, Morel-Kopp MC, Roddie C, Aboud M, Ward CM. Reduced fibrinolysis and increased fibrin generation can be detected in hypercoagulable patients using the overall hemostatic potential assay. J Thromb Haemost. 2007;5(3):528–34. https://doi.org/10.1111/j.1538-7836.2006.02362.x.
134. Johansson PI, Svendsen MS, Salado J, Bochsen L, Kristensen AT. Investigation of the thrombin-generating capacity, evaluated by thrombogram, and clot formation evaluated by thrombelastography of platelets stored in the blood bank for up to 7 days. Vox Sang. 2008;94(2):113–8. https://doi.org/10.1111/j.1423-0410.2007.01011.x.
135. Kawasaki J, Katori N, Kodaka M, Miyao H, Tanaka KA. Electron microscopic evaluations of clot morphology during thrombelastography. Anesth Analg. 2004;99(5):1440–4. https://doi.org/10.1213/01.ANE.0000134805.30532.59.
136. Rivard GE, Brummel-Ziedins KE, Mann KG, Fan L, Hofer A, Cohen E. Evaluation of the profile of thrombin generation during the process of whole blood clotting as assessed by thrombelastography. J Thromb Haemost. 2005;3(9):2039–43. https://doi.org/10.1111/j.1538-7836.2005.01513.x.
137. Jeger V, Zimmermann H, Exadaktylos AK. Can RapidTEG accelerate the search for coagulopathies in the patient with multiple injuries? J Trauma. 2009;66(4):1253–7. https://doi.org/10.1097/TA.0b013e31819d3caf.
138. Callum JL, Rizoli S. Plasma transfusion for patients with severe hemorrhage: what is the evidence? Transfusion. 2012;52(Suppl 1):30S–7S. https://doi.org/10.1111/j.1537-2995.2012.03621.x.
139. Callum JL, Rizoli S. Assessment and management of massive bleeding: coagulation assessment, pharmacologic strategies, and transfusion management. Hematology Am Soc Hematol Educ Program. 2012;2012:522–8. https://doi.org/10.1182/asheducation-2012.1.522.
140. Harr JN, Moore EE, Ghasabyan A, Chin TL, Sauaia A, Banerjee A, Silliman CC. Functional fibrinogen assay indicates that fibrinogen is critical in correcting abnormal clot strength following trauma. Shock. 2013;39(1):45–9. https://doi.org/10.1097/SHK.0b013e3182787122.

141. Jeger V, Willi S, Liu T, Yeh DD, De Moya M, Zimmermann H, Exadaktylos AK. The rapid TEG a-angle may be a sensitive predictor of transfusion in moderately injured blunt trauma patients. Sci World J. 2012;2012:821794. https://doi.org/10.1100/2012/821794.
142. Schlimp CJ, Solomon C, Ranucci M, Hochleitner G, Redl H, Schochl H. The effectiveness of different functional fibrinogen polymerization assays in eliminating platelet contribution to clot strength in thromboelastometry. Anesth Analg. 2014;118(2):269–76. https://doi.org/10.1213/ANE.0000000000000058.
143. Schlimp CJ, Voelckel W, Inaba K, Maegele M, Ponschab M, Schochl H. Estimation of plasma fibrinogen levels based on hemoglobin, base excess and injury severity score upon emergency room admission. Crit Care. 2013;17(4):R137. https://doi.org/10.1186/cc12816.
144. Kashuk JL, Moore EE, Sawyer M, Wohlauer M, Pezold M, Barnett C, Biffl WL, Burlew CC, Johnson JL, Sauaia A. Primary fibrinolysis is integral in the pathogenesis of the acute coagulopathy of trauma. Ann Surg. 2010;252(3):434–42. https://doi.org/10.1097/SLA.0b013e3181f09191.
145. Kashuk JL, Moore EE, Wohlauer M, Johnson JL, Pezold M, Lawrence J, Biffl WL, Burlew CC, Barnett C, Sawyer M, Sauaia A. Initial experiences with point-of-care rapid thrombelastography for management of life-threatening postinjury coagulopathy. Transfusion. 2012;52(1):23–33. https://doi.org/10.1111/j.1537-2995.2011.03264.x.
146. Ellis TC, Nielsen VG, Marques MB, Kirklin JK. Thrombelastographic measures of clot propagation: a comparison of alpha with the maximum rate of thrombus generation. Blood Coagul Fibrinolysis. 2007;18(1):45–8. https://doi.org/10.1097/MBC.0b013e328011 1a8e.
147. Kellman RM, Losquadro WD. Comprehensive airway management of patients with maxillofacial trauma. Craniomaxillofac Trauma Reconstr. 2008;1(1):39–47. https://doi.org/10.1055/s-0028-1098962.
148. Hackl W, Hausberger K, Sailer R, Ulmer H, Gassner R. Prevalence of cervical spine injuries in patients with facial trauma. Oral Surg Oral Med Oral Pathol Oral Radiol Endod. 2001;92(4):370–6. https://doi.org/10.1067/moe.2001.116894.
149. Mosier JM, Joshi R, Hypes C, Pacheco G, Valenzuela T, Sakles JC. The physiologically difficult airway. West J Emerg Med. 2015;16(7):1109–17. https://doi.org/10.5811/westjem.2015.8.27467.
150. Karmy-Jones R, Jurkovich GJ. Blunt chest trauma. Curr Probl Surg. 2004;41(3):223–380. https://doi.org/10.1016/j.cpsurg.2003.12.004.
151. D'Alessandro A, Kriebardis AG, Rinalducci S, Antonelou MH, Hansen KC, Papassideri IS, Zolla L. An update on red blood cell storage lesions, as gleaned through biochemistry and omics technologies. Transfusion. 2015;55(1):205–19. https://doi.org/10.1111/trf.12804.
152. Almac E, Bezemer R, Hilarius-Stokman PM, Goedhart P, de Korte D, Verhoeven AJ, Ince C. Red blood cell storage increases hypoxia-induced nitric oxide bioavailability and methemoglobin formation in vitro and in vivo. Transfusion. 2014;54(12):3178–85. https://doi.org/10.1111/trf.12738.
153. Watkins GM, Rabelo A, Pizak LF, Sheldon GF. The left shifted oxyhemoglobin curve in sepsis: a preventable defect. Ann Surg. 1974;180(2):213–20.
154. Young JA, Lichtman MA, Cohen J. Reduced red cell 2,3-diphosphoglycerate and adenosine triphosphate, hypophosphatemia, and increased hemoglobin-oxygen affinity after cardiac surgery. Circulation. 1973;47(6):1313–8.
155. Ekeloef NP, Eriksen J, Kancir CB. Evaluation of two methods to calculate p50 from a single blood sample. Acta Anaesthesiol Scand. 2001;45(5):550–2.
156. Raat NJ, Hilarius PM, Johannes T, de Korte D, Ince C, Verhoeven AJ. Rejuvenation of stored human red blood cells reverses the renal microvascular oxygenation deficit in an isovolemic transfusion model in rats. Transfusion. 2009;49(3):427–4. https://doi.org/10.1111/j.1537-2995.2008.02002.x.
157. Middelburg RA, Borkent B, Jansen M, van de Watering LM, Wiersum-Osselton JC, Schipperus MR, Beckers EA, Briet E, van der Bom JG. Storage time of blood products and transfusion-related acute lung injury. Transfusion. 2012;52(3):658–67. https://doi.org/10.1111/j.1537-2995.2011.03352.x.
158. Hampton DA, Wiles C, Fabricant LJ, Kiraly L, Differding J, Underwood S, Le D, Watters J, Schreiber MA. Cryopreserved red blood cells are superior to standard liquid red blood cells. J Trauma Acute Care Surg. 2014;77(1):20–7. https://doi.org/10.1097/TA.0000000000000268.
159. Carden DL, Granger DN. Pathophysiology of ischaemia-reperfusion injury. J Pathol. 2000;190(3):255–66.
160. Hirsiger S, Simmen HP, Werner CM, Wanner GA, Rittirsch D. Danger signals activating the immune response after trauma. Mediat Inflamm.2012;2012:315941.https://doi.org/10.1155/2012/315941.
161. Magna M, Pisetsky DS. The role of HMGB1 in the pathogenesis of inflammatory and autoimmune diseases. Mol Med. 2014. https://doi.org/10.2119/molmed.2013.00164.
162. Moussion C, Ortega N, Girard JP. The IL-1-like cytokine IL-33 is constitutively expressed in the nucleus of endothelial cells and epithelial cells in vivo: a novel 'alarmin. PLoS One. 2008;3(10):e3331. https://doi.org/10.1371/journal.pone.0003331.
163. Bae JS, Rezaie AR. Activated protein C inhibits high mobility group box 1 signaling in endothelial cells. Blood. 2011;118(14):3952–3959. blood-2011-06-360701 [pii]. https://doi.org/10.1182/blood-2011-06-360701.
164. Neal MD, Raval JS, Triulzi DJ, Simmons RL. Innate immune activation after transfusion of stored red blood cells. Transfus Med Rev. 2013;27(2):113–8. https://doi.org/10.1016/j.tmrv.2013.01.001.

165. De Waele JJ, De Laet I, Kirkpatrick AW, Hoste E. Intra-abdominal hypertension and abdominal compartment syndrome. Am J Kidney Dis. 2011;57(1):159–69. https://doi.org/10.1053/j.ajkd.2010.08.034.
166. Buchta C, Felfernig M, Hocker P, Macher M, Kormoczi GF, Quehenberger P, Heinzl H, Knobl P. Stability of coagulation factors in thawed, solvent/detergent-treated plasma during storage at 4 degrees C for 6 days. Vox Sang. 2004;87(3):182–6. https://doi.org/10.1111/j.1423-0410.2004.00552.x.
167. Hess JR, Holcomb JB. Resuscitating PROPPRly. Transfusion. 2015. https://doi.org/10.1111/trf.13118.
168. Chhibber V, Greene M, Vauthrin M, Bailey J, Weinstein R. Is group a thawed plasma suitable as the first option for emergency release transfusion? (CME). Transfusion. 2014;54(7):1751–5. https://doi.org/10.1111/trf.12537.
169. Cooling L. Going from a to B: the safety of incompatible group a plasma for emergency release in trauma and massive transfusion patients. Transfusion. 2014;54(7):1695–7. https://doi.org/10.1111/trf.12730.
170. Mehr CR, Gupta R, von Recklinghausen FM, Szczepiorkowski ZM, Dunbar NM. Balancing risk and benefit: maintenance of a thawed group a plasma inventory for trauma patients requiring massive transfusion. J Trauma Acute Care Surg. 2013;74(6):1425–31. https://doi.org/10.1097/TA.0b013e31828b813e.
171. Agarwal V, Talens S, Grandits AM, Blom AM. A novel interaction between complement inhibitor C4b-binding protein and plasminogen that enhances plasminogen activation. J Biol Chem. 2015;290(30):18333–42. https://doi.org/10.1074/jbc.M114.619494.
172. Stenflo J. A new vitamin K-dependent protein. Purification from bovine plasma and preliminary characterization. J Biol Chem. 1976;251(2):355–63.
173. Schuliga M. The inflammatory actions of coagulant and fibrinolytic proteases in disease. Mediat Inflamm. 2015;2015:437695. https://doi.org/10.1155/2015/437695.
174. Ermert D, Blom AM. C4b-binding protein: the good, the bad and the deadly. Novel functions of an old friend. Immunol Lett. 2016;169:82–92. https://doi.org/10.1016/j.imlet.2015.11.014.
175. Martini WZ, Holcomb JB. Acidosis and coagulopathy: the differential effects on fibrinogen synthesis and breakdown in pigs. Ann Surg. 2007;246(5):831–5. https://doi.org/10.1097/SLA.0b013e3180cc2e94.
176. Marietta M, Franchini M, Bindi ML, Picardi F, Ruggeri M, De Silvestro G. Is solvent/detergent plasma better than standard fresh-frozen plasma? A systematic review and an expert consensus document. Blood Transfus. 2016;14(4):277–86. https://doi.org/10.2450/2016.0168-15.
177. Pitkanen H, Jouppila A, Mowinckel MC, Lemponen M, Patiwael S, Sandset PM, Lassila R, Brinkman HJ. Enhanced thrombin generation and reduced intact protein S in processed solvent detergent plasma. Thromb Res. 2015;135(1):167–74. https://doi.org/10.1016/j.thromres.2014.10.020.
178. Brown LM, Call MS, Margaret Knudson M, Cohen MJ, Trauma Outcomes G, Holcomb JB, Wade CE, Brasel KJ, Vercruysse G, MacLeod J, Dutton RP, Hess JR, Duchesne JC, McSwain NE, Muskat P, Johannigamn J, Cryer HM, Tillou A, Pittet JF, De Moya MA, Schreiber MA, Tieu B, Brundage S, Napolitano LM, Brunsvold M, Brunsvold M, Beilman G, Peitzman AB, Zenait MS, Sperry J, Alarcon L, Croce MA, Minei JP, Kozar R, Gonzalez EA, Stewart RM, Cohn SM, Mickalek JE, Bulger EM, Cotton BA, Nunez TC, Ivatury R, Meredith JW, Miller P, Pomper GJ, Marin B. A normal platelet count may not be enough: the impact of admission platelet count on mortality and transfusion in severely injured trauma patients. J Trauma. 2011;71(2 Suppl 3):S337–42. https://doi.org/10.1097/TA.0b013e318227f67c.
179. Heddle NM, Arnold DM, Boye D, Webert KE, Resz I, Dumont LJ. Comparing the efficacy and safety of apheresis and whole blood-derived platelet transfusions: a systematic review. Transfusion. 2008;48(7):1447–58. https://doi.org/10.1111/j.1537-2995.2008.01731.x.
180. Vamvakas EC. Relative safety of pooled whole blood-derived versus single-donor (apheresis) platelets in the United States: a systematic review of disparate risks. Transfusion. 2009;49(12):2743–58. https://doi.org/10.1111/j.1537-2995.2009.02338.x.
181. Sorensen B, Fries D. Emerging treatment strategies for trauma-induced coagulopathy. Br J Surg. 2012;99(Suppl 1):40–50. https://doi.org/10.1002/bjs.7770.
182. Ahmed S, Harrity C, Johnson S, Varadkar S, McMorrow S, Fanning R, Flynn CM, OR JM, Byrne BM. The efficacy of fibrinogen concentrate compared with cryoprecipitate in major obstetric haemorrhageDOUBLEHYPHENan observational study. Transfus Med. 2012;22(5):344–9. https://doi.org/10.1111/j.1365-3148.2012.01178.x.
183. Ng C, Silliman CC, Pearl G, Smith W, Manco-Johnson M, Wang M. Treatment of refractory hemorrhage with factor XIII in a patient with hemophilia a with inhibitor. Pediatr Blood Cancer. 2013;60(7):E23–5. https://doi.org/10.1002/pbc.24478.
184. Lusher J, Pipe SW, Alexander S, Nugent D. Prophylactic therapy with Fibrogammin P is associated with a decreased incidence of bleeding episodes: a retrospective study. Haemophilia. 2010;16(2):316–21. https://doi.org/10.1111/j.1365-2516.2009.02123.x.
185. Key NS, Negrier C. Coagulation factor concentrates: past, present, and future. Lancet. 2007;370(9585):439–48. https://doi.org/10.1016/S0140-6736(07)61199-4.
186. Hauser CJ, Boffard K, Dutton R, Bernard GR, Croce MA, Holcomb JB, Leppaniemi A, Parr M, Vincent JL, Tortella BJ, Dimsits J, Bouillon B, Group CS. Results of the CONTROL trial: efficacy and safety of recombinant activated factor VII in the management of refractory traumatic hemorrhage. J Trauma. 2010;69(3):489–500. https://doi.org/10.1097/TA.0b013e3181edf36e.

187. Kozek-Langenecker S, Sorensen B, Hess JR, Spahn DR. Clinical effectiveness of fresh frozen plasma compared with fibrinogen concentrate: a systematic review. Crit Care. 2011;15(5):R239. https://doi.org/10.1186/cc10488.
188. Young PP, Cotton BA, Goodnough LT. Massive transfusion protocols for patients with substantial hemorrhage. Transfus Med Rev. 2011;25(4):293–303. https://doi.org/10.1016/j.tmrv.2011.04.002.
189. Levy JH, Greenberg C. Biology of factor XIII and clinical manifestations of factor XIII deficiency. Transfusion. 2013;53(5):1120–31. https://doi.org/10.1111/j.1537-2995.2012.03865.x.
190. Schuster V, Hugle B, Tefs K. Plasminogen deficiency. J Thromb Haemost. 2007;5(12):2315–22. https://doi.org/10.1111/j.1538-7836.2007.02776.x.
191. Sartori MT, Danesin C, Saggiorato G, Tormene D, Simioni P, Spiezia L, Patrassi GM, Girolami A. The PAI-1 gene 4G/5G polymorphism and deep vein thrombosis in patients with inherited thrombophilia. Clin Appl Thromb Hemost. 2003;9(4):299–307.

ICU Management of the Maxillofacial Surgery Patient

5

Julie McNeish and David S. Shapiro

Abstract

Oral and maxillofacial surgery patients may require assessment for their critical care needs or admission to the intensive care unit (ICU) in the perioperative, postinjury, or other acute care settings. Patients who require the intensive care unit may have anatomical concerns, postoperative challenges related to airway patency, or any combination of concomitant trauma, pathology, or comorbid respiratory failure. In order to manage these acutely ill patients, the ICU should be equipped with advanced adjuvants to airway management, experienced providers, and assertive protocols to manage airways, treat infection, and manage the nonsurgical needs. This chapter will provide the foundation for critical care assessment, treatments, and needs in the maxillofacial surgery population.

5.1 Introduction

The intensive care unit (ICU) is an important option for oral and maxillofacial surgery patients in the perioperative, postinjury, or other acute care settings. Patients who require the intensive care unit may have anatomical concerns, postoperative challenges related to airway patency, or any combination of concomitant trauma, pathology, or comorbid respiratory failure. Multiply injured trauma patients with traumatic brain injuries (TBI) often have concomitant maxillofacial trauma and are therefore frequent visitors to the ICU. In addition to TBI, maxillofacial trauma is also associated with a multitude of other injuries, including cervical spine, anterior and lateral neck injuries, and thoracic trauma [1]. Patients with pathologies other than trauma must also be considered for ICU level of care, including odontogenic infections, neoplasia, postoperative after complicated maxillofacial, oral, or dental surgery, and other anatomical considerations [2, 3]. Intensive care of the maxillofacial surgery patient is most frequently limited to major traumatic injuries, postoperative care, or acute care in the setting of airway compromise. Primary attention

J. McNeish, D.M.D., M.D.
Division of Oral and Maxillofacial Surgery, School of Dental Medicine, University of Connecticut, Farmington, CT, USA

D.S. Shapiro, M.D., F.A.C.S., F.C.C.M. (✉)
Department of Surgery, Saint Francis Hospital & Medical Center, Hartfort, 06107 Connecticut, USA
e-mail: davidscottshapiro@gmail.com

© Springer International Publishing AG 2018

E.M. Ferneini, J.D. Bennett (eds.), *Perioperative Assessment of the Maxillofacial Surgery Patient*,
https://doi.org/10.1007/978-3-319-58868-1_5

must be given to airway management. The ICU should be equipped with advanced adjuvants to airway management.

5.2 Risk Assessment for ICU

A multitude of scoring systems and physiological assessments exist to aid providers in the decision to admit or maintain patients to the ICU. The acute physiology and chronic health evaluation (APACHE), the simplified acute physiology score (SAPS), mortality prediction model (MPM), 3-day recalibrating ICU outcomes (TRIOS), and organ dysfunction and infection system (ODIN) have each been developed and revised to predict outcomes based on disease severity. Though each score is distinct, they share the commonality of predicting outcomes based on variables at different intervals during admission. Additionally, other scoring systems including the logistic organ dysfunction score (LODS), multiple organ dysfunction score (MODS), and sequential organ failure assessment (SOFA) each can offer predictions on survival based on the degree of organ failure or organ system dysfunction. Scoring systems have improved management of the ICU patient, although it is important to note that they cannot and should not be used solely to predict which patient should benefit from an ICU admission [4]. No calculation or algorithm can replace a provider's opinion that a patient would be best managed in the ICU. Ultimately, each ICU may develop specific guidelines to best triage patients, prepare nursing and other bedside providers, and help guide providers with admission to and transfer from the ICU.

Additional clinical risk factors for patients who may require ICU after any oral or maxillofacial surgery include significant immunosuppression, poorly controlled diabetes mellitus, obstructive sleep apnea, alcohol abuse [5], existing cancer, history of recent radiation therapy, and severe malnutrition. Patients with multiple comorbidities should also be considered.

There is a paucity of evidence specifically on oral and maxillofacial surgery patients who require an ICU stay; however orthopedic, TBI, and other populations serve as surrogates. The most common reason for transition to ICU level of care is acute respiratory failure, including airway failure, within the first 48 h postoperatively or in the initial 48 h of hospitalization postinjury. Similar to the above mentioned risk factors, patients may be predisposed to require ICU care during their hospitalization if comorbid conditions include chronic respiratory failure with or without oxygen dependence, obstructive sleep apnea, chronic kidney disease, or patients who chronically imbibe illicit drugs or alcohol. Other factors that have been associated with the need for ICU care include prolonged anesthesia time, larger procedures, postoperative opioid requirements, and increased blood loss [6].

Airway compromise is the most common diagnosis leading to ICU care and often occurs in the setting of submandibular or other soft tissue infection and multiple facial fractures. The concern alone for airway compromise in patients with significant trismus, closed reduction requiring significant manipulation, the requirement for postoperative wired occlusion, and other situations should be sufficient to warrant ICU care.

5.3 Critical Communication

As in any interdisciplinary patient care scenarios, communication is the cornerstone of safe, high-quality care, safe, and deliberate care. Critical concerns about antibiotic stewardship, planned maxillary mandibular fixation, unclear postoperative airway plans, concomitant respiratory failure, need for reoperation, ventilator-associated infection, enteral nutrition, pressure ulcers, and unexpected airway loss are all anticipated in this patient population, and frank discussions about the risk and preemptive planning are important.

Upon delivery of a patient to the ICU, handover of care should include the following information:

- Patient identification and description (name, medical record number, age, admitting weight, and primary diagnosis; also include primary healthcare contact information).
- Description of the procedure(s) performed including the indication and history of present

illness/injury and complications during the procedure, including any plans to return to the operating room; reconstructive procedures of the oral and maxillofacial structures occasionally call for free or pedicle-based flaps—details of the flap site and care are important.
- Allergies and reactions.
- Medication reconciliation, including home medications, intraoperative vasoactive agents, antibiotics, blood products, and any anticipated need, include anxiolytics, analgesics, and continued antimicrobial therapy.
- Existing intravenous, enteral, and urinary access, as well as surgical drain sites and management plans.
- Concerns or restrictions on extubation from the maxillofacial surgical team and/or anesthesiology team regarding airway management or other findings noted, mouth care, pin sites, wires, or other hardware.
- Tools for bedside care including wire cutters for emergency use, contact information for the covering surgical providers, feeding access (which ideally should have been discussed prior to the case starting), and discharge planning concerns that can be addressed early in the stay; emergency tracheostomy supplies are also an important consideration.

5.4 Airway

Airway management in the maxillofacial surgery patient is discussed elsewhere but must be a consideration in the postinjury, perioperative, and other critical care settings. Maxillofacial patients are often intubated on presentation but can also present with delayed airway loss in the preoperative, peri-injury, and postoperative settings. There are several considerations when attempting to secure the airway in any of these patients. Each patient should be evaluated with the primary diagnosis in mind (trauma, infection, etc.) and the effects on the airway, potential difficulties in mask ventilation and or endotracheal intubation, concern for cervical spine immobilization, risk of regurgitation and aspiration, significant bleeding, and the type of procedure being done, specifically if maxilla-mandibular fixation will be required either during and or maintained at the end of the procedure [7].

Complex procedures often require the availability of multimodality airway management techniques. These techniques may occur preoperatively or concomitantly with the maxillofacial procedures. In patients who are suspected to require an advanced airway for a longer period of time or who will remain in closed reduction, a tracheostomy may be indicated. When utilized, sutures placed to secure the tracheostomy phalange to the skin of the neck should be left for a maximum of 3 days to minimize pressure-associated skin injury. In other cases where a long-term airway is not needed, a nasal airway is contraindicated or unachievable, and if the patient's facial fracture pattern requires maxillary-mandibular fixation, a submental airway can be used. Submental airways permit unobstructed access to the oral cavity and can help to avoid tracheostomy. Following airway management with orotracheal intubation using a reinforced or armored tube a tunnel is created in the floor of the mouth leading to an incision at the midpoint between the chin and the angle of the mandible, usually positioned off midline. An armored tube is used to prevent kinking of the tube as it traverses a sharp angle from the oral cavity to the hypopharynx. The armored tube is passed from within the mouth through the incision after the conduit adapter is removed and delivered through the skin to reconnect to the ventilation tubing. Extubation is performed via a reversal of these steps. Mandibular instability is a contraindication. Complications of this surgical airway include damage to structures inclusive of the neuromuscular (lingual nerve, marginal mandibular branch of the facial nerve), as well as damage to the submandibular gland duct and the sublingual gland which can result in a salivary fistula [6, 8].

Any surgical procedure in proximity to the airway can result in problems after extubation. Many advocate for delay of extubation, but this is likely unnecessary provided precautions and a well-planned management scheme is discussed. It is imperative for the anesthesia and surgical team to make extubation decisions in concert. Further, the surgical team should remain in the operating theater and proceed with the patient to the next level of care, ready to proceed with a surgical airway if needed. Airway edema, soft tissue swelling, hematoma, active bleeding, and foreign bodies may all contribute to a threatened airway in the postoperative setting [9]. Periglottic injury and swelling may result from any number of intraoral, laryngeal, or esophageal monitoring devices. Intraoral manipulation with bite blocks, suction tips, or manipulation devices may all result in laryngeal, pharyngeal, esophageal, tracheal, temporomandibular joint, or nasal injuries [10].

Airway compromise must be addressed quickly and with a well-established protocol. Difficult airway supplies, experienced providers, and a surgical backup are each important. The most common critical care errors that result in mortality of trauma patients have been related to airway and respiratory management [17]. Expertise from anesthesiology colleagues is paramount, but contributions from the maxillofacial surgery team are imperative to address, with, for instance, patients who are wired in occlusion, who must have wire cutters available to avoid delay in establishing transoral airway access.

Table 5.1 Indications for emergency airways

Procedural indications for emergency airway
1. Three total attempts at endotracheal intubation, including at least one by the anesthesiology attending
2. Prolonged time has elapsed since start of rapid sequence induction and injection of induction agents
3. Oxygen saturation falls to <65% during airway management, after the first or second attempt
4. Rapid desaturation or difficult maintaining oxygen saturation while bagging
5. Anesthesiology attending decides additional intubation attempts would be futile

5.4.1 Methods of Emergency Airway Management

No matter where the airway compromise occurs, endotracheal intubation remains the gold standard to secure the airway in the emergency setting. In patients who cannot undergo endotracheal intubation, a surgical airway may be the only means of airway control. Indications for an emergency surgical airway are listed in Table 5.1 [12]. In these situations, a surgical cricothyrotomy may be performed as per the ATLS guidelines. Conversion to a formal tracheostomy should be endeavored soon after cricothyrotomy, if not immediately. Although the ATLS guidelines suggest that cricothyrotomy is an easier and safer procedure, data at Level I Trauma centers show that tracheostomies are more commonly performed when an advanced airway is indicated in this setting. Tracheostomy in the emergent or urgent setting may be performed with traditional open technique or may be performed in the dilational percutaneous method. Though many providers prefer bronchoscopic visualization to perform percutaneous tracheostomy in the elective setting, anatomical needle insertion with aspiration of air may be sufficient in experienced hands to perform the dilational method in the emergent setting. The percutaneous method has gained popularity in the elective setting, increasing the availability of experienced providers [11]. Of note, cricothyrotomy is sometimes preferred in patients with obesity due to easy identification of superficial cricothyroid membrane [12]. Additionally, blind percutaneous dilational tracheostomy (without bronchoscopy) can also be safely performed in experienced hands.

5.4.2 Bedside Airway Management

All advanced airways need to be managed with care and attention. Every person on the team should be aware of the details of the airway for each patient, including when and why the airway was placed. In addition to being well informed, emergency equipment should be easily accessible. Each room or area should have access to extra tubes that are the size-matched to the patient. Other adjuvants to airway management include video-assisted direct laryngoscopy, intubation-compatible bronchoscopy, laryngeal mask airways, nasotracheal intubation, and surgical airway management. A list of equipment that should be available can be seen in Table 5.2.

Table 5.2 Equipment recommended for emergency airway management

• Oral airways	• Laryngoscopes	• Suction tips and tubing
• Nasal airways	• Indirect optical intubators and other adjuvants	• Nonsterile scissors
• Laryngeal mask airways	• Fiber-optic scope	• Sterile gloves
• Oxygen masks	• Endotracheal tubes	• Sutures
• Bag masks	• Bougies or tube exchangers	• Dressings
• Capnography	• Cricothyrotomy set	• Tape
• Intubation medications	• Tracheostomy set	• Tracheostomy collars
• Laryngeal mask airways	• Tracheostomy tubes	• Percutaneous tracheostomy kit

It is important to approach respiratory distress in patients according to their advanced airway needs. Respiratory distress in the intubated patient is most commonly due to pneumonia, fluid overload, or insufficient sedation/analgesia. Atelectasis and poor recruitment, secretions and mucus plugging, or other sources of lobar underventilation may contribute. In the postoperative or postinjury patient, pneumothorax, pneumonia, acute respiratory distress syndrome, airway bleeding, and pulmonary embolism may also be included. Primary therapies for these diagnoses are many, but should not result in manipulation of the existing airway.

Endotracheal cuff dysfunction, tube occlusion, right main stem intubation, and self-extubation are situations requiring replacement of the airway. In these settings, the existing tube should be either withdrawn or replaced, and this should be completed over a tube changer to avoid inadvertent complete loss of airway. Rapid sequence intubation with direct laryngoscopy, while the mainstay, may not be possible given any recent history of oral and maxillofacial surgery. If the tube replacement cannot be completed with the aid of bedside equipment such as a tube exchanger, direct laryngoscopy, or fiber-optic scope, the placement of a laryngeal mask airway (LMA) may be considered but is always a temporizing measure [13]. Use of unstructured or unrigid tubing (e.g., endotracheal suction) to exchange an airway is not recommended, as the softness of the tube results in bending of the conduit leading to either false passage placement or loss of the airway completely.

For tracheostomy patients who are experiencing respiratory distress and or desaturations, it is important to first assess the existing airway for patency, the orotracheal or nasotracheal route for possible intubation, and the tracheostomy itself/knowledge of the tracheostomy type (i.e., cuffed or uncuffed, fenestrated or unfenestrated, etc.) is important. If the patient is breathing spontaneously, it is important to apply high-flow oxygen to both tracheostomy and oral sites while in the process of assuring airway security. The tracheostomy site should be assessed for patency. Speaking valves, plugs, or other attachments should be removed and the tube accessed with a suction catheter for clearance, and possibly with a tube exchanger if another airway is at the ready. Obturators, internal cannulae, valves, and humidification devices each can become occluded with concretions resulting in obstruction. The tube exchanger could be used to both investigate patency and replace the tube. Occasionally, a tracheostomy cuff is noted to be partially herniated from the trachea, causing a tilt or turn of the airway. Deflation of the balloon and reinsertion may be endeavored but should be performed with caution and over a tube changer [14]. Although high-flow oxygen can be applied to the tracheostomy site initially without complication, the site should not be hand ventilated until it is proven to be a patent airway. Ventilation through a displaced tube can result in subcutaneous emphysema which can worsen access to the neck.

The algorithm for addressing respiratory distress and desaturations in laryngectomy patients is similar. The important difference here is that there should be no consideration regarding upper airway access, and orotracheal and nasotracheal routes no longer exist. When ventilating both the tracheostomy and laryngectomy patient via the stoma, a pediatric face mask or LMA can be applied to the skin to aid in oxygen delivery and ventilation until a definitive airway can be placed.

5.5 Trauma

Traumatic injury is the most common cause of death for persons under 40 years old. Nonfatal trauma is associated with a high volume of injury-related disability and cost. Maxillofacial injuries are often concomitant with other injuries, especially traumatic brain injuries. A complete physical exam is important after a known injury presents, and a high index of suspicion is paramount in the assessment of injured patients. Anyone with lacerations of face chin, high neck, anterior scalp, or temple should be considered for imaging of the bony face.

Craniofacial traumatic injuries are commonly limited to nasal bone fractures and cranial vault fractures, encompassing nearly 70% of all injuries [15]. Mandible (13%), zygoma (13%), orbit (3%), and maxilla (2%) make up the remainder. Soft tissue injuries primarily comprise of predominantly lacerations (41%), abrasions (23%), hematomas (23%), and contusions (11%). The majority of maxillofacial injuries are associated with five main injury mechanism categories: activities of daily living (nearly 40%), sports (31%), violence (10%), traffic crashes (5%), and occupational injuries (2%), with predominantly a blunt trauma mechanism. Those in the category of "activities of daily living" sustained mostly dental trauma, while those in automobile collisions experienced facial bone fractures and soft tissue injuries more often. Similar to other traumatic injuries, maxillofacial injuries are most common in patients 15–40 years old. Fractures of the maxilla, nasal bones, and zygomatic are the most common injuries and concomitant subdural and subarachnoid hemorrhage are noted in 10–20% of patients sustaining injuries. Although less concerning, extradural hematomas are the most common head injury (22%), followed closely be subdural hemorrhage (SDH) (17%) and subarachnoid hemorrhage (SAH) (14%) [16]. Craniofacial trauma is also associated with cervical spine injury and cranial nerve injury. These injury patterns may require frequent neurological assessments that require ICU admission depending on a hospital's policies.

As mentioned previously, maxillofacial trauma can adversely affect the airway. Hutchinson reports six particular situations:

1. Posterior inferior displacement of a fractured maxilla parallel to the inclined plane of the base of the skill may block the nasopharyngeal airway.
2. Bilateral fracture of anterior mandible, known as a "bucket handle" fracture, may result in the fractured symphysis and tongue to slide posterior and obstruct the oropharynx.
3. Fractured or exfoliated teeth, bone fragments, blood, and secretions as well as foreign bodies, such as dentures, debris, and shrapnel, can block the airway anywhere along the oral pharynx and larynx, in addition to becoming aspirated.
4. Hemorrhage from distinct vessels in open wounds. This scenario is commonly seen with grossly displaced mandible fractures which result in soft tissue bleeding which can result in a sublingual or other soft tissue hematoma [17]. Hemorrhage can also be seen due to severe nasal or nasopharyngeal bleeding, and the complex blood supply of the nose may contribute to airway obstruction.
5. Soft tissue swelling and edema which result from trauma of the head and neck may cause delayed airway compromise.
6. Trauma of the larynx and trachea may cause swelling and displacement of structures such as the epiglottis, arytenoid cartilages, and vocal cords, thereby increasing risk of cervical airway obstruction.

Another consideration in airway management is with nasoorbitoethmoid injuries and upper-third facial fractures that are associated with skull base fractures. These pose a risk for displacement of endotracheal tubes into the frontal lobe if attempting nasal intubation [17].

In addition to airway management, there is often concern for preoperative and postoperative infection in patients with severe soft tissue injury and multiple open fractures. Based on the evidence available, there is minimal support for postoperative antibiotics for fractures in any facial third. Support exists for preoperative antibiotics for comminuted open mandible fractures and perioperative antibiotics for all facial fractures. The literature reports antibiotics should not be routinely used, but there are clinical scenarios where they should be considered: contamination of fracture sites from sinuses, intraoral exposure, and any delay in treatment. Although no strong evidence exists for the use of antibiotics, surveys from providers depict a different story where antibiotics are routinely used in both preoperative and postoperative setting [18]. Each patient should be evaluated individually, and facial fractures should continue to be considered as a potential source of infection as there have been several cases reports of meningitis following ORIF of panfacial fractures [19].

5.6 Odontogenic Infections

Severe odontogenic infections often follow an unpredictable course. Outpatient therapeutics may be sufficient for the majority of patients, but some progress to life-threatening infection and require aggressive surgical therapy to manage [2]. A high index of suspicion should enable the provider in the emergency department, office, or urgent care setting to recognize an advancing infection. Antibiotics are the mainstay of therapy, but surgical management may result in postoperative ICU stay.

Odontogenic infections often begin with primary decay and evolve through the pulp and into the bony periodontal ligament when untreated. Infection can spread through the ligament into the bony implant surface and subsequently into the subperiosteal region. Maxillary periapical abscesses may progress into canine space or the infratemporal space and the periorbital structures, presenting as cellulitis. Cavernous sinus thrombosis may be among the rare but sinister complications of this progression. Maxillary and mandibular periapical abscesses may both track into the buccal or parotid space. Mandibular periapical abscesses can progress into the sublingual, submandibular, and masticator (masseteric, pterygoid, and temporal) spaces, and any mandibular abscess may further descend into lateral pharyngeal spaces, resulting in infection progressing along the carotid sheath, retropharyngeal space, and mediastinum, where more septic features may be exhibited. Airway compromise can result from pharyngeal progression. In addition to local spread, hematogenous spread can lead to thrombophlebitis, bacteremia, involvement of prosthetic joint or valves, and systemic sepsis [17]. Physical exam findings may be innocuous until late in presentation, which may feature submental or submandibular tenderness, stiff neck, trismus, and septic shock [17, 20].

Ludwig's angina (infection of bilateral submandibular, sublingual, submental spaces) is an airway emergency due to the frequent impending airway loss. In patients who are maintaining their airway but are brought to the OR for drainage, extubation should be thought about carefully, as history suggests that patients typically develop further post-op swelling [17]. In patients with Ludwig's, tracheostomy is a relative contradiction due to difficulty from associated neck edema and due to the associated risk of causing spread to the mediastinum when the neck and pretracheal tissues are involved.

Regardless of what space they involve, many of these patients will go to the operating room for incision and drainage, placement of drains, and extraction of necessary teeth under general anesthesia. Depending on the extent of swelling and trismus, the anesthesia team may choose to utilize awake nasal fiber-optic intubation. In all such cases, the surgeon should be prepared to perform a rescue tracheostomy.

5.7 Nutrition

Critically ill patients are often unable to take nourishment by mouth due to intubation, gastrointestinal obstruction, or functional ileus. In the patient with maxillofacial injuries or surgery, volitional feedings may be impossible for the added reasons of reconstruction or difficulty with mastication. In the early phases of acute illness, injury, or in the immediate postoperative period, deficits of caloric intake can quickly reach the point of muscle loss via a catabolic state that is associated with significantly morbidity [21]. Patients with chemotherapy, radiation treatments, or who have been malnourished for prolonged periods are at further risk for early catabolism. Other patient populations at further risk for malnutrition are geriatric, diabetic, and those with impairments in nutrient bioavailability, such as short gut syndrome, IBD, and other comorbidities [22].

In all maxillofacial patients, nutrition is imperative for wound healing. Studies have shown that a healthy person needs 30–35 kcal/kg of body weight each day. When patients are undergoing wound healing, there is an increase in the daily caloric requirement to 35–40 kcal/kg due to the increase in cell proliferation, protein synthesis, and enzyme activity. Caloric requirements are usually met predominately by carbohydrates. Macronutrients include proteins, carbohydrates, lipids, and essential fats. Where fats and triglycerides allow for epidermal and dermal tissue to develop, proteins contribute the amino acids that serve as the building blocks for tissue growth, cell renewal, and cell repair. Patients with protein malnutrition will have impaired hemostasis, inflammation and granulation tissue formation, cell proliferation, and tissue reorganization and normalization. Protein malnutrition can be made worse when the total number of calories is low, as the body will resort to using the body's muscle stores for energy.

Patients who present with a subacute or chronic condition should be evaluated for malnutrition and considered for preoperative nutritional support. Patients can be evaluated by asking about weight loss and serum albumin levels. If patients are found to have moderate or severe malnutrition and the surgical intervention can be delayed, preoperative nutrition should be considered for 7 days to optimize the patient. Early supplementation with enteral nutrition remains an important therapeutic measure in the care of injured patients and those patients who undergo reconstruction for oral cancers [23, 24].

Nutritional supplementation may be provided via nasogastric, orogastric, nasojejunal, or other enteral access routes, depending upon the nature of the surgical procedure. Placement of enteral access should be considered in the operative planning phase and discussed in the preoperative setting. When mandibulo-maxillary fixation is considered, nasogastric decompression is important in the immediate postoperative period, and nasojejunal access is desirable for the patient with a postoperative stay anticipated to be longer than a few days. Enteral feedings can safely be provided early in the postoperative course. Early postoperative enteral nutrition has been associated with significant improvements in infection, lengths of stay, and possibly reduced mortality [25]. Whether it is preoperative or postoperative nutritional supplementation, nutritional status should be assessed weekly with serum protein markers: pre-albumin and transferrin. Although albumin is used as a preoperative marker, due to its half-life of 18–21 days, it is an inaccurate marker for further nutritional status [24].

Conclusion

Different scoring systems and physiological assessments are available to aid providers in the decision to admit or maintain oral and maxillofacial surgery patients to the ICU. Once admitted, airway compromise, if present, must be addressed quickly and with a well-established protocol. Difficult airway supplies, experienced providers, and a surgical backup are all important factors for appropriate airway management. Providing adequate and early postoperative nutrition in these critically ill patients will optimize their care and improve our patient outcomes.

References

1. Alves LS, Aragao I, Sousa MJC, Gomes E. Pattern of maxillofacial fracures in severe multiple trauma patients: a 7 year prospective study. Braz Dent J. 2014;25(6):561–4.

2. Ylijoki S, Suuronen R, Jousimies-Somer H, Meurman JH, Lindqvist C. Differences between patients with or without the need for intensive care due to severe odontogenic infections. J Oral Maxillofac Surg. 2001;59(8):867–72.
3. Zemplenyi K, Lopez B, Sardesai M, Dillon JK. Can progression of odontogenic infections to cervical necrotizing soft tissue infections be predicted? Int J Oral Maxillofac Surg. 2017;46(2):181–8.
4. Vincent J-L, Moreno R. Clinical review: scoring systems in the critically ill. Crit Care. 2010;14(2):207.
5. Yadav SK, Mandal BK, Karn A, Sah AK. Maxillofacial trauma with head injuries at a tertiary care hospital in Chitwan, Nepal; clinical, medico-legal, and critical care concerns. Tur J Med Sci. 2012;42(Sup 2):1505–12.
6. Melamed R, Boland LL, Normington JP, et al. Postoperative respiratory failure necessitating transfer to the intensive care unit in orthopedic surgery patients: risk factors, costs, and outcomes. Perioper Med. 2016;5:19.
7. Barak M, Bahouth H, Leiser Y, El-Naaj IA. Airway management of the patient with maxillofacial trauma: review of the literature and suggested clinical approach; Biomed Res Int. 2015;2015:724032.
8. MacInnis E, Baig M. A modified submental approach for oral endotracheal intubation. Int J Oral Maxillofac Surg. 1999;28(5):344–6.
9. Popat M, Mitchell V, Dravid R, Patel A, Swampillai C, Higgs A. Difficult airway society guidelines for the management of tracheal extubation. Anaesthesia. 2012;67:318–40.
10. Domino KB, Posner KL, Caplan RA, Cheney FW. Airway injury during anesthesia: a closed claims analysis. Anesthesiology. 1999;91:1703–11.
11. Suri S, Goyal K, Chowdhury T. Role of percutaneous tracheostomy in emergent difficult airway conditions: an update. OA Anaesth. 2013;1(1):8.
12. Dillon JK, Christensen B, Fairbanks T, Jurkovich G, Moe KS. The emergent surgical airway: cricothyrotomy vs tracheotomy. Int J Oral Maxillofac Surg. 2013;42:204–8.
13. Mahmood NA, Chaudry FA, Azam H, Ali MI, Khan MA. Frequency of hypoxic events in patients on a mechanical ventilator. Int J Crit Illn Inj Sci. 2013;3(2):124–9.
14. McGrath BA, Bates L, Atkinson D, Moore JA. Multidisciplinary guidelines for the management of tracheostomy and laryngectomy airway emergencies. Anaesthesia. 2012;67:1025–41.
15. Hussain K, Wijetunge D, Grubnic S, Jackson I. A comprehensive analysis of craniofacial trauma. J Trauma. 1994;36(1):34–47.
16. Gasner R, Tuli T, Hachl O, Rudisch A, Ulmer H. Cranio-maxillofacial trauma: a 10 year review of 9543 cases with 21,067 injuries. J Craniomaxillofac Surg. 2003;31(1):51–61.
17. Morosan M, Parbhoo A, Curry N. Anaesthesia and common oral and maxilla-facial emergencies. Contin Educ Anaesth Crit Care Pain. 2012;12(5):257–62.
18. Mundinger GS, Borsuk DE, Okhah Z, et al. Antibiotics and facial fractures: evidence-based recommendations compared with experience-based practice. Craniomaxillofac Trauma Reconstr. 2015;8(1):64–78.
19. Lai Y-W, Yi-Chia W, Lee S-S, Lai C-S. Meningitis and hydrocephalus secondary to panfacial fracture repair in a traumatic brain injury patient. Kaohsiung J Med Sci. 2013;29(2):116–8.
20. Bali RK, Sharma P, Gaba S, Kaur A, Ghanghas P. A review of complications of odontogenic infections. Natl J Maxillofac Surg. 2015;6(2):136–43.
21. Alberda C, Gramlich L, Jones N, et al. The relationship between nutritional intake and clinical outcomes in critically ill patients: results of an international multicenter observational study. Intensive Care Med. 2009;35:1728–37.
22. Dryden SV, Shoemaker WG, Kim JH. Wound management and nutrition for optimal wound healing. Craniomaxillofac Trauma. 2013;21(1):37–47.
23. Miller KR, Smith JW, Harbrecht BG, Benns MV. Early enteral nutrition in trauma: is there still any doubt? Current Trauma Reports. 2016;2(2):73–8.
24. McAuley D, Barry T, McConnell K, Smith J, Stenhouse J. Early feeding after free flap reconstruction for oral cancer. Br J Oral Maxillofac Surg. 2015;53(7):618–20.
25. McClave SA, Martindale RG, Vanek VW, McCarthy M, et al. Guidelines for the provision and assessment of nutritional support therapy in the adult critically ill patient. JPEN. 2009;33(3):277–316.

6 Nutritional Care of the Maxillofacial Surgical Patient

Jennifer Hartwell

Abstract

Nutritional care is an important aspect of caring for our maxillofacial surgery patient. Consultation with a dietitian should be an essential part of the comprehensive. Careful operative planning, with consideration given to the potential need for durable enteral access, should always be addressed. This chapter will review the nutritional assessment, status, and therapy which are essential in optimizing the surgical care of our patient.

6.1 Introduction

General physical, social, and emotional well-being is inextricably tied to appropriate and balanced nutrition. Patients who have maxillofacial injuries or pathology will often have disruptions in their ability to eat as they previously did. Special consideration should be given to the assessment and support of the maxillofacial patient to optimize their nutrition and restore their ability to return to volitional oral intake, to the degree to which their pathology will allow. Appropriate assessment and thoughtful intervention will provide nutritional support to the patient and will optimize outcomes.

J. Hartwell, M.D., F.A.C.S.
Department of Surgery, IU Health/Methodist Hospital, Indianapolis, IN, USA
e-mail: jhartwell@iuhealth.org

6.2 Nutritional Assessment

Patients who present for consideration of head, neck, and facial surgery may, by nature of their disease, be in some state of malnutrition prior to evaluation. Dysphagia or other medical comorbidities may limit the patient's ability to maintain adequate volitional intake. As such, in the comprehensive evaluation of the patient with a head and neck disease or injury, consideration should be given to nutritional status. Malnutrition has been associated with increased risk for infection, poor wound healing, immunocompromise, increased length of hospital stay, increased mortality, and increased hospital costs [1, 2]. Assessing for and documenting the presence and degree of malnutrition will highlight opportunities throughout the spectrum of care to address and improve nutrition for optimal outcomes: preoperative, intraoperative, postoperative, and even nonoperative.

© Springer International Publishing AG 2018

E.M. Ferneini, J.D. Bennett (eds.), *Perioperative Assessment of the Maxillofacial Surgery Patient*,
https://doi.org/10.1007/978-3-319-58868-1_6

A thorough history and physical exam should be conducted making note of any recent weight loss, or loss of appetite, subjective feelings of weakness or diminished capacity to complete activities of daily living, or generalized fatigue. Loh et al. found that unintentional weight loss was a strong predictor of malnutrition in cancer patients with an odds ratio (OR) of 3.22 [3]. Weight loss of 10 lb over a 6-month period or weight loss of greater than 10% body weight is predictive of poor clinical outcomes [4, 5]. Patients with a body mass index (BMI) $\leq$ 18.5 kg/m^2 are considered underweight and likely suffer from protein-calorie malnutrition [6]. Of particular interest in the maxillofacial surgery candidate, periodontal disease may also be a clue for malnutrition risk.

A query of the patient's typical eating habits will identify deficiencies of protein, kilocalories, fat, carbohydrates, calcium, vitamin C, and B vitamins, among others. Clinicians should ask screening questions about eating disorders such as anorexia and bulimia; question the patient about special or restrictive diets such vegetarian, vegan, or fad diets; assess for risk factors for protein-calorie malnutrition due to social or emotional barriers; inquire about any history of depression, anxiety, or inadequate access to food due to living circumstances such as dependence on a caregiver; and obtain a comprehensive list of the patient's medications, including over-the-counter medications and all supplements.

Determining the presence and degree of malnutrition can be a difficult endeavor. There is no particular lab test that will clinch the diagnosis of malnutrition, nor direct the clinician to appreciate the degree of the problem. A more detailed discussion of laboratory measures will follow, but in general, measurement of albumin levels suffers from lack of sensitivity and specificity for malnutrition, as the value may be low due to other disease states such as nephrotic syndrome and liver disease. Prealbumin has a short half-life and may be affected by short-term changes in inflammatory states or injury, thus being an unreliable marker for global nutrition status. Indeed, the laboratory analysis, physical exam, and complete history will all be required to work in concert to understand the patient's nutrition status.

There are several tools available to the clinician to aid in the assessment of malnutrition, which vary in length, ease of use, and reliability, validity, and accuracy. However, a recent analysis of the available tools suggests that the NRS-2002 and MNA-SF may be more reliable than many others [7]. In fact, data exists to suggest that NRS-2002 [8] performs well in head and neck cancer patients to identify nutritional risk and malnourished patients [9]. These tools are illustrated in Figs. 6.1 and 6.2, respectively.

Once a patient has been identified as malnourished, or at risk for malnourishment, by the aforementioned methods, the patient should be referred to a dietitian for a specialized assessment and plan for intervention and treatment.

A multidisciplinary team should be involved in the creation of the nutrition care plan. The surgeon should supply information about anticipated anatomic considerations or the intention to place a tracheostomy, enteral feeding access, oral wires, or any other hardware that could influence the oral phase of nutrition; the dietitian will provide information specific to the energy and protein needs of the patient; the speech pathologist will be integral in making recommendations for the ordering of a diet within the limits of safety after a swallowing evaluation; nursing staff can provide information about the habits of a patient who is currently hospitalized, such as food preferences, and the percentage of kilocalories consumed. Finally, the patient and family will also provide important information about food aversions, allergies, and cultural or religious restrictions.

6.2.1 Sarcopenic Obesity

Recognition of malnutrition in the cachectic or underweight patient may be more obvious, but recently attention has been drawn to the malnourished obese patient. Known as sarcopenic obesity, these patients are both overweight and undernourished. By definition, patients who are sarcopenic have a loss of muscle mass greater than two standard deviations below the mean as measured by bioelectrical impedance. Obesity is

Nutritional Risk Screening (NRS 2002)

Table 1: Initial screening		Yes	No
1	Is BMI <20?		
2	Has the patient lost weight within the last 3 months?		
3	Has the patient had a reduced dietary intake in the last week?		
4	Is the patient severely ill ? (e.g. in intensive therapy)		

Yes: If the answer is 'Yes' to any question, the screening in Table 2 is performed.
No: If the answer is 'No' to all questions, the patient is re-screening at weekly intervals. If the patient e.g. is scheduled for a major operation, a preventive nutritional care plan is considered to avoid the associated risk status.

Table 2: Final screening

Impaired nutritional status		Severity of disease (≈ increase in requirements)	
Absent **Score 0**	Normal nutritional status	Absent **Score 0**	Normal nutritional requirements
Mild **Score 1**	Wt loss >5% in 3 mths or Food intake below 50-75% of normal requirement in preceding week.	Mild **Score 1**	Hip fracture* Chronic patients, in particular with acute complications: cirrhosis*, COPD*. *Chronic hemodialysis, diabetes, oncology.*
Moderate **Score 2**	Wt loss >5% in 2 mths or BMI 18.5 - 20.5 + impaired general condition or Food intake 25-50% of normal requirement in preceding week	Moderate **Score 2**	Major abdominal surgery* Stroke* *Severe pneumonia, hematologic malignancy.*
Severe **Score 3**	Wt loss >5% in 1 mth (>15% in 3 mths) or BMI <18.5 + impaired general condition or Food intake 0-25% of normal requirement in preceding week in preceding week.	Severe **Score 3**	Head injury* Bone marrow transplantation* *Intensive care patients (APACHE>10).*
Score:	+	**Score:**	**= Total score:**
Age	if ≥ 70 years: add 1 to total score above		**= age-adjusted total score:**

Score ≥3: the patient is nutritionally at-risk and a nutritional care plan is initiated

Score < 3: weekly rescreening of the patient. If the patient e.g. is scheduled for a major operation, a preventive nutritional care plan is considered to avoid the associated risk status.

NRS-2002 is based on an interpretation of available randomized clinical trials. * indicates that a trial directly supports the categorization of patients with that diagnosis. Diagnoses shown in *italics* are based on the prototypes given below.

Nutritional risk is defined by the present **nutritional status** and risk of impairment of present status, due to **increased requirements** caused by stress metabolism of the clinical condition.

A nutritional care plan is indicated in all patients who are
1) severely undernourished (score =3),
2) severely ill (score = 3),
3) moderately undernourished + mildly ill (score 2 +1), or
4) mildly undernourished + moderately ill (score 1 + 2).

Prototypes for severity of disease
Score = 1: a patient with chronic disease, admitted to hospital due to complications. The patient is weak but out of bed regularly. Protein requirement is increased, but can be covered by oral diet or supplements in most cases.
Score = 2: a patient confined to bed due to illness, e.g. following major abdominal surgery. Protein requirement is substantially increased, but can be covered, although artificial feeding is required in many cases.
Score = 3: a patient in intensive care with assisted ventilation etc. Protein requirement is increased and cannot be covered even by artificial feeding. Protein breakdown and nitrogen loss can be significantly attenuated.

Fig. 6.1 (NRS-2002)

defined by body mass index (BMI) ≥ 30 kg/m^2. Patients meeting criteria for both definitions, then, are considered to have sarcopenic obesity, literally understood as patients having too little muscle mass relative to their body size [10]. These patients are in a pro-inflammatory state,

Mini Nutritional Assessment

MNA®

Nestlé NutritionInstitute

Last name: First name:

Sex: Age: Weight, kg: Height, cm: Date:

Complete the screen by filling in the boxes with the appropriate numbers. Total the numbers for the final screening score.

Screening

A Has food intake declined over the past 3 months due to loss of appetite, digestive problems, chewing or swallowing difficulties?
0 = severe decrease in food intake
1 = moderate decrease in food intake
2 = no decrease in food intake ☐

B Weight loss during the last 3 months
0 = weight loss greater than 3 kg (6.6 lbs)
1 = does not know
2 = weight loss between 1 and 3 kg (2.2 and 6.6 lbs)
3 = no weight loss ☐

C Mobility
0 = bed or chair bound
1 = able to get out of bed / chair but does not go out
2 = goes out ☐

D Has suffered psychological stress or acute disease in the past 3 months?
0 = yes 2 = no ☐

E Neuropsychological problems
0 = severe dementia or depression
1 = mild dementia
2 = no psychological problems ☐

F1 Body Mass Index (BMI) (weight in kg) / (height in m)^2
0 = BMI less than 19
1 = BMI 19 to less than 21
2 = BMI 21 to less than 23
3 = BMI 23 or greater ☐

IF BMI IS NOT AVAILABLE, REPLACE QUESTION F1 WITH QUESTION F2.
DO NOT ANSWER QUESTION F2 IF QUESTION F1 IS ALREADY COMPLETED.

F2 Calf circumference (CC) in cm
0 = CC less than 31
3 = CC 31 or greater ☐

Screening score
(max. 14 points) ☐☐

12-14 points:	Normal nutritional status
8-11 points:	At risk of malnutrition
0-7 points:	Malnourished

Ref. Vellas B, Villars H, Abellan G, et al. *Overview of the MNA® - Its History and Challenges.* J Nutr Health Aging 2006;10:456-465.
Rubenstein LZ, Harker JO, Salva A, Guigoz Y, Vellas B. *Screening for Undernutrition in Geriatric Practice: Developing the Short-Form Mini Nutritional Assessment (MNA-SF).* J. Geront 2001;56A: M366-377.
Guigoz Y. *The Mini-Nutritional Assessment (MNA®) Review of the Literature - What does it tell us?* J Nutr Health Aging 2006; 10:466-487.
Kaiser MJ, Bauer JM, Ramsch C, et al. *Validation of the Mini Nutritional Assessment Short-Form (MNA®-SF): A practical tool for identification of nutritional status.* J Nutr Health Aging 2009; 13:782-788.

® Société des Produits Nestlé, S.A., Vevey, Switzerland, Trademark Owners

© Nestlé, 1994, Revision 2009. N67200 12/99 10M

For more information: www.mna-elderly.com

Fig. 6.2 (MNA-SF)

have resistance to insulin, and are at risk for rapid functional decline, development of comorbid-/obesity-related conditions, and even mortality [10]. These patients have specialized nutrition requirements to aid in preservation of lean body mass while decreasing overweight status. The clinician should suspect sarcopenic obesity in patients with BMI $\geq$ 30 kg/m^2 with a reported decrease in functional capacity, and they should be promptly referred to a dietitian.

6.3 Nutrition Requirements

The prevailing goal of nutrition support in the care of the patient with head, neck, or facial pathology is to preserve current lean body mass and provide a means to deliver adequate energy and nutrients to support immune function and prevent complications due to malnourishment.

The unstressed, otherwise healthy individual requires 20–35 kcal/kg/day [11]. However, the injured or critically ill patient may require the upper end of this range, 30–35 kcal/kg/day, or more. Protein requirements may also be markedly increased in critically ill patients. Whereas the recommended requirement for healthy adults is 0.8 g/kg/day, septic patients require 1.5 g/kg/day and trauma and burn patients require up to 2 g/kg/day [12]. After total caloric and protein needs are calculated based on the clinical situation, the exact makeup of the diet can be determined using a guideline for ratios of carbohydrate/lipid/protein of approximately 50%, 20–30%, and 15–20%, respectively [13]. Additionally, vitamins and trace elements are essential to maintain metabolism and cellular activity. There are 13 vitamins that are considered essential in the human diet. These include the eight B vitamins (thiamin, niacin, riboflavin, folate, vitamin B6, vitamin B 12, biotin, and pantothenic acid) as well as vitamin C and the fat-soluble vitamins A, D, E, and K. Trace elements include iron, zinc, copper, manganese, selenium, iodine, chromium, fluoride, and molybdenum [14], the specific doses of which are beyond the scope of this chapter. Most patients who eat a healthy, balanced variety of foods will meet the Recommended Dietary Allowance (RDA) without supplementation. However, patients with altered intake, malabsorption, critical illness, or cancer may have increased requirements of various vitamins and will require alterations of their diet or supplements to meet their daily demands. These needs can be fulfilled by volitional oral intake, tube feedings, dietary supplements, parenteral nutrition, or a combination thereof.

6.4 Route of Nutrition

6.4.1 Enteral Nutrition

Perhaps one of the most challenging aspects of providing adequate nutrition to the patient with maxillofacial pathology is determining an appropriate route of nutrition. Some patients will have mechanical obstruction from an oral mass; loss of dentition may limit tolerance to certain foods; and changes in taste and appetite frequently reduce a patient's ability to maintain adequate nutrition. Trauma patients may have temporary restrictions of their oral intake due to injury, surgery, or placement of oral devices or hardware. Radiation and chemotherapy frequently cause dysphagia, odynophagia, and mucositis. As a result, intolerance to oral diets should be anticipated, and there is evidence to suggest that prophylactic gastrostomy tubes should be considered in these patients [15, 16].

If it is determined that a patient will be unable to sustain adequate volitional intake, an enteral access device should be considered. There are several types of devices available. If it is thought that the patient will need only a short course of supplemental enteral nutrition (<4 weeks), a temporary nasogastric or nasoenteric device can be safely placed at the beside or with the assistance of an endoscopist or under fluoroscopy. If longer-term feeding (>4–6 weeks) is required, a more durable device should be placed, such as a percutaneous endoscopic gastrostomy (PEG) tube or a surgically placed gastrostomy or jejunal tube. Additional considerations include the patient and family's ability to care for the type of device chosen and an evaluation of any contraindications to device placement such as disturbed facial anatomy precluding blindly placing nasogastric tubes or a patient with altered intra-abdominal anatomy due to prior surgery. Relative contraindications to some transabdominal devices include ascites, coagulopathy, gastroparesis, or patients at high risk for aspiration. There is some concern over the risk of tumor implantation via the "pull" technique of PEG placement in which the device is pulled through the mouth and esophagus and then seated in the stomach [17]. This can be ameliorated by utilizing the "push technique" method in which a series of dilators are used to facilitate a percutaneous tract from the anterior abdominal wall, thereby eliminating the process of pulling the tube through a cancerous oral field. If this is a concern, the technique to be utilized should be discussed with the surgeon or proceduralist completing the PEG placement. A summary of access devices can be found in Table 6.1. In patients with gastroparesis or who are at risk for aspiration, combined gastrojejunal enteral access devices may be of benefit as they allow simultaneous gastric decompression and jejunal feeding. Alternatively, if gastric decompression is not required, a surgical or percutaneous jejunostomy tube can be considered. All enteral access devices can be considered temporary as bedside removal can be accomplished for any device after the goals of care have been met and the tube is no longer needed.

6.4.2 Parenteral Nutrition

For patients who simply cannot tolerate enteral nutrition (EN) due to complications such as high output fistulas, complete bowel obstructions, or critically ill patients who require a prolonged period of nil per os (NPO) status, total parenteral nutrition (TPN) should be considered. Pre- or postoperative TPN has been shown to benefit patients with moderate to severe malnutrition, as those patients with the lowest visceral protein stores are more likely to suffer adverse outcomes around the time of surgery and experience delayed wound healing [18].

Total parenteral nutrition (TPN) in the perioperative period is indicated for patients identified as severely malnourished at baseline and who are believed to require the parenteral nutrition for a period of at least 7–14 days in order to achieve protein and calorie goals. However, the risks of TPN cannot be overstated. TPN is a high-alert medication, and much of the safety recommendations surrounding its prescription, administration, and monitoring are derived from literature regarding the safety of other high-alert medications such as chemotherapy [19]. The use of TPN is associated with increased infectious complications, particularly in immunocompromised patients [18]. The use of TPN requires the establishment of central venous access, with all of its attendant risks such as infection, bleeding,

Table 6.1 Types of enteral access devices

Device	Indication	Contraindication	Benefit	Complications
Nasogastric tube	Short-term need	Mid-face trauma, nasal surgery, skull base fracture, esophageal varices	Can be placed at bedside, easy to remove	May become dislodged, less comfortable, may not be indicated for home use
Nasoenteric tube	Short-term need, gastroparesis	Same as nasogastric tube	May reduce aspiration risk	Same as nasogastric tube
PEG	Long-term need	Ascites, coagulopathy, abdominal wall pathology (fistula, ostomy), gastroparesis	Can be placed under light sedation, can bolus feed	Dislodgement can be catastrophic, clogged tube may require replacement
Surgical gastrostomy	Long-term need	Same as PEG	Can be placed if anatomy not amenable for PEG, can bolus feed	Same as PEG, requires surgery
Surgical jejunostomy	Long-term need, gastroparesis	Same as PEG	Reduced aspiration risk	Intestinal obstruction, cannot bolus feed

iatrogenic pneumothorax, and dislodgement. Patients receiving TPN are also at risk for hyperglycemia and electrolyte abnormalities, for which frequent monitoring is required.

While the provision of adequate nutrition is essential for the maxillofacial surgery patient to heal, EN is always preferred to TPN whenever it is feasible, as EN has been shown to promote more favorable outcomes in terms of infection, organ failure, and hospital length of stay [20].

6.5 Specific Diets

6.5.1 General Diet

For patients who have no apparent restrictions or contraindications to volitional oral intake, they should be encouraged to eat ad libitum. Patients should be counseled to eat a variety of foods consistent with the goals of providing their daily calorie, protein, vitamin, and trace element requirements as previously described. However, simply advising a patient to eat a variety of foods will often leave the patient falling short of meeting their daily needs. According to the National Health and Nutrition Examination Survey (NHANES), 87% of Americans fail to reach the recommended goals for vegetable intake; 75% eat too little fruit; and 86% eat too little dairy to meet their daily nutrient and vitamin needs [21]. Patients should be specifically advised to increase their fruit, vegetable, whole grain, and lean meat intake while also decreasing their consumption of foods with added sugars, fats, and sodium, both preoperatively and postoperatively [21].

6.5.2 Dysphagia Diets

Patients who have an injury or lesion of the mouth or face may not be able to safely tolerate a general diet. If there is any concern about the ability of the patient to safely eat, a swallow evaluation by a trained speech pathologist should be requested. Disorders of swallowing are categorized according to the phase that is affected: oral, pharyngeal, or esophageal. Disorders of any phase place the patient at risk of aspiration. For example, patients with disruptions of the oral phase (bolus control) may aspirate thin liquids more than thickened liquids; however, patients with derangements of the pharyngeal phase may tolerate thin liquids better than thickened liquids or soft foods in which they may experience retention of the bolus with the latter [22]. As it cannot always be judged on physical exam and history alone, a formal evaluation, including a videofluorographic swallowing study, is advised if there is any suspicion of risk for aspiration.

6.5.3 Oral Supplements

There are a variety of enteral formulations intended for use as oral supplements for patients who cannot achieve their protein, calorie, or nutrient needs via a standard oral diet. Examples include Boost® (Nestle S.A., Vevey, Switzerland) and Ensure® (Abbott Nutrition, Lake Forest, IL, USA). Most products are constituted to provide approximately 40–60% of kilocalories from carbohydrates, 15–25% from protein, and 15–35% from fat [23]. Their efficacy has mainly been studied in older adults. Available studies suggest that there may be a benefit in terms of weight gain and reduced mortality in undernourished elderly patients [24]. Patients should be encouraged to persist in their efforts to eat a balanced diet of whole foods, but oral supplements may augment the patient's ability to achieve their nutrition goals in the short term while recovering from injury or surgery.

6.6 Monitoring of Nutrition Status and Therapy

6.6.1 Fluid Balance and Electrolytes

A primary goal of a balanced diet or adequate enteral or parenteral nutrition is to maintain euvolemia and electrolytes within normal limits. Starvation and injury can both exacerbate retention of salt and water [25]. Excessive resuscitation, or hypervolemia, leads to edema and ultimately can result in cardiac and respiratory failure, delayed wound healing, infectious complications, and impaired gut function [26]. The daily evaluation of the intake and outputs (urine, drains, feces, emesis, etc.) of the patient can aid in achieving net-even fluid balance.

6.6.2 Weight

As previously discussed, weight loss of 10% of body weight or an unintentional 10 lb weight loss over 6 months is a strong predictor of poor clinical outcomes. Comparing patients treated with concurrent chemoradiation therapy (CCRT), the progression-free group had an ideal body weight (IBW) of 118% (72–193) compared to the group with progression, IBW 101.5% (73–163) ($p = 0.02$) [27]. Additional studies have shown similar results that underweight patients fare worse than their normal weight or overweight counterparts [28, 29]. Goals of therapy for nutrition support in regard to weight include achieving a normal weight for height prior to surgery and supporting the patient for weight maintenance during treatment.

In the hospitalized patient, weight will increase with large volumes of fluid administration and may be the first clue to volume overload. Conversely, weight loss ≥5% body weight is associated with prolonged hospital length of stay [30]. Again, maintenance of euvolemia and pre-hospital weight are essential goals for optimal outcomes.

6.6.3 Caloric Adequacy

Patients with wounds that are in the active healing phase require energy in the range of 30–35 kcal/kg/day [31]. While hospitalized, calculations of caloric intake can be made using available data in the patient's chart, taking into account all kilocalories delivered via dextrose containing intravenous fluids, sedative medications such as propofol (1.1 kcal/mL), enteral nutrition, and parenteral nutrition, the calculation of kilocalories delivered to a patient eating ad libitum is more problematic and is often reported as a percentage of a meal eaten rather than total calories. In this case, when the patient is tolerating approximately 60–75% of their prescribed oral intake, it is presumed they will be successful with continuing to advance toward their nutrition goals and initiation of enteral or parenteral nutrition is likely not warranted [32].

6.6.4 Nutrient Deficiency and Wound Healing

While patients experience alterations in the quantity and nature of their diet in the perioperative period, they will be at increased risk for deficiencies of specific nutrients. Nutrition support is essential for adequate wound healing. The adequate provision of kilocalories, protein, and important nutrients such as vitamins A, B, and C, as well as the trace elements selenium, zinc, copper, and manganese, is required [33]. Laboratory analysis, a thorough history, and a complete physical exam will lead the astute clinician to suspect deficiencies and take steps to correct them. In the postoperative period, electrolytes should be monitored daily until stable. A complete blood count with differential will expose anemia. In particular, attention should be given to the micronutrients listed in Table 6.2 as they are all essential for optimal wound healing. Additionally, research indicates that amino acid (AA) supplementation with arginine and glutamine may improve wound healing. While randomized controlled trials are lacking to confirm the exact dose, timing, and role of these AA, supplementation in the noncritically ill patient may be beneficial [33].

6.6.5 Laboratory Evaluation

In the patient being evaluated for elective surgery, serum albumin levels may be useful as a prognostic indicator. Lower preoperative serum albumin is associated with an increased risk of wound infections and mortality in patients with head and neck cancer [35, 36]. However, mea-

Table 6.2 Signs of nutrient deficiencies [34]

Nutrient	Common sources	Signs of deficiency
Iron	Meat, seafood, broccoli, enriched breads	Microcytic anemia, fatigue, reduced intellectual performance
Zinc	Meat, seafood, greens, whole grains	Diarrhea, altered taste and smell, alopecia, decreased immunity
Vitamin A	Milk, eggs, dark greens, yellow-orange vegetables	Night blindness, dry eyes, decreased immunity
Vitamin E	Vegetable oils, wheat germ, peanuts	Hemolytic anemia, inhibit platelet aggregation, ataxia, weakness
Vitamin K	Liver, green leafy vegetables, broccoli, peas, green beans	Bleeding, osteoporosis/increased fractures
Vitamin C	Citrus fruits, tomatoes	Fatigue, scurvy, anemia, bleeding gums, petechiae, perifollicular hemorrhage, cork screw hair, poor dentition

surement of serum albumin and prealbumin in the critically ill or injured patient must be interpreted with caution as these proteins are acute phase reactants that fluctuate with the systemic inflammatory response [36, 37]. If it is uncertain the degree to which inflammation is playing a role in the hypoalbuminemic patient, a C-reactive protein may be measured; if this value is elevated, then inflammation is likely contributing to the decreased albumin and the conclusion that the patient is malnourished or not progressing with nutrition therapy may be erroneous [36]. While nitrogen balance has also been used to measure protein delivery, this measure too falls short in its ability to predict outcomes [36]. In summary, there is no particular lab value that can guide the clinician. Instead, monitoring of these values, in addition to the measurement of electrolytes and hematologic and coagulation profiles, the physical exam, and overall clinical progression all work in concert to bring understanding of the adequacy of nutrition therapy.

6.7 Complications

As with any intervention, there can be both anticipated and unanticipated complications of medical nutrition therapy. As prevention is the best method to avoid complications, if the clinician is aware of common or serious complications, care can be taken during the initial period of management to reduce the risk of misadventure.

6.7.1 Nausea and Vomiting

Medications such as opioids and chemotherapeutic medications, as well as general anesthesia, can cause significant nausea and vomiting. Postoperative nausea and vomiting (PONV) should be anticipated, and standing orders for its treatment should be provided routinely as part of admission or postoperative orders. Persistent nausea and vomiting may require the placement of a nasogastric (NG) tube for decompression and prevention of aspiration. Depending on the maxillofacial pathology, NG tube placement may be contraindicated for concern over a tissue repair or facial fracture pattern risking inadvertent intracranial malpositioning of the tube [38].

6.7.2 Aspiration

Awake patients eating ab libitum will be at risk for aspiration due to mechanical alterations or obstruction as previously discussed. Despite the best evaluation and recommendations by specialized speech pathologists, all patients remain at risk for some degree of aspiration and should be monitored for tolerance of their diet and signs and symptoms of aspiration. While coughing, choking, and hypoxia are clear and profound symptoms of dysphagia and aspiration, the clinician should be aware of more subtle signs such as drooling, a hoarse voice, a "wet voice," frequent throat clearing, and unexplained fever [39].

While most patients will tolerate gastric tube feedings without complication, concern over aspiration persists, particularly in the critically ill patient. Placing the enteral access device into the small bowel can reduce the risk of aspiration, and the more distal the tube, the further the risk is reduced. An acute episode of hypoxia in a patient receiving enteral nutrition or who has an episode of emesis should prompt the clinician to suspect acute aspiration. A chest x-ray should immediately be obtained, deep endotracheal suctioning performed, and consideration given for formal bronchoscopy [40].

6.7.3 Access Complications

Any access device, enteral or vascular, can become dislodged at any time, due to tension, patient agitation, and manipulation or inadvertently being caught while moving or transporting a patient. Enteral access devices, whether temporary, such as a nasoenteric tube, or durable such as a PEG, should be monitored at least daily. The location of the tube at the skin level should be noted using the standard measurement markings on the device. Changes in the level of the device should prompt an investigation. An x-ray confirms the placement of many devices, and contrast enhanced x-ray can confirm the enteral location of tubes such as a PEG tube. One of the most dreaded complications of gastric tubes is the "buried bumper syndrome." Though relatively rare, noted only in 1.5–8.8% of patients with such tubes [41], it can be lethal. If placed under tension over a long period of time (weeks to months), the bumper of the device slowly erodes through the gastric wall and subsequently through the abdominal wall muscles and subcutaneous tissue. The result is delivery of intraperitoneal tube feedings, or feedings into the soft tissue, leading to peritonitis, or necrotizing soft tissue infection, respectively. Both complications can lead to sepsis and death [41]. A much more common complication of enteral access devices is clogging, which can be prevented by routine use of water flushes and thoroughly crushing any medication to be given through the tube. Tubes unable to be flushed with water or saline can be unclogged using an instillation of pancreatic enzymes [42, 43].

Vascular access devices can become dislodged in many of the same ways: being caught on other equipment, placed under tension, or manipulated by the patient. Similar to enteral devices, daily monitoring of the location of intravenous lines should be documented. Lines suspected of being malpositioned should have their location confirmed via x-ray prior to additional use. If in the proper location, clotted lines can be instilled with alteplase which has an efficacy of up to 93% in unclogging the device [44].

Central venous access devices can serve as a nidus for catheter-related deep vein thrombosis (CRDVT). In a recent study of medical intensive care unit patients, the risk for CRDVT in peripherally inserted central venous catheters (PICCs) and centrally inserted central venous catheters (CICCs) was 4 and 1%, respectively [45]. While the risk is low, a CRDVT may commit the patient to a course of therapeutic anticoagulation which may be costly and carries the risk of bleeding in the short term after surgery. All central venous lines should be monitored daily for erythema, and the limb drained by the vein where the access device lies should be examined for swelling which will alert the clinician to look for a CRDVT by ultrasound.

6.7.4 Infections

Infections can be a devastating complication for any patient. Proper nutrition has been shown to reduce infections, organ failure, and mortality in a variety of patients [46–48]. Patients can suffer from infections of the surgical wound or other infections inherent in any type of surgery such as pneumonia, urinary tract infections, *Clostridium difficile* diarrhea, or intravenous line infections. Localized cellulitis may be treated topically or with a course of antibiotics. More extensive necrotizing soft tissue infections will require removal of the access device and surgical debridement of devitalized tissue.

Use of parenteral nutrition through a central venous line places the patient at particular risk for line infections and bacteremia [49]. Fevers or erythema around the central line site should prompt an investigation of the vascular access device; blood cultures should be obtained per the hospital protocol, and prompt initiation of antibiotics should ensue [50].

6.8 Summary

Patients with maxillofacial pathology have a complex set of nutrition needs due to increased nutritional demand after injury or surgery, consideration of comorbid conditions, and disruption of the normal route of eating. Consultation with a dietitian should be an essential part of the comprehensive care of the patient. Careful operative planning, with consideration given to the potential need for durable enteral access, should always be addressed. As the patient progresses through the course of care, nutritional needs and tolerance to the planned diet can change. As such, the dynamic nature of the nutrition plan should continually be readdressed. Efficacy of the prescribed nutrition therapy will be evidenced by a healing patient, with maintenance of weight, euvolemia, normal laboratory values, and progression toward return to baseline functional status.

References

1. Correia MI, Waitzberg DL. The impact of malnutrition on morbidity, mortality, length of hospital stay and costs evaluated through a multivariate model analysis. Clin Nutr. 2003;22(3):235–9.
2. Lim SL, Ong KC, Chan YH, Loke WC, Ferguson M, Daniels L. Malnutrition and its impact on cost of hospitalization, length of stay, readmission, and 3-year mortality. Clin Nutr. 2012;31(3):345–50.
3. Loh KW, Virens MR, Gerritsen A, Borel Rinkes IH, van Hillegerberg R, Schippers C, Steenhagen E, Ong TA, Moy FM, Molenaar IQ. Unintentional weight loss is the most important indicator of malnutrition among surgical cancer patients. Neth J Med. 2012;70(8):365–9.
4. Stanley KE. Prognostic favctors for survival in patients with inoperable lung cancer. J Natl Cancer Inst. 1980;65:25–32.
5. Dewys WD, Begg C, Lavin PT, Band PR, Bennett JM, Bertino JR, Cohen MH, Douglass HO Jr, Engtrom PF, Ezdinli EZ, Horton J, Johnson GJ, Moertel CG, Oken MM, Perlia C, Rosenbaum C, Silverstein MN, Skeel RT, Sponzo RQ, Tormey DC. Prognostic effect of weight loss prior to chemotherapy in cancer patients. Eastern Cooperative Oncology Group. Am J Med 1980;69(4):491–497.
6. Centers for Disease Control. Healthy Weight. About Adult BMI. https://www.cdc.gov/healthyweight/assessing/bmi/adult_bmi/. Accessed 14 Oct 2016.
7. Skipper A, Ferguson M, Thompson K, Castellanos VH, Porcari J. Nutrition screening tools: an analysis of the evidence. JPEN. 2012;36:292–8.
8. Kondrup J, Allison SP, Elia M, et al. ESPEN guidelines for nutrition screening 2002. Clin Nutr. 2003;22(4):415–21.
9. Orell-Kotikangas H, Osterlund P, Saarilahti K, Schwab U, Makitie AA. NRS-2002 for pre-treatment risk screening and nutritional status in head and neck cancer patients. Support Care Cancer. 2015;23(6):1495–502.
10. Stenholm S, Harris TB, Rantanen T, et al. Sarcopenic obesity-definition, etiology, and consequences. Curr Opin Clin Nutr Metab Care. 2008;11(6):693–700.
11. American Society for Parenteral and Enteral Nutrition Board of Directors and the Clinical Guidelines Task Force. Guidelines for the use of parenteral and enteral nutrition in adult and pediatric patients. J Parenter Enter Nutr. 2002;26(Suppl 1):SA22.
12. Young LS, Kearns LR, Schoepfel SL, Clark NC. Protein. In: Mueller CM, editor. The A.S.P.E.N. adult nutrition support Core curriculum. 2nd ed. Silver Spring: A.S.P.E.N; 2012. p. 94.
13. Wooley JA, Frankenfield D. Energy. In: Mueller CM, editor. The A.S.P.E.N. adult nutrition support Core curriculum. 2nd ed. Silver Spring: A.S.P.E.N; 2012. p. 23.
14. Clark SF. Vitamins and trace elements. In: Mueller CM, editor. The A.S.P.E.N. adult nutrition support Core curriculum. 2nd ed. Silver Spring: A.S.P.E.N; 2012. p. 123, 139–140.
15. Nguyen N, North D, Smith H, et al. Safety and effectiveness of prophylactic gastrostomy tubes for head and neck cancer patients undergoing chemoradiation. Surg Oncol. 2006;15:199–203.
16. Chang J, Gosling T, Larsen J, et al. Prophylactic gastrostomy tubes for patients receiving radical radiotherapy for head and neck cancers: a retrospective review. J Med Imaging Radiat Oncol. 2009;53:431–2.
17. Foster J, Filocamo P, Nava H, et al. The introducer technique is the optimal method for placing percutaneous endoscopic gastrostomy tube in head and neck cancer patients. Surg Endosc. 2007;(6):897–901.
18. Mirtallo JM, Patel M. Overview of parenteral nutrition. In: Mueller CM, editor. The A.S.P.E.N. adult nutrition support Core curriculum. 2nd ed. Silver Spring, MD: A.S.P.E.N; 2012. p. 240.
19. Ayers P, Adams S, Boullata J, et al. A.S.P.E.N. parenteral nutrition safety Consensus recommendations. JPEN. 2014;38(3):296–333.
20. McClave SA, Taylor BE, Martindale RG, et al. Guidelines for the provision and assessment of nutrition support therapy in the adult critically ill patient: Society of Critical Care Medicine (SCCM) and American Society for Parenteral and Enteral Nutrition (A.S.P.E.N.). JPEN. 2016;40(2):159–211.
21. https://health.gov/dietaryguidelines/2015/guidelines/chapter-2/current-eating-patterns-in-the-united-states/. Accessed 10 Oct 2015.
22. Palmer JB, Drennan JC, Baba M. Evaluation and treatments of swallowing impairments. Am Fam Physician. 2000;61(8):2453–62.
23. Cresci G, Lefton J, Esper DH. Enteral formulations. In: Mueller CM, editor. The A.S.P.E.N. Adult

nutrition support Core curriculum. 2nd ed. Silver Spring: A.S.P.E.N; 2012. p. 189.
24. Milne AC, Potter J, Vivanti A, et al. Protein and energy supplementation in elderly people at risk for malnutrition. Cochrane Database Syst Rev. 2009;15:CD003288.
25. Allison S. Fluid, electrolytes and nutrition. Clin Med. 2004;4:573–8.
26. Granado RCD, Mehta RL. Fluid overload in the ICU: evaluation and management. BMC Nephrol. 2016;17:109.
27. Platek ME, Myrick E, McCloskey SA, et al. Pretreatment weight status and weight loss among head and neck cancer patients receiving definitive concurrent chemoradiation therapy: implications for nutrition integrated treatment pathways. Support Cancer Care. 2013;21(10):2825–33.
28. Arthur AE, Peterson KE, Rozek LS, et al. Pretreatment dietary patterns, weight status, and head and neck squamous cell carcinoma prognosis. Am J Clin Nutr. 2013;97(2):360–8.
29. Karnell LH, Sperry SM, Anderson CM, Pagedar NA. Influence of body composition on survival in patients with head and neck cancer. Head Neck. 2016;38(Suppl 1):E261–7.
30. Allard JP, Keller H, Jeejeebhoy KN, et al. Decline in nutritional status is associated with prolonged hospital length of stay in hospitalized patients admitted for 7 days or more: a prospective cohort study. Clin Nutr. 2016;35(1):144–52.
31. Bergstrom N, Bennett MA, Carson CE, et al. Treatment of pressure ulcers: clinical practice guidelines. Rockville: US Department of Health and Human Services, Public Health Service, Agency for Health Care Policy and Research; 1994.
32. McClave SA, Martindale RG, Vanek VQ, McCarthy M, et al. Guidelines for the provision and assessment of nutrition support therapy in the adult critically ill patient: Society of Critical Care Medicine (SCCM) and American Society for Enteral and Parenteral Nutrition (A.S.P.E.N.). JPEN. 2009;33(3):277–316.
33. Stechmiller JK. Wound healing. In: Mueller CM, editor. The A.S.P.E.N. Adult nutrition support core curriculum. 2nd ed. Silver Spring: A.S.P.E.N; 2012. p. 349.
34. Clark S. Vitamins and trace elements. In: Mueller CM, editor. The A.S.P.E.N. adult nutrition support core curriculum. 2nd ed. Silver Spring: A.S.P.E.N; 2012. p. 121–39.
35. Danan D, Shonka DC Jr, Selman Y, et al. Prognostic value of albumin in patients with head and neck cancer. Laryngoscope. 2016;126(7):1567–71.
36. Jensen GL, Hsiao PY, Wheeler D. Adult nutrition assessment tutorial. JPEN. 2012;36(3):267–74.
37. Ferrie S, Allman-Farinelli M. Commonly used "nutrition" indicators do not predict outcome in the critically ill: a systematic review. Nut Clin Prac. 2013;28(4):463–84.
38. Fremstad JD, Martin SH. Lethal complication from insertion of nasogastric tube after severe basilar skull fracture. J Trauma. 1978;18(12):820–2.
39. Malhi H. Dysphagia: warning signs and management. Br J Nurs. 2016;25(10):546–9.
40. Metheny NA. Preventing respiratory complications of tube feedings: evidenced-based practice. Am J Crit Care. 2006;15(4):360–9.
41. Blumenstein I, Shastri Y, Stein J. Gastroenteric tube feedings: techniques, problems, and solutions. World J Gastroenterol. 2014;20(26):8505–24.
42. Dandeles LM, Lodolce LE. Efficacy of agents to prevent and treat enteral feeding tube clogs. Ann Pharmacother. 2011;45(5):676–80.
43. Marcuard SP, Stegall KS. Unclogging feeding tubes with pancreatic enzyme. JPEN. 1990;14(2):198–200.
44. Ng R, Li X, Tu T, Cemba CP. Alteplase for treatment of occluded peripherally inserted central catheters: safety and efficacy in 240 patients. J Vasc Interv Radiol. 2004;15(1):45–9.
45. Nolan ME, Yadav H, Cawcutt KA, Cartin-Ceba R. Complication rates among peripherally inserted central venous catheters and centrally inserted central venous catheters in the medical intensive care unit. J Crit Care. 2016;31(1):238–42.
46. Waitzberg DL, Saito H, Plank LD, et al. Postsurgical infections are reduced with specialized nutrition support. World J Surg. 2006;30(8):1592–604.
47. de Luis DA, Culebras JM, Aller R, Eiros-Bouza JM. Surgical infection and malnutrition. Nutr Hosp. 2014;30(3):509–13.
48. Plochl W, Pezawas L, Artemiou O, et al. Nutritional status, ICU duration and ICU mortality in lung transplant patients. Intensive Care Med. 1996;22(11):1179–85.
49. O'Connor A, Hanly A, Francis E, et al. Catheter related blood stream infections in patients receiving parenteral nutrition: a prospective study of 850 patients. J Clin Med Res. 2013;5(1):18–21.
50. Han Z, Liang SY, Marschall J. Current strategies for the prevention and management of central line associated blood stream infections. Infect Drug Resist. 2010;3:147–63.

7 Fluids and Transfusion During Maxillofacial Surgery

Issa Rezek and Antoine M. Ferneini

Abstract

Adequate fluid resuscitation is a keystone in optimizing outcomes of our maxillofacial surgical patients. Both insufficient and excess fluid delivery can lead to increased postoperative complications. In the current practice, the notion is to always start with crystalloids as the first-line fluid choice. Colloids have no place in office-based minor oral and maxillofacial surgical procedures and may have utility only in the setting of long and/or invasive maxillofacial surgical procedures where significant blood loss is anticipated and advanced monitoring of blood pressure and/or urinary output is available. Surgical blood loss is replaced in a 3:1 ratio of crystalloid to blood loss and a 1:1 ratio if colloid is administered. This chapter will review the fluid and electrolyte balance of our surgical patients. An individualized assessment of every patient and every procedure is the most important factor in improving our patients' safety and outcomes.

7.1 Introduction

The perioperative period is characterized by a wide range of disturbances to the normal physiology of the human body, spanning from minimal to no effect in ambulatory elective procedures to significant compromise of multiple organ systems in the more complicated, emergent ones. Aside from the multiple factors affecting hemodynamic imbalances that are specific to the disease process, the surgical procedure, or the patient's baseline characteristics, there are absolute hemodynamic effects that happen with every procedure whenever sedation or general anesthesia is induced. These effects are usually pronounced as changes in the vascular tone and permeability with subsequent fluid shifts and potential electrolyte imbalances, which occasionally might become life-threatening [1, 2]. For instance, both propofol and inhalational anesthetic agents, which together are considered the

I. Rezek, M.D.
Department of Surgery, Yale University School of Medicine, New Haven, CT, USA

A.M. Ferneini, M.D., F.A.C.S. (✉)
Division of Vascular Surgery, Yale-New Haven Hospital/St. Raphael Campus, New Haven, CT, USA

Connecticut Vascular Center PC, North, CT, USA
e-mail: aferneini@ctvascularcenter.com

© Springer International Publishing AG 2018

E.M. Ferneini, J.D. Bennett (eds.), *Perioperative Assessment of the Maxillofacial Surgery Patient*,
https://doi.org/10.1007/978-3-319-58868-1_7

mainstay choice for anesthesia induction and maintenance in the majority of our surgical patients, cause reduction in systemic vascular resistance [3, 4]. The physiological response to the vascular resistance drop is a subsequent increase in cardiac work to maintain adequate blood pressure and perfusion, which creates an extra workload on the heart that can become deteriorating to a coronary artery disease patient. Fluids are usually given to expand the circulatory volume upon anesthesia induction, but generous fluid administration is problematic in a congestive heart failure or a kidney failure patient. Care should be taken to achieve appropriate fluid balance in order to maintain adequate perfusion, avoid volume overload, and prevent significant electrolyte imbalances. Understanding the perioperative fluid shifts and the appropriate steps of management is a key factor in improving the surgical outcomes of our patients.

Intravenous fluids nowadays are administered in almost every parenteral sedation and general anesthetic [5]. Fluids are used not only for hemodynamic support as mentioned above but also as a carrier for medication administration such as intravenous anesthetic medications and antibiotics. Traditionally, the majority of oral and maxillofacial surgery (OMFS) patients are young and healthy. With the ever-expanding scope of the specialty, however, more surgically extensive procedures are increasingly being performed on more medically complex patients. Therefore, it is essential to have basic understanding of fluid management in the practice of OMFS, which starts with understanding the physiology of fluid distribution and the available fluid products to guide the clinical choice.

7.2 Total Body Water and Fluid Compartments

The total body fluid comprises about 60% of the adult male weight and about 50% of the adult female weight. Thinking of the body fluids in compartments helps explain the fluid and electrolyte imbalances and the subsequent clinical manifestations that follow anesthesia induction. It also guides the selection of the appropriate resuscitative fluid when indicated.

Body fluid compartments can be divided into intracellular and extracellular. The intracellular compartment makes up 2/3 of the total body fluid. The extracellular compartment is further divided into interstitial and intravascular compartments. The intravascular compartment makes up 1/4 of the extracellular fluid, which translates into 1/12 of the total body fluid. Since fluids are administered intravascularly, it is substantial to understand the determinant factors that guide fluid distribution through the compartment barriers under different physiological conditions. This explains why 500 mL of colloid fluid will result in more intravascular volume expansion than with 1 L of crystalloid.

The general rule is that water molecules move across membranes to achieve an osmotic equilibrium. While cellular and capillary membranes are freely permeable to water, this does not apply to other molecules (electrolytes) whether secondary to their size or electrical charge. These molecules are then termed effective osmoles. The most important solutes in the serum that drive its osmolality are sodium, urea, and glucose. Serum osmolality is calculated using the following formula:

Serum osmolality (mOsm/kg) = 2*(Na + K) + (BUN/2.8) + (glucose/18).

Normal serum osmolality ranges between 275 and 290 mOsm/kg. Increases in osmolality stimulate the thirst sensation via the hypothalamus, which also produces antidiuretic hormone (ADH) that increases renal reabsorption of free water. Decreases in osmolality stimulate free water loss on the other hand.

The limited membranous permeability to particular molecules creates driving forces across the membranes, namely, Starling forces [6]. Permeability of the capillaries is affected by the following: the capillary hydrostatic pressure and the interstitial oncotic pressure on one end, both of which facilitate filtration to the interstitial space, and the capillary oncotic pressure and the interstitial hydrostatic pressure on the other end, both of which facilitate filtration back into the intravascular space. While the former set of

Table 7.1 Theoretical proportional distribution of 1 L of each commonly utilized resuscitation solutions across the body fluid compartments

1000 mL	Extracellular compartment Intravascular (mL)	Extracellular compartment Interstitial (mL)	Intracellular compartment (mL)
Colloid (blood, albumin)	1000	0	0
Lactated Ringer's	250	750	0
Normal saline	250	750	0
½ normal saline	166	500	333
¼ normal saline	125	375	500
5% dextrose in water	83	250	666

forces dominates in the arterial end of the capillary bed, the latter dominates in the venous end.

As mentioned, cellular membranes are generally permeable to water and small, nonpolar molecules. Transport of such molecules is usually passive, energy-free, and dependent on the concentration gradient. The transport of larger protein molecules or charged particles however, particularly sodium and potassium ions, is controlled by specialized channels that can function against the concentration gradient. The activation of such channels requires energy in a mechanism termed active transport [7]. Based on the abovementioned principles, Table 7.1 summarizes the theoretical proportional distribution of commonly utilized resuscitation solutions across the body fluid compartments.

7.3 Electrolytes

7.3.1 Sodium

The body sodium content is a major determinant of the osmolality and body fluid volume. The normal concentration ranges between 135 and 145 mEq/L. Sodium concentration disturbances manifest clinically with neurological symptoms including headache, lethargy, confusion, seizure, or even coma as well as cardiovascular effects from impacting the body fluid volume.

Both hypernatremia and hyponatremia can be present concomitantly with hypovolemia, euvolemia, or hypervolemia.

Hypovolemic hypernatremia is usually seen in dehydration from limited free water intake or gastrointestinal tract (GI) loss. Euvolemic hypernatremia occurs in diabetes insipidus, whether central or peripheral, given the free water loss in urine. Hypervolemic hypernatremia is usually iatrogenic.

Hypervolemic hyponatremia occurs in congestive heart failure, chronic renal insufficiency, nephrotic syndrome, and cirrhosis. The drop in plasma protein concentration, whether from the poor synthesis or renal loss, results in interstitial fluid expansion and subsequently increases ADH secretion. Euvolemic hyponatremia occurs in the syndrome of inappropriate ADH secretion (SIADH) or increased water intake. Hypovolemic hyponatremia is the most common form of hyponatremia postoperatively. It is secondary to fluid loss and further redistribution of the extracellular fluid in the surgical site, which is termed "third spacing."

Hypernatremia is treated by calculating the free water deficit by using the following formula:

Free water deficit = [(Serum Na − 140)/140] × 0.6 × weight (Kg).

Half of the calculated water deficit is then replaced over the first 24 h and the rest subsequently. Water can be replaced by either enteral intake by mouth or via feeding tube free water flushes or intravenously. Commonly used solutions are ½ normal saline for mild to moderate cases and D5 water for symptomatic hypernatremia.

Euvolemic or hypervolemic hyponatremia is usually managed by fluid restriction. Hypovolemic hyponatremia requires slow correction with isotonic saline solution for mild to moderate cases. Hypertonic saline solution (3% NaCl) is reserved for severe hyponatremia manifesting with neurological deficits.

It is important to note that correcting sodium concentration abnormalities must happen gradually unless the patient was symptomatic. Serum sodium should not be corrected more rapidly than 0.25 mEq/L/h in hyponatremia cases in order to avoid central pontine myelinolysis. Similarly, concentration should not be reduced more than 0.5 mEq/L/h in hypernatremia to avoid cerebral edema [8–10].

Symptoms of sodium imbalance are neurologic and dependent not only on the sodium concentration but also the rapidity of change. Symptoms associated with hyponatremia reflect an underlying cerebral edema and range from nausea and malaise to lethargy, headache, obtundation, or even seizure. Coma was reported in some cases of severe abrupt hyponatremia. Due to cerebral adaptation, chronic hyponatremia usually presents with less severe symptoms and might even be asymptomatic and discovered on routine laboratory work.

Abrupt hypernatremia results in decrease in brain volume that manifests with subarachnoid hemorrhage or focal neurological deficits. Resulting symptoms include lethargy, irritability, seizure, or coma. Likewise, chronic hypernatremia results in cerebral adaptation that makes symptoms mild or not existent.

7.3.2 Potassium

The normal plasma potassium concentration ranges between 3.5 and 5 mmol/L. Ninety-eight percent of the human body potassium resides intracellularly, which explains the clinically significant hyperkalemia that issues from rhabdomyolysis and tumor cell lysis and also explains pseudo-hyperkalemia which is a lab error resulting from the lysis of red blood cells in the collection tube of a blood sample.

Hypokalemia is common in the postoperative period. It can result from dilution with resuscitation with non-potassium-containing fluids, such as normal saline. It can also result from GI tract or kidney loss as well as alkalosis and high insulin levels. Hyperkalemia happens in acute renal failure, acidosis, insulin deficiency, and cellular lysis. The latter is notable in ischemia–reperfusion injuries such as post-revascularization of an acutely ischemic limb or in trauma patients following extensive muscular injuries. It is important to note also that postoperative hyperkalemia can result from utilizing succinylcholine during anesthesia induction. Succinylcholine is a depolarizing agent used for muscle relaxation/paralysis perioperatively.

Among the symptoms that may result from potassium concentration disturbances, including fatigue, weakness, confusion, and ileus, the most significant are cardiac arrhythmias. Hyperkalemia, particularly when acute as opposed to the tolerated chronic hyperkalemia in chronic renal failure, can result in ventricular arrhythmias. Electrocardiographic (ECG) changes may include peaked T waves, QRS widening, shortened QT intervals, and ventricular ectopy. Hypokalemia on the other hand can result in atrial arrhythmias. Possible ECG changes include flat T or U waves.

Hypokalemia is managed by replenishment of potassium using potassium chloride, either orally or intravenously depending on the severity of the deficit. It is important to note that hypokalemia is frequently associated with acidemia and hypomagnesemia. When present, hypomagnesemia should be corrected before hypokalemia. Acidemia correction should take place after potassium correction in order to avoid the rapid intracellular shift of potassium that can worsen a pre-existing hypokalemia.

Mild hyperkalemia (<5.5 mEq/L) can be managed with dietary modification or stopping the offending medication (such as NSAIDS or ACE inhibitors). If the elevation is chronic, patients may benefit from gastrointestinal cation exchangers such as kayexalate. Treatment should become more aggressive in chronic kidney disease patients or patients with oliguria.

Moderate hyperkalemia (5.5–6.5 mEq/L) is usually approached based on the clinical picture. Aggressive interventions are usually needed for patients with underlying cardiac rhythm disorders in cases of abrupt increase in potassium levels or ongoing mechanism that predisposes to hyperkalemia such as crush injury and tumor lysis syndrome where tissue breakdown results in significant release of intracellular potassium or ongoing gastrointestinal bleed that results in increased potassium reabsorption. Dialysis should be considered for mild or moderate hyperkalemia particularly with uptrending values.

Severe hyperkalemia (>6.5 mEq/L) treatment includes stabilizing the cardiac cellular membrane by giving intravenous calcium such as calcium gluconate or citrate and giving intravenous insulin and dextrose to drive potassium to the intracellular compartment.

7.3.3 Calcium

Calcium is the electrolyte that has the highest amount in the human body. Ninety-nine percent of human calcium is located in the bones. The normal serum calcium concentration ranges between 8.5 and 10.5 mg/dL. Serum calcium concentration is regulated by the parathyroid hormone (PTH), vitamin D, and, to a lesser extent, calcitonin that is secreted from the thyroid medullary cells (C cells). About half of the circulating calcium is bound to plasma proteins, mainly albumin. The bound calcium is biologically inactive as opposed to the active ionized calcium. Patients with malnutrition or hypoalbuminemia should either have their ionized calcium checked or their total calcium corrected for the albumin deficit for a meaningful clinical interpretation, which can be calculated using the following formula:

Corrected calcium (mg/dL) = serum calcium (mg/dL) + 0.8(4-serum albumin (g/dL)).

Hypocalcemia occurs in hypoparathyroidism, vitamin D deficiency, malnutrition, and dilution from administering large amounts of intravenous fluids. Other causes include pancreatitis and rhabdomyolysis. Hypomagnesemia and hyperphosphatemia can result in hypocalcemia as well. Acute hypocalcemia used to occur as a result of rapid blood transfusion, which usually is buffered by the calcium-chelating agent: citrate. With the newer preservation techniques, this event is becoming less common. Hypercalcemia, on the other end, occurs in hyperparathyroidism, immobility secondary to chronic hospitalization, and some malignancies. Hypercalcemia is a known side effect of thiazide and lithium.

Hypocalcemia presents with perioral and fingertip numbness and tingling as well as muscle spasms and hyperreflexia (which are detected clinically by Trousseau's and Chvostek's signs, respectively). Hypocalcemia can manifest as prolonged QT intervals and ventricular arrhythmias as well.

Symptoms of hypercalcemia include nausea, vomiting, constipation, lethargy, and mental status changes. It rarely results in coma. Chronic hypercalcemia can also result in kidney stones or nephrogenic diabetes insipidus. Hypercalcemia can cause short QT intervals on EKG.

Hypocalcemia is managed by oral or intravenous replenishment. Oral forms include calcium carbonate and calcium gluconate. Intravenous forms include calcium gluconate and calcium chloride, the latter of which has a higher concentration of elemental calcium if rapid correction is indicated, but it requires administration through a central venous access. Concomitant hypomagnesemia and hypophosphatemia should be corrected first. Hypercalcemia is managed by calcium intake restriction for mild cases and addressing the underlying cause such as mobilizing the patient when appropriate. Severe hypercalcemia, or hypercalcemic crisis, usually requires fluid resuscitation with normal saline and diuretics. Chronic hypercalcemia is managed with bisphosphonate and calcitonin.

7.3.4 Magnesium

The normal serum magnesium concentration ranges between 1.4 and 2 mEq/L. Hypomagnesemia may result from dilution postoperatively or poor intake and high GI loss. Hypermagnesemia can result from trauma or burns as well as prolonged dialysis, but this is a rare disorder.

Hypomagnesemia can result in some neurological symptoms such as hyperreflexia and weakness, but the most feared presentation is ventricular arrhythmias (torsades de pointes). Hypomagnesemia can complicate hypokalemia and hypocalcemia. This is why it is necessary to replenish magnesium when addressing these electrolyte abnormalities. Hypermagnesemia can result in sedation and loss of reflexes as well as cardiac arrhythmias.

Replenishment for hypomagnesemia is usually performed using oral or intravenous magnesium sulfate. Hypermagnesemia is managed by giving normal saline and loop diuretics. In cases of arrhythmias in the setting of hypermagnesemia, intravenous calcium gluconate is usually administered.

7.3.5 Phosphorus

Normal serum phosphate concentration ranges between 2.2 and 4.7 mg/dL. Hypophosphatemia can result in cardiac and respiratory failure and some neurological symptoms including weakness, seizure, and confusion. It results from poor intake. It can also result from increased renal excretion such as with hyperparathyroidism. A common postoperative scenario for hypophosphatemia is refeeding syndrome, particularly with malnourished patients. Refeeding drives phosphate into the cells to compose adenosine triphosphate molecules, the main energy carrier in human cells.

In contrary, hyperphosphatemia results from increased intake or decreased renal excretion such as in hypoparathyroidism or renal failure patients. Excess phosphate chelates calcium resulting in symptoms of hypocalcemia.

Hypophosphatemia is managed by replenishment, either intravenously or orally depending on the severity of the deficit. Hyperphosphatemia is managed by giving normal saline and acetazolamide. Acute or severe cases may require dialysis.

7.4 Acid–Base Balance

Acid–base balance is important to secure the appropriate physiological environment needed for living cells to function adequately. Consideration to this aspect is essential in directing the perioperative resuscitation. The acid–base balance is maintained via various buffering mechanisms to achieve an adequate concentration of hydrogen ion (H^+). The normal range for the H^+ concentration in the extracellular compartments is 28–42 mmol/L, but is not directly reported and implicated in clinical practice [8]. Instead, the pH, which is the negative algorithm of the [H^+], is utilized in clinical settings. The physiological arterial pH is 7.38–7.42 [8]. Increased H^+ results in decreased pH and acidemia, whereas decreased H^+ results in increased pH and alkalemia. When an acid–base disturbance results from a change in plasma [HCO_3^-], it is termed a metabolic acid–base disorder. Whereas when it results from a change in [pCO_2], then it is called a respiratory acid–base disorder [11].

Acids in the human body formulate from the oxidation of dietary carbohydrates, fats, and amino acids in the form of CO_2 or other nonvolatile endogenous acids such as sulfuric and phosphoric acids. Acids also form in nonphysiological conditions such as starvation which results in the production of keto acids and hypoperfusion which result in the production of lactic acid. Bases on the other end are produced from anionic amino acids (aspartate and glutamate).

The mainstay physiological mechanism of maintaining the acid–base balance is the renal secretion of excessive acids as well as reabsorption and generation of HCO_3^-. However, this process takes hours to days to complete. Acute changes in pH are compensated initially by buffer systems both in the plasma and intracellularly as well as by the lungs until the kidneys manage the disequilibrium if the patient has an appropriate kidney function. This explains why some kidney disorders result in metabolic acidosis.

The most important buffer system in the plasma is the bicarbonate/carbon dioxide (HCO_3^-/CO_2). It functions by either donating or attaining a proton, which explains why HCO_3^- is consumed in metabolic acidosis. Another buffer system is disodium phosphate/monosodium phosphate ($Na_2HPO_4^{2-}/NaH_2PO_4^-$) which functions mainly by regulating intracellular pH. Erythrocytes contain the important hemoglobin (Hb) system, reduced Hb (HHb^-), and oxyhemoglobin (HbO_2^{2-}).

Ventilation is another line of defense in the face of acid–base disturbance. It functions by modulating CO_2 expelling in response to changes in arterial pH. Ventilation is controlled by chemoreceptors located in the medulla centrally as well as the carotid body and the aortic arch. Decreased pH (i.e., increased $[H^+]$) stimulates ventilation (particularly the respiratory rate) which decreases pCO_2. The respiratory response to acid–base changes usually takes few hours to complete. The respiratory correction of an acid–base disturbance is usually partial and does not necessarily succeed in returning pH to the normal range.

7.5 Effective Circulating Volume

The goal of circulatory support is to achieve adequate perfusion, which is a function of the circulatory volume and the pressure combined. While directly intervening on the cardiac contractility and vascular tone is indicated in some scenarios by introducing inotropes and/or vasopressors, the majority of cases get effective circulatory support by managing the circulating volume. The goal of perioperative resuscitation is to reach and maintain effective circulating volume. The effective circulating volume is defined as the intra-arterial fluid volume that is required to achieve adequate tissue perfusion when an acceptable degree of vascular tone exists. This measure is dependent on multiple patient-specific factors such as the cardiac function, body habitus, and the presence of peripheral arterial disease, which makes identifying a unified formula for the adequacy of resuscitation more challenging. Instead, adequate resuscitation is judged by the clinical appearance, vital signs, and urine output as well as laboratory measures such as creatinine and lactic acid normalization.

7.6 Volume Control

A major determinant of fluid volume is the body sodium content, which directly affects the extracellular compartment volume by means of changes in renal fluid and sodium clearance. Renal sodium excretion is regulated via multiple physiological circuits that are initiated by pressure receptors in the periphery, which sense significant changes in the intravascular volume. One of the major regulatory circuits is the renin–angiotensin–aldosterone system. Angiotensin II, the active form of angiotensin, and aldosterone both promote sodium renal reabsorption. The juxtaglomerular cells in the wall of the afferent glomerular arteriole are pressure receptors that get triggered by renal hypoperfusion and secrete renin. Further, Macula densa cells, which are located in the distal convoluted tubule and can detect the tubular fluid sodium concentration, stimulate the juxtaglomerular cells to release renin with low sodium concentration. The aorta and carotid sinus also have pressure receptors that are triggered by low blood pressure and, in response, increase the sympathetic tone as well as renin release.

On the other end, increased intravascular volume is sensed by the cardiac atria which secrete the atrial natriuretic peptide and the cerebral ventricular lining that secrete the brain natriuretic peptide. The natriuretic peptides are vasodilators and promote sodium urinary excretion.

7.7 Fluid and Electrolyte Therapy

The goal of fluid management is to restore and maintain the effective circulating volume and correct any underlying electrolyte abnormality that results from the fluid disturbance or from the correction process itself. The general rule of fluid replacement is to give back the lost volume as estimated by the clinical and laboratorial measurements or the invasive monitoring devices when applicable such as pulmonary artery and central venous catheters. When euvolemia is thought to have been achieved, patients can usually maintain adequate volume from oral (per os (PO)) intake alone. If patients need to remain NPO, then maintenance intravenous fluids are usually administered to replace the physiological sensible and insensible loss on top of the expected third spacing that accompanies surgery. A common rule for maintenance fluid administration is the 4:2:1, which entails administering 4 mL/kg/h for the first 10 kg of the body weight, 2 mL/kg/h for the second 10 kg of the body weight, and 1 mL/kg/h for every kilogram beyond 20 kg. The "body weight" in the above formula was studied in patients whose weights were close to their ideal body weight. It is known that, in overweight patients, the ratio of adipose tissue/ muscular tissue increases. Adipose tissue content of water is less than of the muscular tissue rendering it less accurate to apply the 4:2:1 rule on the actual body weight for obese patients. Instead, many clinicians adopt the "adjusted body weight" as a more practical measure to estimate the need for maintenance intravenous fluids. Adjusted body weight is calculated by the following formula:

Adjusted body weight = ideal body weight + 0.4 * (actual body weight – ideal body weight).

The ideal body weight is estimated by one of these formulas:

Male: Ideal body weight = 50 kg + 2.3 * (actual height – 60 in).

Female: Ideal body weight = 45.5 kg + 2.3 kg * (actual height – 60 in).

The fluid amount obtained from the formula is arbitrary and has to be tailored to the patient's specific medical conditions such as in congestive heart failure or dialysis patients.

A recent review in the NEJM [12] defined the "ideal resuscitation fluid" as one that "produces a predictable and sustained increase in intravascular volume, has a chemical composition as close as possible to that of extracellular fluid, is metabolized and completely excreted without accumulation in tissues, does not produce adverse metabolic or systemic effects, and is cost-effective in terms of improving patient outcomes." Since such ideal fluid is not available for clinical use, it is important to understand the physiological effect of each of the available options in order to guide the decision-making when facing different clinical scenarios.

7.7.1 Crystalloids

Crystalloids are aqueous solutions that contain small molecular weight particles. These particles could be organic (lactate, acetate, dextrose) or inorganic (sodium, chloride, potassium, magnesium) [2]. The crystalloid solution may be prepared to be isotonic, hypotonic, or hypertonic. Crystalloids, in theory, tend to distribute in the intravascular and the interstitial compartments but spare the intracellular compartment if the solution was isotonic. The most common isotonic crystalloid solutions are normal saline and lactated Ringer's.

Normal saline (0.9% NaCl) contains 154 mEq/L of NaCl and has a pH of 4.5. Lactated Ringer's has a lower concentration of Na^+ and Cl^- (130 mEq/L and 109 mEq/L, respectively). Lactated Ringer's contains additional solutes, which are potassium at 4 mEq/L, calcium at 2.7 mEq/L, and bicarbonate at 28 mEq/L. Such composition makes lactated Ringer's less acidic as compared to normal saline (pH of 6.5) rendering it a slightly preferable choice in severely acidotic patients. Normal saline may be better suited for patients with metabolic alkalosis or with hyperkalemia or hypercalcemia. Excessive amount of normal saline can result in hyperchloremic metabolic acidosis.

Maintenance fluids are usually given in the form of ½ normal saline (0.45% NaCl) with or without additional dextrose (usually 5%). There are some available products that combine additional amount of potassium chloride (20 or 40 mEq/L) to replenish the mandatory daily loss of potassium. Table 7.2 summarizes the composition of the most common crystalloid solutions utilized in clinical practice.

7.7.2 Colloids

Colloids are crystalloid solutions that contain large molecular weight particles. These particles do not diffuse freely through the vascular barrier, thus creating an oncotic pressure and causing the colloid fluid to remain in the intravascular compartment completely, at least in theory. It is known now that other factors, such as vascular endothelial integrity in a generalized inflammatory response, may affect the colloid distribution. The most commonly administered colloids in clinical practice are albumin and blood products.

Table 7.2 The composition of the most common crystalloid solutions utilized in clinical practice

	PH	Na+	K+	Cl⁻	Ca2+	HCO³⁻	Dextrose (g)
Normal saline	4.5	154	0	154	0	0	0
½ normal saline	4.5	77	0	77	0	0	0
¼ normal saline	4.5	34	0	34	0	0	0
Hypertonic saline 3%	4.5	513	0	513	0	0	0
Lactated Ringer's	6.5	130	4	109	2.7	28	0
5% dextrose in water	5.0	0	0	0	0	0	50

To a lesser extent, dextran and hydroxyethyl starch have been utilized. We will discuss the administration of blood products in more details.

7.8 Blood Product Transfusion

While still prevalent in the practice of military trauma surgery, whole blood transfusion has a very limited role in managing the civilian population. Instead, separated blood components that were extracted using soft/hard spin are utilized to address the patient's specific hematological disorder, whether related to the hemoglobin level, platelets, or coagulation factors. It should be stressed that transfusion therapy should be directed by the symptoms and the clinical picture (e.g., active bleeding, symptomatic anemia) instead of being dictated solely by cutoff numbers since liberal transfusion is not without complications.

The volume of one unit of whole blood is 500 mL. Using soft spin, blood components are separated into 250 mL of red blood cells (which defines the one unit of packed red blood cells—PRBCs). The remaining 250 mL can be further separated on hard spin to 50 mL of platelets and 200 mL of plasma. Plasma can be frozen at −18° C, the so-called fresh frozen plasma (FFP), or can further be thawed at 1°–6° C to isolate 15 mL of cold-insoluble precipitates, thus named cryoprecipitate, which is rich in clotting factors such as von Willebrand factor, factor XIII, fibronectin, and, most significantly, fibrinogen.

PRBCs are stored at 4° C with citrate-based buffers and have a shelf life of 35–42 days depending on the used buffer. Citrate chelates calcium to prevent extracorporeal clotting of the stored blood. Transfusion of multiple units, such as in the massive transfusion protocol, runs the risk of clinically significant hypocalcemia from the introduced load of citrate. Transfusion with one unit of PRBC is expected to increase the hemoglobin by 1 g/dL and the hematocrit by 3%.

Platelets are stored at room temperature on gentle shakers and have a shelf life of 5 days. FFP, as mentioned earlier, is frozen at −18° C and has a shelf life of about 1 year. Cryoprecipitate is then thawed when needed and then stored at room temperature, to be used within 6 h.

7.8.1 Indications for Transfusion

Restrictive transfusion strategy has been recommended by recent guidelines [13–15] based on the findings from established clinical trials that suggested restrictive transfusion to be at least as effective as to the liberal transfusion for critically ill patients. Further, the American College of Physicians recommended in 2013 to use a restrictive red blood cell transfusion strategy (trigger hemoglobin threshold of 7–8 g/dL compared with higher hemoglobin levels) in hospitalized patients with coronary heart disease (grade: weak recommendation, low-quality evidence), contrary to the former trend toward liberally treating anemia in this patient population [16].

Platelet transfusion is indicated for active bleeding with significant hemodynamic instability or life-threatening active bleeding, such as intracranial hemorrhage, in cases of thrombocytopenia or platelet dysfunction such as patients on aspirin or clopidogrel. In the absence of active bleeding, platelet transfusion is indicated at various thresholds, ranging between 10 K and 100 K count per microliter, depending on the planned surgical procedure and the presence of an underlying hematological disorder. For the vast majority of minor OMFS cases, platelet transfusion is rarely indicated if the platelet count was more than 50 K. For major maxillofacial surgical procedures or more involved outpatient cases, a platelet count over 100 K is usually recommended.

FFP is indicated for correcting coagulation factor deficits or reversing anticoagulant medications such as warfarin. INR (international normalized ratio) is an important measure to follow the response to FFP transfusion but should not be dictating the need to transfuse in the absence of active bleeding. Cryoprecipitate is usually indicated for fibrinogen levels below 100 mg/dL or some cases of von Willebrand disease. A common clinical scenario for transfusing cryoprecipitate in nonactively bleeding patients is thrombolysis treatment which can result in consumptive hypofibrinogenemia.

7.8.2 Complications of Transfusion

Transfusion-associated risks have drastically decreased after immunological advancements that identified compatibility complexes as well as potential precipitators to a severe immune response. Despite its controversy, leukoreduction, which entails washing out PRBC from donor's white blood cells, is practiced in the majority of US blood banks. The reduction in the recipient's exposure to the donor's histocompatibility complex carried on white cell membranes is thought to minimize subsequent complications. Furthermore, blood products are usually cross-matched to minimize the risks for hemolytic reactions. Yet, there continue to be cases of allo-sensitization and less common antibodies that may result in transfusion-related acute lung injury (TRALI), fever, allergic reactions, or even significant hemolytic reactions. Other potential risks of transfusion include volume overload and hypothermia. The risk of infection is becoming rare with an incidence of one to hundreds of thousands of transfusions. The only exception is bacterial contamination which is encountered more frequently with platelet transfusion given the need to store at room temperature. The incidence of bacterial contamination for platelet transfusion is estimated to be 1:1000–1:100,000.

7.9 Summary and Conclusion

Adequate fluid resuscitation is a keystone in optimizing outcomes of our surgical patients. Both insufficient and excess fluid delivery can lead to increased postoperative complications [5, 17, 18]. In the current practice, the notion is to always start with crystalloids as the first-line fluid choice [19]. Colloids have no place in office-based minor oral and maxillofacial surgical procedures and may have utility only in the setting of long and/or invasive maxillofacial surgical procedures where significant blood loss is anticipated and advanced monitoring of vital signs and/or urinary output is available [19]. Surgical blood loss is replaced in a 3:1 ratio of crystalloid to blood loss and a 1:1 ratio if colloid is administered [1]. For most office-based oral and maxillofacial surgical procedures, insensible and urinary losses are negligible. Adequate resuscitation is usually assessed by normalizing tachycardia and hypotension and measuring urine output and lactic acid level. As always, individualized assessment of every patient and every procedure takes precedence over the abovementioned general rules.

References

1. Stoelting RK, Miller RD. Basics of anesthesia. 5th ed. Philadelphia, PA: Churchill Livingstone Elsevier; 2007.
2. Morgan GE, Mikhail MS, Murray MJ. Clinical anesthesiology. 4th ed. New York, NY: McGraw-Hill Companies; 2006.
3. Onder M, Babacan A, Bozkirli F, Somunkiran B, Gunaydin S, Karadenizli Y. The effect of propofol on systemic vascular resistance during cardiopulmonary bypass: a comparative study with thiopentone. Rinsho Kyobu Geka. 1994;14(4):317–20.
4. Loushin MK. The effects of anesthetic agents on cardiac function. In: Iaizzo PA, editor. Handbook of cardiac anatomy, physiology, and devices. Totowa, NJ: Humana Press; 2005. p. 171–80.

5. Doherty M, Buggy DJ. Intraoperative fluids: how much is too much? Br J Anaesth. 2012;109:69–79.
6. Scallan J, Huxley VH, Korthuis RJ. Capillary fluid exchange: regulation, functions, and pathology. San Rafael, CA: Morgan & Claypool Life Sciences; 2010.
7. Hall JE. Guyton and hall textbook of medical physiology. 12th ed. Philadelphia, PA: Saunders Elsevier; 2011.
8. Reddi AS. Fluid, electrolyte and Acid-Base disorders: clinical evaluation and management. 1st ed. New York, NY: Springer; 2014.
9. Adrogue HJ, Madias NE. Hyponatremia. N Engl J Med. 2000;25(342):1581–9.
10. Cameron JL. Current surgical therapy. 11th ed. Philadelphia, PA: Elsevier Saunders; 2014.
11. Adrogue HJ, Madias NE. Management of life-threatening acid-base disorders. N Engl J Med. 1998;338:26–34, 107–111.
12. Myburgh JA, Mythen MG. Resuscitation fluids. N Engl J Med. 2013;369(13):1243–51.
13. Villanueva C, Colomo A, Bosch A, et al. Transfusion strategies for acute upper gastrointestinal bleeding. N Engl J Med. 2013;368:11–21.
14. Carson JL, Brooks MM, Abbott JD, et al. Liberal versus restrictive transfusion thresholds for patients with symptomatic coronary artery disease. Am Heart J. 2013;165:964–71.
15. Hajjar LA, Vincent JL, Galas FR, et al. Transfusion requirements after cardiac surgery: the TRACS randomized controlled trial. JAMA. 2010;304:1559–67.
16. Qaseem A, Humphrey LL, Fitterman N, Starkey M, Shekelle P, Clinical Guidelines Committee of the American College of Physicians. Treatment of anemia in patients with heart disease: a clinical practice guideline from the American College of Physicians. Ann Intern Med. 2013;159(11):770–9.
17. Bellamy MC. Wet, dry or something else? Br J Anaesth. 2006;97:755–7.
18. Holte K, Sharrock NE, Kehlet H. Pathophysiology and clinical implications of perioperative fluid excess. Br J Anaesth. 2002;89:622–32.
19. Saraghi M. Intraoperative fluids and fluid Management for Ambulatory Dental Sedation and General Anesthesia. Anesth Prog. 2015;62(4):168–76.

8 Imaging for Maxillofacial Surgery

Kristine Mosier

Abstract

The perioperative imaging assessment of maxillofacial surgery patients encompasses a broad range of conditions. This chapter will focus on the imaging assessment in the setting of trauma, non-traumatic emergencies, and oncology and will use numerous case examples to illustrate how different imaging modalities are utilized.

8.1 Trauma

Imaging evaluation of the trauma patient is broadly divided into the initial evaluation of injury and the postoperative evaluation of surgical intervention and complications.

8.1.1 Initial Evaluation

Following stabilization, imaging evaluation in the hospital environment is performed using conventional multidetector computerized tomography (MDCT). MDCT allows rapid and accurate assessment of bone and soft tissue injury including acute vascular injury while maintaining stable positioning and without the need for magnet compatible components or devices. Typically in the setting of head and facial trauma, the CT examination will include scans covering the head, facial bones, and cervical spine without intravenous contrast. These are performed separately but contiguously using different scan parameters to optimize imaging of each anatomical region. The noncontrast head CT is obtained to assess either open or closed head injury and is acquired in the axial plane typically using 2–4 mm thick slices with coverage extending from the vertex to the orbits. The images are acquired with soft tissue algorithms windowed specifically to assess brain parenchyma and the presence of blood. Bone algorithms are also acquired. Magnetic resonance imaging (MRI) of the head is generally reserved for the detection of cerebral ischemic sequelae of acute injury, injuries that require early medical or intervention or close neurologic monitoring, or those for which prognostic information is required for hospital management or rehabilitative planning [1, 2].

K. Mosier, D.M.D., Ph.D.
Department of Radiology, Indiana University School of Medicine, Indianapolis, IN, USA
e-mail: kmosier@iupui.edu

© Springer International Publishing AG 2018

E.M. Ferneini, J.D. Bennett (eds.), *Perioperative Assessment of the Maxillofacial Surgery Patient*,
https://doi.org/10.1007/978-3-319-58868-1_8

Imaging of the facial bones and temporal bones is performed using thin-section MDCT images acquired in the axial plane, typically 1–2 mm for facial bones and 0.6–0.8 mm for temporal bones. Additional soft tissue algorithms are applied for facial bones. Multiplanar (coronal and sagittal) reformats are generated from the axial data. In addition, for multi-buttress or complex facial bone fractures, three-dimensional volumetric data sets are generated to assist in the planning of surgical reduction.

8.1.2 Head Trauma

The imaging goals in acute head trauma are to assess the presence and extent of primary and associated secondary injuries. Primary injuries include open or closed skull fractures, extra-axial blood collection, intraparenchymal brain injuries such as hemorrhage, contusion or shear injury, and the presence of intracranial air or foreign body. Secondary injuries are those that result from the primary injury and include brain/brainstem herniation, midline shifts, edema, hypoxia, and vascular compromise. Other secondary effects occurring in the subacute or chronic time period include infection and seizure. Figures 8.1 and 8.2 illustrate several features of primary and secondary brain injury in the acute setting. The images are of a 24-year-old patient involved in a motor vehicle collision (car under semitrailer) with extended extraction time. Figure 8.1 shows the appearance of open head injury with multiple skull fractures, tearing of bridging cortical veins that results in subdural hematoma, contusion of the brain parenchyma from direct force on the brain, and subarachnoid hemorrhage. Extra-axial and subarachnoid collections of blood and edema within the brain cause shifting of the midline and loss of the normal CSF space of the basilar cisterns. Injuries such as these clearly necessitate

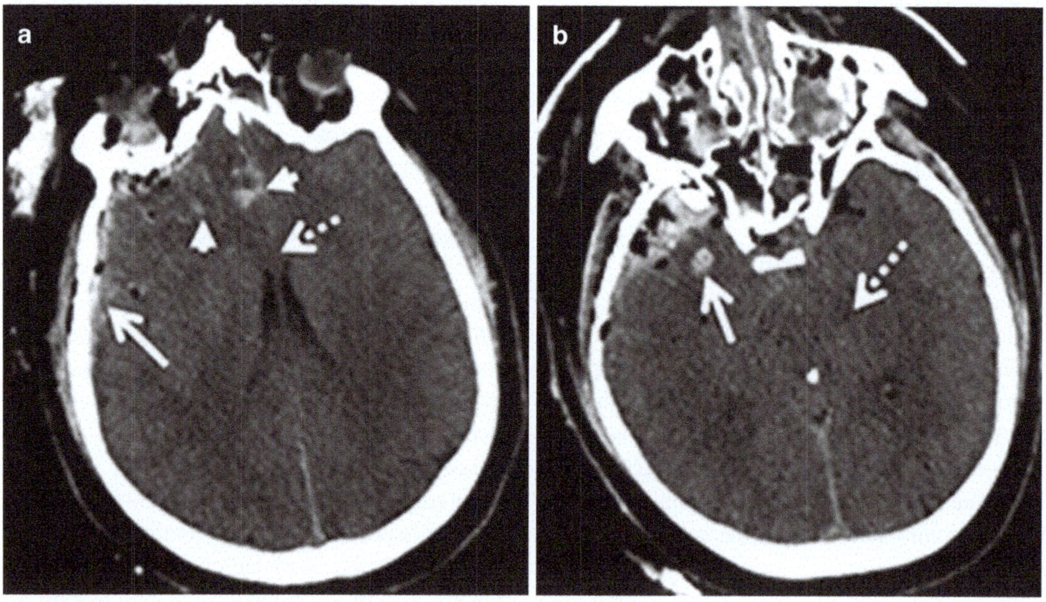

Fig. 8.1 (**a**) Noncontrast head CT in a patient with multiple frontal bone and skull base fractures shows multiple hypodense foci that represent intracranial air (pneumocephalus), acute subdural hemorrhage (*arrow*), midline shift (*dashed arrow*), and contusion and subarachnoid hemorrhage (*arrowheads*). (**b**) A more inferior image in the same patient shows hemorrhagic contusion or shear injury (*arrow*) and effacement of the basilar cisterns with subtle hyperdensity that represents additional subarachnoid hemorrhage (*dashed arrow*)

emergent neurosurgical intervention. The subacute and chronic sequelae of primary and secondary injury may result in an anoxic-ischemic event with infarction and subsequent necrosis of the cortex, ultimately leading to loss of brain parenchyma (encephalomalacia) (Fig. 8.2).

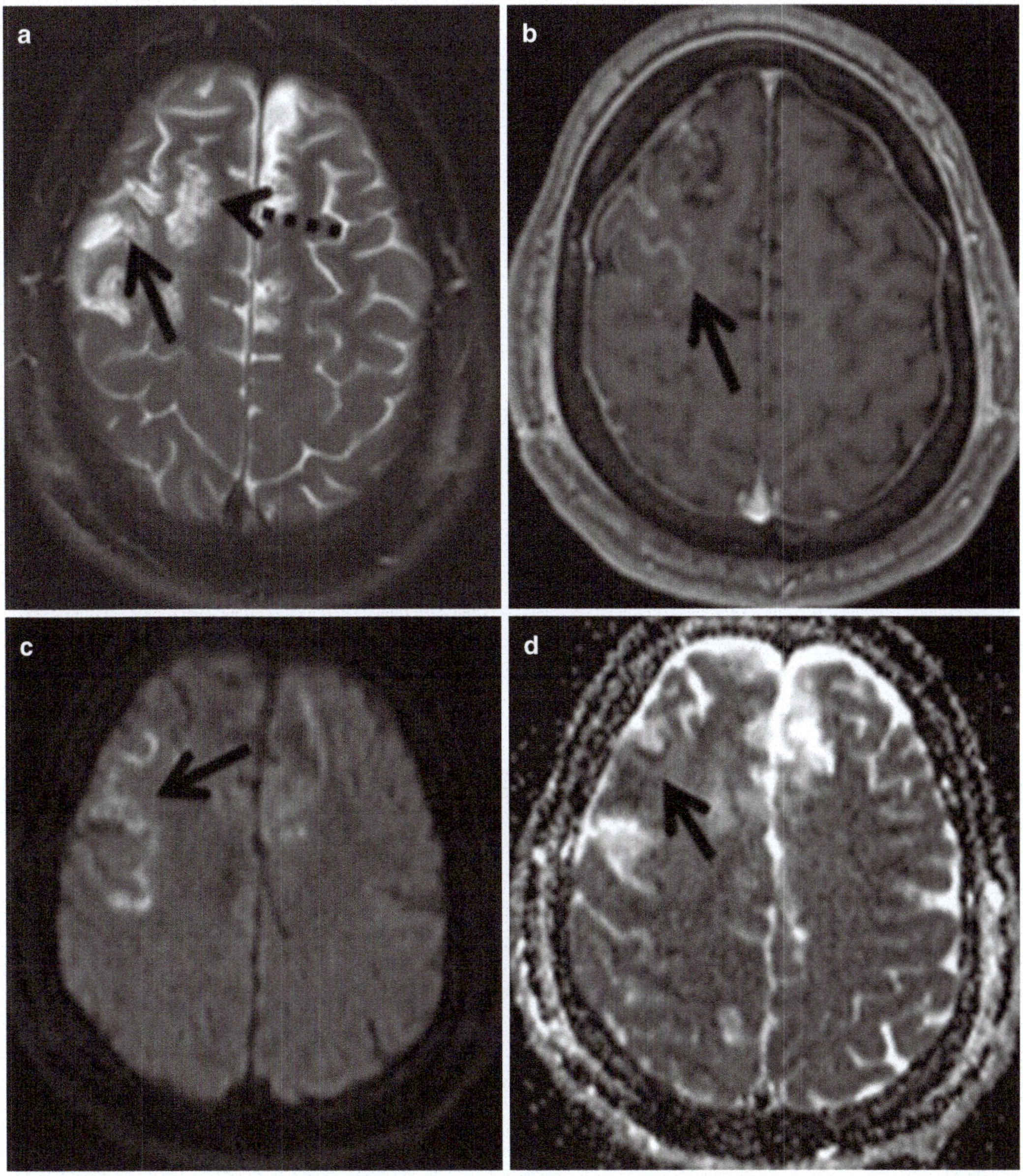

Fig. 8.2 (**a**) Axial T2-weighted MR image of the patient in (Fig. 8.1) obtained approximately 45 days after the CT images. There is T2 hyperintensity in both the cortex of the frontal lobe (*arrow*) and the deep white matter (*dashed arrow*). (**b**) Axial contrast-enhanced T1-weighted SPGR images reveal that the cortex enhances (*arrow*), but the deep white matter does not. This suggests cortical laminar necrosis in the enhancing area and encephalomalacia in the non-enhancing area. (**c**) Axial diffusion (DWI) shows the area of enhancement to be hyperintense (*arrow*) suggesting restricted diffusion. (**d**) Restricted diffusion is confirmed on this Axial ADC map as the hyperintense areas on the DWI image become dark (*arrow*). This supports cortical laminar necrosis and infarction

8.1.3 Skull Base and Facial Bone Trauma

Fractures of the skull base usually result from an impact of considerable force with over 90% the result of blunt trauma, most frequently from motor vehicle accidents. Skull base fractures are frequently associated with intracranial injury and often multiple facial bone fractures [3–5]. The role of imaging is to identify the extent of osseous, intracranial, orbital, and extracranial soft tissue injury, identify vital structures at risk, and aid in the planning of surgical treatment as well as prevention of complications.

Imaging assessment of the skull base is accomplished as described previously with thin-section CT acquired in bone algorithm with multiplanar reformats and 3D volumetric reconstructions as needed. Cerebral spinal fluid (CSF) leaks are common after fractures of the cribriform plate, fovea ethmoidalis, and temporal bones. These leaks can be evaluated with CT cisternography techniques in which CT imaging of the skull base or temporal bones is performed following the intrathecal administration of contrast.

Imaging assessment of cranial vault, skull base, and facial bone fractures is systematically approached using the categorization adopted by the AOCMF in 2014. That is, the skull base is divided into nine segments with left and right sides: anterior skull base consisting of the frontal bone and sinus, orbital roof and lesser wing of the sphenoid, the central skull base consisting of the cribriform plate and planum sphenoidale (central anterior), sella and parasellar regions (central middle) and the clivus (central posterior), the middle skull base including the sphenoid bone, greater wing of the sphenoid and temporal bone, and the posterior skull base including the parietal and occipital bones [6, 7].

Skull base fractures involving the anterior cranial fossa are additionally classified as frontobasal fractures, classified according to involvement of the frontal bone, nasoorbitoethmoid complex, cribriform plate and planum sphenoidale, or orbit and squamous temporal bone [8–10]. Fractures of the anterior cranial vault, owing to their relationship with the frontal and ethmoid sinuses, are frequently associated with pneumocephalus (Fig. 8.3). Pneumocephalus may lead to tension pneumocephalus in which trapped intracranial air leads to increased intracranial pressure and subsequent neurological decline.

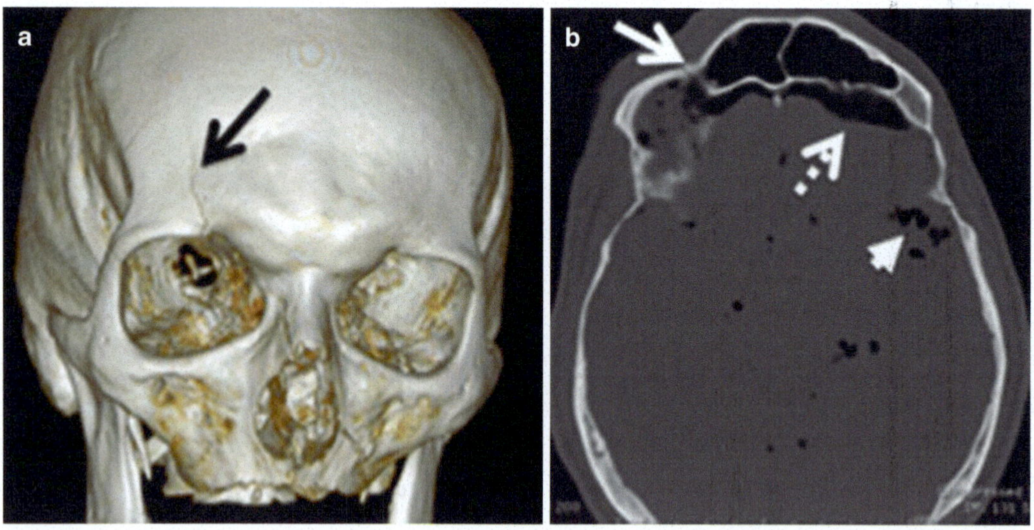

Fig. 8.3 (**a**) 3D volumetric CT reconstruction shows a type I frontobasal fracture as linear noncomminuted fracture through the right frontal bone (*arrow*) in this patient following a motor vehicle accident. (**b**) Axial CT with bone algorithm shows the small fracture through the frontal bone (*arrow*). Despite the small size of the fracture, there is significant extra-axial pneumocephalus (*dashed arrow*) as well as subarachnoid and intraparenchymal air (*arrowhead*). This patient is at considerable risk for developing tension pneumocephalus

Fractures of the middle cranial fossa are more likely to be associated with vascular injury, known as blunt cerebrovascular injury (BCVI), and include carotid dissection, intramural hematoma and thrombus, pseudoaneurysm formation, occlusion, and very rarely transection with extravasation (Fig. 8.4), [11, 12]. Recognition of BCVI is paramount to management of patients with skull base fractures as estimates place the risk of mortality and morbidity from these injuries at approximately 25–60% [12–16]. Depending on the severity of injury, BCVIs are treated with antithrombotic therapy and/or endovascular therapy. Importantly, even lower-grade vascular injuries have a propensity to evolve in the subacute period, and thus close follow-up vascular imaging in the form of CTA, MRA, or conventional digital subtraction angiography (DSA) is recommended [17]. Vascular consequences to middle fossa fracture also include traumatic carotid-cavernous fistula (CCF) in which a high-flow fistula is formed between the cavernous sinus and cavernous carotid artery. Suspected CCF is best evaluated with CTA or DSA techniques. In addition to vascular injury, fractures of the middle cranial fossa and central skull base are associated with cranial nerve injuries, including the optic nerve, as well as cranial nerves III, IV, V, and VI, leading to the potential complication of Horner's syndrome. Similarly, fractures involving the temporal bones and posterior fossa are subject to ossicular injury, carotid and vertebrobasilar BVCI, cranial nerve VII–XII injury, mastoid CSF leaks and meningoencephalocele, and craniocervical junction and cervical spine injury [18].

Fractures of the facial buttresses most often arise following high-speed impact and as such are usually found with motor vehicle accidents. Fractures of the midface and maxillofacial complex are traditionally classified according to the LeFort classification, established on the recognition of the maxillary and pterygoid bones as the critical unifying elements of the transverse and vertical midface buttresses. The transverse buttresses include the squamous temporal bone and zygomatic arch, superior maxilla, orbital rim and floors, and nasofrontal junction superiorly and, inferiorly, the inferior maxilla and palate. In the mandible, the transverse buttresses are composed of the alveolar crest and inferior border. The vertical buttresses include the lateral buttress formed by the frontal bone, zygomaticofrontal suture, lateral orbital rim, zygomaticomaxillary suture, and zygoma into the maxillary tuberosity. Medially the vertical buttress is formed by the frontal bone and nasofrontal junction, medial orbital wall, piriform rim, and anterior nasal spine. The pterygoid plates constitute the posterior elements of both the medial and lateral vertical buttresses. While utilization of the LeFort system aids in an understanding of where frac-

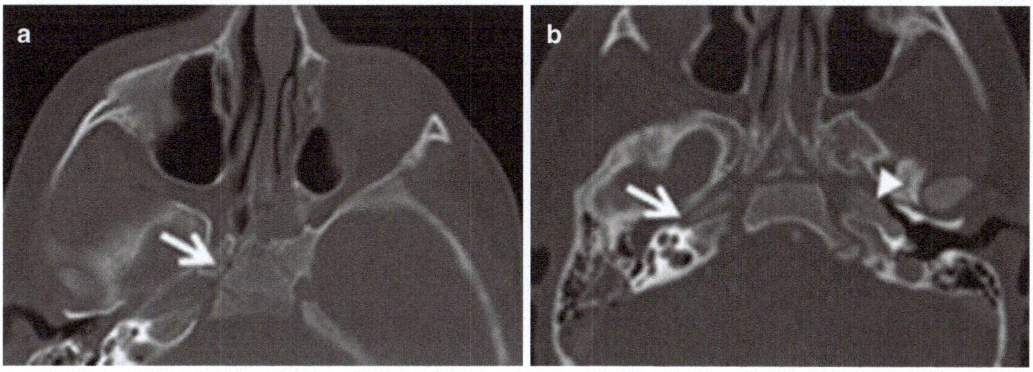

Fig. 8.4 (**a**) Axial bone CT of a 6-year-old male following head trauma from a dropped television shows a noncomminuted fracture through the right sphenoid and clivus (*arrow*) that extends to the foramen lacerum and carotid canal. (**b**) Axial CTA reveals dissection of the horizontal petrous carotid (*arrow*). The narrowed contrast column is due to an intramural hematoma. Compare this to the normal contrast in the contralateral petrous carotid (*arrowhead*)

tures will occur and the consequences of instability, it is worth noting that the majority of midface/maxillofacial fractures do not fall into a specific LeFort classification. The facial and skull base buttresses provide the osseoarchitectural integrity of the craniofacial skeleton; fractures disrupting the major buttresses then result in free-floating segments and disruption of the normal horizontal and vertical facial dimension. The LeFort III fractures result in craniofacial disjunction and therefore involve fractures of the superior medial and lateral maxillary buttresses (nasofrontal junction, orbital floor and lateral wall, zygomaticofrontal suture, zygomaticosphenoid suture) and zygomatic arch (Fig. 8.5). In the LeFort III, the involvement of the zygomatic complex along with the pterygoid plates is the defining feature separating the entire facial skeleton from the skull base. The LeFort II fractures separate the midface from the cranial base and thus similarly involve pterygomaxillary junction fractures as well as fractures of the frontomaxillary suture and nasofrontal junction, medial orbital wall and orbital rim, and zygomaticomaxillary suture, but without involvement of the zygoma (Fig. 8.6). LeFort I fractures involve fractures through the pterygoid plates, piriform rim, medial and lateral walls of the maxilla, and nasal septum and as such separate the entire maxilla from the remaining facial skeleton (Fig. 8.7) [19, 20].

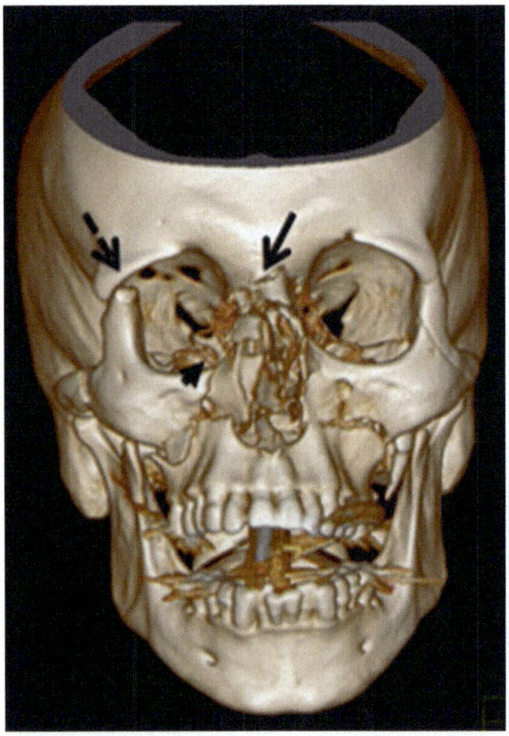

Fig. 8.5 Volumetric 3D CT rendering of patient who sustained multiple facial bone fractures following a motor vehicle accident. The comminuted fractures of the nasomaxillary junction (*arrow*) extend through the medial orbital wall and orbital floor (*arrowhead*). The fracture through the frontal process of the zygoma (*dashed arrow*) completes this LeFort III fracture and illustrates the separation of the facial skeleton from the skull base. This patient also has bilateral LeFort I fractures (Fig. 8.7)

8.1.4 Orbital Trauma

Trauma to the orbits usually involves blunt force that may result in soft tissue injury, fracture of the bony orbital vault, or both. Imaging of orbital injury is best accomplished with noncontrast head and facial bone CT, with 3D volumetric ren-

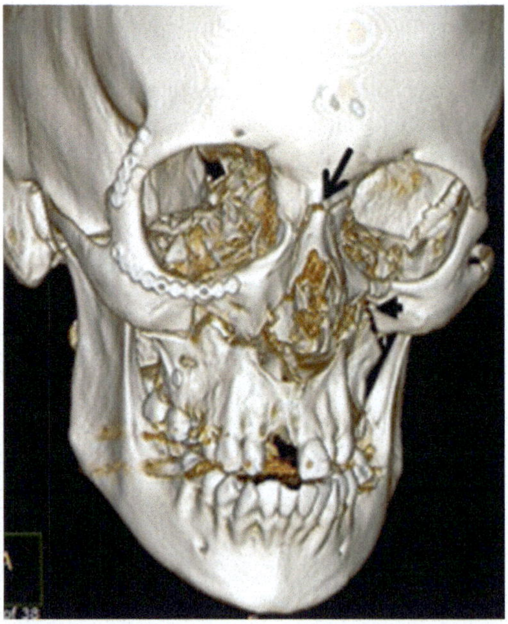

Fig. 8.6 Volumetric 3D CT rendering shows a left LeFort II fracture with fracture through the nasomaxillary junction (*arrow*) and through the medial orbit and orbital rim (*arrowhead*). Fractures extending through the posterior orbital floor are not well visualized in this rendering. The 3D rendering facilitates visualization of how this type of fracture mobilizes the midface

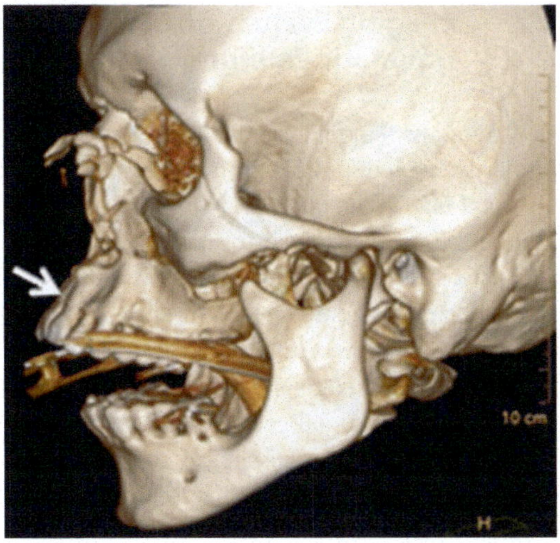

Fig. 8.7 Volumetric 3D CT rendering of the patient in (Fig. 8.5). The sagittal view better illustrates the rotation and anterior mobilization of the maxilla (*arrow*) with a LeFort I fracture

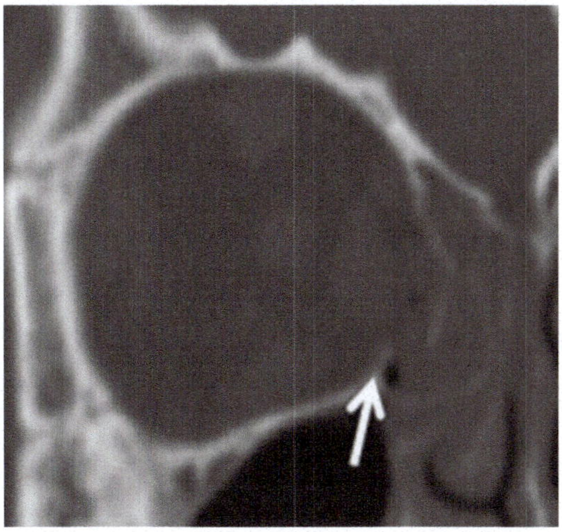

Fig. 8.8 Coronal CT with bone algorithm shows fracture of the inferomedial orbital strut (*arrow*) in this patient with medial orbital blow out fractures

dering generally reserved for cases in which fractures involve the buttresses. MR imaging of the orbits is generally not indicated in the evaluation of trauma, except to assess the presence of known or suspected organic or nonmetallic foreign body.

Fractures of the orbital roof frequently have associated subperiosteal hematomas and may have associated intracranial injuries including subdural or epidural hematomas. Medial orbital wall fractures typically have bony fragments displaced either intraorbitally or into the ethmoid sinuses. Displacement of bony fragments may impinge upon the medial rectus producing diplopia; however, even without frank bone fragment impingement, surrounding subperiosteal hematoma involving the extraocular muscles may also result in diplopia. Medial wall fractures, in addition, introduce intraorbital air from the ethmoid sinuses into the orbit, which in sufficient quantity can contribute to increased intraorbital pressure. Of particular importance are fractures involving the inferomedial orbital strut (Fig. 8.8). The inferomedial orbital strut is at the junction between the medial orbital wall and the orbital floor, often containing ethmoid air cells (Haller cells). Suspensory ligaments to the globe attach here wherein disruption produces significant diplopia. Diplopia is similarly associated with orbital floor blow out fractures when fracture fragments, or associated subperiosteal hematoma, involve the inferior rectus muscles. Orbital floor fractures may also involve the infraorbital foramen and canal. Particularly in pediatric patients, trauma or stimulation to V2 or V1, increased pressure on the globe or traction of the extraocular muscles may generate the oculocardiac reflex resulting in profound bradycardia (Fig. 8.9) [21–23].

Traumatic soft tissue injuries to the globe and orbit span a spectrum from minor injuries of the cornea to avulsion of the globe, injury, compression, or entrapment of the extraocular muscles and the optic nerve, retrobulbar hematoma, and orbital compartment syndromes. Injuries to the globe are classified as partial- or full-thickness wounds depending on the degree of violation of the cornea, sclera, or retinal layers [24]. Full-thickness disruption of the eyewall by blunt force produces a globe rupture, which occurs at one of three locations: the limbus, the attachment of the extraocular muscles, or at the optic nerve head. Globe rupture most commonly occurs at the limbus or the attachment of the extraocular muscles resulting in extravasation of vitreous from the posterior segment. On imaging, the ruptured globe has a characteristic flattened appearance (the "flat tire" appearance) that is the result of vitreal extravasation (Fig. 8.10). Other traumatic injuries to the globe commonly seen include traumatic cataract and less commonly traumatic retinal or choroidal detachment and

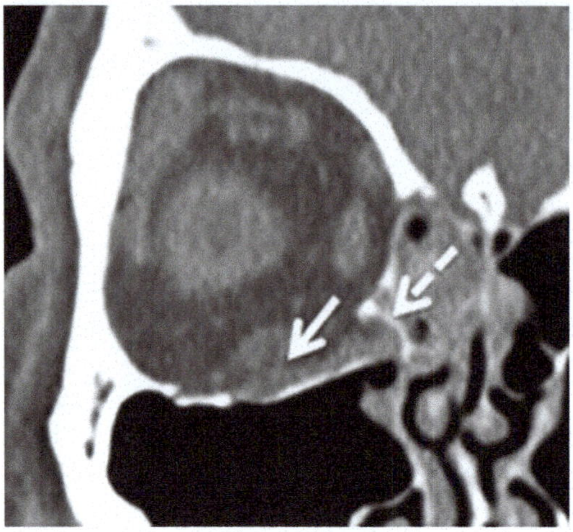

Fig. 8.9 Coronal CT with soft tissue window shows a fracture of the orbital floor with subperiosteal hematoma tethering the inferior rectus (*arrow*) and involving the infraorbital foramen. This patient developed a sinus bradycardia with a HR of 50 on admission to the ER. Note the additional fracture of the inferomedial orbital strut (*dashed arrow*)

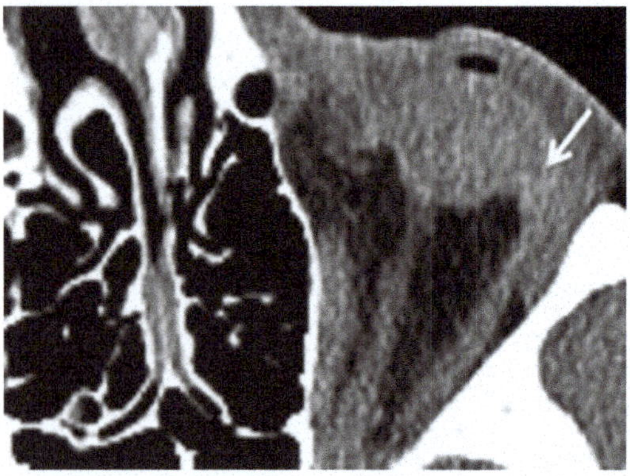

Fig. 8.10 Axial CT with soft tissue window demonstrates the flattened appearance of a globe rupture involving the insertion of the rectus muscles (*arrow*)

hemorrhage. Intraorbital foreign bodies are assessed with noncontrast CT as most are hyperdense or metallic typically arising from motor vehicle accidents and include metal, glass, or stone material or nonaccidental trauma from industrial or workshop environments. As discussed previously, MR imaging for foreign bodies is performed only after the presence of ferromagnetic foreign bodies is excluded by CT imaging and is used to assess the presence and extent of post-septal organic materials.

8.2 Imaging Evaluation of Non-traumatic Emergencies

Non-traumatic emergencies in the head and neck primarily include infection and acute airway obstruction. The imaging evaluation of infection in the head and neck is performed with contrast-enhanced CT. A separate acquisition with bone algorithm is generally not required as the raw data can be windowed for either bone or soft tissue. The goal of imaging is to identify the source of the infection (odontogenic, sinonasal, middle/ear mastoid, salivary gland, etc.) and the extent of infection as well as the degree of airway compromise if applicable.

8.2.1 Oral Cavity Infection

Cross-sectional imaging of oral cavity infection is indicated when there is known or suspected extra-alveolar extension into soft tissue, significant sinonasal extension or extension into the orbit, and/or airway compromise. Evaluation should be performed with contrast-enhanced CT as present cone beam CT (CBCT) techniques do not permit soft tissue algorithms.

Ludwig's angina is a fulminant cellulitis involving the bilateral sublingual and submandibular spaces resulting in severe airway compromise. Ludwig's angina most often arises secondary to apical periodontitis involving the mandibular teeth but may also arise secondary to trauma or ductal obstruction from sialolithiasis. Figure 8.11 demonstrates how the fluid collection and cellulitis in the sublingual and submandibular spaces produce the airway compromise.

Necrotizing fasciitis is another fulminant infectious complication of dental infection that without prompt debridement has a high morbidity and mortality. Necrosis in the deep spaces of the neck may spread inferiorly to the mediastinum or may result in carotid erosion or thrombosis or internal jugular vein thrombophlebitis. Necrotizing fasciitis is more commonly seen in diabetics or patients with immune compromise but may also be seen even in otherwise healthy patients. Figure 8.12 illustrates how a relatively

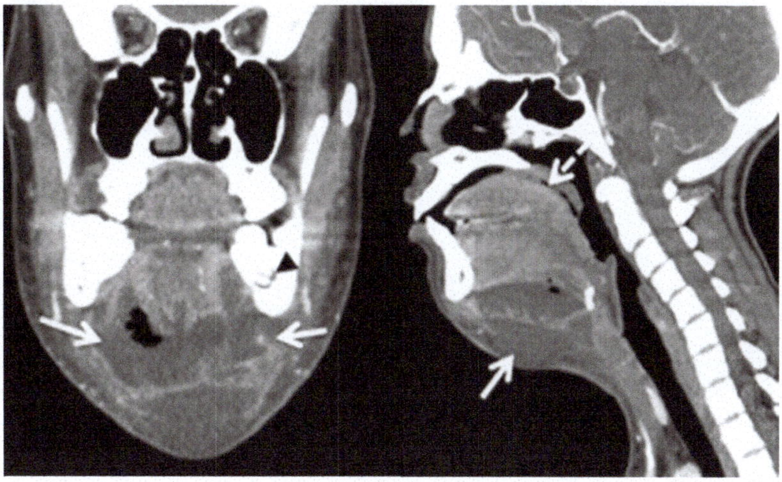

Fig. 8.11 Contrast-enhanced coronal (*left*) and sagittal (*right*) CT images in a patient with Ludwig's angina arising from apical periodontitis involving the left mandibular second molar (*black arrowhead*). Fluid and abscess in the bilateral sublingual and submandibular spaces (*white arrow*) displace the tongue superiorly and posteriorly (*dashed arrow*) compromising the oral airway

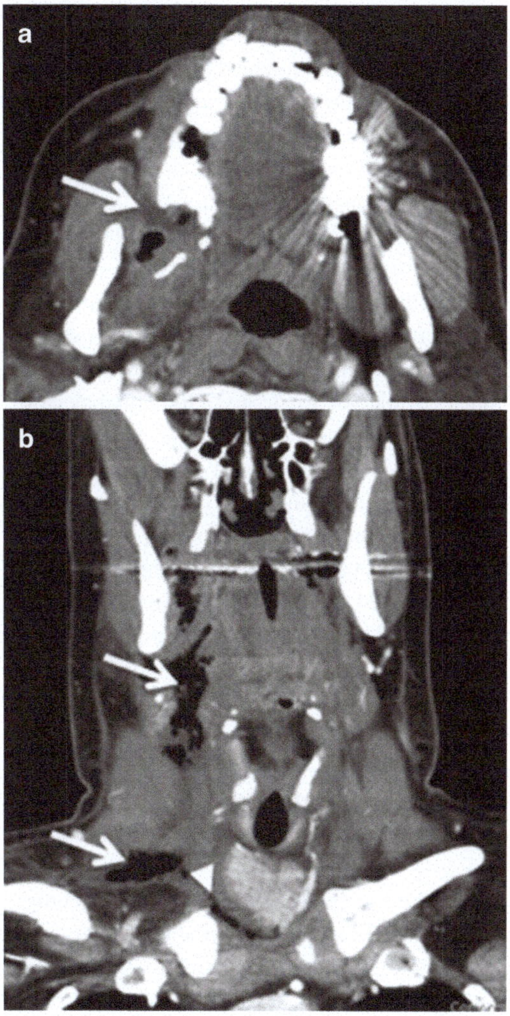

Fig. 8.12 Contrast-enhanced axial (**a**) and coronal (**b**) CT in a patient s/p exodontia of tooth number 1 three days prior. (**a**) Note the small fluid collection (*arrow*) around the right maxillary tuberosity and small focus of gas more posteriorly in the medial pterygoid. (**b**) The coronal image reveals extensive gas collection descending in and around the carotid space (*arrows*) and through the visceral space (*arrowhead*) to the anterior mediastinum

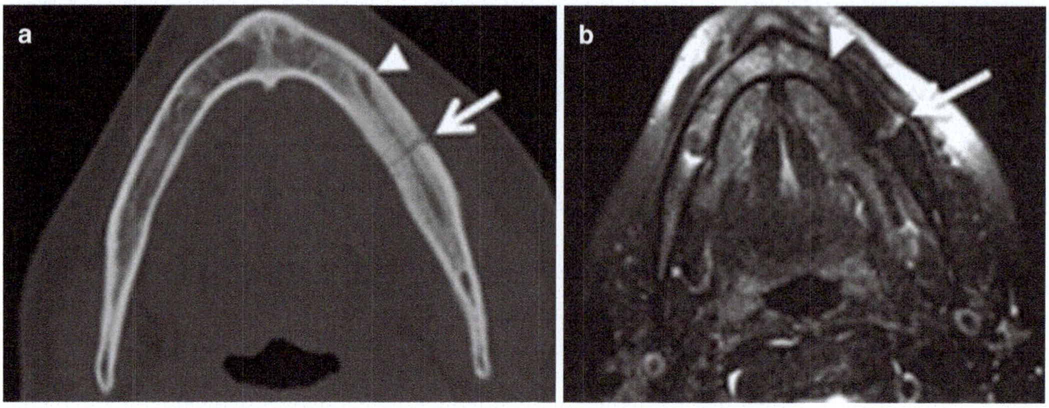

Fig. 8.13 (**a**) Axial bone CT in a patient with MRONJ following exodontia of a left mandibular first molar. There is extensive sclerosis of the left body of the mandible and a pathologic fracture (*arrow*). The anterior margin of involved bone appears to be at about the mental foramen (*arrowhead*). (**b**) Axial T2-weighted MRI from the same patient a few days later shows widening of the pathologic fracture (*arrow*). The extensive T2-hypointense signal in the left body of the mandible represents the nonviable bone that extends to the area of the canine (*arrowhead*)

minor dental infection may spread through the deep spaces to the mediastinum. On imaging, necrotizing fasciitis is distinguished from cellulitis by the degree of gas present and the degree to which the deep spaces of the neck are involved.

Other nonemergent infectious or inflammatory conditions of the maxilla and mandible that may require pre- or postoperative imaging evaluation include osteomyelitis, medication-related osteonecrosis of the jaws (MRONJ), and osteoradionecrosis. There are a number of imaging techniques available to assess the presence of infection or necrosis in the jaws, including CT, MRI, three-phase bone scan with Tc-99 MDP, positron emission tomography (PET), and single photon emission computed tomography (SPECT) [25, 26]. However CT and MR imaging are preferentially used in the preoperative setting to assess the degree of cortical and cancellous involvement in order to determine resection margins (Fig. 8.13).

8.3 Benign and Malignant Lesions of the Oral Cavity

The imaging evaluation of the majority of benign and malignant lesions of the oral cavity typically begins with contrast-enhanced CT as this is the most cost-effective and less motion-sensitive technique to assess the soft tissue characteristics and extent of the tumor as well as the integrity and involvement of the maxillary or mandibular alveolus. A complete discussion of CT or MR imaging of benign and malignant odontogenic lesions is beyond the scope of this chapter; refer to References [27, 28].

Benign lesions of the oral cavity may be developmental in origin with the most common lesions including ranulas, dermoid, epidermoids, or venous vascular malformations. Benign neoplasms may arise from the submandibular, sublingual, or minor salivary glands, lipomas arising from fat within the oral cavity, or neurogenic or vascular lesions. The goal of imaging is to identify the extent of the lesion and invasion into adjacent structures. Figure 8.14 illustrates how contrast-enhanced CT clearly defines these benign lesions. Contrast-enhanced MRI is employed when further soft tissue characterization is needed or to identify vascular components (Fig. 8.15).

The majority of malignant lesions arising in the oral cavity arise from mucosa and as such are squamous cell carcinomas, with malignant sublingual, submandibular, or minor salivary gland carcinomas and lymphomas more uncommon. Malignant lesions in the pediatric population also include sarcomas, typically rhabdomyosarcomas. The goal of imaging in the setting of malignant

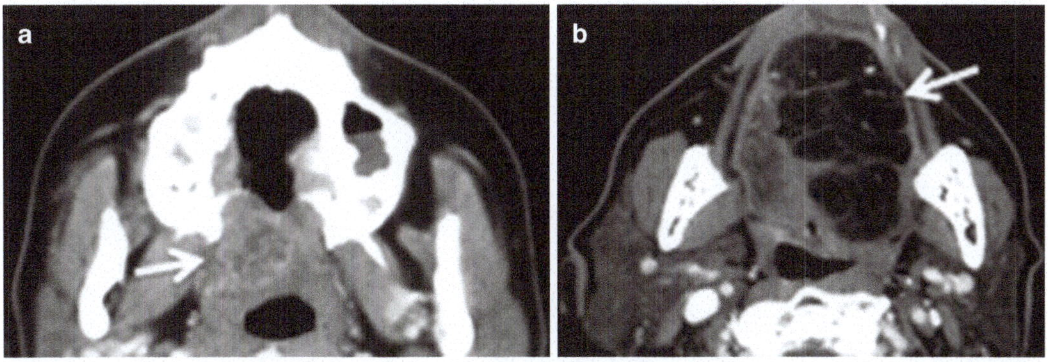

Fig. 8.14 (**a**) Axial contrast-enhanced CT of a patient with a benign mixed tumor (pleomorphic adenoma) of the right soft palate (*arrow*). The lobulated heterogeneous appearance on CT is characteristic of this lesion. The margins are clearly defined as a thin rim of enhancement. (**b**) Axial contrast-enhanced CT of a patient with a large lipoma within the oral tongue (*arrow*). The CT attenuation characteristics readily distinguish this as a fat-containing lesion and demonstrate the defined margins of this benign neoplasm

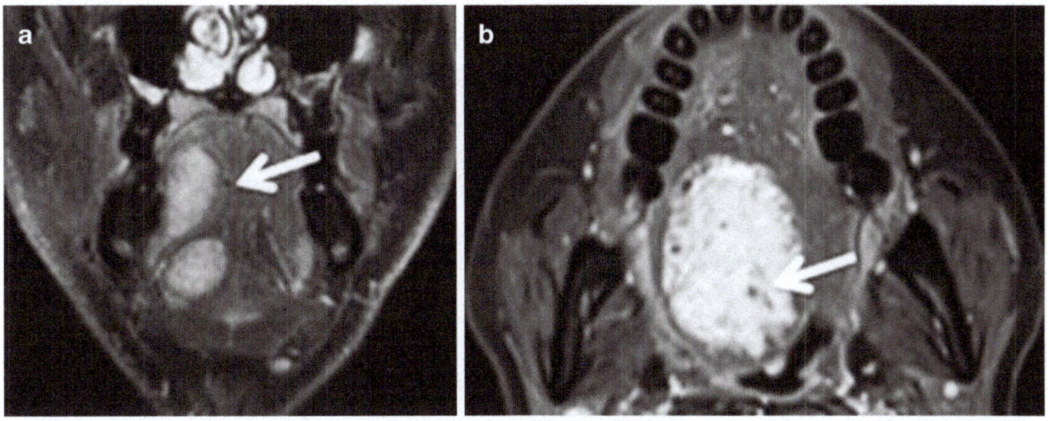

Fig. 8.15 (**a**) Coronal contrast-enhanced MRI with fat saturation shows an enhancing lobulated mass in the oral tongue. The degree of homogenous contrast enhancement and defined margin at the genioglossus and intrinsic tongue muscles (*arrow*) reveals the benign neurogenic nature of this schwannoma. (**b**) Axial contrast-enhanced MRI with fat saturation shows an avidly enhancing mass in the oral tongue of a different patient. The flow voids (*arrow*) within the lesion identify this as a vascular lesion. Hemangioma

disease is not to identify the lesion as most are easily identified on physical examination. Rather the goal of imaging is to identify the extent of the primary lesion and, if applicable, identify nodal and distant metastasis. Imaging is critical to properly staging lesions so that appropriate oncologic management may be instituted. In squamous cell carcinomas of the oral cavity, the most critical elements for staging are the depth of invasion of the tongue, involvement of extrinsic tongue muscles, invasion of the mandible or maxilla, and extension into adjacent sites, e.g., masticator space, oropharynx, sinonasal cavity, etc. Figure 8.16 illustrates how two lesions of the same dimension in the oral tongue have different staging based on local extension. Smaller oral cavity lesions may be obscured by streak artifact from dental restorations although new CT techniques such as dual-energy CT offer promise of improved streak artifact reduction [29]. Susceptibility artifacts from restorations and motion artifact limit the use of contrast-enhanced MRI in the evaluation of oral cavity lesions; nevertheless, improved soft tissue resolution may

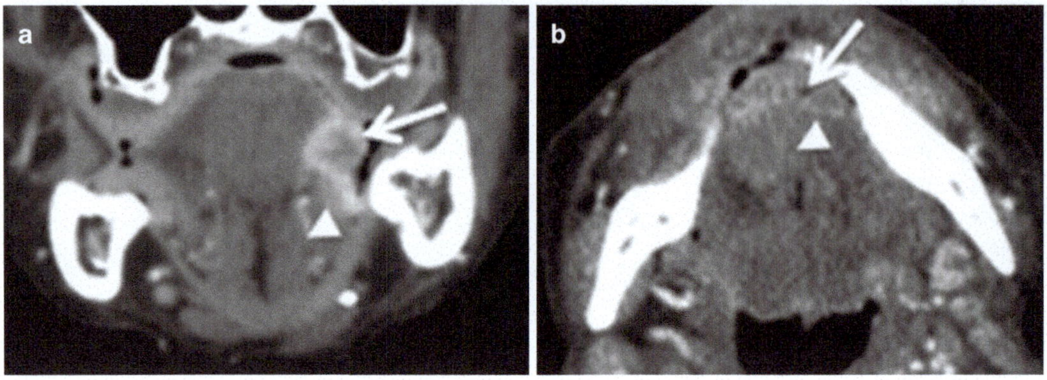

Fig. 8.16 (**a**) Coronal contrast-enhanced CT shows an enhancing lesion involving the left ventral oral tongue and floor of mouth (*arrow*) that on biopsy showed squamous cell carcinoma. Note that there is no involvement of the genioglossus muscle (*arrowhead*), making the T staging T2 by dimension. (**b**) Axial contrast-enhanced CT in a different patient with squamous cell carcinoma shows the enhancing mass involving the ventral oral tongue and floor of the mouth (*arrow*) that by dimension is T2. In this patient, however, extension into the genioglossus (*arrowhead*) upstages the lesion to T4

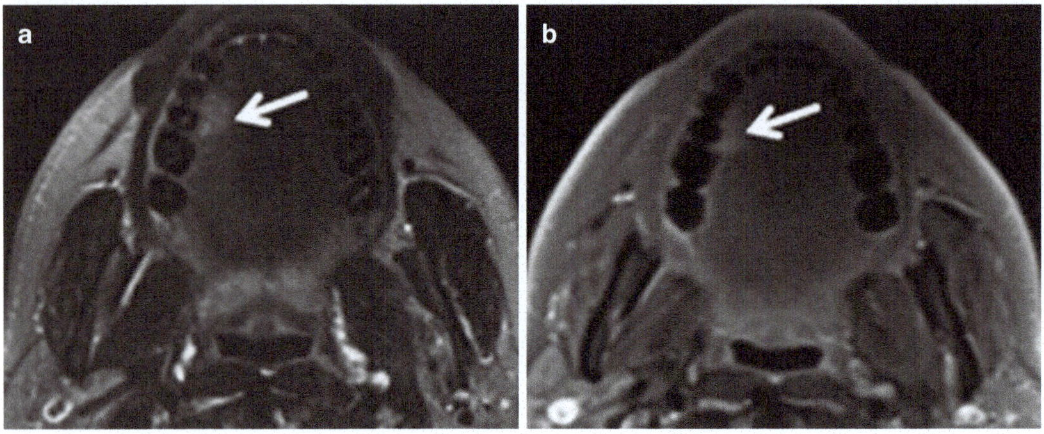

Fig. 8.17 Axial T2-weighted (**a**) and contrast-enhanced (**b**) images in a patient with squamous cell carcinoma of the oral tongue (*arrows*) show that this lesion is limited to the intrinsic tongue muscles

identify smaller lesions (Fig. 8.17), and moreover, MR is essential to identifying perineural extension of disease. PET-CT is employed to identify nodal metastasis that may not be evident based on size criteria and to identify distant metastasis, e.g., lung or osseous metastasis. PET-CT also may identify primary lesions that are inconspicuous on physical exam or conventional CT imaging (Fig. 8.18). Lastly, in the setting of malignant oral cavity lesions, CT angiography (CTA) is generally reserved to assess the viability of flap donor sites.

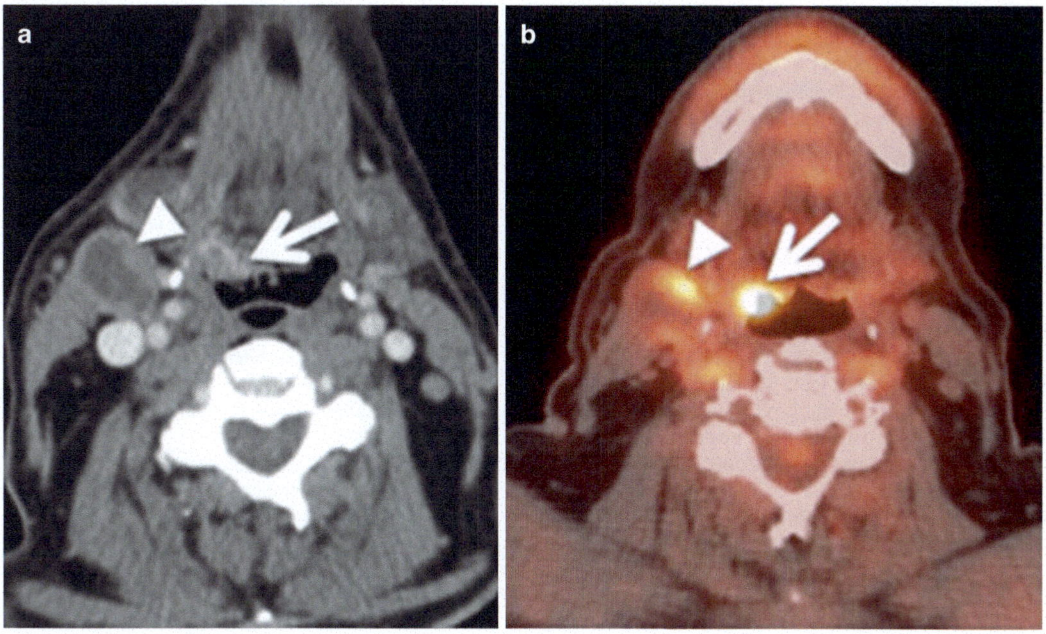

Fig. 8.18 (**a**) Axial contrast-enhanced CT of a patient with squamous cell carcinoma of the right base of the tongue (*arrow*) and partially necrotic nodal metastasis to a right level IIa lymph node (*arrowhead*). Note that the mild asymmetric enhancement is the only feature that suggests the malignant identity of this lesion compared to the normal lingual tonsils on the remaining base of tongue. (**b**) PET-CT of the same patient shows that avid fluorodeoxyglucose (FDG) uptake in the primary at the base of the tongue makes the lesion much more conspicuous (*arrow*) and reveals the extent of necrosis versus viable metastatic deposits in the lymph node (*arrowhead*)

Conclusion

CT with or without contrast remains the essential imaging technique in the workup of trauma, non-traumatic emergencies, and in the evaluation of benign and malignant disease with MRI, PET, and other nuclear medicine techniques playing a complimentary role to add additional information.

References

1. Wintermark M, Sanelli PC, Anzai Y, et al. Imaging evidence and recommendations for traumatic brain injury: conventional neuroimaging techniques. J Am Coll Radiol. 2015;12:e1–e14.
2. Roguski M, Morel B, Sweeney M, et al. Magnetic resonance imaging as an alternative to computed tomography in select patients with traumatic brain injury: a retrospective comparison. J Neurosurg Pediatr. 2015;15:529–34.
3. Alvi A, Doherty T, Lewen G. Facial fractures and concomitant injuries in trauma patients. Laryngoscope. 2003;113:102–6.
4. Fraioli RE, et al. Facial fractures: beyond Lefort. Otolaryngol Clin N Am. 2008;41(1):51–76.
5. Samii M, et al. Skull base trauma: diagnosis and management. Neurol Res. 2002;24(2):147–56.
6. Buitrago-Téllez CH, Schilli W, Bohnert M, et al. A comprehensive classification of craniofacial fractures: postmortem and clinical studies with two- and three-dimensional computed tomography. Injury. 2002;33:651–68.
7. Dileva A, et al. The comprehensive AOCMF classification: skull base and cranial vault fractures–level 2 and 3 tutorial. Craniomaxillofac Trauma Reconstr. 2014;7(Suppl 1):S103–13.

8. Madhusudan G, et al. Nomenclature of frontobasal trauma: a new clinicoradiograhic classification. Plast Reconstr Surg. 2006;117(7):2382–8.
9. Manson PN, et al. Frontobasal fractures: anatomical classification and clinical significance. Plast Reconstr Surg. 2009;124(6):2096–106.
10. Baugnon KL, Hudgins PA. Skull Base fractures and their complications. Neuroimaging Clin N Am. 2014;24(3):439–66.
11. Biffl W, Moore EE, Offner PJ, et al. Blunt carotid arterial injuries: implications of a new grading scale. J Trauma. 1999;47(5):845–53.
12. Nace SR, Gentry LR. Cerebrovascular Trauma. Neuroimaging Clin N Am. 2014;24(3):487–512.
13. Berne JD, Norwood SH, McAuley CE, et al. The high morbidity of blunt cerebrovascular injury in an unscreened population: more evidence of the need for mandatory screening protocols. J Am Coll Surg. 2001;192(3):314–21.
14. Biffl WL, Moore EE, Ryu RK, et al. The unrecognized epidemic of blunt carotid arterial injuries: early diagnosis improves neurologic outcome. Ann Surg. 1998;228(4):462–70.
15. Biffl WL, Moore EE, Elliott JP, et al. The devastating potential of blunt vertebral arterial injuries. Ann Surg. 2000;231(5):672–81.
16. Miller PR, Fabian TC, Croce MA, et al. Prospective screening for blunt cerebrovascular injuries: analysis of diagnostic modalities and outcomes. Ann Surg. 2002;236(3):386–93.
17. Biffl WL, Ray CE Jr, Moore EE, et al. Noninvasive diagnosis of blunt cerebrovascular injuries: a preliminary report. J Trauma. 2002;53(5):850–6.
18. Katzen JT, Jarrahy R, Eby JB, et al. Craniofacial and skull base trauma. J Trauma. 2003;54:1026–34.
19. Winnegar BA, Murillo H, Tantiwongkosi B. Spectrum of critical imaging finding in complex facial skeletal trauma. Radiographics. 2013;33:3–19.
20. Lo Casto A, Priolo GD, Garufi A, et al. Imaging evaluation of facial complex strut fractures. Semin Ultrasound CT MRI. 2012;33:396–409.
21. Sires BS, Stanley RB, Levine LM. Oculocardiac reflect caused orbital floor trapdoor fracture: an indication for urgent repair. Arch Ophthalmol. 1998;116(7):955–6.
22. Kim BB, Qaqish C, Frangos J, Caccemese JF. Oculocardiac reflex induced by an orbital floor fracture: report of a case and review of the literature. J Oral Maxillo Surg. 2012;70:2614–9.
23. Fahling JM, McKenzie LK. Oculocardiac reflex as a result of Intraorbital trauma. J Emerg Med. 2017;52(4):557–8. https://doi.org/10.1016/j.jemermed.2016.08.022.
24. Kuhn F, Morris R, Witherspoon CD, et al. A standardized classification of ocular trauma. Ophthalmology. 1996;103:240–3.
25. Fukumitsu N, et al. What can be identified by 3-phase bone scintigraphy in patients with chronic osteomyelitis of the mandible? Ann Nucl Med. 2010;24(4):287–93.
26. Schuknecht B, Valvanis A. Osteomyelitis of the mandible. Neuroimaging Clin N Am. 2003;13(3):605–18.
27. Mosier KM. Lesions of the jaw. Semin Utrasound CT MRI. 2015a;36:444–50.
28. Mosier KM. Magnetic resonance imaging of the maxilla and mandible. Signal characteristics and features in the differential diagnosis of common lesions. Top Magn Reson Imaging. 2015b;24:23–37.
29. Srinivasan A, Hoeffner E, Ibrahim M, et al. Utility of dual-energy CT virtual keV monochromatic series for the assessment of spinal transpedicular hardware-bone interface. AJR Am J Roentgenol. 2013;201:878–83.

9 Chest X-Ray Interpretation

Elie Tony Nader

Abstract
Historically, a chest X-ray is the first thoracic imaging modality used in the medical field to detect chest diseases. It is fast, painless, and easy to use. Chest X-ray imaging is currently considered the most common diagnostic tool used in the clinical setting. This includes perioperative work-up of the maxillofacial surgery patient. In this chapter, we emphasize a step-by-step approach to read a chest X-ray to help diagnose and monitor diseases, including pneumonia, congestive heart failure, pulmonary edema, lung cancer, and pneumothorax.

9.1 Technical Advances in Chest Radiography [1]

Chest radiographs are produced by radiation which passes through the body, producing a shadow of the anatomy inside, resulting in the image. Given that body structure absorbs X-rays at different extents, the bone appears white as it has high absorption, tissue appears gray as it has less absorption, and air appears black as it has very low absorption. Usually fat looks dark gray on the image.

The radiologic technologist must review each image for the following:

- Correct patient and examination information
- Brightness/contrast
- Exposure indicator
- Processing errors
- Required anatomy
- Positioning accuracy
- Artifacts

The first form of digital imaging, digital subtraction angiography, was introduced in 1977 and put to clinical use in 1980 [2].

Image quality in chest radiography depends on multiple fundamental parameters including image density, contrast, special resolution, and image noise.

E.T. Nader, M.D.
Division of Pulmonary and Critical Care Medicine, Norton Community Physicians Group, Norton, VA, USA
e-mail: elie.nader@yahoo.com

© Springer International Publishing AG 2018

E.M. Ferneini, J.D. Bennett (eds.), *Perioperative Assessment of the Maxillofacial Surgery Patient*,
https://doi.org/10.1007/978-3-319-58868-1_9

9.2 Interpretation [3, 4]

The first step in Chest X-ray interpretation is to determine whether the study is a standard or portable chest radiograph. The standard chest radiograph consists of two views: posteroanterior (PA) view and a lateral view. For the PA view, patient stands in front of the X-ray source, facing the cassette or digital receptor, with the front of the chest against the cassette. Portable X-rays, typically performed on patients in the ICU, are anteroposterior (AP) views, with the patient's back lying against the cassette or receptor plate. Lateral views are typically not performed as part of a routine portable exam due to higher radiation exposure and lack of a moving grid as well as limited mobility of the patient. The PA view should be obtained whenever possible due to better image quality.

Always check the film label to verify patient's name, age, and sex.

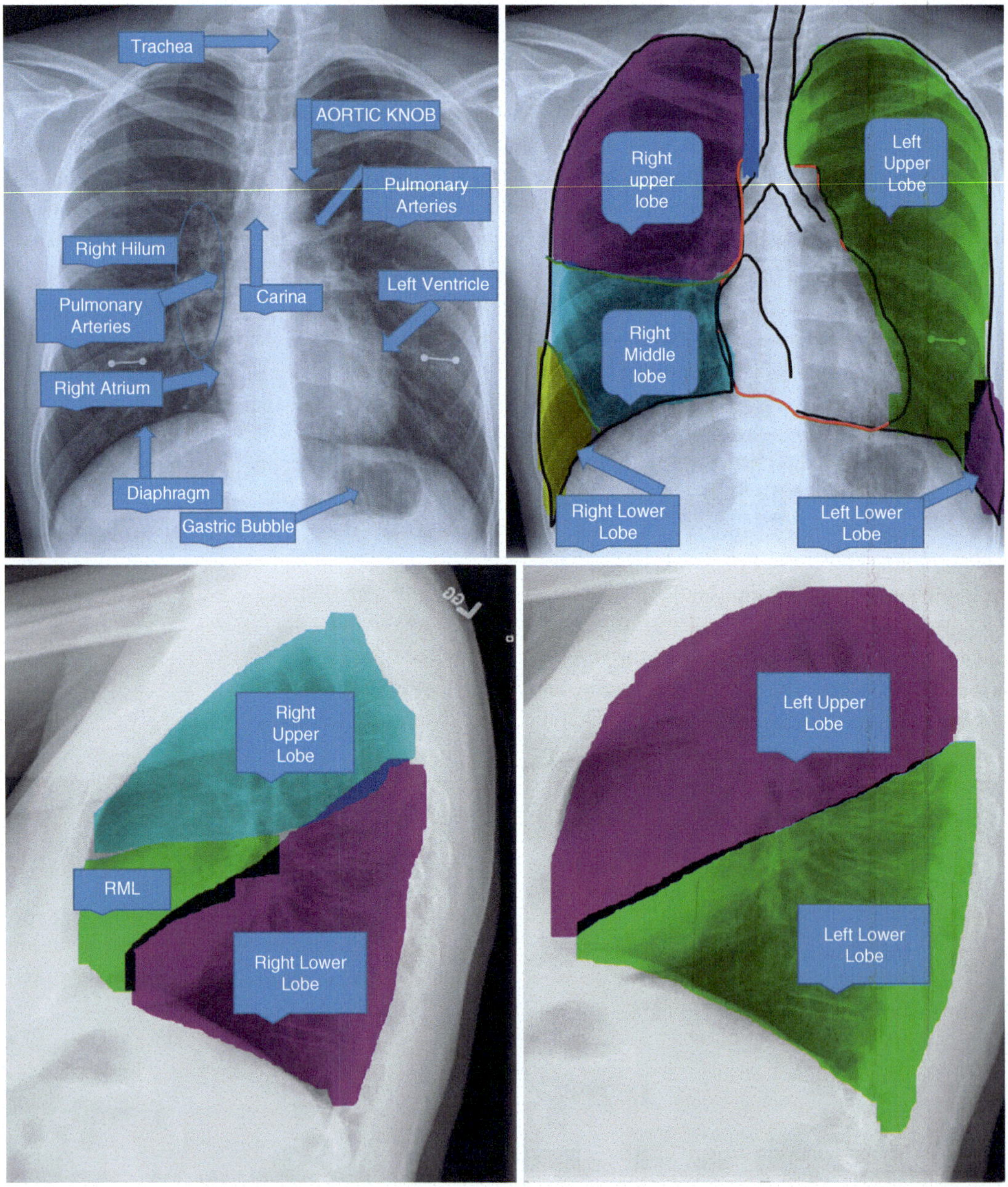

The second step is to determine the film orientation, which requires familiarity with anatomy. While the technologist should label the film as right and left sides, the reader should confirm this by review of basic anatomy. The heart, gastric bubble, and aortic knob are left-sided structures unless the patient has situs inversus. Rotation on the frontal images can be determined by looking for symmetrical spacing of the clavicles relative to the spinous processes and symmetry in size of the chest cavities bilaterally. Rotation on the lateral images can be determined by assessing the ribs which should nearly superimpose bilaterally.

The third step in interpretation of the chest X-ray is to assess technical quality. In general, one should be able to identify the outline of the vertebral bodies within the heart shadow. If the film is under penetrated (underexposed), the thoracic vertebrae will not be visible through the heart.

Interpretation of the radiograph for detection of pathology begins as follows:

9.2.1 Skeletal Structures

Any abnormality in the bone structures would be incidental as X-ray film is obtained with a technique optimized for detection of pathology of the lungs, pleura, and mediastinal structures.

- **Scapulae**: In the PA and lateral view, to avoid superimposition upon the upper lung fields, patient should stand with hands on hips, palms out, and elbows forward, rotating the scapulae to the sides.
- **Clavicles**: Symmetrical spacing of the clavicles on either side of the sternum means there is no rotation of the chest; even mild rotation will result in significant degree of asymmetry.
- **Ribs**: Assessment of the degree of inspiration can be performed by counting the number of ribs to the level of the diaphragm. Carefully identify the first rib at its anterior junction with the manubrium, follow it backward to the spine, then count down the number of posterior ribs. Always compare both sides for symmetry, and look for any fractures or other focal abnormalities.

  The number of ribs identified helps determine how much lungs are inflated. In PA view, if nine posterior ribs are visible, the film was taken in inspiration, while six anterior ribs would qualify as a good film in full inspiration. Visualization of ten or more posterior ribs above the diaphragm typically indicates hyperinflation. On an expiration film, we expect to see fewer than nine posterior ribs; the lung bases will be less well seen, the diaphragms will be elevated and more rounded, and the heart will be larger in its transverse diameter. Emphysema and pneumothorax are better visualized on an expiration film.

9.2.2 Soft Tissues Structures

These include the chest wall, neck and mediastinum, muscle structures, diaphragm bilaterally, and breasts.

Identify the trachea within the neck looking for narrowing, compression, or deviation. If the epiglottis is visible, evaluate for swelling. Check for foreign bodies.

9.2.3 Cardiac Border

The size of the heart reflects underlying chamber enlargement, hypertrophy, or pericardial effusion. The heart is considered enlarged when the transverse diameter of the heart on a PA film is more than 50% or more than 60% on AP films. At the same time, the physician should check for any prosthetic valve, evidence of prior cardiac surgery, or cardiac calcifications.

9.2.4 Pleural Effusion and Pneumothorax

Checking the costophrenic angles on each chest X-ray is essential to rule out a pleural effusion, blunting of the angle reflects small effusion, while larger effusion is usually well visualized.

One should differentiate between lung collapse and large pleural effusion by checking if there is any mediastinal shift. Lateral chest X-ray is especially helpful in identifying a pleural effusion since small effusions will first be visible in the posterior costophrenic sulci (Figs. 9.1, 9.2 and 9.3).

9.2.5 Fields and Fissures

The chest radiograph is considered the first imaging step to assess for pulmonary infiltrates including interstitial or alveolar edema. The presence of bronchograms is useful in identifying consolidation, which may be indicative of pneumonia but can also be seen in atelectasis and some neoplasms (Fig. 9.4).

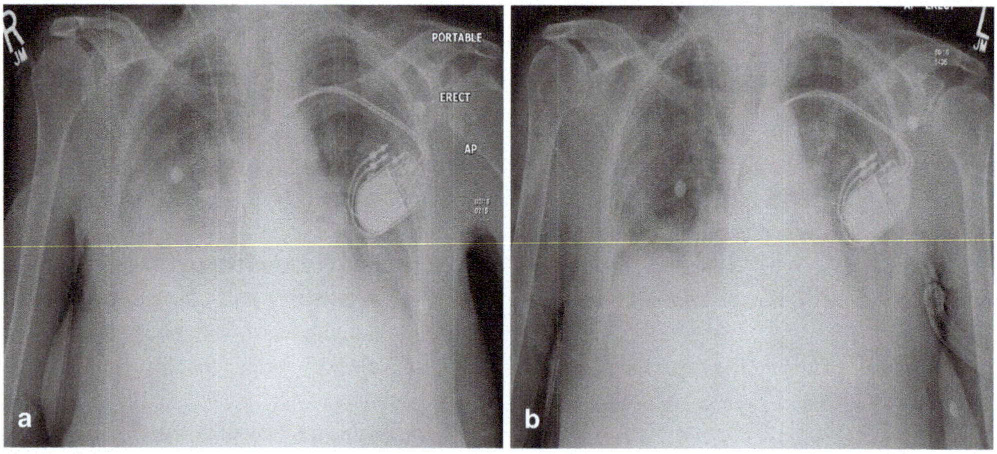

Fig. 9.1 A 72-year-old male patient admitted with the complaint of shortness of breath. (**a**) AP projection: central line in the right internal jugular, pacemaker with multi leads, the heart is mildly enlarged, the lungs mildly hypoinflated, increased opacity in the right mid- and lower lobe with layering bilateral pleural effusion (*right* more than *left*). (**b**) Post-thoracentesis showed decreased in pleural effusion on the right without evidence of pneumothorax

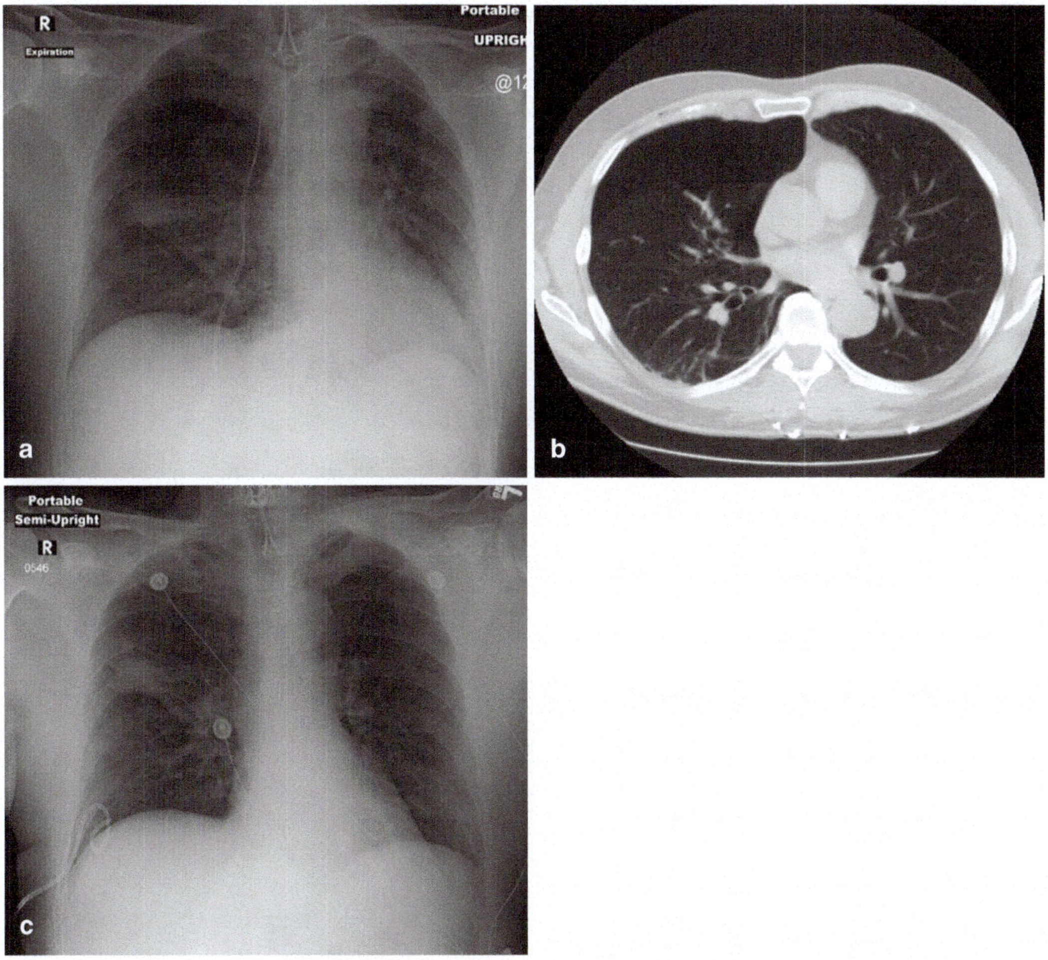

Fig. 9.2 (**a**) A large right apical pneumothorax, with the lung measuring 7.2 cm from the chest wall apex, there is a mild shift of the mediastinum to the left. Opacity in the right upper lobe is noted. (**b**) CT scan of the chest showed a large right apical pneumothorax with compressive atelectasis. (**c**) Pneumothorax resolved after small-bore chest tube placement

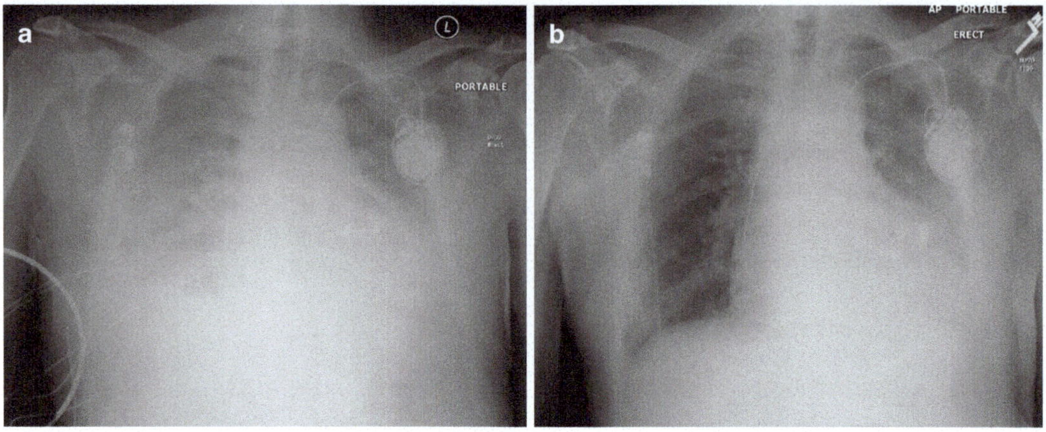

Fig. 9.3 A 86-year-old male patient presented with shortness of breath (**a**) chest X-ray upon admission showed: intact bony structures. The heart is enlarged with a single-lead pacemaker. There are mediastinal sternal wire sutures. Haziness throughout both the right and left hemithorax with bilateral pleural effusion right more than left. (**b**) Post-thoracentesis: AP chest X-ray showed improvement of aeration in the lungs with some residual airspace opacity especially on the left. There is a minimal residual right and mild-to-moderate left residual layering pleural effusion

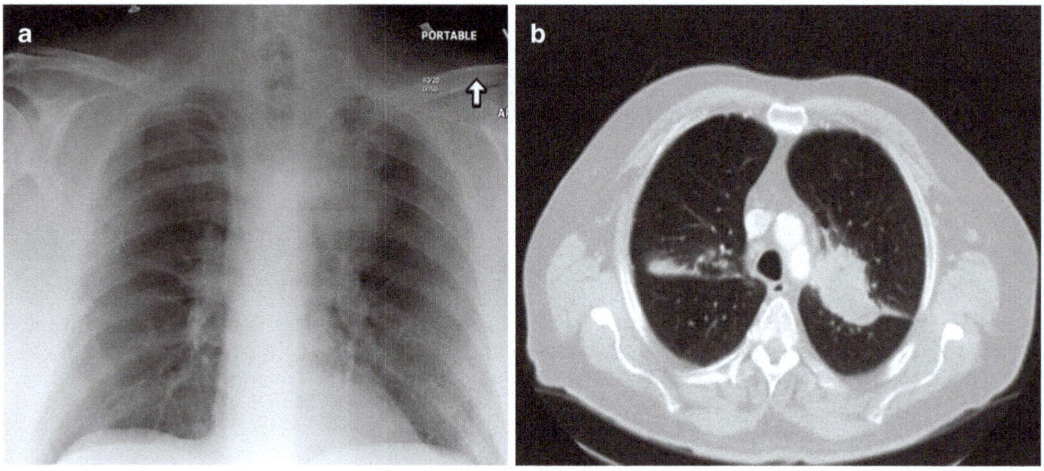

Fig. 9.4 A 76-year-old male patient admitted with shortness of breath, found to have a left upper lobe mass. (**a**) Chest X-ray AP showed masslike opacity in the left peripheral and left suprahilar lung. (**b**) CT scan chest showed large left upper lobe mass partially invading the left mediastinum

9.2.6 Diaphragm

Flattening of diaphragms is seen in asthma or COPD. Slight elevation of the right hemidiaphragm relative to the left is considered physiologic due to liver position; more severe pathological elevation is seen in diaphragm paralysis or lung collapse. Crescent sign which reflects air under the diaphragm may be an indication for bowel perforation and need for emergent surgical intervention (Fig. 9.5).

9.2.7 Hila and Mediastinum

The chest X-ray is considered essential as a quick tool in the setting of acute coronary syndrome. A widened or enlarged mediastinum in the setting

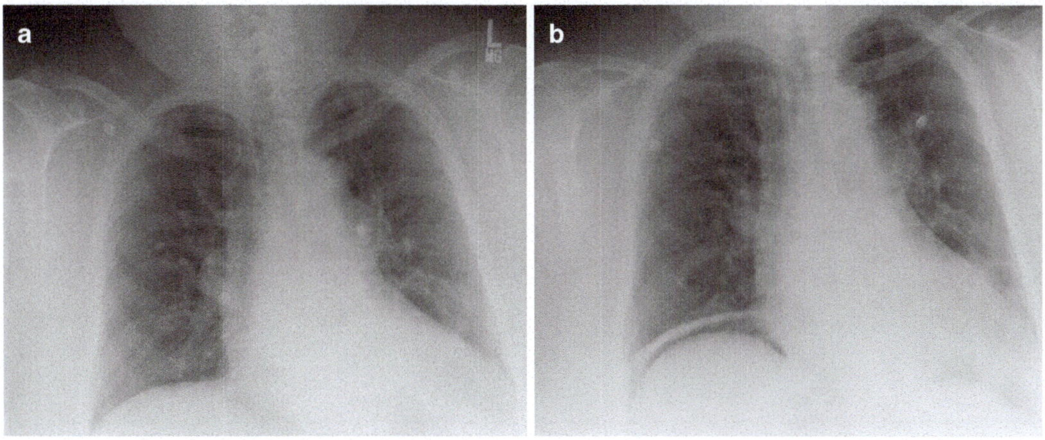

Fig. 9.5 A 56-year-old female patient is admitted for diverticulitis. (**a**) AP CXR upon admission. (**b**) AP CXR after 12 h. Chest X-ray showed right crescent sign, which reflects free air in the abdomen; differentials include iatrogenic or bowel perforation requiring urgent intervention. *NB*: Enlarged heart and mediastinum could be overestimated in AP chest X-rays

of chest pain can be an alarming sign and indication to rule out aortic dissection.

Evaluation of mediastinal shift and tracheal deviation is considered essential in the setting of "white-out" of a hemithorax to differentiate lung collapse versus large pleural effusion. In the former, the trachea will be deviated toward the same side of the white hemithorax, while in pleural effusion, the trachea and mediastinum will be pushed away from the opacified side.

Enlarged mediastinum, in the setting of a PA film, should prompt to rule out an underlying malignancy, lymphadenopathy, aortic aneurysm, and other space-occupying lesions (Fig. 9.6).

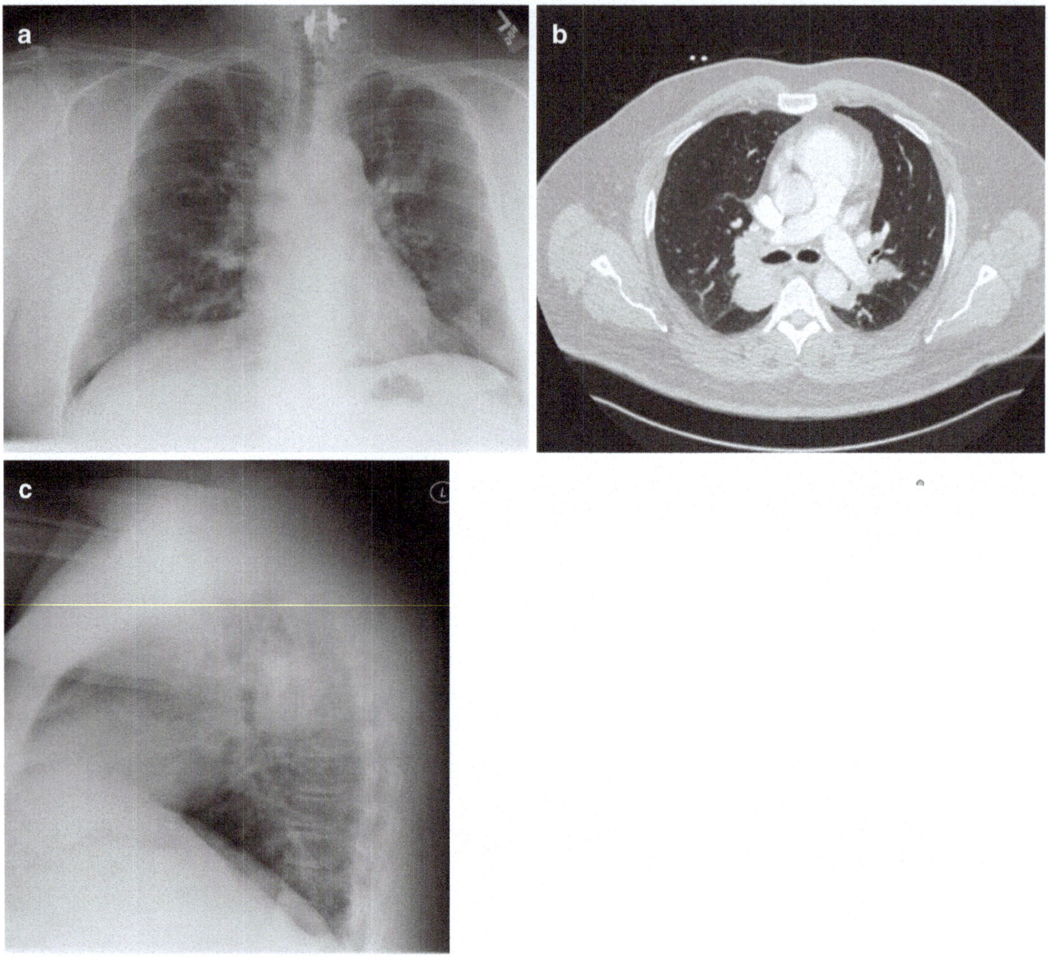

Fig. 9.6 (**a**) CXR (PA and LA). There is a masslike opacity better seen on the lateral view likely in the left suprahilar region. There is also some fullness in the azygos region on the right. (**b**) CT Chest: Conglomerate of masses within bilateral peri-hilar regions and lung parenchyma with narrowing of the main stem bronchi with bilateral lung nodules, some with endobronchial location. (**c**) Patient was diagnosed with metastatic renal cell carcinoma

Conclusion

A chest X-ray is a fast and painless diagnostic tool to aid in the interpretation of chest abnormalities. If used in the right clinical scenario, it can provide a quick and painless way to identify urgent conditions such as aortic dissection, pneumothorax, acute pulmonary edema, and foreign body aspiration (coins, metallic bodies, etc.). Clinical correlation remains essential to avoid misinterpretation and subsequently misdiagnosis.

References

1. MacMahon H, Vyborny C. Technical advances in chest radiography. AJR Am J Roentgenol. 1994;163(5):1049–59.
2. Herrmann TL, Fauber TL, Gill J. Best practices in digital radiography. Albuquerque, NM: American Society of Radiologic Technologists; 2012. https://www.asrt.org/docs/defaultsource/publications/whitepapers/asrt12_bst-pracdigradwhp_final.pdf. Accessed 2 12 2016.
3. Robin Smithuis and Otto van Delden. Chest X-Ray-basic interpretation. http://www.radiologyassistant.nl/en/p497b2a265d96d/chest-x-ray-basic-interpretation.html.
4. How to read a CXR. www.isradiology.org/isr/docs_books/anatomy/Chapter3.pdf.

10 Peri-Operative Infection Control in Maxillofacial Surgery

Julie Ann Smith

Abstract

Healthcare-associated infections are a major preventable cause of significant morbidity of patients receiving care in a healthcare facility. These include surgical site infections, central line-associated bloodstream infections, ventilator-associated pneumonia, and catheter line-associated urinary tract infections. This chapter will discuss concepts in the prevention and management of these infections. There will be focused discussion on antibiotic prophylaxis for specific oral and maxillofacial surgery procedures.

10.1 Healthcare-Associated Infections

Healthcare-associated infections (HAI) are a major preventable cause of morbidity of healthcare facility patients. During the past decade, there has been an increased focus on prevention. On any day, 1 in 25 hospitalized patients has at least one type of HAI [1]. During 2011, it is estimated that there were approximately 722,000 HAI in US hospitals (4% of hospitalized patients) and 75,000 patients died of HAI. The most recent Centers for Disease Control (CDC) data is derived from a 2011 survey of 183 hospitals and 11,290 patients [1, 2]. Of these patients, 452 (4%) had one or more HAI (infections not present at the time of admission to the hospital). Of 504 infections identified, pneumonia and surgical site infections (SSIs) were the most common, each comprising 21.8% of HAI. Gastrointestinal infection comprised 17.1%, urinary tract infection 12.9%, primary bloodstream infection 9.9%, and eye, ear, nose, throat, or mouth infection comprising 5.6% [2]. Less common infections included the lower respiratory tract, skin/soft tissue, cardiovascular, bone/joint, central nervous system, reproductive tract, and systemic. Device-associated infections accounted for 25.6% of HAI (an improvement likely related to an increased focus on this source over the previous decade). Of the GI tract infections, 70.9% were related to *Clostridium difficile*, and *C. Difficile* was the most common pathogen associated with

J.A. Smith, D.D.S., M.D., M.C.R., F.I.C.D.
Willamette Dental Group, Portland, OR, USA

Department of Oral and Maxillofacial Surgery, Oregon Health and Science University, Portland, OR, USA
e-mail: jusmith@willamettedental.com

© Springer International Publishing AG 2018

E.M. Ferneini, J.D. Bennett (eds.), *Perioperative Assessment of the Maxillofacial Surgery Patient*, https://doi.org/10.1007/978-3-319-58868-1_10

HAI (12.1% of HAI). The task force appointed by the Society for Healthcare Epidemiology of America and the Infectious Diseases Society of America Standards and Practice Guidelines Committee published recommendations for the prevention of common HAI in acute care hospitals and published a compendium in 2008 with an update in 2014 [3, 4]. The 2008 Compendium addressed four HAI: central line-associated bloodstream infections (CLABSI), ventilator-associated pneumonia (VAP), catheter-associated urinary tract infections (CAUTIs), and SSI. Two organism-specific categories were included: methicillin-resistant *Staphylococcus aureus* (MRSA) and *Clostridium difficile*. The 2014 Compendium added targeted improvement in hand hygiene. The National and State Healthcare-Associated Infections Progress Report published by the CDC reported several improvements between 2008 and 2014 including a 50% reduction in CLABSI, a 17% decrease in SSI in select procedures, an 8% decrease in *C. difficile* infections (from 2011 to 2014), and a 13% decrease in MRSA bacteremia (from 2011 to 2014) [5]. Although not all oral and maxillofacial surgery patients are at risk for these types of infections, all surgeons should understand the risk factors of HAI and how to prevent HAI. The following sections summarize the major recommendations to prevent HAI. For further details, the reader is referred to the 2014 Compendium update [4].

10.1.1 Compendium Recommendations to Decrease HAI

10.1.1.1 Central Line-Associated Bloodstream Infection (CLABSI)

Occasionally, head and neck surgery patients require a central line and are at risk for a CLABSI. The prevention of CLABSI includes precautions to be taken before, during, and after insertion of the central line. ICU patients over 2 months of age should be bathed daily with a chlorhexidine preparation [4]. At the time of central line insertion, an alcohol-chlorhexidine solution should be used for skin preparation. The femoral vein is to be avoided, especially in the obese. Ultrasound guidance is recommended for internal jugular catheter insertion. In adults, antiseptic- or antimicrobial-impregnated central venous catheters are recommended. Maximum sterile barriers should be used during central venous catheter (CVC) placement. Catheters should be removed once they are no longer necessary. In patients older than 2 months, chlorhexidine-containing dressings should be used. With non-tunneled CVCs, the site should be cleaned with chlorhexidine and transparent dressings changed every 5–7 days. Gauze dressings should be changed every 2 days. Additionally, dressings should be changed immediately if loose, damp, or soiled [4].

10.1.1.2 Ventilator-Associated Pneumonia (VAP)

To decrease the risk of VAP, noninvasive positive-pressure ventilation (NIPPV) should be used instead of intubation whenever possible. Intubated patients should be extubated as soon as possible. If not contraindicated, sedation should be interrupted once per day so that spontaneous breathing trials and assessment for extubation may be performed. Interventions which decrease pooling of secretions superior to the endotracheal tube cuff should be used in patients intubated for more than 48 h. Head-of-bed elevation had been recommended in 2008 with moderate evidentiary support, but in the 2014 update, it received a low quality of evidence rating [3, 4]. Interventions which may decrease VAP include oropharynx selective decontamination, providing oral care with chlorhexidine and mechanical tooth brushing (low evidence). Administration of prophylactic antibiotics has moderate evidentiary support that it may lower the risk of VAP, but its effect on length of mechanical ventilation, hospital length of stay, or mortality is unknown [3, 4].

10.1.1.3 Catheter-Associated Urinary Tract Infection (CAUTI)

In order to reduce CAUTI, catheters should only be inserted when necessary and removed as soon as possible. The use of bladder scanners and intermittent catheterization should be considered whenever possible. The following recommendations have a low level of evidence supporting them, but they do make sense: as small a catheter as possible should be used to decrease urethral trauma, and catheters should only be placed by trained, dedicated personnel [3, 4].

10.1.1.4 Surgical Site Infection (SSI)

Antibiotic prophylaxis should be administered based on evidence-based standards and guidelines. Specific recommendations for oral and maxillofacial surgery will be discussed forthcoming. Hair should not be removed from surgical sites unless its presence interferes with the procedure. Hair should be removed with hair trimmers and not razors. Blood glucose should be controlled during the postoperative period. Perioperatively, a minimum core temperature of 35.5 °C should be maintained. To maximize tissue oxygenation, supplemental oxygen should be administered during and immediately after surgery in which mechanical ventilation was used. The skin should be prepped with alcohol-containing solutions whenever possible. Methods of moderate evidentiary value include performing *S. aureus* screening, decolonizing patients with anti-staphylococcal agents preoperatively for high-risk procedures (certain orthopedic and cardiothoracic procedures), and using antiseptic wound lavage [3, 4].

10.1.1.5 Hand Hygiene (Surgeon)

In general, hand hygiene should be performed with either an alcohol-based rub or an antimicrobial or nonantimicrobial soap. When hands are visibly soiled, hand hygiene should be performed with either antimicrobial or nonantimicrobial soap. Hospitals are to monitor hand hygiene compliance and implement multimodal strategies for maintaining adherence. In caring for patients with known or suspected norovirus or *C. difficile* infection, besides exercising contact precautions, care providers should wash their hands with soap and water after seeing these patients [4].

10.1.1.6 Methicillin-Resistant *Staphylococcus aureus* (MRSA)

In order to control and prevent MRSA, hospitals are expected to conduct MRSA risk assessments and to monitor and implement an active surveillance testing (AST) program. If healthcare providers are epidemiologically associated with a cluster of MRSA infections, they are to be screened for MRSA infection or colonization. As part of the AST, MRSA-colonized patients may be recommended to receive targeted decolonization therapy. A recommendation with a high amount of evidence is that ICU patients should be treated with universal decolonization. The use of gowns and gloves when treating all ICU patients received moderate evidentiary support [3, 4].

10.1.1.7 *Clostridium difficile*

Most strategies described in the Compendium to prevent *C. difficile* infection (CDI) received only low or moderate evidentiary support. Basic strategies for reducing CDI include the use of contact precautions for infected patients, appropriate use of antimicrobials, and cleaning and disinfecting environment and equipment with sporicidal disinfectant or diluted sodium hypochlorite. Patients with diarrhea should be treated with contact precautions while *C. difficile* testing is pending (low evidence). Contact precautions should continue even if the patient becomes asymptomatic and should continue until hospital discharge (low evidence). During CDI outbreaks, hand hygiene should be performed with soap and water after leaving the room of a patient with CDI [3, 4].

10.1.2 Focus on Surgical Site Infections

Surgical site infections still comprise a significant proportion of HAI (21.8%) [2]. Surgical site infections are identified as either superficial incisional SSI, deep incisional SSI, or organ/space SSI [6]. Superficial incisional SSI includes only the skin or subcutaneous tissue, excluding suture abscesses. A deep incisional SSI involves the fascia and muscle. An organ/space SSI is an infection of any organ or space that was opened up during surgery. The timeline for development of an SSI is within 30 days of the procedure, or within 1 year if an implant had been placed [6]. The most common organisms include a patient's own endogenous flora, most commonly including *Staphylococcus aureus*, coagulase-negative *Staphylococcus*, *Escherichia coli*, and *Enterococcus* [6]. Risk factors for developing an SSI include diabetes/poor glucose control, steroid use or altered immune response, nicotine use, malnutrition or obesity, extremes of age, coexisting infections, perioperative transfusions, and prolonged hospitalization [6]. A highly supported method of prevention is the appropriate administration of prophylactic antibiotics. Four proven interventions targeting modifiable risk factors for SSI include appropriate administration of prophylactic antibiotics, appropriate hair removal, postoperative normothermia, and glucose control [6]. These subjects and other interventions for reducing SSI will be discussed herein.

10.1.2.1 Prophylactic Antibiotics

The use of antibiotic prophylaxis in the prevention of surgical site infections is well established in orthopedic and general surgery. Antibiotic prophylaxis refers to the administration of antibiotics prior to contamination by surgical incision, given with the intention of preventing infection. Bowater et al. reviewed a set of meta-analyses of antibiotic prophylaxis including 4809 patients who underwent 23 different types of surgery in 250 clinical trials and concluded that antibiotic prophylaxis is an effective method to prevent wound infection [7]. This meta-analysis did not find a relationship between the level of cleanliness of the case and the effectiveness of antibiotic prophylaxis. This study was in support of the use of antibiotic prophylaxis, but the authors noted that the study did not take into account antibiotic side effects, effect on microbial resistance, and antibiotic prophylaxis cost-effectiveness [7].

Appropriate antibiotic prophylaxis includes proper timing of administration and correct antibiotic selection and dose. To achieve adequate tissue concentration, parenteral prophylactic antibiotics should be administered 30 minutes prior to incision [8, 9]. Multiple studies have shown no additional benefit in administering antibiotics for longer than 24 h, and doing so may increase the risk of developing antibiotic resistance [9]. If the length of surgery extends beyond the half-life of the antibiotic administered, the antibiotic should be redosed. Some authors recommend that an additional dose of antibiotics should be given if the length of the procedure is one to two times the half-life of the antibiotic or in cases of substantial blood loss [10]. For most head and neck surgeries, cefazolin is the routine prophylactic antibiotic, and clindamycin is used in patients allergic to penicillin or cephalosporins [9]. Generally, there is no support for administration of antibiotics after closure of the surgical incision, nor is there support for the routine administration of three doses of antibiotics [9].

10.2 Antibiotic Prophylaxis in Oral and Maxillofacial Surgery

10.2.1 Orthognathic Surgery

The infection rate associated with orthognathic surgery is generally low. Alpha et al. found a range of a 3.4–33.3% infection rate of mandibular osteotomies reported throughout the literature [11]. In their retrospective review of 301 orthognathic surgery patients, Kim et al. found an infection rate of 1% [12]. Chow et al. found that 7.4% of complications were infections in a retrospective review of 2910 orthognathic procedures [13]. They found that having both jaws operated upon significantly increased the risk of developing an infection, with 92.7% of the infected patients having had maxillary and mandibular surgery. Compared to patients who received both preoperative and postoperative antibiotics, those who had received only one preoperative antibiotic dose had a significantly higher rate of infection. The duration of postoperative antibiotics (2–14 days) did not significantly impact the infection rate. In Chow et al.'s study, administration of both preoperative and postoperative antibiotics resulted in a lower infection rate than administration of only preoperative antibiotics. They concluded that a single preoperative dose of antibiotics was not recommended for prophylaxis for orthognathic surgery. The optimal duration of postoperative antibiotics was not clear, but it was felt that at least two postoperative days may be useful [13]. The ideal antibiotic prophylaxis regimen for orthognathic surgery is not entirely clear-cut.

Zijderveld et al. performed a randomized, double-blind, placebo-controlled study comparing single preoperative doses of amoxicillin/clavulanic acid versus cefuroxime versus placebo [14]. They found that the infection rate was 11.1% in the amoxicillin/clavulanic acid group, 17.6% in the cefuroxime group, and 52.6% in the placebo group. They concluded that a single preoperative dose of antibiotics significantly reduced the risk of infection. There was not a significant difference between the two antibiotics studied, but the power of the study may have been too low to demonstrate a significant difference between the two [14].

Fridrich et al. performed a prospective study of 30 orthognathic surgery patients comparing perioperative antibiotics to 1 week of postoperative antibiotics [15]. No significant difference in infection rates was demonstrated between the two groups, supporting that prolonged periods of postoperative antibiotics are not indicated over perioperative dosing.

Lindeboom et al. evaluated antibiotic dosing in their prospective randomized study of prophylactic antibiotic use in 70 patients undergoing bilateral sagittal split osteotomies [16]. Patients were randomized to receive intravenous clindamycin via either single preoperative dosing or 24 h dosing. The preoperative dose was administered 15 min prior to incision, and postoperatively, patients received either clindamycin or placebo every 6 h for 24 h. The infection rate in patients receiving only preoperative antibiotics was 5.6%, and it was 2.8% in those receiving antibiotics for 24 h postoperatively in addition to the preoperative dose. The difference between these two dosing schedules was not significant, and the authors concluded that long-term antibiotic prophylaxis was not necessary in orthognathic surgery.

Overall, the evidence is not crystal clear, but the use of at least perioperative prophylactic antibiotics in preventing infection in orthognathic surgery seems appropriate. The ideal duration of postoperative antibiotics is not clear, but there is no evidence in support of a prolonged duration of postoperative antibiotics [17]. The most prudent approach seems to be to provide a preoperative intravenous antibiotic 30 min prior to incision with redosing at appropriate time intervals during the surgery, without postoperative antibiotics.

10.2.2 Facial Fractures

Mandibular fractures have a higher rate of infection than maxillary fractures. The highest rate of infection is associated with compound fractures, either open to the mouth or those with teeth in the line of fracture. Subcondylar fractures rarely get infected [18]. Chole and Yee performed a randomized controlled trial on patients undergoing either open or closed treatment of facial fractures and compared the use of perioperative antibiotics to no antibiotics [18]. The intervention group received one preoperative and one postoperative dose of cefazolin, and the control group did not receive any antibiotics. 8.9% of patients in the antibiotic group developed infection, and 42.3% of patients in the control group developed infection, demonstrating a significant reduction in infection in the patients who received antibiotics. All infections occurred in the mandible at either the parasymphysis or angle. This beneficial effect of prophylactic antibiotics was significant only for open reductions. Additionally, there was no significant difference between the infection rate of fractures that were treated in a closed manner (with or without antibiotics) versus fractures treated open and in which prophylactic antibiotics were given. The authors concluded that prophylactic antibiotics were beneficial in open treatment of mandibular angle or parasymphysis fractures [18].

Andreasen et al. [19] performed a systematic review of the use of prophylactic antibiotics in facial fractures, which included the Chole and Yee study [18]. Their review included four randomized studies published between 1975 and 1988, none of which met the criteria of a randomized controlled trial. The authors found that open treatment of fractures increased the risk of postoperative infection. They concluded that in treating compound mandibular fractures, especially via an open approach, prophylactic antibiotics were strongly indicated to reduce the risk of postoperative infection and appear to reduce the infection risk approximately threefold [19].

In facial trauma, it is clear that mandible fractures, especially open fractures, have a much higher infection rate than midface fractures. Open treatment increases the risk of infection compared to closed treatment. It is appropriate to administer one dose of preoperative antibiotics and subsequent doses during surgery in open treatment of facial fractures, and despite this precaution, there still may be a slightly higher risk of infection in the treatment of mandible fractures. If there is a delay before treatment of an open mandible fracture, it is reasonable to start oral antibiotics until the patient can undergo surgery.

10.2.3 Third Molars

The use of prophylactic antibiotics in third molar surgery has been thoroughly studied. Most literature does not favor using antibiotic prophylaxis in third molar extractions. Alveolar osteitis, while not related to bacterial infection, occurs in approximately 25–30% of mandibular third molar extractions [20]. The reported incidence of postoperative infection after third molar extraction ranges from 1% to 12% [21, 22]. A guiding principle of antibiotic prophylaxis is that there should be a significant risk of infection associated with the procedure. Since third molar extraction has such a low infection rate, antibiotic prophylaxis may not be indicated.

In Piecuch et al.'s retrospective review of 2134 patients who underwent removal of 6713 third molars, patients underwent one of six different types of treatment: no antibiotics, perioperative systemic antibiotics, topical tetracycline powder in the socket, perioperative systemic antibiotics plus topical tetracycline, postoperative antibiotics, and postoperative antibiotics plus topical tetracycline [23]. The overall infection rate was low—3.5%. The infection rate of maxillary third molars was only 0.27%. Only for mandibular impactions were there any significant differences between interventions. For erupted mandibular third molars, topical tetracycline resulted in a significant reduction in infection compared to no antibiotic use. For soft tissue impacted third molars, there were no significant differences found among any of the treatment groups. For partial bony impactions, systemic perioperative antibiotics and topical tetracycline significantly reduced the infection rate. Further, topical tetracycline appeared to be more effective than systemic perioperative antibiotics in preventing infection in partial bony impaction extractions. In full bony impactions, systemic antibiotics and topical tetracycline reduced infection, with topical tetracycline being more efficacious than systemic perioperative antibiotics. This study was limited by the fact that it was retrospective and not randomized. The degree of impaction seems to affect the infection rate, and different impaction types respond to different prophylactic techniques. The authors believed their results supported the use of prophylactic antibiotics in some form to prevent infection after mandibular third molar extraction. However, it is important to note the overall low incidence of infection may not warrant antibiotic prophylaxis.

Sekhar et al. evaluated systemic antibiotics for third molar prophylaxis in their prospective, randomized, double-blind, controlled study of 125 patients having asymptomatic mandibular third molars removed [24]. Patients received either placebo, a single preoperative dose of metronidazole, or 5 days of postoperative metronidazole. Patients were examined 6 days postoperatively and evaluated for pain on postoperative days 2–6, interincisal opening, the presence or absence of purulence, or alveolar osteitis. There were no significant differences between the study groups for these parameters. The authors concluded that antibiotic prophylaxis did not reduce morbidity in mandibular third molar removal.

Poeschl et al. studied a population of 288 patients who underwent removal of 528 impacted mandibular third molars in a prospective randomized trial [25]. Patients received either no antibiotics, amoxicillin/clavulanic acid for 5 days postoperatively, or clindamycin for 5 days postoperatively. All patients performed a preoperative chlorhexidine rinse. Any hematoma that formed was released on postoperative day 2. Patients whose third molars were partially erupted had iodoform gauze placed in the socket at the time of surgery which was removed on postoperative day 2. Patients were evaluated on postoperative days 2–10 and at 4 weeks for the following: change in interincisal opening compared to baseline, infection, alveolar osteitis, pain, and side effects. There was no significant difference between the treatment interventions regarding the incidence of infection or alveolar osteitis, interincisal opening, or pain. Most cases of alveolar osteitis (69.6%) were associated with partially erupted third molars. The authors concluded that during extraction of asymptomatic third molars, routine postoperative oral antibiotics are not recommended.

In contrast, Arteagoitia et al. found significantly decreased inflammatory and infectious complications when patients who underwent removal of one mandibular third molar received postoperative amoxicillin/clavulanate in their prospective double-blind placebo-controlled randomized clinical trial including 494 patients [26]. Patients received either no antibiotics or 4 days of postoperative amoxicillin/clavulanic acid. The socket was irrigated with chlorhexidine upon completion of the procedure. Patients rinsed with chlorhexidine three times per day for 7 days postoperatively. Infection or inflammation occurred in 1.9% of the antibiotic group and in 12.9% of the no antibiotics group—a significant difference. Without the use of postoperative antibiotics, the relative risk ratio for inflammatory complications was 0.15, and the number needed to treat to prevent one infectious/inflammatory complication was 10. The authors questioned whether it was appropriate to provide antibiotics to all patients just to prevent these complications. They felt clinical judgment was most important and noted that older patients had greater risks of infectious/inflammatory complications.

Ataoglu et al. studied 150 patients undergoing extraction of maxillary and mandibular third molars [27]. Patients were randomized to receive either no antibiotic, 5 days of preoperative amoxicillin/clavulanic acid, or 5 days of postoperative amoxicillin/clavulanic acid. Patients were evaluated for swelling, infection, alveolar osteitis, interincisal opening, and pain on postoperative days 2–7. No significant difference between the three treatment groups was demonstrated, and the authors concluded that in third molar surgery, routine antibiotic prophylaxis is not indicated.

Halpern et al. evaluated the use of intravenous prophylactic antibiotics prior to third molar removal in their placebo-controlled, double-blind, randomized clinical trial of 118 patients [28]. Preoperative intravenous penicillin (clindamycin in penicillin allergic patients) was compared to placebo. Assessment outcomes were postoperative inflammation and surgical site infection. The preoperative antibiotic group had no infections or postoperative inflammatory complications, and the placebo group had an 8.5% ($p = 0.03$) infection rate and no alveolar osteitis. All infections were in sites of partial complete bony impactions requiring bone removal. The authors concluded that intravenous prophylactic antibiotics decreased surgical site infections and the number needed to treat to prevent an infection was 12. A limitation of this study may be its small sample size.

Kaczmarzyk et al. performed a prospective, randomized, double-blind, placebo-controlled trial including 86 patients undergoing third molar removal [29]. There were three treatment groups: single-dose preoperative oral clindamycin versus preoperative single-dose clindamycin plus postoperative clindamycin for 5 days versus placebo. On postoperative days 1, 2, and 7, patients were evaluated for facial swelling, trismus, lymphadenopathy, systemic temperature, alveolar osteitis, and subjective pain assessment. The authors found no significant difference among the groups related to postoperative inflammatory complications, and they concluded the use of prophylactic antibiotics during removal of third molars was not supported. However, the sample size was small.

Ren et al. performed a thorough meta-analysis examining alveolar osteitis and surgical site infection [22]. Randomized controlled clinical trials of antibiotic use during third molar extractions published between 1974 and 2007 were included. There were 2932 patients randomized in 16 trials which reported alveolar osteitis (AO) as an outcome. AO occurred in 6.2% of patients who received preoperative systemic antibiotics and in 14.4% of patients who did not receive preoperative antibiotics. The number needed to treat to prevent one occurrence of AO was 13. There was a statistically significant reduction of AO for mandibular third molars when preoperative systemic antibiotics were used, but postoperative antibiotics did not statistically significantly decrease the incidence of AO. There were 2396 patients in 12 clinical trials reporting surgical site infection as an outcome. Surgical site infection occurred in 4% of patients who received antibiotics, and it occurred in 6.1% of patients who did not. The number needed to treat to prevent one infection was 25. Their meta-analysis suggested it was most effective to administer antibiotics 30–90 min prior to surgery and to continue them for 3–5 days afterward. It was felt that a single preoperative dose was as effective as multiday dosing. Antibiotics given after surgery had started were not effective in preventing infection or AO. Ultimately, the authors concluded that when deciding whether to provide preoperative antibiotics, one must weigh the risks versus benefits. The results were not meant to represent a rigid guideline for antibiotic prophylaxis. It was concluded to be a reasonable choice to administer penicillin 1 h prior to surgical extraction of impacted mandibular third molars. It was recommended that the decision to provide postoperative antibiotics should be based upon risk factors for infection such as history of smoking, the presence of poor oral hygiene, and advanced age.

These are just a few of the studies which have looked at this question, and it is likely best to follow Arteagoitia et al.'s [26] recommendations and use clinical judgment. Prophylactic antibiotics should be more seriously considered in patients believed to be predisposed for infection, such as older patients, or in removal of partial or complete bony impacted mandibular third molars. In true antibiotic prophylaxis, the dose must be administered before surgery, so a high tissue concentration is achieved prior to surgical contamination [17]. Postoperative antibiotics have not been demonstrated to significantly reduce infections in third molar surgery.

The use of chlorhexidine rinses to decrease the risk of AO in third molar surgery has also been studied extensively. Caso et al. performed a meta-analysis including seven RCTs which they divided into two groups: one group of two studies of preoperative chlorhexidine rinses and one group of five studies which examined rinsing on the day of surgery and for several days postoperatively [30]. There was no reduction in AO in the group in which only preoperative rinses were used. Of the studies in which preoperative and postoperative rinses for several days were used, 3 of the 5 studies showed a significant reduction in AO. Limitations of the meta-analysis are that slightly different rinsing protocols were used and differing definitions of AO were used. The minimum number of days postoperative rinsing should be performed to significantly reduce AO was unable to be determined. Postoperative chlorhexidine rinses do seem to decrease the risk of AO, but the ideal protocol is yet to be determined. Although not as common as antibiotic resistance, there has been reported resistance to chlorhexidine of strains of *P. aeruginosa*, *P. mirabilis*, *E. coli*, *P. stutzeri, and S. marcescens* [31].

10.2.4 Skin Care

10.2.4.1 Hair Removal

Preoperative hair removal has been believed to decrease the incidence of SSI. However, a recent Cochrane review by Tanner et al. did not find evidence to support preoperative hair removal to reduce SSIs [32]. It was recommended that if hair had to be removed preoperatively, it should be removed using clippers instead of a razor since there were fewer SSIs when clippers were used. The use of a razor in the operating room or the night before surgery may cause microscopic cuts which may harbor bacteria, and this practice is discouraged [10]. Various studies support that SSIs are lowest when no hair is removed preoperatively, and infection rates are highest when hair is removed with a razor rather than clippers. Consequently hair removal should be avoided, but if absolutely necessary, it should be removed using clippers, and most studies support that if hair is removed, it should be done immediately prior to surgery [9].

10.2.4.2 Skin Preparation (Patient)

The most commonly used skin preparation products include alcohol-based solutions, chlorhexidine gluconate, and iodophors (e.g., povidone-iodine). Alcohol has excellent germicidal activity against bacteria, viruses, and fungi but is flammable and lacks residual germicidal activity. Chlorhexidine and povidone-iodine both effectively reduce bacterial counts on contact with the skin and have excellent activity against skin structure bacteria, but chlorhexidine has longer-lasting activity. Iodophors can be inactivated by contact with blood or serum, so the prep should be allowed to dry before incision. Furthermore, even small concentrations of povidone-iodine (0.5%) can be toxic to fibroblasts and keratinocytes and should never be used on open wounds or in postoperative dressings [10]. Alcohol is frequently added to chlorhexidine or povidone-iodine to augment antiseptic properties. Certain prep solutions such as those that contain alcohol or chlorhexidine should not be used on the face because they can cause serious eye injuries. The following prep solutions should never be used on the face: iodophor 0.7%/isopropyl alcohol 74% (Duraprep), chlorhexidine gluconate 4% (Hibiclens), chlorhexidine gluconate 2%/isopropyl alcohol 70% (Chloraprep), or alcohol 73%/zinc pyrithione (Actiprep) [33]. Ear damage may also occur with these solutions so their use should be avoided around the ears. Chlorhexidine-containing products should not come into contact with the meninges. The use of povidone-iodine is contraindicated in those allergic to iodine or younger than 2 months old. Solutions safe to use in the head and neck region include povidone-iodine 7% scrub/10% paint (Scrub Care) or chloroxylenol 3% (Technicare). Povidone-iodine 7% scrub/10% paint is used by first applying the scrub (carefully avoiding the eyes) and then blotting the skin dry with a sterile towel after 5 min. The paint is then applied and allowed to dry. Chloroxylenol is applied to the skin and either blotted with a sterile towel or allowed to air-dry [33]. When sites distant from the head and neck are also prepped, one should use a chlorhexidine gluconate-containing solution for the distant prep site due to its superior length of activity.

There is no scientific evidence that preoperative bathing with an antiseptic will decrease SSI risk. Preoperative showering with chlorhexidine has been shown to decrease the number of organisms on the skin in comparison to soap and water or povidone-iodine [9]. Various meta-analyses have examined the effectiveness of a preoperative shower in reducing the incidence of SSI. Webster and Osborne evaluated six trials including 10,007 patients comparing preoperative bathing with either 4% chlorhexidine gluconate, bar soap, or placebo versus no bathing [34]. There was no support for chlorhexidine gluconate bathing to decrease the risk of SSI. Chlebicki et al. performed a meta-analysis including 16 trials and 17,932 patients [35]. Chlorhexidine gluconate did not significantly reduce SSI compared to soap, placebo, or no shower or bath. Considering these results, there is no support for preoperative bathing with chlorhexidine gluconate to reduce the risk of SSI.

The critical care and obstetric literature supports the use of iodophor-impregnated drapes (Ioban) to reduce wound contamination, but it does not seem to reduce the risk of SSI [10]. Its use also has been shown to decrease wound contamination in orthopedic surgery but without a decrease in wound infection [10]. In head and neck surgery, the use of these drapes would only be practical for use on distant surgical sites, such as the anterior iliac crest.

InteguSeal is a cyanoacrylate microbial sealant applied to the skin after initial prep with either an iodophor or chlorhexidine gluconate. On contact with skin, it forms a barrier which prevents migration of flora and seals any microabrasions on the skin. It has activity for several days and has not been associated with any local or systemic toxicity. Wilson performed a corporation-funded multicenter randomized trial of 177 patients undergoing inguinal hernia repair comparing InteguSeal to 10% povidone-iodine [36]. The incidence of wound contamination with use of the sealant was 53% and was 68.7% with povidone-iodine—a significant difference. A randomized controlled prospective study was performed by Iyer et al. on patients undergoing coronary bypass grafting from bilateral lower extremities [37]. In each patient, one leg was prepped conventionally, and the other leg was prepped with the sealant. At 5 days, wounds were assessed for signs of infection, and microbiological swabs were obtained from each leg. The study was stopped prematurely after the participation of 47 patients because of significant results. The infection rate in legs treated with the sealant was 2.1%, and in conventionally prepped legs, it was 25.5%. There were 13 positive cultures from sealant-treated legs and 22 positive cultures from conventionally treated legs. The authors concluded that the sealant reduced SSIs, was easy to use, and was not toxic to the skin [37]. Waldow et al., however, found different results in a nonrandomized study examining 998 patients undergoing elective cardiac surgical procedures via a median sternotomy [38]. Patients received a prep which either included or excluded InteguSeal. Postoperative mediastinitis and SSI incidence were not found to be significantly different between the two groups, and the authors did not support the use of cyanoacrylate sealant to reduce the incidence of SSI [38]. InteguSeal is not recommended for use in areas where there may be contact with mucous membranes or the eyes and should not be used on the skin with signs of active infection. Given the findings of the Iyer study, one may wish to consider a cyanoacrylate sealant as part of their prep of sites distant from the head and neck.

10.2.4.3 Skin Preparation (Surgical Team)

The skin scrubs available for the surgical team are similar to those used for patient preparation. There have been a number of studies on this subject, and an overall conclusion may seem difficult to interpret, but essentially, aqueous alcohol rubs are well tolerated and are just as effective as traditional chlorhexidine or povidone-iodine scrubs and have better compliance rates [10]. Aly and Maibach compared a 2 min scrub using chlorhexidine gluconate versus povidone-iodine versus chloroxylenol and evaluated skin bacterial counts immediately after scrubbing as well as at 3–6 h later [39]. Chlorhexidine use was associated with significantly reduced bacterial counts compared to both povidone-iodine and chloroxylenol at all three time points. A more recent study by Parienti et al. compared use of an aqueous alcohol solution (preceded by a non-antiseptic hand wash) to scrubbing with 4% povidone-iodine or 4% chlorhexidine [40]. The primary end point was SSI at 30 days. The use of the alcohol solution did not significantly reduce SSI compared to the povidone-iodine or chlorhexidine. However, the aqueous alcohol was better tolerated and had better compliance than the traditional scrubs. This small sampling of the available studies may seem confusing, but essentially, chlorhexidine gluconate seems to provide longer antibacterial coverage than povidone-iodine, and aqueous alcohol provides just as effective antibacterial coverage. Therefore, when choosing a method for scrubbing in, one should remember that aqueous alcohol is fully effective as long as gross contamination has already been removed. If a more traditional method of scrubbing is preferred, a combination of alcohol with chlorhexidine gluconate is superior to chlorhexidine gluconate alone, which is superior to povidone-iodine.

10.2.5 Temperature Control

During anesthesia, heat is lost from radiation (the biggest contributor to heat loss), evaporation, convection, and conduction [6]. Core body temperature can drop 1.6 °C during the first hour of a general anesthetic [41]. Perioperative hypothermia has been associated with increased cardiac events, greater blood loss and transfusion requirements, increased hospital stay length, and an increased risk of SSI [6, 9, 42, 43]. Kurz et al. performed a double-blind study of 200 patients undergoing colorectal surgery who were randomized to intraoperative hypothermia (34.7+/−0.6 °C) or intraoperative normothermia (36.6+/−0.5 °C) [44]. The study was terminated early due to significant results, a 19% wound infection rate in the hypothermia group versus a 6% infection rate in the normothermia group. Lowering core temperature 2 °C below normal resulted in tripling wound infection rates and increased the length of hospital stay by 20% [44]. The hypothermic patients did have a greater transfusion requirement, but according to their multivariate regression analysis, the transfusion requirement did not independently increase the risk of SSI. Flores-Maldonado et al. excluded patients receiving perioperative transfusions in their study of 290 cholecystectomy patients randomized to either hypothermia (35.4+/−0.4 °C) or normothermia (36.2+/−0.2 °C) [45]. The incidence of SSI was 11.5% in the hypothermic group, and it was 2% SSI in the normothermic group. Hypothermia is felt to increase the risk of SSI because it decreases perfusion (and therefore oxygenation) and also reduces neutrophil function because it reduces superoxide radical production [42, 43]. The best supported methods for maintaining intraoperative normothermia include the use of forced air warmers and warmed intravenous fluids [41]. Although the anesthesia team usually ensures patient normothermia, it is essential for the surgeon to be aware of the importance of maintaining perioperative normothermia.

10.2.6 Oxygenation

Adequate oxygen tension at a wound increases superoxide production by neutrophils, leading to greater bacterial destruction. Adequate oxygen tension is also believed to be essential in collagen and epithelium development [43]. Consequently, some theorize that hyperoxia may reduce SSI. The results of studies examining this question are controversial. Greif et al. performed a prospective randomized trial in 500 patients undergoing colorectal surgery [46]. Patients were randomized to receive either an FiO_2 of 80% or an FiO_2 of 30% intraoperatively and during the postoperative 2 h. 5.2% of the 80% FiO_2 patients and 11.2% of the 30% FiO_2 patients developed surgical site infections, which was a significant difference. There have been some studies which did not demonstrate a beneficial effect of hyperoxygenation; however, each of these studies had some weaknesses, such as low power, or inclusion of nonstandardized surgeries [9]. To this author's knowledge, there have been three meta-analyses published on this subject. Each concluded that hyperoxia does decrease the risk of wound infection, especially during colorectal surgery. However, additional study is warranted [47–49]. There has not been sufficient study on hyperoxygenation in head and neck surgery to determine its impact in this population. Generally, it is believed to be of benefit to provide supplemental oxygen on induction and during surgery. Postoperatively, supplemental oxygen seems to be beneficial as well, but the appropriate length of time it should be administered for has not been determined [9, 43].

10.2.7 Glucose Control

The effects of hyperglycemia upon the immune response are well known: decreased white blood cell number, decreased chemotaxis and phagocytosis, and impaired complement binding to bacterial surfaces. Several studies have shown increased morbidity and mortality in critically ill hyperglycemic patients—even in those who were nondiabetics [43, 50]. Van den Berghe et al. performed a prospective, randomized controlled trial of 1548 surgical intensive care unit patients on mechanical ventilation [50]. Patients received either intensive insulin therapy or conventional glucose management at the time of ICU admission. With intensive insulin therapy, an insulin infusion was started once blood glucose reached 110 mg/dl and a blood glucose of 80 to 110 mg/dl was maintained. With conventional therapy, blood glucose was maintained between 180 and 200 mg/

dl. After being discharged from the ICU, all patients received conventional therapy. Intensive insulin therapy reduced mortality during the ICU stay—it was 4.6% with intensive management and 8% with conventional management. The most significant mortality reduction was due to the impact of intensive insulin management on multisystem organ failure due to sepsis. In-hospital bloodstream infections were reduced by 46% due to intensive insulin therapy [50]. Furnary et al. studied 2467 matched diabetics undergoing open-heart surgery managed with one of these two glucose control protocols with a goal of keeping blood glucose below 200 mg/dl: sliding-scale intermittent subcutaneous insulin injections versus a continuous insulin infusion [51]. Patients who had intermittent insulin had a 2% deep sternal wound infection rate, and those who had continuous insulin infusion had a 0.8% infection rate, which was a significant difference. The impact of hyperglycemia has not been studied extensively in the head and neck surgery population, but close glucose monitoring is likely to be beneficial in this population. Certainly, hypoglycemia should be avoided. A glucose target of 180 mg/dl or less during the perioperative period is felt to be prudent [9].

10.2.8 Tissue Damage

The risk of SSI with the use of electrocautery is controversial. Ji et al. used a rat model for abdominal surgery, finding that incisions created with electric surgical knives have a significantly higher risk of wound infection [52]. Some surgeons believe that electrocautery use is a risk factor for poor wound healing, SSI, and worsened scarring. Several human studies, however, have not demonstrated a higher risk of SSI with cautery use. Kearns et al. performed a randomized prospective trial of 100 patients undergoing a midline laparotomy incision [53]. Patients were randomized to either have all layers of the incision performed with a scalpel or have all layers of the incision performed with diathermy. Between the two groups, there was not a statistically significant difference in wound complications. The use of diathermy did result in a statistically significantly decreased blood loss, shorter open incision time, decreased postoperative pain during the first 48 hours, and a decreased need for morphine during the first 5 postoperative days. Shamim completed a randomized controlled trial of 369 patients undergoing elective or emergent general surgery randomized to have their incisions performed with either a scalpel or diathermy [54]. The findings were similar to those of Kearns et al. in that the patients who had scalpel-created incisions experienced statistically significantly longer open incision time, increased blood loss, and more pain during the first 48 h postoperatively. There was not a statistically significant difference between the two groups' length of hospital stay, length of time for completion of wound healing, or postoperative complication rate according to wound classification. Neurosurgery patients undergoing 177 neurosurgical procedures were studied by Sheikh [55]. Each patient served as his own control by having each of their incisions performed half by steel scalpel and half by microneedle electrocautery. Incision locations included the scalp, neck, abdomen, trunk, and extremities. The incision portions that were electrocautery created took less time and had less blood loss. Electrocautery was concluded to be a safe and effective technique to create neurosurgical incisions, and it was recommended that it especially be considered for cases with potentially critical blood loss risk, such as in pediatric patients. As the aforementioned studies demonstrate, the concern that electrocautery may increase the risk for SSI has not been validated, so electrocautery should be considered whenever necessary to reduce blood loss.

10.2.9 Topical Antibiotics/Irrigation

Wound irrigation is typically performed to clean or decontaminate a wound or to decrease risk of infection. Irrigation is delivered via either high- or low-pressure pulse irrigation or simply via a syringe. It may consist of only saline or may contain antibiotics such as bacitracin, cephalosporins, aminoglycosides, glycopeptides, and chloramphenicol [56]. Additionally, materials containing antibiotics may be placed in a wound and later removed surgically, or antibiotic-containing resorbable materials may be placed. Most studies have focused on cardiothoracic, general, and orthopedic surgery patients. Chlorhexidine and povidone-iodine solutions have been found to be ineffective wound irrigants and are potentially harmful to wounds [9]. A believed benefit of surgical site irrigation is the ability to deliver a high antibiotic concentration to an infected site in which local physiologic changes may decrease effectiveness of systemic antibiotics [56]. Topical antibiotics are associated with limited systemic absorption, so theoretically, there should be a lower likelihood of the development of antibiotic resistance, although this has been debated [56, 57]. However, there has been insufficient research to provide a standard recommendation for surgical wound irrigation with or without antibiotics [56, 57].

The use of antibiotics in irrigation is controversial. Some believe that the length of time of contact between the antibiotic and bacteria is too short to allow for effective antibacterial activity [57]. Additionally, Barnes et al. reported that there have been cases of anaphylaxis and tissue irritation from topical antibiotics [57]. McHugh et al. performed a review of the literature examining antibiotic irrigation in various types of surgery [56]. They found that in abdominal surgery, the evidence only supported using antibiotic irrigation in laparotomy patients who were morbidly obese. On the contrary, they found an increased risk of infection in colorectal surgery patients who had antibiotic-impregnated sponges placed. In orthopedic surgery, there was evidence supporting the use of antibiotic-impregnated bone cement in joint replacement patients, but the effectiveness of antibiotic irrigation or antibiotic beads was not fully clear. In cardiothoracic surgery, there have been two large studies evaluating the efficacy of gentamicin/collagen sponges applied to sternotomy incisions. The results were equivocal, with one study supporting this technique and the other study not supporting this technique to reduce sternal wound infection. In dermatologic surgery, they found that there was no support for the use of topical antibiotics in skin grafting of burn patients. In ocular surgery, studies have demonstrated a statistically significant reduction in endophthalmitis when antibiotics are administered into the anterior chamber of the eye or in a subconjunctival manner [56]. Based on the studies of the use of antibiotic irrigation in other surgical specialties, its use in head and neck surgery really needs to be evaluated by a well-designed randomized controlled prospective study before a clear recommendation can be made. There has been some debate as to whether surfactants such as castile soap and benzalkonium chloride should be added to irrigation to enhance effectiveness. Surfactants interfere with bacteria's adherence to tissues. Surfactants are effective in removing bacteria from the surface of the bone, titanium, and steel, but some studies have shown that surfactants may cause hemolysis, impaired clotting and healing, and skin irritation [57]. Currently, in head and neck surgery, there does not seem to be sufficient evidence to support using surfactants in wound irrigation.

Irrigation can be delivered in either a pulsatile or continuous manner using high pressure (15–35 psi) or low pressure (1–15 psi) [57]. Most studies of high-pressure versus low-pressure irrigation come from the orthopedic surgery literature. High-pressure pulsatile irrigation appears to be more effective in debridement of foreign material and bacteria, but has had significant drawbacks including the potential for more tissue damage, and has been linked to impaired immune response and can cause deeper seeding of bacteria into the tissue or bone [10, 57, 58]. Therefore, the use of high-pressure irrigation should be reserved for wounds in which bacterial contamination is so severe that the increased risk is worth the potential benefit [57]. The literature has been equivocal on whether pulsatile irrigation is more effective than continuous [57]. The optimal volume of irrigation has not been determined [10, 57, 58]. In head and neck surgery, high-pressure irrigation is unlikely to be used except potentially during scalp wound care. When caring for scalp wounds, one must carefully weigh the risk of bacterial seeding of the skull versus the potential benefit of high-pressure debridement of a heavily contaminated wound.

10.2.10 Drains

Drains are often placed to decrease hematoma formation and, thus, reduce risk of an infection. Closed suction drains are preferred to simple drains because there may be retrograde bacteria movement when simple drains are used [9, 10]. Drains should be used only when necessary and removed as soon as possible, since prolonged use is associated with an increased risk of SSI [59]. The orthopedic surgery literature does not demonstrate a difference in infection rates, hematomas, extremity swelling, or the need for reoperation when drains are used, and therefore, the routine use of drains in elective orthopedic surgery has not been supported [10]. In fact, some studies have demonstrated drain use to be associated with an increased need for transfusion [10]. In head and neck surgery, the use of drains to treat infections is definitely supported. However, in non-infection cases, one should carefully consider the necessity of a drain, and when placing a drain, only a closed suction drain should be used.

10.2.11 Transfusions

Compromised tissue oxygenation may increase the risk of infection, and a blood transfusion may be necessary to ensure adequate tissue oxygenation. On the other hand, blood transfusions stimulate a clinically significant immune response which may increase the risk of an infection, and the transfusion itself has a small risk of transmitting an infection. It is theorized that white blood cells release inflammatory mediators during the storage of blood and white blood cells in the transfused product might downregulate the recipient's immune system [60]. To decrease this risk, many US medical centers perform universal leukoreduction of red blood cell stock [61]. There is a lower risk of infection when leukocyte-depleted products are used [9, 62]. In cardiac surgery patients, there is evidence of a higher risk of mortality when non-leukoreduced transfusions are performed [9]. Frietsch et al. studied whether leukoreduction decreases the risk of infection [63]. They studied leukoreduced autologous transfusions versus non-leukoreduced autologous transfusions and did not find a statistically significant difference in postoperative infection rate or median length of hospital stay [63]. However, this study was performed in patients undergoing autologous transfusions and may not be generalizable to other populations. Studies have shown that the increased risk of infection is proportional to the volume of blood transfused and to the length of time the blood was stored prior to transfusion [9, 61]. The storage life of packed red blood cells is up to 42 days. Weinberg et al. retrospectively studied trauma patients who were given at least 1 unit of leukoreduced red blood cells during the first 24 hours of their hospitalization [61]. They found that transfusion of >/= 3 units of "old" blood (stored for 14 days or longer) significantly increased the risk of death compared to >/= 3 units of "young" blood (stored for less than 14 days) [61]. In head and neck surgery, the benefit of providing a transfusion should outweigh the risk of infection. The risk associated with transfusions should be reduced by minimizing the volume of blood transfused, using leukoreduced blood products, and ensuring that transfused blood has been stored for less than 2 weeks.

Conclusions

Perioperative infection control is complex and has been well studied, but there are still many unanswered questions. Recent advances during the last decade have definitely reduced the incidence of HAI. There are many interventions that might reduce the risk of surgical site infections, but there are certain factors that are proven to reduce surgical site infections that are relatively easy to implement. The most important factors appear to be the appropriate administration of prophylactic antibiotics, appropriate hair removal, postoperative glucose control, and maintenance of perioperative normothermia. If a head and neck surgeon focuses on these efforts and remembers the increased risks associated with blood transfusion, especially of older stored blood, then he or she will already be optimizing the care of surgical patients.

References

1. https://www.cdc.gov/hai/surveillance/. Accessed 12 Mar 2017.
2. Magill SS, Edwards JR, Bamberg W, et al. Multistate point-prevalence survey of health care-associated infections. NEJM. 2014;370:1198–208.
3. Yokoe DS, Mermel LA, Anderson DJ, et al. A compendium of strategies to prevent healthcare-associated infections in acute care hospitals. Infect Control Hosp Epidemiol. 2008;29:S12–21.
4. Yokoe DS, Anderson DJ, Berenholtz SM, et al. A compendium of strategies to prevent healthcare-associated infections in acute care hospitals: 2014 updates. Infect Control Hosp Epidemiol. 2014;35(8):967–77.
5. https://www.cdc.gov/HAI/pdfs/progress-report/hai-progress-report.pdf. Accessed 12 Mar 2017.
6. Galway UA, Parker BM, Borkowski RG. Prevention of postoperative surgical site infections. Int Anestheiol Clin. 2009;47(4):37–53.
7. Bowater RJ, Stirling SA, Lilford RJ. Is antibiotic prophylaxis in surgery a generally effective intervention? Testing a generic hypothesis over a set of meta-analyses. Ann Surg. 2009;249(4):551–6.
8. Condon RE, Wittmann DH. The use of antibiotics in general surgery. Curr Probl Surg. 1991;28:807–949.
9. Alexander JW, Solomkin JS, Edwards MJ. Updated recommendations for control of surgical site infections. Ann Surg. 2011;253:1082–93.
10. Fletcher N, Sofianos D, Berkes MB, et al. Prevention of perioperative infection. J Bone Joint Surg Am. 2007;89:1605–18.
11. Alpha C, O'Ryan F, Silva A, Poor D. The incidence of postoperative wound healing problems following sagittal ramus osteotomies stabilized with Miniplates and Monocortical screws. JOMS. 2006;64:659–68.
12. Kim SG, Park SS. Incidence of complications and problems related to Orthognathic surgery. JOMS. 2007;65:2438–44.
13. Chow LK, Singh B, Chiu WK, Samman N. Prevalence of postoperative complications after Orthognathic surgery: a 15-year review. JOMS. 2007;65:984–92.
14. Zijderveld SA, Smeele LE, Kostense PJ, Tuinzing DB. Preoperative antibiotic prophylaxis in Orthognathic surgery: a randomized, double-blind, and placebo-controlled clinical study. JOMS. 1999;57:1403–6.
15. Fridrich KL, Partnoy BE, Zeitler DL. Prospective analysis of antibiotic prophylaxis for Orthognathic surgery. Int J Adult Orthodon Orthognath Surg. 1994;9(2):129–31.
16. Lindeboom JA, Baas EM, Kroon FH. Prophylactic single-dose administration of 600 mg clindamycin versus 4-time administration of 600 mg clindamycin in Orthognathic surgery: a prospective randomized study in bilateral mandibular sagittal ramus osteotomies. Oral Surg Oral Med Oral Pathol Oral Radiol Endod. 2003;95:145–9.
17. Laskin DM. The use of prophylactic antibiotics for the prevention of postoperative infections. Oral Maxillofac Surg Clin North Am. 2003;15:155–60.
18. Chole RA, Yee J. Antibiotic prophylaxis for facial fractures. Arch Otolaryngol Head Neck Surg. 1987;113:1055–7.
19. Andreasen JO, Jensen SS, Schwartz O, Hillerup Y. A systematic review of prophylactic antibiotics in the surgical treatment of maxillofacial fractures. JOMS. 2006;64:1664–8.
20. Blum IR. Contemporary views on dry socket (alveolar osteitis): a clinical appraisal of standardization, Aetiopathogenesis and management: a critical review. Int J Oral Maxillofac Surg. 2002;31:309–17.
21. Zeitler DL. Prophylactic antibiotics for third molar surgery: a dissenting opinion. JOMS. 1995;53:61–4.
22. Ren YF, Malmstrom HS. Effectiveness of antibiotic prophylaxis in third molar surgery: a meta-analysis of randomized controlled clinical trials. JOMS. 2007;65:1909–21.
23. Piecuch JF, Arzadon J, Lieblich SE. Prophylactic antibiotics for third molar surgery: a supportive opinion. JOMS. 1995;53:53–60.
24. Sekhar CH, Narayanan V, Baig MF. Role of antimicrobials in third molar surgery: prospective, double blind, randomized, placebo-controlled study. Br J OMFS. 2001;39:134–7.
25. Poeschl PW, Eckel D, Poeschl E. Postoperative prophylactic antibiotic treatment in third molar surgery—a necessity? JOMS. 2004;62:3–8.
26. Arteagoitia I, Diez A, Barbier L, Santamaria G, Santamaria J. Efficacy of amoxicillin/clavulanic acid in preventing infectious and inflammatory complications following impacted mandibular third molar extraction. Oral Surg Oral Med Oral Pathol Oral Radiol Endod. 2005;100:E11–8.
27. Ataoglu H, Oz GY, Candirli C, Kiziloglu D. Routine antibiotic prophylaxis is not necessary during operations to remove third molars. Br J OMFS. 2008;46:133–5.
28. Halpern LR, Dodson TB. Does prophylactic Administration of Systemic Antibiotics Prevent Postoperative Inflammatory Complications after Third Molar Surgery? JOMS. 2007;65:177–85.
29. Kaczmarzyk T, Wichlinski J, Stypulkowska J, Zaleska M, Panas M, Woron J. Single-dose and multi-dose clindamycin therapy fails to demonstrate efficacy in preventing infectious and inflammatory complications in third molar surgery. Int J Oral Maxillofac Surg. 2007;36:417–22.
30. Caso A, Hung LK, Beirne OR. Prevention of alveolar Osteitis with Chlorhexidine: a meta-analytic review. Oral Surg Oral Med Oral Pathol Oral Radiol Endod. 2005;99:155–9.
31. Russell AD. Bacterial resistance to disinfectants: present knowledge and future problems. J Hosp Infect. 1998;43:S57–68.
32. Tanner J, Woodings D, Moncaster K. Preoperative hair removal to reduce surgical site infection. Cochrane Database Syst Rev. 2006;2:CD004122.
33. Digison MB. A review of anti-septic agents for Peri-operative skin preparation. Plast Surg Nurs. 2007;27(4):185–9.

34. Webster J, Osborne S. Meta-analysis of preoperative antiseptic bathing in the prevention of surgical site infection. Br J Surg. 2006;93:1335–41.
35. Chlebicki MJ, Safdar N, O'Horo JC, et al. Preoperative Chlorhexidine shower or bath for prevention of surgical site infection: a meta-analysis. Am J Infect Control. 2013;41:167–73.
36. Wilson SE. Microbial sealing: a new approach to reducing contamination. J Hosp Infect. 2008;70(S2:11–4.
37. Iyer A, Gilfillan I, Thakur S, et al. Reduction of surgical site infection using a microbial sealant: a randomized trial. J Thorac Cardiovasc Surg. 2011;142:438–42.
38. Waldow T, Szlapka M, Hensel J, et al. Skin sealant InteguSeal has no impact on prevention of postoperative Mediastinitis after cardiac surgery. J Hosp Infect. 2012;81:278–82.
39. Aly R, Maibach HI. Comparative antibacterial activity of a 2-minute surgical scrub with Chlorhexidine Gluconate, Povidone-iodine, and Chloroxylenol sponge-brushes. Am J Infect Control. 1988;16:173–7.
40. Parienti JJ, Thibon P, Heller R, et al. Hand-rubbing with an aqueous alcoholic solution vs traditional surgical hand-scrubbing and 30-day surgical site infection rates. A randomized equivalence study. JAMA. 2002;288:722–7.
41. Forbes SS, McLean RF. Review article: the Anesthesiologist's role in the prevention of surgical site infections. Can J Anesth. 2013;60:176–83.
42. Sessler DI. Complications and treatment of mild hypothermia. Anesthesiology. 2001;95:531–43.
43. Mauermann WJ, Nemergut EC. The Anesthesiologist's role in the prevention of surgical site infections. Anesthesiology. 2006;105(2):413–21.
44. Kurz A, Sessler DI, Lenhardt R, et al. Perioperative Normothermia to reduce the incidence of surgical-wound infection and shorten hospitalization. NEJM. 1996;334(19):1209–15.
45. Flores-Maldonado A, Medina-Escobedo CE, Rios-Rodriguez HM, et al. Mild perioperative hypothermia and the risk of wound infection. Arch Med Res. 2001;32:227–31.
46. Greif R, Akca O, Horn EP, et al. Supplemental perioperative oxygen to reduce the incidence of surgical-wound infection. NEJM. 2000;342(3):161–7.
47. Chura JC, Boyd A, Argenta PA. Surgical site infections and supplemental perioperative oxygen in colorectal surgery patients: a systematic review. Surg Infect. 2007;8:455–61.
48. Qadan M, Akca O, Mahid SS, et al. Perioperative supplemental oxygen therapy and surgical site infection: a meta-analysis of randomized controlled trials. Arch Surg. 2009;144:359–66.
49. Al-Niaimi A, Safdar N. Supplemental perioperative oxygen for reducing surgical site infection: a meta-analysis. J Eval Clin Pract. 2009;15:360–5.
50. den Berghe V, Wouters P, Weekers F, et al. Intensive insulin therapy in critically ill patients. NEJM. 2001;345:1359–67.
51. Furnary AP, Zerr KJ, Grunkemeier GL, et al. Continuous intravenous insulin infusion reduces the incidence of deep sternal wound infection in diabetic patients after cardiac surgical procedures. Ann Thorac Surg. 1999;67(2):352–60.
52. Ji GW, Wu YZ, Wang X, et al. Experimental and clinical study of influence of high-frequency electric surgical knives on healing of abdominal incision. World J Gastroenterol. 2006;12(25):4082–5.
53. Kearns SR, Connolly EM, McNally S, et al. Randomized clinical trial of diathermy versus scalpel incision in elective midline Laparotomy. Br J Surg. 2001;88:41–4.
54. Shamim M. Diathermy vs. scalpel skin incisions in general surgery: double-blind, randomized clinical trial. World J Surg. 2009;33:1594–9.
55. Sheikh B. Safety and efficacy of Electrocautery scalpel utilization for skin opening in neurosurgery. Br J Neurosurg. 2004;18(3):268–72.
56. McHugh SM, Collins CJ, Corrigan MA, et al. The role of topical antibiotics used as prophylaxis in surgical site infection prevention. J Antimicrob Chemother. 2011;66:693–701.
57. Barnes S, Spencer M, Graham D, et al. Surgical wound irrigation: a call for evidence-based standardization of practice. Am J Infect Control. 2014;42:525–9.
58. Anglen JO. Wound irrigation in musculoskeletal injury. J Am Acad Orthop Surg. 2001;9:270–1.
59. McHugh SM, Hill ADK, Humphreys H. Intraoperative technique as a factor in the prevention of surgical site infection. J Hosp Infect. 2011;78:1–4.
60. Gunst MA, Minei JP. Transfusion of blood products and nosocomial infection in surgical patients. Curr Opin Crit Care. 2007;13:428–32.
61. Weinberg JA, McGwin G, Griffin RL, et al. Age of transfused blood: an independent predictor of mortality despite universal Leukoreduction. J Trauma. 2008;65:279–84.
62. Friese RS, Sperry JL, Phelan HA, et al. The use of Leukoreduced red blood cell products is associated with fewer infectious complications in trauma patients. Am J Surg. 2008;196:56–61.
63. Frietsch T, Karger R, Scholer M, et al. Leukodepletion of autologous whole blood has no impact on perioperative infection rate and length of hospital stay. Transfusion. 2008;48:2133–42.

11 Peri-Operative Pain Management in Maxillofacial Surgery

Joseph E. Cillo Jr.

Abstract

Oral and maxillofacial surgery procedures are known to cause acute postoperative pain. Effective management of acute postoperative pain is critically important for physiological and psychological stability. The goal of effective postoperative pain management is to reduce or eliminate pain and discomfort with a minimum of side effects. Inadequate management of acute postoperative pain is a potential source of complications and a significant cause of decreased quality of life. Preemptive and perioperative medication administration and multimodal postoperative therapy have been shown to be effective in postoperative acute pain management following oral and maxillofacial surgery procedures.

11.1 Introduction

Acute postoperative pain is a significant source of morbidity that if not managed properly may have deleterious effects on the patient. According to the *American Society of Anesthesiologists Task Force on Acute Pain Management* [1], acute pain is defined as pain that is present in a surgical patient after a procedure which may result from either procedural trauma or procedure- related complications. Pain management in the perioperative setting refers to actions before, during, and after a surgical procedure that are intended to reduce or eliminate acute postoperative pain. Numerous studies in the general surgery literature have given credence to the effectiveness of proper perioperative pain management.

Acute postoperative pain from oral and maxillofacial surgical procedures is a well-known phenomenon that frequently occurs after third molar removal [2, 3] maxillofacial trauma repair [4, 5], orthognathic surgery [6, 7], and dental implant placement [8–10]. The incidence and severity of acute postoperative pain has been

J.E. Cillo Jr., D.M.D., M.P.H., Ph.D., F.A.C.S.
Division of Oral and Maxillofacial Surgery, Drexel University College of Medicine, Allegheny General Hospital, Allegheny Health Network, Pittsburgh, PA, USA
e-mail: jecdna@aol.com

© Springer International Publishing AG 2018

E.M. Ferneini, J.D. Bennett (eds.), *Perioperative Assessment of the Maxillofacial Surgery Patient*,
https://doi.org/10.1007/978-3-319-58868-1_11

shown to have a direct bearing on the patient-perceived outcomes and satisfaction of their surgical procedure [11, 12]. While most patients who undergo surgical procedures experience acute postoperative pain, a wide review of evidence suggested that less than half of patients report adequate postoperative pain relief [13]. Ineffectual perioperative pain management may lead to a discernable reduction in desirable clinical and psychological outcomes and patients' overall quality of life while effective management may result in improved patient outcomes and increased patient satisfaction [14]. There are many preoperative, intraoperative, and postoperative intervention and management strategies available that aid in the reduction and management of acute postoperative pain. Suitable perioperative pain management may enhance earlier patient mobility, reduce postoperative narcotic consumption, decrease admission rates for intractable pain management, and may lessen potential complications such as ileus, urinary retention, and need for fluid management [15]. Given the negative aspects of patient-perceived outcomes and quality of life issues combined with the potential deleterious consequences of inadequate postoperative pain management, the effective utilization of perioperative pain management becomes evident. The underlying premise that optimal management begins in the preoperative period with an assessment of the patient and development of a plan of care tailored to the individual and the surgical procedure involved [13].

The predictors of acute postoperative pain are determined by degree of preoperative pain, anxiety, age, and type of surgery, while postoperative analgesic consumption is determined by type of surgery, age, psychological stress, and genotype [16]. Genotype has been shown to play a large role in opioid sensitivity [17]. Gene-wide association studies in individuals that have undergone oral surgery have found that specific genes are involved in individual variation responses to analgesic onset and maximum pain rating. This individualized concept of acute postoperative pain has led to a more personalized treatment of pain management [17–19].

11.2 Preemptive Analgesia

Different strategies for perioperative pain management have been employed at the pre-, inter- and postoperative time points. The goal of preoperative administration of analgesics by any route will seek to decrease acute postoperative pain by the maximization of systemic drug levels. This is generally competed in protocols that utilize preemptive analgesia to alleviate acute postoperative pain. Interoperative local administration of medications at the surgical site will tend to minimize systemic exposure and accentuate analgesic efficacy. Preemptive analgesia is a treatment initiated prior to and effective during a surgical procedure with the purpose to decrease or eliminate the physiological consequences of nociception triggered by the surgical procedure. A "protective effect" based on the pharmacological modalities of the medication used (centrally or peripherally acting, anti-inflammatory, antiallodynic, or antihyperalgesic properties) is utilized to effectively block or decrease the passage of surgically triggered nociception to alleviate postoperative pain and diminish narcotic consumption through these pharmacological modalities that may modify the physiological pain and increasing threshold for nociception [20]. The theory being that diminishment of transmission of surgically triggered nociception to the brain may decrease acute postoperative pain perception. It has the potential to be more effective than similar postoperative analgesic treatments owing to the "protective" effect on the nociceptive pathway blockage by pharmacological means [21].

The physiological basis of preemptive analgesia is complex and involves modification of the pain pathways that seeks to alleviate or prevent acute postoperative pain. The majority of clinical studies in oral and maxillofacial surgery postoperative pain management have been conducted for third molar surgery [22–26]. The production of noxious stimuli in surgical procedures produces neurogenic and inflammatory mediators that may propagate postoperative pain. The gate control theory of pain [27] is the idea that physical pain is not a direct result of activation of pain receptor neurons, but rather its perception is modulated by interaction between different neurons. If the neurogenic and inflammatory mediators produced during surgery can be blocked or reduced prior to being perceived by the patient as pain, then there may be a decrease in postoperative pain which may ultimately lead to a decrease opioid consumption and improved quality of life. Another theory asserts that the administration of analgesic prior to stimuli would prevent the establishment of central sensitization from incisional injury (only during the surgical period) and prevent the establishment of central sensitization from incisional and inflammatory injury (during the surgical and early postoperative periods) [28].

There have been numerous medications that have been given preoperatively to attenuate postoperative pain following oral and maxillofacial surgery. Clinical studies in preemptive analgesia for acute postoperative pain management in oral and maxillofacial surgery have included tramadol [29, 30], bupivacaine [22, 23], ketamine [26], diclofenac sodium [31, 32], and nonsteroidal anti-inflammatory medications (ketorolac [33, 34] and ibuprofen [35–37] and selective COX-2 inhibitors etoricoxib [38] and celecoxib [39, 40]).

Preemptive use of ketorolac 30 mg intravenously [41] or intramuscularly [33], oral tramadol 50 mg [42] or 100 mg [43], tramadol 25 mg, and meloxicam 7.5 mg [44] have been shown to reduce the severity of the postoperative sequelae of impacted mandibular third molar surgery. Similar successful results have been found with naproxen, meloxicam, acetaminophen, and rofecoxib [45]. In major maxillofacial surgery, pregabalin [46] alone or in combination with celecoxib [40] has been shown to have a preemptive analgesic effect that lowered postoperative narcotic consumption and perceived patient pain in orthognathic surgery.

11.2.1 Multimodal Versus Single Agent Postoperative Pain Management

A Cochrane review revealed that there is a large body of reliable evidence on the analgesic efficacy of both single and combination doses of analgesics that may produce effective and often long-lasting analgesia at relatively low doses [47]. Combinations have included both narcotic and nonnarcotic medications that, unlike single medication therapies, appear to have a synergistic quality in acute postoperative pain management. These combinations of medications are believed to have an additive analgesic efficacy to combine an efficacious dose of a nonopioid with a dose of an opioid sufficient to produce additive analgesia without a substantial increase in the incidence of adverse effects [48].

Combining drugs or combining different routes of administration of the same drug can increase the intensity and duration of analgesic effect. Combinations that target both peripheral and central pain pathways have different onset times and durations of action. Different sites of action can enhance an analgesic's capacity to minimize pain, and additive and synergistic effects may allow for lower doses [49, 50].

Prescription of opioid-containing analgesic such as hydrocodone with acetaminophen is often given upon completion of many oral and maxillofacial surgery procedures. Numerous clinical trials into both single and multimodal analgesics for management of perioperative pain have been conducted. A Cochrane review revealed a large body of reliable evidence on the analgesic efficacy of both single and combination doses of oral analgesics that produce effective and often long-lasting analgesia at relatively low doses [47]. Combinations generally include both narcotic and nonnarcotic medications that, unlike single medication therapies, appear to have a synergistic quality in acute postoperative pain management. These combinations of medications are believed to have an additive analgesic efficacy to combine an efficacious dose of a nonopioid with a dose of an opioid sufficient to produce additive analgesia without a substantial increase in the incidence of adverse effects [51].

11.3 Patient-Controlled Analgesia

Patient-controlled analgesia (PCA) allows patients to self-administer intravenous (IV) analgesics by means of a computer-controlled pump that administers the preprogrammed dose on demand by the individual. PCA is believed to improve on traditional as needed intravenous and/or oral methods of acute postoperative pain management through superior titration of analgesic medications that address individual pain needs based on pharmacokinetic and pharmacodynamic variation. Advantages of PCA over traditional opioid analgesics administration methods include the autonomy and increased psychologic satisfaction of individualized analgesia administration, less sedation because of drug titration, elimination of delay in the decision to medicate for pain, decreased staff time for patient care, elimination of painful intramuscular injections, and rapid onset of analgesia [51, 52].

As age, gender, and psychological distress (anxiety) may influence postoperative pain medication consumption, an evaluation of the relationship between these in major maxillofacial surgery found preoperative anxiety directly influenced postoperative PCA morphine consumption [53]. Preoperative anxiolytic administration may help reduce postoperative PCA opioid consumption. Similarly, in a prospective randomized double-blind clinical study for acute postoperative pain management that followed orthognathic surgery with demographic, surgical time, fentanyl used, and gender-matched groups, PCA morphine was found to be superior compared to codeine and as effective as naproxen with fewer overall side effects compared to both. Some reports, however, indicate that there is no benefit from morphine PCA in the management of acute postoperative pain from major maxillofacial surgery [54].

11.4 Nonsteroidal Anti-Inflammatory Medications (NSAID)

Nonsteroidal anti-inflammatory drugs (NSAIDs) are a drug class that provide, at lower doses, analgesic and antipyretic effects and, in higher doses, anti-inflammatory effects. Most NSAIDs inhibit the activity of cyclooxygenase-1 (COX-1) and cyclooxygenase-2 (COX-2) and thereby the synthesis of pain mediators prostaglandins and thromboxanes. Inhibition of COX-2 produces anti-inflammatory, analgesic, and antipyretic effects, while inhibition of COX-1 may cause gastrointestinal bleeding and ulcers. Both nonselective NSAIDs and COX-1 inhibitors may increase the risk of stomach and intestinal ulceration and may increase the likelihood of bleeding ulcers. The most common NSAIDs involved in clinical investigations in acute postoperative pain management from oral and maxillofacial surgery procedures have been aspirin, ibuprofen, ketorolac, and celecoxib.

11.4.1 Aspirin

Aspirin, also known as acetylsalicylic acid (ASA), is an NSAID medication used to treat mild to moderate acute postoperative pain and inflammation. Aspirin works through irreversible inactivation of the cyclooxygenase (COX) to suppress the synthesis of prostaglandins and thromboxanes. Aspirin is known to produce increased bleeding through specific irreversible blockage of thromboxane A_2 in platelets with an inhibitory effect on platelet aggregation.

In several randomized double-blind controlled clinical trials to assess the analgesic efficacy in acute postoperative pain management from extraction of impacted third molars, administration of ASA compared with placebo [55], the addition of acetaminophen compared to placebo [56], and the addition of codeine compared to placebo or tramadol [57] produced no significant reduction in pain. The administration of aspirin in these studies resulted in unwanted side effects such as increased intraoperative bleeding, increased postoperative bleeding, hematoma, ecchymosis, and swelling. Considering the increased incidence of postoperative side effects coupled with no significant decrease in acute postoperative pain, the administration of preoperative aspirin is not recommended.

11.4.2 Ibuprofen

Ibuprofen is a synthetic nonsteroidal anti-inflammatory drug (NSAID) widely used as an analgesic and anti-inflammatory agent. It is a nonselective inhibitor of cyclooxygenase (COX), an enzyme required to convert arachidonic acid to prostaglandin H2 (PGH2) which produces hyperalgesia and pyrexia in the body. It is the single most common nonnarcotic medications prescribed for perioperative pain management in oral and maxillofacial surgery [58].

Clinical studies into the timing of dosing of ibuprofen have seen mixed results. As a single-drug modality, the preoperative use of ibuprofen did not show reduction in pain, facial swelling, and trismus after impacted lower third molar extraction when compared to the postoperative administration of the ibuprofen [59]. As a single agent in acute postoperative pain management, ibuprofen 400 mg has also been shown to be superior to acetaminophen 1000 mg following third molar removal [60–62].

Combination drug therapy with ibuprofen and the addition of either a narcotic or nonnarcotic has been shown to have a greater analgesic efficacy than either medication alone. In a systematic review and meta-analysis of randomized clinical trials, ibuprofen 400 mg with oxycodone HCL 5 mg had a superior additive analgesic efficacy for acute postoperative pain control after third molar surgery [63]. The additive analgesic effect of this combination has been shown to be superior to other drug combinations to include oxycodone 5 mg/acetaminophen 325 mg, hydrocodone 7.5 mg/acetaminophen 500 mg[1], or placebo [64]. In addition, the analgesic effect of the combination of ibuprofen 400 mg with 40 mg codeine was found to provide more effective postoperative acute pain management than ibuprofen 400 mg alone following removal of impacted mandibular third molars, but with higher incidence of adverse events than ibuprofen alone.

Combining ibuprofen with nonnarcotic medications has proven to be as effective, if not superior to combinations with narcotic medications without untoward complications or addiction potential. The combination of ibuprofen 400 mg and acetaminophen (APAP) 1000 mg has been shown to provide better postoperative analgesia than either drug alone (at the same dose), with a smaller chance of needing additional analgesia over an 8-h period with minimal side effects [65]. Similarly, several randomized controlled clinical trials have also indicated that ibuprofen-APAP combinations provide greater acute postoperative pain relief than either medication alone after third molar extractions [66]. These studies have shown that combinations of ibuprofen and APAP tend to be more effective in management of acute postoperative pain, with fewer side effects, than many currently available opioid-containing formulations.

11.4.3 Naproxen

Naproxen is an NSAID in the same class as ibuprofen. It is a nonselective COX inhibitor used successfully as an anti-inflammatory for moderate pain in oral and maxillofacial surgery [67]. Naproxen analgesic efficacy has been found to have superior analgesic efficacy to ibuprofen [68] and similar efficacy to another NSAID, oxaprozin [69], in perioperative pain management following impacted third molar surgery.

11.4.4 Ketorolac

Ketorolac is an NSAID generally used to treat moderate to severe pain through inhibition of prostaglandins synthesis. Ketorolac is available in oral (tablet or capsule), intramuscular/intravenous, and nasal spray forms. In a single-dose double-blind, placebo-controlled study, 10 mg of oral ketorolac was found to provide better pain relief with fewer side effects than hydrocodone/acetaminophen following moderate pain from extraction of impacted mandibular third molars [70]. A preoperative intravenous dose of ketorolac 30 mg has been shown to produce less immediate postoperative pain and increased the median

[1] 500-mg dosing of acetaminophen is no longer available.

interval to the rescue medication by 2 h in subjects that had extraction of impacted mandibular third molars under intravenous anesthesia [71]. Ketorolac nasal spray was an effective treatment for moderate to moderately severe short-term pain from third molar removal compared to hydrocodone/acetaminophen (APAP), oxycodone/APAP, oxycodone/ibuprofen, and tramadol HCl/APAP [72]. In combination therapy, effective pain relief and fewer days on medications that followed dental extractions was demonstrated with a combination of 10 mg ketorolac and 15 mg codeine compared with either drug alone [73].

11.4.5 Celecoxib

Celecoxib is a highly selective cyclooxygenase-2 (COX-2) inhibitor that primarily inhibits the isoform of cyclooxygenase to reduce inflammation and moderate to severe pain in adults. As a sole agent for perioperative pain management, this medication has been used widely in the oral surgery literature. Administration of celecoxib that followed oral surgical procedures resulted in a quick onset of action that was effective in the management of acute postoperative pain [74] with greater longevity [75]. It was found to be a superior sole analgesic following third molar surgery compared to prednisolone [76], ibuprofen [39], and placebo [77] and to have equal clinical analgesic efficacy to loxoprofen [75]. A randomized, double-blind, placebo-controlled, prospective clinical trial of patients who underwent minor oral surgical procedures and received either a preoperative oral dose of 200 mg celecoxib, 400 mg ibuprofen, or placebo showed that celecoxib had statistically significant superior analgesic effects on all measures of analgesic efficacy, including overall analgesic effect, time to onset of effect, peak pain relief, and duration of effect [39]. Another randomized double-masked crossover clinical trial conducted on 20 patients who underwent mucoperiosteal flap surgery with preoperative administration of celecoxib found that perceived patient pain was statistically significantly lower with celecoxib compared to placebo [78]. Following maxillomandibular advancement surgery for obstructive sleep apnea in middle-aged adult patients, a one-time preoperative oral dose of celecoxib combined with pregabalin was shown to have decrease postoperative PCA and oral opioid consumption and perceived patient pain [40].

11.4.6 Intravenous NSAIDs

Intravenous NSAIDs have shown to be a very effective medication in the alleviation of acute postoperative pain. Intravenous ketorolac is indicated for short term (less than 5 days) of acute moderately severe pain. It has been shown to have a very high analgesic efficacy when given either preoperatively [79, 80], as a preemptive analgesic [81], and postoperatively for acute postoperative pain after third molar surgery [82, 83]. As these medications are inhibitors of platelet aggregation, there always remains the issue of excessive intraoperative and postoperative bleeding. However, numerous clinical studies in adult and pediatric general and head and neck surgery have revealed that the intravenous administration of either ketorolac or ibuprofen provided excellent postoperative analgesia with no increased risk of postoperative bleeding [84–90].

A major concern for the use of NSAIDs for the management of acute postoperative pain has been the potential for these medications to affect bone healing. Most of these concerns have come from data from animal and laboratory studies and case reports. A systematic review of the literature revealed the limitations in the current understanding of the effects of NSAIDs on bone healing due to the lack of high-quality well-controlled clinical human studies [91]. It was concluded from this review that withholding NSAIDs did not have any proven scientific benefit to patients and may even cause harm by increasing narcotic requirements in cases in which these medications might be beneficial for pain management.

11.5 Narcotics

Narcotics are opioid substances that act on opioid receptors directly on the central nervous system (CNS) to decrease both chronic and acute pain. Either alone or in combination with other medications, narcotics are frequently prescribed after oral and maxillofacial surgery procedures. There are a variety of administration routes that narcotics may be delivered including oral, intravenous, intramuscular, and nasal. Oral narcotics oxycodone and hydrocodone combined with APAP are the most prescribed medication for postoperative pain in North America [92]. The most common intravenous narcotics used in the management of acute postoperative pain following oral and maxillofacial surgery procedures include morphine, meperidine, and tramadol.

11.5.1 Tramadol

Tramadol hydrochloride is a synthetic, centrally acting analgesic with a chemical structure similar to codeine and morphine that allows it low affinity for opioid receptors but with a low addiction potential and good effectiveness for management of moderate to severe acute postoperative pain [34]. As a monoamine reuptake inhibitor, tramadol acquires its analgesic effect from the modification of the transmission of pain impulses though blockage of transporters for the monoamine neurotransmitters serotonin, norepinephrine, and/or dopamine [93]. The side effects of tramadol (constipation, nausea, and vomiting) tend to be more attenuated and acceptable than those of traditional opioids [94].

Tramadol has been administered by several routes for the management of acute postoperative pain from third molar extraction. These have included oral [95], intramuscular [96], intravenous, subcutaneously, and nasally. Clinical studies have revealed that the intravenous route is superior to the oral route [97] in postoperative pain management for third molar removal.

Tramadol has also been studied extensively as both a single agent and in combination with other medications [98]. As a single agent, tramadol has not been shown to produce an effective treatment for acute postoperative pain following dentoalveolar surgery [99]. A meta-analysis of published randomized, double-blind, clinical trials that compared the analgesic efficacy and safety of tramadol with that of nonsteroidal anti-inflammatory drugs (NSAID) revealed that a single dose of tramadol was not as effective or as safe as NSAID in management of acute postoperative pain from third molar removal [95]. Additionally, as a single agent, tramadol is less effective than butorphanol [100], ketorolac [34, 96], lysine clonixinate 91, diclofenac [31], and locally applied ketamine [101]. When administered locally to the surgical site in addition to a systemic dose, tramadol may extend the duration of anesthetic effect and improve the quality of postoperative analgesia following third molar extractions [102].

Tramadol in combination with another medication has a better efficacy in acute perioperative pain management. The combination of tramadol and APAP is superior to either medication alone with respect to pain relief, duration of action, and time to onset [103]. A single-center, double-blind, parallel-group, placebo- and active-controlled study in adults after third molar removal found that the combination of tramadol and APAP provided more effective and rapid analgesia with better tolerability compared to hydrocodone and APAP [104].

11.5.2 Oxycodone/Hydrocodone

The combination of oxycodone and APAP or ibuprofen are some of the most commonly prescribed medications for the management of moderate to severe pain after oral and maxillofacial surgery procedures. In numerous clinical trials, the combinations of these medications, such as oxycodone 5 mg/ibuprofen 400 mg [64], hydrocodone 7.5 mg/ibuprofen 200 mg [105], and hydrocodone 7.5 mg/APAP 500 mg[1] [106], have been shown to be effective in providing effective postoperative analgesia following oral and maxillofacial surgery.

11.6 Anticonvulsant Medications

There have been a variety of medications successfully utilized in the perioperative pain management in oral and maxillofacial surgery. These have included nicotine nasal spray [107], submucosal injections of dexamethasone [108], and even green tea mouthwash [109]. Anticonvulsant medications have also been used to treat both acute and chronic neuropathic pain. Administration of anticonvulsants is nonaddictive that may be effective in the management of postoperative pain. The most common medications investigated in this category were oral pregabalin and local administration of clonidine.

11.6.1 Pregabalin

Pregabalin is an oral anticonvulsive medication known to have antiallodynic and antihyperalgesic properties useful for treating neuropathic pain in adults. Pregabalin binds to and modulates the alpha-two-delta subunit of the voltage-dependent calcium channel in the central nervous system exerting its intended effect to reduce neuropathic pain. The analgesic efficacy of pregabalin administration has been shown in many clinical trials in both general and oral surgery as it has been found to reduce acute postoperative pain, opioid consumption, and opioid-related adverse effects. In a efficacy pain trial with impacted mandibular third molar removal, pregabalin reduced the requirement for rescue medication and resulted in more constant pain control, with fewer peaks of pain intensity [110]. Additionally, 300 mg pregabalin given after third molar removal showed statistically significant differences in pain reduction, pain intensity difference, and pain relief intensity difference compared to placebo and a significantly longer duration of analgesia compared to ibuprofen [111]. The postoperative administration of 75 mg pregabalin was also found to provide more effective analgesia after third molar surgery under local anesthesia when compared to the same dose given preoperatively [112].

As single-drug therapy in major maxillofacial surgery, a preoperative 150 mg oral dose of pregabalin decreased postoperative opioid consumption in the first 24 h after double-jaw surgery [46]. When used in multimodal drug therapy, a combination of 150 mg of pregabalin and 300 mg of celecoxib given orally 1 h prior to adult maxillomandibular advancement for sleep apnea produced significant reduction in both intravenous and oral narcotic consumption and patient-perceived pain in the immediate and 7-day postoperative period [40].

11.7 Clonidine

Clonidine is classified as a centrally acting α_2 adrenergic agonist and imidazoline receptor used to treat a variety of conditions including hypertension and certain pain conditions. Clonidine has been advocated as an adjunct to local anesthetic to aid in postoperative pain management. In double-blind randomized clinical trials, the influence of the admixture of clonidine and lidocaine administered for either infiltrative or nerve block anesthesia for dentoalveolar surgery on postoperative analgesia and hemodynamic stability was studied [113–115]. In these studies, the need for postoperative pain medication was significantly lower in the clonidine group with less postoperative analgesic consumption and no significant difference in hemodynamic stability when compared with epinephrine, even in poorly controlled hypertensive patients.

11.8 Local Administration of Medications

Local administration of medications at surgical sites has long been a modality in perioperative pain. Administration of local anesthetic either prior to incision or after closure has the intention to provide a decrease in acute postoperative pain. Similarly, the premise behind the local administration of medications, such as opioids, at the surgical site is based on the demonstration that specific receptors exist in the peripheral nervous system that may also offer prolonged postoperative analgesia in the ambulatory surgical patient.

11.8.1 Local Anesthetics

There are mixed results from the clinical literature that administration of local anesthetic helps with perioperative pain management. Tuffin et al. [116] found that administration of bupivacaine at the time of removal of impacted third molars may result in reduction of early patient-perceived postoperative pain and reduction of postoperative opiate requirements without significant patient-perceived prolonged anesthetic unpleasantness. Similarly, both Gordon et al. [117] and Nayyar et al. [118] also found a reduction in postoperative pain and analgesic requirement with preoperative bupivacaine injections and extended duration local anesthetic agents such as liposomal bupivacaine placed directly in or in the vicinity of the extraction socket [119]. Conversely, however, Tordoff et al. [120] found no significant difference in postoperative pain from preoperative lidocaine injections, while Campbell and Kendrick [23] found similar results with preoperative bupivacaine injections for control of postoperative pain after extraction of lower third molars. Specifically, Campbell et al. [23] found that the pre-incision administration of local anesthesia did not appear to have any advantage over its postoperative administration in extraction of impacted third molar teeth.

Harvesting iliac crest bone is a common technique in oral and maxillofacial surgery and has been shown to be a source of pain and morbidity. A considerable amount of investigation has been conducted in acute postoperative pain management with local anesthetics delivered either by bolus, continuous infusion, or topically after iliac crest bone harvest. Numerous studies have found that a continuous local infusion of bupivacaine at the iliac crest may help in alleviate bone graft-related pain beyond the perioperative period [121–124], decrease the length of hospitalization [125]. When given as a bolus following iliac crest bone graft harvest, those who received postoperative bupivacaine experienced delayed onset of postoperative pain [126, 127], earlier ambulation, and earlier return to normal daily activity compared to those who received no local anesthesia [127]. Conversely, this was not seen in a similar study of a bolus of bupivacaine that had no significant difference on postoperative pain and gait disturbance compared to no local anesthesia [128]. Locally applied bupivacaine-soaked gel foam at an iliac bone graft harvest site did reduce postoperative parenteral opioid use [129]. While bupivacaine has been the most common anesthetic investigated due to its long duration of action, other long-acting local anesthetics have also been evaluated. Kukidome et al. [130] found that both 0.2% ropivacaine and 0.25% levobupivacaine provided comparable analgesic effects in continuous infiltration anesthesia delivered via a multiple-hole catheter after iliac bone grafting.

11.8.2 Local Medication Administration

Opioid-sparing strategies include the use of locally delivered medications alone or added to local anesthetic to improve acute postoperative pain management. The addition of buprenorphine, a semisynthetic opioid, to 0.5% bupivacaine with epinephrine 1:200,000 used for intraoral nerve blocks for minor oral surgery was shown to provide a threefold increase in the duration of postoperative analgesia, with complete analgesia persisting 30 h beyond the duration provided by the local anesthetic alone in vast majority of patients evaluated [131]. Similarly, the admixture of clonidine, a centrally acting alpha-agonist hypotensive agent that is used to treat a variety of illnesses including certain pain conditions, with local anesthetic at the site of third molar extractions revealed a significantly decreased need for postoperative pain medication with no significant difference in intraoperative hemodynamic changes in systolic, diastolic, and mean arterial pressure [132]. Locally applied morphine to the surgical site after third molar removal did not provide any benefit in acute postoperative pain compared to placebo [133].

Administration of nonsteroidal anti-inflammatory drugs (NSAIDs) such as ibuprofen or ketoprofen [134] to a peripheral site of tissue injury results in greater analgesia compared to oral administration of the same drugs. Some adjuncts to local anesthetics for peripheral blockade have been proposed to enhance the quality and duration of anesthesia and postoperative analgesia, such as antidepressants [135], and opioids [136] such as tramadol [137, 138].

11.9 Acetaminophen

Acetaminophen, also known as propacetamol or N-acetyl-p-aminophenol (APAP), is a medication that has analgesic and antipyretic properties. Its therapeutic effects are like nonsteroidal anti-inflammatory drugs, as it is thought to act primarily in the central nervous system to increase the pain threshold by inhibition of both isoforms of cyclooxygenase, COX-1, COX-2, and COX-3 enzymes involved in prostaglandin synthesis. However, APAP lacks the anti-inflammatory, antiplatelet, and gastric ulcerative effects of NSAIDs. It is a common and effective ingredient in commonly prescribed oral medications given individually or in combination with other medications, usually an opioid, for management of acute postoperative pain [66]. A 1000 mg fast-dissolving APAP tablet was found to have significantly superior analgesic effect, faster analgesic onset, and longer duration of pain relief compared to 500 mg fast-dissolving APAP and conventional oral 650 mg APAP after third molar surgery [139]. APAP may also be administered intravenously and shown to be very effective in the management of acute postoperative pain [140]. In repeated intravenous doses (2 g followed by 1 g), APAP has a significant analgesic effect that is indistinguishable from that of morphine administered IM (10 mg followed by 5 mg) with better tolerability after third molar surgery [141]. The 2-g starting dose of IV APAP has been shown to have superior analgesic efficacy and similar safety to the recommended dose of 1 g in terms of magnitude and duration of analgesic effect for postoperative pain after third molar surgery [142].

Conclusion

Numerous clinical studies have been conducted to establish the most effective perioperative pain management in oral and maxillofacial surgery to include single and multimodal medication of various route administration. In multimodal administration, drug combinations that include both opioid and nonopioid medications have shown to be the most effective in the management of acute postoperative oral and maxillofacial pain. However, while the mainstay of postoperative analgesia has been opioid centered, there is mounting clinical evidence to support a multimodal approach with the intent to reduce opioid side effects (such as nausea and ileus) and addiction. Effective utilization of nonopioid medications in either a preemptive analgesia strategy or postoperative medication regimen may decrease the need for opioid consumption and improve patient quality of life and decrease addiction potential. Intravenous and patient-controlled analgesia are highly effective in the early postoperative hospital period; they tend to be problematic outside the hospital or office setting. Clinical investigations have also revealed that several predictive factors are important in determining an individual's response to perioperative pain management. The most important of these may be the genetic predisposition of the individual to respond to pharmacological therapy. This should lead to future endeavors that target personalized therapy that will provide the most effective and appropriate therapy in the management of acute postoperative pain in oral and maxillofacial surgery patients.

References

1. American Society of Anesthesiologists Task Force on Acute Pain Management. Practice guidelines for acute pain management in the perioperative setting: an updated report by the American Society of Anesthesiologists Task Force on acute pain management. Anesthesiology. 2012;116(2):248–73. https://doi.org/10.1097/ALN.0b013e31823c1030.

2. Lago-Méndez L, Diniz-Freitas M, Senra-Rivera C, Gude-Sampedro F, Gándara Rey JM, García-García A. Relationships between surgical difficulty and postoperative pain in lower third molar extractions. J Oral Maxillofac Surg. 2007;65(5):979.
3. Garcia A, Gude Sampedro F, Gandara Rey J, Gallas Torreira M. Trismus and pain after removal of impacted lower third molars. J Oral Maxillofac Surg. 1997;55(11):1223.
4. Bentley MW, Stas JM, Johnson JM, Viet BC, Garrett N. Effects of preincisional ketamine treatment on natural killer cell activity and postoperative pain management after oral maxillofacial surgery. AANA J. 2005;73(6):427–36.
5. Niemi L, Tuominen M, Pitkänen M, Rosenberg PH. Comparison of parenteral diclofenac and ketoprofen for postoperative pain relief after maxillofacial surgery. Acta Anaesthesiol Scand. 1995;39(1):96–9.
6. Phillips C, Blakey G 3rd, Jaskolka M. Recovery after orthognathic surgery: short-term health-related quality of life outcomes. J Oral Maxillofac Surg. 2008;66(10):2110–5. https://doi.org/10.1016/j.joms.2008.06.080.
7. Phillips C, Blakey G 3rd. Short-term recovery after orthognathic surgery: a medical daily diary approach. Int J Oral Maxillofac Surg. 2008;37(10):892–6. https://doi.org/10.1016/j.ijom.2008.07.005.
8. Bryce G, Bomfim DI, Bassi GS. Pre- and post-operative management of dental implant placement. Part 1: management of post-operative pain. Br Dent J. 2014;217(3):123–7. https://doi.org/10.1038/sj.bdj.2014.650.
9. Nolan R, Kemmoona M, Polyzois I, Claffey N. The influence of prophylactic antibiotic administration on post-operative morbidity in dental implant surgery. A prospective double blind randomized controlled clinical trial. Clin Oral Implants Res. 2014;25(2):252–9. https://doi.org/10.1111/clr.12124.
10. Pani SC, AlGarni B, AlZain LM, AlQahtani NS. Assessment of the impact of stress and anxiety on pain perception in patients undergoing surgery for placement of their first dental implant. Oral Health Dent Manag. 2014;13(2):464–8.
11. Carr DB, Goudas LC. Acute pain. Lancet. 1999;353(9169):2051–8.
12. Leykin Y, Pellis T, Ambrosio C. Highlights in post-operative pain treatment. Expert Rev Neurother. 2007;7(5):533–45.
13. Chou R, Gordon DB, de Leon-Casasola OA, et al. Management of Postoperative Pain: a clinical practice guideline from the American pain society, the American Society of Regional Anesthesia and Pain Medicine, and the American Society of Anesthesiologists' committee on regional anesthesia, executive committee, and administrative council. J Pain. 2016;17(2):131–57. https://doi.org/10.1016/j.jpain.2015.12.008.
14. Glowacki D. Effective pain management and improvements in patients' outcomes and satisfaction. Crit Care Nurse. 2015;35(3):33–41. https://doi.org/10.4037/ccn2015440.
15. Vadivelu N, Mitra S, Narayan D. Recent advances in postoperative pain management. Yale J Biol Med. 2010;83(1):11–25.
16. Ip HY, Abrishami A, Peng PW, Wong J, Chung F. Predictors of postoperative pain and analgesic consumption: a qualitative systematic review. Anesthesiology. 2009;111:657–77. https://doi.org/10.1097/ALN.0b013e3181aae87a.
17. Nishizawa D, Fukuda K, Kasai S, Al e. Genome-wide association study identifies a potent locus associated with human opioid sensitivity. Mol Psychiatry. 2014;19(1):55–62. https://doi.org/10.1038/mp.2012.164.
18. Yoshida K, Nishizawa D, Ichinomiya T, Ichinohe T, Hayashida M, Fukuda K, Ikeda K. Prediction formulas for individual opioid analgesic requirements based on genetic polymorphism analyses. PLoS One. 2015;10(1):e0116885. https://doi.org/10.1371/journal.pone.0116885.
19. Fukuda K, Hayashida M, Ide S, Saita N, Kokita Y, Kasai S, Nishizawa D, Ogai Y, Hasegawa J, Nagashima M, Tagami M, Komatsu H, Sora I, Koga H, Kaneko Y, Ikeda K. Association between OPRM1 gene polymorphisms and fentanyl sensitivity in patients undergoing painful cosmetic surgery. Pain. 2009;147(1–3):194–201. https://doi.org/10.1016/j.pain.2009.09.004.
20. Kelly DJ, Ahmad M, Brull SJ. Preemptive analgesia I: physiological pathways and pharmacological modalities. Can J Anaesth. 2001;48(10):1000–10.
21. Woolf CJ, Chong MS. Preemptive analgesia—treating postoperative pain by preventing the establishment of central sensitization. Anesth Analg. 1993;77:362.
22. Campbell WI, Kendrick RW, Ramsay-Baggs P, McCaughey W. The effect of pre-operative administration of bupivacaine compared with its postoperative use. Anaesthesia. 1997;52(12):1212–6.
23. Campbell WI, Kendrick RW. Pre-emptive analgesia using local anaesthesia: a study in bilaterally symmetrical surgery. Br J Anaesth. 1997;79:657–9.
24. Campbell WI, Kendrick RW, Fee JP. Balanced pre-emptive analgesia: does it work? A double-blind, controlled study in bilaterally symmetrical oral surgery. Br J Anaesth. 1998;81:727.
25. Bridgman JB, Gillgrass TG, Zacharias M. The absence of any pre-emptive analgesic effect for non-steroidal anti-inflammatory drugs. Br J Oral Maxillofac Surg. 1996;34:428.
26. Lebrun T, Van Elstraete AC, Sandefo I, et al. Lack of a pre-emptive effect of low-dose ketamine on postoperative pain following oral surgery. Can J Anaesth. 2006;53:146.
27. Melzack R, Wall PD. Pain mechanisms: a new theory. Science. 1965;150:971.
28. Kissin I. Preemptive analgesia. Anesthesiology. 2000;93:1138.
29. Eriksson L, Tegelberg A. Analgesic efficacy and clinical acceptability of adjunct pre-emptive intrave-

nous tramadol in midazolam sedation for third molar surgery. Oral Maxillofac Surg. 2012;17:193.
30. Eriksson LB, Tegelberg Å. Safety of adjunct pre-emptive intravenous tramadol with midazolam sedation for third molar surgery. Oral Maxillofac Surg. 2015;19(4):353–9. https://doi.org/10.1007/s10006-015-0502-9.
31. Pandit MK, Godhi S, Lall AB. Preoperative intravenous tramadol versus diclofenac for preventing postoperative pain after third molar surgery: a comparative study. J Maxillofac Oral Surg. 2011;10(4):306–9. https://doi.org/10.1007/s12663-011-0250-9.
32. Shah AV, Arun Kumar KV, Rai KK, Rajesh Kumar BP. Comparative evaluation of pre-emptive analgesic efficacy of intramuscular ketorolac versus tramadol following third molar surgery. J Maxillofac Oral Surg. 2013;12(2):197–202. https://doi.org/10.1007/s12663-012-0420-4.
33. Shah AV, Arun Kumar KV, Rai KK, Rajesh Kumar BP. Comparative evaluation of pre-emptive analgesic efficacy of intramuscular ketorolac versus tramadol following third molar surgery. J Maxillofac Oral Surg. 2013;12(2):197–202. https://doi.org/10.1007/s12663-012-0420-4.
34. Gopalraju P, Lalitha RM, Prasad K, Ranganath K. Comparative study of intravenous tramadol versus ketorolac for preventing postoperative pain after third molar surgery--a prospective randomized study. J Craniomaxillofac Surg. 2014;42(5):629–33. https://doi.org/10.1016/j.jcms.2013.09.004.
35. Lustenberger FD, Grätz KW, Mutzbauer TS. Efficacy of ibuprofen versus lornoxicam after third molar surgery: a randomized, double-blind, crossover pilot study. Oral Maxillofac Surg. 2011;15(1):57–62. https://doi.org/10.1007/s10006-010-0255-4.
36. Lau SL, Chow RL, Yeung RW, Samman N. Pre-emptive ibuprofen arginate in third molar surgery: a double-blind randomized controlled crossover clinical trial. Aust Dent J. 2009;54(4):355–60. https://doi.org/10.1111/j.1834-7819.2009.01162.x.
37. Morse Z, Tump A, Kevelham E. Ibuprofen as a pre-emptive analgesic is as effective as rofecoxib for mandibular third molar surgery. Odontology. 2006;94(1):59–63.
38. Costa FW, Soares EC, Esses DF, Silva PG, Bezerra TP, Scarparo HC, Ribeiro TR, Fonteles CS. A split-mouth, randomized, triple-blind, placebo-controlled study to analyze the pre-emptive effect of etoricoxib 120 mg on inflammatory events following removal of unerupted mandibular third molars. Int J Oral Maxillofac Surg. 2015;44(9):1166–74. https://doi.org/10.1016/j.ijom.2015.06.012.
39. Al-Sukhun J, Al-Sukhun S, Penttila H, et al. Preemptive analgesic effect of low doses of celecoxib is superior to low doses of traditional nonsteroidal anti-inflammatory drugs. J Craniofac Surg. 2012;23:526.
40. Cillo JE Jr, Dattilo DJ. Pre-emptive analgesia with pregabalin and celecoxib decreases postsurgical pain following maxillomandibular advancement surgery: a randomized controlled clinical trial. J Oral Maxillofac Surg. 2014;72(10):1909–14. https://doi.org/10.1016/j.joms.2014.05.014.
41. Gopalraju P, Lalitha RM, Prasad K, Ranganath K. Comparative study of intravenous tramadol versus ketorolac for preventing postoperative pain after third molar surgery--a prospective randomized study. J Craniomaxillofac Surg. 2014;42(5):629–33. https://doi.org/10.1016/j.jcms.2013.09.004.
42. Pozos-Guillen A, Martinez-Rider R, Aguirre-Banuelos P, Perez-Urizar J. Pre-emptive analgesic effect of tramadol after mandibular third molar extraction: a pilot study. J Oral Maxillofac Surg. 2007;65(7):1315–20.
43. da Costa Arajo FA, de Santana ST, de Morais HH, Laureano Filho JR, de Oliveira E Silva ED, Vasconcellos RJ. Comparative analysis of pre-emptive analgesic effect of tramadol chlorhydrate and nimesulide following third molar surgery. J Craniomaxillofac Surg. 2012;40(8):e346–9. https://doi.org/10.1016/j.jcms.2012.01.018.
44. Isiordia-Espinoza MA, Sanchez-Prieto M, Tobas F, Reyes-Garcia JG, Granados-Soto V. Pre-emptive analgesia with the combination of tramadol plus meloxicam for third molar surgery: a pilot study. Br J Oral Maxillofac Surg. 2012;50(7):673–7. https://doi.org/10.1016/j.bjoms.2011.12.003.
45. Sener M, Ozgur Pektas Z, Yilmaz I, Turkoz A, Uckan S, Donmez A, Arslan G. Comparison of preemptive analgesic effects of a single dose of nonopioid analgesics for pain management after ambulatory surgery: a prospective, randomized, single-blind study in Turkish patients. Curr Ther Res Clin Exp. 2005;66(6):541–51. https://doi.org/10.1016/j.curtheres.2005.12.001.
46. Ahiskalioglu A, Ance A, Aksoy M, Yalcin E, Ahiskalioglu EO, Kilinc A. Effects of a single-dose of pre-Emptive Pregabalin on postoperative pain and opioid consumption after double-jaw surgery: a randomized controlled trial. J Oral Maxillofac Surg. 2016;74(1):53.e1–7. https://doi.org/10.1016/j.joms.2015.09.008.
47. Moore RA, Derry S, Aldington D, Wiffen PJ. Single dose oral analgesics for acute postoperative pain in adults-an overview of Cochrane reviews. Cochrane Database Syst Rev. 2015;(9):CD008659. https://doi.org/10.1002/14651858.CD008659.pub3.
48. Dionne RA. Additive analgesic effects of oxycodone and ibuprofen in the oral surgery model. J Oral Maxillofac Surg. 1999;57(6):673–8.
49. Mehlisch DR, Sollecito WA, Helfrick LF. Multicenter clinical trial of ibuprofen and acetaminophen in the treatment of postoperative dental pain. J Am Dent Assoc. 1990;121:257.
50. Kehlet H, Dahl JB. The value of "multimodal" or "balanced analgesia" in postoperative pain treatment. Anesth Analg. 1993;77:1048.
51. Ma CSJ, Lin D. Patient controlled analgesia: drug options infusion schedules and other considerations. Hosp Formul. 1991;26:198.

52. Miller RD. Anesthesia. New York, NY: Churchill Livingstone; 1990.
53. Geha H, Nimeskern N, Beziat JL. Patient-controlled analgesia in orthognathic surgery: evaluation of the relationship to anxiety and anxiolytics. Oral Surg Oral Med Oral Pathol Oral Radiol Endod. 2009;108(3):e33–6. https://doi.org/10.1016/j.tripleo.2009.05.027.
54. Precious DS, Multari J, Finley GA, McGrath P. A comparison of patient-controlled and fixed schedule analgesia after orthognathic surgery. J Oral Maxillofac Surg. 1997;55(1):33–9.
55. Hepso HU, Lokken P, Bjornson J, Godan HC. Double-blind crossover study of the effect of acetylsalicylic acid on bleeding and post-operative course after bilateral oral surgery. J Clin Pharmacol. 1976;10:217–25.
56. Skelbred J, Lokken P. Acetylsalicylic acid vs. paracetamol, effects on post-operative course. Eur J Clin Pharmacol. 1977;12:257–69.
57. Moore PA, Crout RJ, Jackson DL, Schneider LG, Graves RW, Bakos L. Tramadol hydrochloride: analgesic efficacy compared with codeine, aspirin with codeine, and placebo after dental extraction. J Clin Pharmacol. 1998;38(6):554–60.
58. Moore PA, Nahouraii HS, Zovko JG, Wisniewski SR. Dental therapeutic practice patterns in the U.S. II. Analgesics, corticosteroids, and antibiotics. Gen Dent. 2006;54(3):201–7.
59. Aznar-Arasa L, Harutunian K, Figueiredo R, Valmaseda-Castellon E, Gay-Escoda C. Effect of preoperative ibuprofen on pain and swelling after lower third molar removal: a randomized controlled trial. Int J Oral Maxillofac Surg. 2012;41(8):1005–9. https://doi.org/10.1016/j.ijom.2011.12.028.
60. Bailey E, Worthington HV, van Wijk A, Yates JM, Coulthard P, Afzal Z. Ibuprofen and/or paracetamol (acetaminophen) for pain relief after surgical removal of lower wisdom teeth. Cochrane Database Syst Rev. 2013;(12):CD004624. https://doi.org/10.1002/14651858.CD004624.pub2.
61. Bailey E, Worthington H, Coulthard P. Ibuprofen and/or paracetamol (acetaminophen) for pain relief after surgical removal of lower wisdom teeth, a Cochrane systematic review. Br Dent J. 2014;216(8):451–5. https://doi.org/10.1038/sj.bdj.2014.330.
62. Ferraiolo DM, Veitz-Keenan A. Ibuprofen is superior to paracetamol for pain relief following third molar removal. Evid Based Dent. 2014;15(4):106–7. https://doi.org/10.1038/sj.ebd.6401059.
63. Au AH, Choi SW, Cheung CW, Leung YY. The efficacy and clinical safety of various analgesic combinations for post-operative pain after third molar surgery: a systematic review and meta-analysis. PLoS One. 2015;10(6):e0127611. https://doi.org/10.1371/journal.pone.0127611.
64. Litkowski LJ, Christensen SE, Adamson DN, Van Dyke T, Han SH, Newman KB. Analgesic efficacy and tolerability of oxycodone 5 mg/ibuprofen 400 mg compared with those of oxycodone 5 mg/acetaminophen 325 mg and hydrocodone 7.5 mg/acetaminophen 500 mg in patients with moderate to severe postoperative pain: a randomized, double-blind, placebo-controlled, single-dose, parallel-group study in a dental pain model. Clin Ther. 2005;27(4):418–29.
65. Derry CJ, Derry S, Moore RA. Single dose oral ibuprofen plus paracetamol (acetaminophen) for acute postoperative pain. Cochrane Database Syst Rev. 2013;24(6):CD010210. https://doi.org/10.1002/14651858.CD010210.pub2.
66. Moore PA, Hersh EV. Combining ibuprofen and acetaminophen for acute pain management after third-molar extractions: translating clinical research to dental practice. J Am Dent Assoc. 2013;144(8):898–908.
67. Sisk AL, Grover BJ. A comparison of preoperative and postoperative naproxen sodium for suppression of postoperative pain. J Oral Maxillofac Surg. 1990;48(7):674–8.
68. Kiersch TA, Halladay SC, Koschik M. A double-blind, randomized study of naproxen sodium, ibuprofen, and placebo in postoperative dental pain. Clin Ther. 1993;15(5):845–54.
69. Kara IM, Polat S, Inci MF, Gamay C. Analgesic and anti-inflammatory effects of oxaprozin and naproxen sodium after removal of impacted lower third molars: a randomized, double-blind, placebo-controlled crossover study. J Oral Maxillofac Surg. 2010;68(5):1018–24. https://doi.org/10.1016/j.joms.2009.09.094.
70. Fricke J, Halladay SC, Bynum L, Francisco CA. Pain relief after dental impaction surgery using ketorolac, hydrocodone plus acetaminophen, or placebo. Clin Ther. 1993;15(3):500–9.
71. Gutta R, Koehn CR, James LE. Does ketorolac have a preemptive analgesic effect? A randomized, double-blind, control study. J Oral Maxillofac Surg. 2013;71(12):2029–34. https://doi.org/10.1016/j.joms.2013.06.220.
72. Niebler G, Dayno J. Effect size comparison of ketorolac nasal spray and commonly prescribed oral combination opioids for pain relief after third molar extraction surgery. Postgrad Med. 2016;128(1):12–7. https://doi.org/10.1080/00325481.2016.1126185.
73. Garibaldi JA, Elder MF. Evaluation of ketorolac (Toradol) with varying amounts of codeine for postoperative extraction pain control. Int J Oral Maxillofac Surg. 2002;31(3):276–80.
74. Aoki T, Ota Y, Mori Y, Otsuru M, Ota M, Kaneko A. Analgesic efficacy of celecoxib in patients after oral surgery: special reference to time to onset of analgesia and duration of analgesic effect. Oral Maxillofac Surg. 2016;20(3):265–71. https://doi.org/10.1007/s10006-016-0565-2.
75. Yamashita Y, Sano N, Shimohira D, Danjo A, Goto M. A parallel-group comparison study of celecoxib

with loxoprofen sodium in third mandibular molar extraction patients. Int J Oral Maxillofac Surg. 2014;43(12):1509–13. https://doi.org/10.1016/j.ijom.2014.09.002.

76. Moghaddamnia AA, Nosrati K, Mehdizadeh M, Milani S, Aghvami M. A comparative study of the effect of prednisolone and Celecoxib on MMO (maximum mouth opening) and pain following removal of impacted mandibular third molars. J Maxillofac Oral Surg. 2013;12(2):184–7. https://doi.org/10.1007/s12663-012-0401-7.
77. Saito K, Kaneko A, Machii K, Ohta H, Ohkura M, Suzuki M. Efficacy and safety of additional 200-mg dose of celecoxib in adult patients with postoperative pain following extraction of impacted third mandibular molar: a multicenter, randomized, double-blind, placebo-controlled, phase II study in Japan. Clin Ther. 2012;34(2):314–28. https://doi.org/10.1016/j.clinthera.2012.01.004.
78. Pilatti GL, Andr_e dos Santos F, Bianchi A, et al. The use of celecoxib and dexamethasone for the prevention and control of postoperative pain after periodontal surgery. J Periodontol. 2006;77:1809.
79. Ong KS, Tan JM. Preoperative intravenous tramadol versus ketorolac for preventing postoperative pain after third molar surgery. Int J Oral Maxillofac Surg. 2004;33(3):274–8.
80. Claseman TS, Foley WL, Davis RD, Morrison JW, Palmore CA, Murchison DF. A clinical evaluation of the analgesic efficacy of preoperative administration of ketorolac and dexamethasone following surgical removal of third molars. Anesth Prog. 1998;45(3):110–6.
81. Ong KS, Seymour RA, Chen FG, Ho VC. Preoperative ketorolac has a preemptive effect for postoperative third molar surgical pain. Int J Oral Maxillofac Surg. 2004;33(8):771–6.
82. Christensen K, Daniels S, Bandy D, Ernst CC, Hamilton DA, Mermelstein FH, Wang J, Carr DB. A double-blind placebo-controlled comparison of a novel formulation of intravenous diclofenac and ketorolac for postoperative third molar extraction pain. Anesth Prog. 2011;58(2):73–81. https://doi.org/10.2344/0003-3006-58.2.73.
83. Gopalraju P, Lalitha RM, Prasad K, Ranganath K. Comparative study of intravenous tramadol versus ketorolac for preventing postoperative pain after third molar surgery--a prospective randomized study. J Craniomaxillofac Surg. 2014;42(5):629–33. https://doi.org/10.1016/j.jcms.2013.09.004.
84. Chin KR, Sundram H, Marcotte P. Bleeding risk with ketorolac after lumbar microdiscectomy. J Spinal Disord Tech. 2007;20(2):123–6.
85. Gan TJ, Candiotti K, Turan A, Buvanendran A, Philip BK, Viscusi ER, Soghomonyan S, Bergese SD, Intravenous Ibuprofen Surgical Surveillance Trial Investigational Sites. The shortened infusion time of intravenous ibuprofen, part 2: a multicenter, open-label, surgical surveillance trial to evaluate safety. Clin Ther. 2015;37(2):368–75. https://doi.org/10.1016/j.clinthera.2014.12.006.
86. Gwirtz KH, Kim HC, Nagy DJ, Young JV, Byers RS, Kovach DA, Li W. Intravenous ketorolac and subarachnoid opioid analgesia in the management of acute postoperative pain. Reg Anesth. 1995;20(5):395–401.
87. Houck CS, Wilder RT, McDermott JS, Sethna NF, Berde CB. Safety of intravenous ketorolac therapy in children and cost savings with a unit dosing system. J Pediatr. 1996;129(2):292–6.
88. Bergese SD, Candiotti K, Ayad SS, Soghomonyan S, Gan TJ, Intravenous Ibuprofen Surveillance Trial Investigational Sites. The shortened infusion time of intravenous ibuprofen part 1: a multicenter, open-label, surveillance trial to evaluate safety and efficacy. Clin Ther. 2015;37(2):360–7. https://doi.org/10.1016/j.clinthera.2014.12.004.
89. Moller PL, Juhl GI, Payen-Champenois C, Skoglund LA. Intravenous acetaminophen (paracetamol): comparable analgesic efficacy, but better local safety than its prodrug, propacetamol, for postoperative pain after third molar surgery. Anesth Analg. 2005;101(1):90–6.
90. Southworth S, Peters J, Rock A, Pavliv L. A multicenter, randomized, double-blind, placebo-controlled trial of intravenous ibuprofen 400 and 800 mg every 6 hours in the management of postoperative pain. Clin Ther. 2009;31(9):1922–35. https://doi.org/10.1016/j.clinthera.2009.08.026.
91. Marquez-Lara A, Hutchinson ID, Nuñez F Jr, Smith TL, Miller AN. Nonsteroidal anti-inflammatory drugs and bone-healing: a systematic review of research quality. JBJS Rev;4(3), 2016. pii: 01874474-201603000-00005. doi:https://doi.org/10.2106/JBJS.RVW.O.00055.
92. Mutlu I, Abubaker AO, Laskin DM. Narcotic prescribing habits and other methods of pain control by oral and maxillofacial surgeons after impacted third molar removal. J Oral Maxillofac Surg. 2013;71:1500.
93. Rosenberg M, Carroll F, Negus S. Effects of monoamine reuptake inhibitors in assays of acute pain-stimulated and pain-depressed behavior in rats. J Pain. 2013;14(3):246–59. https://doi.org/10.1016/j.jpain.2012.11.006.
94. Scott RF. A double-blind comparison of nalbuphine and meperidine hydrochloride as intravenous analgesics in combination with diazepam for oral surgery outpatients. J Oral Maxillofac Surg. 1987;45(6):473–6.
95. Isiordia-Espinoza MA, de Jesús Pozos-Guillén A, Aragon-Martinez OH. Analgesic efficacy and safety of single-dose tramadol and non-steroidal anti-inflammatory drugs in operations on the third molars: a systematic review and meta-analysis. Br J Oral Maxillofac Surg. 2014;52(9):775–83. https://doi.org/10.1016/j.bjoms.2014.05.005.

96. Isiordia-Espinoza MA, Pozos-Guillen A, Martinez-Rider R, Perez-Urizar J. Comparison of the analgesic efficacy of oral ketorolac versus intramuscular tramadol after third molar surgery: a parallel, double-blind, randomized, placebo-controlled clinical trial. Med Oral Patol Oral Cir Bucal. 2016;21(5):e637–43.
97. Ong CK, Lirk P, Tan JM, Sow BW. The analgesic efficacy of intravenous versus oral tramadol for preventing postoperative pain after third molar surgery. J Oral Maxillofac Surg. 2005;63(8):1162–8.
98. Perez-Urizar J, MartÃnez-Rider R, Torres-Roque I, Garrocho-Rangel A, Pozos-Guillen A. Analgesic efficacy of lysine clonixinate plus tramadol versus tramadol in multiple doses following impacted third molar surgery. Int J Oral Maxillofac Surg. 2014;43(3):348–54. https://doi.org/10.1016/j.ijom.2013.08.003.
99. Collins M, Young I, Sweeney P, Fenn GC, Stratford ME, Wilson A, Harris M. The effect of tramadol on dento-alveolar surgical pain. Br J Oral Maxillofac Surg. 1997;35(1):54–8.
100. Hassan SS, Ahmed A, Rai M, Kalappa TM. Analgesic efficacy of tramadol and butorphanol in mandibular third molar surgery: a comparative study. J Contemp Dent Pract. 2012;13(3):364–70.
101. Gönül O, Satilmiş T, Ciftci A, Sipahi A, Garip H, Göker K. Comparison of the effects of topical ketamine and tramadol on postoperative pain after mandibular molar extraction. J Oral Maxillofac Surg. 2015;73(11):2103–7. https://doi.org/10.1016/j.joms.2015.05.012.
102. Pozos AJ, MartÃnez R, Aguirre P, Pérez J. Tramadol administered in a combination of routes for reducing pain after removal of an impacted mandibular third molar. J Oral Maxillofac Surg. 2007;65(8):1633–9.
103. Medve RA, Wang J, Karim R. Tramadol and acetaminophen tablets for dental pain. Anesth Prog. 2001;48(3):79–81.
104. Fricke JR Jr, Karim R, Jordan D, Rosenthal N. A double-blind, single-dose comparison of the analgesic efficacy of tramadol/acetaminophen combination tablets, hydrocodone/acetaminophen combination tablets, and placebo after oral surgery. Clin Ther Jun. 2002;24(6):953–68.
105. Ziccardi VB, Desjardins PJ, Daly-DeJoy E, Seng GF. Single-dose vicoprofen compared with acetaminophen with codeine and placebo in patients with acute postoperative pain after third molar extractions. J Oral Maxillofac Surg. 2000;58(6):622–8.
106. Forbes JA, Bates JA, Edquist IA, Burchfield WH, Smith FG, Schwartz MK, Kit V, Hyatt J, Bell WE, Beaver WT. Evaluation of two opioid-acetaminophen combinations and placebo in postoperative oral surgery pain. Pharmacotherapy. 1994;14(2):139–46.
107. Yagoubian B, Akkara J, Afzali P, Alfi DM, Olson L, Conell-Price J, Yeh J, Eisig SB, Flood P. Nicotine nasal spray as an adjuvant analgesic for third molar surgery. J Oral Maxillofac Surg. 2011;69(5):1316–9. https://doi.org/10.1016/j.joms.2010.07.025.
108. Freda NM, Keenan AV. Moderate evidence to recommend submucosal injection of dexamethasone in reducing post-operative oedema and pain after third molar extraction. Evid Based Dent. 2016;17(2):58–9. https://doi.org/10.1038/sj.ebd.6401174.
109. Eshghpour M, Mortazavi H, Mohammadzadeh Rezaei N, Nejat A. Effectiveness of green tea mouthwash in postoperative pain control following surgical removal of impacted third molars: double blind randomized clinical trial. Daru. 2013;21(1):59. https://doi.org/10.1186/2008-2231-21-59.
110. Olmedo-Gaya MV, Manzano-Moreno FJ, Galvez-Mateos R, GonzÃ¡lez-Rodriguez MP, Talero-Sevilla C, Vallecillo-Capilla M. Oral pregabalin for postoperative pain relief after third molar extraction: a randomized controlled clinical trial. Clin Oral Investig. 2016;20(7):1819–26. https://doi.org/10.1007/s00784-015-1657-3.
111. Hill CM, Balkenohl M, Thomas DW, Walker R, Mathé H, Murray G. Pregabalin in patients with postoperative dental pain. Eur J Pain. 2001;5(2):119–24.
112. Cheung CW, Choi WS, Leung YY, Lui F, Ng JK, Hei-Ho AM, Irwin MG. A double-blind randomized crossover study to evaluate the timing of pregabalin for third molar surgery under local anesthesia. J Oral Maxillofac Surg. 2012;70(1):25–30. https://doi.org/10.1016/j.joms.2011.03.056.
113. Brkovic B, Gardasevic M, Roganovic J, Jovic N, Todorovic L, Stojic D. Lidocaine+clonidine for maxillary infiltration anaesthesia: parameters of anaesthesia and vascular effects. Int J Oral Maxillofac Surg. 2008;37(2):149–55.
114. Brkovic B, Todorovic L, Stojic D. Comparison of clonidine and epinephrine in lidocaine anaesthesia for lower third molar surgery. Int J Oral Maxillofac Surg. 2005;34(4):401–6.
115. Patil PM, Patil SP. Is clonidine an adequate alternative to epinephrine as a vasoconstrictor in patients with hypertension? J Oral Maxillofac Surg. 2012;70(2):257–62. https://doi.org/10.1016/j.joms.2011.07.011.
116. Tuffin JR, Cunliffe DR, Shaw SR. Do local analgesics injected at the time of third molar removal under general anaesthesia reduce significantly post-operative analgesic requirements? A double-blind controlled trial. Br J Oral Maxillofac Surg. 1989;27(1):27–32.
117. Gordon SM, Dionne RA, Brahim J, Jabir F, Dubner R. Blockade of peripheral neuronal barrage reduces postoperative pain. Pain. 1997;70:209–15.
118. Nayyar MS, Yates C. Bupivacaine as pre-emptive analgesia in third molar surgery: randomised controlled trial. Br J Oral Maxillofac Surg. 2006;44(6):501–3.
119. Hersh EV, Moore PA. Comment on controlling dental post-operative pain and the intraoral local delivery of drugs. Curr Med Res Opin. 2015;31(12):2185–7. https://doi.org/10.1185/03007995.2015.1109504.

120. Tordoff SG, Brossy M, Rowbotham DJ, James JN, James R, Raphael JH. The effect of pre-incisional infiltration with lignocaine on postoperative pain after molar teeth extraction under general anaesthesia. Anaesthesia. 1996;51:585–7.
121. Singh K, Phillips FM, Kuo E, Campbell M. A prospective, randomized, double-blind study of the efficacy of postoperative continuous local anesthetic infusion at the iliac crest bone graft site after posterior spinal arthrodesis: a minimum of 4-year follow-up. Spine (Phila Pa 1976). 2007;32(25):2790–6. https://doi.org/10.1097/BRS.0b013e31815b7650.
122. Puri R, Moskovich R, Gusmorino P, Shott S. Bupivacaine for postoperative pain relief at the iliac crest bone graft harvest site. Am J Orthop (Belle Mead NJ). 2000;29(6):443–6.
123. Hahn M, Dover MS, Whear NM, Moule I. Local bupivacaine infusion following bone graft harvest from the iliac crest. Int J Oral Maxillofac Surg. 1996;25(5):400–1.
124. Saikrishna D, Sujit S, Sheetal KR. Use of a modified epidural catheter for analgesia after iliac crest bone procurement. J Maxillofac Oral Surg. 2009;8(3):254–6. https://doi.org/10.1007/s12663-009-0062-3.
125. Sbitany H, Koltz PF, Waldman J, Girotto JA. Continuous bupivacaine infusion in iliac bone graft donor sites to minimize pain and hospitalization. Cleft Palate Craniofac J. 2010;47(3):293–6. https://doi.org/10.1597/09-049.1.
126. O'Neill KR, Lockney DT, Bible JE, Crosby CG, Devin CJ. Bupivacaine for pain reduction after iliac crest bone graft harvest. Orthopedics. 2014;37(5):e428–34. https://doi.org/10.3928/01477447-20140430-52.
127. Hoard MA, Bill TJ, Campbell RL. Reduction in morbidity after iliac crest bone harvesting: the concept of preemptive analgesia. J Craniofac Surg. 1998;9(5):448–51.
128. Barkhuysen R, Meijer GJ, Soehardi A, Merkx MA, Borstlap WA, BergÃ SJ, Bronkhorst EM, Hoppenreijs TJ. The effect of a single dose of bupivacaine on donor site pain after anterior iliac crest bone harvesting. Int J Oral Maxillofac Surg. 2010;39(3):260–5. https://doi.org/10.1016/j.ijom.2009.10.015.
129. Gamli M, Dalgic A, Ornek D, Horasanli E, Kilci O, Un C, Dikmen B. Evaluation of the efficacy of bupivacaine soaked in Gelfoam(Â®) at the iliac crest bone graft site. Rev Bras Anestesiol. 2012;62(6):811–8. https://doi.org/10.1016/S0034-7094(12)70181-2.
130. Kukidome H, Matsuura N, Kasahara M, Ichinohe T. Continuous postoperative pain control using a multiple-hole catheter after iliac bone grafting: comparison between ropivacaine and levobupivacaine. Int J Oral Maxillofac Surg. 2016;45(4):454–9. https://doi.org/10.1016/j.ijom.2015.09.010.
131. Modi M, Rastogi S, Kumar A. Buprenorphine with bupivacaine for intraoral nerve blocks to provide postoperative analgesia in outpatients after minor oral surgery. J Oral Maxillofac Surg. 2009;67(12):2571–6. https://doi.org/10.1016/j.joms.2009.07.014.
132. Bernard JM, Macaire P. Dose-range effects of clonidine added to lidocaine for brachial plexus block. Anesthesiology. 1997;87:277.
133. Moore UJ, Seymour RA, Gilroy J, Rawlins MD. The efficacy of locally applied morphine in post-operative pain after bilateral third molar surgery. Br J Clin Pharmacol. 1994;37(3):227–30.
134. Dionne RA, Gordon SM, Tahara M, et al. Analgesic efficacy and pharmacokinetics of ketoprofen administered into a surgical site. J Clin Pharmacol. 1999;39:131.
135. Strumper D, Durieux ME. Antidepressants as long-acting local anesthetics. Reg Anesth Pain Med. 2004;29:277.
136. Bazin JE, Massoni C, Bruelle P. The addition of opioids to local anaesthetics in brachial plexus block: the comparative effects of morphine, buprenorphine and sufentanil. Anesthesia. 1997;52:858.
137. Kapral S, Gollmann G, Waltl B, et al. Tramadol added to mepivacaine prolongs the duration of an axillary brachial plexus blockade. Anesth Analg. 1999;88:853.
138. Robaux S, Blunt C, Viel E, et al. Tramadol added to 1.5% mepivacaine for axillary brachial plexus block improves postoperative analgesia dose-dependently. Anesth Analg. 2004;98:1172.
139. Yue Y, Collaku A, Brown J, Buchanan WL, Reed K, Cooper SA, Otto J. Efficacy and speed of onset of pain relief of fast-dissolving paracetamol on postsurgical dental pain: two randomized, single-dose, double-blind, placebo-controlled clinical studies. Clin Ther. 2013;35(9):1306–20. https://doi.org/10.1016/j.clinthera.2013.07.422.
140. Moeller C, Pawlowski J, Pappas AL, Fargo K, Welch K. The safety and efficacy of intravenous ketorolac in patients undergoing primary endoscopic sinus surgery: a randomized, double-blinded clinical trial. Int Forum Allergy Rhinol. 2012;2(4):342–7. https://doi.org/10.1002/alr.21028.
141. Van Aken H, Thys L, Veekman L, Buerkle H. Assessing analgesia in single and repeated administrations of propacetamol for postoperative pain: comparison with morphine after dental surgery. Anesth Analg. 2004;98(1):159–65.
142. Juhl GI, Norholt SE, Tonnesen E, Hiesse-Provost O, Jensen TS. Analgesic efficacy and safety of intravenous paracetamol (acetaminophen) administered as a 2-g starting dose following third molar surgery. Eur J Pain. 2006;10(4):371–7.

12 Chronic Medications and Maxillofacial Surgery

James Omlie and Andrew Herlich

Abstract

The decision to continue or stop using chronic medication is maybe controversial, and it is important to understand the current guidelines utilizing evidence-based medicine. The controversy lies within the limited evidence regarding many medications and the importance of strategizing medication management on an individual basis. Much of what we do is in the gray zone. The more complicated patients take many medications. As patient' disease states change, this influences when, where, and how a surgery is planned and how medications are administered. We have put a "bottom line" at the beginning of each section to facilitate a quick decision when necessary.

12.1 Cardiovascular Medications

12.1.1 Beta-Blockers

Bottom line: Continue beta-blockers through the day of surgery. Do not initiate beta blockade acutely prior to the surgical procedure. There is no data for the initiation of beta blockade in head and neck surgery. In the case of an urgent procedure, it is recommended to proceed without beta blockade in communication with a cardiologist, anesthesiologist, surgeon, and the patient.

Chronic use of beta-blockers is associated with certain disease states, such as ischemic heart disease and congestive heart failure. There has been considerable debate as to whether one should be started on a beta-blocker prior to major noncardiac surgery given certain risk factors; however, it is generally agreed that those on chronic therapy or being treated post cardiovascular/cerebrovascular event should be continued on that medication [1–3]. Beta-blockers reduce ischemia by reducing myocardial oxygen demand, which has a net effect greater than the decreased perfusion. Additionally, patients with atrial fibrillation are treated with this medication

J. Omlie, D.D.S., M.D. (✉)
Department of Oral and Maxillofacial Surgery, University of Pittsburgh Medical Center, Pittsburgh, PA, USA
e-mail: omliejj@upmc.edu

A. Herlich, D.M.D., M.D., F.A.A.P
Department of Anesthesiology, University of Pittsburgh School of Medicine, Pittsburgh, PA, USA

© Springer International Publishing AG 2018

E.M. Ferneini, J.D. Bennett (eds.), *Perioperative Assessment of the Maxillofacial Surgery Patient*,
https://doi.org/10.1007/978-3-319-58868-1_12

for rate control, which has been shown to be more efficacious than rhythm control [4]. Patients who have been taking this class of medication for more than a short time span have an upregulation of beta receptors. Abrupt withdrawal of these medications can result in significant morbidity and mortality due to the high risk of ischemia [5]. Continuous use of beta-blockers during the perioperative period demonstrated significantly less morbidity and mortality at 30 days and 1 year postoperatively compared to those who discontinued use during the perioperative period [6]. The POISE trial and several other studies have shown that initiating β-blockers in noncardiac surgery resulted in total mortality and stroke [7, 8]. Additionally, a 2014 meta-analysis looked at 16 randomized controlled trials (RCTs) and a cohort study with 12,000 patients in which a beta-blocker was started within 24 hours of noncardiac surgery showing a 30% increase in the 30-day risk of all-cause mortality [8]. If any questions arise in a patient with recent cardiovascular, cerebrovascular events, and the surgery can be postponed, a discussion among a cardiologist, anesthesiologist, surgeon, and patient must be had to properly plan any therapy with class of medication.

12.1.2 Alpha-2 Agonists

Bottom line: Continue alpha-2 agonists due to high risk of rebound hypertension with acute withdrawal. Do not initiate therapy prior to procedure.

Alpha-2 agonists, such as clonidine, have the potential to reduce the high catecholamine state associated with surgery. The POISE-2 trial examined the initiation of clonidine preoperatively in noncardiac surgery in over 10,000 patients. This study showed increased incidence of clinically significant hypotension and nonfatal cardiac arrest with no improvement in all-cause mortality and myocardial infarction [9]. Patients already on this antihypertensive therapy should continue use during the perioperative period due to rebound hypertension when the medication is withdrawn abruptly [10, 11]. Coordination among a cardiologist, anesthesiologist, surgeon, and patient is recommended if patient cannot be administered pills in the postoperative period. If PO intake is not an option, transdermal patches can be used, but this must be initiated 3 days prior to surgery with communication among the team.

12.1.3 Calcium Channel Blockers

Bottom line: Continue calcium channel blockers (CCBs) through the morning of surgery.

Patients on CCBs are more likely to have several comorbidities that contribute to postoperative complications such as diabetes mellitus, peripheral vascular disease, and COPD [12, 13]. This patient population is generally less healthy, and there are theoretical and evidence-based benefits of CCBs in improving perioperative ischemia by treating the balance of myocardial oxygen supply and demand. CCBs theoretically improve this balance through negative inotropic, negative chronotropic, afterload reducing, and coronary vasodilator properties [12]. There are no reported interactions with anesthetics or acute withdrawal syndromes (exception of coronary vasospasm with coronary revascularization procedures). A meta-analysis showed reduced ischemia and atrial arrhythmias in patients undergoing noncardiac surgery, as well as decreased incidence of major end points (CHF, MI, and death) with CCB use [12]. There are reports of minor intraoperative hypotension when beta-blockers and CCBs were taken concomitantly; however, these responded to small boluses of ephedrine without any adverse outcomes [14]. There have been several reports and studies documenting the possible interaction between CCBs and increased propensity for bleeding. Theoretically there is thought to be a CCB-mediated inhibition of platelet aggregation and of protective vasoconstriction [15]. However, these studies are largely inconclusive due to shortcomings of the respective studies due to patient population and possible protective beta-blocker effect in those with GI bleeds. Two studies in patients undergoing cardiac surgery failed to demonstrate similar results with 1 cohort study involving 5157 patients receiving nimodipine intraoperatively [15–17]. CCBs should be continued due to the theoretical benefit, lack of evidence showing CCB-related adverse cardiovascular events, and contradictory findings as to whether they increase bleeding risk.

12.1.4 ACE Inhibitors and Angiotensin II Receptor Blockers

Bottom line: The decision to continue or discontinue the morning of surgery should be individualized to the patient and type of procedure. This should be discussed with the prescribing physician, anesthesiologist, surgeon, and the patient. Patients on multiple antihypertensive medications and/or being treated for congestive heart failure will likely need to have this medication continued through the day of surgery. It is important to remember that the therapeutic effect of ACE inhibitors (ACEI) and angiotensin II receptor blockers (ARBs) is typically observed several weeks after initiation of therapy.

The management of patients on ACE inhibitors or angiotensin II receptor blockers in the perioperative period has been a subject of controversy due to multiple confounding factors. The mechanism of action is blunting of the renin-angiotensin-aldosterone system (RAAS), which theoretically can result in prolonged hypotension during surgery. Several studies have documented this effect requiring treatment with pressors, especially patients receiving both an angiotensin blocker and a diuretic [18, 19]. There are varying results in those undergoing cardiac, vascular, or noncardiac surgery with earlier studies showing increased hypotensive events (typically a systolic BP < 90 mmHg), 30-day mortality [20, 21], and acute kidney injuries (AKIs) in the vascular and cardiac surgery groups. However, in the noncardiac surgery population, a recent study had shown increased perioperative hypotension in those continuing their ACEI or an ARB. A recent study showed an increased incidence of all-cause mortality within 30 days following noncardiac surgery with 12.9% of those continuing their medication and 12% of those withholding [22, 23]. This study by Roshanov et al. had a significantly smaller study size in comparison to Turan et al. with 4802 patients and 18,000 patients, respectively, and the larger study from the Cleveland Clinic demonstrated no difference in hypotensive events and no association with in-house hospital complications or increased 30-day mortality [24]. Additionally, nonrandomized studies show a possible myocardial protective effect [25]; however, there is conflict whether ACEI increase the risk of AKI with many of these studies examining a patient population undergoing cardiac surgery [26, 27]. Understandably, there is a lot of contradictory evidence with data showing continuing ACEI up to the morning of surgery increases perioperative hypotension but reduces the incidence of post-op hypertension. For a patient on multiple antihypertensive medications, it is justifiable to continue the medication. There is also limited evidence for increased risk of MI or death in noncardiac surgical patients, with the exception of the recent VISION study [19, 22, 24]. Patients taking this medication should be asked for any history of idiopathic angioedema due to the speed and idiosyncratic behavior of this reaction which is potentially dangerous given the danger to the airway. If this history is confirmed, the medication should be discontinued and the procedure postponed. It is okay to continue perioperatively especially in patients with CHF and hypertension (multiple medications). Overall recommendation is to individualize the decision-making based on the medical history, other cardiac medications, and the type of surgery and anesthesia planned [2].

12.1.5 Diuretics

Bottom line: Recommend holding the medication the morning of surgery due to increased risk of hypotension and hypokalemia and the ability to achieve quick diuresis using IV medications. Continue medication if taken for severe CHF (multiple doses of diuretic a day); and if possible the surgery should be handled in a hospital setting in coordination with the prescribing physician, anesthesiologist, surgeon, and patient.

Diuretics are often prescribed for patients with CHF and hypertension according to the latest JNC criteria. The major concern regarding the use of this class of medication, notably thiazide and loop diuretics, is the potential for hypokalemia with risk of perioperative arrhythmias and hypovolemia [28]. Understandably, there is a concern for perioperative hypotension given that anesthetic agents cause systemic vasodilation resulting in hypotension. Given the additional volume reduction with diuretic use, this effect could theoretically be augmented. Interestingly, an RCT showed no difference in intraoperative hypotension, vasopressor use, or volume of fluid administration between those who continued loop diuretics the day of surgery and those who did not (Khan et al. 2010). A downside of preoperative diuretic use is the risk of an AKI. A study involving 2725 subjects looked at the incidence of AKIs in patients receiving diuretics, ACEI/ARBs, or nothing, which resulted in a post-op odds of 2.07 of an AKI in the group taking diuretics [26].

Unfortunately, the data is limited on whether diuretics should be discontinued, especially in an ambulatory setting. It is recommended to withhold the morning of surgery due to the risk of hypotension and AKI and the ability to achieve quick diuresis if needed. Additionally, some office-based surgical centers may not have the ability to adjust if pressor drips are needed in a nonresponsive hypotensive episode. Therefore, the risks of each patient and especially the reason why they are on a diuretic should play into the proper selection of surgical environment.

12.1.6 Statins

Bottom line: Continue statins throughout the perioperative period if patient is already on this medication. Additionally, consider preprocedural initiation of statin therapy in any adult >45 with more than one cardiovascular risk factor [29].

HMG-CoA reductase inhibitors (statins) have been shown to prevent vascular events through several different mechanisms. Studies have demonstrated plaque stabilization, reduction of inflammation, and decreased thrombogenesis, and this pleiotropism is of benefit in the perioperative period. Pleiotropic effects of a drug are actions that are different from what the agent was specifically developed [30]. Another novel pleiotropic effect that has been ascribed to statins is the underlying antithrombotic effect due to decreases in the RBC lipid composition, causing increased RBC deformability and in turn decreased RBC aggregation [31]. Several studies have shown improved outcomes in more invasive procedures. A systematic review of observational studies demonstrated a reduction in postoperative acute coronary syndrome and mortality [32]. Several randomized trials of perioperative statin use for patients undergoing vascular surgery or procedures with high risk for cardiovascular complications showed decreased incidence of complications [33–35]. Statin therapy should be continued for patients throughout the perioperative period and consideration for those with at least one risk factor and over the age of 40 to initiate statin therapy [29]. It is wise to continue statin therapy; however, it is important to recognize that patients can develop side effects. If symptoms of muscle pain develop, the medication should be stopped, especially with the potential risk of rhabdomyolysis.

12.2 Pulmonary Agents

12.2.1 Inhaled Beta-Agonists and Anticholinergics

Bottom line: Inhaled beta-agonists, anticholinergics, and inhaled corticosteroids should be continued throughout the perioperative period. It is crucial to find out the level of control, and if an asthmatic uses rescue inhaler greater than 2× a week, the patient is under poor control and requires optimization depending on the urgency of surgery.

There are several inhaled medications used to treat COPD and/or asthma. It is recommended to continue the patient's beta-agonists (albuterol, salmeterol, formoterol) and/or anticholinergics (ipratropium, tiotropium) throughout the morning of surgery. This has been shown to reduce the incidence of post-op pulmonary complications and therefore should be continued perioperatively [36–38]. If the patient is unable to use the metered dose inhaler, the drugs can be administered via a nebulizer or circuit when the patient is intubated. It is recommended to continue inhaled bronchodilators, anticholinergics, and glucocorticoids throughout the perioperative period if the patient is able to do so. Additionally, the use of bronchodilator therapy prophylactically has likely benefit especially in the presence of a wheeze or decreased breath sounds [39]. However, if a patient has these symptoms showing poor control of pulmonary disease, it is essential to consider canceling the case to achieve better disease control if possible.

12.2.2 Theophylline

Bottom line: Discontinue theophylline the night before surgery due to limited protective effects and potential for adverse events.

Theophylline is used to treat COPD and asthma with its dual mechanism of action as a phosphodiesterase inhibitor and nonselective adenosine receptor antagonist. This medication does not have rescue efficacy in a COPD exacerbation, and there is no data supporting protective effects in the perioperative period [40]. There is high risk for DDIs due to multiple medications affecting the metabolism of theophylline causing either subtherapeutic or toxic levels. Toxic levels have been shown to cause arrhythmias and neurotoxicity. Theophylline should be discontinued preoperatively due to limited efficacy in preventing adverse outcomes in the perioperative period and the high risk of toxic levels secondary to drug-drug interactions (DDIs).

12.2.3 Glucocorticoids

Bottom line: Oral glucocorticoids should be continued through the morning of surgery, especially if being used for optimization of COPD and/or asthma. Stress doses should be given in the same manner whether pulmonary or nonpulmonary, and the approach should be the same. Discussion among the physician managing patient's asthma, anesthesiologist, surgeon, and patient is important to coordinate proper therapy.

Systemic glucocorticoids are reserved for the treatment of patients with poorly controlled asthma in hopes of reversing and/or stabilizing inflammation [41]. In addition to inhaled β2 agonists and inhaled steroids, pediatric patients are given oral prednisolone (1 mg/kg/day with maximum dose of 60 mg) 3–5 days before surgery or oral dexamethasone (0.6 mg/kg with maximum dose of 16 mg) [42–44]. If the child or adult is already taking chronic steroid medication, the dose needs to be increased 5 days before surgery [45]. The risk of discontinuing steroid use in a patient with chronic management is precipitation of adrenal insufficiency if abruptly withdrawn. Studies have shown that the incidence of wound infection associated with the use of perioperative steroids has been shown to be low [46]. It is recommended to continue chronic therapy of systemic steroids with consideration of a stress dose given the strength and time frame of treatment as recommended in Section 14.3 glucocorticoid stress dosing. Additionally, patients may require supplementation to stabilize poor control; however, this patient population should have their surgery postponed if possible to achieve optimization.

12.2.4 Leukotriene Inhibitors

Bottom line: Continue use of leukotriene inhibitors perioperatively due to control of asthmatic symptoms, as well as no withdrawal or interactions with anesthetics.

Leukotriene inhibitors are a novel agent that help control asthma, but are not used as a rescue drug for acute therapy. Interestingly, these medications have a relatively short half-life, but the control of asthmatic symptoms and pulmonary function lasts weeks following discontinuation if oral intake was interrupted [47]. There have been no reported interactions with anesthetic medications as well as no withdrawal syndromes. There is no parenteral substitution, but if the patient cannot tolerate PO medications, the effects on asthma symptoms and pulmonary function will continue for weeks. Therefore, missing a dose or two is not a critical issue.

12.3 Endocrine Agents

12.3.1 Glucocorticoids

Bottom line: Ascertain dosage and time period of use, and continue the current dosage with consideration of a stress dose. The old recommendations of stress dose steroids are controversial with many recent studies showing that it is not supported by evidence [48–50], and discussion among the medical team is important.

Surgery is one of the most potent activators of the stress response, which activates the hypothalamic-pituitary-adrenal (HPA) axis resulting in increased ACTH and cortisol levels. Patients on chronic steroids blunt this response with decreased levels of ACTH and at minimum need continue their glucocorticoid medication. Baseline cortisol secretion in patients not taking steroid medications is 8–10 mg/day and increases to 50 mg/day during minor surgery or illness [51]. Major noncardiac surgery stress response can vary from 75 to 100 mg/day and can reach 200–500 mg/day with major trauma [48, 52]. Patients who have been taking glucocorticoids less than 3 weeks, those receiving a morning dose less than 5 mg/day of prednisone for any length of time, and those being treated with less than 10 mg of prednisone a day every other day are not considered to have suppression of the HPA axis and do not require supplementation [53–56]. For patients who have taken greater than 20 mg/day for 3 or more weeks and/or Cushingoid appearance, it is wise to assume HPA axis suppression and an increased perioperative dose may be necessary. Patients taking 5–20 mg prednisone for 3 or more weeks may have HPA suppression, and additional testing may be necessary. At minimum these patients should continue their current dose. Recommendations for stress dose revolve around the type of surgery. For minor procedures the usual morning dose should be taken. For surgeries with moderate surgical stress (total joint replacement, lower extremity revascularization), take usual morning dose with 50 mg hydrocortisone IV before the procedure and 25 mg IV every 8 h for 24 h. For major procedures that should be performed at a tertiary care center (esophagogastrectomy, open heart surgery), take the usual morning dose with 100 mg hydrocortisone IV prior to procedure followed by 50 mg IV every 8 h for the first 24 h. This dose should be tapered by half per day until the maintenance dose is reached.

Understandably, stress dose supplementation is controversial with several recent studies showing that patients continuing their current corticosteroid dose the morning of surgery is enough to compensate for the HPA axis suppression. It takes up to 18 months for the HPA axis to recover following therapy [57, 58]. However, the goal is to mitigate risk of an adrenal crisis and hypotensive collapse, and it is recommended to follow current guidelines in discussion with the prescribing physician, anesthesiologist, surgeon, and patient [48, 49].

12.3.2 Diabetic Medications

Bottom line: Joint management strategy with patient's primary care physician (PCP) and/or endocrinologist, anesthesiologist, surgeon, and the patient. Continue metformin and basal insulin the day of surgery. For consistency have the patient bring their own glucometer. The location of where to perform the procedure depends on the complexity of the surgery and the complexity of patient disease.

The management of patients with diabetes is complex, and this patient population will be frequently encountered due to current health trends. The first step in management is the assessment of the patient's diabetes: type, medications, and usual level of blood glucose control [59]. This background helps achieve perioperative goals to avoid hypoglycemia (most severe, can induce arrhythmias, or other cardiac events, transient neurocognitive deficits), prevent ketoacidosis/hyperosmolar states, maintain fluid and electrolyte balance, and avoid marked hyperglycemia. This is best achieved in coordination with the patient's prescribing physician. The caveat to recommendations in the literature in most consensus strategies is by expert opinion and personal experience. Strategies have not been proven to optimally reduce outcomes of morbidity, mortality, and hospital length of stay [60, 61]. The decision of which regimen to utilize and when is predicated on individual patients, hospital resources, and clinician's judgment.

Patients that have type 2 diabetes managed with diet alone typically do not require therapy. Supplemental short-acting insulin may be needed preoperatively if the patient has a blood glucose read of over 150 mg/dL on the glucometer. However, this target blood glucose measurement varies depending on control. Those with type 2 diabetes on oral hypoglycemic/non-insulin injectables should continue their medication until the morning of surgery with the exception of metformin [62]. Sulfonylureas increase the risk of hypoglycemia, and metformin was previously thought to potentially cause lactic acidosis, but it has been shown that the overall benefits from the medication outweigh the relatively uncommon risk [50]. Other medications which should be discontinued the morning of surgery include thiazolidinediones which worsen fluid retention and peripheral edema, sodium-glucose cotransporter 2 (SGLT2) inhibitors that increase risk of hypovolemia (AKI, euglycemic DKA), and dipeptidyl peptidase IV (DPP-IV) inhibitors and glucagon-like peptide-1 (GLP-1) analogs which can alter GI motility. Dulaglutide is a new medication that is used for treatment of type 2 diabetes. This medication involves subcutaneous injections every 2 weeks, and studies examining this medication in comparison to other modalities showed less hypoglycemic events when used alone or with non-insulin secretagogue therapy [63]. Most medications can be restarted after surgery when patient resumes eating.

Patients with type 1 or insulin-dependent type 2 diabetes have their medications adjusted according to length of procedure and type of insulin regimen. For procedures less than 2 h, patients can continue subcutaneous insulin perioperatively. If a minor, early morning procedure is planned (delayed breakfast), patients taking once daily long-acting insulin or insulin pump can continue basal insulin regimen. However, if the patient has history of low-glucose measures, recommend reduction of basal dose by 10–20%.

If there is a planned morning procedure where the patient will miss meals in the morning and lunch, or late-day procedures, the patient should omit their short- or rapid-acting insulin (lispro, aspart, glulisine). Patients taking two types of insulin (intermediate or long and rapid or short acting) give 1/2–1/3 of usual morning dose of intermediate- or long-acting insulin. Patients on an insulin pump should continue their basal infusion rate perioperatively. There should be consideration for administering dextrose containing IV solution 75–125 mL/h that is recommended by several studies [64–69]. Patients with frequent hypoglycemia or low-end normal blood glucose reduce nighttime dose by 10–20% of the long-acting insulin. Moreover, basal metabolic demands utilize one-half of an individual's insulin regardless of PO status, which is why it is necessary to administer insulin even in the absence of oral intake. If a long complex procedure is planned that may require IV insulin, it is best to reconsider the setting of the elective surgery.

If ambulatory surgery is performed, patients should bring their own glucometer with them to check their blood sugar before and after the procedure to see if IV fluids need to be changed. Appointments should be kept short and staged if necessary. If the patient is on insulin or a combination of oral medication and insulin, it would be wise to perform the procedure in a hospital

Insulin Comparison Chart

Insulin Name (Trade)	When does it start working? (onset)	When will the effect be the greatest? (peak)	How long will it lower blood glucose? (duration)	Notes for Use	MGH Formulary Availability*
Rapid Acting Analogs					
Lispro (HumaLOG™)	<15 minutes	30-90 minutes	3-5 hours	If mixing with NPH, rapid acting insulin (clear formulation) should be drawn into syringe first. Mixture should be given immediately to avoid effects on peak action.	Nonformulary
Aspart (NovoLog™)	<15 minutes	30-90 minutes	3-5 hours		3 mL FlexPen®
Glulisine (Apidra™)	<15 minutes	30-90 minutes	3-5 hours		Nonformulary
Short Acting					
Regular (Novolin R™ or Humulin R™)	0.5-1 hour	2-4 hours	4-8 hours	If mixing with NPH, short acting insulin (clear formulation) should be drawn into syringe first. Mixture should be given immediately to avoid effects on peak action.	3 mL vial 20 mL vial (500 units/mL)—*restricted*
Intermediate Acting					
NPH (NovoLIN N™ or HumuLIN N™)	1-2 hours	4-10 hours	10-18 hours	Cloudy formulation.	3 mL vial
Long Acting Analogs					
Glargine (Lantus™)	1-2 hours	No peak	20-24 hours	Do not mix with other insulin formulations.	3 mL SoloStar® pen
Detemir (Levemir™)	1-2 hours	Relatively flat	Up to 24 hours (dose-dependent)	Both glargine and detemir are clear formulations.	3 mL FlexPen®
Combinations					
NovoLIN 70/30 or HumuLIN 70/30	0.5-1 hour	2-10 hours	10-18 hours	70% NPH +30% regular insulin. Insulin action includes 2 peaks (1 from each formulation). Cloudy formulation.	3 mL vial
NovoLog Mix 70/30 or HumaLOG Mix 75/25 or 50/50	<15 minutes	1-2 hours	10-18 hours	Insulin action includes 2 peaks (1 from each formulation). <u>Novolog Mix (cloudy formulation)</u>: aspart protamine 70% + aspart 30% <u>Humalog mix (cloudy formulation)</u>: 75/25=75% lispro protamine + 25% lispro 50/50=50% lispro protamine + 50% lispro	10 mL vial—*HumaLOG Mix 75/25 only*

*All insulin preparations are 100 units/mL except concentrated regular insulin U500 containing 500 units/mL.
Onset, Peak, and Duration may vary considerably in different people.
Insulin analogs and analog mix formulations are available in prefilled pens:

- KwikPen® is a disposable pen manufactured for Lilly products including HumaLOG® and HumaLOG® Mix.
- FlexPen® is a disposable pen manufactured for Novo Nordisk products including NovoLog® and Levemir®.
- SoloSTAR® pen is a disposable pen manufactured for Sanofi products including Lantus® and Apidra®.

Fig. 12.1 Insulin comparison chart [70]

setting and/or consider bringing an anesthesiologist to the ambulatory center (Fig. 12.1).

12.3.3 Drugs Used for Thyroid Disease

Bottom line: Patients with poorly controlled hyperthyroidism and hypothyroidism must have their elective procedure delayed until better control is achieved. Patients must continue taking their medication through the morning of surgery.

Most patients who have well-treated thyroid disease do not need special consideration prior to surgery. It is those with undiagnosed or poorly treated thyroid conditions that must be identified for optimization and delay of the planned procedure until this is achieved.

Patients with hypothyroidism receive thyroid hormone replacement, and these patients do not carry an increased risk of perioperative morbidity. No special treatment is required other than continuation of their chronic thyroid hormone replacement [71]. Additionally, the half-life of T4 is almost 7 days; therefore, parenteral T4 is usually not needed. If the patient cannot eat for 5–7 days, consider IV or IM T4 at 80% of the oral dose. If patient presents with severe hypothyroidism (myxedema coma, altered mental status, pericardial effusion) or moderate hypothyroidism, the procedure must be delayed until the condition is treated. In the event of an urgent procedure, it is recommended to supplement with both T3 and T4.

Patients with hyperthyroidism are treated with methimazole, propylthiouracil, thionamides, and sometimes beta-blockers. Severe or moderate symptoms (atrial fibrillation, palpitations, tachycardia, tremulousness, anxiety, and heat intolerance) [72] must be detected during the consultation due to potential for life-threatening complications, such as thyroid storm [73]. If the patient has well controlled and/or treated hyperthyroidism, it is okay to proceed with the planned procedure with the patient taking their respective medication the morning of surgery.

12.3.4 Oral Contraceptives

Bottom line: Continue oral contraceptive (OCP) therapy through the morning of surgery if patient is undergoing a low-risk procedure. If the medication is used in an older female who smokes, and is undergoing a major operation, it is recommended to consider discontinuing the medication 4–6 weeks prior to the day of surgery.

The use of OCPs is the most frequent cause of thrombosis in young women due to the high frequency of use. Females who are older (>30 years of age) and smoke have an even higher risk of thromboembolism; however, even those in a lower-risk population undergoing major surgery are at risk. The OCPs with higher estrogen content (>35 mcg) tend to have greater risk of thromboembolism than those with lower content [74]. If the decision is made to discontinue OCP use, it should be stopped 4–6 weeks prior to surgery, especially in those undergoing moderate- to high-risk procedures. Patients who continue their OCP and require reversal of the non-depolarizing muscle-blocking agents with sugammadex must be advised to use other methods of contraception due to the binding of hormone by the reversal agent [75].

12.4 Medications Affecting Hemostasis

Bottom line: Consult with hematologist and PCP if patient is on these medications, and these medications require a more involved procedure, and it would be best accomplished in the hospital. Bridging therapy is becoming less necessary.

The goal when deciding how to manage antithrombotic medications is balancing the risk of intraoperative and post-procedural bleeding with continued treatment against the thrombotic risk with cessation of therapy. The challenge is determining how to manage a patient with moderate-to-high risk of thromboembolism undergoing a high-risk procedure. Assessment of thrombotic risk should identify atrial fibrillation, mechanical heart valves and/or recent venous thromboembolism, cancer, and coronary stents. If there is a history of atrial fibrillation, a CHADS2 score or a CHA2DS2-VASc score must be obtained as well as determining whether the tachyarrhythmia is valvular in nature or not [76]. The CHADS2 score or a CHA2DS2-VASc score is on a 6-point and a 9-point scale, respectively, and the higher the score, the greater the thrombotic risk. Valvular atrial fibrillation indicates the coexistence of severe valvular heart disease, and these patients are at greater risk for thromboembolism than those with nonvalvular atrial fibrillation [76]. Patients with mechanical mitral valves, caged-ball or tilting disk aortic valves, or multiple prosthetic valves present a high risk for thromboembolism. History of recent deep vein thrombosis (DVT) less than 3 months ago and history of severe thrombophilia (protein C, protein S, or antithrombin deficiency; antiphospholipid syndrome, homozygous for factor V Leiden) present a high risk for thromboembolism [76]. Other factors with greater concern for thromboembolism are cancer and recent coronary stent placement. Cancer creates an increased risk of thrombosis with cancer-specific prothrombotic therapy, hormonal therapy, angiogenesis inhibitors, radiotherapy, and/or presence of indwelling catheters [77]. Recent revascularization procedures with placement of stents require dual antiplatelet for the first 6 weeks and 1 year for bare metal stents and drug-eluting stents, respectively; and any procedures planned during this time period must be of the urgent or emergent nature only. Any elective surgery within a year of revascularization procedures with stent placement should ideally be postponed until 12 months [78]. Ultimately, patients in the high-risk group should have any elective surgeries postponed and the care coordinated with their PCP, hematologist, anesthesiologist, and surgeon. Most of the patients should have their procedures in a hospital setting.

Estimation of the bleeding risk considers the type of procedure and additional risk factors such as antithrombotic agents, active cancer and chemotherapy, a history of bleeding, and reinitiation of antithrombotic therapy within 24 h following surgery. It can be difficult to estimate bleeding risk with a procedure because grades of bleeding severity are not standardized across surgical subspecialties [79]. However, procedures that can result in intracranial, intraspinal, intraocular, retroperitoneal, intrathoracic, or pericardial bleeding are considered high risk with these locations being classified as major [76, 79].

Patients that fall within the high thrombotic risk category typically require bridging therapy. The three main categories are mechanical heart valve, nonvalvular atrial fibrillation, and/or venous thromboembolism. Mechanical heart valves that involve mitral valve replacement, two or more mechanical valves, and non-bileaflet aortic-valve replacement with other risk factors (stroke, TIA, intracardiac thrombus, cardioembolic event increase risk) indicate required bridging. Nonvalvular atrial fibrillation with prior stroke or embolic event, cardiac thrombus, or CHADS2 score $\geq$ 4 (prior stroke, TIA, intracardiac thrombus, cardioembolic event increase risk) requires bridging if antithrombotic therapy is stopped. Venous thromboembolism for the past 3 months or severe thrombophilia should be coordinated with bridging therapy if antithrombotic is discontinued [76].

The timing of antithrombotic medication interruption will be discussed below for each class of medication. Again, the decision to discontinue, bridge, or continue the antithrombotic medication must consider the risk of thromboembolism versus the risk of periprocedural bleeding. If a patient is at high risk, it is best coordinated with the medical and the surgery performed in a hospital setting.

12.4.1 Aspirin

Bottom line: Low-dose aspirin should be discontinued the morning of surgery if it is the only antithrombotic medication being administered. If patient is taking aspirin for dual antiplatelet therapy (DAPT) or more complex medical conditions, discussion with the prescribing physician, anesthesiologist, surgeon, and patient is required. If patient has bare metal stent (BMS) or drug-eluting stent (DES), it is recommended to postpone treatment if within 6 weeks and 1 year, respectively, of stent placement.

Low-dose aspirin has been shown to prevent myocardial infarction and major vascular events and is part of the dual antiplatelet therapy utilized after stent placement in revascularization procedures [80]. The concern during surgery is aspirin irreversibly inhibits platelet aggregation which can increase blood loss during surgery; however, low-dose aspirin alone does not substantially increase the risk of clinically important bleeding following an invasive procedure [81]. However, the POISE-2 trial involving 10,010 patients showed that the administration of aspirin before surgery and throughout the early postsurgical period, there was no significant effect on the rate of composite death or nonfatal MI, but there was an increased risk of major bleeding [82]. Moreover, if a patient is on single therapy low-dose aspirin, it is recommended to discontinue use 7–10 days prior to the morning of surgery [76, 82].

In more complex patients receiving DAPT, the decision to continue or discontinue aspirin therapy should utilize the regimen weighing risks of thromboembolism versus increased bleeding and in discussion with the medical time. This patient population should have their surgery in a hospital setting.

Patients with recent percutaneous coronary intervention (PCI) really should have an elective procedure until stable; however, those on DAPT should be approached on a case-by-case basis. Consideration of the type of surgery and risk of bleeding, the urgency of the surgery, and length of time from stenting all play into whether one of the medications can be stopped prior to surgery. This decision involves a discussion among the PCP, cardiologist, surgeon, and anesthesiologist.

For elective, noncardiac surgery in stented patients before 1 full year and the risk of bleeding requiring interruption of full DAPT, the P2Y12 inhibitor should be discontinued as brief as possible. Aspirin therapy should be continued because of the increased risk of stent thrombosis. Minor surgical and dental procedures usually do not require discontinuing DAPT. Clopidogrel/ticagrelor, prasugrel, and ticlodipine should be stopped 5, 7, or 10–14 days prior to procedure depending on expected bleeding intraoperatively [76]. Following surgery, it is recommended to give a 300 mg clopidogrel loading dose as soon as possible.

12.4.2 P2Y12 Receptor Blockers

Bottom line: Patients on this medication typically should not have an elective procedure prior to 12 months of DAPT. It is recommended to postpone surgery and in urgent/emergent situations discuss discontinuing the medication with the medical team.

Clopidogrel, prasugrel, ticagrelor, and ticlodipine are P2Y12 receptor blockers that are used to treat patient with prior cerebrovascular events, recent acute coronary syndromes, or recent PCI or PVI with stenting [83]. Although the risk of stent thrombosis is low with cessation of clopidogrel, it is still increased and can be fatal. Elective surgery should be postponed for a minimum period (BMS, 6 weeks; DES, 12 months) in coordination with the prescribing physician and the surgical/anesthesia team. A study looking at perioperative bleeding in 10,000 patients with 2010 of those continuing clopidogrel showed that the bleeding risk in these patients undergoing peripheral artery or carotid surgery was low with little difference in comparison to those with no antiplatelet therapy or aspirin alone [84].

Patients who have complete minimum duration of DAPT, the P2Y12 receptor blocker may be stopped, surgery performed, and restarting therapy following the procedure. Again, if within minimum DAPT time frame, it is recommended to consult the treating cardiologist, surgeon, and anesthesiologist and plan for surgery at a center with 24-h interventional cardiology coverage. If bleeding risk outweighs that of thrombosis, in coordination with the medical team, discontinue the P2Y12 receptor blocker for as brief of a time period as possible with continuation of aspirin therapy. Discontinue clopidogrel and ticagrelor discontinued at least 5 days before surgery [85], prasugrel at least 7 days, and ticlopidine 7–10 days prior to the morning of surgery [76].

12.4.3 Nonsteroidal Anti-inflammatory Drugs

Bottom line: NSAIDs are used acutely the day of surgery or following surgery are effective in multimodal postoperative pain control. The problem occurs when a patient takes the medication chronically, which the potential for renal toxicity and an antiplatelet effect exists.

NSAIDs have a reversible inhibition of COX-1 and COX-2. Results in decreased production of thromboxane A2 (TxA2) leading to increased bleeding perioperatively, however, may reduce the risk of thromboembolic events similar to aspirin [86]. Although celecoxib has greater COX-2 inhibition which has less antiplatelet effect, there is still potential for renal toxicity and risk for adverse cardiovascular effects [87]. It is recommended to discontinue chronic NSAID use 3 days before the morning of surgery. The duration of the antiplatelet effect was shown to normalize within 24 h in healthy individuals [88]. The recommendations regarding chronic use of NSAIDs are controversial, and distinguishing between intermittent uses of acute pain will help guide management.

12.4.4 Warfarin

Bottom line: Patients on warfarin should have the need for elective surgery critically evaluated; and a discussion with the prescribing PCP, hematologist, anesthesiologist, surgeon, and the patient is recommended.

Warfarin is a vitamin K antagonist used to reduce the risk of thromboembolism by inhibiting synthesis of factors II, VII, IX, and X. Resolution of therapy is determined by testing PT/INR with 93% of patients having an INR ≤ 1.5 [89]. Conversely, it takes several days for warfarin to become therapeutic again, which may require bridging in patients with high thromboembolic risk as discussed at the beginning of this section.

If the decision is made to discontinue therapy for more than a minor surgical procedure, it is recommended to stop warfarin 1–8 days prior to the morning of surgery depending on INR and patient characteristics [76]. Other recommendations are to standardize to discontinue 5 days prior to elective surgery and checking the PT/INR day before procedure. If INR >1.5, low dose oral vitamin K can be given and the INR rechecked the following day. The goal is to achieve an INR ≤1.5 especially for procedures with high bleeding risk (neurosurgery—intracranial, spinal, ophthalmologic, urologic) and when using neuraxial anesthesia [90]. The biological half-life is 36–24 h, and observed time period for PT/INR to normalize is 4–6 days [91]. Urgent/emergent procedures require preoperative administration of FFP and Vitamin K. Overall, it is estimated that patients are subtherapeutic for 8 days (4 prior and 4 post-surgery). Bridging is reserved for those at very high risk and of thromboembolism (recent stroke, mechanical heart valve, CHADS2 score of 5 or 6). LMWH started 3 days prior to procedure. In the patient unable to tolerate oral medications (trauma, head and neck cancer patients, postoperative ileus), continue use of bridging agent. Once adequate hemostasis is achieved, resume warfarin with postoperative bridge. Douketis et al. recommend restarting therapy 12–24 h postoperatively, and it can take up to 10 days to attain full anticoagulation (INR >2.0) [92]. These decisions must be made through comanagement of the patient, and the proper environment for surgery is likely at a hospital-based facility.

12.4.5 Factor Xa Inhibitors (Rivaroxaban, Apixaban, Edoxaban)

Bottom line: Critically examine the need for discontinuing medication for an elective surgery using the guidelines provided weighing high risk for thrombosis versus high bleeding risk. Discussion with the prescribing PCP, hematologist, anesthesiologist, surgeon, and the patient is recommended.

Factor Xa inhibitors are relatively new medications in comparison to warfarin. They have shorter half-lives and are easier to discontinue and resume rapidly. However, there is no specific antidote creating a problem in trauma patients and those that need a quick procedure. These medications irreversibly block the enzymatic function of factor Xa converting prothrombin to thrombin. If the decision is made to discontinue the mediation, it is recommended to stop apixaban 1–2 days and rivaroxaban ≥1 day, respectively, prior to the morning of surgery with longer interval for high bleeding risk procedures [76]. The elimination half-time which is 5-9 hours is rolonged in a patient with renal disease and the period in which the anticoagulant should be discontinued must be adjusted when considering the renal insufficiency. The patient may require longer intervals for those with very high bleeding risk (neuraxial anesthesia). For most dentoalveolar procedures, the medication need not be discontinued. These drugs must be used with caution in patients on dual inhibitors CYP-3A4 and P-glycoprotein (ketoconazole, ritonavir), and dose change or alternative medication is considered. Bridging therapy is used in those falling into the high risk of thromboembolism or unable to take oral medications (head and neck procedures, intestinal ileus, GI surgery). Once hemostasis is achieved, again use caution if following a procedure with high bleeding risk restarting on post-op day (POD) 3 and can restart on POD 1 for low bleeding risk.

12.4.6 Factor IIa Inhibitors (Dabigatran)

Bottom line: Critically examine the need for discontinuing medication for an elective surgery using the guidelines provided weighing high risk for thrombosis versus high bleeding risk. Discussion with the prescribing PCP, hematologist, anesthesiologist, surgeon, and the patient is recommended.

Dabigatran is a direct thrombin inhibitor often used to treat atrial fibrillation. Similar to other novel oral anticoagulants, it is difficult to monitor the therapeutic, and there is a lack of reversal agents. The decision to discontinue dabigatran must be based on the same issues of weighing the risk of thromboembolism versus risk of bleeding. For most dentoalveolar surgery, the medication need not be discontinued. If the medication is discontinued, it should be stopped 1–2 days prior to the morning of surgery in patients with normal renal and 3–5 days in those with a creatinine clearance <50 mL/min [76]. Bridging should be used only in patients with high risk of thromboembolism and/or require extended interruption, especially given the rapid onset and offset reducing the overall need for bridging. The medication can be resumed after hemostasis, however, given relatively fast onset use caution in patients with higher risk of bleeding due to their surgery. It is recommended to delay resumption for 2–3 days following procedures with high risk for bleeding.

12.5 Psychotropic Agents

Management of psychotropic agents varies with the class of drug and the severity of mental illness. There is a shortage of good evidence-based data to support decision-making [93]. In general, these medications should be continued especially in patients with serious or unstable mental illness due to risk of psychiatric decompensation. Additionally, several medications cannot be administered parenterally in an acute decompensation.

12.5.1 Tricyclic Antidepressants

Bottom line: Decision to continue TCAs should be made on a case-by-case basis depending on the severity of depression and the risk of arrhythmias.

TCA management is unclear given the lack of evidence-based recommendations. These medications lower the seizure threshold and possess significant anticholinergic, antihistaminic, and alpha-1 blocking properties unlike newer agents. Acute withdrawal of TCAs is associated with insomnia, headache, increased salivation, and sweating. These medications can augment the pressor effects used intraoperatively, but it is generally safe with local anesthetics containing epinephrine. These medications are associated with serotonin syndrome when given in combination with tramadol and meperidine as described in Chapter 13 on DDIs. Most expert opinion, textbooks, and literature recommend continuing use in the perioperative period; however, the FDA has warnings for continuing use and recommends cessation prior to elective surgery [93]. The risk for an acute exacerbation and/or withdrawal can outweigh the potential adverse effects, especially in those without cardiac disease. However, if the decision is made to discontinue the medication, it should be stopped 7–14 days prior to the morning of surgery.

12.5.2 Selective Serotonin Reuptake Inhibitors (SSRIs)

Bottom line: SSRIs should be continued through the morning of surgery; however, the type of procedure (neurosurgery) and a patient on aspirin/DAPT tapering of the SSRI should be considered.

SSRIs have been shown to potentially increase bleeding risk due to effects on platelet aggregation, especially in those taking NSAIDs [94, 95]. Yet, several other studies involving orthopedic surgery, open heart procedures, and plastic surgery showed no increased bleeding risk [96, 97]. Cessation of SSRIs can exacerbate depression and other mood disorders and can take as long as 3 weeks to leave the system. Additionally, the half-life of SSRIs varies significantly. Acute withdrawal of short-acting medications can result in patient discomfort due to discontinuation syndrome (dizziness, chills, muscle aches, and anxiety). Given the risk of exacerbation of mood disorders, acute withdrawal syndrome, and the discrepancies in studies showing bleeding risk, it is recommended to continue SSRIs through the morning of surgery. In procedures with greater bleeding risk and if patient is on DAPT, SSRIs should be discontinued preoperatively with involvement of the psychiatrist and/or PCP with another medication considered during the perioperative period.

12.5.3 Selective Norepinephrine Reuptake Inhibitors (SNRI) and Bupropion

Bottom line: SNRIs should be continued through the morning of surgery; however, the type of procedure (neurosurgery) and a patient on aspirin/DAPT tapering of the SNRI should be considered.

SNRIs should be managed similar to SSRIs. There is limited data regarding use. A retrospective study of 4136 patients undergoing CABG demonstrated increased risk of renal dysfunction and prolonged ventilation, but bleeding and long-term mortality were no different [96]. Patients on SNRIs, like bupropion, should continue use, but the anesthesiologist and surgeon should avoid use of pseudoephedrine due to potential DDIs.

12.5.4 Monoamine Oxidase Inhibitors (MAOIs)

Bottom line: Management of MAO inhibitors requires close collaboration between the anesthesiologist and psychiatrist. They should be continued the morning of surgery if the anesthesiologist is comfortable with MAO inhibitor safe procedures and if the patient is at risk of a major depressive syndrome. Continue medications for patients taking MAOIs for intractable narcolepsy. Otherwise, the medication should be discontinued 2 weeks before elective surgery.

MAO inhibitors are less often prescribed but are still used in refractory mood disorders where withdrawal and acute exacerbations are a significant problem. MAOIs cause accumulation of biogenic amines in CNS and PNS neurons, and the administration of ephedrine can result in severe hypertensive crisis. Avoid use of anticholinergics (dextromethorphan) and meperidine due to risk of serotonin syndrome. Type II reactions inhibit hepatic enzymes resulting in prolonged respiratory depression in patients taking opiates. Use of epinephrine containing LAs is overall safe as well as benzodiazepines, inhalational anesthetic agents, and NSAIDs [98]. Safe anesthetic techniques have been implemented for patients unable to discontinue MAOIs, which involves avoiding certain medications, such as meperidine and dextromethorphan as well as cautious use of sympathomimetics [99, 100]. Overall decision in continuing medication must involve collaboration of the patient, anesthesiologist, and psychiatrist. If anesthesiologist is comfortable with MAOI, safe procedures and/or patient is at high risk for exacerbation of depressive syndrome. If aforementioned criteria are not met, cessation of MAOI is 2 weeks prior to procedure with transition to TCA or SSRI for the perioperative period. If continued, close monitoring for any intraoperative interactions.

12.5.5 Mood-Stabilizing Agents (Lithium and Valproate)

Bottom line: Both lithium and valproate should be continued the morning of surgery. The risk of a manic episode outweighs the inherent interactions and physiologic effects of these agents.

Lithium has several issues that must be recognized when performing elective surgery. Lithium decreases release of neurotransmitters and can prolong the effect of neuromuscular blockers. Narrow therapeutic index, therefore risk for toxicity (maintained renal function, interactions with diuretics, NSAIDs, ACEIs, and serotonergic drugs). Chronic use has effects on thyroid function, which has been shown to cause goiter and hypothyroidism as well as linked to autoimmune thyroiditis and hyperthyroidism [101]. Up to 20% of patients taking lithium have diabetes insipidus. Maintain euvolemia and normal serum sodium through polydipsia. Risk of volume depletion and hypernatremia is due to limited access to free water in the perioperative period. Valproate has several DDIs that should be recognized including NSAIDs and some antibiotics. Lithium should be continued in the perioperative period with closed attention to fluid and electrolyte monitoring as well as checking thyroid function.

12.5.6 Antipsychotics

Bottom line: The decision to continue or withhold antipsychotic medications should be made on a case-by-case basis. The risk of acute psychosis must be verse; adverse drug events should be considered when making these decisions. Complex patients on multiple medications communicate with prescribing psychiatrist, patient (if competent), and/or caregiver.

Patients with schizophrenia require chronic treatment with antipsychotics. These medications are valuable in the perioperative period in controlling acute psychoses. However, use of typical and atypical antipsychotics has been linked to increased risk of sudden cardiac death [102]. The atypical antipsychotics act at several receptors in addition to the D2 receptor and have been shown to prolong the QT interval as well as arrhythmias [98]. The efficacy of these medications in controlling perioperative psychoses or delirium is apparent in the literature. A randomized controlled trial involving 495 patients at risk for delirium undergoing total joint replacement had significant reduction in incidence of delirium with use of olanzapine (decreased from 40 to 1%). More patients were able to return home instead of rehabilitation facilities [103]. Another study examining prophylactic haloperidol use in ICU patients following noncardiac surgery had decreased incidence of postoperative delirium, and mean number of days to onset and mean number of delirium free days were increased [104]. The decision to continue or discontinue should be made on an individual basis, and those at risk for exacerbation of psychoses should have their medication generally continued. There is some disagreement on management with Attri et al. 2012 and Peck et al. 2010 recommending communication among the medical team and the prescribing physician with continuation of the medication. Current up-to-date recommendations suggest holding in patients with EKGs showing QT prolongation with consideration of shorter-acting and low-dose antipsychotics with consultation of the psychiatrist [105]. The concern is the potentiation of sedative and hypotensive effects of anesthetics and opiates. Additionally, monitoring for extrapyramidal side effects and neuroleptic malignant syndrome is critical. However, in patients with the potential for these adverse events, they should be managed in the hospital setting.

12.5.7 Psychostimulants

Bottom line: Psychostimulants should be discontinued the morning of surgery due to low risk of temporarily discontinuing the medication.

Medications used to treat ADHD can increase risk for hypertension and arrhythmias, lower the seizure threshold, and interact with perioperative medications [105]. Per packaging guidelines there is risk of severe hypertension when methylphenidate is used in conjunction with halogenated anesthetics. However, a case series found no adverse effects when amphetamines continued on the day of surgery, but no pressor support is required in these patients [106]. The data is lacking when considering how to manage these patients. There is low risk of adverse events in the non-abusing patient, but there is potential for cardiovascular interactions depending on whether pressor support is needed or an intravascular interaction. It is recommended to discontinue the medication the morning of surgery in the ambulatory setting with special consideration in the pediatric patient and their ability to cooperate prior to any planned anesthetic.

12.6 Chronic Opioid Therapy

Bottom line: Patients on chronic opioid therapy require individualized perioperative analgesic measures. It is recommended to continue most medications to treat the tolerance and utilize multimodal pain treatment for acute analgesic control.

Opioid tolerance typically requires a higher amount of medication, and to optimize pain control, consultation with a pain management specialist may be necessary. Multimodal analgesic strategy utilizing regional modalities as well as systemic non-opioid medications (NSAIDs, acetaminophen, gabapentin, ketamine, or lidocaine) should be considered in the individualized treatment plan. Often the baseline level of therapy should be maintained during the perioperative period with addition of multimodal therapy. If patient is unable to resume oral intake, a fentanyl patch can be substituted as necessary for postoperative pain, but this must be planned with a pain management specialist.

12.6.1 Methadone

Bottom line: Patients should continue methadone through the morning of surgery with the use of additional opioid therapy as needed for acute pain [107]. Delay surgery if within the first 2 weeks of therapy due to high risk of potentially fatal events [108–112].

Methadone is commonly used to treat opioid dependence due to its long half-life, less euphoria, and other opioid-associated side effects. It is also used in the setting of chronic pain treatment as well. Thirty percent of prescription-related deaths are associated with methadone therapy, and the largest proportion of methadone-associated deaths fall into the induction phase (first 2 weeks). This is attributed to overestimation of the patient's tolerance to opioids [108–112]. The drug-gene interaction involving the CYP2B6 polymorphisms influences oral administration (addiction/chronic pain) more than IV (intraoperative). Oral bioavailability is high, and those receiving repeat doses (steady state) versus single doses have more variability in metabolism with this drug-gene interaction, which has potential for oversedation if not recognized. The timing of methadone therapy must be known prior to any planned procedures, and within the first 2 weeks, the elective surgery must be delayed. Patients should continue the usual dose of methadone through the morning of surgery. This can be given orally or the usual dose cut in half for IV administration. Breakthrough pain is treated with additional opioids as needed (PO, IV, PCA). These patients are still at risk for serious side effects due to unequal efficacy at receptor sites. As the analgesic effects require more medication, the respiratory depression is worsened. If there is concern for oversedation and monitoring is required, the patient should have their procedure scheduled in a hospital setting.

12.6.2 Buprenorphine

Bottom line: The decision to continue or withhold buprenorphine should be individualized and in coordination with the prescribing physician. The medication is typicallyy continued in surgeries with minimal postoperative pain, but more invasive procedures require consideration of other analgesic modalities.

Patients taking this medication for narcotic addiction or chronic pain present a challenge for postoperative pain control. It is a semisynthetic opioid which acts as a partial mu-receptor agonist (1000× affinity of morphine) and antagonistic at the kappa receptor. There are two different preparations: one has buprenorphine and the other also contains naloxone as well. Multimodal therapy with other opioid medications may not be as effective due to the high affinity for opioid receptor, which can decrease the efficacy of other opioid medications [113]. There is a ceiling effect for analgesia and respiratory depression in comparison to methadone, which can increase respiratory depression. Bryson et al. recommends two different strategies for acute pain control. The first strategy involves surgery with minimal postoperative pain with continuation of buprenorphine and maximizes use of non-opioid analgesia with utilization of regional anesthesia if possible. The second strategy involves surgery with anticipated moderate to severe postoperative pain. It is important to coordinate with prescribing clinician; if possible discontinue 72 h before surgery and transition to another opioid [107]. If possible, the utilization of regional anesthesia and non-opioid medications is recommended, and IV opioids should be used for breakthrough pain. Resumption of therapy should be coordinated with the prescribing physician when acute post-op pain has resolved.

12.7 Drugs of Abuse (Chronic Tobacco/Alcohol)

12.7.1 Chronic Tobacco Use

Bottom line: Advise patient to stop smoking at least 8 weeks before the planned procedure; however, there should be no smoking cessation within a week of surgical date due to stunned cilia and increased mucous production.

Chronic tobacco use increases the risk of postoperative pulmonary complications and wound infections [114–116]. If patients are evaluated far enough in advance (optimally at least 8 weeks), the patient should be advised to stop smoking [117]. Abstinence at least 8 weeks prior to surgical date will allow the greatest recovery of endobronchial cilial mucus clearance. Although there isn't a consensus on the exact time period, if the patient is to have surgery within a week of the surgical date, the patients should continue their habit. Acute withdrawal can precipitate increased mucous production and decreased clearance due to stunned cilia; however, several meta-analyses showed improved outcomes regardless of the stop date [114–116].

12.7.2 Chronic Alcohol Use

Bottom line: Elective surgeries should be postponed in the active chronic alcoholic due to bleeding risk, increased anesthetic requirement, and risk for acute withdrawal. Each patient should be assessed on an individual basis.

Alcoholic patients present a particular problem given the reliance on patient history and the need for further testing to determine presence of liver disease or coagulopathies. Patients with a history of alcoholic hepatitis are absolutely contraindicated for elective procedures, and the surgery should be postponed for at least 12 weeks for a repeat liver biopsy to show resolution. These patients present a particular problem with anesthetic plans in an ambulatory surgical center due to risk of adverse events upon emergence, increased anesthetic requirement, as well as the risk of acute withdrawal. Patients with a history of alcoholism have a higher risk of emergence delirium, and the elderly have increased incidence of cognitive decline following surgery in the setting of chronic alcoholism [118, 119]. Overall recommendation is to communicate with the patient, physician, and anesthesiologist to determine extent of abuse, any existing liver disease or dilated cardiomyopathy, and the necessity of the planned procedure.

Conclusion

Perioperative management of chronic medications must be assessed on an individual basis as regards their medical history, type of procedure, medication list, and the communication among the medical team (surgeon, anesthesiologist, internal specialist, and PCP). Several chronic medications have limited evidence supporting withholding or continuing use, and the healthcare professional must keep up to date with changing recommendations while keeping in mind the individualized approach.

References

1. Engelhard K. Anaesthetic techniques to prevent perioperative stroke. Curr Opin Anesthesiol. 2013;26(3):368–74.
2. Fleisher LA, Fleischmann KE, et al. ACC/AHA guideline on perioperative cardiovascular evaluation and Management of Patients Undergoing Noncardiac Surgery: a report of the American College of Cardiology/American Heart Association task force on practice guidelines. Circulation. 2014;130:e278–333.
3. Fleischmann KE, Beckman JA, et al. 2009 ACCF/AHA focused update on perioperative Beta blockade: a report of the American College of Cardiology Foundation/American Heart Association task force on practice guidelines. JACC. 2009;54(22):2102–28.
4. January CT, Wann SL, et al. Clinical practice guideline: 2014 AHA/ACA/HRS guideline for the

Management of Patients with atrial fibrillation: executive summary: a report of the American College of Cardiology/American Heart Association task force on practice guidelines and the Heart Rhythm Society. J Am Coll Cardiol. 2014;64:2246–80.
5. Lefkowitz RJ, Caron MG, Stiles GL. Mechanisms of membrane-receptor regulation. Biochemical, physiological, and clinical insights derived from studies of the adrenergic receptors. N Engl J Med. 1984;310(24):1570.
6. Wallace AW, Au S, Cason BA. Association of the pattern of use of perioperative β-blockade and postoperative mortality. Anesthesiology. 2010;113:794–805.
7. POISE Study Group, Devereaux PJ, Yang H, et al. Effects of extended-release metoprolol succinate in patients undergoing non-cardiac surgery (POISE trial): a randomized controlled trial. Lancet. 2008;371(9627):1839.
8. Bouri S, Shun-Shin MJ, Cole GD, Mayet J, Francis DP. Meta-analysis of secure randomized controlled trials of β-blockade to prevent perioperative death in non-cardiac surgery. Heart. 2014;100(6):456.
9. Devereaux PJ, Sessler DI, et al. Clonidine in patients undergoing noncardiac surgery. N Engl J Med. 2014;370(16):1504.
10. Hart GR, Anderson RJ. Withdrawal syndromes and the cessation of antihypertensive therapy. Arch Intern Med. 1981;141(9):1125–7.
11. Bruce DL, Croley TF, Lee JS. Preoperative clonidine withdrawal syndrome. Anesthesiology. 1979;51(1):90.
12. Wijeysundera DN, Beattie WS. Calcium channel blocker for reducing cardiac morbidity after noncardiac surgery: a meta-analysis. Anesth Analg. 2003;97(3):634.
13. Wijeysundera DN, Beattie WS, Rao V, et al. Calcium antagonists are associated with reduced mortality after cardiac surgery: a propensity analysis. J Thorac Cardiovasc Surg. 2004;127(3):755–62.
14. Smith I, Jackson I. Beta-blockers, calcium channel blockers, angiotensin converting enzyme inhibitors and angiotensin receptor blockers: should they be stopped or not before ambulatory anaesthesia? Curr Opin Anesthesiol. 2010;23:687–90.
15. Kizer JR, Kimmel SE. Epidemiologic review of the calcium channel blocker drugs. An up-to-date perspective on the proposed hazards. Arch Intern Med. 2001;161(9):1145.
16. Grodecki-De Franco P, Steinhubl S, Taylor P, et al. Calcium antagonist use and perioperative bleeding complications: an analysis of 5,157 patients [abstract]. Circulation. 1996;94(suppl):I–476.
17. Mohr JP, Orgogozo JM, Harrison MJG, et al. Meta-analysis of oral nimodipine trials in acute ischemic stroke. Cerebrovasc Dis. 1994;4:197–203.
18. Kheterpal S, Khodaparast O, Shanks A, O'Reilly M, Tremper KK. Chronic angiotensin-converting enzyme inhibitor or angiotensin receptor blocker therapy combine with diuretic therapy is associated with increased episodes of hypotension in noncardiac surgery. J Cardiothorac Vasc Anesth. 2008;22:180–6.
19. Mets B. To stop or not? Anesth Analg. 2015;120(6):1413–9.
20. Miceli A, Capoun R, Flno C, Narayan P, et al. Effects of angiotensin-converting enzyme inhibitor therapy on clinical outcome in patients undergoing coronary artery bypass grafting. J Am Coll Cardiol. 2009;54:1778–84.
21. Railton CJ, Wolpin J, Lam-McCulloch J, Belo SE. Renin-angiotensin blockade is associated with increased mortality after vascular surgery. Can J Anaesth. 2010;57:736–44.
22. Roshanov P, Rochwerg B, Patel A, Salehian O, et al. Withholding *versus* continuing angiotensin-converting enzyme inhibitors or angiotensin II receptor blockers before noncardiac surgery: an analysis of the vascular events in noncardiac surgery patlents cOhort evaluatioN Propective cohort. Anesthesiology. 2017;126:16–27. Article in Press Accessed 18 Nov 19.
23. London MJ. Perioperative Administration of Angiotensin-Converting Enzyme Inhibitors or angiotensin II receptor blockers: do we have enough "VISION" to stop it? Anesthesiology. 2017;126(1):1–3. Article in Press Accessed 18 Nov 16.
24. Turan A, You J, Shiba A, Kurz A, Saager L, Sessler DI. Angiotensin converting enzyme inhibitors are not associated with respiratory complications or mortality after noncardiac surgery. Anesth Analg. 2012;114:552–60.
25. Drenger B, Fontes ML, Mioa Y, et al. Patterns of use of perioperative angiotensin-converting enzyme inhibitors in coronary artery bypass graft surgery with cardiopulmonary bypass: effects on in-hospital morbidity and mortality. Circulation. 2012;126(3):261.
26. Tagawa M, Ogata A, Hamano T. Pre- and/or intra-operative prescription of diuretics, but not renin-angiotensin-system inhibitors, is significantly associated with acute kidney injury after non-cardiac surgery: a retrospective cohort study. PLoS One. 2015;10(7):e0132507.
27. Yacoub R, Patel N, Lohr JW, Rajagopalan S, Nader N, Arora P. Acute kidney injury and death associated with renin angiotensin system blockade in cardiothoracic surgery: a meta-analysis of observational studies. Am J Kidney Dis. 2013;62:1077–86.
28. Wolf A, McGoldrick KE. Cardiovascular Pharmacotherapeutic considerations in patients undergoing anesthesia. Cardiol Rev. 2011;19(1):12–6.
29. Chou R, Dana T, Blazina I, Daeges M, Jeanne TL. Statins for prevention of cardiovascular disease in adults evidence report and systematic review for the US preventive services task force. JAMA. 2016;316(19):2008–24.
30. Davignon J. Beneficial cardiovascular pleiotropic effects of statins. Circulation. 2004;109(23):III39–43.
31. Xian-Yu JB, Feng JF, Chen YC, Yang YW. Effects of simvastatin and atorvastatin on biochemical

and hematological markers in patients with risk of cardiovascular diseases. Int J Clin Exp Med. 2015;8(8):13983–9.
32. Kapoor AS, Kanji H, Buckingham J, Devereaux PJ, McAlister FA. Strength of evidence for perioperative use of statins to reduce cardiovascular risk: systemic review of controlled studies. BMJ. 2006;333(7579):1149. Epub 2006 Nov 6 Accessed on 15 Nov 16.
33. Schouten O, Boersma E, Hoeks SE, et al. Fluvastatin and perioperative events in patients undergoing vascular surgery. N Engl J Med. 2009;361(10):980.
34. Dunkelgrun M, Boersma E, Schouten O, et al. Bisoprolol and fluvastatin for the reduction of perioperative cardiac mortality and myocardial infarction in intermediate-risk patients undergoing noncardiovascular surgery: a randomized controlled trial (DECREASE-IV). Ann Surg. 2009;249(6):921.
35. Durazzo AE, Machado FS, Ilkeoka DT, et al. Reduction in cardiovascular events after vascular surgery with atorvastatin: a randomized trial. J Vasc Surg. 2004;39(5):967.
36. Celli BR, MacNee W, ATS/ERS Task Force. Standards for the diagnosis and treatment of patients with COPD: a summary of the ATS/ERS position paper. Eur Respir J. 2004;23(6):932.
37. Licker M, Schweizer A, Ellenberger C, Tschopp JM, Diaper J, Clergue F. Perioperative medical management of patients with COPD. Int J Chron Obsrtuc Pulmon Dis. 2007;2(4):493–515.
38. Cm H, Galvango SM Jr. Patients with chronic pulmonary disease. Med Clin North Am. 2013;97(6):1095–107.
39. Woods BD, Sladen RN. Perioperative considerations for the patient with asthma and bronchospasm. Br J Anaesth. 2009;103(supplemental):i57–65.
40. Vestbo J, Hurd SS, Agusti AG, et al. Global strategy for the diagnosis, management, and prevention of chronic obstructive pulmonary disease: GOLD executive summary. Am J Respir Crit Care Med. 2013;187(4):347–65.
41. Rajesh MC. Anaesthesia for children with bronchial asthma and respiratory infections. Indian J Anaesth. 2015;59(9):584–8.
42. Zachary CY, Evans R. Perioperative management for childhood asthma. Ann Allergy Asthma Immunol. 1996;77:468–72.
43. Liccardi G, Salzillo A, De Blasio F, D'Amato G. Control of asthma for reducing the risk of bronchospasm in asthmatics undergoing general anesthesia and/or intravascular administration or radiographic contrast media. Curr Med Res Opin. 2009;25:1621–30.
44. von Ungern-Sternberg BS, Boda K, Chambers NA, et al. Risk assessment for respiratory complication in paediatric anesthesia: a prospective cohort study. Lancet. 2010;376:773–83.
45. Tirumalasetty J, Grammer LC. Asthma, surgery, and general anesthesia: a review. J Asthma. 2006;43:251–4.
46. FW S, Beckman DB, Yarnold PA, Grammer LC. Low incidence of complications in asthmatic patients treated with preoperative corticosteroids. Allergy Asthma Proc. 2004;25(5):327–33.
47. Reiss TF, Chervinsky P, Dockhorn RJ, Shingo S, Seidenberg B, Edwards TB. Montelukast, a once-daily leukotriene receptor antagonist, in the treatment of chronic asthma: a multicenter, randomized, double-blind trial. Montelukast research study group. Arch Intern Med. 1998;158(11):1213.
48. Young SL, Coulthard P, Wrzosek A, Supplemental A. Perioperative steroids for surgical patients with adrenal insufficiency. Cochrane Database Syst Rev. 2012;12:CD005367.
49. de Lange DW, Kars M. Perioperative glucocorticoid supplementation is not supported by evidence. Eur J Intern Med. 2008;19(6):461–7.
50. MacKenzie R, Goodman SM. Stress dose steroids: myths and perioperative medicine. Curr Rheumatol Rep. 2016;18:47.
51. Lamberts SW, Bruining HA, de Jong FH. Corticosteroid therapy in severe illness. N Engl J Med. 1997;337(18):1285.
52. Chernow B, Alexander HR, Smallridge RC, Thompson WR, et al. Hormonal responses to graded surgical stress. Arch Intern Med. 1987;147(7):1273–8.
53. Cooper MS, Stewart PM. Corticosteroid insufficiency in acutely ill patients. N Engl J Med. 2003;348(8):727.
54. Axelrod L. Perioperative management of patients treated with glucocorticoids. Endocrinol Metab Clin North Am. 2003;32(2):367–83.
55. Ackerman GL, Nolsn CM. Adrenocortical responsiveness after alternate-day corticosteroid therapy. N Engl J Med. 1968;278(8):405.
56. Fauci AS. Alternate-day corticosteroid therapy. Am J Med. 1978;64(5):729.
57. LaRochelle GE, LaRochelle AG, Ratner RE, Borenstein DG. Recovery of the hypothalamic-pituitary-adrenal (HPA) axis in patients with rheumatic disease receiving low-dose prednisone. Am J Med. 1993;95(3):258–64.
58. Livanou T, Ferriman D, James VH. Recovery of hypothalamo-pituitary-adrenal function after corticosteroid therapy. Lancet. 1967;2(7521):856–9.
59. Vann MA. Perioperative management of ambulatory surgical patients with diabetes mellitus. Curr Opin Anesthesiol. 2009;22:718–24.
60. Joshi GP, Chung F, Vann MA, et al. Society for Ambulatory Anesthesia consensus statement on perioperative blood glucose management in diabetic patients undergoing ambulatory surgery. Anesth Analg. 2010;111(6):1378.
61. Dhataruya K, Levy N, Kilvert A, et al. NHS diabetes guideline for the perioperative management of the adult patient with diabetes. Diabet Med. 2012;29(4):420–33.
62. McCormack J, Johns K, Tildesley H. Metformin's contraindications should be contraindicated. JAMC. 2005;173(5):502–4.

63. Jendle J, Grunberger G, et al. Efficacy and safety of dulaglutide in the treatment of type 2 diabetes: a comprehensive review of the dulaglutide clinical data focusing on the AWARD phase 3 clinical trial program. Diabetes Metab Res Rev. 2016;32:776–90.
64. Hirsch IB, McGill JB. Role of insulin in management of surgical patients with diabetes mellitus. Diabetes Care. 1990;13(9):980.
65. Peters A, Kerner W. Perioperative management of the diabetic patient. Exp Clin Endocrinol Diabetes. 1995;103(4):213.
66. Metchick LN, Petit WA Jr, Inzucchi SE, et al. Inpatient management of diabetes mellitus. Am J Med. 2002;113(4):317.
67. Marks JB. Perioperative management of diabetes. Am Fam Physician. 2003;67(1):93.
68. Smiley DD, Umpierrez GE. Perioperative glucose control in the diabetic or nondiabetic patient. South Med J. 2006;99(6):580.
69. Hoogwerf BJ. Perioperative management of diabetes mellitus: how should we act on evidence? Cleve Clin J Med. 2006;73(Suppl 1):S95.
70. MGH Insulin Comparison Chart. http://ww4.mgh.org/Physicians/Formulary%20Documents/Insulin%20Comparison%20Chart.pdf. Accessed on 28 Nov 16.
71. Bennett-Guerrero E, Kramer DC, Schwinn DA. Effect of chronic and acute thyroid hormone reduction on perioperative outcome. Anesth Analg. 1997;85:30–6.
72. Frost L, Vestergaard P, Mosekilde L. Hyperthyroidism and risk of atrial fibrillation or flutter. Arch Intern Med. 2004;164:1675–9.
73. Vickers P, Garg KM, Arya R, Godha U, Mathur P, Jain S. The role of selective beta 1-blocker in the preoperative preparation of thyrotoxicosis: a comparative study with propranolol. Int Surg. 1990;75(3):179.
74. Vandenbroucke JP, Rosing J, Bloemenkamp KW, Middeldorp S, Helmerhorst FM, Bouma BN, Rosendal FR. Oral contraceptives and the risk of venous thrombosis. N Engl J Med. 2001;344(20):1527.
75. Smart A, Gallagher J. Clinicians and women's learning package on Sugammadex (Bridion) and hormonal contraceptives. Aust Nurs Midwifery J. 2015;22(9):52.
76. Baron TH, Kamath PS, McBane RD. Management of Antithrombotic Therapy in patients undergoing invasive procedures. N Engl J Med. 2013;368(22):2113–24.
77. McBane RD, Wysokinski WE, Daniels PR, et al. Periprocedural anticoagulation management of patients with venous thromboembolism. Arterioscler Thromb Vasc Biol. 2010;30:442–8.
78. Kleinman NS. Grabbing the horns of a dilemma: the duration of dual antiplatelet therapy after stent implantation. Circulation. 2012;125:1967–70.
79. Schulman S, Elbazi R, Zondag M, O'Donnell M. Clinical factors influencing normalization of prothrombin time after stopping warfarin: a retrospective cohort study. Thromb J. 2008;16:15.
80. Baigent C, Blackwell L, Collins R, et al. Aspirin in the primary and secondary prevention of vascular disease: collaborative meta-analysis of individual participant data from randomized trials. Lancet. 2009;373:1849–60.
81. Carmignani L, Picozzi S, Bozzini G, et al. Transrectal ultrasound-guided prostate biopsies in patients taking aspirin for cardiovascular disease: a meta-analysis. Transfus Apher Sci. 2011;45: 275–80.
82. Devereaux PJ, Mrokbrada M, Sessler DI, et al. Aspirin in patients undergoing noncardiac surgery. N Engl J Med. 2014;370(16):1494–503.
83. Patrono C, Coller B, Dalen JE, FitzGerald GA, Fuster V, Gent M, Hirsh J, Roth G. Platelet-active drugs: the relationship among dose, effectiveness, and side effects. Chest. 2001;119(1 suppl):39s.
84. Stone DH, Goodney PP, Schanzer A, Nolan BW, Adams JE, et al. Clopidogrel is not associated with major bleeding complications during peripheral arterial surgery. J Vasc Surg. 2011;54(3):779–84.
85. Dweck MR, Cruden NL. Noncardiac surgery in patients with coronary artery stents. Arch Intern Med. 2012;172(14):1054–5.
86. Beattie WS, Warriner CB, Etches R, Badner NH, Parsons D, et al. The addition of continuous intravenous infusion of ketorolac to a patient-controlled analgesic morphine regimen reduced postoperative myocardial ischemia in patients undergoing elective total hip or knee arthroplasty. Anesth Analg. 1997;84(4):715.
87. Trelle S, Reichenbach S, Wandel S, Hildebrand P, Tschannen B, Villiger PM, Egger M, Juni P. Cardiovascular safety of non-steroidal anti-inflammatory drugs: network meta-analysis. BMJ. 2011;342:c7086.
88. Goldenberg NA, Jacobson L, Manco-Johnson MJ. Brief communication: duration of platelet dysfunction after a 7-day course of ibuprofen. Ann Intern Med. 2005;142(7):506.
89. BRIDGE: Study Investigators. Bridging anticoagulation: is it needed when warfarin is interrupted around the time of a surgery or procedure? Circulation. 2012;126:1630–9.
90. Healy JS, Eikelboom J, Douketis J, Wallentin L, Oldgren J, RE-LY Investigators. Periprocedural bleeding and thromboembolic events with dabigatran compared with warfarin: results from the randomized evaluation of long-term anticoagulation therapy (RE-LY) randomized trial. Circulation. 2012;126(3):343.
91. White RH, McKittrick T, Hutchinson R, Twitchell J. Temporary discontinuation of warfarin therapy: changes in the international normalized ration. Ann Intern Med. 1995;122(1):40.
92. Douketis JD, Spyropoulos AC, Spencer FA, et al. Perioperative management of antithrombotic

therapy: antithrombotic therapy and prevention of thrombosis, 9th ed: American College of Chest Physicians Evidence-Based Clinical Practice Guidelines. Chest. 2012;141(2 suppl):e326S.
93. Huyse FJ, Touw DJ, van Schijndel RS, de Lange JJ, Slaets JP. Psychotropic drugs and the perioperative period: a proposal for a guidance in elective surgery. Psychosomatics. 2006;47(1):8.
94. Labos C, Dasgupta K, Nedjar H, Turecki G, Rahme E. Risk of bleeding associated with combined use of selective serotonin reuptake inhibitors and antiplatelet therapy following acute myocardial infarction. CMAJ. 2011;183(16):1835.
95. Auerbach AD, Vittinghoff E, Maselli J, Pekow PS, Young JQ, Lindenauer PK. Perioperative use of selective serotonin reuptake inhibitors and risks for adverse outcomes of surgery. JAMA Intern Med. 2013;173(12):1075–81.
96. Tully PJ, Cardinal T, Bennetts JS, Baker RA. Selective serotonin reuptake inhibitors, venlafaxine and duloxetine are associated with in hospital morbidity but not bleeding or late mortality after coronary artery bypass graft surgery. Heart Lung Circ. 2012;21(4):206–14.
97. Xiong GL, Jiang CRM, Shaw LK, Smith PK, et al. Safety of selective serotonin reuptake inhibitor use prior to coronary artery bypass grafting. Clin Cardiol. 2010;33(6):E94–8.
98. Attri JP, Bala N, Chatrath V. Psychiatric patient and anaesthesia. Indian J Anaesth. 2012;56(1):8–13.
99. Stack CG, Rogers P, Linter SP. Monoamine oxidase inhibitors and anaesthesia. A review. Br J Anaseth. 1988;60(2):222.
100. Peck T, Wong A, Norman E. Anaesthetic implications of psychoactive drugs. Continuing education in Anaesthesia, critical care and pain. Br J Anaesth. 2010;10(6):177–81.
101. Barbesino G. Drugs affecting thyroid function. Thyroid. 2010;20(7):763.
102. Ray WA, Chung CP, Murray KT, Hall K, Stein CM. Atypical antipsychotic drugs and the risk of sudden cardiac death. N Engl J Med. 2009;360(3):225.
103. Larsen KA, Kelly SE, Stern TA, Bode RH Jr, Price LL, Hunter DJ, Gulczynski D, et al. Administration of olanzapine to prevent postoperative delirium in elderly joint-replacement patients: a randomized controlled trial. Psychosomatics. 2010;51(5):409.
104. Wang W, Li HL, Wang DX, Zhu X, Li SL, Yao GQ, et al. Haloperidol prophylaxis decreases delirium incidence in elderly patients after noncardiac surgery: a randomized controlled trial. Crit Care Med. 2012;40(3):731–9.
105. Muluk V, Cohn SL, and C Whinney. Perioperative medication management. UpToDate. 2016. Accessed on 3 Nov 2016.
106. Fischer SP, Schmiesing CA, Guta CG, Brock-Utne JG. General anesthesia and chronic amphetamine use: should the drug be stopped preoperatively? Anesth Analg. 2006;103(1):203.
107. Bryson EO. The perioperative management of patients maintained on medications used to manage addiction. Curr Opin Anesthesiol. 2014;27:359–64.
108. Srivastava A, Kahan M. Methadone induction doses: are our current practices safe? J Addict Dis. 2006;25(3):5–13.
109. Shields LB, Hunsaker JC, Corey TS, et al. Methadone toxicity fatalities: a review of medical examiner cases in a large metropolitan area. J Forensic Sci. 2007;52(6):1389–95.
110. Center for Substance Abuse Treatment (CSAT). Medication-assisted treatment for opioid addiction in opioid treatment programs. In: Treatment improvement protocol [TIP] series 43. HHS publication no. (SMA) 08–4214. Rockville, MD: CSAT, Substance Abuse and Mental Health Services Administration; 2008.
111. Modesto-Lowe V, Brooks D, Petry N. Methadone deaths: risk factors in pain and addicted populations. J Gen Intern Med. 2010;9:898.
112. Webster LR, Cochella S, Dasgupta N, et al. An analysis of root causes for opioid-related overdose deaths in the United States. Pain Med. 2011;12:S26–35.
113. Orman JS, Keating GM. Buprenorphine/naloxone: a review of its use in the treatment of opioid dependence. Drugs. 2009;69(5):577–607.
114. Mastracci TM, Carli F, Finley RJ, Muccio S, Warner DO. Members of the evidence-based reviews in surgery group. Effect of postoperative smoking cessation interventions on postoperative complications. J Am Coll Surg. 2011;212(6):1094.
115. Thomsen T, Villebro N, Moller AM. Interventions for preoperative smoking cessation. Cochrane Database Syst Rev. 2010;7:CD002294.
116. Warner DO. Perioperative abstinence from cigarettes: physiologic and clinical consequences. Anesthesiology. 2006;104(2):356.
117. Smetana GW, Lawrence VA, Cornell JE. American College of Physicians. Preoperative pulmonary risk stratification for noncardiac surgery: systematic review for the American college of physicians. Ann Intern Med. 2006;144(8):581.
118. Sousa G, Pinho C, Santos A, Abelha FJ. Postoperative delirium in patients with history of alcohol abuse. Rev Esp Anestesiol Reanim. 2017;64(4):214–22.
119. Hudetz JA, Iqbal Z, Gandhi SD, et al. Postoperative cognitive dysfunction in older patients with a history of alcohol abuse. Anesthesiology. 2007;106(3):423–30.

13 Ethical Dimensions of Maxillofacial Surgery

Lawrence P. Garetto and Odette M. Aguirre

Abstract

All interactions between doctor and patient, as well as interactions among doctors, have an ethical dimension. This chapter reviews the various domains of ethics in healthcare, including professional ethics, clinical ethics and professional standards. The chapter will also explore ethical issues associated with the profession, stages of care, and specific patient situations such as caring for minors, the incompetent adult, and the adult with compromised decisional capacity.

13.1 Introduction

Surgeons, like all members of the healthcare team, belong to an ethical community, and all interactions between doctor and patient, as well as interactions among members of the healthcare team, have an ethical dimension. It is an inescapable fact that an ethical dimension is never not present. To consider otherwise would be to do great harm to the professional nature of the responsibility in caring for another human being. For anyone accepting the role as doctor, there are additional obligations above what is expected of a layperson that one must assume [1]. Principal among these is the well-cited prima facie[1] duty to put a patient's needs before those of the doctor and, by analogy, society's needs before those of the profession [2–5]. Yet, despite how often we say this and how commonly it is taught, it is still an aspirational goal or ideal because in practicality, it is not always possible to do so. Although aspirational goals are essential to maintain high standards for any profession, there is also a need to recognize when they are not being met and to continually evaluate the nature of work and the behavior of the profession to attempt to do so.

L.P. Garetto, Ph.D. (✉)
Department of Oral Pathology, Medicine and Radiology, Indiana University School of Dentistry, Indianapolis, IN, USA

Charles Warren Fairbanks Center for Medical Ethics, IU Health Methodist Hospital, Indianapolis, IN, USA
e-mail: lgaretto@iu.edu

O.M. Aguirre, D.D.S., M.S., M.P.H.
Department of Biomedical and Applied Sciences, Indiana University School of Dentistry, Indianapolis, IN, USA

[1]The term prima facie *was* delineated by philosopher W.D. Ross (1877–1971) to mean duties that obligate us to act certain ways, assuming everything else is equal. These duties can be overridden by other considerations.

© Springer International Publishing AG 2018

E.M. Ferneini, J.D. Bennett (eds.), *Perioperative Assessment of the Maxillofacial Surgery Patient*,
https://doi.org/10.1007/978-3-319-58868-1_13

The concept of ethics in professional life has to do with the "should I" question. The advanced technical training of surgeons (knowledge and skill), the modern technology available at hand, and the unbalanced relationship due to the power differential between doctor and patient in need [6] always set up a "should I" vs. "can I" deliberation. In many instances, these two questions will be unmistakably concordant, and there is not a driving need to spend time distinguishing between them. But for some circumstances, the "should I" question must be considered as an intentional and deliberative act prior to any "can I" hands-on action. The ability to recognize an ethical issue when one is present is termed *ethical sensitivity*. As such, in order to recognize that reflection is a necessary step to address the "should I" question, and before action is taken, a surgeon must appreciate that an ethical issue is present and of a nature that requires deliberation. In this vein and for the purposes of this chapter, we simplify defining ethics as *reflecting on right behavior*.

13.2 Domains of Ethics in Healthcare

Ethics in healthcare can be subdivided into different domains. We define three somewhat related areas in this chapter: *professional ethics*, *professional standards*, and *clinical ethics*.

13.2.1 Professional Ethics

The most commonly discussed area of ethics in dentistry as a whole is *professional ethics*. In general, it is the first topic presented to new dental students and focuses on the unique relationship that healthcare providers hold with society. Professional ethics describes obligations that are different, and in many ways elevated, for members of a profession than for the laity (society in general). As mentioned above, the concept of an unwritten "societal contract" describing the prima facie duty to put a patient's needs above those of the provider (and society's needs above those of the profession) embodies this branch of ethics. The focus of professional ethics is "outward" on patients in general (i.e., society), not on the profession itself (we define that as the domain of *professional standards*).

An often-debated professional obligation within dentistry is the duty to ensure fair treatment and just allocation of scarce health resources. It is outside the scope of this chapter to delve into social justice concerns and access to care issues beyond noting that they are important elements of the prima facie duty to society that the dental profession must concern itself through reflection, discussion, and especially advocacy.

Finally, *professional ethics* does not get "into the weeds" in addressing specific ethical dimensions present in caring for a particular patient. That is the realm of *clinical ethics* discussed below. Codes of ethics, professional advisory opinions, and other statements about professional obligations are certainly focused on the domain of *professional ethics* but also contain sections that govern intra-professional relationships (addressing *professional standards*).

13.2.2 Professional Standards

A second domain of healthcare ethics is focused on *professional standards*. This is an "inward" focus of the profession on itself and describes the responsibilities that a clinician has to self and other members of the profession in maintaining appropriate professionalism, competency, and accepted standards of care. This area encompasses the important responsibility of peer review and self-regulation. The relative independence of a profession to self-regulate is not a right, but rather a privilege granted by society. This privilege is dependent on society's belief that professionals are trustworthy, and to retain trustworthiness, professionals must meet the obligations expected by society. As long as practitioners judged inadequate by their *peers* are dealt with by the profession itself, the trust that patients place in the profession is maintained [5, 7]. In the absence of *competent* self-regulation, erosion of trust occurs, and professional independence cannot be assured. The obligation to self-regulation is a hallmark attribute that characterizes a true profession from other occupations with the moniker of "professional." It is by no means a simple task, and it is compromised when perceptions arise that the self-regulation is self-serving and "protectionist" to the profession at the expense of the public. When this happens, the privilege to self-regulate may be compromised or subsumed by others outside the profession.

In hospital-based oral surgery environments, the maintenance of professional standards is governed by committees whose membership may consist of both physicians and hospital-based dentists. State boards of dentistry and national organizations like the American Association of Oral and Maxillofacial Surgeons (AAOMS) also play an important role by producing, maintaining, and disseminating ethical codes and rules that highlight both aspirational and judicial guidelines for their members (e.g., state practice acts, AAOMS Code). By their nature, these codes and rules evolve over time as science and technology changes, but the core principles and values upon which they are based are enduring [2, 3].

13.2.3 Clinical Ethics

Where *professional ethics* describes the obligations of a profession to patients in general (i.e., the public or society), *clinical ethics* is focused on the relationship of a clinician with a specific patient and encompasses the ethical dimension of care that is unique to the contextual circumstances of that patient's situation. Clinical ethical issues are most vividly apparent when there is some sort of conflict with, or concern about, a patient. An example would be when a clinician cares for a patient who does not have decisional capacity. In such a situation, it is likely that neither ethical nor perhaps the legal ability to achieve informed consent is possible without a more complex relationship involving a surrogate participating in the decision process. Given such a circumstance, the pathway to proceeding with care is more complex than for a patient with full decisional capacity. A failure to recognize the ethical implication in such a situation is termed *ethical insensitivity* and may result in inappropriate care.

In general, clinical ethical issues are encompassed in four somewhat discreet areas: (1) medical/dental issues, (2) patient preferences, (3) quality-of-life issues, and (4) contextual or "other factors" that impact the care of the patient [8]. Clinical ethical issues can range from very common (e.g., a patient who does not speak the same language as the clinician providing care) to unusual (e.g., an outpatient presenting with an "out-of-hospital" *do not resuscitate* directive). Examples of clinical ethical issues or circumstances are shown in Table 13.1.

Table 13.1 Clinical ethical dimensions of patient care

Confidentiality
• Who has access to the patient's private information?
Informed consent
• Who may appropriately give consent?
Decisional capacity and competence
• Is the patient able to make their own decisions?
Surrogate decision-making
• Is the surrogate making decisions with the best interest of the patient evident?
Respect for patient autonomy vs. nonmaleficence dilemma
• Is the patient requesting treatment that is inappropriate from the dentist's perspective?
Abuse
• What is the threshold for reporting?
Patient behavioral issues
• Is the safety of patient, clinician, or staff endangered due to the patient's behavior?
Lack of patient resources
• Are access to care issues limiting patient autonomy?
Conflict between clinicians
• What is the impact on patient care?
Conflict within families
• Is there disagreement about a treatment plan by a noncustodial parent?
Communication issues
• Are there language comprehension obstacles, or impairment of the patient's, vision/hearing?
"Difficult" patient
• Is the patient uncooperative? Does the patient have limited mouth opening?
Emergency management
• What is the impact of unscheduled patients on other patients?

13.3 The AAOMS Code of Professional Conduct

The AAOMS Code of Professional Conduct is a collection of ethical duties recognized by the association that offers guidance on issues that surgeons may face during the exercise of the specialty. Members' observance of these ethical standards forms the basis of the social contract between the profession and the public. Similar to other ethical codes, the AAOMS Code is not a static document, as it would be impossible to consider and advocate courses of action for the variety of clinical encounters that oral surgeons will come across. However, it constitutes a valuable framework to help support ethically-sound decisions with due consideration given to patient needs and applicable laws. The Code urges fellows and members of the association to "seek to achieve the highest level of ethical conduct in relations with their patients, their peers and the public" (AAOMS Code, A.1) [3] and encourages oral and maxillofacial surgeons to "safeguard their patients, their profession and the public by ensuring that care is rendered only by persons who are professionally competent and of good moral character" (AAOMS Code, A.1 and E.1) [3]. Both of these requirements, competence and moral character, have clear ethics components. Competence, or acquiring and maintaining knowledge and skills, is essential to do no harm to patients, the very definition of the ethical principle of nonmaleficence. Good moral character, on the other hand, is harder to outline, although it can be conceptualized as a person's disposition to think, feel, and behave in an ethical manner. To better understand the attributes of moral character, a model with three interrelated elements has been proposed: (1) the motivation to do good, avoid doing harm, and treat others fairly; (2) the capacity and ability to effectively self-regulate; and (3) the value placed on a positive moral identity (i.e., being a good person). It can be hypothesized that possessing a high level of these three key elements will result in good moral character [9]. However, even with these elements in place, good moral character may not guarantee ethical behavior especially if there is a poor understanding or recognition of professional identity. As such, consultation with ethics codes and applying a model for ethical decision-making are useful.

13.4 Making Decisions and Dealing with Dilemma

Making decisions from an ethics perspective is similar to clinical decision-making. Numerous models are available in the literature to assist healthcare providers with this task. The American College of Dentists' *Ethics Handbook for Dentists* succinctly cites three models as well as the principles and values on which they are based [4]. All decision-making starts with the premise that ethical sensitivity has enabled the identification of the issue about which a decision must be made. In the absence of this sensitivity, a decision-making process cannot be applied because no problem is ever identified. Subsequently, and in various orders, the models all contain steps addressing (1) option thinking as to the different possible solutions to the problem (2) recognition of professional principles and values that apply, (3) evaluation of contextual factors specific to the case, and finally, (4) assessment of "benefits vs. burdens" for each option that should lead to a concordant choice of solution. Many times, the second largest impediment (after insensitivity) in addressing a situation is a failure to identify more than the most obvious of options. One strategy to expand the scope of available options is to think first about the two ends of the spectrum and identify the most conservative approach (sometimes that may be the option of "do nothing") and then identify the most "aggressive" approach. By considering those two solutions as "bookends," other options that are less conservative and less aggressive can be identified. This requires reflection and deliberation but, with practice, becomes a habituated strategy. A stepwise decision-making model is shown in Table 13.2.

While these models are useful for critically considering any clinical decision with ethical

Table 13.2 Ethical decision-making model derived from Ozar [10]

Steps
1. Identify the ethical dimension or concern present in the situation
2. Identify potential solutions for dealing with the situation
3. What are the professional principles and values related to the situation?
4. What specific contextual factors are present in the case (e.g., finances, family issues, decisional capacity)?
5. Of the options identified (in #2 above) and based on #3 and #4, what are the benefits and burdens of each option? Which options would be ethically appropriate and which are ethically inappropriate?
6. Choose the "best" option under the circumstances and implement it

dimensions (and remembering the premise that all clinical decisions in caring for a patient contain an ethical component), such a logic process is essential when dealing with situations involving conflict or an ethical dilemma. In ethics, a dilemma can be defined as a "conflict of rights" and usually involves ethical principles that may be at odds, such as respecting a patient's autonomy vs. not doing harm. More generally, dilemmas represent having to choose between alternatives, each of which may present only a partial benefit to the situation at hand, and none of which are free of burdens. Some might phrase this as choosing the "least worst" option.

One strategy that ethicist David Ozar [10] has proposed is using a values-based approach in considering how to respond to situations where any decision would elevate one principle above another. The five ethical principles (autonomy, nonmaleficence, beneficence, justice, and veracity) accepted by the dental profession are prima facie duties and not hierarchical. Conversely, Ozar's *Central Values of Dental Practice* (Table 13.3) are ranked in order of relative importance. To place a lower rank value above one of higher rank would be to act inappropriately. Using a *central values*-based approach may help to identify an appropriate course of action in dilemma situations when ethical principles are in conflict with each other.

Table 13.3 Ozar's Central Values of Dental Practice [10]

1. The patient's life and general health
2. The patient's oral health
3. The patient's autonomy
4. The dentist's preferred patterns of practice
5. Aesthetic values
6. Efficiency in the use of resources

13.5 Ethical Dimensions in Oral and Maxillofacial Surgery

The remainder of this chapter is organized into two sections, ethical issues associated with (1) the profession and (2) the patient. While these sections identify common ethical issues that an oral surgeon may encounter in practice, creating a comprehensive list and analysis is not possible because of the myriad contextual factors present in the care of unique patients.

13.5.1 Ethical Issues Associated with the Profession

During the course of exercising their specialty, oral surgeons may confront some of the same ethical dilemmas as other dentists and general surgeons. In general, there has been a surge in ethical dilemmas encountered due to the progression of scientific knowledge, the introduction of new technologies, improvements in accepted procedures, scrutiny of existing clinical practices (such as the prophylactic extraction of third molars), increase in patient expectations, and changes in organization and financing of the healthcare system [11]. Oral surgeons might even face some dilemmas more often due to the nature of a practice where most patients come through referral from other dentists. The success of the oral surgeon's practice is reliant not only on providing competent patient care but also on showing respect and empathy for patients, establishing trust, and on maintaining good and lasting relationships that ensure future referrals.

The oral and maxillofacial surgeon's ethical responsibilities are present at all stages of patient care (perioperative, intraoperative, and

Table 13.4 Examples of ethical issues at different stages of patient care

Stage of patient care	Examples of ethical issues
Handoff from general practitioner	Patient acceptance
	Patient involvement
	Informed consent
	Confidentiality
	Proper handling of records
	Differing opinions with other dental practitioners
Presurgical	Recognizing scope of practice
	Consultation
	Emergency services
Surgical	Competence
	Performing procedure for the first time
	Recognizing limitations
	Practicing within scope of practice
	Identity of clinician performing surgery
	Starting or withholding treatment
	Continuing or withdrawing treatment
	Overtreatment
	Delegation of patient care
	Supervision of staff
	Complications and errors
	Impairment (self and peer)
Postsurgical	Managing complications and errors
	Proper and timely patient discharge
	Patient abandonment
Handoff back to general practitioner	Communication of findings to referring dentist
	Patient without referring dentist
	Patient refusing to return to referring dentist
	Justifiable criticism
	Handling of incidental findings

postoperative), independently of the type of surgery (elective, urgent, major, or minor). Ethical duties of involving the patient in decision-making (autonomy), preventing and minimizing harm (nonmaleficence), protecting patient's welfare (beneficence), fair treatment (justice), and honest communication (veracity) will be ever present during all interactions with the patient and the referring dentist. Yet, there are some steps with specific ethical implications for the professional specialty when one follows a patient's journey from a general practitioner to an oral and maxillofacial surgeon (Table 13.4). These stages of care are (1) handoff from the general practitioner, (2) presurgical, (3) surgical, (4) postsurgical, and (5) handoff back to the general practitioner.

13.5.1.1 Handoff from the General Practitioner

The first step in the ethical handling of a patient referral is acceptance without discrimination. Upholding the ethical principle of justice means that patients cannot be denied services based on their race, creed, sex, national origin, or religion or solely because they are infected with a bloodborne pathogen (ADA Code: Justice 4.A and 4.A.1; AAOMS Code, F.3 and F.3.00) [2, 3].

Another ethical principle of relevance at this point of the patient's journey is that of respect for autonomy and patient's right to self-determination. While it may be reasonably expected that the referring dentist has explained to the patient the motive for the referral, the oral and maxillofacial surgeon must obtain specific informed consent from the patient. This will ensure that a competent patient can be involved in meaningful decision-making by being informed of the preoperative diagnosis, proposed treatment, expected benefits, and potential risks (ADA Code: Autonomy 1.A; AAOMS Code, B.1 and B.2) [2, 3]. The amount of information given to the patient will depend on the procedure and its risks. If residents or trainees will be involved in surgical procedures, the patient should also be informed and must give consent (AAOMS Code, B.2.00) [3, 12]. Another aspect of patient autonomy relevant at this stage is the duty to properly handle patient records, safeguarding privacy and confidentiality to protect patient welfare (ADA Code: Autonomy 1.B.2; AAOMS Code, B.1 and B.3) [2, 3].

After patient handoff, the oral surgeon faces obligations toward the referring dentist as well. These are based on effective communication, which is essential for the benefit of the patient. Communication may pose an ethical dilemma when there are differences in opinion with the referring dentist or with other surgeons about the recommended treatment. These must be resolved to ensure the best patient care. Ethical handling of differing opinions may require pursuing consultation with other experts to avoid harming the patient (nonmaleficence), promoting the patient's welfare (beneficence), communicating truthfully (veracity), and not communicating differences of opinion in a manner that unjustly suggests mistreatment (justice). After being informed of all options, the patient must also participate in decision-making (autonomy).

Once the oral surgeon has accepted a patient, a doctor-patient relationship based on trust, mutual respect, and cooperation must be established (AAOMS Code, H.3) [3]. It is worthwhile exploring how this relationship varies from the one that the patient has with the referring dentist. From the perspective of the patient, the relationship with the oral surgeon must be quickly created under circumstances that can be stressful as there may be pain or fear about undergoing the proposed surgical procedure. A special bond can be created in this particular context as a result of the surgeon's task to address a clinical need that justifies a surgical intervention (the "rescue" of the patient from a problem), the immediacy afforded by the surgical procedure ("proximity"), the surgery itself (the "ordeal"), and the outcome (the "aftermath") [13]. In the oral surgeon's viewpoint, the relationship with the referred patient will likely be temporary but will involve a high level of responsibility and intensity with a patient that is particularly vulnerable. This is why an additional characteristic of the surgical relationship, "presence," is essential and must be evident not only by the surgeon's physical presence but also by the commitment and responsiveness to the patient's needs through all stages of the surgical experience [13].

13.5.1.2 Presurgical Stage

As mentioned previously, the AAOMS Code of Professional Conduct encourages oral and maxillofacial surgeons to safeguard their patients, their profession, and the public by ensuring that care is provided only by professionally competent clinicians (AAOMS Code, E.1) [3]. To provide the most appropriate care and cause no harm to the patient, oral surgeons have the responsibility to maintain knowledge, training, and skills current (ADA Code: Nonmaleficence 2.A; AAOMS Code, C.2) [2, 3]. Furthermore, the AAOMS Code specifies that the preoperative evaluation and diagnosis must be performed by the oral surgeon, according to the standard of care (AAOMS Code, B.2.00 and C.1.01) [3] and avoiding unnecessary or substandard services (AAOMS Code, F.1) [3].

To protect the patient's welfare, a comprehensive preoperative evaluation is needed. This should include a complete and careful assessment of medical history, physical examination, and appropriate diagnostic tests to determine the best surgical plan and patient management strategy. Respect for the principle of nonmaleficence may compel the oral surgeon to seek consultation with the patient's treating physician regarding other systemic disorders that could affect surgical procedures and outcomes (ADA Code: Nonmaleficence 2.B) [2]. Perioperative risk assessment is of utmost importance especially in elderly, pediatric, or medically complex patients. Observation and assessment of the mental status of the patient must be part of the initial evaluation, to determine decisional capacity and because undergoing surgery can be an emotionally charged experience.

If, at this stage of care, it is determined that the patient requires emergency treatment, ethics guidelines state that the oral surgeon should either make reasonable arrangements for care of the patient or treat the emergency and refer the patient back to their own general practitioner (ADA Code: Justice 4.B; AAOMS Code, F.1.00 and G.1.01) [2, 3]. The surgeon should inform the other dentist of the condition found and the treatment provided (AAOMS Code, G.1.01) [3]. Sometimes a patient might reach out to an oral surgeon for emergency treatment without having been referred. In this case, there is still an ethical obligation to provide or arrange for needed care, and upon completion of treatment, the surgeon must inform the patient if there is further dental therapy required (ADA Code, Justice 4.B; AAOMS Code, G.1.01) [2, 3]. If the patient referred himself or herself to the oral surgeon for treatment that is not emergent (such as the desire to have implants placed), the oral surgeon is advised to seek consultation with other dental practitioners or specialists to ensure comprehensive care [14].

13.5.1.3 Surgical Stage

Among general surgeons, there is recognition that common ethical dilemmas pertaining to the exercise of the profession include uncertainty about starting vs. withholding treatment, hesitation about continuing vs. withdrawing treatment, and the possibility of overtreatment [11]. The dilemma of whether to start or withhold treatment may be faced when working with patients that have advanced oral cancer or in situations where patient survival is unlikely (e.g., emergency and trauma cases). The predicament of whether to continue or withdraw treatment comes up in cases of advanced oral cancer as well, when initial or additional surgery can result in complications, pain, suffering, and decreased quality of life. Finding the optimal level of treatment for patients with advanced cancer or elderly patients with severe physical or mental illness is a related ethical dilemma. Oral surgeons must be aware of not recommending or performing interventions that will not benefit the patient in the long run. Furthermore, there is recognition that, in an attempt to extend patients' lives, the surgeon might end up overtreating and lengthening the patients' pain and suffering instead. The decision to continue to provide treatment, at the risk of overtreating, may be based on a respect for patient autonomy (patient preference or surrogate decision-maker choice), but it also could be the result of the clinician avoiding the hard decision to abstain from further care when benefit to the patient is unlikely [11]. Note that Ozar's [10] *Central Value* of patient's life and general health must be rightly placed above all other considerations and a decision to go from curative to palliative care may be necessary. The responsibility to provide appropriate end-of-life care is firmly based on the ethical principles of beneficence (by promoting patient welfare), nonmaleficence (by refraining from harming the patient either by failing to treat or by providing unwanted or unhelpful therapy), autonomy (by respecting patient's wishes, within boundaries of accepted treatment), and veracity (by communicating truthfully with the patient) [15].

Once it is decided that care will be rendered, several ethical concerns can emerge when selecting and performing a surgical procedure. The oral surgeon must uphold the principle of nonmaleficence and avoid harming the patient by maintaining knowledge and skills current, recognizing competence and limitations, and only performing procedures within the scope of practice (ADA Code: Nonmaleficence 2.A; AAOMS Code, C.1.00) [2, 3]. A significant issue impacting competence and skills may be the identity of the clinician performing the surgery. While it is acceptable to delegate part of the patient's care to associates, residents, or assistants, the responsibility for supervising personnel and making sure the patient's care is within practice standards falls squarely on the oral surgeon's shoulders. The patient must have been fully informed about whether or not the surgeon would be the one performing the procedure and consent obtained if surgery would be performed by an assistant under the oral surgeon's active supervision (AAOMS Code, B.2.00 and C.1.02) [3]. All oral surgeons will be in the position of performing a certain procedure for the first time, whether because they are in the beginning stages of their career or because a novel procedure is indicated. Both these events must be guided by the ethical principles of nonmaleficence, veracity, and autonomy. Nonmaleficence dictates that the oral surgeon must not execute untested procedures, must not perform procedures before having proper training, and should not perform them without close supervision and active participation from an experienced surgeon. The ethical duty of veracity prescribes that the oral surgeon has an obligation to communicate truthfully with the patient about providers that will participate in the surgery and the innovative aspects of the planned procedure (AAOMS Code, B.2.00) [3, 16]. Finally, respect for patient autonomy and patient involvement is vital, so that proper informed consent can be obtained (ADA Code: Autonomy 1.A; AAOMS Code, B.2 and B.2.00) [2, 3].

Self-care is intertwined with the oral surgeon's ability to practice. Respect for the principle of nonmaleficence requires that if the surgeon is impaired due to abuse of controlled substances, alcohol, or other chemical agents, clinical practice must be limited to protect patients and staff. As well, an oral and maxillofacial surgeon has the ethical obligation to address peer impairment and urge impaired colleagues to seek treatment and to report such behavior to the local well-being committee or to an appropriate dental organization (ADA Code: Nonmaleficence 2.D; AAOMS Code, D.1, D.2) [2, 3].

During surgical procedures, there may be unforeseen complications or medical errors that will necessitate urgent or unanticipated action. The oral surgeon will have to show good judgment and clinical skills to handle such adverse events. And, in the absence of a health proxy, the ethical oral surgeon must also demonstrate familiarity with the patient's wishes and preferences, as obtaining true informed consent from a patient that is unconscious, is sedated or has impaired judgment will be impossible.

13.5.1.4 Postsurgical Stage

Postoperative care must be provided by the oral and maxillofacial surgeon according to accepted treatment parameters (AAOMS Code, C.1.01) [3]. The oral surgeon must continue to care for the patient during the postoperative period, including addressing and treating complications, managing pain, preserving the patient's well-being, and discharging the patient with comprehensive and tailored instructions. If care has begun, the surgeon cannot discontinue it until completed. In cases where the surgeon must discontinue treatment, the patient must be given ample time to contact and obtain services of another oral and maxillofacial surgeon (ADA Code: Nonmaleficence 2.F; AAOMS Code, F.2 and F.2.00) [2, 3] without endangering patient life and general health or oral health. During this stage of care, the oral surgeon needs to properly handle disclosure of complications and errors; this will entail communicating honestly and truthfully with the patient, the referring dentist, and other relevant care providers, thereby honoring the ethical principle of veracity.

13.5.1.5 Handoff Back to General Practitioner

Once surgical treatment has been completed, the oral surgeon shall return the patient to the referring dentist or to the dentist of record for future care. If there is no referring dentist, the surgeon must inform the patient of whether there is need for further dental treatment. Ethical dilemmas may arise if the surgeon fails to communicate clinical findings to the referring dentist, or if the surgeon overlooks the responsibility to ensure that the patient is informed about having to consult a dentist for further treatment.

Another ethical dilemma may arise if the patient objects to returning to the referring dentist and asks for a recommendation for a new dentist instead. To handle this matter ethically, the surgeon must uphold the ethical principles of justice, nonmaleficence, and autonomy. This will involve trying to elucidate the reason behind the patient's desire and determining if the patient's request is justifiable. If after communicating with the referring dentist to privately discuss the patient's concerns the surgeon feels that the patient will be best served by returning to the referring dentist, the patient must be encouraged to do so. On the other hand, communication with the referring dentist may pose an ethical dilemma when the surgeon observes defective or inappropriate dental work in a patient. If the surgeon is concerned with the care that the patient has received from the referring dentist, then it is ethically appropriate to offer recommendations for other general practitioners [17]. The oral surgeon is not exempt from the duty to participate in self-regulation of peers and the profession and has a duty to report to the appropriate reviewing organization continuous faulty treatment by a dental colleague, in accordance with the principle of justice. The oral surgeon should contact the previous dentist to inquire about circumstances surrounding this patient's treatment. Patients should also be truthfully informed of the condition of their oral health without judgmental or derogatory comments about prior treatment (ADA Code: Justice 4.C and 4.C.1) [2].

A current issue of concern is how to ethically handle incidental findings, especially with the advent of newer technologies that may provide a wealth of information and may show conditions out of the scope of practice of the oral surgeon that require interpretation from a trained expert. Expectations and obligations will vary depending on the significance of the incidental finding; responsibilities are due not only to the referring dentist but most especially to the patient. Respect for patient autonomy and beneficence dictates that the patient's informed consent records the patient's desires about how and whether incidental findings will be shared to allow other health practitioners to address potential problems [18, 19].

13.5.2 Ethical Issues Associated with the Patient

The domain of *clinical ethics* focuses on the ethical dimension of care for a specific patient. Any patient, by the individual nature of their situation and condition, has healthcare needs that may be generally similar to other patients presenting with the same surgical need, but contextually, they always have uniqueness as well. Ethically, it is the elements that are unique to each patient that require assessment so as to be able to provide care that is truly in that patient's best interest. But, it is not just the technical provision of care that must be specifically focused on the patient. Rather, the patient must be adequately and appropriately prepared for care by the surgeon in advance of hands-on action.

13.5.2.1 The Nature of the Relationship Between Surgeon and Patient

The relationship of oral surgeon and patient is inherently different from the patient's relationship with their own general dentist. The most prominent difference is related to the duration of the relationship. As was discussed above, the relationship of a patient with the oral surgeon is generally of a much shorter duration than that with their general practitioner. As well, the relationship is much more focused on a specific problem than on comprehensive oral care. Oral surgery by a specialist is a means to carry out a component of the patient's needs identified by the referring dentist in their process of providing comprehensive care. From the patient's perspective, the need to establish a relationship with another care provider is likely an added burden (e.g., mentally, financially) adding more anxiety to that already present due to their health needs. Because anxiety is a recognized factor affecting the decisional capacity of patients [20], the more consequential the nature of the patient's clinical condition, the greater the need for the surgeon to develop a meaningful relationship to help maximize the patient's decision-making and, as such, their autonomy.

13.5.2.2 The Nature of Consent

The "informed" nature enabling consent or refusal of treatment by a patient is not just a signature on a form, but rather a process. Similar to any care provider, there is an ethical obligation for surgeons to work to maximize the autonomy of a patient by enabling them to understand the nature of the proposed care, its benefits and risks, as well as the quality-of-life dimensions associated with doing or not doing a procedure. There is an added obligation in surgical circumstances where the patient must be intentionally incapacitated by pharmacologic agents to perform the surgery. During surgical care, once it begins and before it ends, the surgeon alone makes decisions about care because the patient may not have the ability to participate in decisions during that time. The required work by the surgeon during the presurgical stage, if adequately comprehensive, prepares the patient for expected courses of events and for routine "adjustments" because of circumstances that may be encountered during the surgical period. But, no further consent or interaction may be possible once a patient is anesthetized and an unexpected (especially if emergent) event arises. The surgeon must be ethically sensitive to the inequality of power during such a situation and recognize that the fiduciary obligation to put the patient's needs first becomes an actual duty rather than a prima facie duty.

13.5.2.3 Caring for Minors and Incompetent Adults

Ethically and legally, there are similarities when caring for (1) minor patients who have not reached the age for legal consent or (2) adults who have been legally determined to be incompetent for medical decision-making. Competence is a legal state that, under current law, is granted to individuals at the age of majority (or earlier with legal emancipation) and can be removed from an adult only through a judicial process. In these care situations, the patients themselves cannot give consent (in the legal sense), but depending on age or degree of incapacity, they may be able to *assent* to a plan of care. In both these patient groups, someone other than the patient is acknowledged as the legal guardian, and in this role, they are the de facto surrogate decision-maker.

In the case of an incompetent adult, there will be specific documentation naming the guardian appointed by the court. With minors, unless specific documentation naming a court-appointed guardian is present, guardianship may be appropriately assumed to be the child's parent(s). It is essential that a surgeon specifically identify the legal guardian prior to proceeding with care of patients who are not autonomous decision-makers.

Beyond those already described, there are additional ethical obligations in caring for patients in these groups. It is also necessary for surgeons to not only work to achieve informed consent by the surrogate but to also assess whether decisions by the surrogate are appropriately focused on maintaining or improving the health of the patient. It is beyond the scope of this chapter to fully discuss the elements and types of surrogate decision-making (see Torke et al. 2008 [21] for in-depth review). But, in situations where the surrogate's decision (or their decision-making) is assessed *by the clinician* to <u>not</u> be in the patient's best interest, consideration must be given to contacting child or adult protective service law enforcement divisions as those decisions may be construed as a form of abuse or neglect (ADA Code: Beneficence 3.E and 3.E.1; AAOMS Code, E.4) [2, 3]. This action is obligatory by both ethical and legal standards, and the challenge for any clinician is the need to come to decision as to what action by the surrogate would be beyond a threshold and require reporting. Such an action is also obligatory when patients in this category present with signs of neglect relative to their life and general health.

13.5.2.4 Caring for Adults with Compromised Decisional Capacity

Incompetent patients are a distinct category and are identifiable by the presence of a formally appointed, legally designated guardian. Many patients with deficits in decision-making or memory have not been through a legal process and formally declared incompetent. As such, it is important to distinguish between *competence* and *capacity*. As mentioned above, *competence* is a legal state. The decisional *capacity* of a patient should be assessed by any clinician interacting with the patient prior to hands-on treatment. Decisional capacity involves multiple abilities, all of which must be present for patients to make reasoned decisions regarding treatment. The patient must have the ability to (1) declare a preference or choice (i.e., to reach a decision), (2) understand relevant information to the degree necessary to make the choice, (3) appreciate their situation and the likely consequences of treatment vs. no treatment, and (4) employ logic or rational thought in reaching a decision given pertinent information about their situation [20].

Every clinician must be ethically sensitive to the relative ability of a patient to make decisions involving their own health [22]. This does not always take the form of a formal assessment process, but rather may simply be as a result of conversation in which the patient simply does not seem "quite all there." While a formal diagnosis of compromised decisional capacity should be performed by a physician (and many physicians refer such assessments to psychiatrists), non-physician clinicians are still ethically obligated to assess whether a patient's decision-making is appropriate prior to moving forward with care to assure that the consent to proceed was made with adequate understanding [23].

There are many circumstances including extreme anxiety, drug impairment (legal or otherwise), alcohol abuse, congenital cognitive impairment, degenerative cognitive disorders, and other conditions that result in compromised decisional capacity. In non-emergent situations, if, in the assessment of the surgeon preparing to provide care to a patient, it is not clear that the patient possesses adequate decisional capacity, then a pause is necessary to consider "next steps." The level of concern by the surgeon about the capacity of the patient should be in direct proportion to the gravity of the decision to be made and the criticality of the situation. While the ethical obligations involving the care of such patients touch on all the ethical principles, the foremost duty is to put concern about the patient's life and general health above all else. Patients in a state of decisional incapacity represent a vulnerable population, and even though legal guardianship is not in force, extreme care and consultation should be taken prior to proceeding with treatment.

Conclusion

Oral and maxillofacial surgeons occupy a highly esteemed, trusted, and privileged position within the dental specialties and society as a whole. Attainment of complex and technically difficult skills is essential for patient care. However, development of sensitivity necessary to recognize the ethical dimensions in every clinical interaction is as imperative an ability as the advancement of technical expertise and clinical experience. Due to the nature of surgical care, ethical dilemmas will arise and will challenge relationships with patients and other care providers. Addressing ethical dimensions of patient care helps fulfill the clinician's obligations to individual patients, the profession, and society. An ethically mindful oral surgeon is habitually aware of the responsibility of caring for patients in a competent manner but also reflects and acts to deliver humane care that benefits patients and provides for optimal outcomes.

References

1. Cruess SR, Cruess RL. Professionalism must be taught. BMJ. 1997;315(7123):1674–7.
2. American Dental Association. ADA Principles of Ethics and Code of Conduct. 2016.
3. American Association of Oral and Maxillofacial Surgeons. Code of Professional Conduct. 2014.
4. American College of Dentists. Ethics Handbook for Dentists. 2016.
5. Welie JVM. Is dentistry a profession? Part 3. Future challenges. J Can Dent Assoc. 2004;70(10):675–8.
6. Jones JW, McCullough LB, Richman BW. Introduction: a primer on surgical ethics. The ethics of surgical practice. New York: Oxford University Press, Inc; 2008. p. 3–11.
7. Irvine D. The performance of doctors. I: professionalism and self regulation in a changing world. BMJ. 1997;314(7093):1540–2.
8. Jonsen AR, Siegler M, Winslade WJ. Clinical ethics: a practical approach to ethical decisions in clinical medicine. 6th ed. New York: McGraw-Hill; 2006.
9. Cohen TR, Morse L. Moral character: what it is and what it does. In: Brief AP, Staw BM, editors. Research in organizational behavior. Amsterdam: Elsevier; 2014.
10. Ozar DT, Sokol DJ. Dental ethics at chairside: professional principles and practical applications. 2nd ed. Washington, DC: Georgetown University Press; 2002.
11. Torjuul K, Nordam A, Sørlie V. Action ethical dilemmas in surgery: an interview study of practicing surgeons. BMC Med Ethics. 2005;6:7.
12. Adedeji S, Sokol DK, Palser T, McKneally M. Ethics of surgical complications. World J Surg. 2009;33(4):732–7.
13. Little JM. Ethics in surgical practice. Br J Surg. 2001;88(6):769–70.
14. Wentworth RB. What are specialists' ethical obligations when treating patients who refer themselves? J Am Dent Assoc. 2009;140(3):364–5.
15. Daniel R, Mitchell JJ, Gates PE. End-of-life issues for the oral and maxillofacial surgeon. Oral Maxillofac Surg Clin North Am. 2010;22(4):519–25.
16. Moore FD. Ethical problems special to surgery: surgical teaching, surgical innovation, and the surgeon in managed care. Arch Surg. 2000;135(1):14–6.
17. Foy PJ. What ethical considerations are involved when a patient requests recommendations for a new

general dentist from a specialist? J Am Dent Assoc. 2012;143(2):174–5.
18. Hupp JR. Cone-beam computed tomography incidental findings-a cause for worry? J Oral Maxillofac Surg. 2013;71(7):1157–8.
19. Friedlander AH, Bertolami CN. The ethics of managing incidental findings: implications and challenges for the profession. J Am Dent Assoc. 2014;145(9):910–1.
20. Leo RJ. Competency and the capacity to make treatment decisions: a primer for primary care physicians. Prim Care Companion J Clin Psychiatry. 1999;1(5):131–41.
21. Torke AM, Alexander GC, Lantos J. Substituted judgment: the limitations of autonomy in surrogate decision making. J Gen Intern Med. 2008;23(9):1514–7.
22. Buchanan A. Mental capacity, legal competence and consent to treatment. J R Soc Med. 2004;97(9):415–20.
23. Van TT, Chiodo LK, Paunovich ED. Informed consent and the cognitively impaired geriatric dental patient. Tex Dent J. 2009;126(7):582–9.

14 Medicolegal Aspects of Maxillofacial Surgery

Brendan Faulkner, Patrick J. Kennedy, Elisabeth M. Swanson, Sean M. Stokes, and James R. Hupp

Abstract

Before and after maxillofacial surgery, the goal should be to do careful and regularly updated patient assessments and to have clear and open communications with the patient that are well-documented. During surgery, monitoring, controlling, and documenting the patient's anesthetic course and any surgical emergencies are critical. All of this reflects quality care fostering patient safety and will legally protect the surgeon as well.

All surgical procedures carry the potential for patient harm which may lead to a claim of medical negligence. However, between 1992 and 2014, the rate of malpractice claims paid on behalf of physicians in the United States declined substantially.[1]

The risk of legal claims against a maxillofacial surgeon, in general, is low relative to other surgical specialists. This chapter offers suggestions on how the risk can be further reduced through systematic, well-documented perioperative assessment of the patient.[2]

Before and after maxillofacial surgery, the goal should be to do careful and regularly updated patient assessments and to have clear and open communications with the patient that

[1] Schaffer AC, Jena AB, Seabury SA, Singh H, Chalasani V, Kachalia A. Rates and Characteristics of Paid Malpractice Claims Among US Physicians by Specialty, 1992–2014. JAMA Intern Med. Published online March 27, 2017. doi:https://doi.org/10.1001/jamainternmed.2017.0311. This database study linked National Practitioner Data Bank claims data with physician specialty and found that the overall rate of claims paid on behalf of physicians deceased by 55.7% from 1992 to 2014. Mean compensation amounts and the percentage of payments exceeding $1 million increased during that time, with wide differences in rates and characteristics across specialties.

[2] All discussions of clinical practices are from a legal (nonclinical) perspective only.

B. Faulkner, Esq. (✉) • P.J. Kennedy, Esq.
E.M. Swanson, Esq. • S.M. Stokes, Esq.
RisCassi & Davis P.C., Hartford, CT, USA
e-mail: BFaulkner@riscassidavis.com

J.R. Hupp, D.M.D., M.D., J.D., M.B.A., F.A.C.S.
Journal of Oral Maxillofacial Surgery,
Fairfield Glade, TN, USA

Emeritus of Oral-Maxillofacial Surgery, School of Dental Medicine, East Carolina University, Greenville, NC, USA

© Springer International Publishing AG 2018

E.M. Ferneini, J.D. Bennett (eds.), *Perioperative Assessment of the Maxillofacial Surgery Patient*,
https://doi.org/10.1007/978-3-319-58868-1_14

are well-documented. During surgery, monitoring, controlling, and documenting the patient's anesthetic course and any surgical emergencies are critical. All of this reflects quality care fostering patient safety and will legally protect the surgeon as well.

14.1 Preoperative Patient Assessment

Obtaining and documenting a patient's medical history and physical examination findings, as well as appropriate laboratory and imaging results are essential to developing an effective treatment plan. Even where the patient's primary care physician has performed a history and physical examination, it is the oral and maxillofacial surgeon's responsibility to determine whether further assessment is necessary.[3] The preoperative assessment should also include a thoughtful and open discussion with the patient and, when appropriate, with his or her family. (This topic is more fully covered in Part 1, Chap. 2).

By identifying factors that increase a patient's surgical risk, the maxillofacial surgeon is positioned to formulate strategies to reduce the risk (or to recommend that the patient to delay or not undergo the procedure). When documenting the level of risk (e.g., low, moderate, high), the surgeon should keep in mind comorbidities, namely, other factors that increase the risk of complications, morbidity, and/or mortality. Incomplete information, or failure to properly appreciate the significance of it, increases the risk of a malpractice claim. The failure to learn all of patient's prescription and non-prescription medications, for example, can have disastrous consequences.

The surgeon should also consider scheduling higher-risk patients at times and on days when there is no time pressure. For example, the serum glucose of type I diabetic patients is easier to manage earlier in a day when they have been required to adjust their insulin and calorie intake.

14.1.1 Medical History

Patient completion of an easy to understand and concise questionnaire is the beginning of a thorough assessment of a patient's medical history. Several forms are available online from well-respected facilities and other institutions that can be readily adapted to the surgeon's particular practice.

The goals of preparing a complete medical history should include searching for perioperative cardiac, pulmonary, and infectious complications and extensive inquiry into the patient's medication history.[4]

Recent use of particular medications may seem insignificant to some patients, while in fact such medication use would have important clinical ramifications (e.g., with anticoagulants, aspirin, nonsteroidal anti-inflammatories, supplements, herbals, and over-the-counter medications). The surgeon should ask direct questions about this in the interview.

Surgical patients should also be asked to detail their allergies, surgical, anesthesia history, and their daily activities as evidence of their functional status.[5]

The particular risks of the surgical procedure under consideration should be kept in mind throughout this process.

[3] *Parameters of Care: Clinical Practice Guidelines for Oral and Maxillofacial Surgery, Patient Assessment.* AAOMS ParCare 2012 (PAT-1). This is one of eleven clinical sections included in AAOMS PARCARE 2012, which is a living document, which is available at http://www.mfch.cz/doc/ParCare2012%20Complete.pdf. As defined therein, "Parameters of care" is a phrase used to describe an organized range of accepted patient management strategies, including guidelines, criteria, and parameters. The American Association of Oral and Maxillofacial Surgeons (AAOMS), the professional organization, is representing more than 9000 oral and maxillofacial surgeons in the United States.

[4] Zambouri A. Preoperative evaluation and preparation for anesthesia and surgery. *Hippokratia*. 2007; 11(1):13–21.

[5] *Id.*

14.1.2 Physical Examination

The clinical assessment, like the medical history, should also be thorough and recorded in detail. If the patient's primary care physician recently performed a complete history and physical examination, the surgeon may use that data to help him or her do a more focused history and physical related to the planned surgery and anesthesia. Although this does not need to be conducted by the oral or maxillofacial surgeon performing the procedure,[6] it must be obtained and reviewed by the surgeon prior to the procedure. Note that brief chart notes may allow a picture of substandard care to be painted in a subsequent malpractice lawsuit. So the surgeon should carefully document the presurgical patient evaluation(s) performed.

A thorough physical exam may provide important documentation regarding a patient's physical and mental condition prior to the procedure, particularly as they relate to the planned procedure. This information may prove critical if the patient later claims they had physical symptoms prior to the procedure that were contraindications for such a procedure or if the patient later claims symptoms were caused by the procedure. In either situation, documentation of the physical exam will provide important documentation for refuting such claims. If the patient refuses a complete physical exam, or any part of a physical exam, this too should be documented.

14.1.3 Establish a Definitive Diagnosis Prior to Treatment

When diagnosing and managing patients with diseases of the oral and maxillofacial region, it is important to include documentation of the differential diagnosis reached and how each condition reasonably likely to be present was ruled out. It is better to have considered and reasonably ruled out a condition, than to have not even considered a condition that would typically be on an oral and maxillofacial surgeon's maxillofacial surgeon's differential diagnosis. If this is not well-documented, in an ensuing claim for alleged malpractice, the surgeon will be hard-pressed to argue that it occurred but was not documented. This is particularly important when doing revision surgery since a patient may have problems such as nerve deficits that preexist the planned revision surgery. Thus, documentation of the patient's presurgical physical status is critical.

Only after each possible diagnosis on the differential has been ruled out, should the oral and maxillofacial surgeon proceed with treatment, although in some situations the surgery is required to help establish the diagnosis. Attempting to establish a definitive diagnosis prior to major surgery will eliminate both the risk of missing a more severe diagnosis that had not been thoroughly ruled out and the risk of overtreating a patient who would have been better served with more conservative measures. Either situation could lead to dissatisfied patients.

Once a definitive diagnosis has been reached, a patient must be thoroughly educated on all treatment options.

14.1.4 Medical Record

The oral and maxillofacial surgeon is responsible for ensuring the completeness of the patient's medical record, which is also considered a legal document. It cannot be overemphasized that the patient's medical history, physical exam, differential diagnosis, and the discussions regarding treatment options must be thoroughly recorded in the medical records. Medical records (and their metadata) are often at the heart of medical negligence claims and the ability to successfully defend those claims.

14.1.4.1 General Considerations

Thorough, accurate, legible records are a boon to quality of care and decrease the likelihood of claims. They protect patients and doctors alike. A medical negligence attorney reviewing a case is less likely to become involved where the record includes detailed, well-reasoned notes. When

[6] http://www.aaoms.org/images/uploads/pdfs/parcare_assessment.pdf (PAT-7)

malpractice claims are made, thorough record-keeping will protect the surgeon from the adage "if it's not documented, it didn't happen."

It is also good practice to document a patient's ability to participate in care and that he or she understands all aspects of treatment, medications[7] prescribed and their contraindications, postsurgical instructions, the follow-up plan, and how to get in touch with the surgeon or a person covering for the surgeon after hours.

Outlining the reason(s) supporting the decision to perform a procedure should be recorded. Often these reasons reflect the risk-benefit analysis. Such documentation will help substantiate the need for the procedure. It will also show the use of clinical judgment. In a lawsuit claiming harm due to continuing a medication during the procedure, for example, the surgeon's assertion that he/she discussed this issue with the patient will be significantly stronger if reflected in the record. In addition, if the surgeon obtained information from the patient's other doctors or consultants, those notes should also be included in the patient's presurgical records.

14.1.4.2 Electronic Medical Records

An electronic medical record (EMR) is a digital version of a patient's medical record. Medical practices often use a fillable or menu-driven electronic forms to create patient medical records. While there are benefits to such a system, the medical provider will need to resist the urge to simply check boxes and copy and paste from earlier records. Copying and pasting (or "cloning") is an attractive option in a busy surgical office or practice, but adequately documenting a patient's present complaints and symptoms is critical to ensuring the highest quality of care and safeguarding against future claims. It is always obvious to experienced professionals when medical records have simply been copied and pasted.

14.1.4.3 Patient Safety Risks of Electronic Medical Records

That electronic medical records (EMRs) pose certain risks to patient safety has become clear over time but has not generated the attention these risks deserve. Issues with unclear or misleading preprogrammed options and drop-down menus, as well as typographical errors, and overuse of the cut-and-paste function have resulted in patient harm. Likewise, injuries and deaths have been linked to medication management, clinical documentation, diagnostic imaging, and clinical decision support systems, as well as data-to-narrative functions, within EMRs.

In light of these concerns, when reviewing an EMR, the oral and maxillofacial surgeon must review it critically, using medical judgment. If a box has been checked that does not make sense in context of the patient's overall presentation, that portion of the record should be examined more closely.

It is important that medical providers recognize the fallibility of EMRs, the margin of error when using fillable forms, and use medical judgment when reviewing them. EMR systems typically provide areas for the clinician to type in comments or other prose documentation, and these should be used in addition to check box or menu-driven portions of the EMR.[8]

14.1.4.4 EMRs in Litigation

Mandatory EMR systems that record information about access to an EMR reflect that information by way of audit trails or logs and revision histories. An audit trail is a record, in chronological order, of who accessed an electronic medical record system. It will have several details about each access (who, what, where, when, etc.).[9] It

[7]Opioids, anticoagulants, and other medications can pose liability risks that are beyond the scope of this chapter. *See* CDC Guideline for Prescribing Opioids for Chronic Pain, Dowell, D., MD; Haegerich, T. Ph, Chou, R., MD. MMWR Recomm Rep 2016; 65:1–49. Opioid Abuse in Chronic Pain—Misconceptions and Mitigation Strategies, Volkow, N., M.D., and McLellan, A.T., Ph.D., N Engl J Med 2016; 374:1253–63. In general, if there is any question regarding a patient's current medications, the physician should be quick to obtain a medical consult and to document it in the record.

[8]For a good discussion of this topic, *see generally* Byyny RL. The tragedy of the electronic health record. Pharos Alpha Omega Alpha Honor Med Soc 2015; 78:2–5.

[9]Biomedical Informatics: Computer Applications in Health Care and Biomedicine 815 (Edward H. Shortliffe and James J. Ciminino eds., 4th ed., 2013).

also shows any person changing, correcting, supplementing, altering, or amending the record. Accesses of the audit trail itself will likewise be shown in what is referred to as a disclosure. A revision history chronologically lists document or data versions showing all changes.

Malpractice claims can be won or lost based on the evidence in an audit trail, revision history, and similar evidence because jurors tend to credit computer-generated data over testimony of witnesses who may have an interest in the outcome of the case.

In the event of adverse incidents, special care must be taken to preserve the complete record, including radiographs, treatment, and account notes, as well as informed consent documents. Never change the record.[10] If the record is incorrect, EMR systems have methods for adding supplemental information to an existing record and describe why the existing record is in error. However, no attempt should be made to delete any portion of the record later found to be inaccurate.

14.1.4.5 HIPAA

Medical records are subject to the Health Insurance Portability and Accountability Act Regulations (HIPAA). HIPAA offers very broad privacy protections to patients. Under HIPAA, a clinician has a duty to safeguard any information pertaining to a patient's treatment, which extends to even disclosing the identity of a patient. Surgeons need to be particularly vigilant not to breach their duties under HIPAA when a patient asserts a claim. Particularly if the surgeon's care is not the subject of a claim, HIPAA prohibits the clinician from having unauthorized communications with anyone, including attorneys.

While HIPAA ensures a patient's right to privacy, other federal law ensures a patient's access to records. If a patient makes a request for medical records, either individually or through an attorney with a duly executed HIPAA authorization form, the clinician must release those records.

14.1.5 Communication

14.1.5.1 Communication with Patient

From both a quality of care and a risk mitigation perspective, the value of communicating with the patient clearly cannot be overstated. Clients commonly seek the advice of medical negligence attorneys complaining of communication failures with their doctors.

Communication between surgeon and patient is critical to establishing trust, rapport, and confidence in the relationship. As a result of open and honest discussion with the surgeon, the patient should have reasonable expectations for his or her postsurgical appearance and function, as well as the risks involved. This is critically important. If possible, this should also be discussed with the patient's family present. The prudent practitioner will listen closely and reflectively to the patient, pay close attention to his or her family, and make a clear note of the discussion. An open dialogue will lead to a relationship of trust and partnership. An important part of communication is listening. Often, looking at or entering information into the electronic medical record impedes quality listening. Disclosing any conflicts is also essential.

All communications with a patient (including e-mail, phone calls, texting, etc.) should be documented clearly, thoroughly, and in a timely manner. This should be the subject on ongoing staff training and a written policy and procedure.

When poor or unplanned outcomes do arise, quietly listening while the patient explains his or her dissatisfaction is good practice, as are concerns for the patient and regret of the outcome. The surgeon should discuss what steps can be taken to help mitigate the patient's concerns. These types of communication, as opposed to avoidance or confrontation, are generally appreciated and make it less likely the patient's family will ever consult a lawyer specializing in medical negligence.

[10] Parameters of Care: *Clinical Practice Guidelines for Oral and Maxillofacial Surgery, Patient Assessment.* AAOMS ParCare 2012 (PAT-1).

14.1.5.2 Apologizing to the Patient

There may be occasions when a surgeon feels morally compelled to offer an apology. Additionally, studies have shown that apologizing to patients when an error occurs, or there is a bad outcome, may help to encourage settlement or reduce the amount of compensation sought by a patient.[11] However, recent studies also show that apologizing when a patient does not know an error occurred may actually be the impetus for a claim.[12] While apologizing is an important part of interpersonal relationships, legally, a clinician apology may have negative consequences. At trial, a defendant's words can be offered by the opposite side as an admission. In other words, if a doctor apologizes to a patient, it may be presented at trial as an admission of wrongdoing.

Recognizing the legal jeopardy into which a heartfelt apology may place a doctor, many state legislatures have enacted laws protecting apologies from being offered as admissions of wrongdoing at trial. Thirty-five states and the District of Columbia have such laws.[13] The laws on clinician apologies however vary from state to state, and many contain subtle nuances that demand close attention to the wording of an apology. For example, in Maine an apology may be protected, but if it is accompanied by an admission of fault, that fault admission is admissible.[14] If a medical error does occur, or there is a bad outcome, and a surgeon feels compelled to offer an apology, risk management and legal counsel in the state of the incident must be consulted regarding the potential evidentiary admissibility of an apology at trial.

[11]Nicole Saitta and Samuel D. Hodge, *Efficacy of a Physician's Words of Empathy: An Overview of State Apology Law,* The Journal of America Osteopathic Association, Vol. 112, 302–306 (2012).

[12]Benjamin J. McMichael, R. Lawrence Van Horn, and W. Kip Viscusi *Sorry Is Never Enough: The Effect of State Apology Laws on Medical Malpractice Liability Risk*, 15 (Dec, 10, 2016), available at https://ssrn.com/abstract=2883693.

[13]Nicole Saitta and Samuel D. Hodge, *Efficacy of a Physician's Words of Empathy: An Overview of State Apology Law,* The Journal of America Osteopathic Association, Vol. 112, 302–306 (2012).

[14]*Id.*

Despite the possible legal implications of an apology, practically speaking, the effect of a medical provider's sincere apology and willingness to take responsibility at trial can be important. Often, large verdicts come as a result a jury's desire to punish a wrongdoer who is unconcerned with the consequences of their actions. A sympathetic, likeable, and humble defendant may leave a lasting impression on a jury.

14.1.5.3 Communication with Other Medical Care Providers

Miscommunications during handoffs or between medical care providers when responsibility for a patient is transferred are known to be a significant cause of medical errors. Such an error could occur, for instance, if providers do not discuss information about a diagnostic test during a shift change. Cross-covering clinicians present the most significant risk for an adverse event related to a handoff error.

A systemized handoff communications process (bundled communication and training tools) was shown to reduce medical errors by 23% and preventable adverse events by 30%. A key component of this system is an oral handoff process centered around the "I-PASS" mnemonic referring to illness severity (if there is any concern that a patient is at risk of deteriorating, this should be clearly communicated), patient summary (exam findings, laboratory data, and clinical changes), action list (written out by bullet points or numerically), situation awareness and contingency planning ("if/then" statements), and synthesis by receiver (e.g., read-back).[15] Timely, clear, and concise written communication regarding patient information is also important to avoiding handoff errors.

As with the patient, listening carefully to other doctors, nurses, and physician assistants minimizes harm as well. A recent analysis found that 30% of all claims involve a communication failure and that provider-provider communication

[15]*See* www.ipasshandoffstudy.com. A specific toolkit for perioperative handoffs is available at www.aorn.org/PracticeResources/ToolKits/PatientHandOffToolKit/.

failures are more likely to lead to payments in lawsuits than problems with provider-patient communication.[16]

14.1.6 Informed Consent

Each person has a right to decide what to do with their body, including in the medical context. The basic principle is that doctors must give patients the important facts necessary to make an intelligent decision.

According to the American Medical Association, informed consent includes providing the patient with the diagnosis, the nature and purpose of the procedure, the risk and benefits of the treatment or procedure, alternatives (including their risks and benefits), and the risks and benefits of not receiving treatment.

Many claims against surgeons involve inadequate communication during the consent process. Both verbal and written communication is important to preventing claims arising out of the failure to provide the patient with adequate information. Furthermore, failure to adequately document the informed consent discussion of risks or alternatives is also a common cause of claims that can be easily avoided.

The informed consent discussion should be a continuing process focused on the sharing of information about the treatment or procedure, including any uncertainty about it. It should convey the necessary facts while building a bond between the doctor and patient. Informed consent should not be thought of as a piece of paper but the foundation of a trusting doctor-patient relationship.

A thoughtful informed consent discussion will bridge the gap between what the patient does not know and may be anxious about and the surgeon's knowledge. The patient should understand that he or she and the maxillofacial surgeon are going to cooperate in an effort to improve the health or function. Information on videos about the patient's condition and surgery are commonly available. They can be useful but should be considered a supplement but not a substitute to an in-person discussion of the planned surgery between the surgeon and the patient.

The patient must understand the full range of possible outcomes, and this understanding should be documented. Tell patients the best, worst, and most likely possible outcomes of the procedure, so they can decide whether it is worth the risks. Use common words and encourage patients to take notes, ask questions, and summarize their understanding. Additionally, studies have shown written warnings provided to patients significantly improves their understanding of warnings.

When multiple surgical choices are presented, the option with the least risk should be offered. Sometimes this includes a no treatment option. Under such circumstances, the records should reflect an offer of no treatment was made and rejected by the patient.

Informed consent should include a documented explanation of indicated complications such as pain, swelling, bleeding, infection, temporary or permanent nerve damage, and death. With respect to risk of nerve injuries, in particular, an informed consent form (and discussion) specifically identifying the potential for numbness and functional limitations is advisable. Consider the use of individualized informed consent forms for specific procedures. Additionally, the plan for postoperative pain control, venous thromboembolism prophylaxis, antibiotics, and substitution of and return to current medications should all be discussed preoperatively.

The patient's expectations will be realistic if the informed consent discussion is thoughtful. This will also serve to militate against a malpractice claim. Reassure, but do not overpromise results. In fact, under-promising may be a better approach.

In some situations, part of the informed consent discussion may have to include telling the patient that other surgeons are more experienced with the procedure under consideration. Be aware that some malpractice lawyers subpoena the surgeon's volume of cases involving the procedure at issue from the hospitals where the surgeon has

[16]Malpractice Risks in Communication Failures, 2015 Annual Benchmarking Report. CRICO Strategies.

privileges to determine the accuracy of the surgeon's representations as to his or her level of experience.

Not mentioning a doctor's financial incentive or conflict, a safer alternative surgical option or the availability of more qualified surgeons can all be problems for the defendants in lawsuits. The bottom line is that the surgeon must always put the patient's interests first, and the informed consent discussion should be well-documented.

14.1.7 Intraoperative Assessment

The surgeon is considered the "captain of the ship" in the operating room. Therefore, he or she must be aware of everything affecting patient safety and the success of the operation. Although the clinician providing the patient's anesthesia is responsible for properly delivering that service, the surgeon is expected to intervene if he/she believes the anesthesia care being provided is not completely satisfactory. The same is true for nursing services. The surgeon should keep himself/herself apprised of the patient's vital signs, intraoperative laboratory results, blood loss, fluid replacement, possible breaks in aseptic technique, and other aspects of the patient's overall clinical situation.

Studies have shown the value of surgical check lists and pre-incision time-outs. Most hospital operating rooms require use of such patient safety approaches. Prior to wound closure, a sponge count and check that any other materials are accounted for is important. If any question arises, intraoperative imaging should be considered.

14.1.8 Postoperative Assessment and Practice

The postoperative assessment of the patient is an important part of the patient's record.

The first postoperative assessment of the patient provides an important baseline against which the patient's future condition will be assessed. It should include the individualized postoperative plan, the patient's cardiac and respiratory status, and his or her mental status.

The procedure note should be completed in a timely fashion, preferably immediately following surgery. This allows postsurgical providers to have the information needed to effectively carry out their responsibilities. Operative notes should be dictated and signed within 24 h of the procedure.

It is important for the surgical site to be inspected and the results documented, preferably by the surgeon. Patient management in the postoperative unit should also include documented monitoring of vital signs, assessment of oxygen saturation, ability to urinate, and input/output records.

For outpatient surgery with sedation or general anesthesia, patients must meet minimum safe discharge criteria as determined by an accepted scoring tool. Provide written postoperative instructions to the patient. Include the phone number to call in case of a problem.

Patients should be educated on what is considered "excessive" bleeding, and the importance of contacting the surgeon or calling 911 should be stressed. In addition to the provision of written instructions to the patient, the record should reflect that the patient was informed about early signs of postoperative problems such as an infection.

Same day follow-up calls for patients at high risk of postoperative bleeding are good care and will prevent patients from feeling neglected. For this reason, frequent follow-up is also a good practice. Every time a patient is reviewed, there must be a clear clinical note.

All concerns or complaints must be promptly investigated and addressed no matter how seemingly insignificant. An experienced plaintiff's lawyer will point out that the standard of care requires a doctor who cares. By the same token, following a mistake, a good rapport (as opposed to arrogance or indifference) may have considerable influence.

14.1.9 Medical Negligence

The civil justice system provides accountability which in turn drives the development of systems, policies, procedures, and guidelines to ensure patient safety.

The laws governing medical negligence claims vary from state to state. For instance, some states have a pre-suit requirement of filing a "good faith certificate." Others require that the case be presented to a medical malpractice tribunal first.

In general, the basic requirements of proof by a party filing a medical negligence claim are establishing the existence of a patient-doctor relationship, a breach of the standard of care, and damages caused by such breach. The standard of care is established through qualified experts testifying as to the prevailing practice, or, in other words, what a reasonably prudent, similarly trained surgeon would do under similar circumstances. Based on all of the testimony and documentary evidence presented, the jury is charged with determining whether it is more likely than not that there was a breach of the standard of care. If there was, the next determination is whether the plaintiff suffered harm as a result of the breach of the standard care which more likely than not would have been avoided had the standard of care been met. In some circumstances, depending on state law, a patient who has lost a significant chance of a better outcome as a result of medical malpractice may also be entitled to compensation.

A plaintiff who has been injured as a result of medical malpractice can recover compensatory damages consisting of past and future economic harm (e.g., medical bills and lost wages) and non-economic damages for past and future pain and suffering caused by the medical error.

14.1.9.1 Discovery in Medical Malpractice Cases

Discovery is the process through which the parties to litigation obtain information, documentary evidence, and testimony from the opposing party and, on occasion, from third parties.

As noted previously, the patient's record and all electronic metadata (e.g., audit log, revision history, etc.) are often the most important evidence in a claim for medical malpractice. This information will be exchanged as part of the discovery process. Additionally, the surgeon's continuing education records are often the subject of discovery in malpractice suits, as are employment agreements.

At some point in the litigation, the defendant surgeon will likely have to give a deposition, which is simply testimony under oath in the form of a question-and-answer session by the plaintiff's attorney. The session is transcribed by a court reporter and may be videotaped. The attorney assigned to defend the surgeon in the case will spend a significant amount of time preparing the surgeon for his or her deposition including reviewing documents and discussing likely topics and questions. The plaintiff's attorney may also depose other individuals who participated in the patient's care including office staff and operating room personnel. The surgeon's attorney will also attend the depositions to help insure that the plaintiff's attorney is following proper procedures and asking relevant questions. The surgeon's attorney will also depose the patient and, in some cases, others claiming an injury due to the surgeon's actions.

14.1.9.2 The Odds of Successfully Defending Against a Claim of Malpractice Claim Are Generally in the Defense's Favor

If and when the maxillofacial surgeon is eventually sued for malpractice, the odds are significantly in the surgeon's favor. PIAA, the insurance trade association representing medical professional liability insurance companies, risk retention groups, and other similar entities, has reported that 70% of the claims closed within its collaborative database (containing hundreds of thousands of closed medical and dental claims and suits) have no indemnity payment. The odds are even better for the clinician when the medical record is clear, detailed, thorough, and contemporaneous with treatment.

Additionally, trials in malpractice claims are rare. Most cases are settled before trial for a number of reasons. Because these cases are time-intensive and expensive for the attorneys bringing them, experienced counsel place a premium on careful case selection. It is simply not a good business practice for a plaintiff's lawyer to get involved in a case that the lawyer does not feel has a strong chance of being resolved favorably to the plaintiff. Additionally, the stakes are typically high, and both sides usually have an opportunity to mitigate their risk through a compromise settlement.

14.1.9.3 Insurance

Medical malpractice or professional liability insurance provides an amount of money from which to pay settlements or adverse judgments in such liability claims. The legal term for this is indemnification. Professional liability coverage also pays for legal representation in the context of such claims.

The prudent practitioner should also consider purchasing a third type of coverage, which applies to defending the insured in proceedings by the state board of medical examiners and is not typically included in standard malpractice policies. Likewise, it is important to be aware of so-called wasting policies in which the limits of liability for indemnification are reduced by the amount spent on defense costs.

In the event of an adverse event, bad outcome, or dissatisfied patient that the surgeon believes *may* lead to a claim, the professional liability carrier should be notified as soon as possible. The liability insurer also has a duty on behalf of its insured to investigate and preserve evidence.

14.1.9.4 Consent to Settle

Most medical professional liability policies have a "consent to settle" clause that gives the surgeon veto power over the decision to settle a lawsuit. It may be in the clinician's best interest to settle if there is a risk of an excess judgment for which he might be held personally responsible, but there can be strong countervailing considerations as well such as report of the settlement to a national database and feared damage to reputation. The risk of an excess judgment, however, can be virtually eliminated by purchasing adequate liability coverage. In the unlikely event there is a risk of an excess judgment at some point, the surgeon would be wise to retain personal counsel (separate from the defense provided by the insurer) to provide advice as to the best course of action. Finally, with respect to consent to settle provision, the clinician should be aware of so-called hammer clauses which apply to the situation in which the insurer wants to settle a claim, but the clinician will not consent. If there is such a provision, and the case is eventually resolved by way of judgment or settlement for more than the insurer was willing to settle for when the clinician would not consent, then the clinician will be responsible the excess amount and attorney's fees (depending on the policy language).

14.1.10 Common Claims Against the Maxillofacial Surgeon

While medical errors are the third leading cause of death in the United States (behind heart disease and cancer), claiming at least 251,000 lives every year,[17] and it is estimated that 40,000 patients per day are injured because of medical errors,[18] malpractice claims remain rare.

Nationwide, approximately 85,000 medical malpractice cases are filed annually. In Connecticut, there were 250 malpractice cases filed in 2015 across all medical specialties. By way of reference, Connecticut has approximately 3.5 M residents and more than 35 hospitals. At one of those hospitals that year, Yale New Haven Hospital, there were 78,529 inpatient visits and 1,204,666 outpatient encounters.

Successful claims are rarer still, as noted previously.

[17] Makary Martin A, Daniel Michael. *Medical error—the third leading cause of death in the US*. BMJ 2016; 353:i2139.

[18] Agency for Healthcare Research and Quality. *HealthGrades seventh annual patient safety in American hospitals study*. Golden, CO: Healthgrades, Inc., 2010.

14.1.10.1 Wrong-Site Extractions

Wrong-site extractions continue to be a leading source of malpractice claims against oral and maxillofacial surgeons and were recently suspected to be on the rise.[19] Poor communication between clinicians has been found to be a leading cause of wrong-site extractions.[20] Prior to taking out a tooth that has no obvious reason to be removed, the surgeon should take extra measures to make certain that they are removing the correct tooth.

14.1.10.2 Failure to Diagnose Cancer

Studies of closed medical negligence claims regarding maxillofacial surgery indicate that claims for failure to diagnose oral cancer are increasing.[21]

In order to mitigate this risk, all of the diagnostic scans must be read to avoid missing any pathology. The careful examination of the tissue of the oral cavity should not be rushed. Patients should be questioned about risk factors such as past tobacco and alcohol use that the patient may not have included in the written questionnaire.

14.1.10.3 Nerve Injuries

The risk of nerve injuries varies depending on the procedure.[22] Preventable nerve injuries in the course of lower third molar extractions commonly lead to claims, as do similar injuries in implant procedures. In general, the greater the degree of impairment from the nerve injury, the greater the likelihood is that a patient will at least consult with a lawyer. When important anatomic structures are at risk, accurate and precise preoperative imaging and preoperative bone measurements are needed.

When nerve injuries do occur and the surgeon does not have expertise in nerve assessment, referrals for microsurgical evaluation should be made without hesitation once it is clear that nerve function is not rapidly returning. Failure to make such referrals is a common cause of malpractice claims and may also lead to a claim for punitive damages.

14.1.10.4 Anesthesia Errors

Anesthesia, when administered by the maxillofacial surgeon, can also be the source of malpractice claims.

Some of the most serious clinical and legal problems relate to airway management errors resulting in hypoxic injury, as well as problems from anesthesia interactions with other medications. An oral and maxillofacial surgeon is held to the same standard of care as an anesthesiologist.[23] Thus, careful patient selection and the appropriate choice of anesthetic technique help minimize foreseeable problems. Following nationally recognized monitoring strategies and regular updating of one's knowledge in the area of ambulatory anesthesia are also important. Additionally, any staff members who may be called upon to assist in a medical or anesthetic emergency should receive training in the recognition and means of assisting in managing office emergencies. Good documentation of the anesthetic portion of a procedure is just as important as documenting other aspects of the patient's care.

14.1.10.5 Implant Surgeries

Implant placement surgeries have a higher relative risk of malpractice claim. These commonly relate to nerve injuries but may also relate to problems in implant positioning or other aspects of treatment planning that lead to esthetic or functional problems. Careful assessment of

[19] Oral and Maxillofacial Surgeons National Insurance Company. At: www.ds4dds.com/omsnic/Pages/default.aspx Accessed: March 31, 2017.

[20] Paleg O, Givot N, Halamish-Shani T, Taicher S. *Wrong tooth extraction; root cause analysis*. Quintessence Intl 2010; 41 (10):869–72.

[21] Melrose RJ. *Failure to diagnose pathology: an avoidable complication in oral and maxillofacial surgery*. Oral Maxillofac Surg Clin North Am. 2011 Aug; 23(3):465–73. doi: https://doi.org/10.1016/j.coms.2011.04.008.

[22] *See*, e.g., Marei HF. *Medical litigation in oral surgery practice: Lessons learned from 20 lawsuits*. J Forensic Leg Med. 2013 May; 20(4):223–5. doi: https://doi.org/10.1016/j.jflm.2012.09.025. Epub 2012 Sep 27.

[23] It is important to know the state regulations with respect to acceptable delegation of duties in this respect. Consultation with counsel in the state where the surgeon's practice is based is advisable.

potential implant sites via inspection, imaging, and, when indicated, mounted casts helps avoid errors that may lead to litigation. In addition, it is important to have a close working relationship with the restorative dentist to help avoid errors due to miscommunications or inconsistent statements made to the patient.

14.1.10.6 Medication Errors

New medications are continuously being introduced to the market, so it is imperative for the maxillofacial surgeon to keep his or her knowledge current. Several "apps" are available for ready reference and allow the surgeon to understand all patient medication, even if they are new to the market. A quick call to or conversation with the pharmacist may also be prudent if any doubts exist. Review of drug safety sheets for combining medications should be documented when adverse drug-drug or drug-disease interactions exist. The failure to promptly respond to a patient's adverse drug interaction can also be the basis of liability.

14.1.11 Policies, Procedures, and Guidelines

The Institute of Medicine defines clinical practice guidelines as "statements that include recommendations intended to optimize patient care that are informed by a systematic review of evidence and an assessment of the benefits and harms of alternative care options." In general, they make sure the knowledge that has been developed by the medical profession is applied consistently and correctly.

Depending on the nature of the maxillofacial surgeon's practice, a number of guidelines may pertain. For example, clinical practice guidelines cover the management of patients with third molar teeth, prevention of wrong-site tooth extraction, and the administration of anesthesia in outpatient facilities.

One of the methods used to assess a patient's presurgical risk is the classification of the American Society of Anesthesiologists (ASA). Thorough patient assessment allows for assignment of an ASA physical status to all surgical patients according to the most recent guidelines.

14.1.11.1 General Considerations

In general, clinical practice guidelines reflect minimum safety standards with which healthcare professionals are expected to comply. Most of these guidelines are based on an examination by experts across various specialties of the current data within the paradigm of evidence-based medicine.

Clinical practice guidelines typically evaluate and synthesize the highest quality evidence and most current data about diagnosis, risk/benefit assessment, and treatment. Committees of experts sift through the scientific literature and offer clear recommendations for clinical decision-making. Among the goals of clinical practice guidelines are to standardize medical care, improve patient safety, and to reduce risk. Studies have demonstrated that the use of such guidelines is an effective way of achieving those goals.

The federal government has a searchable database of clinical practice guidelines (www.guidelines.gov), and there are several other convenient tools to access guidelines such as Epocrates and Smart Medicine. Note that the American Association of Oral and Maxillofacial Surgeons has promulgated clinical practice guidelines for patient assessment that provide a useful organizational structure for the process.

Additionally, hospitals have their own policies, procedures, and protocols, which are often based on consensus guidelines. Policies are purposeful plans of action directed toward a risk or issue of concern. Procedures are specific sets of practices to be followed when specific circumstances arise. Protocol is essentially synonymous with procedure. As a condition of privileges, a hospital typically requires a doctor to abide by hospital and medical staff policies and procedures.

14.1.11.2 Policies, Procedures, and Clinical Practice Guidelines in Litigation

Policies and procedures, clinical practice guidelines, and other minimum patient safety standards also come into play frequently in litigation concerning malpractice allegations. Most often, the plaintiff is relying on policies and guidelines to demonstrate a breach of the standard of care. Occasionally, the defense claims that compliance with practice guidelines is proof that there was *not* a breach. These claims are considerably less persuasive than the former. Additionally, the source and history of a practice guideline must always be considered.

When used in litigation, clinical practice guidelines, policies, and procedures can be persuasive evidence of the standard of care and a breach thereof. In a case with competing well-qualified experts, juries often want to know, "where is it written down?"

14.1.12 Concluding Thoughts: Practice Tips for Decreasing Risk of Malpractice Claim

In sum, any practiononer should keep these practical tips in mind to help reduce the risk of legal claims.

14.1.12.1 Communicate Effectively

Dissatisfaction with communication commonly undergirds medical negligence claims.

Be transparent. Fully explain the potential for bad outcomes despite good care. Anger commonly motivates patients to seek the advice of malpractice attorneys. If their expectations are reasonable from the outset, they are less likely to be angered by a bad outcome.

14.1.12.2 Document Timely and Thoroughly

Good documentation is also critical to avoiding professional negligence claims. Meticulous notes provide a window into a surgeon's decision-making and often shield the competent surgeon from malpractice claims. Conversely, poor note-taking will often lead to litigation as the plaintiff's attorney is duty-bound to fill in the gaps that led to a poor outcome. Even the surgeon who believes that he/she has met the standard of care may be done by poor note-taking as memory may fade by the time she is asked to recite the decision-making process.

14.1.12.3 Err on the Side of Safety

Deciding not to perform surgery is one of the most important decisions a surgeon makes. Likewise, choosing the course of treatment that presents the lowest level of risk is almost always in the patient's best interests.

14.1.12.4 Know What You Don't Know

Do not hesitate to have a colleague review a case or assist in surgery for any reason.

14.1.12.5 Promptly Investigate and Address Postoperative Problems (Yourself, If at All Possible)

Inadequate postsurgical follow-up commonly leads to an unsatisfied patient who may be more likely to consult with an attorney as a result.

14.1.12.6 Review All Adverse Events for Lessons Learned

The occasional failure is always a chance to learn. Similarly, an annual risk assessment of the clinician's practice is advisable.

Part 2

Medical Management of the Surgical Patient

15 Cardiovascular Disease and Maxillofacial Surgery

Yulanka Castro-Dominguez and Andre Ghantous

Abstract

Patients undergoing noncardiac surgeries can be at risk of significant cardiovascular events. The preoperative cardiovascular evaluation constitutes a set of tools to help identify patients are at higher risk of events who may benefit from specific strategies to optimize their outcome. In this chapter, we first discuss the initial clinical evaluation which includes obtaining medical history, physical examination, and functional status assessment. Second, we address current models for risk stratification and recommended management based on assessed risk. Third, how to determine if further and which cardiac testing is needed to further elucidate the risk. Finally, we discuss appropriate management and optimization of patients with cardiac conditions, from medications to coronary revascularization.

15.1 Introduction

Patients undergoing noncardiac surgeries can be at risk of significant cardiovascular events. This risk is related to patient- and surgery-specific characteristics. The purpose of the preoperative cardiac evaluation is to evaluate current cardiac status, identify patients who might be at elevated risk of complications from surgery, and recommend strategies that may influence outcomes. It also provides the patient and healthcare providers with additional information regarding the benefit-to-risk ratio related to the procedure, hence aiding in informed decisions.

15.2 Clinical Evaluation

At the time of the initial evaluation, the clinician needs to query about symptoms, such as angina, dyspnea, syncope, palpitations, and edema. Also, inquire about history of cardiac disease or significant comorbidities including coronary artery or valvular disease, heart failure, hypertension, diabetes, chronic kidney disease, and cerebrovascular or peripheral artery disease.

Y. Castro-Dominguez, M.D.
A. Ghantous, M.D., F.A.C.C. (✉)
Division of Cardiology, Department of Internal Medicine, Yale University School of Medicine, New Haven, CT, USA
e-mail: Andre.Ghantous@ynhh.org

© Springer International Publishing AG 2018

E.M. Ferneini, J.D. Bennett (eds.), *Perioperative Assessment of the Maxillofacial Surgery Patient*,
https://doi.org/10.1007/978-3-319-58868-1_15

During this initial questioning, the clinician should be able to identify the presence of unstable symptoms or cardiac conditions that place the patient at very high risk of complications, such as recent myocardial infarction (MI), unstable angina, decompensated heart failure, significant arrhythmias, or hemodynamically significant valvular heart disease. In these patients, surgery should be deferred until optimization of cardiac condition.

Patients who require an emergency surgery or procedure in which life or a limb is threatened are already at increased risk of perioperative cardiovascular complications. In these cases, there is no room for an extensive evaluation of a patient's cardiovascular profile, and in most cases, the benefit of proceeding with surgery outweighs the risk of waiting to perform additional testing. Postoperative management of possible cardiovascular repercussions should be the focus in at-risk patients.

Additionally, functional status is evaluated. Functional capacity is a reliable predictor of perioperative cardiac events and is determined based on the patient's ability to perform certain daily tasks. It is expressed in terms of metabolic equivalents (METs), where 1 MET is the resting oxygen consumption. It is further classified as excellent (>10 METs), good to moderate (10 to 4 METs), or poor (<4 METs) (see Table 15.1). Patients with poor functional status (<4 METS) are at higher risk of perioperative complications.

Table 15.1 Estimated energy requirements for various activities

1 to 4 METs
Eat, dress, or use the toilet
Walk on level ground at 2–3 mph
Golfing with a cart
4 to 10 METs
Climb a flight of stairs or hill
Walk on level ground at 4 mph
Perform heavy work around the house, such as moving heavy furniture or scrubbing floors
Running a short distance
>10 METs
Participate in strenuous sports such as swimming, singles tennis, football, basketball, and skiing

Conversely, highly functional asymptomatic patients are at much lower risk and can generally proceed with surgery without further cardiovascular testing [1].

Physical examination includes measurement of blood pressure in both arms, evaluation of jugular venous pulsation (JVP), auscultation of the heart for murmurs or gallops and lungs for rale, and examination of the extremities for edema and pulses. Significant findings include elevated JVP, severe aortic stenosis murmur, pulmonary edema, or S3 gallops.

15.3 Risk Stratification

15.3.1 Risk Prediction Models

The Revised Cardiac Risk Index (RCRI) developed in 1999 by Lee et al. is the best validated and most widely used scoring system when estimating preoperative risk (Table 15.2) [2]. It incorporates six independent predictors of major cardiac complications: high-risk type of surgery, history of ischemic heart disease, history of congestive heart failure, history of cerebrovascular disease, preoperative treatment with insulin, and preoperative serum creatinine > 2.0 mg/dL. This risk stratification system predicts outcome but also identifies patients who need additional testing or medical interventions.

Another commonly used risk score is the American College of Surgeons' National Surgical Quality Improvement Program risk (ACS-NSQIP) model. This is a more complex model with the potential to provide a procedure-specific estimate of major adverse cardiovascular events. However, it has yet to have external validation [3]. The model calculator is available online.

15.3.2 Management Based on Risk

Low-risk patients—patients with an estimated risk of complications <1% are deemed low risk and require no additional cardiovascular testing prior to surgery.

Table 15.2 Revised Cardiac Risk Index

Six independent predictors of major cardiac complications
High-risk type of surgery (examples include vascular surgery and any open intraperitoneal or intrathoracic procedures)
History of ischemic heart disease (history of MI or a positive exercise test, current complaint of chest pain considered to be secondary to myocardial ischemia, use of nitrate therapy, or ECG with pathological Q waves; do not count prior coronary revascularization procedure unless one of the other criteria for ischemic heart disease is present)
History of HF
History of cerebrovascular disease
Diabetes mellitus requiring treatment with insulin
Preoperative serum creatinine >2.0 mg/dL (177 micromol/L)
Rate of cardiac death, nonfatal myocardial infarction, and nonfatal cardiac arrest according to the number of predictors
No risk factors—0.4 percent (95% CI: 0.1–0.8)
One risk factor—1.0 percent (95% CI: 0.5–1.4)
Two risk factors—2.4 percent (95% CI: 1.3–3.5)
Three or more risk factors—5.4 percent (95% CI: 2.8–7.9
Rate of myocardial infarction, pulmonary edema, ventricular fibrillation, primary cardiac arrest, and complete heart block
No risk factors—0.5 percent (95% CI: 0.2–1.1)
One risk factor—1.3 percent (95% CI: 0.7–2.1)
Two risk factors—3.6 percent (95% CI: 2.1–5.6)
Three or more risk factors—9.1 percent (95% CI: 5.5–13.8)

Adapted from Lee TH, Marcantonio ER, Mangione CM, Thomas EJ, Polanczyk CA, Cook EF, et al. Derivation and prospective validation of a simple index for prediction of cardiac risk of major noncardiac surgery. Circulation. 1999;100(10):1043–9

High-risk patients—patients with a risk of complications >1% may require further cardiovascular testing or optimization.

In those higher risk patients, we then assess their functional capacity as recommended per the 2014 American College of Cardiology/American Heart Association guidelines for preoperative cardiovascular evaluation. In patients who can achieve >4 METs in their daily living activities, no further cardiac testing is needed. In those whose functional capacity is poor or unknown, additional testing may be indicated only if it will impact decision-making or perioperative care (see Fig. 15.1).

15.4 Preoperative Cardiac Testing

Prior to proceeding with further cardiac testing in an asymptomatic patient, the purpose of testing and how it might change management must be carefully considered. In most cases, preoperative coronary evaluation will not impact medical management. However, ischemic evaluation may provide useful information for decision-making in a case where the risk-benefit ratio for elective surgery is uncertain or when lower risk surgical interventions are an option.

15.4.1 Electrocardiogram

A 12-lead ECG is recommended for patients with known coronary artery disease, arrhythmia, structural heart disease, and peripheral arterial or cerebrovascular disease, unless the patient is going for low-risk surgery. A preoperative ECG can be considered in asymptomatic patients with no history of heart disease but is rarely useful in those undergoing low-risk surgeries.

15.4.2 Echocardiogram

Routine use of echocardiography prior to surgery carries no benefit and is not indicated. It may be beneficial in specific circumstances, such as patients with symptoms suggestive of undiagnosed heart failure or those with history of heart failure and a change in symptoms. It is also reasonable in patients with suspected or known moderate to severe valvular heart disease if there has been a change in clinical status. Patients with left ventricle systolic dysfunction have an increased risk of perioperative complications, particularly postoperative heart failure, and may benefit of medical optimization prior to surgery.

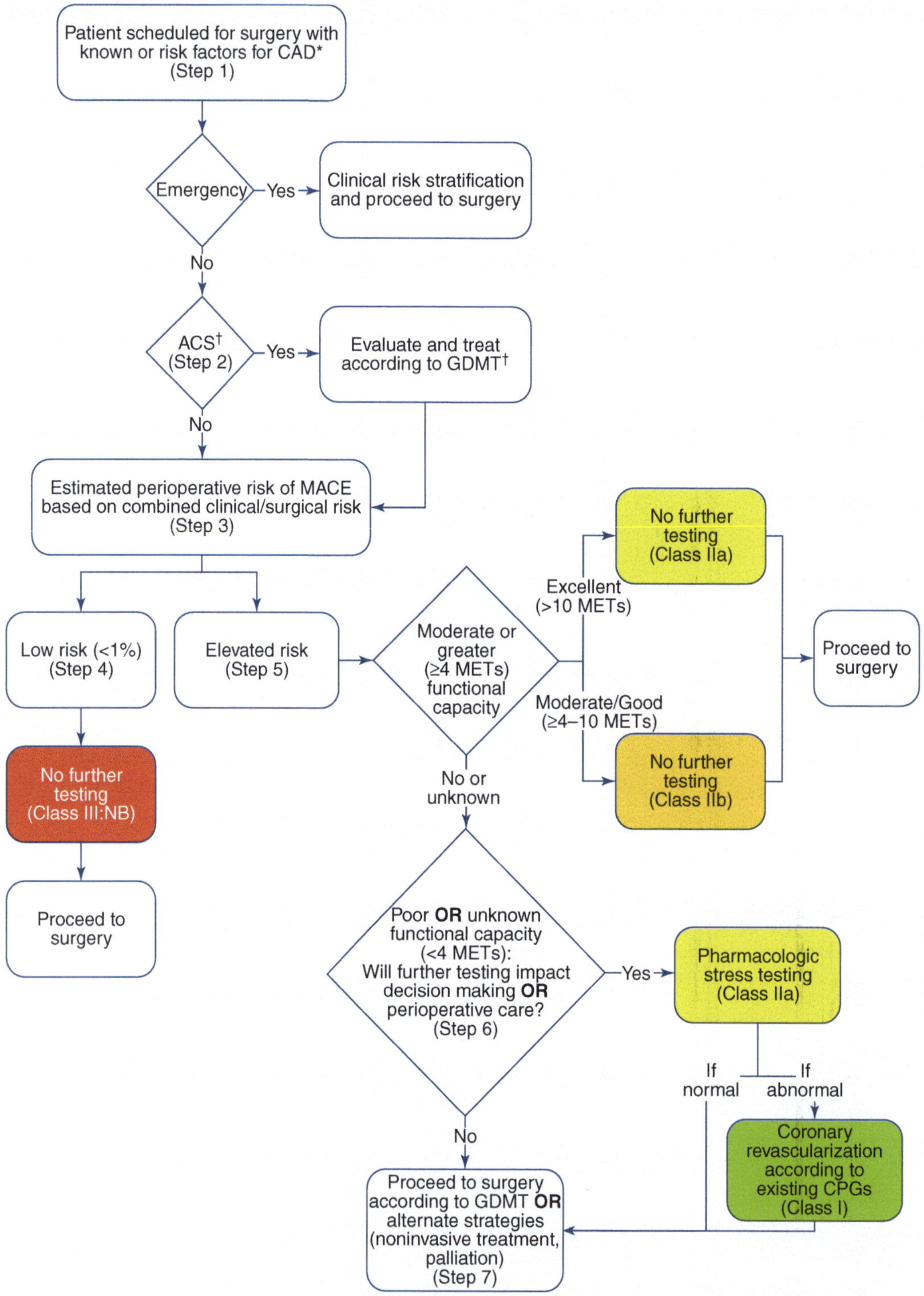

Fig. 15.1 Stepwise approach to perioperative cardiac assessment. CAD, coronary artery disease; ACS, acute coronary syndrome; GDMT, guideline-directed medical therapy; MACE, major adverse cardiac events; MET, metabolic equivalent; CPG, clinical practice guideline. Reproduced with permission (*to be requested*) from Fleisher LA, Fleischmann KE, Auerbach AD, Barnason SA, Beckman JA, Bozkurt B, et al. 2014 ACC/AHA guideline on perioperative cardiovascular evaluation and management of patients undergoing noncardiac surgery: a report of the American College of Cardiology/American Heart Association Task Force on practice guidelines. Journal of the American College of Cardiology. 2014;64(22):e77–137

15.4.3 Stress Testing

Patients who are deemed low risk and those who have elevated risk but had good functional capacity (>4 METs) can proceed with surgery without stress testing. Stress testing should be reserved for patients who based on the results of these tests could potentially be considered for angiography and revascularization regardless of the proposed surgery.

There are different modalities for stress testing, such as exercise ECG, exercise or pharmacological stress echocardiogram, and exercise or pharmacological nuclear stress testing.

Exercise, when feasible, is the preferred modality of stress testing because it not only provides information about ischemia but also an objective assessment of functional capacity. In patients who cannot exercise, pharmacological stress testing is available. Stress testing with imaging is indicated when patients are unable to exercise and when baseline ECG is abnormal.

Exercise ECG—indicated in patients who are able to exercise and have a normal baseline ECG. Exercise induces ischemia as the coronary vessels that have stenosis are unable to maintain adequate blood flow related to myocardial oxygen demand. At adequate workload, ST-segment changes are measured and number of leads involved. Advantages are that it provides additional diagnostic and prognostic information, such as exercise capacity, blood pressure and heart rate response, and provoked symptoms. It should not be used if baseline ECG is abnormal (LBBB, paced rhythm, ST-segment depressions).

Stress echocardiogram—provides information on wall motion abnormalities which indicates areas at risk of myocardial ischemia. It also allows evaluation of ventricular and valvular function. Dobutamine, used in those who cannot exercise, increases myocardial oxygen demand and provokes ischemia due to insufficient perfusion in a myocardial segment provided by a stenotic vessel. Stress echocardiogram with dobutamine should be avoided in patients with severe hypertension, hypotension, or significant arrhythmias.

Nuclear stress testing—single-photon emission computerized tomography (SPECT) and positron emission tomography (PET) imaging take advantage of the relative differences in coronary blood flow with stress. In the coronary arteries, areas distal to a stenosis are already maximally dilated at rest. When exposed to a vasodilator (adenosine, dipyridamole, regadenoson), normal coronary arteries without stenosis vasodilate and receive more blood flow compared to those already maximally vasodilated stenotic areas. A radioactive tracer (thallium, technetium) is initially injected and taken up by the myocardium, and images are obtained at rest. Then, with exercise or vasodilator stress, a second injection is given. Tracer is again distributed with blood flow and, therefore, less tracer is distributed to the myocardial region supplied by a stenotic vessel. This relative difference in flow between stress and rest tomographic images is seen as a perfusion defect and is indicative of coronary artery disease.

A normal study has an excellent negative predictive value for perioperative complications. Conversely, the presence of moderate to large areas of myocardial ischemia is associated with increased risk of perioperative MI and death.

15.5 Preoperative Coronary Revascularization

There is no evidence to support routine coronary revascularization before noncardiac surgery with the intention to reduce perioperative risk of cardiac events. Multiple studies have addressed the role of "prophylactic" preoperative revascularization in asymptomatic patients prior to noncardiac surgery and have shown no improvement in survival or postoperative outcomes [4]. Patients with asymptomatic ischemia on stress testing or with stable coronary artery disease do not seem to benefit from preoperative revascularization. Yet some authors argue that patients with high-risk features on stress testing may benefit from revascularization.

Furthermore, revascularization is recommended before noncardiac surgery in cases where revascularization would be indicated regardless of the planned surgery. These include acute coronary syndromes and stable angina with left main disease or significant three-vessel disease where intervention may lead to improved long-term survival.

In patients where revascularization is indicated and noncardiac surgery is time sensitive, a strategy of balloon angioplasty or bare-metal stent placement should be considered. This owing to recommended waiting times prior to surgery are much shorter in the abovementioned compared to waiting times for drug-eluting stents. Patients who undergo coronary artery bypass grafting (CABG) should wait at least 4 weeks before proceeding with noncardiac surgery.

15.6 Perioperative Medical Therapy

15.6.1 Beta-Blockers

The use of beta-blockers perioperatively is associated with a reduction in cardiac events, including cardiovascular death, myocardial infarction, and cardiac arrest. However, beta-blocker use is also associated with harm with increased rates of bradycardia, stroke, hypotension, and total mortality. Therefore, beta-blockers should not be started routinely perioperatively in patients without indications for receiving long-term beta-blocker therapy.

For patients identified as having an indication for long-term beta-blocker therapy, such as systolic heart failure, arrhythmias, stable angina, or prior MI, beta-blockers should be started preferably more than 1 week before surgery to allow titration. For patients who have moderate- to high-risk ischemia in preoperative testing or three or more RCRI factors, starting a beta-blocker at least 1 day prior to surgery is reasonable after careful consideration of potential adverse effects. Beta-blockers should not be started on the day of surgery.

In patients who are already receiving long-term beta-blockers for recommended indications, these should be continued perioperatively.

15.6.2 Statins

Statin therapy is known to reduce long-term cardiovascular events in at-risk patients and likewise carries a protective effect on cardiac complications during noncardiac surgery. The benefits of statins are related to their pleiotropic effects, primarily reducing inflammation and stabilizing coronary plaques.

Patients with coronary artery disease or who otherwise meet indications for statin therapy should be started on a statin prior to surgery. In addition, patients undergoing vascular surgery may benefit from initiation of statins. Finally, statins should be continued perioperatively in those already on statin therapy long term.

15.6.3 Antiplatelet Therapy

In patients who are taking aspirin for primary or secondary prevention of cardiovascular disease who have not had previous coronary stenting, aspirin can be held 5–7 days before surgery. However, when the risks of potential increased cardiac events outweigh the risks of surgical bleeding, it may be reasonable to continue it.

In patients who have undergone percutaneous coronary intervention (PCI), perioperative management of antiplatelet therapy requires careful consideration of the risks of adverse cardiac events with early discontinuation and the risks of bleeding with maintenance of therapy (see Fig. 15.2). The risk of stent thrombosis in the perioperative period is highest in the first 4–6 weeks after stent implantation. Premature discontinuation of dual antiplatelet therapy (DAPT—aspirin and $P2Y_{12}$ receptor inhibitor) in this early period is a strong risk factor for stent thrombosis.

The ideal waiting time before proceeding with nonurgent surgery after PCI should be at least 12 months after drug-eluting stent placement, 4–6 weeks after bare metal stent placement, and 2–4 weeks after balloon angioplasty. In cases of patients who had drug-eluting stent placement and surgery is needed prior to 12 months, cardiology consultation is warranted for the management of the dual antiplatelet, which can be influenced

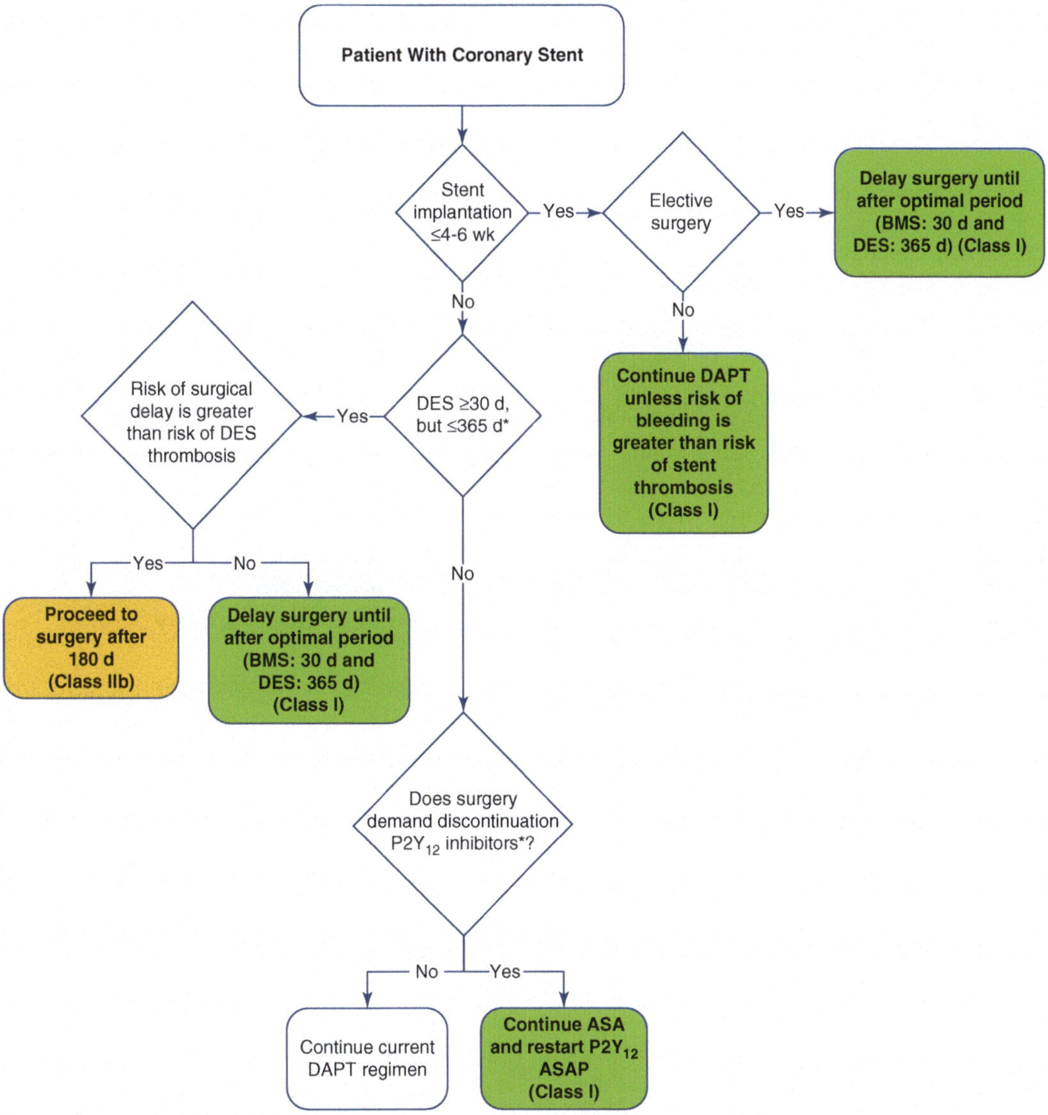

Fig. 15.2 Algorithm for antiplatelet management in patients with PCI and noncardiac surgery. ASA indicates aspirin; ASAP, as soon as possible; BMS, bare-metal stent; DAPT, dual antiplatelet therapy; DES, drug-eluting stent; and PCI, percutaneous coronary intervention. Reproduced with permission (*to be requested*) from Fleisher LA, Fleischmann KE, Auerbach AD, Barnason SA, Beckman JA, Bozkurt B, et al. 2014 ACC/AHA guideline on perioperative cardiovascular evaluation and management of patients undergoing noncardiac surgery: a report of the American College of Cardiology/American Heart Association Task Force on practice guidelines. Journal of the American College of Cardiology. 2014;64(22):e77–137

by the generation of drug-eluting stents used since the newer generation are relatively safer.

If a patient needs urgent surgery prior to the above recommended times, DAPT should be continued unless the relative risk of bleeding outweighs the benefit of the prevention of stent thrombosis.

If surgery demands discontinuation of the $P2Y_{12}$ inhibitor, aspirin should be continued. The $P2Y_{12}$ inhibitor should be restarted when the risk of major bleeding has passed. There is no evidence that starting anticoagulants or antithrombotic during this period reduces risk of stent thrombosis.

15.7 Management of Cardiac Conditions Perioperatively

15.7.1 Valvular Heart Disease

Valvular lesions can have different implications for perioperative risk and management depending on their hemodynamic severity. Patients with suspected significant valvular lesions based on history or physical exam should undergo echocardiogram to evaluate severity and effects on left ventricular function and pulmonary pressures. Overall, stenotic lesions carry a higher risk of morbidity and may require periprocedural intervention to reduce surgical risk, while regurgitant lesions are better tolerated and can usually be managed medically.

Severe *aortic stenosis* significantly increases perioperative mortality, and symptomatic patients should be considered for aortic valve replacement (AVR), either surgical (SAVR) or transcatheter (TAVR). In selected symptomatic patients, percutaneous aortic valvuloplasty can be performed as a short-term bridge through noncardiac surgery. However, in patients that are asymptomatic where noncardiac surgery is needed, elevated-risk surgery can be performed with appropriate intraoperative and postoperative hemodynamic monitoring [5].

Patients with severe *mitral stenosis* that meet indications for valvular intervention should have mitral valvuloplasty or open commissurotomy before elective noncardiac surgery. If valvuloplasty is not favorable or if the noncardiac surgery is an emergency, then noncardiac surgery can be performed using appropriate intraoperative hemodynamic monitoring. Strategies during perioperative period should be focused in avoiding tachycardia and hypotension and careful monitoring of intravascular volume.

Severe *aortic and mitral regurgitation* are better tolerated than stenotic lesions, yet these lesions do carry a higher risk of perioperative complications. In asymptomatic patients with severe regurgitant lesions, elective noncardiac surgery can be performed with the appropriate hemodynamic monitoring. Main goals during perioperative period would be to optimize diuretic therapy and reduce afterload.

Patients with *prosthetic valves* who are on oral anticoagulation may need to have interruption of the anticoagulation prior to noncardiac surgery. In cases where the procedure has minimal to no risk of bleeding, it may be reasonable to continue anticoagulation perioperatively. When interruption of oral anticoagulation is needed, bridging with heparin is indicated for patients with (1) a mechanical valve in the mitral position and (2) prosthetic aortic valve with one or more risk factors, such as atrial fibrillation, previous thromboembolism, heart failure, and hypercoagulable condition, or an older-generation prosthetic aortic valve.

15.7.2 Heart Failure and Cardiomyopathy

Heart failure remains a significant risk factor for adverse cardiac events, including death after noncardiac surgery. However, when patients with heart failure are optimized and stabilized prior to surgery they are less likely to have adverse outcomes perioperatively. In cases where patients are acutely decompensated (depending of urgency of noncardiac surgery), postponing surgery and proceeding only after patient has been stabilized should be considered. The goals of optimization include restoring normal oxygenation, optimizing volume status, improving end-organ perfusion, and identifying underlying etiology or precipitating factor.

Patients with hypertrophic obstructive cardiomyopathy undergoing noncardiac surgery need careful monitoring of volume status and hemodynamics since perioperative hemodynamic fluctuations may be poorly tolerated. Conditions that can reduce left ventricle filling and thereby increase outflow obstruction include volume loss, hypotension, decrease in preload, tachycardia, and increase in contractility. Arterial vasodilators, over diuresis and inotropic agents if needed should be used with close monitoring due to possibility of increasing dynamic outflow obstruction and further decrease cardiac output.

15.7.3 Arrhythmias

Cardiac arrhythmias occur commonly in the postoperative period especially in older patients, and their effects vary depending on the etiology of the arrhythmia and hemodynamic significance. Frequent ventricular premature beats and asymptomatic non-sustained ventricular tachycardia are not associated with increased perioperative risk. Depending on the nature and acuity of the arrhythmia, investigation of possible underlying cardiopulmonary disease, drug toxicity, myocardial ischemia, or metabolic disturbances should be considered.

Symptomatic and hemodynamically significant arrhythmias are managed similarly to the non-operative setting but should be focused in identifying and addressing underlying cause.

15.7.4 Permanent Pacemakers and Implantable Cardioverter-Defibrillators (ICDs)

Pacemakers and ICDs have important implications for perioperative management. The presence of a cardiovascular implantable device invariably means the presence of underlying cardiac disease, such as arrhythmias or cardiomyopathy. Moreover, electrocautery with monopolar and, rarely, bipolar systems may interfere with pacemakers. Before an elective surgery, the surgical team should communicate with the clinician following the device in advance for recommendations regarding device reprogramming. Device reprogramming can include changing pacing to an asynchronous mode and inactivating ICD tachytherapies. In certain models application of a magnet over the device can be done to inactivate ICD. Identifying the manufacturer of the pacemaker or ICD permits quick access to specialist advice and company assistance.

Conclusion

The goals of the preoperative cardiovascular evaluation are to assess individual patient risk prior to surgery and to determine which patients may benefit from interventions that can meaningfully decrease this risk. By following the current recommended guidelines, the decision tree becomes more clear, avoiding unnecessary testing in low-risk patients and implementing strategies to optimize patients at higher risk of complications.

References

1. Fleisher LA, Fleischmann KE, Auerbach AD, Barnason SA, Beckman JA, Bozkurt B, et al. 2014 ACC/AHA guideline on perioperative cardiovascular evaluation and management of patients undergoing noncardiac surgery: a report of the American College of Cardiology/American Heart Association task force on practice guidelines. J Am Coll Cardiol. 2014;64(22):e77–137.
2. Lee TH, Marcantonio ER, Mangione CM, Thomas EJ, Polanczyk CA, Cook EF, et al. Derivation and prospective validation of a simple index for prediction of cardiac risk of major noncardiac surgery. Circulation. 1999;100(10):1043–9.
3. Bilimoria KY, Liu Y, Paruch JL, Zhou L, Kmiecik TE, Ko CY, et al. Development and evaluation of the universal ACS NSQIP surgical risk calculator: a decision aid and informed consent tool for patients and surgeons. J Am Coll Surg. 2013;217(5):833–42.e1-3.
4. McFalls EO, Ward HB, Moritz TE, Goldman S, Krupski WC, Littooy F, et al. Coronary-artery revascularization before elective major vascular surgery. N Engl J Med. 2004;351(27):2795–804.
5. Agarwal S, Rajamanickam A, Bajaj NS, Griffin BP, Catacutan T, Svensson LG, et al. Impact of aortic stenosis on postoperative outcomes after noncardiac surgeries. Circulation. 2013;6(2):193–200.

16 Pulmonary Disease and Maxillofacial Surgery

Daniel McNally

Abstract

This chapter will discuss the prevalence, pathophysiology, and manifestation of pulmonary disease. The chapter will review preoperative assessment including preoperative testing in order to determine anesthetic risk and risk stratification. Perioperative management including patient optimization and how to manage chronic medications as well as airway management, what medications are indicated, pain management, and potential problems and complications are described for each specific disease process.

16.1 Medical Disease

16.1.1 Pathophysiology

Pulmonary disorders can be divided into three broad categories: obstructive diseases, restrictive diseases, and disorders of the pulmonary vascular system. Fortunately, these categories, based on pathophysiology, are generally equally useful in identifying an appropriate clinical approach to the problem.

The most common disorders are the obstructive diseases. Obstruction refers to limitation in airflow through the "conducting airways" which include the trachea, bronchi, and bronchioles, ending just before the alveoli. These are disorders in which there is increased airway resistance, which may be on the basis of airways narrowed by bronchospasm, or by inflammation, or by the loss of supporting structural tissues around the airways so that the otherwise normal intrathoracic pressures during expiration cause flow limitation on a mechanical basis.

These obstructive disorders cause impairment by increasing the work of breathing required to move air through narrow airways with increased resistance, as well as by altering the distribution of airflow to various regions in the lung, upsetting the balance between ventilation of alveoli and perfusion of alveoli that is necessary to achieve efficient transfer of oxygen into the bloodstream. Many of the obstructive disorders also have an inflammatory component, where airway edema may contribute to narrowing, and

D. McNally, M.D.
Department of Medicine, Division of Pulmonary, Critical Care and Sleep Medicine, University of Connecticut School of Medicine, Farmington, CT, USA
e-mail: mcnally@uchc.edu

© Springer International Publishing AG 2018

E.M. Ferneini, J.D. Bennett (eds.), *Perioperative Assessment of the Maxillofacial Surgery Patient*,
https://doi.org/10.1007/978-3-319-58868-1_16

inflammatory cells may accumulate in the airway, further narrowing it and causing increased resistance.

The obstructive disorders include a cluster of pulmonary diseases called "chronic obstructive pulmonary disease" (COPD). This is not a single disorder, but rather a collective term for a group of disorders that share the mechanism of airflow obstruction, but have distinct mechanisms and distinct definitions. The three most common disorders included under the label COPD include chronic bronchitis, emphysema, and chronic persistent asthma.

The definition of chronic bronchitis is largely historical. It includes individuals with chronic sputum production. For epidemiologic purposes, this has been defined as productive cough on most days during at least 3 months out of the last 2 years, but for clinical purposes, a similar and general "do you bring up phlegm most days?" is more appropriate. Bronchial mucosal surfaces which have been damaged by irritants such as cigarette smoke or following a viral illness frequently react to that stimulus by proliferation of mucus-producing glandular cells in an effort to protect and heal those surfaces. This is frequently an ineffective strategy, since the system of cilia on bronchial epithelial cells may have been damaged, and the patient may be unable to effectively clear mucus from the airway. The result is that airborne particles, colonizing microorganisms, and the increased volume of mucus are all trapped in the airways, leading to plugging, increased resistance, and abnormal gas exchange.

The definition of asthma is a functional one: reversible airway obstruction. This may occur on the basis of environmental allergens, inhaled irritants including occupational exposures, or as the sequelae of inflammation triggered by a viral infection. At least early in the disease process, this obstruction may be quite reversible. Constriction of bronchial smooth muscle and airway edema together cause increased airway resistance and increased work of breathing, as well as alterations in the distribution of ventilation that can lead to inefficient gas exchange. In recent years, we have come to understand that individuals with asthma usually have a quality called "bronchial hyperreactivity" which may persist even between attacks of asthma and bronchospasm. In bronchial hyperreactivity, irritant stimuli, even cold air, can trigger an episode of bronchoconstriction. That same individual, if not exposed to a specific trigger, may be both asymptomatic and have normal airflow and be identified only if tested following exposure to a specific trigger. While most asthma continues to be quite reversible, some individuals with chronic or repeated episodes may have changes in the bronchial system where inflammation, edema, smooth muscle hypertrophy, and bronchoconstriction persist even long after a triggering stimulus has been removed. This has been termed "bronchial remodeling" reflecting the structural changes of increased inflammatory cells, increased mucus production, and bronchial muscle thickening that are often seen. These individuals may have what can be termed chronic persistent asthma and deserve to be thought of under the label COPD.

Emphysema is defined as dilation and destruction of the distal airspace. Either through an enzyme deficiency or much more commonly through the damaging effects of cigarette smoking, neutrophils are attracted to the alveoli and release proteolytic enzymes which damage the alveolar septal walls. At the same time, in the case of cigarette smoking, the natural protective mechanisms preventing this proteolytic damage are inhibited. The result is destruction of alveolar walls and the formation of bullae, large open cyst-like spaces. The net result is the loss of alveolar surface area for gas exchange. At first thought, this process, involving the alveoli, may not seem to be an obstructive disease. However, the alveolar walls are the supporting structures around the bronchial system, and when destroyed the normal intrathoracic pressures can now compress the bronchial system, causing increased resistance and reduced airflow. The remnants of the alveolar spaces, overfilled with air which cannot exit through the narrowed bronchial system, become dilated, forming the bullae.

In addition to these individual disorders, some individuals may have multiple mechanisms at work, causing overlap. For example, many individuals will have emphysema, as well as excess mucus production, and legitimately fit the definition of chronic bronchitis as well. Less common problems that may legitimately be considered as obstructive diseases include bronchiectasis where secretion clearing is hindered by destructive changes in the bronchial system. Lastly, individuals may have structural abnormalities causing airflow obstruction, such as vocal cord paralysis or a tumor impinging the bronchial system.

This last idea, obstruction of the larger diameter upper airway conducting system, is particularly important as the mechanism underlying obstructive sleep apnea. Individuals with obstructive sleep apnea may have structural issues such as obesity, a floppy or an enlarged soft palate, large tonsils, or a narrow jaw, which combined with the reduced muscle tone in the pharyngeal airway muscles noted during sleep lead to episodes of airway obstruction, followed by stress related to hypoxemia, hypercapnia, and the increased work of breathing itself, culminating in an arousal at the central nervous system level that causes a partial or complete awakening from sleep as the obstruction is relieved. The arousal, beneficial though it is in terminating the apnea, when repeated frequently through the night causes fragmented sleep and ultimately excessive daytime sleepiness.

Restrictive lung disorders are those in which there is simply less lung, either in terms of lung surface area, the volume of air within the alveolar space, or the volume of air exchanged between the alveolar space and the environment in the act of ventilation, as oxygen is delivered to the bloodstream and carbon dioxide removed. Restrictive lung disease can occur in situations where there is literally nothing wrong with the lung, such as neuromuscular disease where muscle weakness leads to inadequate ventilation and accumulation of carbon dioxide, or sedative drug overdose where the respiratory control centers are inhibited. There are a wide variety of diseases which can produce inflammation or scarring of the alveolar surfaces. These include interstitial pneumonias related to medications or toxic exposures, hypersensitivity pneumonitis related to exposure to organic dusts in the environment, as well as multiple diseases where the lung is just another site of a systemic inflammatory process such as rheumatoid arthritis or systemic lupus. Some restrictive lung disorders may begin as an inflammatory process, which can either go on to resolve or lead to fibrosis and irreversible loss of function.

The alveoli in the lung represent a unique environment where the capillaries are closely exposed to the inspired air, with only a capillary wall cell and an alveolar epithelial cell separating them. This close apposition is part of what makes the transfer of oxygen normally so efficient, but leads to poor oxygen transfer when inflammation or scarring alter the distribution of blood flow or the inspired air. Good oxygen transfer requires matching of the distribution of ventilation and the distribution of blood flow, at a fairly microscopic level, and when ventilation perfusion is not well matched, hypoxemia results. The lung normally has the ability to change the regional distribution of both ventilation and perfusion, allowing the oxygen transfer process to adjust in response to localized problems such as a mucous plug or a small area of pneumonia which reduce ventilation by reducing perfusion and maintaining the overall balance to distribution of both. The combination of this autoregulation process and the natural, generous reserve of lung tissue we are born with allows the lung to continue to provide adequate oxygenation for the body needs even in the face of a surprising level of alveolar inflammation and damage. The processes that cause restrictive lung disease can interfere with that ventilation perfusion matching.

In addition to the effects on oxygen transfer, restrictive lung disease can have a substantial effect on the work of breathing. Without any change in airway resistance, the inflammatory and fibrotic processes in the alveolar space will change the mechanical performance of the lung tissue, reducing its compliance. Reduced compliance means an increase in the pressure and total work required to bring air into the alveolus because the lung has become increasingly stiff. This increased work of breathing can lead to respiratory failure just as much as the increased resistance of the obstructive diseases.

Problems which affect the pulmonary vascular space will often behave very much like restrictive disorders affecting the alveoli. They may cause mismatch between ventilation and perfusion with resulting hypoxemia. In addition, by increasing the resistance in the pulmonary capillaries, the cardiac output may be reduced, leading to inadequate delivery of oxygen to the tissues even though the oxygen content of a given quantity of blood is normal. This is often accompanied by increased pressures in the pulmonary vascular system, including increased pressures in the right heart. The right ventricle is meant to be a low-pressure system, especially in comparison to the left ventricle. When increased pulmonary resistance causes increased right-sided pressures, a large and hypertrophied right ventricle may develop and affect the left ventricle which will then fill poorly, leading to reduced cardiac output. This underscores an important distinction between the words hypoxia and hypoxemia. Hypoxemia refers to the oxygen content of a given quantity of blood. This is important, but unless there is adequate cardiac output to deliver that quantity of blood, hypoxia, at the tissue level, will result, and this is the crucial value we try to maintain.

In addition to problems causing increased pulmonary vascular resistance and maldistribution of blood flow, the pulmonary alveolar space can be "flooded" as pulmonary edema. This can occur as congestive heart failure, where problems of poor contractility or valvular heart disease can lead to increased pressure in the pulmonary capillary space with resulting outpouring of fluid into the alveolus. This results in areas without ventilation, while perfusion continues, causing ventilation perfusion mismatch and hypoxemia. This process is referred to as shunt, because blood flowing through the lungs is never exposed to the inspired gases. As a result, shunt hypoxemia is "refractory" and does not improve significantly when the inspired concentration of oxygen is increased. At the same time, the flooding of the pulmonary alveolar space leads to a washing out of surfactant. Surfactant is normally present in the alveolus to reduce surface tension and allow alveoli of different sizes to coexist at the same distending pressure. When washed away, alveoli will tend to close, further diminishing ventilation to those regions and making reinflation of the lung more difficult. In addition to the hydrostatic forces at work in congestive heart failure, many processes which cause acute lung injury and inflammation will produce a leakiness of the pulmonary capillary surface and non-cardiogenic pulmonary edema. This can arise in the context of severe pulmonary infection or through the mechanism of sepsis from distant infections.

16.1.2 Prevalence

Respiratory disorders are fairly common. The prevalence of chronic obstructive lung disease averages about 6% of the population, although it is less than half of that in younger individuals and more than twice as common in older individuals [1]. Much of it is related to cigarette smoking, which varies significantly by region, gender, and age group. Not all of this disease is recognized, and only about half of the population who would fit a reasonable definition of chronic obstructive lung disease are in fact recognized as having it and receiving a medication to treat it. Asthma also varies significantly depending upon worldwide location, but in the United States has a prevalence of about 8% [2]. The prevalence of restrictive lung disease is significantly less. Taking idiopathic pulmonary fibrosis as an example, it has a prevalence of only about 0.064% [3]. Obstructive sleep apnea has a prevalence ranging from 4 to 12% depending upon the age group studied and the definition of the disorder [4], but analysis of large populations suggests that only about 1 out of 5 individuals with obstructive sleep apnea have been diagnosed.

16.1.3 Manifestations of Disease

The cardinal manifestations of pulmonary diseases include dyspnea, cough, and wheezing. Dyspnea is the sensation of breathlessness, very much a subjective complaint. We often note objective findings like tachypnea or use of accessory muscles in breathing that suggest to us an individual is dyspneic, but the ultimate measure is the individual's perception of difficulty breathing. Dyspnea does not correlate well with hypoxemia, and in fact individuals can be comfortable but quite hypoxemia or quite short of breath but have normal oxygen levels. Increased work of breathing, and the sensation of having to do additional work in order to move air in and out of the lungs, perceived through the usual proprioreceptive mechanisms, is a much greater stimulus to dyspnea than hypoxemia alone. Lung stiffness, measured as a reduction in compliance or change in volume divided by change in pressure as we move air in and out of the lungs, is also a major factor in dyspnea. This is in addition to the fact that it takes more work to move air in and out of stiff lungs, since stimulation of stretch receptors within the lung, even in the absence of a change in actual work of breathing, can produce a sensation of dyspnea. Many individuals faced with increased work of breathing such as this will shift to a pattern of rapid shallow breathing, taking a greater number of breaths with smaller tidal volumes at the steepest portion of the curve defining the relationship between lung volume change and pressure change. Taking rapid shallow breaths at the steepest portion of that curve, where compliance is the highest, reduces their work of breathing.

Cough is normally a beneficial reflex. It is one of the mechanisms which allows clearance of unwanted or injurious material from the airway. The alveolar space is maintained and protected by alveolar macrophages which can engulf and remove material, as well as our nonspecific inflammatory system and the specific antibodies and lymphocytes of our allergic immune system. The respiratory bronchioles and smaller bronchi are protected by the mucociliary escalator, where islands of mucus are produced, catch particulate and other potentially injurious material and organisms, which are then propelled upward in the bronchial system by movement of the microscopic cilia. Many respiratory disorders which affect the bronchial system damage the mucociliary escalator and as a result leave the patient unable to clear secretions appropriately. This leads to more irritation and inflammation, to which the body's typical response is to generate more mucus, which in turn only aggravates the problem further.

Lastly, cough is the physical reflex by which accumulations of these mucus islands are raised and eliminated from the airway. Cough is an appropriate response to clear the secretions, but when the quantity of secretions is excessive, or when our ability to generate adequate flow of air to raise this material is compromised, then individuals may have an ineffective cough mechanism because of either obstructive or restrictive disorders. In the obstructive case, increased airway resistance limits the velocity of airflow needed to raise material, while in restrictive disorders the total volume of air available to push secretions out may be diminished. Patients with restrictive disorders may have normal expiratory flows in relative terms, but the total air available to raise secretions is diminished. Some individuals with restrictive disorders will have a nonproductive cough based on irritation of receptors near the small airways and the interstitial space between alveoli without any bronchial abnormality.

Wheezing is a high-pitched continuous sound usually associated with expiration and very typical of diminished airflow from obstruction. Because of the relationship between intrathoracic pressure outside of the alveoli pushing air out and air pressure around the bronchi tending to close the airways and diminish flow, most problems producing noise in expiration arise from abnormalities involving the conducting airways inside the lungs. Although wheezing does refer to this quality of sound when heard through a stethoscope by a physician, most patients will recognize wheezing and describe it accurately. It suggests a problem within the lungs related to obstruction of flow. On the other hand, noisy sounds during inspiration, because of the relationship between the pressure within the extrathoracic upper airways and the pressure in the environment surrounding the patient, suggest a problem of obstruction occurring at the extrathoracic level. These are typically labeled as stridor and are also something that is reported by patients as often as heard through a stethoscope.

It may seem counterintuitive not to put hypoxemia near the top of the list for manifestations of pulmonary disease. However, hypoxemia may be surprisingly independent of the degree of respiratory distress showed by an individual and generally must be measured by pulse oximetry or other techniques to be identified. Patients who have become significantly hypoxemic in a gradual fashion may show surprisingly little in terms of signs and symptoms, even to the point where pulmonary vasoconstriction induced by the hypoxemia has produced right heart failure. Identification of hypoxemia by cyanosis is distinctly unreliable, since demonstration of cyanosis requires about 5 g of unoxygenated hemoglobin per 100 mL of blood to produce the characteristic blue color. Individuals with significant anemia may not survive long enough to reach a low enough oxygen saturation to achieve 5 g of unoxygenated hemoglobin and thus never manifest cyanosis.

Hypercapnia can also be surprisingly inconsistent in terms of the symptoms it is associated with. Hypercapnia can produce reduced responsiveness, and certainly any patient with significant underlying lung disease who presents with obtundation needs to be evaluated with arterial blood gas measurement for elevated levels of CO2. However, some individuals who have increased work of breathing are able to readjust their respiratory control centers and allow the level of CO2 in the blood to gradually rise. The result is a higher gradient of CO2 from the bloodstream to the environment, which allows the elimination of carbon dioxide and maintenance of a stable CO2 level with less total ventilation and as a result less work. Not all patients with lung disease are able to make this compromise, but those who can, termed "CO2 retainers," benefit from reduced work of breathing. Most individuals can compensate for the elevated CO2 level by retaining bicarbonate and maintaining a normal pH. However, making this adaptation to allow the PCO2 to rise, and benefiting from doing less work, also implies the individual has a less robust ability to compensate for any additional demands on his work of breathing. Those individuals who have elevated PCO2, particularly when it has occurred gradually and is not accompanied by hypoxemia, may have little change in mental status.

Respiratory diseases presenting as chest pain are generally limited to those causing inflammation or reaction at the surface of the lung, since only the parietal pleural surfaces have pain fibers. Pain is typically described as "pleuritic" when it varies in intensity with respiratory effort and timing. Even the most typical pain which becomes worse with a deep breath or a cough, and is commonly labeled pleuritic, may not arise from the pleura. Pain involving the chest wall musculature and bony and cartilaginous structures can produce that same sort of pain, so any complaint of pleuritic pain must include consideration of all of the parts of the chest wall "bellows" system as possible causes.

In considering the overall picture of a patient presenting with pulmonary disease, we often use the phrase "respiratory distress." Respiratory distress is a gestalt evaluation that includes a number of factors:

- Is the patient tachypneic, which would suggest that they have an inefficiency in gas exchange or have shifted to a rapid shallow pattern of breathing because of respiratory muscle fatigue or stiff lungs?
- Is the patient using accessory muscles, which would suggest work of breathing greater than the capability of the diaphragm alone to support?
- Does the patient have audibly noisy breathing, which can suggest restricted airflow or turbulence arising from bronchospasm or increased airway secretions?
- Is there discoordination between the movement of the abdomen and the chest? In normal respiration, as the diaphragm descends both the abdomen and chest move outward with inspiration. When there is significant respiratory muscle weakness, particularly of the lower intercostal muscles, the lower chest segments may move inward, paradoxically, during inspiration.
- Does the patient have increased heart rate or blood pressure suggesting increased sympa-

thetic activity in response to diminished delivery of oxygen to the tissues?
- Does the patient have altered mental status, which may reflect significant hypoxemia and hypercapnia?

At the same time, an appropriate assessment of overall respiratory distress requires an estimate of where the patient is in the natural history of his disease and in the unfolding history of any current exacerbation. Are the current symptoms a significant change from the patient's usual condition? Does the patient have reserves?

16.1.4 Anesthetic Risks

The interaction between anesthesia and the respiratory system creates some specific problems which can aggravate the pathophysiology of pulmonary diseases. Foremost among them is the reduction in functional residual capacity that occurs with anesthesia. Functional residual capacity is the volume of air left in the lung at the end of expiration. It is the volume of air that keeps alveolar units open and functional, so that the next inspiration will deliver air in a uniform fashion, allowing good matching between perfusion and ventilation and thus good oxygenation. Individuals ventilated at a constant volume, without sighs and without changes in position, will gradually lose functional residual capacity as the effectiveness of surfactant diminishes over time and alveolar units may close. Although we usually think of atelectasis as a macroscopic phenomenon where regional reduction in ventilation leads to collapse of lung segments or lobes, this loss of functional residual capacity is micro-atelectasis. This loss of functional residual capacity is an even greater problem in procedures where the abdomen or thorax may be entered and diaphragmatic function affected.

Sedating and general anesthetic agents will defeat the normal protective reflexes involving the bronchi and the upper airways, and with loss of cough, the ability of the conducting airways to clear secretions raised by the mucociliary escalator is diminished. Postoperative analgesia will produce the same problem, potentially leading to macro-atelectasis. The normal airway has a remarkable ability to clear irritants and microorganisms from the lower respiratory tract, but in the face of altered protective reflexes and atelectasis, there may be not just mismatch of ventilation and perfusion, but infection with a significant inflammatory response potentially affecting the whole patient.

Sedating and general anesthetic agents, as well as analgesics, are likely to affect ventilatory drive. During the procedure the patient is typically under close monitoring to determine when respiratory drive is adequate and the patient can be expected to resume control of their own ventilation and maintain an appropriate CO2 level. However, particularly in patients with chronic obstructive lung disease who may be "CO2 retainers," the balance between the timing of medication, the course of the procedure, and the return of their respiratory drive can be challenging. The same problem occurs in patients who have received neuromuscular blockade. The usual assessments used in determining if sufficient strength has returned may underestimate how much respiratory muscle weakness may affect both ventilation and oxygenation for a patient with underlying respiratory disease. Many patients with chronic obstructive lung disease and other disorders have greatly increased work of breathing and must use accessory muscles of respiration including intercostal and shoulder girdle muscles to maintain adequate and uniform ventilation. They do not have the reserve that the ordinary patient has and may require a greater margin in time or alterations in dose to be sure adequate strength has returned.

In patients with long-standing hypoxemia, or where the pulmonary vascular bed has been altered through mechanisms that would include fibrosis or thromboembolic disease, patients may have increased right heart pressures and right ventricular dysfunction from pulmonary hypertension. In those patients, the vasodilator effects of many common anesthetic agents may affect the right-sided circulation, leading to reduced filling of the right ventricle. Those individuals may be dependent upon an "overfilled" right ventricle to maintain an adequate cardiac output and may show significantly diminished forward output if they become hypovolemic, even in relative terms, during anesthesia.

Patients with obstructive sleep apnea are most at risk for airway compromise, hypoxemia, and catastrophic events in the postoperative period, particularly when receiving opiate analgesics. However, a subset of patients with obstructive sleep apnea may have airways which are difficult to manage during induction of general anesthesia, and knowledge of or suspicion of obstructive sleep apnea mandates appropriate preparation and monitoring during intubation.

16.2 Preoperative Assessment

16.2.1 Preoperative Evaluation

The preoperative evaluation should begin with an assessment of the patient's exercise capacity. Although multiple factors can affect this, including conditioning and cardiac and musculoskeletal disease, having an idea of what the limits are on the patient's activity provides a starting point to assess the patient's pulmonary reserve. Starting with an open-ended questions such as "what is the most physically demanding thing you can do?" allows you to understand this from the patient's perspective. The second question should then be "what sensation is it that makes you stop when you do something strenuous?" If the patient's answer is shortness of breath, then it may be reasonable to conclude the limitation is respiratory. At times patients will have difficulty describing what stops them, and offer terms such as "fatigue," but then further questions can be directed asking where they feel it and what do other people see or hear when they reach a stopping point. Although in the laboratory we use oxygen consumption, measured in metabolic equivalents or "mets" as a reflection of work done or actual energy used, it is easier to question patients based on activities of daily living. This allows patients to be divided into three broad categories: individuals whose most strenuous activity is what we would commonly recognize as recreational exercise or home activity such as yard work, a middle category of patients whose most strenuous activity are the core activities of daily living like grocery shopping or cleaning inside the home, and the most limited group whose most strenuous activity are basic self-care issues like dressing and toileting. If these limitations appear to be on the basis of dyspnea, individuals in the middle and worst category will be at increased risk for perioperative problems related to the respiratory disease.

The next issue is to understand what the natural history of the patient's disease is and whether there has been any recent deterioration that would put the patient at increased risk. Asking the patient to compare their exercise tolerance and dyspnea to what they were capable of a year earlier may be helpful, as well as asking whether or not they feel they are better or worse than their "usual." It is helpful at this point to look for any current problems that may have worsened their functional status. This could include signs of infection such as increased or purulent secretions or fever, manifestations of congestive heart failure including orthopnea or nocturnal awakenings with breathlessness, and looking to see if the patient has findings suggesting that more than one respiratory process at work. Individuals with obstructive disease may have abrupt deterioration if they develop concurrent restriction from chest wall pain or weight gain. Patients with restrictive disorders may deteriorate if they develop concurrent obstruction, even as simple as an episode of acute bronchitis with increased purulent secretions and airflow limitation related to the body's inflammatory response to that infection.

A search for nocturnal symptoms can be particularly helpful. Because bronchial smooth muscle tone may be greater at night, and because following a period of immobility and reduced secretion clearing during sleep patients may have an added burden of material they need to raise, an individual reporting nighttime symptoms may be at increased risk even if they have little to report during the daytime. It is also important to look for increased use of medications to relieve symptoms, since in some cases the effectiveness of these drugs will allow the patient to continue to maintain a good level of function despite the fact that their underlying respiratory disease is worsening.

The patient's symptoms of cough and production of secretions may be helpful in assessing the patient's severity and predicting the likely response to perioperative stresses. Individuals who raise secretions in mild or moderate quantity and feel better after they do so may be at less risk for perioperative issues than a patient who clearly has secretions but is unable to raise them, or who feels little benefit when they do raise them. The character of the secretions in terms of color may be less helpful, since more chronic secretions or material from patients who are dehydrated may be darker or ominously colored. A patient whose secretions are thick and viscous may have a greater risk for airway plugging and ventilation perfusion mismatch particularly if their volume status moves to the drier end of the spectrum during the perioperative period.

There are a number of useful screening tools to help in identifying patients at risk for obstructive sleep apnea. The simplest of these is the "STOP-BANG" tool [5] which takes eight basic items and helps to categorize the patient as at low, medium, or high risk for having obstructive sleep apnea (see Table 16.1).

Some basic historical questions should be part of this preoperative review. This would include whether the patient has ever had difficulty involving intubation or anesthesia, including prolonged intubation or requirement for reintubation, with prior procedures. A patient with known lung disease who has required intubation in the past should be viewed as being at higher risk. It is often helpful to ask the patient when they were last hospitalized, how often they have gone to the hospital or the emergency room, and how often and how recently have they been treated with corticosteroids in the past. Patients who have been treated with supplemental oxygen, from that sole observation, deserve additional attention. Patients treated with very low flow rates of supplemental oxygen at rest may develop greater hypoxemia when faced with the changes in ventilation perfusion matching from atelectasis or airway plugging. Even though many patients on supplemental oxygen are not CO2 retainers, being on supplemental oxygen should serve as a caution that this patient could have abnormalities in terms of their respiratory drive and their sensitivity to increased work of breathing and the effect of medications on their respiratory drive.

Physical examination for patients with respiratory disease centers on auscultation of the chest. The first step is listening for the ordinary breath sounds generated by air movement in the large airways. The bilateral nature of lungs is particularly helpful here, since it is easy to make a comparison, region by region, to identify asymmetry, absence, or alterations in breath sounds that may identify lung which is collapsed and unventilated leading to absent sounds, or areas where the quality of the breath says has changed suggesting consolidation, or filling of alveoli with fluid, or inflammatory or infectious material. Second is listening for the adventitious sounds not usually present in normal lung. These include high-pitched continuous sounds or wheezes, which reflect increased resistance and airflow limitation of the bronchi, fine crackles which may reflect fluid in alveoli, course crackles which may reflect sticky secretions in smaller airways, and rhonchi which are low-pitched continuous sounds arising from airway secretions. Lastly, it can be helpful to ask the patient to perform a forced expiration, taking in a maximum breath and forcing it out as quickly and completely as possible through an open mouth. At one level this is a poor man's pulmonary function test, since most patients with normal airflow can expel a maximum vital capacity breath in 3 seconds or

Table 16.1 The STOP-BANG Questionnaire

Snoring?	BMI > 35
Tired?	Age > 50
Observed apnea?	Neck size >16 in.
Pressure (hypertension)	Gender = male
Risk of obstructive sleep apnea	
Low: 0 to 2 "yes" answers	
Medium: 3 or 4 "yes" answers	
High: 5 to 8 "yes" answers OR 2 or more and BMI > 35 OR 2 or more and neck >16	

From Chung 2016

less while patients with obstruction may take significantly longer. This maneuver may bring out unappreciated symptoms such as wheezing or cough that may reflect airway irritability and secretions. It also provides an insight to the patient's ability to take in a maximal breath and forcefully expel it. While this maneuver seems quite simple, it requires a motivated patient with adequate strength, a working chest bellows to allow both the full inspiration and forceful expiration, and a lack of significant airway obstruction. These factors look at respiratory function in an integrated fashion which nicely mimics the demands the patient will face during the perioperative period.

16.2.2 Pre-procedure Testing

In cases where clinical assessment suggests serious pulmonary disease, it may be helpful to have pulmonary function testing to confirm or refute that assumption. Pulmonary function testing can measure expiratory flow rates, as an assessment of obstruction, and lung volumes and diffusion capacity, allowing measurement of restrictive disease. The diffusion capacity uses carbon monoxide as the surrogate measure to assess the transfer of oxygen from the alveolar space into the bloodstream. This measurement is sensitive not just to the quantity of lung present but also to alterations in its vascular supply. Pulmonary function testing results are evaluated against predicted values usually calculated based on the patient's gender, height, and age. Obviously, perfectly normal patients may vary from this predicted value. In precise terms, we use the standard error of the estimate from the regression equation used to calculate the predicted value, but as a simple shorthand normal patient, values are largely within ±20% of the predicted. Pulmonary function testing reports typically present a bewildering array of values. However, it is possible to narrow down the data to a more limited set of values (summarized in Table 16.2) which can be linked to the pathophysiology that affects the perioperative period [6].

Table 16.2 Useful pulmonary function test results in predicting perioperative pulmonary risks

Measure	Warning criteria	Function measured
FEV1	<1 L	Effective cough volume
Maximum voluntary ventilation	<50% predicted	Overall chest bellows function
pCO2	>45 mmHg	Adequate control of ventilation

From Tisi 1987

The forced expiratory volume in 1 s, the FEV1, is the most commonly used measure of lung function, available on simple handheld spirometers as well as more complex equipment available in a hospital laboratory. It is the volume of air expired in the first second during a forceful effort after a full inspiration. It can be reduced both in restrictive and obstructive disorders. We frequently look at the FEV1 in relationship to the forced vital capacity, the total amount of air expired in this maximal effort. This FEV1/FVC ratio is useful in determining if obstruction is present. If the FEV1/FVC ratio is less than 70%, or somewhat lower in elderly patients, then obstruction is present. If the FEV1 is reduced, but the FEV1/FVC ratio is normal or high, then in relative terms there is no obstruction, and these findings would suggest restriction.

For the purposes of perioperative assessment, however, one can take a simpler approach. As the FEV1 is reduced, whether from obstruction or restriction, the patient will have increasing difficulty in generating an adequate amount of air to clear secretions during the process of coughing. In a simple way, one can consider the FEV1 to be a "cough volume," and patients with a reduced FEV1 from either mechanism are likely to have difficulty maintaining uniform ventilation and clearing secretions.

Second, we will frequently ask the patient to take the largest and most forceful breaths possible, inspiring and expiring, for 10 s. This is then multiplied by 6 to calculate the maximum possible ventilation in liters per minute that this patient could possibly generate, called the maximum voluntary ventilation, MVV. It is a theoretical concept, since no patient is likely to maintain that great level of effort for an entire minute, and if they did, the increase ventilation would likely result in hypocapnia and the associated symptoms of hyperventilation. This test is a composite measure of how the chest bellows works. It requires strength, adequate lung volumes, and a lack of obstruction to generate a maximal result. This measure is sometimes criticized because it requires good patient cooperation, strength, and effort to achieve a maximal result. However, all of those qualities are exactly the factors required to avoid respiratory compromise in the perioperative period. A patient with weakness, a lack of motivation, or pain hindering effort will have a compromise in this value just as much or sometimes more than a patient with serious obstructive or restrictive lung disease.

Third, in patients where there is concern that there respiratory control centers may not function normally, measurement of pCO2, the partial pressure of carbon dioxide, in arterial blood may be helpful. Pulse oximetry has allowed us to measure arterial oxygen saturation easily and noninvasively, but arterial pCO2 remains the definitive standard in measuring the patient's ventilatory response. A pCO2 of 45 or higher, particularly in a patient who is not acutely decompensating, suggests that their respiratory control center has adapted to increased work of breathing and allowed the pCO2 to rise in the interest of a lower requirement for total minute ventilation. This patient is at risk for having an inadequate respiratory drive during the postoperative period and potentially requiring prolonged ventilatory support. This high work of breathing applies to both patients with severe obstructive and restrictive disorders, usually appearing late in the course of the disease. Similar information can be obtained by looking at the bicarbonate level on a blood chemistry study, but bicarbonate levels can be affected by multiple other factors including fluid intake and output, diuretics, and renal function. Measurement of pCO2 provides an unambiguous picture. Some clinicians may argue for inclusion of other values, most commonly a measurement of oxygenation. However, while providing supplemental oxygen is relatively easy, compensating for a patient whose ventilatory drive is inadequate increases the complexity of care required.

A chest X-ray should be considered for patients who are elderly, have more advanced disease, or have other comorbidities. The chest X-ray provides information about the severity of the disease that is complementary to what pulmonary function testing may reveal, particularly for the degree of involvement by fibrosis or emphysema. It also provides a baseline that may be useful during the perioperative time to accurately identify what is new disease and what is old disease, which can be essential in identifying complications. Although CT scanning, particularly when done with high resolution, can provide more detailed information, including distinguishing potentially reversible inflammation from more irreversible fibrosis, that usually belongs as part of the ongoing care of the patient rather than a preoperative evaluation.

16.2.3 What to Do About Chronic Medications?

A review of the patient's current medication use can be helpful in identifying the patient's problems and their severity. Inhaled medications for the obstructive disorders include inhaled steroids taken further anti-inflammatory effect and inhaled bronchodilators. These medications are most commonly given by an inhaled route, using either a propellant-driven metered dose inhaler or a dry powder inhaler. Both devices require patient education to achieve optimal delivery. Propellant-driven metered dose inhalers are frequently used with a spacer which increases the distance between the canister opening and the patient by a small amount, reducing the amount of drug deposited in the mouth and improving the amount delivered to the lungs. These inhaled drugs are commonly used because, for a given amount of beneficial response in the airways, the systemic effects and potential side effects are reduced compared to what they would be with an oral medication. While there are a large number of agents available, they can be summarized into smaller groups based on their mechanisms, as indicated in Table 16.3 which includes both generic and brand names. Knowing what the patient has been treated within the past can be helpful in identifying prior diagnoses.

Table 16.3 Common respiratory medications by class, with generic and brand names

Respiratory Medications	
Short-acting beta-agonist bronchodilators	
Albuterol	Proventil Proair Ventolin
Levalbuterol	Xopenex
Albuterol/ipratropium	Combivent Duoneb
Epinephrine	Asthmanefrin Bronkaid Primatene
Long-acting beta-agonist bronchodilators	
Salmeterol	Serevent
Olodaterol	Striverdi
Vilanterol	
Formoterol	Perforomist Foradil
Indacaterol	Arcapta
Arformoterol	Brovana
Short-acting anticholinergic bronchodilators	
Ipratropium	Atrovent
Long-acting anticholinergic bronchodilators	
Tiotropium	Spiriva
Umeclidinium	Incruse
Aclidinium	Tudorza
Inhaled corticosteroids	
Beclomethasone	Qvar
Budesonide	Pulmicort
Fluticasone	Flovent Arnuity
Flunisolide	Aerobid Aerospan
Mometasone	Asmanex
Ciclesonide	Alvesco
Phosphodiesterase inhibitor bronchodilator	
Theophylline	
Aminophylline	
Leukotriene inhibitors/antagonists	
Montelukast	Singulair
Zafirlukast	Accolate
Zileuton	Zyflo
Antibody against interleukin-5	
Reslizumab	Cinqair
Mepolizumab	Nusala
Antibody against IgE	
Omalizumab	Xolair
Combination products	
Vilanterol (beta-agonist)/ umeclidinium (anticholinergic)	Anoro

Table 16.3 (continued)

Respiratory Medications	
Tiotropium (anticholinergic)/ olodaterol (beta-agonist)	Stiolto
Vilanterol (beta-agonist)/ fluticasone (corticosteroid)	Breo
Mometasone (corticosteroid)/ formoterol (beta-agonist)	Dulera
Budesonide (corticosteroid)/ formoterol (beta-agonist)	Symbicort
Fluticasone (corticosteroid)/ salmeterol (beta-agonist)	Advair
Anti-inflammatory and immunomodulatory	
Corticosteroids prednisone methylprednisolone	
Cyclophosphamide	Cytoxan
Azathioprine	Imuran
Mycophenolate	Cellcept
N-acetylcysteine	
Nintedanib	Ofev
Pirfenidone	Esbriet Pirfenex Pirespa
Drugs for pulmonary hypertension	
Pulmonary arterial vasodilators	
Epoprostenol (continuous infusion)	Flolan Veletri
Iloprost (inhaled)	Ventavis
Treprostinil (oral or parenteral)	Tyvaso Remodulin Orenitram
Endothelin receptor antagonists	
Bosentan	Tracleer
Macitentan	Opsumit
Ambrisentan	Letairis
Adenylyl cyclase inhibitors	
Sildenafil	Revatio Viagra
Tadalafil	Cialis Adcirca
Calcium channel blockers	
Diltiazem	Cardizem
Nifedipine	Procardia
Amlodipine	Norvasc
Soluble guanylate cyclase stimulator	
Riociguat	Adempas

Many patients with milder obstructive disease will need only an inhaled bronchodilator to use when symptoms develop. However, when patients typically need this "rescue" medication on a daily basis, they should be on an anti-inflammatory medication to reduce the underlying bronchial hyperreactivity and inflammation that leads to bronchospasm, and often on a regularly scheduled bronchodilator. Finding out how often the patient needs their rescue inhaler and how regular they are in use of their regularly scheduled medications provides important insights into the severity of their disease. In general, patients on inhaled medications should continue before and during the perioperative period. A patient who needs rescue medication on a daily or greater basis is probably undertreated in terms of the long-term, scheduled medications.

Some patients will receive their inhaled medication using an air-powered nebulizer device. While this may have been done because of the patient's poor technique using inhalers or at the patient's request, in general patients with nebulizers are sicker. The devices do provide a higher dose of medication, although there is nothing intrinsically different about the response that could not be matched by more puffs of inhaled medication.

Not all medications given orally necessarily carry a greater side effect profile. The oral leukotriene inhibitors have very few side effects. This is not true for oral or systemic steroids. Patients who have been on chronic steroids are likely to have more significant disease and will need a decision and a plan as part of their preoperative assessment about whether or not the steroid dose can be reduced, or whether the severity of the patient's disease requires continued therapy. There are a small number of patients who continue to take oral bronchodilator therapy, with theophylline or, even more rarely, oral albuterol. In order to achieve a beneficial effect, the level in the systemic circulation is much more likely to reach a point where it produces side effects and symptoms. These drugs with their sympathomimetic properties may contribute to tachycardia and cardiac irritability during anesthesia, and whenever possible their discontinuance with the substitution of an inhaled bronchodilator regimen prior to the procedure is preferable.

Patients with restrictive lung disorders may be receiving corticosteroids or other immunomodulatory medications. In general these medications will need to be continued through the perioperative period, with plans made for alternate route of delivery if oral feeding is not possible. For patients with pulmonary vascular disorder, the need to have a plan for how their medications will be continued through the perioperative period is crucial, since discontinuance of the medications can result in worsening right heart failure, and when done abruptly can be life-threatening.

Patients who are anticoagulated for pulmonary vascular disorders, including pulmonary thromboembolism, need a plan for "bridging" using a short-acting agent in many cases. If the patient is on a long-term anticoagulant with a longer duration of affect, they may need to be shifted to a shorter-acting medication, often injected low molecular weight heparin, with that dosing held typically 12–24 h before the procedure. Once the procedure and the risk of further bleeding is over, if the patient is returning to an anticoagulant that takes time to achieve its effect, they may require bridging with immediate acting short duration anticoagulation until the long-term drug is again effective.

16.2.4 Steps to Optimize Patient: Pre-op Preparation

Optimizing the patient preoperatively starts with looking for evidence that their disease has recently changed or worsened. Patients with recent infection, new problems of clearing secretions, noncompliance with therapy, or overuse of rescue medication should have those problems dealt with before surgery, if possible. There is always a balance between the urgency of the surgery and the need for time to allow the patient to be optimized. Because inflammation underlies many of the respiratory issues, a simple change in medication is usually not sufficient, but rather a change in medication and time for it to work is needed. If the patient has signs suggesting infection, antibiotics may be needed. If secretion clearing is a problem, improved humidity in the environmental air, additional fluids, and mucolytic medication such as guaifenesin may be needed.

For many patients, the problem is less the plan of therapy than its implementation. For those patients, getting them to optimize their delivery of inhaled medications through good technique, being sure they are taking the intended number of doses per day, and avoiding specific triggers during the perioperative period is the challenge. This brings up the difficult issue of cigarette smoking. A surprising number of patients with respiratory disease continue to smoke, and although the benefits of smoking cessation in terms of cardiovascular disease and reducing the risk of lung cancer may take months or years to realize, in terms of symptomatic airway disease, the benefits come more quickly. Patients should be unequivocally advised to stop smoking, and since the success rate is significantly higher with nicotine replacement therapy, that should always be included. This will produce a benefit in reducing airway inflammation over the span of a few days and in reducing myocardial irritability and improving the ability to carry oxygen to the bloodstream even more efficiently.

A decision to add systemic steroids should be made if the patient's status represents a marked reduction from their usual, or if their usual baseline starts at a low level. In both cases it will take time for the steroids to work, generally in the range of 4–7 days to see a definitive improvement although some symptoms may improve sooner. The patients who would benefit from this step would include those who are becoming refractory to their rescue bronchodilator, even if reported only on an occasional basis, as well as patients who are symptomatic at rest or having worsening symptoms related to specific triggers which were previously well-tolerated.

16.2.5 What Should Cancel Surgery?

A decision to cancel surgery in many ways parallels the decision to move ahead with systemic corticosteroids. Patients who have failed to respond to a course of corticosteroids as an outpatient, or who are becoming unresponsive to inhaled bronchodilators, which may be manifest as overuse of rescue inhaler more than 4–6 times a day, should be considered for cancelation of their surgery. Evidence of an infection with fever or pneumonic infiltrate identified on X-ray should prompt cancelation.

In the context of restrictive lung diseases, which usually move at a more leisurely pace, the abrupt appearance of greatly worsened dyspnea should prompt cancelation and further investigation. Some of those patients may have a new and distinct process leading to dyspnea, such as pulmonary thromboembolism. Because dyspnea may arise on the basis of pulmonary congestion from cardiac dysfunction, patients with the abrupt appearance of dyspnea should be evaluated for cardiac ischemia. The abrupt the appearance of a symptom, the more it differs from the patient's usual natural history, and the lack of a clear explanation, all add to making a decision to cancel surgery.

16.3 Intraoperative Management

16.3.1 Effect of Anesthesia on Disease

Anesthesia produces changes in pulmonary function through its effects on smooth muscle function, protective reflexes, and the effects of typical operative positioning on ventilation and perfusion. General anesthesia causes loss of the cough reflex that clear secretions as well as laryngeal reflexes which may be beneficial in protecting the upper airways. Muscle relaxation and supine positioning will lead to a reduction in the functional residual capacity and the increased likelihood that micro-atelectasis will cause low ventilation perfusion ratio lung units and pulmonary shunt, where blood flow moves to the lung without making contact with inspired gas.

Even steps as seemingly innocent as preoxygenating the patient leading to a high oxygen concentration in the alveolar space may lead to significantly faster adsorption of gas from unstable, partially closed alveoli and worsening atelectasis.

Reduced effectiveness of the respiratory muscles, particularly the intercostal muscles relative to the diaphragm, leads to alterations in the distribution of ventilation and more mismatch. Respiratory control centers, particularly those driven by hypoxia more than the medullary chemoreceptors driven by CO2 concentration, are diminished, leading to global decreases in ventilation.

16.3.2 What Anesthetic Medications to Use and Not to Use?

Barbiturates and propofol as induction agents will produce significant respiratory control center depression. Some of the barbiturates may increase muscle tone and may transiently lead to greater cough. Ketamine will have less effect on central respiratory drives, and as a smooth muscle dilator, it may reduce bronchospasm and airway pressures. However, in some patients it may increase secretions and salivation, leading to potential airway compromise. Etomidate shares the property of less depression of drive, but may leave more motor tone and more cough. In most cases, for patients where bronchospasm is a significant issue, and potent smooth muscle relaxation is desirable, ketamine may be a reasonable choice. Because of its bronchodilator properties, propofol is a good induction agent in patients with reactive airway and asthmatics.

Inhalational agents used during general anesthesia will as expected reduce respiratory drive and are all strong smooth muscle dilators, producing bronchodilation. Some agents will affect large airways more than small airways, but in general it is a dose-dependent relationship, so that if bronchospasm is an issue, an increased dose will resolve it. The inhalational agents, however, do alter how the mucociliary escalator works, leading to poor secretion clearing and potential plugging with ventilation perfusion mismatch. For some of the inhalational agents which have direct irritant properties, there may be a transient increase in cough, which is generally reduced at higher concentrations. Some agents, such as sevoflurane, do not have as much irritant quality.

16.3.3 Potential Problems

Pulmonary problems which develop abruptly in the operating room usually involve an event leading to sudden hypoxemia, hypercapnia, increased airway resistance, or reduced lung compliance. Some of them may reflect a mechanical problem with the anesthesia hardware or airway equipment, but others will reflect a change in the pathophysiology of the patient.

The abrupt appearance of high airway pressures should raise the concern that resistance or compliance has changed. This can be determined by looking at not just the peak pressure but the plateau pressure during a prolonged inspiratory hold. If the plateau pressure is elevated, this suggests the problem is low compliance and stiff lungs. This can occur with the development of acute lung injury and capillary leak pulmonary edema, often labeled as on a hydrostatic basis from volume overload. However, if the plateau pressure is low but the peak airway pressures are high, this suggests increased resistance. This could occur with a mechanical issue such as tube malpositioning, increase secretions, or bronchospasm.

Intraoperative development of hypoxemia can reflect anything that leads to ventilation perfusion mismatch. This would include acute lung injury and capillary leak pulmonary edema often labeled as adult respiratory distress syndrome. This can be triggered by any of the mechanisms that trigger sepsis, since it reflects an inappropriate and "too global" activation of inflammatory mediators causing changes in the permeability of the alveolar capillary surface. Filling of alveoli with fluid, combined with damage to surfactant, leads to alveolar collapse. This is reversed, with variable success, by use of positive end expiratory pressure or PEEP which will stabilize alveoli. Alveoli can also be filled with infectious or inflammatory material. This can happen abruptly if there is localized infection at one site, and through changes in patient positioning, the infectious/inflammatory material is spread more diffusely to previously healthy lung worsening VQ mismatch.

Intraoperative development of hypercapnia is generally not a function of reduced respiratory drive with reduced minute ventilation since the volume and rate of ventilation is controlled as part of the anesthetic process. However, if there is abrupt development of dead space, regions of lung where there is ventilation without perfusion, then the patient being ventilated with a constant minute value by the anesthesia equipment will become inefficient in clearing carbon dioxide with resulting hypercapnia. This process can occur with the intraoperative occurrence of a pulmonary thromboembolism.

16.3.4 Fluid Management

Excess fluid in the lungs typically first accumulates in the looser connective tissue space around the smaller bronchioles. There it may manifest as wheezing caused by compression of the bronchioles. Changes in lung compliance may also come early and appear as increased airway pressure. Only later in the process will increased alveolar fluid lead to the crackles commonly associated with pulmonary edema. By that point, mismatch between ventilation and perfusion is already well-established, and it will take time for the volume overload leading to this fluid or time for the inflammation-driven capillary leak to resolve. It is important to recognize that the lungs are the principal targets of fluid excess and that patients with underlying lung disease will tolerate the additional lung stiffness and VQ mismatch poorly. This is not the same as arguing that they should be deliberately kept at a low intravascular volume, since that itself will lead to worsening cardiac output and worsening oxygen delivery due to the mechanisms of diminished ventricular filling and increased systemic resistance in the body's effort to maintain arterial pressure, even at the expense of cardiac output. The best approach is to provide the minimum volume the patient requires, but realize that some patients may tolerate this poorly and be prepared to provide appropriate monitoring and support during the immediate postoperative period.

16.4 Postoperative Management

16.4.1 Airway Management

The patient needs to be positioned so they can achieve an adequate inspiration, use their respiratory muscles optimally including allowing the diaphragm to descend without competition from the abdominal space, and be able to generate an effective cough. A check for the ability of the patient to breath around the deflated endotracheal tube, as a way of detecting glottic region edema that may manifest after extubation, should be part of the routine before extubation.

In addition to the typical assessment of patient strength by asking them to lift their head off the pillow and measurement of an exhaled volume to judge readiness for extubation, asking the patient immediately following extubation to demonstrate their cough will give insight into how well they may protect their airway. Because the presence of the endotracheal tube before extubation interferes with glottic closure, it is difficult to evaluate this before extubation. When the patient has a poor cough, suctioning the pharyngeal space has the advantage of preventing raised material from being re-aspirated, as well as stimulating more cough and stronger cough.

Another useful tool to judge which patients may be at risk for airway complications shortly after extubation is to ask the patient to phonate as a way of demonstrating that their vocal cords are not edematous and can move freely. Patients who are unable to phonate may simply have weakness or lack of effort, but the ability to phonate effectively suggests cord edema is not present and does give another measure of their general chest bellows function in being able to move air across the cords. If the patient is unable to phonate, careful examination looking for other evidence of upper airway obstruction, such as intercostal muscle retraction or paradoxical movement of the chest and abdomen, should be performed. Nebulization of racemic epinephrine, typically 0.5 mL of a 2.25% solution, can be given, but does not always work. It is important, however, not to allow a trial of racemic epinephrine to delay taking more definitive action if the patient has severe upper airway obstruction. These actions would include reintubation and, in more extreme cases, creation of a surgical airway.

Patients with obstructive sleep apnea, especially following general anesthesia or when given narcotic analgesia, may manifest their airway obstruction. In distinguishing this from upper airway edema related to hematoma or periprocedural trauma, a key distinction is that obstruction in sleep apnea improves when the patient is sufficiently stimulated to awaken. The patient who shows waxing and waning breathing pattern, with the reduced breath portion terminating in snorting or other signs of an arousal, should be considered to have obstructive sleep apnea. These patients can be treated just as we would in the outpatient setting with continuous positive airway pressure (CPAP) administered by a mask. However, the realization that CPAP creates positive pressure in the nasopharynx and mouth may make this impossible if there is concern that air could be forced into suture lines creating submucosal emphysema and potentially causing infection as oral secretions are forced into those fascial planes. If a patient with suspected or proven obstructive sleep apnea cannot be treated with CPAP, they require close monitoring of end-tidal CO2 levels, oxygenation and cardiac rhythm. Patients who show significant oxygen desaturations or other signs of increased sympathetic activity that may come from the stress of their obstructive events may need to be awakened frequently to reverse these desaturations. The patient should be placed on CPAP as soon as it is possible, since at some point the cumulative effect of their awakenings will force sleep upon them. That may actually put them at greater risk for more severe oxygen desaturations on the second or subsequent postoperative nights when REM sleep may increase as a rebound process, so the goal should be early use of CPAP whenever possible.

Some patients may show a waxing and waning pattern of breathing postoperatively, but not show arousals coincident with a return of airway tone and the initiation of breathing. These patients may have Cheyne Stokes breathing related to alterations in the respiratory control center. They resume breathing after an apnea, or increase breathing during the crescendo portion of the Cheyne Stokes cycling, sometimes without evidence of an arousal. When they do show arousals, the arousals tend to occur at the nadir of the ventilatory efforts. They can be monitored without specific intervention, as long as oxygenation remains adequate, until the residual effects of the anesthesia resolve.

16.5 Postoperative Complications

Atelectasis may be identified on chest radiographs, particularly when seen as thin "plates" of collapsed lung often not following a lobar or segmental pattern, or by evidence of volume loss of the total lung, or it may be suspected based on regionally decreased breath sounds or when fever appears generally after the first postoperative day. The appearance of a new density on chest radiographs, particularly when it does not have the typical picture of consolidation with air bronchograms, combined with increased respiratory distress or fever suggests atelectasis. Atelectasis causes dysfunction by causing decreased regional ventilation to the lung, resulting in ventilation perfusion mismatch and hypoxemia, and also interferes with secretion clearing promoting an environment for infection.

Atelectasis can occur because of pain hindering respiratory movement and chest bellows function, related to bronchospasm or the plugging of the airways with secretions, or as part of the loss of functional residual capacity and alveolar volume associated with the perioperative state and anesthesia. Measures to improve alveolar recruitment such as incentive spirometry and mobilization of the patient, encouraging deeper breaths and cough, are the cornerstones of treatment. Correcting the underlying issue in terms of pain or bronchospasm is also important. Many patients benefit from a brief educational session prior to their surgery, going over the potential postop problems such as atelectasis and teaching them to use incentive spirometry. Mucolytic therapy with agent such as oral guaifenesin or inhaled acetylcysteine may help to speed resolution, but will seldom in themselves correct atelectasis unless the initiating factors are controlled and measures to recruit alveoli are performed on a consistent basis.

If fever develops, and if the radiograph shows localized infiltrate particularly with air bronchograms, the issue may not be just atelectasis, but pneumonia. Hospital-associated pneumonia frequently reflects the flora of the hospital, and knowledge of the typical organisms and antibiotic sensitivities in that hospital is important in selecting therapy. For patients in settings where methicillin-resistant staphylococcal infection or pseudomonas are common organisms, coverage must be adapted to treat for those organisms. For all patients, measures that help with secretion clearing, including humidification of airflow and suctioning that is appropriate, should be included.

Patient who begin to show signs of respiratory distress related to high work of breathing or the end organ effects of hypoxemia and hypercapnia from atelectasis or pneumonia may need ventilatory support. While in the past this would have meant reintubation and mechanical ventilation, now with the ability to use bilevel positive airway pressure delivered with a nasal or full face mask, we can deliver substantial ventilatory support in a relatively noninvasive fashion. Bilevel positive airway pressure as used to deliver noninvasive ventilatory support serves three functions: first, the positive pressure maintains an open upper airway, allowing delivery of ventilation. Second, it accomplishes the work of breathing, moving air into and out of alveoli, exchanging carbon dioxide. Third, the positive pressure at the alveolar level helps to stabilize the alveolar space, reversing some of the changes of atelectasis at both the macroscopic and microscopic levels.

Patients with acute lung injury and adult respiratory distress syndrome will have some degree of ventilation perfusion mismatch, caused by alveolar collapse and loss of surfactant function. In those cases the expiratory pressure is responsible for stabilizing and recruiting alveoli, and the difference between the inspiratory and expiratory pressures serves to compensate for the additional work of breathing imposed by stiff lungs.

Patients who have upper airway obstruction from upper airway edema or submucosal hemorrhage may develop pulmonary edema not based on capillary leak as in adult respiratory distress syndrome or from increased pressure in the pulmonary capillaries causing fluid to transudate into the alveoli as in congestive heart failure, but rather from the negative pressure in the alveoli generated by vigorous efforts to inspire against the obstructive airway. This negative pressure in the alveolar space draws fluid into the alveoli producing "negative pressure" pulmonary edema. Support for these patients starts with correction of the upper airway obstruction, which generally requires reintubation or creation of the surgical airway by way of tracheostomy. Once the obstruction is resolved, the normal mechanisms that clear alveolar fluid into the interstitial space, then into the pulmonary lymphatics, and back into the right side of circulation can resolve the edema. It is important to recognize that these patients generally will not respond to noninvasive positive airway pressure from bilevel PAP until the obstruction is resolved.

Bleeding from the surgical site, or trauma during intubation or extubation, can produce significant hemoptysis. Fortunately, blood is relatively nonirritating and does not produce a significant inflammatory effect or cause alveolar capillary leak. However, aspiration of blood in the airways can cause significant ventilation perfusion mismatch and hypoxemia. The first step in dealing with this is to secure the airway by reintubation.

Patients who show high airway resistance and other findings of bronchospasm such as wheezing sufficient to cause respiratory distress should have a trial of nebulized bronchodilator. If this is effective, it can be repeated as often as every hour for a few hours unless the patient exhibits significant tachycardia or has a history of other serious arrhythmias. A patient who does not respond to inhaled bronchodilator after 2–3 doses of nebulized bronchodilator 20 min apart likely has a significant inflammatory component to their airway obstruction, which will take time to resolve.

These patients need to be in a setting where close observation is provided, since they are likely to need noninvasive ventilatory support by bilevel positive airway pressure to maintain adequate ventilation despite the high airway resistance until a combination of time and anti-inflammatory corticosteroids can reduce the airway inflammation and edema and restore responsiveness to bronchodilators.

Some postoperative patients manifest wheezing not because of airway inflammation and bronchoconstriction but rather because of interstitial edema surrounding small airways and producing bronchiolar narrowing in what was once called "cardiac asthma." This may occur before the patient demonstrates the typical crackles associated with alveolar edema. These patients generally do not show a robust response to bronchodilators, and this possibility should be considered in patients who have a positive fluid balance postoperatively with wheezing unresponsive to treatment.

Since increased mucus production generally accompanies bronchospasm and airway inflammation, patients with wheezing will frequently have continued ventilation perfusion mismatch from airway plugging even after bronchospasm is improved. In fact, hypoxemia from ventilation perfusion mismatch may worsen as bronchospasm resolves, and airway secretions may redistribute causing new areas of reduce ventilation while other areas improve and before changes in perfusion can adjust to the moving plugging. Postoperative patients generally benefit from adequate humidification of inspired oxygen and enough humidification of the environment to avoid airway drying. Corticosteroid therapy will tend to reduce the amount of secretions, as well as reducing airway irritability and edema. In patients where their underlying diagnoses make administration of systemic glucocorticoids problematic, inhaled corticosteroids delivered via nebulizer can reduce airway secretions and improve airflow distribution without an unreasonable burden in terms of steroid side effects.

Conclusion

Perioperative management of the patient with pulmonary disease requires an appropriate preoperative assessment. This allows the patient to be optimized for both anesthetic and surgical intervention. Patients must be diligently monitored and observed throughout the perioperative period to identify and provide early intervention to optimize outcome and avoid potential adverse events.

References

1. Centers for Disease Control. MMWR. 2012;61(46):938.
2. Centers for Disease Control. MMWR. 2011;60(17):547.
3. Raghu G. Incidence and prevalence of idiopathic pulmonary fibrosis. Am J Respir Crit Care Med. 2006;174(7):810–6.
4. Young T, Peppard PE, Gottlief DJ. Epidemiology of obstructive sleep apnea: a population health perspective. Am J Respir Crit Care Med. 2002;165:1217–39.
5. Chung F, Abdullah HR, Liao P. STOP-Bang questionnaire: a practical approach to screen for obstructive sleep apnea. Chest. 2016;149(3):631–8.
6. Tisi GM. Preoperative identification and evaluation of the patient with lung disease. Med Clin N Am. 1987;71(3):399–412.

17 Neurologic Disorders and Maxillofacial Surgery

Pooia Fattahi, Masoud Yeganegi, and Katherine Kedzierski

Abstract

Managing the patient with a neurological disorder remains a challenge to oral and maxillofacial surgeons. Proper preoperative evaluation allows the surgeon to optimize the patient before a surgical procedure. This chapter will discuss the most common neurological disorders, including Parkinson's disease, dementia, epilepsy, multiple sclerosis, and cerebrovascular disease.

17.1 Introduction

Patients with a neurological disorder are seen in our practice on a daily basis. Cerebrovascular disease is common in our patient population. Patients with dementia present a challenge to health-care providers and family members. Alzheimer disease (AD) is the most common form of dementia in the elderly, accounting for 60–80% of cases. Other common neurological disorders include Parkinson's disease, epilepsy, and multiple sclerosis. Proper perioperative management minimizes complications and enhances our patients' safety.

P. Fattahi, M.D. (✉)
Yale University, Department of Neurology and Internal Medicine, CT, USA

Waterbury Neurology, Waterbury CT, USA
e-mail: pooia.fattahi@gmail.com

M. Yeganegi, M.D., M.A.Sc.
Jagiellonian University Medical College, Kraków, Poland

University of Toronto, Institute of Biomaterials and Biomedical Engineering, Toronto, ON, Canada

K. Kedzierski, M.D.
Department of Neurology, Yale University, CT, USA

Waterbury Neurology, Waterbury CT, USA

17.2 Neurological Diseases

17.2.1 Dementia

17.2.1.1 Medical Disease

Either degenerative or nondegenerative disease can cause dementia, which is characterized by symptoms impairing activities of daily life that include memory impairment, cognitive dysfunction in multiple domains, behavior disturbances, and psychiatric manifestations [1, 2]. Associated behavioral and psychological symptoms, such as

© Springer International Publishing AG 2018

E.M. Ferneini, J.D. Bennett (eds.), *Perioperative Assessment of the Maxillofacial Surgery Patient*,
https://doi.org/10.1007/978-3-319-58868-1_17

delusions, hallucinations, sleep disturbances, and mood disorders, usually make dementia patients totally dependent or even bedridden [3]. Alzheimer disease (AD) is the most common form of dementia in the elderly, accounting for 60–80% of cases. As the population ages, the overall burden of dementia is increasing worldwide. In the United States in 2012, an estimated 5.2 million individuals over 65 years of age had AD, a number that is expected to reach 6.7 million by 2025 [4].

The major dementia syndromes include [5]:

- Alzheimer disease (AD)
- Dementia with Lewy bodies (DLB)
- Frontotemporal dementia (FTD)
- Vascular (multi-infarct) dementia (VaD)
- Parkinson's disease with dementia (PDD)

Less common disorders such as progressive supranuclear palsy (PSP) and Huntington disease can also be associated with dementia. Non-neurodegenerative dementias may be reversible, or progression slowed or halted, if the underlying cause can be identified and adequately treated [6]. Most elderly patients with chronic dementia have AD (approximately 60–80%), and many of these patients also have concomitant cerebrovascular disease. The prevalence of VaD is relatively high in blacks, hypertensive persons, and patients with diabetes; some of the reversible dementias (e.g., metabolic dementias) tend to occur in younger individuals. DLB may be as prevalent as VaD in older cohorts of patients [7]. FTD is much less common than AD or VaD. Alcohol-related dementia, chronic traumatic encephalopathy, medication side effects (e.g., antihistamine use), depression, and other central nervous system illnesses (e.g., prion diseases, HIV infection) are responsible for the majority of the remaining chronic dementias. Dementia frequently has more than one cause, particularly as the condition progresses and especially in older persons. In addition, medical illnesses and comorbidities exacerbating poor cognition are common in elderly patients with dementia. The bedside evaluation combined with historical information from a reliable informant provides most of the information needed to ascertain the cause of dementia [8].

Table 17.1 Aspects of cognitive function tested by the Mini-Mental State Examination [11]

Orientation in time
Orientation in place
Repetition of named objects
Repetition of simple phrase
Ability to undertake simple arithmetic
Recall of objects named earlier in the interview
Naming of objects shown by examiner
Execution of simple tasks by written and spoken command
Writing a simple sentence
Copying a simple design

17.2.1.2 Preoperative Assessment

Specific consideration of preoperative risk assessment, early recognition, and appropriate interventions for the perioperative complications of dementia surgical patients is needed to reduce surgical complications and improve postoperative outcomes. Stroke, pneumonia, septicemia, acute renal failure, and urinary tract infection are the major complications that occur significantly more often in dementia patients than controls [9].

It is important to assess the severity of cognitive disturbance. The Mini-Mental State Examination (MMSE) is a test of global cognitive function [10] that can be performed at the bedside. It consists of a series of questions on orientation and simple commands to assess comprehension (Table 17.1). Variations in MMSE allow comparison to be made with time and measure progress following illness or surgery. Performance of a complete MMSE may be difficult to justify in an asymptomatic preoperative patient. However, it is reasonable to assume that a patient who is unable to recall simple information pertaining to time and place (e.g., date or hospital) will score significantly less than the maximum 30 points. Such information may be of serious clinical significance when it comes to predicting the possibility of postoperative confusion [11].

Duggleby and Lander [12] assessed 66 patients after hip arthroplasty for several days, undertaking serial MMSE examinations. Four patients failed to complete the study, for reasons that might arguably be attributable to confusion, and no details of anesthetic technique are recorded. However, the data are striking. More than a quarter of these patients had MMSE scores <26 on the third postoperative day, and, even by day 5, MMSE scores in a few patients failed to return to preoperative levels. These patients were relatively young (mean age 64.8, range 50–80).

17.2.1.3 Postoperative Assessment

Postoperative bleeding, deep wound infection, acute myocardial infarction, and pulmonary embolism did not increase in the dementia group. The reasons that these complications are more prevalent in surgical patients with dementia are unclear and might be multifactorial [9]. The common symptoms of acute renal failure could be nausea and vomiting; elderly patients often have no fever in the early stages of pneumonia, septicemia, and urinary tract infection. These factors usually delay diagnosis [13]. Malnutrition due to eating problems, deconditioning, and febrile episodes could interfere with postoperative pulmonary care quality and result in pneumonia [14]. Acute renal failure or acute kidney injury might originate from multiple factors. Preoperative and postoperative renal protection could be conducted more aggressively by maintaining euvolemia, adequate cardiac output, and renal perfusion and by avoiding nephrotoxins in surgical patients with dementia [15]. Risk factors associated with postoperative pulmonary complications are age older than 70 years, poor nutritional status, pneumonia, cigarette smoking, chronic respiratory disease, three categories of surgery (upper abdominal, thoracic, or emergency), anesthetic time greater than 180 min, and significant intraoperative blood loss [16]. Specific interventions, such as early pulmonary rehabilitation (including lung expansion maneuvers, chest physical therapies, and thromboprophylaxis), have been proven effective in reducing the risk of pulmonary complications after hip fracture surgery [17]. Stroke resulting in neurological deficits also might be neglected by medical personnel if masked by preexisting neurological deficits. To identify the stroke risk group among surgical patients with dementia and deliver optimal intervention for risk factor control would be crucial for prevention of stroke postoperatively [18]. Febrile episode with underlying bacteremia or septicemia is a serious and potentially lethal factor for advanced dementia patients (Table 17.2).

Postoperative cognitive dysfunction (POCD) has been defined for research purposes as deterioration in performance in a battery of neuropsychological tests that would be expected in <3.5% of controls. This dry statistical statement equates to a catastrophic loss of cognitive ability; it is the difference between a person who is capable of living independently and one who is not. POCD can be usefully defined as a long-term, possibly permanent, disabling deterioration in cognitive function following surgery [19] (Table 17.3).

Table 17.2 Postoperative complications and mortality associated with dementia in multivariate logistic regression model [13]

	Adjusted OR (95 % CI)
30-day postoperative mortality	1.56 (1.36–1.78)
Postoperative complications	
Acute myocardial infarction	0.97 (0.82–1.14)
Acute renal failure	1.55 (1.39–1.73)
Deep wound infection	0.87 (0.70–1.08)
Pneumonia	2.44 (2.31–2.58)
Pulmonary embolism	0.99 (0.65–1.50)
Postoperative bleeding	0.98 (0.89–1.09)
Septicemia	2.02 (1.90–2.15)
Stroke	1.66 (1.57–1.75)
Urinary tract infection	1.62 (1.50–1.74)
Any of above	1.93 (1.86–2.00)

Adjusted for sex, age, teaching hospital or not, low income, urbanization, coexisting medical conditions, types of surgery, and anesthesia
OR odds ratios, *CI* confidence intervals

Table 17.3 Predisposing factors for POCD [11]

Early POCD
Increasing age
General rather than regional anesthesia
Increasing duration of anesthesia
Respiratory complication
Lower level of education
Reoperation
Postoperative infection
Prolonged POCD (months postoperatively)
Increasing age only

17.2.2 Epilepsy

17.2.2.1 Introduction

Over 50 million people suffer from epilepsy globally, of whom 30–40% of patients have drug-resistant epilepsy [20]. Epilepsy continues to be a poorly understood disease and subject to a continuously evolving classification scheme. Seizure attacks are unpredictable and often do not have a specific trigger. And thus, it is important to prepare for potential stressors associated with any medical practice and, in this case, oral and maxillofacial procedures. Surgical teams should be adequately prepared to handle seizure events, which can be dangerous for the patient if not handled properly.

Epidemiologically, epilepsy follows a bimodal age distribution, with the highest peak in childhood, particularly in the developing world [21]. In the developed world, incidence is highest in the first few months of life, falling after the first year of life, remaining stable for the first decade and falling again in adolescence. Incidence is lowest in young and middle adulthood but increases during the fifth decade of life, with a significant increase in the sixth decade. Prevalence of self-reported epilepsy is 5.6/1000 (95% CI, 5.1–6.0) in Canada and 6.3/1000 (95% CI, 4.9–7.8) in the United States [21–24]. Epilepsy is more prevalent in low-income households, in which inadequate dental care is also endemic [21–26].

Epilepsy is generally diagnosed when a person has two or more unprovoked seizures separated by at least 24 h. This definition has been expanded to also include cases with one unprovoked (or reflex) seizure and a probability of further seizures similar to the general recurrence risk (at least 60%) after two unprovoked seizures, occurring over the next 10 years [27].

Despite the incidence of seizure events, patients are often not regularly overseen by an appropriate specialist. In a National Health Interview Survey (NHIS), 0.7% of children 6–17 of age were reported to have had at least one seizure in the preceding year. However, only 65% had visited an appropriate medical specialist in the preceding 12 months. It is therefore possible that a patient with a history of seizures reports for an oral and maxillofacial procedure while not being under the care of a specialist. Patients with daily convulsive seizures are of particular concern and may require more advanced monitoring, while nonconvulsive seizures are less dangerous to the patient [23, 28].

Given the unpredictable nature of their condition, epilepsy patients are often considered at risk during medical procedures. The risk of seizures during or following a surgical operation as well as potential pharmacological challenges is of concern. However, it should be noted that the incidence of such complications are fairly low, at around 0.13 cases per dentist per year in Britain according to one study [29]. In another study the incidence of fits or seizures per dentist per year was found to be 0.1 in Scotland and 0.07 in Britain and Wales [29, 30]. No deaths were reported following these events. However, nearly 50% of respondents claimed to not know how to insert an oral airway. Thus there is room for further education and preparation in dealing with emergency situations.

17.2.2.2 Patient and Staff Education

Studies on knowledge of dental and maxillofacial surgeons on how best to deal with epileptic patients can be found sporadically. A 2014 study in Jordan found an incredible lack of knowledge and understanding of epilepsy among dental students in addition to a significant social bias against individuals suffering from epilepsy [31]. A 2009 study in Canada surveying all 288 practicing dentists in London, Ontario, showed much more positive trends, though six percent of all respondents did not think they could safely treat a patient with epilepsy in their offices. Less than half (48.7%) knew that they needed to time a seizure event [32]. Thus despite a positive attitude, access to care for epileptic patient was clearly affected. Results from Hyderabad, India, were encouraging on some key areas and lacking in others [33]. There is a scattered pattern of fear in society toward epileptic patient that has seeped slightly into the medical profession as well. Given that there is a significant positive correlation between periodontal disease and seizure severity, this issue is of importance for patients living with epilepsy [34]. Knowledge and education of medical personnel are crucial to ensuring patients living with epilepsy have adequate access to care.

17.2.2.3 Preoperative Considerations

The most crucial preoperative consideration with epilepsy patients is a thorough and appropriate history tailored to their disease. Several important factors that may help identify individuals who may be more susceptible to having a clinically significant epileptic seizure during a treatment procedure are listed below (see Table 17.4). It is important to communicate to the patient that the reason for such an exhaustive history is simply adequate preparation to ensure the patient does not feel stigmatized (Table 17.5).

The most important risk for perioperative seizures is alterations in the antiepileptic drug (AED) regime. Despite potential presurgical dietary restrictions (e.g., NPO), antiepileptic medication schedules must not be altered. This needs to be clearly communicated to the patient, as they may wrongly assume they cannot take their medications. Prior to most surgical procedures patients are orally hydrated and that can be used as an opportunity to keep up with AED dosages. Changes to medication schedules prior to surgery should be avoided if possible.

Table 17.4 Factors influencing seizure susceptibility

Disease history	Recent exacerbations in seizure frequency, any history of seizures during past procedures
Associated neurological syndromes	History of traumatic brain injury, stroke, brain malformations (Sturge-Weber, tuberous sclerosis), Lennox-Gastaut syndrome (rare), other genetic syndromes (Down's, Fragile X, Rett, Angelman)
Frequency	Daily or weekly occurrence
Triggers	Stress-induced, situational or psychogenic triggers, inadequate sleep or fatigue
Intensity and duration	History of status epilepticus or seizure clusters, focal or convulsive seizures with loss of consciousness
Recent changes	Any changes in medication, missed doses, concurrent medications, or recent GI disturbances that may be unknowingly affecting absorption
Unstable or refractory disease	Currently prescribed and using rescue medication (e.g., benzodiazepines), vagal nerve stimulation device, or on a ketogenic diet

Table 17.5 Risk factors for lowered seizure threshold

Anticonvulsant medication nonadherence
Anticonvulsant withdrawal
Concurrent medication or therapy (e.g., antidepressants, antipsychotics, antihistamines, antibiotics, CNS stimulants)
Anesthetics
Sleep deprivation or disturbance
Emotional or physical stress
Alcohol withdrawal
Hypoglycemia

When it comes to assessing the need for seizure prevention measures, the invasiveness and timing of the procedure is most important. Simple procedures shorter than 30 min usually require no special measures other than a confident and well-prepared staff. However seizures can arise unexpectedly, with or without preceding aura and in some cases due to particular triggers. These may include sleep disturbances or deprivation and stress. There have even been rare reported cases of patients in whom brushing the teeth and in others the mere thought of toothbrushing induces seizures [35, 36]. In patients with stress-induced triggers, prophylactic oral benzodiazepines may be appropriate [37].

According to one study, administration of 10 mg of oral clobazam achieved abolition or reduction of seizures in around half the cases [38]. It is equally important for patients prone to anxiety-induced seizures to be confident in his or her medical team as well. Clobazam should be prescribed by a neurologist or GP and given 30 min prior to the procedure. Oral diazepam (5–10 mg) is another option, which can be prescribed by a dentist prior to the procedure and given two hours before the procedure, though its sedative side effects should be taken into account. Diazepam should be used with caution as it may increase the risk of seizures if used excessively in the long term [39].

Patients following a ketogenic diet are of importance, as there are subject to increase risk for caries [34, 40, 41]. If deemed necessary, rapidly discontinuing a ketogenic diet over weeks rather than months appears to be safe [42]. There is no significant risk of seizure exacerbation overall and only a slightly elevated risk (1.4, $p = 0.01$) for those in whom the diet had resulted in significant (50–99%) seizure reduction [42].

As patients can receive a warning aura before seizures begin, the management of the condition sometimes involves measures to prevent the seizure, once the aura has begun. Vagus nerve stimulation therapy (VNST) in epilepsy employs an implantable electronic device to control severe treatment-resistant epilepsy. Members of the surgical team need to understand the operating principles of VNST in the management of intractable epilepsy including medical devices, interactions, and safety features [43]. Most dental equipments do not interfere with VNST [44]. However, the use of diathermy and cardiac defibrillators may damage the pulse generator [45]. The paddles may need to be placed away from the pulse generator, perpendicular to the pulse generator and the lowest possible and clinically appropriate setting [43]. A small surgical scar under the left collar bone can help determine the position of the pulse generator. The surgical team who implanted the VNST device should be made aware of the upcoming procedure and should communicate with the dental and maxillofacial surgical team to discuss safety. In addition any medication changes when the VNST device is switched off should be discussed. Finally, It is important that the anesthetist and dental team be aware that some laryngopharyngeal dysfunction may be present in these patients with an increased risk of aspiration [46]. Abnormal vocal cord motion may cause partial obstruction with a laryngeal mask airway, and thus alternative airway access may need to be considered [47].

17.2.2.4 Perioperative Considerations

Similar to patients with a history of a cerebrovascular accident, patients with epilepsy are more sensitive to hypoxia than healthy ones. Seizure activity is precipitated more easily and thus hypoxia must be carefully avoided. N_2O is not considered epileptogenic and therefore can be safely administered to patients so long as hypoxia is avoided. Thus, epilepsy does not represent a contraindication to the use of inhalation sedation.

Epileptic patients are also considered candidates for IV moderate sedation. As discussed previously, seizure activity of the patient should continue to be controlled through their regular AED regime. These patients should then easily tolerate almost any technique of sedation. It is in the patients whose seizure activity is not well under control that the IV route can be beneficial. Stress-reduction protocol is recommended in epilepsy patients. Although inhalation sedation may prove effective, the use of intravenous benzodiazepines, particularly midazolam, is recommended as well as previously discussed. Conscious sedation via a benzodiazepine may be indicated due of their anticonvulsant properties [48]. Conscious sedation with midazolam via the intravenous route provides additional anxiolytic and anticonvulsant effects and has been recommended for those with uncontrolled epilepsy [49]. The use of O_2 via nasal cannula or nasal hood is strongly recommended to avoid hypoxia. Light to moderate levels of sedation may be safely achieved in these patients.

General anesthesia (GA) in patients with epilepsy needs special care. General anesthesia has several advantages over IV sedation such as complete control of the airway and is more appropriate for long and intricate operations [28]. However, in patients with poorly controlled epilepsy, general anesthesia can be disadvantageous. GA has an overall mortality of 1 in 220,000 [50]. Seizures can also be triggered by metabolic disturbances and AED discontinuity during post-op and pre-op periods, by metabolic disturbances or hypoglycemic fasting states [51]. It is important to note that seizure-like activity is normal even in healthy patients during induction of and emergence from anesthesia. Many anesthetic drugs have various convulsant and anticonvulsant properties [52]. Enflurane, etomidate, and sevoflurane have been found to increase the likelihood of epileptiform EEG activity [28, 49]. EEG monitoring may be useful in some cases as it may provide early signs of cortical instability and epileptiform activity [37].

Propofol dosage required and time to emerge have been found to be affected in patients undergoing antiepileptic therapy. When using an antiepileptic, the dose of propofol (5.7 ± 1.51 mg/kg/h) in the patient population was significantly lower than without an antiepileptic (6.8 ± 1.27 mg/kg/h) ($P < 0.0001$). The time to emerge in patients given an antiepileptic (29.5 ± 12.5 min) was significantly longer than without an antiepileptic (21.6 min ± 10.0 min) ($P < 0.0001$). These pharmacodynamics effects are related to AED effects on liver metabolism or propofol [53].

17.2.2.5 Acute Management of Complications

While taking a thorough history from the patient, their documented rescue medication should be noted in the event that they have a seizure. Different patients have different degrees of the disease, and it is best to attempt using rescue medication proven in their case.

Calm observation should be the first response to a seizure event, along with airway support and supplemental oxygen as necessary. Restraining the patient should be avoided (unless there is a definite threat to their safety that would require some restraining). Most epileptic seizures are self-limited without a need for further medication intervention [28].

If the seizure has lasted twice as long as the patient's usual seizures, or after 4 min (whichever is sooner), and if patient is non-cannulated, 10 mg buccal or intranasal midazolam may be given. If the patient is cannulated, IV midazolam can be given in 1–2 mg 60 s increments titrated to effect to control the seizure [28].

If a second seizure occurs after administration of midazolam, emergency services and an ambulance must be called. In such a case, an underlying abnormality such as metabolic imbalances or hypoglycemia should be considered.

In seizures longer than 5 min or those that reoccur without the recovery of normal consciousness, emergency services and an ambulance should be called regardless of whether treatment has been possible [28].

17.2.3 Multiple Sclerosis

17.2.3.1 Medical Disease

The pathophysiology of multiple sclerosis is considered to be autoimmune in nature [54]. Given the rapid response of MS symptoms to high-dose steroids, it is suspected that acute edema and its resolution underlie clinical relapse and remission processes [54]. MS results in reversible demyelination at various sites in the CNS. Following chronic inflammation, it may eventually produce scarring (gliosis).

The global prevalence of multiple sclerosis (MS) is approximately 30 per 100,000 (with a range of 5–80). Regionally, the median estimated prevalence of MS is greatest in Europe (80 per 100,000), followed by the Eastern Mediterranean (14.9), the Americas (8.3), the Western Pacific (5), Southeast Asia (2.8), and Africa (0.3) [55]. MS is presumably an autoimmune disease that is two to three times more common in women and often presents in young adulthood. It typically becomes clinically evident between the ages of 15 and 45 years, though it can begin earlier or later [56]. The average onset of MS in patients is 30 years [57].

Common clinical findings found in patients with MS include visual loss, sensory symptoms in one side of the face or limbs, motor weakness, diplopia, gain disturbances, optic neuritis, Lhermitte's sign (an electrical sensation that runs down the back and into the limbs), fatigue, and heat sensitivity [58]. Conduction can occur across partially demyelinated axons but is affected by multiple factors, such as increases in body temperature, an indicator of reduced capacitance of the thinning myelin sheath [59]. The onset of multiple sclerosis is often polysymptomatic.

The disease course and symptomatology of MS are heterogeneous [57]. At initial presentation, MS may be clinically categorized as relapsing-remitting MS (RRMS), secondary progressive multiple sclerosis (SPMS), primary progressive MS (PPMS), or progressive-relapsing multiple sclerosis (PRMS). RRMS is most common and observed in 85–90% of patients. It is characterized by self-limited episodes that develop subacutely, evolving over days or weeks and persisting for days or weeks before gradually dissipating. Recovery of neurologic function is usually complete. SPMS, however, begins as a typical RRMS in which acute episodes become less frequent over time and the patient begins to experience a persistent deterioration in neurologic function independent of any acute attacks [56]. In PPMS, which accounts for 10% of cases, the onset is insidious and the patient experiences a persisting decline in neurologic function in the absence of acute clinical episodes. PRMS begins with a progressive course resembling that of PPMS. However, at some point, occasional clinical episodes are superimposed upon the steadily progressive disease course [56]. These four clinical courses reflect a variable clinical expression, whose underlying disease mechanism has yet to be fully understood. It is generally believed that MS is triggered by environmental factors in a genetically susceptible host that initiate an autoimmune response against the CNS [60]. Clinical outcomes are variable in MS patients; however 50% of all MS patients will require the use of a walking aid within ten years after clinical onset [58].

17.2.3.2 Preoperative Assessment

As MS may result in demyelination across the entire CNS and affect important functional regions, a full neurological workup is a basic requirement. Lesions in the respiratory center of the medulla oblongata and other regions of the spinal cord may lead to respiratory dysfunction in advanced cases. Though vital capacity and total lung volumes may be normal, other pulmonary function parameters such as forced vital capacity and forced expiratory volume may be affected and could be as low as 50% of normal values [61, 62]. A full pulmonary function workup is recommended several weeks prior to surgery, and arterial blood gases can be examined preoperatively to prepare for anesthesia [63]. Alternatively, the patient's ability to exhale deeply and clear pulmonary secretions can be used to assess pulmonary function in lieu of a full pulmonary workup [63]. In addition to respiratory dysfunction, obstructive sleep apnea syndrome (OSAS), central sleep apnea, and insomnia or narcolepsy have also been reported in MS patients [64]. OSAS is likely caused by lesions in higher brain centers that regulate breathing and respiratory muscles but may also be an obesity-related by-product of physical inactivity in MS patients [65]. Lesions in the thoracic spinal cord may also affect autonomic function, which can potentially create hemodynamic instability in some patients [66]. When MS patients are given neuroaxial regional anesthesia, marked hypotension may result [67]. Potential risk of autonomic dysfunction should be considered in MS patients who suffer from preoperative impotence, bladder or bowel dysfunction, vasomotor instability, or syncope. More generally, any stressful procedure may cause an exacerbation, and thus, as a rule, elective surgery should always take place during the remission phase and be avoided during a relapse [63].

Medications used in MS may complicate anesthesia in various ways, some of which have been summarized in Table 17.6. There is little conclusive data on whether MS treatment should be ceased prior to surgery. However, it is known that MS is particularly sensitive to treatment cessation and disease recurrence has been reported days to months after discontinuing treatment [68–70]. In one study, 20% of patients who discontinued their treatment with interferon-β showed a resurgence of disease activity within 30 days [68]. In all studies, relapses were particularly strong in those with already highly active disease. Thus, potential anesthetic risks of medications should be evaluated against the risks of disease recurrence and the necessity for the surgical procedure.

17.2.3.3 Intraoperative Management

Irrespective of anesthetic technique, MS symptoms may worsen perioperatively and postoperatively. More specifically, as has already been

Table 17.6 MS medications and potential anesthetic complications

Medication	Adverse effects[a] with anesthetic significance	Perioperative implications
Corticosteroids	• Hypokalemia • Paresthesia • Impaired glucose tolerance	• Cardiac arrhythmia • Preoperative documentation in regional anesthesia • Hyperglycemia
Interferon-β	• Dyspnea • Flu-like symptoms • Elevated liver enzymes • Abnormal blood counts	• Ventilation complications • Differentiation from true infections • Altered drug clearance, hepatotoxicity • Increased neuroaxial anesthesia risk in cases of thrombocytopenia
Glatiramer acetate	• Respiratory infection • Hypotension • Abnormal blood count • Paresthesia • Laryngospasm	• Airway hyperresponsiveness • Increased drop in blood pressure • Increased neuroaxial anesthesia risk in cases of thrombocytopenia • Preoperative documentation in regional anesthesia • Ventilation access
Natalizumab	• Respiratory infections • Flu-like symptoms • Hepatic insufficiency • Hypotension	• Airway hyperresponsiveness • Differentiation from true infections • Altered drug clearance • Increased drop in blood pressure
Dimethyl fumarate	• Infections	• Fever
Teriflunomide	• Respiratory infections • Flu-like symptoms • Paresthesia • Pharyngitis • Hypertension	• Airway hyperresponsiveness • Differentiation from true infections • Preoperative documentation in regional anesthesia • Establishing an airway • Perioperative blood pressure adjustment
Mitoxantrone	• Respiratory infections • Hepatic insufficiency • Paresthesia • Hypotension • Bradycardia • Acute Heart Failure • Abnormal blood counts	• Airway hyperresponsiveness • Altered drug clearance • Preoperative documentation in regional anesthesia • Increased drop in blood pressure • Increased risk of bradycardia • Hemodynamic complications • Increased neuroaxial anesthesia risk in cases of thrombocytopenia
Fingolimod	• Bradycardia; AV block (with first dose) • Paresthesia • QTc interval risk • Pulmonary function limitations (FEV1, DLCO reduction)	• Bradycardia or asystole risk • Preoperative documentation in regional anesthesia • Risk of increased QT interval in combination with QT-prolonging medications or in patients with high baseline QTc • Ventilation complications
Cyclophosphamide	• Myelosuppression	• Increased neuroaxial anesthesia risk in cases of thrombocytopenia
Baclofen	• Sedation • Hypotension • Paresthesia	• Respiratory depression • Increased drop in blood pressure

AV atrioventricular, *CBC* complete blood count, *IFN* interferon, *LFT* liver function test
[a]Based on manufacturer data, does not include all possible side effects

discussed, MS patients are very susceptible in changes in the environment. Increases in temperature may result in exacerbations of symptoms, otherwise known as Uhthoff's phenomenon. Thus, elevated body temperature is one of the most studied triggers affecting up to 80% of patients [71]. Careful temperature monitoring and control, room temperature modification, and cooling devices may be used in extreme cases, and antipyretics should be considered in infections [72]. Pseudo-relapses (worsening of symptoms due to fever/sepsis) should be differentiated from true disease exacerbation.

Both inhalation and intravenous agents have been used successfully in MS patients. Sevoflurane has been employed without complications [73]. Desflurane and nitrous oxide have also been reported as potentially safe anesthetic agents [74, 75]. As any general increase in stress may potentiate MS symptoms, premedication can be useful with benzodiazepines. Midazolam has been used with minimal effect on thermoregulatory control, though attention should be paid in patients with respiratory compromise [74]. Clonidine has been used without issues as well [76]. Propofol, remifentanil, and fentanyl are acceptable anesthetic agents in patients with MS [73, 77].

When it comes to muscle relaxants, it is crucial to avoid succinylcholine in patients with multiple sclerosis. Although succinylcholine has been used successfully in some patients with MS, there is a significant risk of hyperkalemia particularly during exacerbations [76, 78, 79]. Patients remain at high risk for hyperkalemia for months or years even in the absence of any symptoms such as flaccidity, spasticity, or hyperreflexia. If necessary, rocuronium and vecuronium may be used with sugammadex as an antagonist [80].

Since MS is a disease of the central nervous system, peripheral nerve blocks are not as much of a concern. However, spinal anesthesia has been associated with exacerbation of MS disease [81–83], though any surgery or anesthetic process may lead to exacerbations on account of increased stress. Due to the susceptibility of demyelinated neurons to the neurotoxic effects of local anesthetics, there is an increased risk in postoperative exacerbations [84]. In contrast to intrathecal administration in spinal anesthesia, epidural anesthesia involves lower risk [85].

17.2.3.4 Postoperative Management

Multiple sclerosis patients should be carefully monitored following surgery. Hemodynamic instabilities due to autonomic dysfunction may be observed. Elevated body temperature should be expected and treated aggressively. MS patients with respiratory involvement are at increased risk for airway compromise and care should be given to avoid hypoventilation and atelectasis. As multiple sclerosis patients are more sensitive to neuromuscular blockade, residual effects should be accounted for in the postoperative period. Given that any surgical procedure increases stress, patients should be closely monitored for any evidence of postoperative deterioration, and appropriate intervention should be considered.

17.2.4 Parkinson's Disease

17.2.4.1 Medical Disease

Parkinson's disease is a slowly progressive neurodegenerative disorder that is presently thought to arise from a combination of environmental and genetic factors [86]. It is characterized by the deterioration of the dopaminergic neurons in the substantia nigra pars compacta, SNpc, located in the midbrain. The resultant dopamine deficiency in the basal ganglia leads to significant motor dysfunction. The gold standard for diagnosis has been the presence of SNpc degeneration and Lewy body pathology at postmortem pathological examination, containing abnormal aggregates of α-synuclein protein [86].

The incidence of the disease rises abruptly with age, from 17.4 in 100,000 person years between 50 and 59 years of age to 93.1 in 100,000 person years between 70 and 79 years [87, 88]. Prevalence of Parkinson's disease is higher in Europe, North America, and South America (estimated crude prevalence for all ages: 66–1500 per 100 000, 111–329 per 100 000, and 31–470 per 100 000 [86].The lifetime risk of developing the disease is 1.5% [87, 88]. Men are at an increased risk of getting this disease, with the male-to-female ratio being nearly 3:2 [89]. The median age of onset is 60 years and the mean duration of the disease from diagnosis to death is 15 years [90].

Clinical diagnosis is based on the presence of motor symptoms including resting tremor, rigidity, and bradykinesia. The tremor is present at rest, typically affects one side of the body worse than the other, improves with movement, and typically has a pill rolling appearance. It should be noted that the lack of resting tremor does not necessarily exclude the diagnosis of Parkinson's disease. There are two main clinical phenotypes emerging in Parkinson's disease: those patients whose presentation is tremor predominant versus those with a more marked postural instability and gait disorder. The latter group has an increased risk of cognitive decline and dementia in their later years [91]. The tremor predominant phenotype has been associated with a slower disease progression, less depression, and less apathy [92]. Patients may oftentimes recall that their symptoms were preceded by several years by loss of sense of smell, constipation, pain, fatigue, erectile dysfunction, rapid eye movement (REM) sleep disorder, and mood changes. REM sleep disorder is characterized by the acting of dreams by shouting out, flailing arms and legs, and even falling out of bed. Other sleep disorders can also occur, and patients commonly report sleep fragmentation (difficulty staying asleep) in addition to insomnia.

Following diagnosis, 50% of patients develop dementia within the first 10 years [93]. Anxiety and depression may occur early on in the course of the disease. Patients may also develop hypophonia (softer voice), micrographia (smaller handwriting), and masked facies (diminished facial expression). Autonomic issues like postural hypotension, bladder irritability, and excessive sweating can also occur. Patients' gaits may appear shuffling, have festinating qualities, and sometimes suffer from freezing episodes. Consequently, falls are a major issue. In the later stages of the disease, psychosis can be seen that oftentimes includes visual hallucinations. Finally, the development of dysphagia in end-stage Parkinson's leads to increased risk for aspiration pneumonia.

17.2.4.2 Preoperative Assessment

Largely owing to the disease affecting predominantly elderly populations, patients with Parkinson's disease commonly present for urological, ophthalmological, and orthopedic procedures [94]. Patients with Parkinson's disease may also be presenting for a therapeutic pallidotomy, thalamotomy, or deep brain stimulation surgery. For each patient a routine history, physical examination, and preoperative testing are required, in addition to special consideration to the patient's Parkinson's related systemic issues.

Respiratory complications, especially aspiration pneumonia, are the most common causes of death in PD [95]. An obstructive ventilatory pattern has been seen in up to one third of patients, but this may also be due to preexisting chronic obstructive pulmonary disease [96]. Further, upper airway dysfunction leads to retained secretions, atelectasis, aspiration, and respiratory infection [94]. Other difficulties include postextubation laryngospasm and postoperative respiratory failure [97, 98]. Autonomic nervous system dysfunction can lead to issues with salivation, micturition, gastrointestinal issues, temperature regulation, and cardiovascular control. Cardiac arrhythmias and orthostatic hypotension may occur. Gastrointestinal dysfunction includes constipation, sialorrhea, dysphagia, and esophageal dysmotility. Therefore, in addition to standard testing, it may be prudent to also consider obtaining preoperatively a chest X-ray, pulmonary function testing, arterial blood gas analysis, and an electrocardiogram.

By continuing a patient's home medication regimen, one can help prevent a PD exacerbation or symptoms of overdosing. PD medications are given on strict schedules specific to each patient, and drug administration can be hindered by nothing by mouth status, and therefore planning ahead to minimize medication disruptions will be helpful. If missing multiple doses of PD medications is unavoidable, then dopaminergic agents like apomorphine subcutaneously (with pretreatment with antiemetics) or rotigotine transdermally can be considered [99]. These medications can also be useful since PD patients are at

Table 17.7 MS medications and potential anesthetic complications

Medication	Adverse effects[a] with anesthetic significance	Perioperative implications
Levodopa	• Hypotension • Thrombocytopenia • Upper airway infection • Hypokalemia	• Increased drop in blood pressure • Increased neuroaxial anesthesia risk • Airway hyperresponsiveness • Cardiac arrhythmia
Dopamine agonists (bromocriptine, pramipexole, ropinirole, rotigotine, apomorphine)	• Hypotension • Erythromelalgia (bromocriptine) • Pulmonary fibrosis (bromocriptine) • Increased blood urea nitrogen level (ropinirole) • Skin site reactions (rotigotine) • Valvular heart disease (cabergoline)	• Increased drop in blood pressure • Pain control • Ventilation complication • Altered drug clearance, nephrotoxicity • Preoperative documentation for regional anesthesia • Hemodynamic complications
Monoamine oxidase-B Inhibitors (selegiline, rasagiline)	• Gamma-glutamyl transpeptidase increased, hepatitis (selegiline) • Hyperkalemia (selegiline) • Pneumothorax (selegiline) • Flu-like symptoms	• Altered drug clearance, hepatotoxicity • Cardiac arrhythmia • Ventilation complication and hemodynamic complications • Differentiation from true infections
Anticholinergic agents (trihexyphenidyl, benztropine)	• Paradoxical sinus bradycardia (trihexyphenidyl) • Paralytic ileus (benztropine)	• Bradycardia • Bowel regimen consideration
Amantadine	• Hypotension • Arrhythmia, cardiac arrest	• Increased drop in blood pressure • Hemodynamic complications
Catechol-O-methyl transferase inhibitors (tolcapone, entacapone)	• Liver failure (tolcapone) • Respiratory infections	• Impaired drug clearance, hepatotoxicity • Airway hyperresponsiveness

[a]Based on manufacturer data, does not include all possible side effects

increased risk of developing postoperative ileus [100]. As a result, aggressive bowel regimens are necessary to aid with gastrointestinal motility. It is important to note that abrupt cessation or decrease in dopaminergic drugs can lead to a life-threatening process called parkinsonism-hyperpyrexia syndrome that is akin to neuroleptic malignant syndrome where patients experience altered mental status, autonomic dysfunction, fevers, rigidity, and tremors. Monoamine oxidase-B inhibitors like rasagiline or selegiline should be discontinued 1–2 weeks prior to surgery due to their interaction with opioids and contribution to labile blood pressures and increasing the risk of serotonin syndrome [101]. The various ways in which PD medications can further complicate anesthesia have been summarized in Table 17.7.

17.2.4.3 Intraoperative Management

In patients with Parkinson's disease, there are several considerations that should be kept in mind regarding intraoperative anesthetic and palliative choices. For patients taking levodopa, anesthetic agents like halothane should be avoided due to its sensitization of the heart to catecholamines [94]. Newer inhalational agents like isoflurane and sevoflurane are less arrhythmogenic, but hypotension is still an issue due to hypovolemia, norepinephrine depletion, and autonomic dysfunction [94]. Further, bromocriptine and pergolide can cause excessive vasodilation further exacerbating hypotension [94]. Propofol can aggravate dyskinesias to the point of interfering with the procedure [101]. Opioid-induced muscle rigidity can occur following the use of agents like fentanyl, and this typically responds to neuromuscular block [102]. Morphine at low doses can reduce dyskinesias and at higher doses increase akinesia [103]. The combination of meperidine and selegiline should be avoided due to patients have been reported to get agitated, have muscle rigidity, and have hyperthermia [104]. In ophthalmic procedures, diphenhydramine has been shown to be useful due to its anticholinergic activity suppressing tremor that would otherwise complicate the surgery [105].

Additionally, PD patients' preexisting comorbidities may likewise potentially complicate procedures. Sialorrhea due to impaired swallowing can worsen during sedation, and anesthesia can be ameliorated by glycopyrrolate by mouth and ipratropium spray [99]. Sialorrhea and dysphagia also place PD patients at increased risk of aspiration pneumonia, and therefore intubation may be needed more readily [101].

Another consideration is that some patients with Parkinson's disease may have had deep brain stimulators implanted, and consequently consultation with a movement disorder specialist may be helpful in determining which tests or procedures these devices will need to be turned off for. For instance, electrocautery may damage stimulator leads, and if cauterization is necessary, then bipolar cautery is preferred and the stimulator should be turned off [100]. Currently, there is insufficient data regarding safety of magnetic resonance imaging, and therefore if a patient needs it, it would be wise to consult first with the device manufacturer and radiologist [101].

17.2.4.4 Postoperative Management

Postoperatively, patients with PD are more prone to confusion and hallucinations [106]. Unfortunately, many antipsychotics can also worsen parkinsonism and would be best avoided if possible [101]. Postoperative pain can be treated with high-dose nonsteroidal anti-inflammatory agents due to opioids potentially potentiating delirium and depressing respiratory function. Opioids should be particularly avoided in patients taking monoamine oxidase-B inhibitors due to their serotonin reuptake inhibition [107]. Meperidine is therefore especially contraindicated, although tramadol, methadone, dextromethorphan, and propoxyphene also have weak serotonin reuptake inhibition properties [108]. These interactions can cause agitation, rigidity, diaphoresis, hyperpyrexia, serotonin syndrome, and death [101]. In contrast, morphine, codeine, oxycodone, and buprenorphine do not have serotonin reuptake inhibition issues [108]. Furthermore, monoamine oxidase-B inhibitors inhibit the metabolism of opioids in the liver, thereby potentiating opioid effects and therefore should be held 1–2 weeks prior to surgery [101]. Antiemetic agents like ondansetron and domperidone are preferred due to alternatives like metoclopramide, prochlorperazine, and promethazine causing dopamine antagonistic side effects and associated extrapyramidal side effects [107, 109]. Respiratory issues like reduced cough, bronchospasm, and aspiration pneumonia make incentive spirometry and aspiration precautions pivotal. Providers should be therefore careful in determining when to lift the nothing by mouth status since medications need to be restarted as soon as possible at the risk of developing aspiration pneumonia. Maintaining adequate hydration is important to offset PD autonomic dysfunction like orthostatic hypotension. On a final note, physical therapy ordered early in the hospital course may improve mobility and overall recovery and help prevent deep vein thrombosis, pulmonary embolism, constipation, contractures, pressure ulcers, and pneumonia [101].

17.2.5 Stroke Disease

17.2.5.1 Medical Disease

Cerebrovascular disease is caused by one of several pathophysiologic processes involving the blood vessels of the brain.

- The process may be intrinsic to the vessel, as in atherosclerosis, lipohyalinosis, inflammation, amyloid deposition, arterial dissection, developmental malformation, aneurysmal dilation, or venous thrombosis.
- The process may originate remotely, as occurs when an embolus from the heart or extracranial circulation lodges in an intracranial vessel.
- The process may result from inadequate cerebral blood flow due to decreased perfusion pressure or increased blood viscosity.
- The process may result from rupture of a vessel in the subarachnoid space or intracerebral tissue.

Sudden loss of focal brain function is the core feature of the onset of ischemic stroke. However, patients with conditions other than stroke can present in a similar fashion. The symptoms of brain ischemia may be transient, lasting seconds to minutes, or may persist for longer periods of time. Symptoms and signs remain indefinitely if the brain becomes irreversibly damaged and infarction occurs. Unfortunately, neurologic symptoms do not accurately reflect the presence or absence of infarction, and the tempo of the symptoms does not indicate the cause of the ischemia [110]. Approximately 80% of strokes are due to ischemic cerebral infarction and 20% to brain hemorrhage. There are three main subtypes of brain ischemia: thrombosis, embolism, and systemic hypoperfusion.

Globally, the incidence of stroke due to ischemia is 68%, while the incidence of hemorrhagic stroke (intracerebral hemorrhage and subarachnoid hemorrhage combined) is 32%, reflecting a higher incidence of hemorrhagic stroke in low- and middle-income countries [111]. In the United States, the proportion of all strokes due to ischemia, intracerebral hemorrhage, and subarachnoid hemorrhage is 87%, 10%, and 3%, respectively [112]. Worldwide, stroke is the second most common cause of mortality and the third most common cause of disability. While the incidence of stroke is decreasing in high-income countries, including the United States [113], the incidence is increasing in low-income countries [114]. The overall rate of stroke-related mortality is decreasing in high- and low-income countries, but the absolute number of people with stroke, stroke survivors, stroke-related deaths, and the global burden of stroke-related disability is high and increasing [115]. Men have a higher incidence of stroke than women at younger but not older ages, with the incidence reversed and higher for women by age 75 years and older.

17.2.5.2 Preoperative Assessment

Although rare, stroke is a feared surgical complication, with a mortality rate of up to 26% [115]. The majority of perioperative strokes are embolic [116]. Hypoperfusion is an uncommon mechanism of perioperative stroke, even in patients with carotid artery stenosis [117]. Less common mechanisms of perioperative stroke include hemorrhagic infarction; air, fat, and paradoxical embolism; and arterial dissection due to neck manipulation [116].

By and large, preoperative risk factors are a reflection of the traditional risk factors for stroke in the general population. Female sex, renal insufficiency, pulmonary disease, and preoperative discontinuation of antithrombotic therapy are additional preoperative risk factors [118].

The risk of stroke following general surgery is low (Table 17.8) [119]. By contrast, cardiac, vascular, and neurologic procedures are associated with higher risk [115], reaching 8% for combined procedures (e.g., combined coronary artery bypass grafting [CABG] and valve surgeries) [115] and 13% for patients with prior stroke or transient ischemic attack (TIA) [120]. No validated models are currently available for the prediction of perioperative stroke risk in general surgical patients. A predictive model for assessing the risk of stroke in patients undergoing CABG does exist, using seven preoperative variables of varying weights to arrive at an aggregate

Table 17.8 Risk of perioperative stroke after various surgical procedures [116]

Procedure	Risk of stroke (%)
General surgery	0.08–0.7
Peripheral vascular surgery	0.8–3.0
Isolated CABG	1.4–3.8
Isolated valve surgery	4.8–8.8
Resection of head and neck tumors	4.8
Carotid endarterectomy	5.5–6.1
Combined CABG and valve surgery	7.4
Aortic repair	8.7
Double- or triple-valve surgery	9.7

estimate of risk (Table 5) [121]. This risk must be considered in the context of additional intraoperative and postoperative risk factors and weighed against the benefits of surgery. Many preoperative risk factors, such as advanced age and history of cerebrovascular disease, are nonmodifiable. Nonetheless, a detailed history can meaningfully alter preoperative management. A history of cerebrovascular disease is a strong predictor of perioperative stroke [115, 117–120]. As cerebrovascular reserve remains tenuous in the days and weeks following a stroke, at least 6 months is needed following a stroke or TIA in order to ensure stabilization of the patient's hemodynamic and neurologic status before an elective procedure. Specific questions must be asked to uncover any previously unreported, unrecognized, or inadequately evaluated cerebrovascular symptoms within this 6-month period. Medical management of other preoperative risk factors, such as diabetes and hypertension, must also be optimized.

No validated models are currently available for the prediction of perioperative stroke risk in general surgical patients. A predictive model for assessing the risk of stroke in patients undergoing CABG does exist, using seven preoperative variables of varying weights to arrive at an aggregate estimate of risk (Table 17.9) [121]. This risk must be considered in the context of additional intraoperative and postoperative risk factors and weighed against the benefits of surgery.

Many preoperative risk factors, such as advanced age and history of cerebrovascular disease, are nonmodifiable. A history of cerebrovascular disease is a strong predictor of perioperative stroke [117]. As cerebrovascular reserve remains tenuous in the days and weeks following a stroke, at least 6 months is needed following a stroke or TIA in order to ensure stabilization of the patient's hemodynamic and neurologic status before an elective procedure. Medical management of other preoperative risk factors, such as diabetes and hypertension, must also be optimized. It is generally considered safe to continue anticoagulation in most patients undergoing dental procedures, cataract surgery, arthrocentesis, and diagnostic endoscopy with or without biopsy [122]. Continuing moderate-dose warfarin therapy (international normalized ratio [INR]

Table 17.9 Prediction of perioperative stroke risk in patients

Risk factor	Weighted score
Advanced age	
55–59 years	1.5
60–64 years	2.5
65–69 years	3.5
70–74 years	4.0
75–79 years	4.5
≥80 years	5.5
Urgent	1.5
Emergent	2.5
Female sex	1
Ejection fraction <40%	1.5
Vascular disease[b]	2.0
Diabetes mellitus	1.5
Creatinine > 2mg/dL or dialysis	2.0
Total score	Stroke risk (%)
0–1	0.3
2	0.4
3	0.6
4	0.8
5	1.0
6	1.2
7	1.6
8	2.1
9	2.9
10	5.8
11	9.8
12	>10.0

[a]Undergoing CABG
Nonelective surgery

1.8–2.1) is safe and effective in patients undergoing knee or hip replacement surgery [68]. For more invasive procedures, the rate of perioperative thromboembolic events in high-risk patients on long-term anticoagulant therapy is 0% with bridge therapy using intravenous heparin and 0.6% in the absence of bridge therapy [122]. Thus, current evidence supports the continuation of anticoagulation for some invasive procedures, such as colonoscopy and minor surgeries. If oral anticoagulation must be stopped, bridge therapy with heparin should be used and anticoagulation should be resumed early in the postoperative period [123].

17.2.5.3 Perioperative Considerations

The risk of perioperative stroke depends on patient characteristics [123], the nature and timing of the procedure, and certain complications in the postoperative period, including postoperative atrial fibrillation and hypercoagulability [123].

By and large, preoperative risk factors are a reflection of the traditional risk factors for stroke in the general population. Female sex, renal insufficiency, pulmonary disease, and preoperative discontinuation of antithrombotic therapy are additional preoperative risk factors [122, 123].

Patients with a history of stroke frequently have coexisting vascular disease. Therefore, the overall management aim is protection against further strokes as well as prevention of further damage to other organs. These patients mostly have multiple vessel involvement including the coronary arteries. They are also likely to suffer from other comorbidities such as hypertension and/or diabetes mellitus [124].

Care is required to reduce the incidence of complications potentiated by the presence of focal neurological deficits, as well as those related to coexisting illnesses. Alterations of respiratory control, mechanics, and pattern are common following a CVA and lead to gas exchange abnormalities. Central or obstructive sleep apnea may occur. Immobility can cause further complications such as hypostatic or aspiration pneumonia and venous thromboembolism. Many of these patients would need admission to a critical care areas following surgery for these reasons [125].

Stroke patients may be at increased risk of aspiration due to impaired swallowing, ineffective cough, and reduced gastric emptying [126].

Poor nutritional intake following the stroke may lead to malnutrition and may be associated with poor survival and functional outcomes after the surgery [127].

Conclusion

Perioperative management of the patient with a neurological disorder remains a challenge to the oral and maxillofacial surgeon. Proper and systematic preoperative evaluation allows the surgeon to optimize the patient during the perioperative period. Consultation and communication with the patient's neurologist are recommended in order to optimize our patient's care.

References

1. Ritchie K, Lovestone S. The dementias. Lancet. 2002;360:1759–66.
2. Morris JC, Heyman A, Mohs RC, et al. The consortium to establish a registry for Alzheimer's disease (CERAD). Part I. Clinical and neuropsychological assessment of Alzheimer's disease. Neurology. 1989;39:1159–65.
3. Schwam E, Xu Y. Cognition and function in Alzheimer's disease: identifying the transitions from moderate to severe disease. Dement Geriatr Cogn Disord. 2010;29:309–16.
4. Hebert LE, Scherr PA, Bienias JL, Bennett DA, Evans DA. Alzheimer disease in the US population: prevalence estimates using the 2000 census. Arch Neurol. 2003;60(8):1119.
5. Knopman DS, Boeve BF, Petersen RC. Essentials of the proper diagnoses of mild cognitive impairment, dementia, and major subtypes of dementia. Mayo Clin Proc. 2003;78(10):1290.
6. Clarfield AM. The reversible dementias: do they reverse? Ann Intern Med. 1988;109(6):476.
7. Rahkonen T, Eloniemi-Sulkava U, Rissanen S, Vatanen A, Viramo P, Sulkava R. Dementia with Lewy bodies according to the consensus criteria in a general population aged 75 years or older. J Neurol Neurosurg Psychiatry. 2003;74(6):720.
8. Jorm AF, Fratiglioni L, Winblad B. Differential diagnosis in dementia. Principal components analy-

sis of clinical data from a population survey. Arch Neurol. 1993;50(1):72.
9. Chen T-L, et al. Postoperative adverse outcomes in surgical patients with dementia: a retrospective cohort study. World J Surg. 2012;36:2051–8.
10. Folstein MF, Folstein SE, McHugh PR. Mini-Mental State: a practical method for grading the cognitive state of patients for the clinician. J Psychiatr Res. 1975;12:189–98.
11. Fines DP, Severn AM. Anaesthesia and cognitive disturbance in the elderly. Contin Educ Anaesth Crit Care Pain. 2006;6(1):37–40.
12. Duggleby W, Lander J. Cognitive status and postoperative pain: older adults. J Pain Symptom Manage. 1994;9:19–27.
13. Wolfe M, Almond A, Robertson S, et al. Chronic kidney disease presenting acutely: presentation, clinical features andoutcome of patients with irreversible chronic kidney disease who require dialysis immediately. Postgrad Med J. 2010;86:405–8.
14. Mitchell SL, Teno JM, Kiely DK, et al. The clinical course of advanced dementia. N Engl J Med. 2009;361:1529–38.
15. Brienza N, Giglio MT, Marucci M. Preventing acute kidney injury after noncardiac surgery. Curr Opin Crit Care. 2010;16:353–8.
16. Rock P, Rich PB. Postoperative pulmonary complications. Curr Opin Anaesthesiol. 2003;16:123–31.
17. Lo IL, Siu CW, Tse HF, et al. Preoperative pulmonary assessment for patients with hip fracture. Osteoporos Int. 2010;21:S579–86.
18. Pendlebury ST, Rothwell PM. Prevalence, incidence, and factors associated with pre-stroke and post-stroke dementia: a systematic review and meta-analysis. Lancet Neurol. 2009;8:1006–18.
19. Dijkstra JB, Jolles J. Postoperative cognitive dysfunction versus complaints: a discrepancy in long-term findings. Neuropsychol Rev. 2002;12:1–14.
20. Bindra A, Chouhan RS, Prabhakar H, et al. Perioperative anesthetic implications of epilepsy surgery: a retrospective analysis. J Anesth. 2015;29:229–34.
21. Kotsopoulos IAW, Van Merode T, Kessels FGH, et al. Systematic review and meta-analysis of incidence studies of epilepsy and unprovoked seizures. Epilepsia. 2002;43:1402–9.
22. Tellez-Zenteno JF, Pondal-Sordo M, Matijevic S, et al. National and regional prevalence of self-reported epilepsy in Canada. Epilepsia. 2004;45:1623–9. [cited 27 Aug 2016]. http://doi.wiley.com/10.1111/j.0013-9580.2004.24904.x.
23. Cui W, Kobau R, Zack MM, Helmers S, Yeargin-Allsopp MM. Seizures in children and adolescents aged 6–17 years: United States, 2010–2014. MMWR Morb Mortal Wkly Rep. 64:1209–28. Atlanta 2015. http://search.proquest.com/docview/1732957912?accountid=13567.
24. Annegers JF, Hauser WA, Lee JRJ, et al. Incidence of acute symptomatic seizures in Rochester, Minnesota, 1935–1984. Epilepsia. 1995;36:327–33.
25. Winkler AS, Schaffert M, Schmutzhard E. Epilepsy in resource poor countries–suggestion of an adjusted classification. Epilepsia. 2007;48:1029–30. [cited 30 Aug 2016]. http://www.ncbi.nlm.nih.gov/pubmed/17509005.
26. Chi DL, Rossitch KC, Beeles EM. Developmental delays and dental caries in low-income preschoolers in the USA: a pilot cross-sectional study and preliminary explanatory model. BMC Oral Health. 2013;13:53. [cited 30 Aug 2016]. http://bmcoralhealth.biomedcentral.com/articles/10.1186/1472-6831-13-53.
27. Fisher RS, Acevedo C, Arzimanoglou A, et al. A practical clinical definition of epilepsy. Epilepsia. 2014;55:475–82.
28. Ransford N, Soryal I, McCorry D, et al. Specialist management of routine dental procedures in adults with refractory epilepsy. Br Dent J. 2014;216:403–7. [cited 25 Aug 2016]. http://www.ncbi.nlm.nih.gov/pubmed/24722093.
29. Girdler NM, Smith DG. Prevalence of emergency events in British dental practice and emergency management skills of British dentists. Resuscitation. 1999;41:159–67.
30. Atherton G, McCaul J, Williams S. Medical emergencies in general dental practice in Great Britain. Part 1: their prevalence over a 10-year period. Br Dent J. 1999;186:72–9.
31. Hassona YM, Mahmoud AA, Ryalat SM, et al. Dental students' knowledge and attitudes toward patients with epilepsy. Epilepsy & Behavior: E&B. 2014;36:2–5. [cited 23 Aug 2016]. http://www.ncbi.nlm.nih.gov/pubmed/24835896.
32. Aragon CE, Hess T, Burneo JG. Knowledge and attitudes about epilepsy: a survey of dentists in London, Ontario. J Can Dent Assoc. 2009;75:450.
33. Doshi D, Reddy BS, Kulkarni S, et al. Dentists' knowledge, attitudes and practices toward patients with epilepsy in Hyderabad city, India. Epilepsy Behav. 2012;23:447–50.
34. Costa ALF, Yasuda CL, Shibasaki W, et al. The association between periodontal disease and seizure severity in refractory epilepsy patients. Seizure. 2014;23:227–30.
35. Ott DVM, Kauert A, Holtkamp M. Toothbrushing-induced seizures at onset of cryptogenic partial epilepsy: a case report. J Neurol. 2014;261:432–4.
36. Navarro V, Adam C, Petitmengin C, et al. Toothbrush-thinking seizures. Epilepsia. 2006;47:1971–3.
37. Voss LJ, Sleigh JW, Barnard JPM, et al. The howling cortex: seizures and general anesthetic drugs. Anesth Analg. 2008;107:1689–703.
38. Wolf P. Acute administration of benzodiazepines as part of treatment strategies for epilepsy. CNS Neuroscience and Therapeutics. 2011;17:214–20.
39. Crispian S. Oral and maxillofacial medicine: the basis of diagnosis and treatment. 3rd ed. London, UK: Churchill Livingstone; 2013.

40. Costa ALF, Yasuda CL, França MC, et al. Refractory epilepsy is highly associated with severe dentoalveolar and maxillofacial injuries. Epileptic Disord. 2011;13:61–4.
41. Sharma A, Mathur V. Refractory epilepsy and the ketogenic diet: pathophysiological aspects and possible implications in dental practice. J Indian Soc Pedod Prev Dent. 2011;29:188. http://go.galegroup.com.ezp.lib.rochester.edu/ps/i.do?id=GALE%7CA269739044&sid=summon&v=2.1&u=nysl_ro_rochstru&it=r&p=ITOF&sw=w&asid=3e19dc4e679fbb51d17daadfc7389a24.
42. Worden LT, Turner Z, Pyzik PL, et al. Is there an ideal way to discontinue the ketogenic diet? Epilepsy Res. 2011;95:232–6.
43. Lisowska P, Daly B. Vagus nerve stimulation therapy (VNST) in epilepsy: implications for dental practice. Br Dent J. 2012;212:69–72. [cited 31 Aug 2016]. http://www.nature.com/doifinder/10.1038/sj.bdj.2012.47.
44. Roberts HW. The effect of electrical dental equipment on a vagus nerve stimulator's function. Journal of the American Dental Association. 2002;133:1657–64.
45. Cyberonics: epilepsy patient's manual for vagus nerve stimulation with the model 106 (US); 2015.
46. Banzett RB, Guz A, Paydarfar D, et al. Cardiorespiratory variables and sensation during stimulation of the left vagus in patients with epilepsy. Epilepsy Res. 1999;35:1–11.
47. Bernards CM. An unusual cause of airway obstruction during general anesthesia with a laryngeal mask airway. Anesthesiology. 2004;100:1017–8. [cited 1 Sep 2016]. http://www.ncbi.nlm.nih.gov/pubmed/15087642.
48. Coulthard P, Coulthard P, et al. Oral and maxillofacial surgery, radiology, pathology and oral medicine, vol. 1: Churchill Livingstone; 2013.
49. Malamed SF: Sedation: a clinical guide to a patient. 2010
50. Lagasse RS. Anesthesia safety: model or myth? A review of the published literature and analysis of current original data. Anesthesiology. 2002;97:1609–17.
51. Schauwecker P. The effects of glycemic control on seizures and seizure-induced excitotoxic cell death. BMC Neurosci. 2012;13:94. [cited 1 Sep 2016].
52. Modica P, Tempelhoff R, White PF. Pro- and anticonvulsant effects of anesthetics (Part I). Anesth Analg. 1990;70:303–15.
53. Ouchi K, Sugiyama K. Required propofol dose for anesthesia and time to emerge are affected by the use of antiepileptics: prospective cohort study. BMC Anesthesiol. 2015;15:34. [cited 25 Aug 2016]. http://ovidsp.ovid.com/ovidweb.cgi?T=JS&PAGE=reference&D=prem&NEWS=N&AN=25788855.
54. Hafler DA. Multiple sclerosis. J Clin Invest. 2004;113:788–94.
55. Multiple sclerosis international federation, World Health Organization: ATLAS Multiple Sclerosis Resources in the World. Geneva; 2008.
56. Goodin DS. The epidemiology of multiple sclerosis: insights to disease pathogenesis. Handb Clin Neurol. 2014;122:231–66.
57. Dendrou C, Fugger L, Friese M. Immunopathology of multiple sclerosis. Nat Rev Immunol. 2015;15:545–58.
58. Richards RG, Sampson FC, Beard SM, et al. A review of the natural history and epidemiology of multiple sclerosis: implications for resource allocation and health economic models. Health Technol Assess. 2002;6:1–73.
59. Compston A, Coles A. Multiple sclerosis. Lancet. 2008;372:1502–17.
60. Weiner HL. Multiple sclerosis is an inflammatory T-cell-mediated autoimmune disease. Arch Neurol. 2004;61:1613–5.
61. Mutluay FK, Gürses HN, Saip S. Effects of multiple sclerosis on respiratory functions. Clin Rehabil. 2005;19:426–32.
62. Smeltzer SC, Skurnick JH, Troiano R, et al. Respiratory function in multiple sclerosis. Chest. 1992;101:479–84.
63. Dorotta IR, Schubert A. Multiple sclerosis and anesthetic implications. Curr Opin Anaesthesiol. 2002;15:365–70.
64. Caminero A, Bartolomé M. Sleep disturbances in multiple sclerosis. J Neurol Sci. 2011;309:86–91.
65. Ferini-Strambi L, Filippi M, Martinelli V, et al. Nocturnal sleep study in multiple sclerosis: correlations with clinical and brain magnetic resonance imaging findings. J Neurol Sci. 1994;125:194–7.
66. Aisen M, Arlt G, Foster S. Diaphragmatic paralysis without bulbar or limb paralysis in multiple sclerosis. Chest. 1990;98:499–501.
67. Adamec I, Habek M. Autonomic dysfunction in multiple sclerosis. Clin Neurol Neurosurg. 2013;115:3–9.
68. Siger M, Durko A, Nicpan A, et al. Discontinuation of interferon beta therapy in multiple sclerosis patients with high pre-treatment disease activity leads to prompt return to previous disease activity. J Neurol Sci. 2011;303:50–2.
69. O'Connor PW, Goodman A, Kappos L, et al. Disease activity return during natalizumab treatment interruption in patients with multiple sclerosis. Neurology. 2011;76:1858–65.
70. Havla JB, Pellkofer HL, Meinl I, et al. Rebound of disease activity after withdrawal of fingolimod (FTY720) treatment. Arch Neurol. 2012;69:262–4.
71. Guthrie TC, Nelson D. Influence of temperature changes on multiple sclerosis: critical review of mechanisms and research potential. J Neurol Sci. 1995;129:1–8.
72. Makris A, Piperopoulos A, Karmaniolou I. Multiple sclerosis: basic knowledge and new insights in perioperative management. J Anesth. 2014;28:267–78.

73. Inoue S, Furuya H. Sevoflurane is safe for anesthetic management in patients with multiple sclerosis. Acta Anaesthesiol Taiwan. 2006;44:187–9.
74. Sahin L, Korkmaz HF, Sahin M, et al. Desflurane anaesthesia in a patient with multiple sclerosis in total hip replacement. Arch Med Sci. 2010;6:984–56.
75. Ceyhan A, Uyar ET, Gencay IY, et al. Anesthesia in multiple sclerosis and obstructive sleep apnea: case report and literature review. Journal of Research in Medical Sciences. 2011;16:828–35.
76. Hachenberg T, Schneemilch C. Anesthesia in neurologic and psychiatric diseases: is there a "best anesthesia" for certain diseases? Curr Opin Anaesthesiol. 2014;27:394–402.
77. Lee KH, Park JS, Il LS, et al. Anesthetic management of the emergency laparotomy for a patient with multiple sclerosis: a case report. Korean Journal of Anesthesiology. 2010;59:359.
78. Cooperman LH. Succinylcholine-induced hyperkalemia in neuromuscular disease. JAMA. 1970;213:1867.
79. Levine M, Brown DFM. Succinylcholine-induced hyperkalemia in a patient with multiple sclerosis. J Emerg Med. 2012;43:279–82.
80. Sinikoglu N, Totoz T, Gumus F, et al. Repeated sugammadex usage in a patient with multiple sclerosis: a case report. Wien Klin Wochenschr. 2016;128:71–3.
81. Vandam LD, Dripps RD. Exacerbation of preexisting neurologic disease after spinal anesthesia. N Engl J Med. 1956;255:843–9.
82. Hebl JR, Horlocker TT, Schroeder DR. Neuraxial anesthesia and analgesia in patients with preexisting central nervous system disorders. Anesth Analg. 2006;103:223–8. table of contents
83. Perlas A, Chan VWS. Neuraxial anesthesia and multiple sclerosis. Canadian Journal of Anesthesia/Journal Canadien D'anesthésie. 2005;52:454–8.
84. Bader AM, Hunt CO, Datta S, et al. Anesthesia for the obstetric patient with multiple sclerosis. J Clin Anesth. 1988;1:21–4.
85. Stoelting RK, Hines RL, Marschall KE. Stoelting's anesthesia and co-existing disease. Philadelphia, PA: Elsevier Health Sciences; 2012.
86. Kalia LV. Parkinson's disease. Lancet. 2015;386(9996):896–912.
87. Bower JH, Maraganore DM, McDonnell SDK, Rocca WA. Incidence and distribution of parkinsonism in Olmsted County, Minnesota, 1976–1990. Neurology. 1999;52:1214–20.
88. de Rijk MC, Breteler MM, Graveland GA, et al. Prevalence of Parkinson's disease in the elderly: the Rotterdam Study. Neurology. 1995;45:2143–6.
89. De Lau LML, Breteler MMB. Epidemiology of Parkinson's disease. Lancet Neurol. 2006;5:525–35.
90. Katzenschlager R, Head J, Schraq A, Ben-Shlomo Y, Evans A, Lees AJ. Fourteen-year final report of the randomized PDRG-UK trial comparing three initial treatments in PD. Neurology. 2008;71:474–80.
91. Burn DJ, Rowan EN, Allan LM, Molloy S, O'Brien JT, McKeith IG. Motor subtype and cognitive decline in Parkinson's disease, Parkinson's disease with dementia, and dementia with Lewy bodies. J Neurol Neurosurg Psychiatry. 2006;77:585–9.
92. Rajput AH, Voll A, Rajput ML, et al. Course in Parkinson disease subtypes: a 39 year clinicopathologic study. Neurology. 2009;73(3):206–12.
93. Williams-Gray CH, Mason SL, Evans JR, et al. The CamPaIGN study of Parkinson's disease: 10-year outlook in an incident population-based cohort. J Neurol Neurosurg Psychiatry. 2013;84:1258–64.
94. Nicholson G. Parkinson's disease and anaesthesia. Br J Anaesth. 2002;89(6):904–16.
95. Hoehn MM, Yahr MD. Parkinsonism: onset, progression and mortality. Neurology. 1967;17:427–42.
96. Obenour WH, Stevens PM, Cohen AA, McCutchen JJ. The causes of abnormal pulmonary function in Parkinson's disease. Am Rev Respir Dis. 1972;105:382–7.
97. Backus WW, Ward RR, Vitkun SA, Fitzgerald D, Askanazi J. Postextubation laryngospasm in an unanaesthetised patient with Parkinson's disease. J Clin Anesth. 1991;3:314–6.
98. Easdown LJ, Tessler MJ, Minuk J. Upper airway involvement in Parkinson's disease resulting in postoperative respiratory failure. Can J Anaesth. 1995;42:344–7.
99. Seppi K, Weintraub D, Coelho M, et al. The movement disorder society evidence-based medicine review update: treatments for the non-motor symptoms of Parkinson's disease. Mov Disord. 2011;26:S42–80.
100. Medtronic DBS therapy: information for prescribers. In: Medtronic, editor; 2010. p. 16-17.
101. Katus LL. Perioperative management of patients with Parkinson's disease. Am J Med. 2014;127(4): 275–80.
102. Wand P, Kuschinsky K, Sontag KH. Morphine-induced muscle rigidity in rates. Eur J Pharmacol. 1973;24:189–93.
103. Berg D, Becker G, Reiners K. Reduction of dyskinesia and induction of akinesia induced by morphine in two parkinsonian patients with severe sciatica. J Neural Transm. 1999;106:725–8.
104. Zornberg GL, Alexander Bodkin J, Cohen BM. Severe adverse interaction between pethidine and selegiline. Lancet. 1991;337:246.
105. Stone DJ, Difazio CA. Sedation for patients with Parkinson's disease undergoing ophthalmic surgery. Anesthesiology. 1988;68:821.
106. Golden WE, Lavender RC, Metzer WS. Acute postoperative confusion and hallucinations in Parkinson's disease. Ann Intern Med. 1989;111:218–22.
107. Pfeiffer RF. Gastrointestinal dysfunction in Parkinson's disease. Lancet Neurol. 2003;2:107–16.
108. Gillman PK. Monoamine oxidase inhibitors, opioid analgesics and serotonin toxicity. Br J Anaesth. 2005;95:434–41.
109. Brennan KA, Genever RW. Managing Parkinson's disease during surgery. BMJ. 2010;341:c5718.

110. Caplan LR. Terms describing brain ischemia by tempo are no longer useful: a polemic (with apologies to Shakespeare). Surg Neurol. 1993;40(2):91.
111. Krishnamurthi RV, et al. Global and regional burden of first-ever ischaemic and haemorrhagic stroke during 1990–2010: findings from the Global Burden of Disease Study 2010. Lancet Glob Health. 2013;1(5):e259.
112. Benjamin EJ, et al. Heart disease and stroke statistics-2017 update: a report from the American Heart Association. Circulation. 2017;135:e1.
113. Koton S, et al. Stroke incidence and mortality trends in US communities, 1987 to 2011. JAMA. 2014;312(3):259–68. https://doi.org/10.1001/jama.2014.7692.
114. Feigin VL, et al. Global and regional burden of stroke during 1990–2010: findings from the Global Burden of Disease Study 2010. Lancet. 2014;383(9913):245–54.
115. Wong GY, Warner DO, Schroeder DR, et al. Risk of surgery and anesthesia for ischemic stroke. Anesthesiology. 2000;92(2):425–32.
116. Bucerius J, Gummert JF, Borger MA, et al. Stroke after cardiac surgery: a risk factor analysis of 16,184 consecutive adult patients. Ann Thorac Surg. 2003;75(2):472–8.
117. Limburg M, Wijdicks EF, Li H. Ischemic stroke after surgical procedures: clinical features, neuroimaging, and risk factors. Neurology. 1998;50(4):895–901.
118. Selim M. Perioperative stroke. N Engl J Med. 2007;356(7):706–13.
119. Kam PC, Calcroft RM. Peri-operative stroke in general surgical patients. Anaesthesia. 1997;52(9):879–83.
120. Naylor AR, Mehta Z, Rothwell PM, Bell PR. Carotid artery disease and stroke during coronary artery bypass: a critical review of the literature. Eur J Vasc Endovasc Surg. 2002;23(4):283–94.
121. Charlesworth DC, Likosky DS, Marrin CA, et al. Development and validation of a prediction model for strokes after coronary artery bypass grafting. Ann Thorac Surg. 2003;76(2):436–43.
122. Dunn AS, Turpie AG. Perioperative management of patients receiving oral anticoagulants: a systematic review. Arch Intern Med. 2003;163(8):901–8.
123. Dunn AS, Wisnivesky J, Ho W, Moore C, McGinn T, Sacks HS. Perioperative management of patients on oral anticoagulants: a decision analysis. Med Decis Making. 2005;25(4):387–97.
124. Veenith TV, et al. Perioperative care of a patient with stroke. International Archives of Medicine. 2010;3:33.
125. Rochester CL, Mohsenin V. Respiratory complications of stroke. Semin Respir Crit Care Med. 2002;23:248–60.
126. Schaller BJ, Graf R, Jacobs AH. Pathophysiological changes of the gastrointestinal tract in ischemic stroke. Am J Gastroenterol. 2006;101:1655–65.
127. Dennis M. Nutrition after stroke. Br Med Bull. 2000;56:466–75.

18 Renal Disorders and Maxillofacial Surgery

George Sunny Pazhayattil and Marc Ciampi

Abstract

The kidneys are designed to perform several essential physiologic functions. Renal dysfunction in any form results in significant systemic manifestations in the human body. Patient with kidney dysfunction undergoing any surgical procedure presents unique challenges. Proper understanding of basic pathophysiology of renal disease, appropriate clinical evaluation prior to the surgery, and proper monitoring and care during the intraoperative and postoperative period are integral to achieving good surgical outcomes. This chapter addresses the basic concepts that should guide a surgeon when dealing with a patient with abnormal kidney function. A multidisciplinary approach to care is recommended when managing a patient with any form of kidney dysfunction during the perioperative phase. This involves appropriate consultation with patient's primary care provider, nephrologist, and pharmacist as indicated.

18.1 Overview of Structure and Functions of Kidney

Kidneys are a pair of bean-shaped retroperitoneal organs weighing 140–150 g and measuring 10–12 cm in length. The blood supply to the kidneys is through renal arteries which arise directly from the abdominal aorta. On average, kidneys receive 20% of the cardiac output which represents highest tissue-specific blood flow of all organs in the body (350 mL/min per 100 g tissue) [1]. The nephron is the basic functional unit of the kidney. The nephrons are packed together compactly to make up the kidney parenchyma, and it is estimated that each kidney consists of

G.S. Pazhayattil, M.D., FACP
M. Ciampi, M.D., FACP, FASN (✉)
Quinnipiac University Netter School of Medicine, North Haven, CT, USA

Yale University School of Medicine, New Haven, CT, USA
e-mail: doclife@gmail.com; majciampi@me.com

© Springer International Publishing AG 2018
E.M. Ferneini, J.D. Bennett (eds.), *Perioperative Assessment of the Maxillofacial Surgery Patient*,
https://doi.org/10.1007/978-3-319-58868-1_18

approximately one million nephrons. Each nephron consists of a capillary tuft known as the glomerulus and a series of tubules. The glomerulus serves as the filtration unit which creates the initial ultrafiltrate which is then sequentially modified in the tubules by a complex process involving secretion and absorption of various components. The final product is the urine which then enters the renal pelvis where it is collected by the ureter. The ureter channels it to the bladder from where it is finally excreted.

The kidneys perform multiple essential functions. The primary function of the kidney is filtration and excretion of metabolic end products and toxins. In many instances the kidneys work in partnership with the liver in excreting medications and other drug end products. Kidneys are also the primary organs responsible for regulation of water, electrolyte, and acid-base balance in the body. In addition to these excretory and regulatory functions, kidneys also serve an endocrine role by secreting hormones and enzymes such as renin, angiotensin, erythropoietin, and 1,25-dihydroxyvitamin D3, the active form of vitamin D. Renin and angiotensin, in conjunction with the adrenal hormone aldosterone, play an important role in blood pressure regulation. Erythropoietin is essential for maturation of erythrocytes in the bone marrow, and 1,25-dihydroxyvitamin D3 plays an important role in regulating calcium and phosphate balance.

18.2 Clinical Evaluation of the Kidney

18.2.1 Urinalysis

This is probably the most basic of all tests to evaluate kidney and urinary tract. It is important to realize that the urine collection and handling is important when it comes to reliability of the results. Certain factors could result in false positive findings in urinalysis. Examples include strenuous exercise or menstruation resulting in false positive hematuria. The relevant components of a typical urinalysis are discussed under Table 18.1.

Table 18.1 Urinalysis

Finding	Relevance
Turbidity	Normal urine is usually clear. Turbidity may suggest infection, pyuria, crystalluria, or chyluria
Color	Normal color is light yellow. Darker yellow is usually related to concentrated urine. Red-brown color suggests hematuria, hemoglobinuria, or myoglobinuria
Specific gravity	High specific gravity suggests more concentrated urine. This could suggest volume-depleted state
Detection of heme	Suggests presence of red blood cells (RBCs), free hemoglobin, or free myoglobin
Detection of nitrate and leukocyte esterase	When both are positive, it is usually suggestive of urinary tract infection
Detection of protein	Presence of protein in urine should prompt further evaluation. It should also be noted that common dipstick is not sensitive to assess presence of non-albumin protein such as monoclonal proteins
Glucose	Presence of glycosuria usually represents hyperglycemia with glucose levels more than 180 mg/dL. Glycosuria in the absence of hyperglycemia could signal proximal tubular dysfunction
Microscopy	This valuable tool identifies the presence of cells, urinary casts, crystals, bacteria, and other pathogens

18.2.2 Measuring Renal Clearance

The parameters that are generally described as markers of renal clearance are (1) serum creatinine concentration (SCr), (2) blood urea nitrogen concentration (BUN), and (3) glomerular filtration rate (GFR). Of these markers, BUN and SCr have been the most commonly used parameters to define kidney function. Unfortunately both BUN and SCr are unreliable for measuring renal function due to several reasons. Both these markers are influenced by multiple nonrenal factors such as age, sex, diet, muscle mass, metabolic rate, and hydration status. In a patient with acute kidney injury (AKI) where there is ongoing damage to kidney tissue, relying on SCr is even more misleading for two main reasons. (1) The renal reserve allows for up to 50% loss of functioning nephrons before the SCr starts rising. (2) There is a lag period before the SCr starts to rise. In AKI, the SCr can take several hours or days to reach a new steady state and consequently does not mirror the ongoing decline in kidney function in the acute setting. An actual calculation of GFR by measuring the 24 h urinary clearance of inulin is the gold standard for measuring renal function. Inulin is an inert polysacharide which when administered, is freely filtered by the glomeruli, and is neither reabsorbed nor secreted throughout the rest of the nephron. Unfortunately this is a time consuming, technically challenging and expensive task and is almost never used in clinical situations. On the other hand, a timed (usually 24-h) urine collection to calculate creatinine clearance can be a useful clinical test where an accurate measurement of GFR is required. Once again, the usefulness of the test is limited by required duration of urine collection and the challenges involved in accurate collection of urine over the period of time. Also, creatinine unlike inulin is actively secreted in the tubules resulting in overestimation of GFR calculation. Hence, the clinicians are caught between the unreliability of SCr and the challenges involved in timed urine collection. To address this problem, formulas have been created to calculate GFR estimates (eGFR). These complex formulas use SCr and other clinical parameters such as age, gender, race, and body size. There are several such formulas in use but the most commonly used are the Cockcroft-Gault, the Modification of Diet in Renal Disease Study (MDRD), and CKD Epidemiology Collaboration (CKD-EPI) equations. Many labs include eGFR in their results which help clinicians get a better picture of the renal function. At the time of writing this chapter, there is a great deal of interest in establishing a reliable biomarker to accurately assess renal function during AKI. This continues to be an active area of research, but as of now, none of the biomarkers have been introduced to regular clinical practice.

18.2.3 Proteinuria

In addition to measuring the effectiveness of excretory function of kidneys, in certain situations it is important to monitor the presence of protein in the urine (proteinuria). In normal subjects protein never crosses the glomerular basement membrane (GBM). Hence, proteinuria is a sign of damage to the integrity of GBM. In certain clinical scenarios such as diabetic nephropathy, proteinuria is an early indicator of renal damage. In such situations proteinuria precedes the actual drop in GFR by several months to years. Excessive proteinuria is also a poor prognostic marker for future loss of kidney function. The most common way of detection of proteinuria is on a dipstick urinalysis. This test serves to detect proteinuria but does not reliably quantify it. For quantification of proteinuria a 24 h urine collection is generally considered as the gold standard test. However, as mentioned before, performing a 24 h urine collection has its own drawbacks. Fortunately, evidence supports the use of urine protein-to-creatinine ratio in a random urine sample for quantifying 24 h proteinuria [2]. This simple test closely correlates with the 24 h urinary protein excretion. This is a simple and inexpensive test and should be used as the initial test to quantify proteinuria.

18.2.4 Renal Imaging

In certain clinical scenarios, imaging the kidneys and urinary tract is necessary. A renal ultrasound scan is most frequently employed for this purpose. Ultrasound scanning could detect certain congenital malformations such as congenital solitary kidney, horseshoe kidney, and polycystic kidney disease. In some instances, AKI could be related to obstruction which can be detected on an ultrasound by noticing hydronephrosis, the terminology used for the finding of swollen kidney(s). Employing color Doppler sonography and renal artery duplex scanning can also aid in diagnosis of vascular malformations involving renal arteries or renal veins. When it comes to evaluation of complex cysts or tumors of the kidneys, a computed tomography (CT) or magnetic resonance imaging (MRI) scan is more useful than a renal ultrasound. As will be discussed later, care should be taken before ordering the use of intravenous contrast dye with CT or MRI scans in a patient with compromised renal function. In general we recommend discussing the risks with a nephrologist before using contrast dye in such patients. More advanced imaging techniques such as nuclear scintigraphy can be employed for a more accurate assessment of renal flow and function. The details of these studies are beyond the scope of this chapter.

18.3 Pathophysiology of Renal Disease

Patients with kidney disease can be divided into following broad categories:

1. Patients with AKI but not requiring renal replacement therapy
2. Patients with AKI requiring renal replacement therapy
3. Patients with chronic kidney disease (CKD) but renal replacement therapy has not yet been initiated
4. Patients who have progressed to end stage renal disease (ESRD) and require ongoing dialysis
5. Patients with ESRD in the past but underwent kidney transplantation
6. Patients who have normal renal clearance but manifests critical derangements in electrolytes or acid-base status

18.3.1 AKI

AKI is a clinical syndrome characterized by an acute decline in GFR resulting in decrease in renal clearance and accumulation of waste products and toxins. Several criteria and definitions for AKI exist, but the most widely accepted practical definition is provided by Kidney Disease Improving Global Outcomes (KDIGO) clinical practice guidelines for AKI. According to KDIGO guidelines, definition of AKI is any of the following [3]:

- Increase in SCr by ≥0.3 mg/dL within 48 h
- Increase in SCr to ≥1.5 times baseline, which is known or presumed to have occurred within the prior 7 days
- Urine volume ≤0.5 mL/kg/h for 6 h

The course of AKI differs depending on the clinical scenario. In majority of patients, AKI is reversible with appropriate supportive management without requiring renal replacement therapy. In some patients short-term dialysis may be required while the kidneys recover. In such cases, the appropriate management to treat or alleviate kidney damage should be continued in hopes of renal recovery. On rare occasions a severe case of AKI may lead to ESRD necessitating lifelong renal replacement therapy. AKI in the perioperative period has serious implications, being associated with high mortality, morbidity, and a much more complicated postoperative course. If nonemergent, it is advisable to postpone any surgery until the renal function is stabilized. In any patient with AKI who is undergoing surgery, we recommend the involvement of a nephrologist before the procedure for risk stratification and co-management during the perioperative period.

18.3.2 CKD

Based on National Health and Nutrition Examination Survey (NHANES) report, the prevalence of CKD is around 14% of total US adult population [4]. The prevalence is much higher in individuals aged 60 and older. CKD is increasingly becoming one of the most common chronic conditions worldwide. The two leading causes for CKD are hypertension and diabetes mellitus.

The most simplistic and widely recognized definition of CKD is any alteration of kidney structure or function that is present for more than 3 months, potentially leading to multisystem involvement. Many of the manifestations of CKD could be similar to that of AKI, but the key distinguishing factor is the duration of the disease. The easiest way to determine this is by comparing the patient's current clinical parameters (SCr, eGFR, and proteinuria) to previous available lab results. Table 18.2 reviews the current staging of CKD based on eGFR categories [5]. This staging of CKD which is solely based on GFR categories provides some indication of the severity of the disease, but predicting the actual prognosis will require the knowledge of additional factors such

Table 18.2 Staging CKD

Stage of CKD	GFR (mL/min/1.73 m²)	Description
Stage 1	>90	Kidney damage with normal GFR
Stage 2	60–89	Kidney damage with mild reduction in GFR
Stage 3	30–59	Kidney damage with moderate reduction in GFR
Stage 4	15–29	Kidney damage with severe reduction in GFR
Stage 5	<15	Kidney failure

as the exact etiology of renal disease, presence of histologic and structural abnormalities, degree of proteinuria, and presence of other comorbid conditions.

CKD results in sustained derangements resulting in secondary organ involvement. The most notable effect is on the cardiovascular system. CKD accelerates the process of atherosclerosis, vascular calcification, and left ventricular hypertrophy. The presence of CKD, whether it is manifested by proteinuria or reduced GFR, increases the risk of cardiovascular disease [6]. Other systemic manifestations of CKD include extravascular volume overload due to impaired excretion of salt and water, electrolyte derangements, metabolic acidosis due to impaired excretion of acids, anemia due to deficient production of erythropoietin, and bone-mineral disorders due to dysregulation of calcium and phosphorus balance. Some of the infrequent effects of CKD relevant to readers include increased incidence of oral pathology such as gingival hyperplasia, enamel hypoplasia, and gingival bleeding [7]. In summary, presence of CKD significantly worsens morbidity and mortality risk of the patient. Primary care providers usually detect and guide management of early stages of CKD. A nephrology consultation is required in advanced CKD (beyond stage 3 CKD) or if the presentation of CKD is advanced or rapidly progressive. Findings of proteinuria and hematuria should also be evaluated by a nephrologist.

18.3.3 ESRD

This denotes irrecoverable kidney damage requiring chronic dialysis or a kidney transplant as a consequence of progressive CKD or lack of recovery from AKI. As of 2013 USRDS data estimated there were 661,648 prevalent cases of ESRD; the unadjusted prevalence of this disease was 2034 per million in the US population. Around 100,000 patients are initiated on chronic dialysis each year. Currently, there are three main modalities for chronic dialysis. Hemodialysis arranged at an outpatient dialysis center (in-center hemodialysis) is the commonest modality followed by peritoneal dialysis and home hemodialysis.

Presence of renal dysfunction in any form poses an increased surgical risk and a higher perioperative mortality [8, 9]. Increased risk could be related to various factors as detailed in Table 18.3.

Table 18.3 Factors leading to increased perioperative risk in patients with AKI, CKD, or ESRD and potential implications

Risk factor	Potential implication
Electrolyte derangements	Increases risk for perioperative arrhythmias
Acid-base disorders	Increases risk for perioperative arrhythmias, hypotension and ventilator dependence
Uremic platelet dysfunction	Increases risk for intraoperative and postoperative bleeding
Reduced renal clearance of medications	Increases risk for drug toxicities and drug interactions
Poorly controlled hypertension	Increases risk of adverse cardiovascular events
Poorly controlled volume status	Increases cardiovascular risk, perioperative hypotension, or hypertension and ventilator dependence
Increased association with anemia, malnutrition, inflammation, and cardiovascular comorbidities	Increases overall surgical risk and incidence of perioperative mortality

18.3.4 Kidney Transplant Recipients

Kidney transplantation is the best course of treatment for a patient with advanced CKD or those who have progressed to ESRD [10]. Compared to chronic dialysis, kidney transplantation was associated with reduced risk of mortality and cardiovascular events as well as better quality of life [11]. The key to long-term transplant survival is continued immunosuppression. Transplant recipients are required to continue a complex regimen of immunosuppressive medications for the rest of their life. This strategy aimed at preventing rejection also predisposes the individual to increased rates of infections. Infections are an important cause of morbidity and mortality in kidney transplant recipients. Given the complexity of care, it is strongly recommended that any surgical plans be discussed with patient's transplant team or with patient's nephrologist. Specific perioperative considerations and guidelines for kidney transplant recipients are described below.

- It is recommended that elective surgeries be planned either before the transplantation surgery or 1 year after the transplantation.
- Immunosuppressive medications should be continued without any change unless specifically advised by transplant team. In situations when oral medications cannot be administered, appropriate intravenous substitutions should be made as advised by transplant team.
- In transplant patients who are already on moderate to high dose of prednisone adrenal suppression may be an issue. This warrants consideration of intravenous steroids during the perioperative period.
- Avoid drugs that affect the CYP 3A4 enzyme system to prevent fluctuations of tacrolimus and cyclosporine levels. This could either result in drug toxicity or undertreatment both of which are detrimental. If use of such a drug is unavoidable, the dose of antirejection medications may need to be adjusted. Advice from patient's transplant team is critical in guiding such dose adjustments.
- Knowledge of oral manifestations in transplant patients is important during the preoperative evaluation. Gingival hypertrophy is associated with use of certain antirejection medications particularly cyclosporine and tacrolimus. Immunosuppression and chronic steroid use could also result in infectious or noninfectious ulcers which should be noted and appropriately managed during preoperative period.
- Wound healing is delayed in patients on long-term steroids. Patients who are on antirejection medication sirolimus are also at higher risk for delayed wound healing.

18.4 Before, During, and After Surgery

We have already discussed the specific perioperative considerations in patients with AKI, CKD, ESRD, and kidney transplant recipients in this chapter. Here we will discuss general guidelines involved in assessing and optimizing a patient with renal disease for surgery.

- As with any patient, preoperative assessment begins with a careful history taking and by performing detailed physical examination. The emphasis during this phase is on assessment of blood pressure control, careful evaluation of volume status, and complete documentation of current medications. Ideally all patients with advanced CKD (CKD IV and beyond) should be evaluated by a nephrologist for preoperative assessment.
- Preoperative labs should include a complete blood count and a metabolic panel—sodium, potassium, chloride, blood urea nitrogen, creatinine, calcium, and bicarbonate levels.
- If severe acid-base disturbances are suspected, an arterial blood gas should be obtained to accurately assess the acid-base status. Any significant acid-base abnormality should be addressed before proceeding with any surgery.
- *Optimization of volume status:* A routine chest X-ray could help evaluate fluid status. Evidence of pulmonary congestion on a chest X-ray is usually a sign of volume overload.

Ideally patients should be euvolemic at the time of surgery. In patients who undergo hemodialysis, it is advisable to arrange any surgery on the day after dialysis. If the surgery is emergent, nephrologist should be consulted as early as possible to guide dialysis during perioperative period.

- *Preoperative anemia management:* As mentioned before anemia is frequently associated with renal dysfunction. The goal hemoglobin should be as close to normal range as possible. In most cases, hemoglobin level above 10 g/dL is considered safe for surgery. Preoperative transfusion may be necessary in certain cases. The threshold for ordering transfusion differs depending on the cardiovascular risk. In patients who may need kidney transplantation in the future blood transfusions should be avoided as far as possible to prevent antibody formation. These antibodies may reduce their chances in securing a successful match in the future. In the case of elective surgery in patients with CKD or ESRD, early discussion with nephrologist could result in better utilization of erythropoietin analogues in conjunction with iron supplementation to achieve optimal hemoglobin. This strategy will prevent unnecessary need for blood transfusions during the perioperative period.
- *Preoperative management of hypertension:* The widely accepted goal blood pressure for patients with renal dysfunction is $\leq$130/80. Careful titration of antihypertensive regimen should help achieve this goal.
- *Minimizing bleeding risk*: Uremia can cause platelet dysfunction thereby increasing the risk of perioperative bleeding. This effect is compounded in the presence of antiplatelet agents. Bleeding time is the most sensitive indicator but is seldom performed. In dialysis patients, heparin is commonly used during hemodialysis, and the residual anticoagulant may last for few hours after the dialysis session. Hence it is critical to inform patient's nephrologist and the dialysis team about the timing of surgery so that heparin may be discontinued appropriately. Dialysis should minimize uremia-related platelet dysfunction. In situations when a patient is not receiving dialysis, desmopressin (DDAVP) has been used to correct bleeding times. The usual dose is 0.3mcg/kg IV 1 h prior to surgery [12].
- *Optimizing electrolyte levels*: Most important electrolyte abnormality that results in significant perioperative complications is hyperkalemia. There are no guidelines that definitively state a maximum safe level of potassium prior to induction of anesthesia. In general, it is recommended that the potassium level be with in normal range prior to any surgery requiring general anesthesia. In case of emergency surgery, where this is not possible, continuous intraoperative electrocardiogram (ECG) monitoring and frequent measurement of potassium levels are required. If needed, temporizing medical management can be instituted by anesthesiologist until more definitive management can be pursued. Other electrolytes that should be monitored include sodium, calcium, and magnesium levels.
- *Antibiotic prophylaxis*: It is recommended that patients with ESRD undergoing hemodialysis using a central venous catheter or arteriovenous graft (AVG) receive antibiotic prophylaxis prior to the surgery. In adult patients, a single oral preoperative dose of 2 g amoxicillin or 600 mg clindamycin (in case of penicillin allergy) is recommended [13].
- *Cardiovascular evaluation*: As mentioned before patients with renal dysfunction often have pre-existing cardiac morbidity. Careful preoperative cardiac evaluation is required with emphasis on diagnosing unstable coronary artery disease and presence of congestive heart failure. Any suspicion of cardiac disease should prompt a formal evaluation by a cardiologist.
- *Proper care of vascular access for hemodialysis*: In patients undergoing hemodialysis using arteriovenous fistula (AVF) or arteriovenous graft (AVG), care should be taken to preserve the functioning of these dialysis accesses. This includes avoiding placing a BP cuff on the arm with AVF or AVG and avoiding placement of IV lines and any form of finger sticks to the arm. In patients with an advanced CKD

anticipating dialysis in the future, any IV lines should be placed on the dominant arm there by preserving the non-dominant arm for future AVF or AVG placement. In patients with advanced CKD or with ESRD, placement of peripherally inserted central catheters (PICC) should be avoided to preserve the superficial veins for future dialysis access placement.

- *Proper intraoperative management*: The two main concerns during the intraoperative phase are (1) dose adjustment of medications and (2) intraoperative volume balance and hemodynamics. Common medications that are used during a surgery which require special attention are described under Table 18.4. Intraoperative volume balance requires special attention in patients with renal dysfunction. Intraoperative volume loss and associated hypotension could result in renal hypoperfusion leading to loss of kidney function. This is one of the commonest causes for postoperative AKI. For this reason, intraoperative hypotension should be promptly managed. It is desirable to maintain a mean arterial pressure (MAP) of >60 mmHg throughout the surgery. Intraoperative monitoring of urine output especially during prolonged surgery could give an indication of status of renal perfusion. A decrease in urine output suggests hypoperfusion. The other issue which specifically pertains to dialysis patients is the amount of fluid administered during the intraoperative period. Excessive administration of IV fluids could result in fluid overload in dialysis patients.
- *Postoperative care of patient with renal disease:* During the immediate postoperative phase, the concerns are similar to what we have discussed during the intraoperative phase. The goal is to avoid prolonged periods of hypotension, proper dosing of medications that are cleared by the kidneys, and judicious use of IV fluids. One specific consideration during postoperative pain management is the importance of avoiding NSAIDs. From a nephrology stand point, the main concern during this phase is postoperative AKI. This could manifest as a new AKI in a patient who had normal renal function before the surgery or acute worsening of renal function in a patient with pre-existing CKD. Postoperative AKI is associated with significant morbidity and mortality. Please refer to Sect. 12.4, Chap. 12, for an in-depth review on this topic.

Table 18.4 Special considerations for the use of intraoperative and postoperative medications

Drug	Special considerations
Midazolam	• Dose reduction required in renal dysfunction
Succinylcholine (SCh)	• May be used if *K* <5.5 meq/L • The neuromuscular block caused by SCh may be prolonged • If *K* >5.5 meq/L, use atracurium or cisatracurium
Inhalational anesthetics	• Most inhalational anesthetics are eliminated predominantly via exhalation which makes it safe to use in patients with renal dysfunction • Concerns have been expressed regarding the theoretical renal toxicity of sevoflurane due to its inorganic fluoride ion metabolite. The US Food and Drug Administration (FDA) recommends the use of sevoflurane with fresh gas flow rates at least 1 L/min for exposures up to 1 h and at least 2 L/min for exposures greater than 1 h [14]
Morphine, hydromorphone, meperidine, and codeine	• Avoid use in patients with ESRD because of the risk of accumulation of metabolites • Use fentanyl instead
NSAIDs	• Should be strictly avoided in patients with any form of renal dysfunction
Antibiotics	• Dosing and frequency of antibiotics may need to be adjusted based on the eGFR

Conclusion

Surgical procedures are frequently necessary in patients with renal disorders. The increased morbidity and mortality risk associated with this patient population prompts proper evaluation and preparation. Preoperative management of these patients involves multiple interdependent factors which can be challenging. Perioperative care of these patients should involve a multidisciplinary team approach.

This team includes the patient, family physician, nephrologist, anesthesiologist, and the surgeon.

References

1. Briggs JP, Kriz W, Schnermann JB. Overview of kidney function and structure. In: Primer on Kidney Diseases. 5th ed. Philadelphia: Saunders; 2009. p. 2–18.
2. Schwab SJ, Christensen RL, Dougherty K, Klahr S. Quantitation of proteinuria by the use of protein-to-creatinine ratios in single urine samples. Arch Intern Med. 1987;147(5):943–4.
3. Kellum JA, Lameire N, Aspelin P, Barsoum RS, Burdmann EA, Goldstein SL, Herzog CA, Joannidis M, Kribben A, Levey AS, MacLeod AM, Mehta RL, Murray PT, Naicker S, Opal SM, Schaefer F, Schetz M, Uchino S. Kidney disease: improving global outcomes (KDIGO) acute kidney injury work group. KDIGO clinical practice guideline for acute kidney injury. Kidney Int Suppl. 2012;2(1):1–138. https://doi.org/10.1038/kisup.2012.1.
4. USRDS United States Renal Data System. 2015 USRDS annual data report: epidemiology of kidney disease in the United States. National Institutes of Health, National Institute of Diabetes and Digestive and Kidney Diseases, Bethesda, MD, 2015.
5. KDIGO. Summary of Recommendation Statements. Kidney Int Suppl. 2013;3(1):5–14. doi:https://doi.org/10.1038/kisup.2012.77.
6. Sarnak MJ, Levey AS, Schoolwerth AC, Coresh J, Culleton B, Hamm LL, McCullough PA, Kasiske BL, Kelepouris E, Klag MJ, Parfrey P, Pfeffer M, Raij L, Spinosa DJ, Wilson PW. Kidney disease as a risk factor for development of cardiovascular disease: a statement from the American Heart Association Councils on Kidney in Cardiovascular Disease, High Blood Pressure Research, Clinical Cardiology, and Epidemiology and Prevention. Circulation. 2003;108(17):2154–69. https://doi.org/10.1161/01.cir.0000095676.90936.80.
7. Dioguardi M, Caloro GA, Troiano G, Giannatempo G, Laino L, Petruzzi M, Lo Muzio L. Oral manifestations in chronic uremia patients. Renal Failure. 2016;38(1):1–6. https://doi.org/10.3109/0886022X.2015.1103639.
8. de Mutsert R, Grootendorst DC, Axelsson J, Boeschoten EW, Krediet RT, Dekker FW. Excess mortality due to interaction between protein-energy wasting, inflammation and cardiovascular disease in chronic dialysis patients. Nephrol Dial Transplant. 2008;23(9):2957–64. https://doi.org/10.1093/ndt/gfn167.
9. Kellerman PS. Perioperative care of the renal patient. Arch Intern Med. 1994;154(15):1674–88.
10. Suthanthiran M, Strom TB. Renal transplantation. N Engl J Med. 1994;331(6):365–76. https://doi.org/10.1056/nejm199408113310606.
11. Tonelli M, Wiebe N, Knoll G, Bello A, Browne S, Jadhav D, Klarenbach S, Gill J. Systematic review: kidney transplantation compared with dialysis in clinically relevant outcomes. Am J Transplant. 2011;11(10):2093–109. https://doi.org/10.1111/j.1600-6143.2011.03686.x.
12. Chen KS, Huang CC, Leu ML, Deng P, Lo SK. Hemostatic and fibrinolytic response to desmopressin in uremic patients. Blood Purif. 1997;15(2):84–91.
13. Tong DC, Walker RJ. Antibiotic prophylaxis in dialysis patients undergoing invasive dental treatment. Nephrology (Carlton). 2004;9(3):167–70. https://doi.org/10.1111/j.1440-1797.2004.00245.x.
14. Gentz BA, Malan TP Jr. Renal toxicity with sevoflurane: a storm in a teacup? Drugs. 2001;61(15):2155–62.

19 Gastroenterological and Hepatic Disorders and Maxillofacial Surgery

Sashidhar Sagi and Marwan Ghabril

Abstract

The management of gastrointestinal and hepatic disorders in the perioperative period is driven by considerations of risks related to the specific underlying condition, its treatment, and the impact of either on the efficacy or tolerance and safety of anesthetic agents. This chapter highlights these conditions and summarizes salient aspects of pathophysiology, disease impact, and management considerations in the context of maxillofacial surgery.

Abbreviations

CD	Crohn's disease
CI	Confidence interval
CT	Computed tomography
CTP	Child-Turcotte-Pugh
ERCP	Endoscopic retrograde cholangiopancreatography
GERD	Gastroesophageal reflux disease
HPS	Hepatopulmonary syndrome
IBD	Inflammatory bowel disease
LES	Lower esophageal sphincter
MELD	Model for End-Stage Liver Disease
MRI	Magnetic resonance imaging
OR	Odds ratio
PPH	Portopulmonary hypertension
TNF-α	Tumor necrosis factor-alpha
UC	Ulcerative colitis

S. Sagi, M.D. • M. Ghabril, M.D. (✉)
Division of Gastroenterology and Hepatology, Indiana University School of Medicine, Indianapolis, IN, USA
e-mail: mghabril@iu.edu

19.1 Introduction

Gastrointestinal and hepatic disorders are common in the general population, but the vast majority of common disorders like mild gastroesophageal reflux disease, dyspepsia, irritable bowel syndrome, and non-advanced nonalcoholic liver disease do not affect the perioperative management of maxillofacial surgical patients. Certain disease states, however, warrant unique consideration and specific interventions, and medication management may help in optimizing outcomes. The information related to specific disease states is organized by anatomical organ involvement.

19.2 Esophageal Disorders

Structural and functional disorders of the foregut impair transit of gastroesophageal contents and could lead to dysphagia, regurgitation, and aspiration. Structural esophageal disorders could be developmental anomalies like esophageal atresia,

© Springer International Publishing AG 2018

E.M. Ferneini, J.D. Bennett (eds.), *Perioperative Assessment of the Maxillofacial Surgery Patient*,
https://doi.org/10.1007/978-3-319-58868-1_19

tracheoesophageal fistula (TEF), esophageal webs and rings, and diverticula. Esophageal stenosis could be congenital or acquired. Benign esophageal strictures are most commonly from gastroesophageal reflux disease and involve the distal esophagus. The most common cause of malignant esophageal stricture is esophageal adenocarcinoma.

19.2.1 Pharyngoesophageal Diverticula

19.2.1.1 Zenker's Diverticulum

Zenker's diverticula develop when abnormally high pressures occur during swallowing and lead to protrusion of mucosa through an area of anatomic weakness in the pharynx known as Killian's triangle. Killian's triangle is located posteriorly where the transverse fibers of the cricopharyngeus muscle of the upper esophageal sphincter intersect with the oblique fibers of the inferior pharyngeal constrictor muscle [1]. The estimated prevalence of Zenker's diverticula is between 0.1% and 0.01%. It is more common in men and generally presents in the seventh or eighth decade of life with dysphagia, regurgitation, choking, and aspiration [2]. Barium swallow is the most useful study when this is suspected. The main risk of anesthesia is that of aspiration at induction. The best method to empty the diverticulum is to have the patient express and regurgitate the contents immediately before induction, as even prolonged fasting does not ensure emptying. Cricoid pressure during induction does not prevent aspiration as the opening of the diverticulum is above the level of the cricoid and may actually contribute to aspiration. The safest method of airway management may be awake fiber-optic intubation [3]. Care should be taken to avoid diverticular perforation when passing orogastric and nasogastric tubes.

19.2.1.2 Esophageal Diverticula

These are most commonly located in the middle or distal esophagus and have an estimated prevalence of 0.015% on autopsy studies to 2% of radiology studies in patients with swallowing problems [4]. These diverticula can be divided into two types: traction and pulsion diverticula. Traction diverticula are pulled out by an inflammatory, fibrotic, or neoplastic process outside of the esophagus. Pulsion diverticula are typically located near the diaphragmatic hiatus (epiphrenic diverticula) and are caused by motility disorders [5]. Aspiration precautions and care to avoid perforation when passing orogastric and nasogastric tubes minimize perioperative complications.

Table 19.1 Etiology of esophageal strictures

Benign	Malignant
Eosinophilic esophagitis	Adenocarcinoma
Peptic stricture	Squamous cell carcinoma
Medication-induced stricture	
Schatzki ring	

19.2.2 Esophageal Strictures

Strictures of the esophagus could be benign or malignant (Table 19.1) and typically present with solid food dysphagia, progressing to dysphagia for liquids in severe strictures. Associated regurgitation and weight loss can also occur. Diagnosis is by barium esophagogram and endoscopy. Tissue diagnosis with biopsies and dilation or stenting can be performed at endoscopy for the relief of symptoms. Adequate therapy of the stricture prior to surgery reduces the risk of aspiration.

19.2.3 Esophageal Motility Disorders

Primary and secondary neuromuscular disorders of the esophagus (Table 19.2) present with dysphagia, chest pain, or heartburn. Diagnosis is made by barium esophagogram, endoscopy, and esophageal manometry findings. Optimizing medical management, suctioning the esophageal contents prior to induction of anesthesia, limiting anticholinergic drug use in induction of anesthesia, and using proton pump inhibitors to

Table 19.2 Esophageal motility disorders

Primary	Secondary
Achalasia	Reflux-related dysmotility
Distal esophageal spasm	Scleroderma and other rheumatologic disorders
Hypercontractile (jackhammer) esophagus	Chagas' disease
Hypertensive LES	
Nutcracker (high-pressure) esophagus	

decrease the volume of gastric reflux and prokinetics like metoclopramide and domperidone help decrease the risk of aspiration in the perioperative period.

19.2.4 Gastroesophageal Reflux Disease

Gastroesophageal reflux disease (GERD) is a condition, which develops when the reflux of gastric contents causes troublesome symptoms and/or complications [6]. GERD is prevalent worldwide, particularly in the developed world, and this is increasing because of the epidemic of obesity [7]. The incompetence of the lower esophageal sphincter (LES), esophageal dysmotility, the presence of a hiatal hernia, reflux of gastric and duodenal contents, and increased transdiaphragmatic pressure gradient all play a role in the pathophysiology of GERD. Heartburn and regurgitation are the typical symptoms of GERD. Some patients report dysphagia and less commonly present with noncardiac chest pain. Atypical symptoms include respiratory symptoms such as chronic cough, aspiration pneumonia, pulmonary fibrosis, hoarseness, globus, and dental erosions [8]. GERD is usually diagnosed by careful symptom evaluation, and a trial proton pump inhibitor (PPI) therapy is initiated to confirm the diagnosis [9]. Endoscopy is performed in severe or refractory cases and may help in confirming the diagnosis with findings of esophagitis and exclude other etiologies. However, endoscopy can be normal in up to 60% of patients with GERD confirmed by ambulatory pH monitoring which is considered the gold standard for diagnosis [10]. Lifestyle measures, histamine-receptor antagonists, and PPIs have been the mainstay of therapy of GERD. PPIs are preferred because they are more effective than histamine-receptor antagonists in alleviating symptoms and healing esophagitis [11]. Endoscopic and surgical therapies to augment the LES mechanism are reserved for refractory cases.

In patients at high risk of reflux, precautions to reduce the perioperative risk of aspiration should be undertaken. These include gastric decompression and reduction of gastric secretions with PPIs. Adjunctive therapy with metoclopramide may increase gastric emptying and LES pressure thereby reducing reflux. Avoiding opiates and anticholinergics and anesthetic techniques like induction while awake and cricoid pressure may reduce the risk of aspiration [12].

19.3 Gastric Disorders

19.3.1 Gastroparesis

Gastroparesis is a syndrome of significantly delayed gastric emptying in the absence of mechanical obstruction. Cardinal symptoms include early satiety, postprandial fullness, nausea, vomiting, bloating, and upper abdominal pain. Diabetes and postsurgical, idiopathic, or postviral gastroparesis are the most common associated conditions. Less commonly associated conditions include Parkinsonism, paraneoplastic disease, and scleroderma. Gastric neuromuscular abnormalities, smooth muscle dysfunction, and pylorospasm play a role in the pathophysiology of gastroparesis. Dietary modification to promote gastric emptying and prokinetics like metoclopramide and domperidone help in alleviating symptoms [13]. Perioperative management to reduce the risk of aspiration should include measures as described above for severe GERD along with management of the associated conditions.

19.3.2 Gastric Outlet Obstruction

Congenital and acquired gastric outlet obstruction can present with symptoms similar to gastroparesis. Prolonged vomiting may cause dehydration and hypochloremic-hypokalemic metabolic alkalosis secondary to the loss of gastric juice rich in hydrogen and chloride.

Acquired gastric outlet obstruction can be due to benign causes like peptic ulcer disease, caustic injury, acute and chronic pancreatitis, Crohn's disease, NSAID-induced strictures, annular or ectopic pancreas, and benign polyps and gastroduodenal tumors. Locally advanced primary gastric, pancreatic, and duodenal malignancies or metastatic intra- and extra-abdominal cancers cause malignant GOO. Correction of electrolyte abnormalities, treatment of the underlying cause, and relieving the obstruction by endoscopic balloon dilation for benign obstruction and stenting for malignant obstruction help alleviate symptoms and reduce the perioperative risk of aspiration [14, 15].

19.4 Ileocolonic Disorders

While colonic disease is common, e.g., irritable bowel syndrome, diverticulosis, and adenomatous polyps, these have no impact on anesthesia or technical aspects of maxillofacial surgery. The exception to this is inflammatory bowel disease (IBD), given the inflammatory nature of the condition, its systemic impact, associated extraintestinal disorders, and complexity of its medical management.

19.4.1 Inflammatory Bowel Disease

19.4.1.1 Prevalence and Pathophysiology

Idiopathic inflammatory bowel disease comprises two types of chronic intestinal disorders: Crohn's disease (CD) and ulcerative colitis (UC). Inflammatory bowel disease results from an inappropriate inflammatory response to intestinal microbes in a genetically susceptible host. Inflammatory bowel disease affects approximately 1.4 million Americans, and its peak onset is in persons 15–30 years of age.

Crohn's disease generally involves the ileum and colon, but it can affect any region of the intestine, often discontinuously. Ulcerative colitis involves the rectum and may affect part of the colon or the entire colon (pancolitis) in an uninterrupted pattern. In Crohn's disease, the inflammation is often transmural, whereas in ulcerative colitis the inflammation is typically confined to the mucosa. Crohn's disease can be associated with intestinal granulomas, strictures, and fistulas, but these are not typical findings in ulcerative colitis. Cigarette smoking affects these two diseases differently: smokers are at increased risk for Crohn's disease and tend to have more severe disease, whereas former smokers and nonsmokers are at greater risk for ulcerative colitis. Patients with inflammatory bowel disease are at risk for primary sclerosing cholangitis, ankylosing spondylitis, and psoriasis [16–18].

19.4.1.2 Disease Manifestations

Classically, UC presents with bloody diarrhea, abdominal pain, urgency, and tenesmus. The diagnosis of UC is made on the basis of the typical symptoms, endoscopic evidence of continuous colonic inflammation, which almost always begins in the rectum, and chronic active colitis on colorectal biopsies.

Crohn's disease is a clinical diagnosis that integrates history and physical findings with objective data from imaging and laboratory studies, including histopathology, and should neither be based nor excluded on any one variable or result. Typical symptoms include abdominal pain and cramping and diarrhea with or without blood or mucus. Evidence-based diagnostic techniques for suspected Crohn's disease have been published by the European Crohn's and Colitis Organisation [19].

19.4.1.3 Chronic Medications Used

In UC, disease severity and patient preference dictate the appropriate treatment options that consist of mesalamine, corticosteroids, immunosuppressive drugs like thiopurines and methotrexate, and biologic agents, which are monoclonal antibodies to tumor necrosis factor-alpha (TNF-α) and adhesion molecules.

Treatment of CD is based on disease phenotype, activity, comorbidities, and other individual characteristics of the drug and patient. Corticosteroids, immunosuppressive drugs, and biologic agents used to treat UC are also used in treatment of CD. In most cases, a fast-acting short-term use agent (i.e., steroids or anti-TNF) to achieve rapid symptom relief and disease control is combined with thiopurines or methotrexate for long-term maintenance. Surgery in both UC and Crohn's is reserved for cases where there are complications, neoplasia, or refractoriness to medical therapy.

19.4.1.4 Preoperative Optimization

Regardless of the type of surgery, adequate control of IBD is paramount for the best outcomes, given the systemic nature of the disease. Common extraintestinal complications of IBD include anemia and malnutrition, which need to be addressed to reduce associated perioperative risk. Intravenous iron therapy for iron deficiency anemia and enteral or parenteral nutrition therapy for severe malnutrition may be needed. Exclusive enteral nutrition has been shown to reduce the postoperative septic complications of fistulizing Crohn's disease [20].

Perioperative medication management in IBD has a significant impact on postoperative outcomes.

Aminosalicylates are poorly absorbed and are primarily eliminated by the kidneys. In patients in whom decreased glomerular filtration is more likely (age, >65 years; American Society of Anesthesiologists physical status score, IV or V; revised cardiac risk index score, >2; chronic heart disease), a reasonable approach in the perioperative phase is to discontinue mesalamine a day before surgery with resumption 3 days after surgery [21].

Corticosteroid use in the preoperative period has been shown to increase postoperative complications (odds ratio (OR 1.41), 95% confidence interval (CI) 1.07–1.87), particularly infectious complications (OR 1.68, 95% CI 1.24–2.28), in a dose-dependent manner (OR 2.04 (95% CI 1.28–3.26) [22]. Whenever possible the dose of steroid should be reduced to prednisone < 20 mg/day, or equivalent and routine use of stress-dose steroids should also be avoided [23]. In general, patients receiving 5 mg or less of prednisone each day, alternate-day glucocorticoids, or any dose of glucocorticoids for less than 3 weeks are not considered to have a suppressed hypothalamic-pituitary-adrenal axis and do not require "stress-dose" glucocorticoids. In contrast, patients receiving more than 20 mg/d of prednisone (or its equivalent) for more than 3 weeks or with features of Cushing syndrome should be assumed to have a suppressed hypothalamic-pituitary-adrenal axis and considered for "stress-dose" glucocorticoid supplementation perioperatively [24].

Purine analogs (6-mercaptopurine/azathioprine) are used as steroid-sparing maintenance agents in IBD and bone marrow suppression. Azathioprine is known to be antagonistic to neuromuscular blocking agents. Reversal of neuromuscular blockade produced by d-tubocurarine and increase of the neuromuscular blockade produced by succinylcholine have been described [25]. In patients taking azathioprine with end-stage renal failure undergoing renal transplantation, dose adjustments to increase atracurium by 37%, vecuronium by 20%, and pancuronium by 45% have been suggested. Immunosuppressive therapy with purine analogs does not seem to affect postoperative outcomes [22, 26, 27]. It has been recommended, on the basis of weak evidence and physiologic considerations, that thiopurines be stopped on the day of surgery and resumed 3 days afterward because of their renal elimination and potential for toxic metabolite accumulation [28].

Methotrexate competitively inhibits the enzyme dihydrofolate reductase, impairing DNA synthesis and therefore cellular replication. Concern has been raised about the potential interaction between nitrous oxide used for anesthesia and methotrexate. Patients who receive methotrexate during the immediate postoperative period (within 6 h) after nitrous oxide-based anesthesia often develop severe bone marrow depression and mucositis. However, no quantitative data for dose-effect interactions are available. Existing data do not suggest a significant increase in the risk of perioperative infections or impaired wound healing. Given the lack of data, in patients with a history of previous or severe septic complications, it may be reasonable to discontinue methotrexate 1 week before surgery and resume it no sooner than 1 week after or when the surgical wound has successfully healed [24].

19.4.1.5 Postoperative Outcomes

Multiple studies have been conducted to evaluate the effect of biologic agents on postoperative outcomes in IBD. Infliximab has been the most studied agent with limited or no data on other agents like adalimumab and certolizumab. These studies are limited by multiple confounding factors, such as lack of homogeneity of included conditions (both CD and UC), procedures (with or without anastomoses), disease severity (more complex disease in the group receiving anti-TNF), outcomes (all complications vs. infectious complications), different definitions of complications, and lack of prospective randomized studies. Many retrospective studies have shown no difference in terms of immediate and late (within 30 days) complication rates between patients who were or were not exposed to anti-TNF agents prior to or after surgery. Most evidence suggests that infliximab can be used safely in the perioperative period [23, 24]. However, it may be prudent to schedule elective surgery around the time a dose of the biologic is due and administer the dose as soon as the absence of postoperative infectious complications is confirmed, typically within 2–3 weeks.

19.4.1.6 Thromboembolic Events in IBD

Patients with IBD have long been known to be at increased risk of thromboembolism. In surgical patients with IBD, the overall risk of venous thromboembolism is the sum of many risk factors, ranging from a disease-induced hypercoagulable state, exacerbated by steroid use, malnutrition, anemia, and thrombocytosis, to the risks due to operative characteristics, such as emergency surgery, previous pelvic surgery, length of procedures, and immobility [29]. During the perioperative period, patients with IBD should receive prophylaxis based on American College of Chest Physicians Evidence-Based Clinical Practice Guidelines [30]. However, a recent study demonstrated that standard prophylactic low molecular weight heparin may be insufficient for venous thromboembolism prophylaxis in patients with IBD. An elevated risk of postoperative deep venous thrombosis in patients with UC (OR, 7.4; 95% CI, 1.4–44.4; $P = .017$) has been described despite prophylactic anticoagulation with 4000 IU/d of low molecular weight heparin. The rate of deep venous thrombosis in patients with UC was higher than in patients with colorectal cancer ($P = .009$) [31]. For patients undergoing surgery, prophylaxis with 5000 U of subcutaneous heparin three times daily, 40 mg of subcutaneous enoxaparin once daily, or 2.5–5.0 mg of subcutaneous fondaparinux daily has been recommended [24].

19.5 Pancreatic Disorders

19.5.1 Acute Pancreatitis

The incidence of acute pancreatitis in the United States varies from 4.9 to 73.4 per 100,000 patients. It is an acute inflammatory process of the pancreas with variable involvement of other regional tissues or remote organ systems. Clinically acute pancreatitis is diagnosed when two of the following three criteria are met: (1) symptoms consistent with pancreatitis, (2) a serum amylase or lipase level greater than three times the laboratory's upper limit of normal, and (3) radiologic imaging consistent with pancreatitis, usually using computed tomography (CT) or magnetic resonance imaging (MRI) [32, 33]. Gallstones and alcohol cause a majority of cases. Less common causes include drugs and toxins, hereditary and metabolic disorders like hyperlipidemia and hypercalcemia, infections, trauma, after thoracic or abdominal surgery (postoperative), and post-endoscopic retrograde cholangiopancreatography (ERCP). Severe pancreatitis, characterized by organ failure, can often be associated with cardiac and respiratory failure and adult respiratory distress syndrome requiring mechanical ventilation. Fluid and electrolyte abnormalities from associated renal failure may require dialysis. Enteral nutrition compared to total parenteral nutrition is associated with fewer infectious complications, less multiple organ failure, and lower mortality [34]. Enteral nutrition via a nasojejunal tube is the preferred route although feeding via nasogastric tubes may be non-inferior [33]. Elective maxillofacial surgery should be deferred until organ failure improves significantly or resolves.

19.5.2 Chronic Pancreatitis

Chronic pancreatitis in the clinical context refers to a syndrome of destructive, inflammatory conditions that encompasses the many sequelae of long-standing pancreatic injury. The incidence rate in the United States is approximately 8 per 100,000 with a prevalence rate of about 50 per 100,000. It is more common in men, and most patients diagnosed are above the age of 40 [35]. Histologic changes from the normal pancreatic architecture include irregular fibrosis, acinar cell loss, islet cell loss, and inflammatory cell infiltrates. Diagnosis currently depends on identifying defined clinical, functional, morphologic, and histologic features that characterize the final common pathologic pathway of a variety of pancreatic disorders [36]. Risk factors for chronic pancreatitis are listed in Table 19.3. Characteristic abdominal pain, symptoms and signs of maldigestion, weight loss, and in the late stages with diabetes mellitus are the presenting features. Diagnosis is established in at-risk patients, by documenting pancreatic exocrine insufficiency with low stool elastase or serum trypsin levels and/or changes related to chronic inflammation, fibrosis, and calcification on CT, MRI, magnetic resonance cholangiopancreatography, endoscopic ultrasound, or ERCP. Treatment includes avoiding alcohol and tobacco and nonnarcotic and narcotic analgesics, and if pain persists, in those with a dilated pancreatic duct, endoscopic and surgical therapy can be tried. Pancreatic enzyme replacement therapy corrects symptoms of exocrine insufficiency, including steatorrhea, fat-soluble vitamin, and calcium deficiency and weight loss. In a small case series, jejunal feeding has been shown to improve weight as well as to reduce abdominal pain, GI side effects, and narcotic use and can be used to reduce malnutrition-associated perioperative complications [37].

Table 19.3 Risk factors for chronic pancreatitis

Toxic-metabolic	Idiopathic
• Alcohol	Genetic
• Tobacco	Autoimmune
• Hypercalcemia	Recurrent and severe acute pancreatitis
• Hypertriglyceridemia	Obstruction of the pancreatic duct
• Chronic kidney disease	

19.6 Liver Disorders

The liver plays a vital role in metabolism of coagulation factors, bilirubin, and drugs and/or toxins, as well as in protein synthesis and glucose homeostasis. Patients with liver disease are at an increased risk of complications, morbidity, and mortality with any major surgery, including maxillofacial surgery. Liver disease can be categorized as acute and chronic.

19.6.1 Acute Liver Injury

Acute liver injury frequently presents in otherwise healthy adults in their 30s and can result from hepatotoxicity (drugs or herbal or dietary supplements), viral hepatitis, autoimmune hepatitis, or ischemia [38]. It is characterized by acute increases in liver transaminases which may be asymptomatic and when severe can present with abdominal pain, nausea, vomiting, jaundice, pruritus, clay-colored stool, and dark urine. In its most severe form, acute liver injury leads to fulminant liver failure with accompanying coagulopathy and hepatic encephalopathy, where liver transplantation may be the only lifesaving option. The incidence of acute liver failure is estimated at less than ten cases per million persons per year and is therefore relatively rare [38]. Nevertheless, elective surgery should be postponed in the setting of acute liver injury, and even clinically urgent or emergent surgery should be avoided in patients with fulminant liver failure.

19.6.2 Chronic Liver Disease

Chronic liver disease is much more common than acute liver injury, with an estimated prevalence of approximately 15% in the general adult population in the United States [39]. Liver disease appears to be more prevalent in patients undergoing head and neck surgery (6.8%) compared to other surgeries (3.3%) [40]. Common causes of chronic liver disease include nonalcoholic fatty liver disease, chronic viral hepatitis (hepatitis C infection mostly in the United States, hepatitis B less commonly), and alcohol abuse. Less common causes include autoimmune conditions (autoimmune hepatitis, primary sclerosing cholangitis, primary biliary cholangitis) and inherited metabolic diseases (hereditary hemochromatosis, alpha-1-antitrypsin deficiency, Wilson's disease). These chronic underlying liver conditions are not directly impacted by anesthesia or nonhepatic surgery. However, when they lead to advanced liver fibrosis and cirrhosis, they account for the majority of liver-related postoperative morbidity and mortality.

19.6.2.1 Preoperative Evaluation

In general, chronic liver disease is often asymptomatic, even in the setting of advanced but compensated disease, and, as a result, may not be recognized by the patient or their clinicians. It is important to identify any chronic liver condition ahead of planned surgery, to allow for appropriate evaluation and staging of liver disease, as well as to ensure optimal considerations in anesthesia and postoperative care. This highlights the need for vigilance during preoperative evaluation for risk factors for and potential signs and symptoms of chronic liver disease. These include taking a detailed history of alcohol use and illicit drug use, transfusion history and family history of liver disease. It is also important to query for symptoms of fatigue, edema, abdominal swelling, jaundice, pruritus, and altered mental status. Physical exam findings may include edema, spider angioma, palmar erythema, fluid wave or shifting abdominal dullness, male gynecomastia or testicular atrophy, and muscle wasting. Initial laboratory testing when liver disease is known or suspected should include a complete blood count (may identify thrombocytopenia or pancytopenia reflecting splenomegaly due to portal hypertension), complete metabolic profile and prothrombin time to assess for elevated transaminases, and hyperbilirubinemia, hypoalbuminemia, and coagulopathy to assess for liver synthetic dysfunction. Abdominal imaging by ultrasound is also reasonable in suspected cases of liver disease, which may identify a nodular liver contour of cirrhosis and features of portal hypertension, such as ascites and splenomegaly. When liver disease is established, formal preoperative evaluation by the anesthesiologist performing the anesthesia is recommended, particularly in cases of advanced liver disease. Specific preoperative measures are addressed in relation to individual risk factors discussed below.

19.6.2.2 Liver Disease and Operative Risk

Liver disease, particularly when advanced, poses significant anesthetic and operative challenges with associated risks of bleeding, infection, prolonged hospital stays, deterioration in liver function, and increased mortality. These risks are related to multiple factors that warrant individual consideration.

(a) Limitations in hepatic functional capacity put patients at risk for coagulopathy, hyperbilirubinemia, hypoalbuminemia, and impaired nitrogen metabolism. In advanced disease, this can impact metabolism of neuromuscular blocking agents as well as opiates and benzodiazepines, with undesirably prolonged effects.
(b) Portal hypertension associated with cirrhosis puts patients at risk for (1) ascites or hepatic hydrothorax which may limit pulmonary

vital capacity, (2) esophageal or gastric varices which are asymptomatic but can lead to life-threatening acute upper gastrointestinal bleeding if large and challenged by aggressive volume expansion, and (3) hepatic encephalopathy which can lead to alteration in mental status and coma under stress of infection, gastrointestinal bleeding, dehydration, or sedating medications. Patients with decompensated cirrhosis may require therapeutic paracentesis or thoracentesis, knowledge of presence and size of esophageal or gastric varices, and optimization of treatment of hepatic encephalopathy with lactulose and/or rifaximin. One would not expect collateral vessels that form in the setting of cirrhosis to pose direct risk in relation to the anatomically distinct surgical fields of maxillofacial surgery.

(c) Patients with decompensated cirrhosis have an activated renin-angiotensin system and are at an increased risk for both fluid overload from salt and water retention. They are also at risk of dehydration from over-diuresis and gastrointestinal fluid and electrolyte losses from lactulose therapy. Patients may also be intravascularly depleted despite severe edema, anasarca, or third spacing (e.g., ascites). These patients need serial evaluation and correction of fluid, electrolyte, and acid-base imbalances in the preoperative, intraoperative, and postoperative periods.

(d) Renal dysfunction is common in decompensated cirrhosis and may be multifactorial, with acute kidney injury occurring frequently in hospitalized patients. In most cases the etiology is prerenal, but one must consider potential obstruction uropathy and avoid nephrotoxins such as nonsteroidal anti-inflammatories at all time, with awareness of the nephrotoxic potential of intravenous contrast if given within 2–3 days of planned surgery. Avoiding hypovolemia and splanchnic hypoperfusion and vigilance for postoperative infections or sepsis, which could precipitate hepatorenal syndrome, are key to avoiding renal injury perioperatively.

(e) Cirrhotic cardiomyopathy is an increasingly recognized but poorly understood consequence of end-stage liver disease. It is characterized by a blunted response to pharmacologic or physiologic stress in the absence of decreased resting cardiac output or contractility [41]. This may in part be explained by splanchnic arterial vasodilation and impaired cardiac calcium signaling, with clinical features of high-output cardiac failure. Other cardiac conditions to be aware of in this population include diastolic dysfunction, which may be present in approximately 27–37% of cirrhotics [42, 43], but there is little data on impact on nonhepatic surgery. There are no distinct electrocardiographic abnormalities although QT interval prolongation is common in end-stage liver disease and can be associated with diastolic dysfunction [43]. It would be prudent to obtain baseline electrocardiograms and echocardiograms in patients with no liver disease, particularly in the presence of a hyperdynamic circulation, hypertension, or signs and symptoms of cardiopulmonary compromise.

(f) Coagulopathy and thrombocytopenia are common in patients with end-stage liver disease, which pose a risk for intra- and postoperative bleeding complications. Standard coagulation parameters are uniformly tested in this population including prothrombin time, activated partial thromboplastin time, and occasionally plasma fibrinogen. Common approaches for treating prolonged prothrombin time and INR include vitamin K supplementation (10 mg orally per day) for a week prior to planned surgery and transfusion with fresh frozen plasma and/or cryoprecipitate as needed immediately before surgery. Similarly, thrombocytopenia is commonly addressed with platelet transfusion immediately before surgery. The use of thrombopoietin receptor agonists has undergone preliminary study in patients with chronic liver disease to increase platelet counts prior to elective procedures [44]. Although further study is needed, the approach could be considered in conjunction with an experienced hematologist.

There are no universally agreed-upon thresholds for blood product transfusion in end-stage liver disease prior to surgery. There is evidence however that the standard coagulation parameters may not accurately reflect bleeding risk in these patients [45]. Thromboelastography is an assay that measures clot formation, strength, and dissolution, may better reflect total clotting function, and is used by some centers to guide intraoperative management of blood product transfusion during liver transplantation [45]. At present, there are no uniform guidelines for use of thromboelastography in perioperative care of cirrhotic patients.

(g) Cirrhosis can be associated with a number of pulmonary complications, including the aforementioned ascites and hepatohydrothorax (accumulation of ascites in the pleural space via diaphragmatic defects), which can cause restrictive pulmonary dysfunction by limiting diaphragmatic contraction and lung expansion, respectively. Pulmonary complications of cirrhosis include hepatopulmonary syndrome (HPS) and portopulmonary hypertension (PPH), which are pathophysiologically associated with pulmonary vascular dilation and shunting and pulmonary arteriolar vasoconstriction, respectively.

Hepatopulmonary syndrome is associated with inadequate oxygenation of human due to intrapulmonary shunting. While it is present in approximately 25% of patients with cirrhosis, it is severe (PaO_2 <60 mmHg) in a small subset of patients [46]. Clinically it is marked by exertional dyspnea and platypnea and clinically by orthodeoxia. Significant HPS can be screened for by room air pulse oximetry (threshold <96%) and confirmed by agitated saline contrast echocardiography. There is no meaningful pharmacologic therapy for HPS, and treatment is supportive (oxygen supplementation) to ensure adequate oxygenation. Patients with severe or very severe (PaO_2 <50 mmHg) disease may be expected to require prolonged mechanical ventilation and pulmonary care postoperatively.

Portopulmonary hypertension is defined as pulmonary arterial hypertension (mean arterial pressure > 25 mmHg and pulmonary capillary wedge pressure <15 mmHg) in patients with portal hypertension and no alternative causes. It is present in 2% of patients with portal hypertension [47] and in advanced stages can be associated with right heart failure. When PPH is recognized, patients are treated with vasodilator therapy which may include prostacyclin analogs, phosphodiesterase inhibitors, or endothelin receptor antagonists. These treatments need to be continued throughout the perioperative period, and patients may require intraoperative inhaled nitrous oxide to maintain adequate vasodilation of the pulmonary vasculature. Patients with HPS and PPH should be evaluated preoperatively in conjunction with an experienced pulmonologist.

(h) Patients with advanced liver disease are at risk for muscle wasting and malnutrition associated with increased risk of infections and sepsis, hepatorenal syndrome, and major hepatic complications [48]. While sarcopenia may not be easily reversed, every effort should be made to ensure adequate protein calorie intake prior to surgery, in coordination with a dietitian experienced with this population.

(i) Patients with cirrhosis are considered to be at increased risk of bacterial infection. In a large prospective study, the risk of postoperative infection following non-colorectal abdominal surgery was increased in patients with cirrhosis (OR 2.45) [49]. Vigilance is recommended to rule out clinical and subclinical infections in these patients preoperatively. This should include screening for urinary tract infections, pneumonia, cellulitis, and spontaneous bacterial peritonitis. The latter requires a diagnostic paracentesis with white blood cell count and differential, with a polymorphonuclear cell count of 250 per mm^3 or greater indicating presence of spontaneous bacterial peritonitis.

19.6.2.3 Prediction of Postoperative Mortality in Cirrhosis

The risk of mortality with general anesthesia and surgery is considerable in end-stage liver disease. The 30-day mortality rate after major head and neck surgery in the American College of Surgeons National Surgical Quality Improvement Program (2005–2013) was as high as 14.6% and sixfold higher in patients with advanced liver disease [40]. A number of observational studies identify both the Child-Turcotte-Pugh (CTP) classification (Table 19.4) and the Model for End-Stage Liver Disease (MELD) as important predictors of postoperative mortality in cirrhosis. The CTP classification was described first, and postoperative mortality risk is estimated to range from 10% in class A, 30–31% in class B, and 76–82% in class C cirrhosis [50, 51]. Postoperative mortality is also substantially higher in emergency surgery (44–50%) compared with elective surgery (18–20%) [51, 52]. Postoperative mortality was lower when mainly laparoscopic surgery was performed at an institution with dedicated expertise in liver disease and transplantation [53].

The Model for End-Stage Liver Disease is a mathematical formula based on bilirubin, INR, and creatinine and is used to predict mortality in patients with end-stage liver disease. In more recent studies, MELD was found to be superior to CTP in predicting postoperative mortality [52, 54]. In the largest series from the Mayo Clinic (including 772 patients with cirrhosis undergoing major cardiovascular orthopedic and digestive surgery) MELD, American Society of Anesthesiologist, class, and age predicted mortality [54]. Thirty-day mortality increased linearly with MELD from 5.7% with MELD < 8 to >50% with MELD > 20. The Mayo Clinic maintains an online postoperative risk calculator in patients with cirrhosis based on this study, which can be useful in daily practice [55].

Both CTP and MELD strongly predict postoperative mortality and highlight the importance of advanced liver disease as a major driver of that risk. This underscores the importance for assessing the presence and severity of liver disease, other medical comorbidities, as well as the scope, timing, and urgency of surgery in these patients. A case can easily be made, based on these data and the complexity involved, to defer surgery in patients with decompensated cirrhosis to institutions with expertise in advanced liver disease and transplantation. Importantly, these centers are staffed by hepatologists, anesthesiologists, and other specialists (nephrologists, pulmonologists, cardiologists, neurologists, and infectious disease experts) experienced with this patient population.

19.6.2.4 Intraoperative Care

In addition to the challenges outlined above, a number of factors specific to patients with liver disease may guide the intraoperative care of these patients. These include (1) increased risk of reduced total hepatic blood flow with general anesthesia with resultant liver injury, (2) decreased albumin with reduced drug binding, and (3) impaired metabolism of drugs and associated toxins with prolongation of half-life of anesthetic, sedative, and analgesic drugs. Therefore, the general principles are to avoid hepatic hypoperfusion, preferentially using nonhepatically cleared drugs where possible, and caution with dosing of hepatically metabolized drugs while avoiding potentially hepatotoxic ones.

Table 19.4 The Child-Turcotte-Pugh classification system. Class A (5, 6), B (7–9), C (10–15)

Points	1	2	3
Prothrombin/INR	<1.7	1.7–2.2	>2.2
Albumin (g/L)	>3.5	2.8–3.5	<2.8
Bilirubin (mg/dL)	<2	2–3	>3
Ascites	None	Controlled	Uncontrolled
Hepatic encephalopathy	None	Controlled	Uncontrolled

General anesthesia is associated with decreased portal and hepatic blood flow, even in otherwise healthy individuals, particularly early in the course of anesthesia [56, 57]. Patients with liver disease are at increased risk of hepatic decompensation with the use of general anesthesia, possibly due to baseline cardiovascular changes such as decreased systemic vascular resistance, increase cardiac index, and inadequate compensatory mechanisms to hypovolemia or hemorrhage intraoperatively [56]. Where possible, local anesthesia is preferred to general anesthesia in patients with advanced liver disease.

Of the inhaled anesthetics, isoflurane and newer agents such sevoflurane undergo less hepatic metabolism than halothane and enflurane, and are associated with less systemic vasodilation and negative inotropic effect, and less impact of decreased hepatic perfusion [56]. There is also a much lower risk of hepatotoxicity with isoflurane as compared with halothane, which should be avoided in patients with liver disease [56].

Of the neuromuscular blocking agents, atracurium and cisatracurium are favored in patients with advanced liver disease or buttery obstruction as they are not metabolized by the liver or kidneys [58]. They are preferred over other neuromuscular blocking agents which may have a prolonged effect in patients with liver disease due to diminished plasma pseudocholinesterase activity, increased volume of distribution, and impaired biliary excretion.

Analgesic and sedating agents, such as opiates benzodiazepines and barbiturates, can be expected to have prolonged effect in patients with liver disease due to variable metabolism of these agents. These can lead to prolonged sedation and precipitation of hepatic encephalopathy. Shorter-acting agents are therefore preferred, such as fentanyl, with minimization if not avoidance of benzodiazepines where possible.

19.6.2.5 Postoperative Care

The same principle guiding preoperative and intraoperative care should be applied in postoperative monitoring and management of patients with liver disease. This includes similar attention to the choice of analgesic agents, as well as those frequency considerations, with attention to mental status for signs or symptoms of hepatic encephalopathy. Attention to maintaining adequate intravascular volume and avoidance of nephrotoxins is important to prevent prerenal kidney injury.

Vigilance for infections is important as patients can have an attenuated clinical picture early on an infection. Aggressive care is recommended even in cases of suspected infection until culture results are available. This would include attention to volume status and resuscitation, as well as broad antibiotic coverage to include hospital-acquired infections. Cirrhotic patients with severe sepsis are at an increased risk of adrenal insufficiency or blunted cortisol response to corticotropin. This was described in 50% of such patients in one study, correlating with severity of liver disease, and is associated with worse outcomes [59]. Consideration of stress-dose steroids is important in the setting.

An important aspect of care is providing adequate deep venous thrombosis prophylaxis. Patients with advanced liver disease often have prolonged prothrombin time and have traditionally been considered to have hypocoagulable state as a result. However, objective evidence indicates that these patients are deficient in both pro- and anticoagulant factors [60] and that cirrhosis is not protective against but may increase the risk of venous thrombotic events (hazard ratio 1.7, 95% CI 1.05–2.78) [61]. Therefore, deep venous thrombosis prophylaxis is recommended, even in patients with cirrhosis, and may include unfractionated heparin or low molecular weight heparin provided this is deemed safe from a surgical site bleeding perspective and platelet count is >50,000 per microliter.

Finally, deterioration in liver disease or new decompensation of previously compensated cirrhosis may not develop in the early postoperative period. While there is no clear data to guide this, it is recommended to follow patients with advanced liver disease or cirrhosis for up to 3 months postoperatively for optimal safety.

References

1. van Overbeek JJ. Pathogenesis and methods of treatment of Zenker's diverticulum. Ann Otol Rhinol Laryngol. 2003;112(7):583–93.
2. Sen P, Kumar G, Bhattacharyya AK. Pharyngeal pouch: associations and complications. Eur Arch Otorhinolaryngol. 2006;263(5):463–8.
3. Aouad MT, Berzina CE, Baraka AS. Aspiration pneumonia after anesthesia in a patient with a Zenker diverticulum. Anesthesiology. 2000;92(6):1837–9.
4. Schima W, Schober E, Stacher G, Franz P, Uranitsch K, Pokieser P, et al. Association of midoesophageal diverticula with oesophageal motor disorders. Videofluoroscopy and manometry. Acta Radiol. 1997;38(1):108–14.
5. D'Journo XB, Ferraro P, Martin J, Chen LQ, Duranceau A. Lower oesophageal sphincter dysfunction is part of the functional abnormality in epiphrenic diverticulum. Br J Surg. 2009;96(8):892–900.
6. Vakil N, van Zanten SV, Kahrilas P, Dent J, Jones R, Global Consensus Group. The Montreal definition and classification of gastroesophageal reflux disease: a global evidence-based consensus. Am J Gastroenterol. 2006;101(8):1900–20. quiz 43
7. El-Serag HB, Sweet S, Winchester CC, Dent J. Update on the epidemiology of gastro-oesophageal reflux disease: a systematic review. Gut. 2014;63(6): 871–80.
8. Patti MG. An evidence-based approach to the treatment of gastroesophageal reflux disease. JAMA Surg. 2016;151(1):73–8.
9. Sonnenberg A, Delco F, El-Serag HB. Empirical therapy versus diagnostic tests in gastroesophageal reflux disease: a medical decision analysis. Dig Dis Sci. 1998;43(5):1001–8.
10. Hirano I, Richter JE. Practice parameters Committee of the American College of G. ACG practice guidelines: esophageal reflux testing. Am J Gastroenterol. 2007;102(3):668–85.
11. Labenz J, Malfertheiner P. Treatment of uncomplicated reflux disease. World J Gastroenterol. 2005;11(28):4291–9.
12. Glassman MS, Dozer AJ, Newman LJ. Gastroesophageal reflux in neurologically impaired children: perioperative evaluation and management. South Med J. 1992;85(3):289–92.
13. Camilleri M, Parkman HP, Shafi MA, Abell TL, Gerson L. American College of G. Clinical guideline: management of gastroparesis. Am J Gastroenterol. 2013;108(1):18–37. quiz 8.
14. Kochhar R, Kochhar S. Endoscopic balloon dilation for benign gastric outlet obstruction in adults. World J Gastrointest Endosc. 2010;2(1):29–35.
15. van Halsema EE, Rauws EA, Fockens P, van Hooft JE. Self-expandable metal stents for malignant gastric outlet obstruction: a pooled analysis of prospective literature. World J Gastroenterol. 2015;21(43):12,468–81.
16. Abraham C, Cho JH. Inflammatory bowel disease. N Engl J Med. 2009;361(21):2066–78.
17. Bernstein CN, Wajda A, Blanchard JF. The clustering of other chronic inflammatory diseases in inflammatory bowel disease: a population-based study. Gastroenterology. 2005;129(3):827–36.
18. Loftus EV Jr, Sandborn WJ. Epidemiology of inflammatory bowel disease. Gastroenterol Clin North Am. 2002;31(1):1–20.
19. Van Assche G, Dignass A, Panes J, Beaugerie L, Karagiannis J, Allez M, et al. The second European evidence-based consensus on the diagnosis and management of Crohn's disease: definitions and diagnosis. J Crohns Colitis. 2010;4(1):7–27.
20. Li G, Ren J, Wang G, Hu D, Gu G, Liu S, et al. Preoperative exclusive enteral nutrition reduces the postoperative septic complications of fistulizing Crohn's disease. Eur J Clin Nutr. 2014;68(4):441–6.
21. Borthwick E, Ferguson A. Perioperative acute kidney injury: risk factors, recognition, management, and outcomes. BMJ. 2010;341:c3365.
22. Subramanian V, Saxena S, Kang JY, Pollok RC. Preoperative steroid use and risk of postoperative complications in patients with inflammatory bowel disease undergoing abdominal surgery. Am J Gastroenterol. 2008;103(9):2373–81.
23. Spinelli A, Allocca M, Jovani M, Danese S. Review article: optimal preparation for surgery in Crohn's disease. Aliment Pharmacol Ther. 2014;40(9):1009–22.
24. Kumar A, Auron M, Aneja A, Mohr F, Jain A, Shen B. Inflammatory bowel disease: perioperative pharmacological considerations. Mayo Clin Proc. 2011;86(8):748–57.
25. Dretchen KL, Morgenroth VH 3rd, Standaert FG, Walts LF. Azathioprine: effects on neuromuscular transmission. Anesthesiology. 1976;45(6):604–9.
26. Aberra FN, Lewis JD, Hass D, Rombeau JL, Osborne B, Lichtenstein GR. Corticosteroids and immunomodulators: postoperative infectious complication risk in inflammatory bowel disease patients. Gastroenterology. 2003;125(2):320–7.
27. Colombel JF, Loftus EV Jr, Tremaine WJ, Pemberton JH, Wolff BG, Young-Fadok T, et al. Early postoperative complications are not increased in patients with Crohn's disease treated perioperatively with infliximab or immunosuppressive therapy. Am J Gastroenterol. 2004;99(5):878–83.
28. Rosandich PA, Kelley JT 3rd, Conn DL. Perioperative management of patients with rheumatoid arthritis in the era of biologic response modifiers. Curr Opin Rheumatol. 2004;16(3):192–8.
29. Fleming FJ, Kim MJ, Salloum RM, Young KC, Monson JR. How much do we need to worry about venous thromboembolism after hospital discharge? A study of colorectal surgery patients using the National Surgical Quality Improvement Program database. Dis Colon Rectum. 2010;53(10):1355–60.
30. Douketis JD, Spyropoulos AC, Spencer FA, Mayr M, Jaffer AK, Eckman MH, et al. Perioperative management of antithrombotic therapy: antithrombotic ther-

apy and prevention of thrombosis, 9th ed: American College of Chest Physicians Evidence-Based Clinical Practice Guidelines. Chest. 2012;141(2 Suppl):e326S–50S.
31. Scarpa M, Pilon F, Pengo V, Romanato G, Ruffolo C, Erroi F, et al. Deep venous thrombosis after surgery for inflammatory bowel disease: is standard dose low molecular weight heparin prophylaxis enough? World J Surg. 2010;34(7):1629–36.
32. Banks PA, Bollen TL, Dervenis C, Gooszen HG, Johnson CD, Sarr MG, et al. Classification of acute pancreatitis—2012: revision of the Atlanta classification and definitions by international consensus. Gut. 2013;62(1):102–11.
33. Tenner S, Baillie J, DeWitt J, Vege SS. American College of G. American College of Gastroenterology guideline: management of acute pancreatitis. Am J Gastroenterol. 2013;108(9):1400–15. 16.
34. Al-Omran M, Albalawi ZH, Tashkandi MF, Al-Ansary LA. Enteral versus parenteral nutrition for acute pancreatitis. Cochrane Database Syst Rev. 2010;1:CD002837.
35. Yadav D, Lowenfels AB. The epidemiology of pancreatitis and pancreatic cancer. Gastroenterology. 2013;144(6):1252–61.
36. Etemad B, Whitcomb DC. Chronic pancreatitis: diagnosis, classification, and new genetic developments. Gastroenterology. 2001;120(3):682–707.
37. Stanga Z, Giger U, Marx A, DeLegge MH. Effect of jejunal long-term feeding in chronic pancreatitis. JPEN J Parenter Enteral Nutr. 2005;29(1):12–20.
38. Bernal W, Wendon J. Acute liver failure. New Engl J Med. 2013;369(26):2525–34.
39. Younossi ZM, Stepanova M, Afendy M, Fang Y, Younossi Y, Mir H, et al. Changes in the prevalence of the most common causes of chronic liver diseases in the United States from 1988 to 2008. Clin Gastroenterol Hepatol. 2011;9(6):524–30. e1; quiz e60.
40. Cramer JD, Patel UA, Samant S, Yang A, Smith SS. Liver disease in patients undergoing head and neck surgery: incidence and risk for postoperative complications. Laryngoscope. 2017;127(1):102–9.
41. Donovan CL, Marcovitz PA, Punch JD, Bach DS, Brown KA, Lucey MR, et al. Two-dimensional and dobutamine stress echocardiography in the preoperative assessment of patients with end-stage liver disease prior to orthotopic liver transplantation. Transplantation. 1996;61(8):1180–8.
42. Falletta C, Fili D, Nugara C, Di Gesaro G, Mina C, Baravoglia CM, et al. Diastolic dysfunction diagnosed by tissue Doppler imaging in cirrhotic patients: Prevalence and its possible relationship with clinical outcome. Eur J Intern Med. 2015;26(10):830–4.
43. Karagiannakis DS, Vlachogiannakos J, Anastasiadis G, Vafiadis-Zouboulis I, Ladas SD. Frequency and severity of cirrhotic cardiomyopathy and its possible relationship with bacterial endotoxemia. Dig Dis Sci. 2013;58(10):3029–36.
44. Qureshi K, Patel S, Meillier A. The use of thrombopoietin receptor agonists for correction of thrombocytopenia prior to elective procedures in chronic liver diseases: review of current evidence. Int J Hepatol. 2016;2016:1802932.
45. Stravitz RT. Potential applications of thromboelastography in patients with acute and chronic liver disease. Gastroenterol Hepatol (N Y). 2012;8(8):513–20.
46. Schenk P, Schoniger-Hekele M, Fuhrmann V, Madl C, Silberhumer G, Muller C. Prognostic significance of the hepatopulmonary syndrome in patients with cirrhosis. Gastroenterology. 2003;125(4):1042–52.
47. Hadengue A, Benhayoun MK, Lebrec D, Benhamou JP. Pulmonary hypertension complicating portal hypertension: prevalence and relation to splanchnic hemodynamics. Gastroenterology. 1991;100(2):520–8.
48. Periyalwar P, Dasarathy S. Malnutrition in cirrhosis: contribution and consequences of sarcopenia on metabolic and clinical responses. Clin Liver Dis. 2012;16(1):95–131.
49. Pessaux P, Msika S, Atalla D, Hay JM, Flamant Y. French Association for Surgical R. Risk factors for postoperative infectious complications in noncolorectal abdominal surgery: a multivariate analysis based on a prospective multicenter study of 4718 patients. Arch Surg. 2003;138(3):314–24.
50. Garrison RN, Cryer HM, Howard DA, Polk HC Jr. Clarification of risk factors for abdominal operations in patients with hepatic cirrhosis. Ann Surg. 1984;199(6):648–55.
51. Mansour A, Watson W, Shayani V, Pickleman J. Abdominal operations in patients with cirrhosis: still a major surgical challenge. Surgery. 1997;122(4):730–5. discussion 5–6.
52. Farnsworth N, Fagan SP, Berger DH, Awad SS. Child-Turcotte-Pugh versus MELD score as a predictor of outcome after elective and emergent surgery in cirrhotic patients. Am J Surg. 2004;188(5):580–3.
53. Telem DA, Schiano T, Goldstone R, Han DK, Buch KE, Chin EH, et al. Factors that predict outcome of abdominal operations in patients with advanced cirrhosis. Clin Gastroenterol Hepatol. 2010;8(5):451–7. quiz e58.
54. Teh SH, Nagorney DM, Stevens SR, Offord KP, Therneau TM, Plevak DJ, et al. Risk factors for mortality after surgery in patients with cirrhosis. Gastroenterology. 2007;132(4):1261–9.
55. Mayo Clinic. Post-operative mortality risk in patients with cirrhosis- online calculator.
56. Friedman LS. The risk of surgery in patients with liver disease. Hepatology. 1999;29(6):1617–23.
57. Cowan RE, Jackson BT, Grainger SL, Thompson RP. Effects of anesthetic agents and abdominal surgery on liver blood flow. Hepatology. 1991;14(6): 1161–6.

58. Parker CJ, Hunter JM. Pharmacokinetics of atracurium and laudanosine in patients with hepatic cirrhosis. Br J Anaesth. 1989;62(2):177–83.
59. Tsai MH, Peng YS, Chen YC, Liu NJ, Ho YP, Fang JT, et al. Adrenal insufficiency in patients with cirrhosis, severe sepsis and septic shock. Hepatology. 2006;43(4):673–81.
60. Tripodi A. Hemostasis abnormalities in cirrhosis. Curr Opin Hematol. 2015;22(5):406–12.
61. Ng KJ, Lee YK, Huang MY, Hsu CY, Su YC. Risks of venous thromboembolism in patients with liver cirrhosis: a nationwide cohort study in Taiwan. J Thromb Haemost. 2015;13(2):206–13.

20 Endocrine Disorders and Maxillofacial Surgery

Marconi Abreu and Hassan Khalid

Abstract

Endocrine disorders are frequently seen in patients undergoing maxillofacial surgical procedures. Approximately one-third of those patients are overweight, 10% have diabetes and 5% have a thyroid condition. It is imperative to optimize endocrine conditions as it decreases the perioperative and postoperative morbidity and mortality. This chapter reviews the most common endocrine disorders and helps the surgeon identify preoperatively which patients need simple medication adjustment and which ones require urgent referral to an endocrinologist.

20.1 Obesity

20.1.1 Medical Disease

Obesity is defined as an increase in body fat mass. Body mass index (BMI, kg/m^2) classifies the severity of obesity:

- BMI 25–29.9: Overweight
- BMI 30–34.9: Grade I obese
- BMI 35–39.9: Grade II obese
- BMI ≥ 40: Grade II (morbidly obese)

M. Abreu, M.D. (✉)
Division of Endocrinology, Department of Internal Medicine, University of Texas Southwestern Medical Center, Dallas, TX, USA
e-mail: Marconi.Abreu@UTSouthwestern.edu

H. Khalid, M.D.
Department of Internal Medicine, Texas Tech University at Permian Basin, Odessa, TX, USA

Obesity is not without risk. In the Framingham study, overweight men had a mortality rate 3.9 times greater than the normal weight group [1]. Morbidity and mortality rise sharply when BMI is >30 kg/m^2, and the risk of premature death doubles in individuals with a BMI of >35 kg/m^2 [2].

Obesity is a complex and heritable disorder which results from the interaction among genetic susceptibility, epigenetics, and environment [3, 4]. Fundamentally, these interactions cause an imbalance between caloric consumption and energy expenditure favoring liver formation of free fatty acids and deposit of triacylglycerols in fat cells.

Central obesity (visceral obesity) is defined as a waist circumference >40 inches (102 cm) in men and 35 inches (88 cm) in women. In patients with visceral obesity, fat is deposited inside the abdominal cavity among the internal organs. Unlike peripherally deposited

© Springer International Publishing AG 2018

E.M. Ferneini, J.D. Bennett (eds.), *Perioperative Assessment of the Maxillofacial Surgery Patient*,
https://doi.org/10.1007/978-3-319-58868-1_20

fat, intra-abdominal fat is highly metabolic and plays a role in numerous disease states. It predisposes patients to insulin resistance, elevated levels of triglycerides, decreased levels of high-density lipoprotein cholesterol (HDL), and a higher risk of cardiovascular disease. It is also linked to hypertension, diabetes mellitus, obstructive sleep apnea, fatty liver, and polycystic ovarian syndrome. Patients with increased visceral obesity are at higher risk for developing deep vein thrombosis [5].

Hormones play a role in the way fat deposits in the human body. Testosterone induces visceral fat deposition, while estrogen shifts the metabolism toward subcutaneous fat accumulation. During caloric surplus, females deposit fat below the waistline, while males often accumulate fat centrally. The "pear-shaped" fat distribution mostly seen in females is not associated with metabolic syndrome.

Table 20.1 The obesity surgery mortality risk stratification score

Risk factor	Score
(a)	
BMI > 50 kg/m^2	1
Male	1
Age > 45 years	1
Hypertension	1
Risk factors for pulmonary embolism:	1
Previous venous thromboembolism	
Inferior vena cava filter	
Hypoventilation (sleep-disordered breathing)	
Pulmonary hypertension	
(b)	
	Risk of mortality
Class A: 0–1 points	0.2–0.3%
Class B: 2–3 points	1.1–1.5%
Class C: 4–5 points	2.4–3.0%

(a) Risk factors; (b) risk of mortality
Adapted from DeMaria, E.J., et al. [6]

20.1.2 Preoperative Assessment

Obese patients present a unique set of challenges and require specific perioperative care. All patients scheduled for noncardiac surgery should undergo a comprehensive history and physical exam which includes screening for possible metabolic-related diseases such as hypertension, diabetes mellitus, hyperlipidemia, obstructive sleep apnea, and coronary artery disease prior to surgery. Laboratory evaluation should include at a minimum comprehensive metabolic panel (CMP), complete blood count (CBC), glycosylated hemoglobin A1c (HbA1c), prothrombin time (PT), partial thromboplastin time (PTT), thyroid-stimulating hormone (TSH), lipid profile and resting ECG. If patients have pre-existing medical conditions, their disease state should be optimized prior to surgery.

The obesity surgery mortality risk stratification score (OS-MRS) (Table 20.1) is a validated tool to stratify the mortality risk of obese patients undergoing bariatric surgery [6]. Although not originally intended, it may also be helpful for non-bariatric surgery risk stratification.

The perioperative risk of obese patients undergoing noncardiac surgery depends not only on the presence but also on the functional status of obesity-related comorbidities. Severe OSA is present in 10–20% of patients with BMI > 35 kg/m^2 and is associated with a higher incidence of postoperative hypoxemia, respiratory failure, postoperative cardiac events, and ICU admissions [7]. Untreated OSA raises the risk of patients developing pulmonary hypertension or heart failure. Most OSA patients endure difficult and prolonged intubations because of increased pharyngeal collapsibility and abnormal facial and upper airway morphology [8, 9].

Untreated OSA may progress to obesity hypoventilation syndrome which manifests as daytime hypoventilation, chronic hypercapnia, resting hypoxemia at room air, and compensatory metabolic alkalosis. A serum bicarbonate level of >27 mEq/L in an obese patient without other reasons to have metabolic alkalosis should raise clinical suspicion for this condition. Such patients should be referred to sleep medicine for further work-up and management [10].

Hence, all obese patients should undergo obstructive sleep apnea (OSA) screening using a validated tool such as the STOP-BANG questionnaire prior to surgery (Table 20.2). Patients with higher scores should also undergo polysomnography and be initiated on continuous positive airway pressure therapy prior to surgery if indicated [12].

Obesity is a prothrombotic state. Elevated estrogen levels, due to increased aromatase activity in adipose cells, increase the risk of myocardial infarction and stroke. Mechanical limitation of mobility further increases the risk for deep vein thrombosis [13]. The postoperative incidence of venous thrombotic events (VTE) in obese patients is ten times higher as compared to the risk of postoperative VTE in normal weight individuals [14]. It is recommended that all patients undergoing major surgery receive VTE prophylaxis [15].

Obesity is also linked to increased cardiac intra-operative mortality and morbidity. Obesity-related fatty infiltration of the conducting system predisposes patients to arrhythmias and sudden cardiac death [16].

The FDA has approved several medications for the treatment of obesity. Table 20.3 summarizes the most commonly prescribed medications, their mechanisms of action, surgical implications, and perioperative management of patients while on the therapy.

Table 20.2 STOP-BANG scoring model

1. *S*noring
Do you *s*nore loudly (louder than talking or loud enough to be heard through closed doors)?
Yes No
2. *T*ired
Do you often feel *t*ired, fatigued, or sleepy during daytime?
Yes No
3. *O*bserved
Has anyone *o*bserved you stop breathing during your sleep?
Yes No
4. Blood *p*ressure
Do you have or are you being treated for high blood *p*ressure?
Yes No
5. *B*MI
*B*MI more than 35 kg/m^2?
Yes No
6. *A*ge
*A*ge over 50 years old?
Yes No
7. *N*eck circumference
*N*eck circumference greater than 40 cm?
Yes No
8. *G*ender
*G*ender male?
Yes No
High risk of OSA: answering yes to three or more items *Low risk of OSA:* answering yes to less than three items

Reprinted from *Anesthesiology*, with permission from Lippincott Williams and Wilkins/Wolters Kluwer Health [11]

20.1.3 Intraoperative Management

Anesthetic medications have altered pharmacokinetics and pharmacodynamics in obese patients [17]. Anesthetic dosing based on total body weight (TBW) can result in overdose; therefore, calculation using lean body weight (LBW) is commonly preferred except when using neuromuscular antagonists. LBW directly correlates with cardiac output and better determines early drug distribution kinetics [18]. It also results in a more standardized anesthetic effect across the BMI range [19].

Adipose tissue can temporarily trap lipophilic anesthetic drugs, such as halothane and isoflurane, and release them back into the circulation and central nervous system after their administration prolonging the drug effect. Those with morbid obesity experience this phenomenon more prominently. Newer anesthetics with lower lipid solubility, such as desflurane and sevoflurane, have more favorable characteristics of awakening [20].

20.1.4 Postoperative Management

Postoperative management includes prompt recovery of protective airway reflexes, proper analgesia, respiratory and physical therapy, infection control, and early ambulation. Obese patients are at risk for postoperative prolonged mechani-

Table 20.3 Perioperative management of drugs prescribed to treat obesity

Drug	Mechanism of action	Surgical implications	Comments
Phentermine (generic) Phentermine/topiramate—(Qsymia®)	Releases norepinephrine in central neurons → appetite suppression	Risk for hypertensive crises	Discontinue perioperatively
Orlistat (Xenical®) Orlistat OTC (Ali®)	Partially blocks gastric and pancreatic lipases	Intra-operative diarrhea Fat soluble Vitamin malabsorption (A, D, E, and K) Risk for hepatotoxicity and oxalate stones	Widely accessible to patients (generic) → often missed on medication reconciliation Discontinue perioperatively
Liraglutide (Saxenda®)	Glucagon-like peptide-1 (GLP-1) receptor agonist → glucose-dependent insulin secretion	Nausea and vomiting with drug re-initiation	Hold on the day of surgery Restart once tolerating PO If held > 3 days, restart at lower dose to avoid nausea
Lorcaserin (Belviq®)	Selective 5-HT_{2C} receptor agonist → induce satiety	Interacts with serotonergic drugs (tramadol, SSRIs, SNRIs, etc.)	Risk for serotonin syndrome from drug interaction

cal ventilation and weaning difficulty. Patient should be fully awake before extubation and avoid the supine position. Lung atelectasis reduces inspiratory volume, closes airways sooner, and limits expiratory flow resulting in the development of intrinsic PEEP [21]. The reduced ability to clear secretions raises the risk for nosocomial pneumonia, short-term mortality, and long-term mortality [22].

Those with OSA are at higher risk for developing respiratory depression and arrest following an intravenous opioid analgesic bolus [23]. Patient-controlled opioid analgesia and elevation of the head of the bed to 30–45° while in the post-anesthesia care unit (PACU) reduce postoperative complications from the use of narcotic analgesics [24, 25].

Adequate tissue perfusion postoperatively is essential for proper wound healing, and tissue oxygen partial pressure inversely relates to the risk of infection [26]. Fat tissue expands without concomitant increase in blood flow per cell resulting in relative tissue hypoxia. A group of researchers found that obese patients suffer from wound and tissue hypoxia putting them at increased risk of infection in the perioperative period [27].

20.2 Type 1 and Type 2 Diabetes Mellitus

20.2.1 Medical Disease

Type 1 diabetes mellitus is characterized by autoimmune destruction of the insulin-producing β-cells of the pancreas, usually leading to absolute insulin deficiency. An unknown antigenic stimulus in genetically susceptible individuals triggers T-cell-mediated destruction of the pancreatic β-cells. The rate of β-cell destruction is quite variable, but usually rapid in infants and children and slower when the disease is diagnosed in adulthood [28].

Type 2 diabetes mellitus develops from the combination of insulin resistance and inadequate insulin secretion from the β-cells of the pancreas. The etiology of type 2 diabetes mellitus is multifactorial. Individuals with genetic predisposition will normally develop the disease only after weight gain. The chronic consumption of a calorie-dense diet and reduced physical activity from modern living results in central obesity. This caloric surplus culminates in free fatty acid deposits in the liver and muscle with worsening of insulin resistance. The pancreas initially increases insulin output to meet the increased demand. However, chronic exposure to high oxidative stress from glucotoxicity and lipotoxicity results in β-cell apoptosis and insulin deficiency [29].

The hallmark of diabetes mellitus is elevated plasma glucose. Chronic exposure of tissues to hyperglycemia results in microvascular and macrovascular complications [30]. Severe hypoglycemia and hyperglycemia are major causes of emergency room visits with mortality rates 1.7 times higher in adults with type-2 diabetes mellitus than those without the disease. 28.5% of patients aged 40 and above have retinopathy resulting in loss of vision, with an additional 4.4% having advanced disease that can lead to blindness. Diabetes mellitus caused 44% of all new cases of kidney failure in the United States in 2011 and was responsible for 60% of nontraumatic lower limb amputations among patients aged 20 and above [31]. The illness raises cardiovascular risk by two- to fourfolds.

20.2.2 Preoperative Assessment

Tight blood glucose (BG) control for patients undergoing major surgical procedures is associated with reduced morbidity and mortality and lower rates of wound infection. Limited evidence exists for those considering minor surgical procedures [32–35].

Preoperative evaluation includes a comprehensive history and physical exam, laboratory analysis, and a resting ECG because those with autonomic diabetic neuropathy have a higher risk for silent ischemia, perioperative hypotension, and respiratory arrest. A stress test should follow a suspicious ECG tracing. Laboratories should include a comprehensive metabolic panel, HbA1c, and lipid profile. Patients undergoing elective surgery should have their hypertension and hyperlipidemia optimized preoperatively.

Controlled patients should continue all antidiabetic medications until the day prior to surgery. Metformin and sulfonylureas should be held 24 h prior to the surgical procedure to minimize the risk of lactic acidosis and hypoglycemia, respectively. Other oral medications can be held on the day of the procedure. When prolonged hospitalization is expected, or diabetes is uncontrolled, discontinuation of all oral medications and initiation of insulin therapy preoperatively are recommended. Those already on insulin therapy should continue their home dose of basal insulin and hold their prandial insulin while they are not eating. Those with higher risk for hypoglycemia can have their total daily dose (TDD) reduced by 10–20%. NPH insulin peaks in 4–6 h. To minimize the risk of hypoglycemia while fasting, patients using NPH or premix insulin should instead use detemir or glargine as their basal insulin. Table 20.4 summarizes the difference between the different available insulin preparations in the market, and Table 20.5 provides a

Table 20.4 Insulin onset, peak, and duration

	Onset	Peak	Duration
Basal insulin			
Glargine (Lantus®)	2–4 h	Relatively flat	~24 h
Detemir (Levemir®)	2–4 h	Relatively flat	18–24 h
NPH (Novolin N®)	2 h	4–6 h	10–18 h
NPH (Humulin N®)	2 h	4–6 h	10–18 h
Prandial insulin/correction			
Regular (Novolin®)	30 mins	2–4 h	6–8 h
Aspart (Novolog®)	10–15 mins	1–2 h	3–5 h
Lispro (Humalog®)	10–15 mins	1–2 h	3–5 h
Glulisine (Apidra®)	10–15 mins	1–2 h	3–5 h
Premix insulin			
NPH/Regular 70/30 (Novolin 70/30®)	30 mins	2–4 h	10–18 h
NPH/Regular 70/30 (Humulin 70/30®)	30 mins	2–4 h	10–18 h
NPH/Aspart 70/30 (Novolog 70/30®)	15 mins	1–2 h	10–18 h
NPH/Lispro 75/25 (Humalog 75/25®)	15 mins	1–2 h	10–18 h

Table 20.5 Stepwise approach to optimizing BG with insulin therapy

Goals of therapy:
• Average fasting and preprandial BG ~100–150 for patient with low risk for hypoglycemia
• Average fasting and preprandial BG ~120–180 for patients with higher risk for hypoglycemia (e.g., type 1, CKD, poor appetite, etc.)
Insulin dosing:
• TDD is defined as the total daily dose of insulin required in 24 h
• Patients already on insulin continue their home dose of insulin. Reduce the TDD of insulin by 10–20 % in those at higher risk for hypoglycemia (e.g., elderly, CKD)
• Patient on NPH or premix insulin should convert their TDD to a regime using detemir or glargine as the basal insulin
• In insulin naïve the TDD is usually around 0.3–1.0 units of insulin/kg of bodyweight/day. The initial insulin dose should take into consideration blood glucose levels and body weight. Patients at high risk for hypoglycemia will require a lower starting dose while patients with higher risk for hyperglycemia and with high insulin requirements before the procedure (e.g., obese, septic, on steroids, tube feedings) will require higher starting dose:
– 0.4 units/kg/day is a safe starting total daily dose for most patients [36]
– 50 % of the TDD should be given as basal insulin (detemir or glargine) and 50% of the TDD should be divided equally by the number of meals per day and given as prandial insulin (regular, aspart, lispro, or glulisine) prior to each meal
• Example: 105 kg × 0.4 u/kg/day. TDD = 42 units. 50% as basal = 21 units of basal insulin QD. 50% as prandial = 7 units given 15 min before each meal of prandial insulin
• Increase TDD (both the basal and prandial insulin) each day by 10% if average BG 180–250 mg/dL and by 20% if > 250 mg/dL until BG targets are achieved

-stepwise approach to optimizing BG with insulin therapy perioperatively.

Patients with uncontrolled blood glucose levels should monitor their BG more frequently in the week prior to the elective surgery. If elevated, antidiabetic medications should be titrated until BG levels are between 100 and 180 mg/dL prior to the procedure. All patients with type 1 DM and those with severely uncontrolled type 2 DM should preferably be started on an insulin-glucose drip protocol the night prior to the procedure. The continuous infusion of glucose and insulin has the added advantage of predictable BG levels with low risk for hypoglycemia [37, 38]. Once these patients tolerate enteral nutrition, transition them back to subcutaneous insulin. The first shot of basal insulin should be administered about 2–4 h prior to discontinuing the insulin drip to allow some overlap. Alternatively, if an insulin-glucose drip protocol is not available, basal and bolus insulin therapy can be initiated perioperatively. If adequate preoperative BG control is not achieved, the surgeon should consider postponing the surgery [37] and consulting the endocrinology service for optimization of glycemic control.

It is important to note that providers should not withhold basal insulin in patients with type 1 DM perioperatively. Insulin is often inadvertently withheld in this population due to normoglycemia or for being NPO, increasing the risk for the development of diabetic ketoacidosis. All patients on insulin pump or use U500 insulin as outpatient should be evaluated by the staff endocrinologist before surgery.

20.2.3 Intraoperative Management

Some induction and anesthetic agents can contribute to hypoglycemia. The commonly used induction agent etomidate blocks cortisol synthesis by its action on 11β-hydroxylase, attenuating the hyperglycemic response to surgery [39]. Patient at higher risk for hypoglycemia receiving this agent should be closely monitored. High doses of benzodiazepines and high potency opioids such as fentanyl can decrease pituitary secretion of ACTH, consequently reducing adrenal production of cortisol [40, 41]. Midazolam used in usual sedative doses does not usually contribute to hypoglycemia; however, these effects become prominent when midazolam is used as a continuous IV infusion. Diabetes mellitus reduces the body's ability to clear triglycerides from the circulation. Prolonged use of propofol in patients with diabetes mellitus increases the risk of hyperglycemia, hypertriglyceridemia, and pancreatitis [42].

20.2.4 Postoperative Management

Stress from surgery and anesthesia ignite several metabolic changes in the human body. They increase the body production of catabolic hormones such as cortisol, glucagon, growth hormone, and epinephrine, which in turn stimulate gluconeogenesis, glycogenolysis, and lipolysis. Other postoperative problems include interruption of food intake, altered consciousness which masks the symptoms of hypoglycemia, and poor surgical wound healing. Patients with diabetes mellitus are at increased risk for wound infection, hypoglycemia, hyperglycemia, and ketosis [32, 35]. This risk can be minimized by frequent BG monitoring and by keeping BG levels between 120 and 180 mg/dL postoperatively.

20.3 Hypothyroidism

20.3.1 Medical Disease

Hypothyroidism is the syndrome defined by thyroid hormone deficiency. Primary hypothyroidism is hypothyroidism due to a process within the thyroid gland. Secondary hypothyroidism is hypothyroidism caused by pituitary etiologies. Subclinical primary hypothyroidism is defined by a serum TSH above the upper reference limit with a normal free thyroxine (T4) level, whereas overt disease has elevated TSH (usually > 10 mIU/L) with a subnormal free T4.

Symptoms of overt hypothyroidism include dry skin, cold intolerance, fatigue, muscle cramps, hoarseness, and constipation. In very uncontrolled disease, patients can also display a prolonged ankle-jerk relaxation time, bradycardia, hypothermia, pericardial effusion, and altered mental status. Hashimoto's thyroiditis is the most common cause of primary hypothyroidism and accounts for >95% of all cases. The presence of thyroperoxidase antibodies mediates lymphocytic infiltration and cell-mediated destruction of the thyroid gland leading to a progressive decrease in thyroxine production.

20.3.2 Preoperative Assessment

Preoperative evaluation should start with a comprehensive history and physical exam. Neck discomfort, neck swelling, stridor, dysphagia, hoarseness, or positional dyspnea in patients with hypothyroidism should alert to changes in airway anatomy, which may influence the management of the airway during anesthesia. The physical examination should focus on looking for the presence of a thyroid enlargement (goiter) and the position of the trachea. Reported compressive symptoms, the presence of goiter, or the palpation of a thyroid nodule should prompt evaluation with a neck ultrasound preoperatively. If tracheal deviation is suspected, a CT scan of the neck should be considered.

Despite the relatively high prevalence of thyroid disease in the general population, no evidence exists to support screening for thyroid disease in the asymptomatic patient undergoing surgery. However, all patients with a history of hypothyroidism should have serum TSH level checked preoperatively to evaluate the status of the disease. While TSH is sufficient to evaluate primary hypothyroidism, a free T4 level should also be ordered when central hypothyroidism is suspected as it commonly presents with inappropriately normal TSH and a low free T4.

Patients with uncontrolled hypothyroidism are at risk for delayed weaning from mechanical ventilation; in such patients, surgery should be delayed if possible, until a euthyroid state is achieved to minimize preoperative risk. However, the proper treatment of hypothyroidism prior to urgent procedures is not always possible or practical. Dose adjustments of oral levothyroxine take 4–6 weeks to achieve a new steady state due to its half-life of 7 days.

Patients with controlled hypothyroidism should continue their routine oral thyroid hormone dose through the day of the surgery and afterward [43]. Those with severe hypothyroidism (i.e., bradycardia, hypothermia, altered mental status, or free T4 level <0.5 ng/dL) may have bowel edema which impairs oral levothyroxine absorption [44]. Thus 300–500 mcg bolus should be given IV followed by 1.6 mcg/kg/day of oral levothyroxine in such cases. When oral administration is not possible or desired, levothyroxine can be given IV and should be dosed as 50–80% of the calculated oral dose.

It is important to note that, although rare, patients with either central or primary hypothyroidism are at higher risk for concomitant adrenal insufficiency and, if present, the treatment of hypothyroidism can trigger an adrenal crisis [45]. When dealing with cases of severe hypothyroidism, one must assess the adrenal reserve prior to initiating levothyroxine replacement. If a random cortisol level is <12 mcg/dL, it is important to consider either performing a cosyntropin stimulation test to rule out adrenal insufficiency or empirically treat with hydrocortisone 25 mg Q6-8h intravenously. The clinician should then quickly taper the hydrocortisone dose prior to discharge to 10–15 mg PO q.a.m. and 5 mg q.p.m. and schedule a follow-up visit with an endocrinologist as outpatient to reassess the hypothalamic-pituitary-adrenal (HPA) axis.

20.3.3 Intraoperative Management

Patients with untreated or partially treated hypothyroidism have decreased cardiac output and reduced GFR, which in turn lead to reduced drug clearance [46]. No current guidelines exist on proper adjustments of anesthetic doses, but this alteration in drug pharmacokinetics should be considered when administering anesthesia. Patients with uncontrolled hypothyroidism are intraoperatively prone to hypothermia, bradycardia, augmentation of neuromuscular blockade, and delayed recovery from anesthesia [47]. Use of tranquilizers, narcotics, and hypnotics should be limited.

20.3.4 Postoperative Management

Patients with hypothyroidism are at risk for delayed weaning from mechanical ventilation due to a decreased central drive [48] and respiratory muscle weakness [49]. Therefore, all patients failing extubation, particularly those with associated bradycardia and hypothermia, should be checked for hypothyroidism. A retrospective study found a 3% prevalence of newly diagnosed hypothyroidism in patients admitted to a long-term weaning facility. After thyroid hormone supplementation, 75% of these patients were weaned from mechanical ventilation [50]. Therefore, we recommend rapid correction of hypothyroidism with IV levothyroxine in patients with uncontrolled hypothyroidism failing extubation. Once extubated, patients can resume their oral dose of levothyroxine. If neither bradycardia nor hypothermia is present, no further specific immediate postoperative management or monitoring is required. If the dose of levothyroxine was modified perioperatively, a TSH and free T4 level should be checked 6 weeks later to assure the dose adjustment is appropriate.

20.4 Hyperthyroidism

20.4.1 Medical Disease

Hyperthyroidism is a medical condition defined by thyroid hormone excess. Primary hyperthyroidism is hyperthyroidism due to a process within the thyroid gland. Secondary hyperthyroidism is hyperthyroidism due to a process arising from the pituitary gland. Subclinical hyperthyroidism is defined as a serum TSH level below the lower reference limit with a normal free thyroxine level (T4), whereas in overt disease, the TSH is suppressed (<0.05 mIU/L), with an elevated free T4 level.

Patients with hyperthyroidism can present with moist skin, heat intolerance, fatigue, weight loss, palpitations, dyspnea, insomnia, anxiety, oligomenorrhea, hair loss, and increase in stool frequency. Hyperthermia, jaundice, atrial fibrillation, pulmonary edema, or altered mental status can also be seen in severe cases. Graves' disease is the most common cause of primary hyperthyroidism. In Graves' disease, TSH receptor-stimulating immunoglobulin (TSI) binds to the TSH receptor, continuously promoting thyroxine production and secretion. Toxic multinodular goiter (TMNG), toxic adenoma, and thyroiditis are other common causes of hyperthyroidism.

20.4.2 Preoperative Assessment and Management

Preoperative evaluation of hyperthyroid patients should start with a comprehensive history and physical exam. Symptoms such as neck discomfort, neck swelling, stridor, dysphagia, hoarseness of voice, or positional dyspnea in patients with hyperthyroidism should alert to changes in airway anatomy, which may influence the management of the airway during anesthesia. The presence of exophthalmos, with smooth thyroid enlargement, or a bruit on physical examination is suggestive of Graves' disease. When the diagnosis of Graves' disease is not obvious by physical exam alone, or a nodule is palpated, a nuclear medicine (NM) thyroid uptake and scan should be ordered. A diffuse increase in radioactive iodine uptake in the thyroid scan is suggestive of Graves' disease, while a diffuse decrease in radioactive iodine uptake suggests thyroiditis. When a toxic adenoma is present, the NM thyroid uptake and scan should reveal an area of increased focal update of radioactive iodine with suppressed uptake in the rest of the gland. If the scan showed a pattern of scattered uptake by the thyroid gland, a toxic multinodular goiter should be suspected. A cold nodule appears as a focused area of decreased radioactive iodine uptake on a NM thyroid scan. This finding should be further evaluated with a neck ultrasound preoperatively, as cold nodules could be malignant. Additionally, if the patient reports compressive symptoms, he or she should also be further evaluated with a neck ultrasound prior to the planned procedure.

Despite the relatively high prevalence of thyroid disease in the general population, no evidence exists to support screening for hyperthyroidism in the asymptomatic patient undergoing surgery. However, all patients with known hyperthyroidism should have a serum TSH level checked preoperatively to evaluate the status of the disease.

Patients with subclinical hyperthyroidism can proceed with elective surgery after their heart rate is adequately controlled with beta-blockers. Those with uncontrolled hyperthyroidism should postpone elective procedures until their hyperthyroidism is adequately controlled. During their hospitalization, the endocrinology service should be consulted as these patients are at high risk for thyroid storm, a potentially life-threatening condition, after a stressful event like surgery. Those who are uncontrolled on treatment can have their medications intensified, while treatment naïve patients should start methimazole 20 mg QD-BID. Methimazole is generally preferred over propylthiouracil (PTU) due to less risk of hepatotoxicity and easier dosing due to its longer half-life. The only exception is in the first trimester of pregnancy at which time PTU is the recommended thionamide due a lower, but still present, risk of teratogenicity. Pregnant hyperthyroid patients are generally transitioned to methimazole in the second trimester of pregnancy once the risk of teratogenicity decreases [51]. Thionamides like methimazole and PTU have the potential to cause agranulocytosis and fatal liver failure. Patients should be counseled at every medical visit to seek urgent care if they develop fever, sore throat, or jaundice. If a patient presents in thyroid storm (Table 20.6), he or she should be monitored in the ICU due to the high mortality associated with this condition. In emergent surgical situations, preparation for surgery should be guided by an experienced endocrinologist. The management of thyroid storm and emergent surgery preparation is complex and beyond the scope of this chapter.

Radioactive iodine ablation (RAIA) is the most commonly used curative treatment of hyperthyroidism in the United States and is favored over thyroidectomy. It is usually well tolerated, with a low risk of complications. However, the full effects of the treatment may take up to 6 months to become fully apparent. Consequently, this treatment modality is impractical during the perioperative period.

Table 20.6 Diagnostic criteria for thyroid storm

Diagnostic parameter	Scoring points	Diagnostic parameter	Scoring points
Thermoregulatory dysfunction		**Cardiovascular dysfunction**	
Temperature °F (°C)		*Tachycardia (beats/minute)*	
99–99.9(37.2–37.7)	5	90–109	5
100–100.9 (37.8–38.2)	10	110–119	10
101–101.9 (38.3–38.8)	15	120–129	15
102–102.9 (38.9–39.2)	20	130–139	20
103–103.9 (39.3–39.9)	25	>/=140	25
>/=104.0 (>/=40.0)	30	*Congestive heart failure*	
Central nervous system effects		Absent	0
Absent	0	Mid (pedal edema)	5
Mild (agitation)	10	Moderate (bibasilar rales)	10
Moderate (delirium, psychosis, extreme lethargy)	20	Severe (pulmonary edema)	15
Severe (seizures, coma)	30	*Atrial fibrillation*	
Gastrointestinal-hepatic dysfunction		Absent	0
Absent	0	Present	10
Moderate (diarrhea, nausea/vomiting, abdominal pain)	10	*Precipitating event*	
Severe (unexplained jaundice)	20	Absent	0
		Present	10
A score of 45 or more is highly suggestive of thyroid storm; a score of 25–44 supports the diagnosis; and a score below 25 makes thyroid storm unlikely.			

Adapted with permission from L. Wartofsky [52]

20.4.3 Intraoperative Management

Patients with untreated or partially treated hyperthyroidism have increased cardiac output and increased GFR, which in turn lead to increased drug clearance. No current guidelines exist on the proper adjustment of anesthetic doses, but this alteration in drug pharmacokinetics should be considered when administering anesthesia. Patients with uncontrolled hyperthyroidism are intraoperatively prone to tachycardia, atrial fibrillation, and congestive heart failure.

20.4.4 Postoperative Management

Postoperative management is variable and should be done in accordance with the recommendations of the staff endocrinologist.

20.5 Adrenal Insufficiency

20.5.1 Medical Disease

Adrenal insufficiency (AI) is defined as a diminished secretion of cortisol by the adrenal glands. Primary AI results from a failure of the adrenal gland. The most common etiologies are tuberculosis, adrenalitis due to 21 hydroxylase antibodies, adrenalectomy, or metastasis.

Secondary AI results from a diminished secretion of ACTH by the pituitary. This can be due to suppression of the adrenal gland due to prolonged use of exogenous steroids or conditions causing mass effect into the sellar space such as pituitary adenoma, craniopharyngioma, or infiltrative disease.

Symptoms of adrenal insufficiency include fatigue, lack of appetite, nausea, vomiting, weight loss, and hypoglycemia. Because aldosterone is primarily modulated by the renin-angiotensin system and not influenced by ACTH, patients with secondary AI do not usually show signs of mineralocorticoid deficiency such as hyponatremia or orthostatic hypotension. Melanocyte-stimulating hormone (MSH) and ACTH share the same precursor molecule. Therefore, hyperpigmentation of skin creases, nipples, gums, and lips can be present in primary AI.

20.5.2 Preoperative Assessment and Management

Preoperative evaluation should start with a comprehensive history and physical exam to look for symptoms and physical findings suggestive of AI. No evidence exists to support screening for adrenal insufficiency in the asymptomatic patient undergoing surgery. However, patients with a diagnosis of AI or those who present with signs and symptoms suggestive of adrenal insufficiency should be properly diagnosed and managed perioperatively.

Figure 20.1 shows a stepwise approach in making the diagnosis of AI in the ambulatory setting. In patients not currently on steroids, the initial work-up should include the measurement of cortisol and DHEA-S. Cortisol, if possible, should be checked between 8 and 9 AM when it is commonly at its highest level and less likely to result in the "gray zone" in patients with normal adrenal function. A random cortisol level ≥12 mcg/dL in ambulatory patients excludes adrenal insufficiency, while a level ≤5 mcg/dL is highly suggestive of AI. Levels between 6 and 12 mcg/dL are considered to be in the "gray zone." In those cases, a DHEA-S level ≥54.5 mcg/dL also excludes AI, while lower levels of DHEA-S require further investigation with a cosyntropin stimulation test [53] (Fig. 20.2). Once the diagnosis of AI is established, an ACTH level is helpful to reveal the level of hypothalamic-pituitary-adrenal axis dysfunction. ACTH is invariably elevated in primary AI, whereas it can be low or inappropriately normal in secondary AI.

In response to stress, the adrenal glands increase their cortisol production during anesthesia, surgery, trauma, and critical illness. Traditionally, it is estimated that adults secrete 75–100 mg/day of cortisol in response to major surgery and 50 mg/day in response to minor surgery. Patients with adrenal insufficiency are unable to increase their cortisol production to meet this demand. Those with established adrenal insufficiency are typically on physiologic doses of steroids (15–20 mg of hydrocortisone equivalent/day) chronically and will require at least tripling of their maintenance dose perioperatively [54]. Table 20.7 shows glucocorticoid dose equivalents.

The presence of AI should not postpone or cancel surgery under any circumstance. In patients requiring emergent surgery, or when the proper diagnosis of adrenal insufficiency cannot be established prior to the procedure,

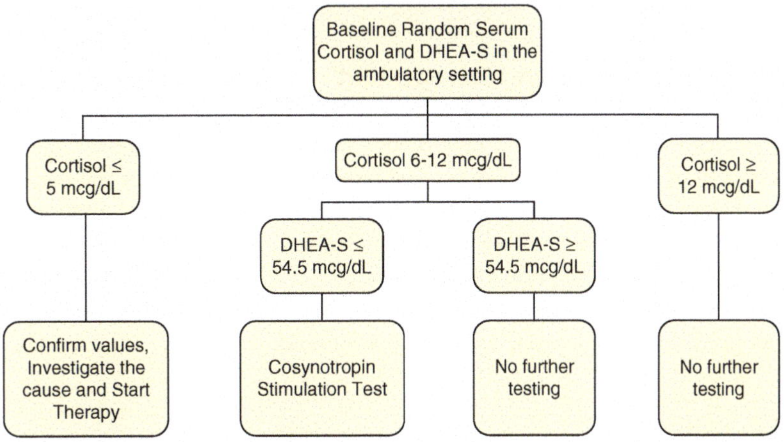

Fig. 20.1 Reprinted from *Endocrine Practice*, with permission from the American Association of Clinical Endocrinologists [53]

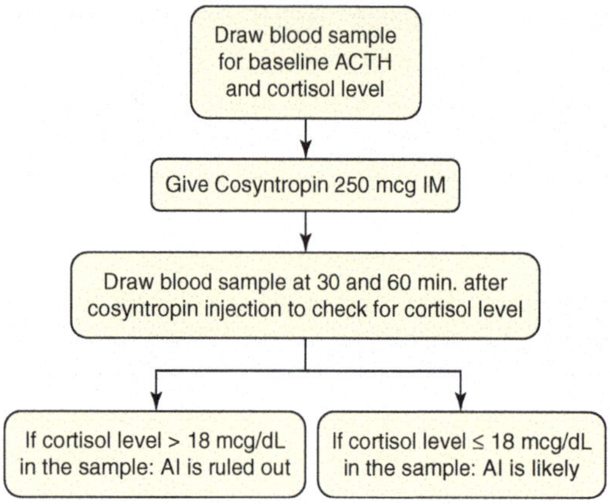

Fig. 20.2 Cosyntropin stimulation test

Table 20.7 Relative potencies of glucocorticoids

Glucocorticoid	Equivalent potency (mg)
Prednisone	5
Prednisolone	5
Hydrocortisone	20
Methylprednisolone	4
Dexamethasone	0.75

stress dose steroids should be started empirically. The clinician can consider giving hydrocortisone 25 mg Q6-8h IV perioperatively in these cases. Other supportive treatments such as IV fluids and/or vasopressors should be given as needed the dose of hydrocortisone should be quickly tapered to 15–20 mg/day prior to discharge [55]. Patients with primary AI also require mineralocorticoid replacement with fludrocortisone 0.05–0.1 mg/day.

20.5.3 Intraoperative Management

Etomidate can suppress the endogenous adrenal synthesis of cortisol in a dose-dependent fashion by inhibiting adrenal mitochondrial 11-β hydroxylase. Patients with AI or those in which the clinician suspects AI should not be given this anesthetic [56].

Patients with primary AI are prone to intraoperative hypotension due to mineralocorticoid deficiency. The clinician should monitor the volume status of these patients closely and resuscitate with normal saline or ringer lactate if needed.

20.5.4 Postoperative Management

When used in very high doses, opioids can suppress the HPA axis at a central level and cause biochemical adrenal insufficiency. This can contribute to postoperative hypotension [57].

To prevent the complications related to the use of supraphysiologic doses of steroids, the drugs should be tapered to preoperative or physiologic doses prior to discharge. Ideally, patients should be on the lowest possible dose of hydrocortisone required to prevent symptoms of AI. Typically, this dose is approximately 15–20 mg/day (usually 10–15 given q.a.m. and 5 mg q.p.m.). The clinician should educate the patients to recognize symptoms of adrenal insufficiency and instruct them to temporarily double the dose during periods of acute illness or if the patients experience a constellation of symptoms including nausea, vomiting, fatigue, lack of appetite, and weight loss. The patients who were not on steroids preoperatively and were empirically started on this medication for the surgical procedure should have their hypothalamic-pituitary-adrenal axis reevaluated by an experienced endocrinologist to assess its long-term need.

Conclusion

Endocrine disorders are frequently seen in patients undergoing maxillofacial surgical procedures. The management of these problems is often straightforward. It is imperative to optimize endocrine conditions as it decreases the perioperative and postoperative morbidity and mortality. This chapter aims to guide clinicians with medical decision making when dealing with common endocrine diseases in order to improve the quality of care delivered to patients undergoing surgery.

References

1. Harris T, et al. Body mass index and mortality among nonsmoking older persons. The Framingham heart study. JAMA. 1988;259(10):1520–4.
2. Garrison RJ, Castelli WP. Weight and thirty-year mortality of men in the Framingham study. Ann Intern Med. 1985;103(6 (Pt 2)):1006–9.
3. Vasconcelos LH, et al. Ion channels in obesity: pathophysiology and potential therapeutic targets. Front Pharmacol. 2016;7:58.
4. Pigeyre M, et al. Recent progress in genetics, epigenetics and metagenomics unveils the pathophysiology of human obesity. Clin Sci (Lond). 2016;130(12):943–86.
5. Redinger RN. The pathophysiology of obesity and its clinical manifestations. Gastroenterol Hepatol (N Y). 2007;3(11):856–63.
6. DeMaria EJ, et al. Validation of the obesity surgery mortality risk score in a multicenter study proves it stratifies mortality risk in patients undergoing gastric bypass for morbid obesity. Ann Surg. 2007;246(4):578–82. discussion 583-4
7. Mutter TC, et al. A matched cohort study of postoperative outcomes in obstructive sleep apnea: could preoperative diagnosis and treatment prevent complications? Anesthesiology. 2014;121(4):707–18.
8. Isono S. Obesity and obstructive sleep apnoea: mechanisms for increased collapsibility of the passive pharyngeal airway. Respirology. 2012;17(1):32–42.
9. Siyam MA, Benhamou D. Difficult endotracheal intubation in patients with sleep apnea syndrome. Anesth Analg. 2002;95(4):1098–102; table of contents.
10. Chau EH, et al. Obesity hypoventilation syndrome: a review of epidemiology, pathophysiology, and perioperative considerations. Anesthesiology. 2012;117(1):188–205.
11. Chung F, et al. STOP questionnaire: a tool to screen patients for obstructive sleep apnea. Anesthesiology. 2008;108(5):812–21.
12. Chung F, et al. High STOP-bang score indicates a high probability of obstructive sleep apnoea. Br J Anaesth. 2012;108(5):768–75.
13. Desciak MC, Martin DE. Perioperative pulmonary embolism: diagnosis and anesthetic management. J Clin Anesth. 2011;23(2):153–65.
14. Parkin L, et al. Body mass index, surgery, and risk of venous thromboembolism in middle-aged women: a cohort study. Circulation. 2012;125(15): 1897–904.
15. Geerts WH, et al. Prevention of venous thromboembolism: American college of chest physicians evidence-based clinical practice guidelines (8th edition). Chest. 2008;133(6 Suppl):381S–453S.
16. Pantanowitz L. Fat infiltration in the heart. Heart. 2001;85(3):253.
17. Janmahasatian S, et al. Quantification of lean bodyweight. Clin Pharmacokinet. 2005;44(10):1051–65.
18. Collis T, et al. Relations of stroke volume and cardiac output to body composition: the strong heart study. Circulation. 2001;103(6):820–5.
19. Dong D, et al. Morbid obesity alters both pharmacokinetics and pharmacodynamics of propofol: dosing recommendation for anesthesia induction. Drug Metab Dispos. 2016;44(10):1579–83.
20. Casati A, Putzu M. Anesthesia in the obese patient: pharmacokinetic considerations. J Clin Anesth. 2005;17(2):134–45.
21. Koutsoukou A, et al. Expiratory flow limitation in morbidly obese postoperative mechanically ventilated patients. Acta Anaesthesiol Scand. 2004;48(9):1080–8.
22. Khuri SF, et al. Determinants of long-term survival after major surgery and the adverse effect of postoperative complications. Ann Surg. 2005;242(3):326–41. discussion 341-3.
23. Cullen DJ. Obstructive sleep apnea and postoperative analgesia: a potentially dangerous combination. J Clin Anesth. 2001;13(2):83–5.
24. Bell RL, Rosenbaum SH. Postoperative considerations for patients with obesity and sleep apnea. Anesthesiol Clin North Am. 2005;23(3):493–500. vii.
25. Etches RC. Respiratory depression associated with patient-controlled analgesia: a review of eight cases. Can J Anaesth. 1994;41(2):125–32.
26. Babior BM. Oxygen-dependent microbial killing by phagocytes (first of two parts). N Engl J Med. 1978;298(12):659–68.
27. Kabon B, et al. Obesity decreases perioperative tissue oxygenation. Anesthesiology. 2004;100(2):274–80.
28. American Diabetes Association. Classification and diagnosis of diabetes. Diabetes Care. 2014;38(Suppl 1):S8.
29. DeFronzo RA. From the triumvirate to the ominous octet: a new paradigm for the treatment of type 2 diabetes mellitus. Diabetes. 2009;58(4):773.
30. UK Prospective Diabetes Study (UKPDS) Group. Intensive blood-glucose control with sulphonylureas or insulin compared with conventional treatment and risk of complications in patients with type 2 diabetes (UKPDS 33). Lancet. 1998;352(9131):837–53.
31. CDC. National diabetes statistics report, 2014. http://www.cdc.gov/diabetes/pubs/statsreport14/national-diabetes-report-web.pdf. Accessed 10 Aug 2016.
32. Risum O, et al. Diabetes mellitus and morbidity and mortality risks after coronary artery bypass surgery. Scand J Thorac Cardiovasc Surg. 1996;30(2):71–5.
33. Thompson BM, et al. Perioperative Management of Patients with Diabetes and Hyperglycemia Undergoing Elective Surgery. Curr Diab Rep. 2016;16(1):2.
34. Thompson J, et al. Metabolic changes in the non-insulin-dependent diabetic undergoing minor surgery: effect of glucose-insulin-potassium infusion. Br J Surg. 1986;73(4):301–4.

35. Mossad SB, et al. Coagulase-negative staphylococcal sternal wound infections after open heart operations. Ann Thorac Surg. 1997;63(2):395–401.
36. Umpierrez GE, et al. Randomized study of basal-bolus insulin therapy in the inpatient management of patients with type 2 diabetes (RABBIT 2 trial). Diabetes Care. 2007;30(9):2181.
37. Marks JB. Perioperative management of diabetes. Am Fam Physician. 2003;67(1):93–100.
38. Bergman SA. Perioperative management of the diabetic patient. Oral Surg Oral Med Oral Pathol Oral Radiol Endodontol. 2007;103(6):731–7.
39. Fragen RJ, et al. Effects of etomidate on hormonal responses to surgical stress. Anesthesiology. 1984;61(6):652–6.
40. Desborough JP, et al. Midazolam modifies pancreatic and anterior pituitary hormone secretion during upper abdominal surgery. Br J Anaesth. 1991;67(4):390–6.
41. Klingstedt C, et al. High-and low-dose fentanyl anaesthesia: circulatory and plasma catecholamine responses during cholecystectomy. Br J Anaesth. 1987;59(2):184–8.
42. Devlin JW, Lau AK, Tanios MA. Propofol-associated hypertriglyceridemia and pancreatitis in the intensive care unit: an analysis of frequency and risk factors. Pharmacotherapy. 2005;25(10):1348–52.
43. Njoku MJ. Patients with chronic endocrine disease. Med Clin North Am. 2013;97(6):1123–37.
44. Holvey DN, et al. Treatment of myxedema coma with intravenous thyroxine. Arch Intern Med. 1964;113:89–96.
45. Graves L 3rd, Klein RM, Walling AD. Addisonian crisis precipitated by thyroxine therapy: a complication of type 2 autoimmune polyglandular syndrome. South Med J. 2003;96(8):824–7.
46. Basu G, Mohapatra A. Interactions between thyroid disorders and kidney disease. Indian J Endocrinol Metab. 2012;16(2):204–13.
47. Lele AV, et al. Severe hypothyroidism presenting as myxedema coma in the postoperative period in a patient taking sunitinib: case report and review of literature. J Clin Anesth. 2013;25(1):47–51.
48. Ambrosino N, et al. Impaired ventilatory drive in short-term primary hypothyroidism and its reversal by L-triiodothyronine. J Endocrinol Invest. 1985;8(6):533–6.
49. Martinez FJ, Bermudez-Gomez M, Celli BR. Hypothyroidism. A reversible cause of diaphragmatic dysfunction. Chest. 1989;96(5):1059–63.
50. Datta D, Scalise P. Hypothyroidism and failure to wean in patients receiving prolonged mechanical ventilation at a regional weaning center. Chest. 2004;126(4):1307–12.
51. Cooper DS, Rivkees SA. Putting propylthiouracil in perspective. J Clin Endocrinol Metab. 2009;94(6):1881–2.
52. Burch HB, Wartofsky L. Life-threatening thyrotoxicosis. Thyroid storm. Endocrinol Metab Clin North Am. 1993;22(2):263–77.
53. Al-Aridi R, Abdelmannan D, Arafah BM. Biochemical diagnosis of adrenal insufficiency: the added value of dehydroepiandrosterone sulfate measurements. Endocr Pract. 2011;17(2):261–70.
54. Bornstein SR, et al. Diagnosis and treatment of primary adrenal insufficiency: an endocrine society clinical practice guideline. J Clin Endocrinol Metab. 2016;101(2):364–89.
55. Marik PE, Varon J. Requirement of perioperative stress doses of corticosteroids: a systematic review of the literature. Arch Surg. 2008;143(12):1222–6.
56. Thompson Bastin ML, Baker SN, Weant KA. Effects of etomidate on adrenal suppression: a review of intubated septic patients. Hosp Pharm. 2014;49(2):177–83.
57. Policola C, et al. Adrenal insufficiency in acute oral opiate therapy. Endocrinol Diabetes Metab Case Rep. 2014;2014:130071.

Check for updates

21 Rheumatologic Disorders and Maxillofacial Surgery

Steven Hugenberg

Abstract

Rheumatologic illnesses encompass a wide variety of conditions that because of systemic inflammation may affect many different organ systems. Chronic inflammation associated with most rheumatologic conditions increases the risk for cardiovascular events, but patients may be asymptomatic. Furthermore, several diseases increase risk for chronic lung diseases, e.g., pulmonary fibrosis and/or pulmonary hypertension. There is a risk of perioperative flares of the underlying disease, especially with crystal-induced conditions such as gout and pseudogout. Anesthesia may be complicated not only by the presence of underlying cardiopulmonary disease but also by cervical spine involvement, particularly in rheumatoid arthritis and ankylosing spondylitis and airway involvement. Use of immunosuppressive medications may increase the risk of perioperative infections, but without them the primary condition could flare which could also result in postoperative complications. Oftentimes, the management of patients with rheumatic diseases requires a multidisciplinary approach.

21.1 Introduction

Patients with rheumatologic conditions present a number of challenges when undergoing surgery [1, 2]. Due to chronic inflammation, most rheumatologic conditions increase risk for cardiovascular events, but preoperatively typical symptoms may not be present. In addition, several diseases may cause chronic lung diseases such as pulmonary fibrosis and/or pulmonary arterial hypertension. There is also a risk of postoperative flares of the underlying disease, especially with crystal-induced conditions such as gout and pseudogout or in patients with inflammatory arthropathy especially if medications are withheld around the time of surgery. Anesthesia may be complicated not only by the presence of underlying cardiopulmonary disease but also by cervical spine disease, particularly in rheumatoid arthritis (RA) and ankylosing spondylitis (AS), or laryngeal/

S. Hugenberg, M.D.
Rheumatology Division, Department of Medicine, Indiana University School of Medicine, Indianapolis, IN, USA
e-mail: shugenbe@iu.edu

© Springer International Publishing AG 2018

E.M. Ferneini, J.D. Bennett (eds.), *Perioperative Assessment of the Maxillofacial Surgery Patient*,
https://doi.org/10.1007/978-3-319-58868-1_21

tracheal involvement (RA, granulomatosis with polyangiitis). Lastly, immunosuppressive medications increase risk of perioperative infections. Most of the literature regarding perioperative management of patients with rheumatologic illnesses is based on joint replacement surgery so one has to extrapolate from that information and it may not be applicable to all patients or procedures. When managing rheumatic disease patients in the perioperative period, the involvement of the rheumatologist is essential, but it is also necessary to do so in a multidisciplinary manner with the inclusion of cardiology, pulmonary and/or nephrology specialists, and perhaps others, depending on the organ involvement the patient has.

A short review of specific diseases will occur followed by a brief general discussion of drug management in the perioperative period.

21.2 Rheumatoid Arthritis (RA)

Pathophysiology: RA is a systemic autoimmune disease for which the exact cause is unknown, but likely contributory factors are a combination of genetic and environmental factors. From a cellular basis, both B and T lymphocytes play a role in causing elaboration of pro-inflammatory cytokines such as tumor necrosis factor alpha (TNFα) and interleukins 1, 6, and 17 (IL-1, IL-6, and IL-17). Characteristic antibodies such as rheumatoid factor (RF) and anti-citrullinated peptide antibody (ACPA) probably have a role in pathogenesis [3, 4].

The inflammatory response, while mostly centered in the synovial membranes of the joints, often leads to system manifestations (Table 21.1).

RA affects approximately 1% of the population, predominantly females [4, 5]. Classically, it causes symmetrical polyarthritis affecting mostly the joints of the hands, wrists, and feet, but large joint involvement is not unusual. About 30–40% of patients have rheumatoid nodules, typically those with a positive RF, which are characteristically located over the olecranon processes and other extensor surfaces. Untreated, RA often causes deformities of the joints (swan neck, boutonniere, ulnar deviation, etc.) with resultant loss of function/disability. The RF is positive in 75% of patients, and the ACPA is positive in approximately the same percentage [4]. However, the RF is less specific for the diagnosis of RA than the ACPA.

Table 21.1 Systemic manifestations of rheumatoid arthritis

Organ system	Manifestations
Skin	Nodules, vasculitis (palpable purpura, nail fold infarctions, digital ischemia
HEENT	Sjogren's syndrome (keratoconjunctivitis sicca, xerostomia), episcleritis, scleritis
Pulmonary	Fibrosis, bronchiolitis obliterans with organizing pneumonia (BOOP), cryptogenic organizing pneumonia (COP)
Hematologic	Anemia of chronic disease, Felty syndrome (neutropenia, splenomegaly, infections), increased risk of lymphoma
Neurologic	Peripheral neuropathy, mononeuritis multiplex due to vasculitis, cervical myelopathy due to C1–C2 subluxation
Cardiac	Pericarditis, increased risk of coronary artery disease (CAD) and congestive heart failure (CHF)

Extra-articular manifestations have a significant impact on morbidity and mortality (Table 21.1).

Most of the risk of anesthesia relates to airway management (cervical spine subluxation, arthritis of the cricoarytenoid joints, or involvement of temporomandibular joints causing decreased ability to open the mouth) [1, 2, 6, 7] and cardiovascular disease, when present.

Preoperative assessment: A thorough history and physical examination are necessary to exclude significant cardiopulmonary disease. Since symptoms may be atypical or minimal, symptoms such as unexplained dyspnea on exertion and/or atypical chest pains should be evaluated with appropriate testing such as cardiac stress test, echocardiogram, chest radiograph (CXR), and/or pulmonary function testing [1, 2].

Patients with known CAD or pulmonary fibrosis should have medical clearance by cardiology or pulmonary, respectively.

Patients with long-standing, usually seropositive, RA may develop subluxation of C1 on C2 placing the patient at risk for spinal cord compression, especially when the neck is flexed. Since the neck is not flexed during direct laryngoscopic endotracheal intubation the risk is relatively low, but movement of the neck should be minimized at the time of surgery. Preoperatively, the patient should have flexion and extension views of the C-spine to detect instability [1, 2]. However, some recommend that in the absence of symptoms of cervical myelopathy (paresthesia, weakness, radicular symptoms) and the decreasing incidence of this finding, screening cervical spine radiographs in all patients are not necessary [6]. However, in patients who have long-standing RA and deformities, preoperative flexion/extension radiographs of the cervical spine should be routinely preformed. Typically, > 4–5 mm of subluxation is considered significant. If present and the patient is asymptomatic, anesthesiologist should be made aware to take appropriate precautions when intubating the patient such as performing with fiber-optic guidance [7]. If the patient has symptoms suggestive of myelopathy, additional imaging (MRI, CT) is necessary, and neurosurgical evaluation should occur before proceeding with surgery.

A small number of patients with RA may have chronic cricoarytenoid arthritis [6, 7]. They often are asymptomatic or on occasion may have hoarseness, dyspnea, or upper airway obstruction. Its presence may make intubation difficult necessitating the use of fiber-optic guidance also.

21.3 Systemic Lupus Erythematosus (SLE)

Pathophysiology: SLE results from a complex, multifactorial interplay between genetic and environmental factors. Immune complex deposition in organs composed of autoantibodies that are thought to have resulted from loss of immune tolerance and dysfunctional immune regulation contributes to the development of disease. Gender, hormones, and the hypothalamic pituitary adrenal axis play a role in susceptibility and manifestations.

The prevalence of SLE is approximately 20–150 per 100,000 [5, 8–10]. The prevalence is influenced by race (about threefold greater in African-Americans compared to white) and sex (female to male ratio 9:1) [11]. Frequency is also greater in Hispanic-Americans, African-Caribbean, and Asians [11].

The manifestations of SLE are myriad and may vary a great deal from one patient to another. Table 21.2 provides a synopsis of these.

Preoperatively, patients with SLE should have a thorough history and physical examination to exclude significant cardiopulmonary disease. If this involvement is established or there is suspicion, appropriate testing and consultations should be obtained for stratification of risk [1, 2]. As in RA, symptoms in lupus patients with cardiovascular disease may be absent or minimal. Typically, those with SLE do not have unusual airway management requirements or precautions. If chronically anticoagulated because of cardiolipin antibody syndrome, warfarin should be stopped 5 days prior to surgery and switched to low

Table 21.2 Major organ manifestations of systemic lupus erythematosus

Organ system	Manifestations
Hematologic	Autoimmune hemolytic anemia, leukopenia, lymphopenia, thrombocytopenia, thrombotic events (cardiolipin antibodies, lupus anticoagulant)
Musculoskeletal	Arthralgia, arthritis, myositis
Skin	Malar rash, discoid rash, photosensitivity, alopecia, subacute cutaneous lupus
Cardiac	Pericarditis, noninfectious (Libman-Sacks) endocarditis, increased risk of coronary artery disease, myocarditis
Pulmonary	Pleuritis/effusion, fibrosis, shrinking lung
Renal	Glomerulonephritis, interstitial nephritis, chronic kidney disease
Neurologic	Seizure, psychosis, peripheral neuropathy, stroke, myositis

molecular weight heparin or unfractionated heparin. These should be stopped 24 and 4 h prior to surgery, respectively [1].

Anesthesia does not impact disease activity. In patients with chronic kidney disease (CKD) or on dialysis, adjustment of drug dosing may be necessary. In addition, close attention should be paid to perioperative fluid management in such patients so as to prevent volume overload and electrolyte abnormalities [7]. Patients with significant pulmonary disease may have greater oxygenation requirements [7].

In the postoperative period, lupus patients with cardiolipin antibody syndrome have increased risk for thrombotic events, specifically deep venous thrombosis (DVT)/pulmonary embolism. If chronically anticoagulated, they should be started on their medication regimen as soon as feasible and safe and appropriate prevention strategies for DVT should be taken until then [1].

21.4 Ankylosing Spondylitis (AS) and the Seronegative Spondyloarthropathies (SpA)

Pathophysiology: Ankylosing spondylitis and the seronegative spondyloarthropathies (psoriatic arthritis [PsA], reactive arthritis, and arthritis associated with inflammatory bowel disease [IBD]) are systemic inflammatory disorders that predominantly affect the entheses, where ligaments, tendons, and capsules attach to the bone. Inflammation of the sacroiliac joints and axial skeleton, causing inflammatory back pain and stiffness, is the hallmark feature. In addition, involvement of peripheral joints and entheses may result in dactylitis (sausage digits), peripheral arthritis, and enthesitis (plantar fasciitis, Achilles tendonitis). These findings occur most frequently in PsA. At the enthesis, inflammation, bone erosion, and syndesmophyte formation occur. In many patients, especially those with spondylitis, HLA B27 may play a role in genetic predisposition. TNFα and IL-17 are the inflammatory cytokines that have a key role in the process [12].

Formation of syndesmophytes in the spine leads to loss of motion and eventually fusion of the cervical, thoracic, and lumbar spines, in severe cases leading to the "bamboo spine." This typically is seen in AS and enteropathic spondylitis; in PsA, the spondylitis and sacroiliitis are somewhat asymmetric [12].

Patients with PsA often have pain and swelling of the distal interphalangeal joints, symmetric polyarthritis, and asymmetric oligoarthritis or, in severe cases, develop arthritis mutilans and telescoping digits and dramatic angulation deformities.

Many patients with SpA have a fused cervical spine, especially AS. Patients with SpA, typically AS, have recurrent acute anterior uveitis (iritis), aortic regurgitation, conduction disturbances, and a restrictive ventilatory defect because chest expansion is limited due to fusion of the articulation of the ribs with the thoracic spine. As with RA and SLE, patients with AS and PsA are at increased risk for CV disease. While the vertebral bodies do not become displaced as in RA, the rigid cervical spine may present special difficulties for endotracheal tube placement.

The prevalence of these conditions is listed in Table 21.3.

As in almost all rheumatologic diseases, while the articular structures and entheses are the prime site of inflammation in SpA, they are all systemic diseases affecting other organ systems such as the eyes, lungs, and heart (Table 21.4).

The intubation of patients with AS and SpA may be challenging due to fusion of the cervical spine [2]. Care should be taken when moving the neck. While the cervical spine may be fused, it is fragile. Sudden or extreme forced motion possi-

Table 21.3 Prevalence of seronegative spondyloar thropathies

Condition	Prevalence per 100,000 [13]
Spondyloarthropathy (SpA), overall	346–1310
Ankylosing spondylitis	520
Psoriatic arthritis	109
Enteropathic arthritis, peripheral	65
Enteropathic arthritis, axial	50–150

Table 21.4 Systemic manifestations of spondyloarthropathies [12]

Organ	Ankylosing spondylitis	Psoriatic arthritis	Reactive arthritis	IBD[a] associated
Eye	Anterior uveitis	Anterior uveitis	Conjunctivitis, uveitis	Uveitis
Lung	Restrictive defect Fibrosis (upper lobe)	X	X	X
Heart	Aortitis/aortic regurgitation Conduction defects Increased risk of CAD	Increased risk of CAD	X	X
Skin	X	Psoriasis	Keratoderma blennorrhagica, circinate balanitis, oral ulcers	Erythema nodosum, Pyoderma gangrenosum
GI/GU	X	X	History of nongonococcal urethritis or bacterial gastroenteritis	Crohn's disease Ulcerative colitis

[a]*IBD* Inflammatory bowel disease; *X* not affected

bly could result in a "chalk stick" fracture resulting in instability of the spine and ensuing myelopathy. Given the limited mobility of the neck, fiber-optic direct laryngoscopy may be necessary to place the endotracheal tube because of the decreased neck mobility [7].

21.5 Crystal-Induced Arthropathies: Gout and Pseudogout

Pathophysiology: Gout and pseudogout are caused by crystals deposited in the synovial tissue and cartilage. Under the correct circumstances, the crystals are phagocytized by polymorphonuclear cells resulting in a severe acute inflammatory response mediated by the inflammasome (IL-1). The crystal associated with gout is monosodium urate (MSU) and with pseudogout, calcium pyrophosphate dihydrate (CPPD). During acute attacks, crystals can be identified by examination of synovial fluid under compensated polarizing light microscopy. MSU crystals are needle-shaped and are strongly negatively birefringent; CPPD crystals are weakly positively birefringent and are rectangular or rhomboid in shape [14].

Both conditions cause acute episodes of monoarthritis with swelling, pain, and redness of the involved joint. Chronic gout can lead to deposition of uric acid in soft tissues (tophi). Either condition can be precipitated by acute illnesses, changes in hydration status, and classically in the postoperative period, typically 1–3 days later. Risk factors for gout include CKD, diuretic use, alcohol use/abuse, and a genetic component. The largest risk factor for pseudogout is aging because of the association of chondrocalcinosis with aging. In addition, there are metabolic conditions associated with pseudogout: hyperparathyroidism, hemochromatosis, hypophosphatasia, and hypomagnesemia.

The prevalence of gout in North America and Western Europe is 1–4%. Men are affected more often than women with a prevalence ratio of 3–4:1 [14]. The prevalence data for pseudogout and CPPD deposition disease is less robust but it is estimated to affect 1/1000 persons and up to 15% of those between the ages of 65 and 74 [14].

There are no major anesthetic risks for patients with gout outside of the risks defined by their comorbid conditions (age, CKD, cardiovascular disease). There are no significant issues with anesthesia, airway establishment, or maintenance.

In the patient with known gout, it is important to maintain their medical management until immediately before surgery and resume it as soon as possible postoperatively. This will reduce the likelihood of an attack after surgery. Urate-lowering drugs (allopurinol, febuxostat, probenecid) are safe to continue. If the patient is on a prophylactic drug such as colchicine, it should be maintained as well to reduce the risk of an acute attack in the perioperative period.

If the patient should suffer an attack of gout or pseudogout after surgery, the most effective and efficient treatment is to use nonsteroidal anti-inflammatory drugs (NSAIDs) if not otherwise contraindicated. A short course of systemic glucocorticoids can be used if NSAIDs are not able to be prescribed. For gout, another acute treatment option is oral colchicine given as a 1.2 mg loading dose followed by another 0.6 mg an hour later. Colchicine is less effective for acute pseudogout but can be tried if there are no other options. Intra-articular steroid injection(s) can also be used in the acute setting if other modalities are contraindicated. In general, management of acute gout or pseudogout in the postoperative setting is best performed by obtaining a rheumatologist or general internal medicine consultation.

21.6 Scleroderma

Scleroderma (SSc) is a systemic disease that causes thickening and fibrosis of the skin and Raynaud's phenomenon as its most noticeable manifestations. However, it is a systemic disease affecting numerous organs, in particular the lungs and kidneys. For classification purposes, scleroderma is usually divided into diffuse cutaneous (dcSSc) and limited cutaneous (lcSSc) because the two types have different manifestations and prognosis.

Pathophysiology: The pathogenesis of SSc is not completely understood. Development of disease in part is related to immune activation, vascular damage, and excess synthesis of extracellular matrix, mostly collagen. At play are activated fibroblasts and endothelial cells.

Scleroderma is rare with an estimated population prevalence of 240 per million. Women are affected four to five times more frequently than men [15, 16].

The clinical manifestations of SSc include Raynaud's phenomenon, sclerodactyly, fibrosis, and thickening of skin of the extremities, trunk, and face. In dcSSC, the skin thickening is proximal to the elbows. Limited scleroderma, which was once referred to as CREST (calcinosis, Raynaud's, esophageal dysmotility, sclerodactyly, telangiectasia) syndrome, typically involves only the skin distal to the elbows and knees. Systemic manifestations include pulmonary fibrosis, pulmonary arterial hypertension, severe gastroesophageal reflux disease (GERD) and gastrointestinal dysmotility, arthritis, myopathy, and scleroderma renal crisis (severe hypertension, acute kidney injury, microangiopathic hemolytic anemia, heart failure, stroke/mental status changes) [17].

Pulmonary fibrosis, which can lead to secondary pulmonary hypertension, and scleroderma renal crisis occur in dcSSc. Pulmonary arterial hypertension in the absence of pulmonary fibrosis occurs more frequently in lcSSc. In addition, involvement of the skin of the chest can lead to a restrictive ventilatory defect in dcSSc.

Preoperatively, careful assessment of pulmonary and cardiac disease is needed. Pulmonary function tests should be performed if the patient has known interstitial lung disease and they have not been checked recently. An echocardiogram, and perhaps even right heart catheterization may needed to assess right ventricular and pulmonary artery pressures if there is concern for pulmonary arterial hypertension. In those with pre-existing fibrotic lung disease and/or pulmonary hypertension, preoperative evaluation and clearance by pulmonary and cardiology are recommended.

Administration of anesthesia does not affect disease, and there are no anesthetics that need to be avoided, but if there is renal dysfunction, drugs that require renal elimination must be properly dosed. Involvement of the skin of the face resulting in diminished oral aperture creates difficulty with endotracheal intubation so using fiber-optic guidance may be necessary. Additionally, patients with severe GERD are prone to aspiration so appropriate precautions should be taken when intubating the patient. Patients should be on proton pump inhibitors preoperatively to reduce gastric pH. Intraoperatively, because of the tautness of skin over the thorax causing decreased pulmonary compliance, higher pressures may be needed to ventilate the patient. Patients with lung disease may be at risk for hypoxemia with respiratory depression so caution should be exercised in using opioids for pain control. In addition, if pulmonary hypertension is present, induction agents that do not increase pulmonary vascular resistance such as etomidate should be used [7].

21.7 Idiopathic Inflammatory Myopathies (IIM) (Dermatomyositis/ Polymyositis)

The inflammatory myopathies are encompassed by polymyositis and dermatomyositis. They are characterized by progressive proximal muscle weakness and elevated muscle enzymes (creatine kinase, lactate dehydrogenase, aspartate aminotransferase, aldolase). Dermatomyositis has characteristic cutaneous finding: Gottron's sign, Gottron's papules, heliotrope rash, and the so-called "V" sign (anterior chest below the neck, shawl sign (across the posterior shoulders and neck) and holster sign (lateral thighs) [18].

Pathophysiology: IIM's result from both the innate and adaptive immune system resulting in an inflammatory response to striated muscle fibers. Histologically, activated T lymphocytes infiltrate the muscle fibers. Release of interferon gamma by these cells also influences pathogenesis [18].

The prevalence of polymyositis is 1/14,000 and dermatomyositis 1/50,000 [13, 18]. Females are affected twice as often as men. African-Americans develop dermatomyositis more often than Caucasians.

Patients with IIM may develop pulmonary fibrosis, and in rare cases hypoventilation from diaphragmatic and intercostal muscle weakness. Dysphagia due to involvement of the pharynx, hypopharynx, and upper one-third of the esophagus which is composed of striated muscle puts patients at increased risk for aspiration.

As the disease affects the skeletal muscle fibers, not the neuromuscular junction, nondepolarizing muscle relaxants and succinylcholine are safe in these conditions [7]. In patients who have pharyngeal/esophageal involvement, one must be cognizant of the risk of aspiration and appropriate preventative actions should be taken [7]. Patients with pulmonary fibrosis may have greater oxygenation requirements and may need prolonged mechanical ventilation.

21.8 Vasculitis

The vasculitides refer to conditions that result in inflammatory change in blood vessels resulting in destruction and necrosis of the vessel wall. These pathological changes can result in stenoses or aneurysms leading to ischemia of the skin and internal organs. Vasculitis is typically classified by the size of the vessel involved; small, medium, and large, and additionally whether the anti-neutrophil cytoplasmic antibody (ANCA) is positive or negative (Table 21.5) [19]. Behcet disease, because its etiopathogenesis is not understood, but has or is associated with vascular disease will be discussed under this heading.

21.8.1 ANCA Associated Vasculitis (AAV)

The AAV are

- Granulomatosis with polyangiitis (GPA)
- Eosinophilic granulomatosis with polyangiitis (EGPA)
- Microscopic polyarteritis (MPA)

21.8.1.1 GPA

GPA, formerly known as Wegener granulomatosis, is a rare multisystem autoimmune disease of unknown etiology. Its hallmark features include necrotizing granulomatous inflammation and pauci-immune vasculitis in small- and medium-sized blood vessels. GPA has an estimated prevalence of 3/100,000 [20].

The pathologic hallmarks of GPA are vasculitis of the small- to medium-sized vessels, "geographic" necrosis, and granulomatous

Table 21.5 Classification and manifestations of systemic vasculitides (adapted from ref. [24])

Vessel size	Disease	Organ(s) affected	Description	Age (years)	Clinical features	Laboratory/serology Other
Small	GPA	Upper and lower respiratory tracts, kidney, skin	Granulomatous inflammation of resp. tract, necrotizing vasculitis of capillaries, venules, arterioles; necrotizing GN	40–50	Pneumonitis, nodular and/or cavitary infiltrates, ulcerations of nasopharynx, sinusitis, saddle nose deformity, subglottic stenosis, pauci-immune necrotizing GN, skin ulcers, palpable purpura, digital ischemia	C-ANCA, PR3 +
	EGPA	Resp. tract, heart, peripheral nerves	Eosinophilic and granulomatous inflammation of resp. tract; necrotizing vasculitis of small-medium vessels	50–60	Allergic rhinitis, asthma, pulm infiltrates often transient, peripheral neuropathy, myocarditis	P-ANCA, MPO + Eosinophilia Possible association with leukotriene inhibitor use
	MPA	Skin, lungs, heart, kidneys	Necrotizing vasculitis of capillaries, venules, arterioles and sometimes small and medium arteries	50–60	Alveolar hemorrhage, palpable purpura, pauci-immune crescentic necrotizing GN	P-ANCA, MPO +
Medium	PAN	Kidneys, visceral organs, peripheral and central nervous systems	Necrotizing inflammation of medium or small arteries	30–40	Fever, wt. loss, HTN, abd. pain, melena, neuropathy, mononeuritis multiplex, renal ischemia but no GN, livedo reticularis	ANCA negative Hep B surface antigen + 8–10%
Large	Takayasu Arteritis	Aorta and major branches, eyes	Granulomatous inflammation of aorta and branches	30–40	Arm claudication, lower blood pressure and weaker pulse in one arm, HTN, visual disturbance	
	GCA (temporal arteritis)	Extra-cranial branches of carotid artery	Granulomatous inflammation extra-cranial branches of carotid a., esp. temporal arteries, may affect aorta and major branches with	60–70	Fever, facial pain, headache, scalp tenderness, visual loss and symptoms due to ischemic optic neuropathy	Association with polymyalgia rheumatica, very high erythrocyte sedimentation rate

inflammation, particularly in the airways. The initial pathologic lesion is that of the granuloma believed to be caused by cellular immune processes [20]. Environmental exposures, including respiratory tract infections, have been implicated as inciting factors for granuloma formation [20].

The presence of ANCAs within neutrophils in the majority of patients with GPA suggests the role of humoral autoimmunity. GPA is usually associated with the presence of diffuse staining cytoplasmic ANCA (C-ANCA) directed against serine proteinase 3 antigen (PR3-ANCA) [20].

The other AAVs include microscopic polyangiitis (MPA), renal-limited vasculitis, and Churg-Strauss syndrome (eosinophilic granulomatous with polyangiitis [EGPA]), all of which are more commonly associated with perinuclear-staining ANCA (P-ANCA) directed against myeloperoxidase (MPO-ANCA).

A pathogenic role for PR3-ANCAs in GPA has been proposed because PR3-ANCA is strongly associated with the disease although this has not been proven definitively.

21.8.1.2 EGPA

EGPA (formerly known as Churg-Strauss syndrome) is a granulomatous small-vessel vasculitis. The cause of this allergic angiitis and granulomatosis is unknown. No data have been reported regarding the role of immune complexes or cell-mediated mechanisms in this disease, although autoimmunity is evident with the presence of hypergammaglobulinemia, increased levels of immunoglobulin E (IgE), rheumatoid factor, and ANCA.

EGPA is a rare systemic necrotizing vasculitis with a prevalence of 1–3/100,000 that affects small-to-medium-sized vessels and is associated with severe asthma and blood and tissue eosinophilia [21]. Key clinical features of EGPA are:

- Asthma (wheezing, expiratory rhonchi)
- Eosinophilia of more than 10% in peripheral blood
- Paranasal sinusitis
- Pulmonary infiltrates (often transient)
- Histological evidence of vasculitis with extravascular eosinophils
- Mononeuritis multiplex or polyneuropathy

21.8.2 Medium Vessel Vasculitis: Polyarteritis Nodosa (PAN)

Polyarteritis nodosa (PAN) is a systemic vasculitis characterized by necrotizing inflammatory lesions that affect medium-sized and small muscular arteries, preferentially at vessel bifurcations, resulting in microaneurysm formation, aneurysmal rupture with hemorrhage, thrombosis, and, consequently, organ ischemia or infarction. It is rare, with an incidence of about 3–4.5 cases per 100,000 population annually [22].

The pathogenesis of polyarteritis nodosa is unknown but it is not immune complex mediated based on measurement of circulating immune complexes and complement levels. While hepatitis B virus is strongly linked with PAN, the role of immune complex-induced disease is confined to HBV-related PAN. The role of immune complexes in non-HBV-related PAN is unclear and has not been identified. Impaired function of endothelial cells may be part of idiopathic PAN or a consequence of it; in HBV-PAN, virus replication may directly injure the vessel wall. Endothelial dysfunction can perpetuate the inflammation through cytokine and adhesion molecule production. HBV-related PAN may occur at any time during the course of acute or chronic hepatitis B infection, although it typically occurs within 6 months of infection [22].

The activity of HBV-PAN does not parallel that of the hepatitis, and symptoms are the same as those of idiopathic PAN. Some studies with small numbers of patients have found that GI manifestations, severe hypertension, renal infarction, and orchiepididymitis are more common in HBV-PAN.

HBV was once the cause of up to 30% of PAN cases. Widespread use of the hepatitis B vaccine has significantly decreased the incidence of HBV-PAN, which is now estimated to account for less than 8% of all PAN cases, mostly in Eastern Asia.

Vascular lesions in medium-sized muscular arteries occur mainly at bifurcations and branch points. Inflammation may start in the vessel intima and progress to include the entire arterial wall, destroying the internal and external elastic lamina, resulting in fibrinoid necrosis. Aneurysms develop in the weakened vessel, carrying a subsequent risk for rupture and hemorrhage. Thrombi may develop at the site of the lesions. As lesions progress, proliferation of the intima or media may result in obstruction and subsequent tissue ischemia or infarction. PAN spares large vessels (the aorta and its major branches), the smallest vessels (capillaries and small arterioles), and the venous system.

21.8.3 Large Vessel Vasculitis: Takayasu Arteritis, Giant Cell Arteritis (Temporal Arteritis)

Takayasu arteritis (TA) is an inflammatory disease of large- and medium-sized arteries, with a predilection for the aorta and its branches. Advanced lesions demonstrate a panarteritis with intimal proliferation [23].

The prevalence TA is 2.6–6.4 persons per million population. It is observed more frequently in patients of Asian or Indian descent. Japanese patients with TA have a higher incidence of aortic arch involvement. In contrast, series from India report higher incidences of abdominal involvement [23]. Approximately 80% of patients with Takayasu arteritis are women; however, the high female-to-male ratio seems to decrease west of Japan. In India, the female-to-male ratio is as low as 1.6:1.

Lesions produced by the inflammatory process can be stenotic, occlusive, or aneurysmal. All aneurysmal lesions may have areas of arterial narrowing. Vascular changes lead to the main complications, including hypertension, most often due to renal artery stenosis or, more rarely, stenosis of the suprarenal aorta; aortic insufficiency due to aortic valve involvement; pulmonary hypertension; and aortic or arterial aneurysm [23].

Congestive heart failure (CHF) is not an uncommon finding. Dilated cardiomyopathy, myocarditis, and pericarditis, all also have been reported but are less frequent than CHF. In patients in whom the pulmonary artery is involved, the right artery appears to be affected more than the left, with those patients developing pneumonia, interstitial pulmonary fibrosis, and alveolar damage [23].

Other pathophysiologic consequences include hypotensive ischemic retinopathy, vertebrobasilar ischemia, microaneurysms, carotid stenosis, hypertensive encephalopathy, and inflammatory bowel disease [23]. Rarely, Takayasu arteritis has also been associated with glomerulonephritis, SLE, polymyositis, polymyalgia rheumatica, rheumatoid arthritis, Still disease, and ankylosing spondylitis.

Giant cell arteritis (GCA), or temporal arteritis, is a systemic inflammatory vasculitis of unknown etiology that occurs in older persons and can result in a wide variety of systemic, neurologic, and ophthalmologic complications. GCA is the most common form of systemic vasculitis in adults [23].

GCA typically affects the superficial temporal arteries, hence the term temporal arteritis. In addition, GCA most commonly affects the ophthalmic, occipital, vertebral, posterior ciliary, and proximal vertebral arteries. It is the involvement of the ophthalmic and posterior ciliary arteries that leads to amaurosis fugax and even vision loss by causing ischemic optic neuropathy. It also affects medium- and large-sized vessels, including the aorta and the carotid, subclavian, and iliac arteries. The prevalence and incidence of GCA increase proportionally to age. Females are more frequently affected than men [23].

Histopathologically, GCA is marked by transmural inflammation of the intima, media, and adventitia of affected arteries, as well as patchy infiltration by lymphocytes, macrophages, and multinucleated giant cells. Mural hyperplasia can result in arterial luminal narrowing, resulting in subsequent distal ischemia [23].

21.8.4 Behcet Disease (BD)

Behcet disease (or syndrome) is a multi-system inflammatory condition that is manifested by recurrent/relapsing episodes of oral aphthous ulcers, genital ulcers, skin lesions, and eye disease. It is a rare condition with a point prevalence estimate of 5.2/100,000 in the United States based on a population-based study [25]. In this patient cohort, 100% had recurrent oral ulcerations and 62% recurrent genital ulcerations. Nearly 70% of the patients were female and the same percentage Caucasian. Behcet disease may affect many different organ systems:

- Skin (85%)—papulopustular lesions (54%), erythema nodosum (46%)
- Arthritis (46%)—poly- or oligoarthritis
- Vascular (23%)—deep venous thrombosis (15%), superficial phlebitis (8%)
- Eye (62%)—anterior uveitis (54%), posterior uveitis (54%), panuveitis (46%), retinal vasculitis (38%)
- Gastrointestinal—abdominal pain, nausea, vomiting
- Neurologic—stroke (15%), aseptic meningitis (8%), migraine

In addition, other vascular manifestations of BD include aneurysms and arterial stenosis. Inflammation of large arteries has been reported to lead to aneurysms and narrowing or occlusion of the vessel.

In regard to anesthesia risk, in severe cases of BD, ulcerations of the oral mucosae can result in severe angular cheilitis such that the oral aperture is reduced and/or scarring of the pharynx creates difficulty with insertion of the endotracheal tube [26, 27]. Therefore, preoperatively, a thorough examination of the mouth and oropharynx should be performed so that appropriate changes in the anesthetic approach can be made if necessary [27].

Preoperative evaluation of patients with vasculitis should include assessment of the organ systems involved the specific disease. As GPA, EGPA, and PAN may all affect renal function, it is necessary to know the serum creatinine and estimated glomerular filtration rate. Ongoing lung disease should be assessed as well, although, in general, elective surgery should not be performed in patients with active vasculitis.

GPA may present some unique challenges to performing anesthesia. If subglottic stenosis is present, it is essential to have otorhinolaryngology assess the severity and activity. A smaller than usual endotracheal tube may be necessary and it may be safer to intubate the patient using fiber-optic laryngoscopy [7]. In severe cases, tracheostomy may be required, although this would not be recommended for the purposes of elective surgery [7]. Extubating patients with subglottic stenosis can result in acute upper airway compromise so the care team should be prepared for emergency upper airway management. Chronic sinusitis and saddle nose deformity may make ventilating with a mask challenging and prohibit nasotracheal intubation [7].

Doses of anesthetics that are predominantly excreted renally need to be adjusted for the patient's renal function [7].

Patients with large vessel vasculitis involving upper extremity arteries could result in difficulty in monitoring blood pressure, and a blood pressure cuff placed on the arm where there is proximal arterial stenosis could restrict blood flow enough to impair perfusion of the digits. Assessment of upper and lower extremity pulses preoperatively is essential.

21.9 Management of Pharmacologic Agents

Most patients with inflammatory rheumatic diseases are on immunosuppressive, biologic anti-inflammatory therapy and/or glucocorticoids. Management of these agents in the perioperative period is outlined in Table 21.6. Most of the information regarding medical therapy is derived from recommendations for patients with rheumatoid arthritis undergoing joint replacement surgery. The evidence for recommendations for immunosuppressive drugs before and after surgery for other diseases is relatively sparse so it is necessary to extract from the literature regarding joint replacement surgery. The American College of Rheumatology (ACR) and the American Association of Hip and Knee Surgeons (AAHKS) recently presented guidelines for drug management in the perioperative period based on a systematic review of the literature [28] which are summarized in Table 21.6.

In patients on chronic glucocorticoid therapy, there has traditionally been a concern about development of acute adrenal insufficiency around the time of surgery mandating the use of stress doses of glucocorticoids. However, current evidence indi-

Table 21.6 Pharmacologic agents for rheumatologic conditions: perioperative recommendations

Drug	Clinical use	Infection risk	Need/when to stop
Hydroxychloroquine	SLE, RA, dermatomyositis	No	No
Sulfasalazine	RA, SpA	No	No
Methotrexate	RA, SLE, SpA, IIM	No	No
Leflunomide	RA		No
Tumor necrosis factor α Inhibitors[a]	RA, SpA	Yes	Hold for surgery, plan surgery 1 week after end of dosing interval (etanercept wk 2; adalimumab wk 3; golimumab wk 5 SQ, wk 9 IV; infliximab wk 5, 7 or 9, certolizumab wk 3 or 5)
Tocilizumab	RA, giant cell arteritis	Yes	Hold for surgery, plan surgery 1 week after end of dosing interval, wk 2 SQ, wk 5 IV
Abatacept	RA	Yes	Hold for surgery, plan surgery 1 week after end of dosing interval (wk 5 IV, wk 2 SQ)
Tofacitinib	RA	Yes	Withhold 7 days in advance
Mycophenolate mofetil	SLE	Possibly	Withhold 7 days prior and restart 3–5 days after, do not hold in severe SLE
Azathioprine	RA, SLE, AAV	Possibly	Withhold 7 days prior and restart 3–5 days after, do not hold in severe SLE
Rituximab	RA, AAV	±	Stop one dosing interval prior to surgery (month 7)
Belimumab	SLE		Hold for surgery, plan surgery 1 week after end of dosing interval (week 5)

[a]Etanercept, infliximab, adalimumab, golimumab, certolizumab

cates there are no significant differences in the hemodynamic profile between patients receiving stress doses of corticosteroids and those receiving only their usual daily dose [28]. In addition, higher doses of glucocorticoids given perioperatively increase the risk of infections and impair wound healing as well as potentially cause hyperglycemia, hypertension, and fluid retention [1]. Therefore, it is recommended that patients on chronic glucocorticoid therapy take it up until the time of surgery and resume at the same dose postoperatively [28].

The panel recommended restarting biologic therapy in patients with RA, SpA, and SLE, for whom their therapy was withheld prior to surgery; a minimum of 14 days after surgery in the absence of wound healing problems, surgical site infection or systemic infection [28].

Conclusion

Rheumatologic conditions are often complex multisystem diseases that require careful consideration when surgery is being planned for patients who have them. Awareness of involvement of the cardiopulmonary, including increased risk of cardiovascular disease, the renal systems, as well as the airway is key to the management of such patients in the perioperative period. Crystal-induced arthropathies are likely to flare in the postoperative period, so it is important to be aware of strategies to prevent and treat exacerbations. In addition, medications used to treat rheumatologic diseases may increase risk of infection, although changes in medications may cause the diseases to flare possibly resulting in delays in recovery and healing. Therefore, a judicious approach to medication management around the time of surgery is key, and those guidelines are outlined in this chapter. The approach to patients with rheumatologic illnesses in the perioperative period often requires an interdisciplinary approach to include the surgical team, anesthesiologist, the rheumatologist, and frequently other medical specialists.

References

1. Veetil Akkara B, Bongartz T. Perioperative care for patients with rheumatic diseases. Nat Rev Rheumatol. 2012;8:32–41.
2. Bissar L, Almoallin H, Alblazi K, Alotaibi M, Alwafi S. Perioperative management of patients with rheumatic diseases. Open Rheumatol J. 2013;7:42–50.
3. Choy E. Understanding the dynamics: pathways involved in the pathogenesis of rheumatoid arthritis. Rheumatology. 2012;51(suppl 5):v3–v11.
4. Erikson A, Canella A, Mikuls T. Clinical features of rheumatoid arthritis. In: Kelley & Firestein's textbook of rheumatology. 10th ed. Philadelphia: Elsevier; 2017. p. 1167–86.
5. Helmick CG, Felson DT, Lawrence RC, et al. Estimates of the prevalence of arthritis and other rheumatic conditions in the United States—part I. Arthritis Rheum. 2008;58:15–25.
6. Vieira E, Goodman S, Tanaka P. Anesthesia and rheumatoid arthritis. Rev Bras Anestesiol. 2011;61:367–75.
7. Ramani R. Skin and musculoskeletal diseases. In: Hines R, Marschall K, editors. Stoelting's anesthesia and co-existing disease. 6th ed. Philadelphia: Elsevier (Saunders); 2012. p. 437–65.
8. Chakravarty E, Bush T, Manzi S, et al. Prevalence of adult systemic lupus erythematosus in California and Pennsylvania in 2000: estimates obtained using hospitalization data. Arthritis Rheum. 2007;56:2092–4.
9. Dall'Era M, Wofsy D. Clinical features of systemic lupus erythematosus. In: Kelley & Firestein's textbook of rheumatology. 10th ed. Philadelphia: Elsevier; 2017. p. 1345–67.
10. Danchenko N, Satia J, Anthony M. Epidemiology of systemic lupus erythematosus: a comparison of worldwide disease burden. Lupus. 2006;15:308–15.
11. Pons-Estel G, Alarcon G, Scofield L, et al. Understanding the epidemiology and progression of systemic lupus erythematosus. Semin Arthritis Rheum. 2010;39:257–68.
12. Van der Linden S, Brown M, Kenna T, Maksymowych W, Robinson P. Ankylosing spondylitis. In: Kelley & Firestein's textbook of rheumatology. 10th ed. Philadelphia: Elsevier; 2017. p. 1256–74.
13. Lawrence RC, Felson DT, Helmick CG, et al. Estimates of the prevalence of arthritis and other rheumatic conditions in the United States—part II. Arthritis Rheum. 2008;58:26–35.
14. Al-Ashkar F. Gout and pyrophosphate deposition disease. 2016. http://www.clevelandclinicmeded.com/medicalpubs/diseasemanagement/rheumatology/gout-and-pseudogout/. Accessed Dec 2016.
15. Barnes J, Mayes M. Epidemiology of systemic sclerosis: incidence, prevalence, survival, risk factors, malignancy, and environmental triggers. Curr Opin Rheumatol. 2012;24:165–70.
16. Mayes M, Lacey J Jr, Beebe-Dimmer J, et al. Prevalence, incidence, survival, and disease characteristics of systemic sclerosis in a large US population. Arthritis Rheum. 2003;48:2246–55.
17. Wigley F, Boin F. Clinical features and treatment of scleroderma. In: Kelley & Firestein's textbook of rheumatology. 10th ed. Philadelphia: Elsevier; 2017. p. 1424–1460.e.5.
18. Kanneboyina N, Galdue H, Lundberg I. Inflammatory diseases of muscle and other myopathies. In: Kelley & Firestein's textbook of rheumatology. 10th ed. Philadelphia: Elsevier; 2017. p. 1461–88.
19. Stone J. Classification and epidemiology of systemic vasculitis. In: Kelley & Firestein's textbook of rheumatology. 10th ed. Philadelphia: Elsevier; 2017. p. 1512–9.
20. Chung S, Monach P. ANCA associated vasculitis. In: Kelley & Firestein's textbook of rheumatology. 10th ed. Philadelphia: Elsevier; 2017. p. 1541–58.
21. Groh M, Pagnoux C, Baldini C, Bel E, Bottero P, Cottin V, et al. Eosinophilic granulomatosis with polyangiitis (Churg-Strauss) (EGPA) Consensus Task Force recommendations for evaluation and management. Eur J Intern Med. 2015;26(7):545–53.
22. Lugmani R. Polyarteritis nodosa and related disorders. In: Kelley & Firestein's textbook of rheumatology. 10th ed. Philadelphia: Elsevier; 2017. p. 1559–70.
23. Hellman D. Giant cell arteritis, polymyalgia rheumatica, and takayasu's arteritis. In: Kelley & Firestein's textbook of rheumatology. 10th ed. Philadelphia: Elsevier; 2017. p. 1520–40.
24. Sharma P, Sharma S, Baltaro R, Hurley (2011) Systemic vasculitis. Amer Fam Physician. 83:556–565.
25. Calamia K, Wilson F, Icen M, et al. Epidemiology and clinical characteristics of Behçet's disease in the US: a population-based study. Arthritis Rheum. 2009;61:600–4.
26. Bhalerao P, Patil V, Page N. A case of Behcet's disease posted for surgery: anaesthetic implications. Indian J Anaesth. 2015;59:517–9.
27. Turner M. Anaesthetic difficulties associated with Behcet's syndrome. Brit J Anaesth. 1972;44:100–2.
28. Goodman S, Springer B, Guyatt G, et al. American College of Rheumatology/American Association of hip and knee surgeons guideline for the perioperative management of antirheumatic medication in patients with rheumatic diseases undergoing elective total hip or total knee arthroplasty. Arthritis Care Res; 2017;69:1111–24.

22 Hematologic Disorders and Maxillofacial Surgery

Michele Obeid, Joelle El Amm, and Hady Ghanem

Abstract

One of the most dreaded complications that can complicate surgeries in general, maxillofacial surgeries being one of them, is bleeding. The risk of bleeding should be thoroughly assessed initially by the surgeon, but also by the anesthesiologist in the preoperative setting, and in some situations by the expert opinion of a hematologist. This assessment relies in a major part on a careful history and physical examination, taking into account documentation about possible prior spontaneous and traumatic or surgical bleeding as well as a careful review of all medications that can interfere with hemostasis. This initial step has to be completed by basic laboratory work-up to check the major pathways of primary and secondary hemostasis and requires in some situations a more elaborate work-up in the case of a suspected hemostatic disorder. In the present chapter, we will review the situations that have to be taken into account while assessing a patient in the preoperative setting and present guidance for managing these disorders.

22.1 Introduction

The preoperative hematologic assessment relies heavily on excellent exploration of previous surgical history, anticoagulant medications being used, family history, and general history of easy bruising or excessive bleeding. When indicators of hematologic dysfunction have been identified, appropriate laboratory tests such as CBC, PT, PTT, bleeding time, or fibrin split products define the severity of the condition. Possible guidance of a hematology specialist and a proper perioperative planning are needed in such situations.

M. Obeid, M.D. • J. El Amm, M.D. • H. Ghanem, M.D. (✉)
Division of Hematology and Oncology, Lebanese American University, School of Medicine, Beirut, Lebanon
e-mail: hady.ghanem@umcrh.com

22.2 Anemia

According to the World Health Organization (WHO), anemia is defined as a hemoglobin concentration less than 13 g/dL in males and 12 g/dL

© Springer International Publishing AG 2018

E.M. Ferneini, J.D. Bennett (eds.), *Perioperative Assessment of the Maxillofacial Surgery Patient*,
https://doi.org/10.1007/978-3-319-58868-1_22

in females [1]. Preoperatively, anemia is the most common hematologic laboratory abnormality encountered. It is estimated that about one-third of patients assessed in the preoperative setting have been found to have anemia [2]. In the setting of perioperative medicine, there is considerable evidence of an association between preoperative anemia and surgical morbidity and mortality [3, 4].

Before performing any invasive procedure, the surgeon estimates the risk for bleeding and assesses the possibility of abnormal bleeding because this can have devastating effects on outcome. A good history taking and physical examination help the surgery team and the anesthesiologist to have a good idea about what to expect perioperatively. Symptoms of anemia can be very vague such as malaise, dyspnea, palpitations, pallor, and cyanosis. Other signs and symptoms as easy bruising, excessive bleeding with previous surgery or trauma, history of hematuria, hematochezia, melena, hemarthroses, or muscle hematoma necessitate further evaluation. Physical examination should focus on identifying any lymphadenopathy, hepatomegaly, or splenomegaly. In addition, physical exam signs of petechiae, purpura, ecchymoses, and mucosal bleeding are clues that require exploration. Rectal and pelvic exams should be performed for the presence of blood. In many cases, anemia is incidentally found on laboratory tests, which can guide us toward identifying the cause of the anemia and identifying bleeding abnormalities such as a platelet disorder (quantitative or qualitative) or a coagulation disorder (inherited or acquired) [2].

The decision to transfuse a patient preoperatively depends on the estimated blood loss for the surgical procedure proposed and the consideration of the underlying risk factors for ischemic heart disease.

Patient with normovolemic anemia and low cardiac risk undergoing a procedure with small expected blood loss can be managed safely without transfusion tolerating hemoglobin levels of 6 or 7 g/dL. Those with hemoglobin levels greater than 10 g/dL rarely require a transfusion [5].

There is an increasing body of evidence to suggest that the use of restrictive transfusion thresholds is non-inferior to liberal transfusion thresholds [6]. Therefore, although preoperative anemia is common and associated with a worse patient outcome, blood transfusion may not be the most appropriate solution, as it may actually increase morbidity.

The main causes of anemia in the general population are related to iron deficiency, vitamin B12 and folate deficiency, renal failure, and anemia of chronic disease. It is imperative to diagnose the cause of anemia and direct treatment of anemia depending on its cause.

22.3 Von Willebrand Disease

Von Willebrand disease (VWD) is the most common inherited bleeding disorder affecting up to 1% of the population resulting in surgical and nonsurgical bleeding risks. This autosomal dominant disease manifests as easy bruisability, epistaxis, and significant oral surgical bleeding. VWD results from quantitative and qualitative defects in the von Willebrand factor, an important protein in hemostasis. The von Willebrand factor binds to platelet glycoprotein Ib to allow for adherence of the platelet to subendothelial surface proteins. VWD can be divided into three different categories: type 1 VWD having a partial deficiency of the factor, type 2 with a qualitative defect within the protein, and type 3 having a severe deficiency of the total protein complex. A ristocetin cofactor assay directly relays the activity of von Willebrand factor because it will only agglutinate with platelets with properly functioning von Willebrand factor. In addition, factor VIII levels are often found to be deficient in VWD patients because factor VIII and von Willebrand factor share an intimate association.

Basically, the treatment of VWD depends on the type of von Willebrand disease. Most type 1 and some type 2 patients respond to desmopressin acetate at a dosage of 0.3 μg/kg infused over 30 min stimulating the release of von Willebrand factor from endothelial cells and raising the plasma level of the von Willebrand factor and factor VIII by three to five times. Repeated administration of desmopressin in proximity may lead to tachyphylaxis; therefore, no more than once daily and no more than three consecutive daily administrations are acceptable.

Patients who do not respond to desmopressin may require pooled human plasma. Careful postoperative clinical assessment is obligatory to determine further treatment in patients known to have VWD. Several products available in the United States and approved by the FDA contain intact vWF such as Humate-P, Alphanate, and Wilate. These plasma-derived products contain vWF and factor VIII in varying ratios and used in those with a severe dysfunction of the factor or those undergoing a more invasive procedure with a high risk of bleeding [7, 8].

22.4 Sickle Cell Syndromes

Sickle cell anemia is one of the most common hemoglobinopathies affecting 10% of all African-Americans living in the United States. This disease occurs as a result of a genetic mutation substituting a valine for glutamic acid in the sixth position of the beta chain of the hemoglobin molecule. This results in an alteration in the shape of the erythrocyte when the hemoglobin is deoxygenated leading to anemia, chronic hemolysis, and vascular occlusion.

The sickle cell trait (heterozygous state) creates very few surgical or anesthesia risks. On the other hand, the disease (homozygous state) is of significant importance when planning a surgical procedure. Perioperative management is focused on hydration, excellent oxygenation, and keeping abnormal hemoglobin S levels below 30–50% while keeping normal hemoglobin A levels greater than 8–10 g/dL.

22.5 Hemophilia

Hemophilia is an inherited bleeding disorder. It results from either decreased levels of factor VIII (known as hemophilia A) or factor IX (hemophilia B). The prevalence of hemophilia is approximately 1 in 5000 males with up to 90% having a deficiency in factor VIII and about 10% having a deficiency in factor IX. Hemophilia can be mild, moderate, or severe. Patients with severe hemophilia have a factor level of less than 1%. Factor levels between 1% and 5% correspond to moderate hemophilia, and for mild hemophilia, factor levels are between 5% and 35%. The classic clinical signs of a patient with hemophilia are bruising, muscle and joint hemorrhage, and excessive bleeding after trauma or surgical procedures.

The treatment for hemophilia is replacement of factors VIII or IX done through purified plasma-derived concentrate or more recently recombinant factor concentrates. Surgical procedures require preoperative doses of factor concentrations to allow for adequate control of postoperative bleeding. Factor VIII is given with an initial loading dose of 50 units/kg, followed by 25 units/kg every 12 h to reach the minimum factor VIII level of 30%. Factor IX is dosed at 100 units/kg loading dose followed by 25 units/kg every 12 h to maintain a minimum level of 25–30%. Occasionally, in mild cases or after minor procedures, the use of desmopressin (DDAVP) can raise the levels of factor VIII that allow for adequate hemostasis. For minor surgery, a level of factor VIII or IX of 50% or more would be sufficient, whereas in major procedures, an 80–100% level of factor VIII or factor IX is required [7, 9].

22.6 Platelet Function Disorders

Platelet disorders are usually divided into two categories: defects of function or number of platelets or both. Patients with platelet function disorders present usually with similar symptoms regardless of the defect. They present with mucocutaneous bleeding similar to patients with vWD. The two most commonly available tests of platelet function are the platelet aggregation assays and the PFA-100. The PFA-100 has limitations in that it is affected by both hemoglobin level and platelet count and has limited sensitivity. Platelet aggregometry is the most specific test for platelet function. Both tests can be affected by several medications [10].

22.7 Thrombocytopenias

The normal range for platelet levels is between 150 and 400 × 109/L. The platelets are routinely synthesized by the bone marrow and then destroyed by the spleen. Normally, only one-third of all the circulatory platelets are sequestered by the spleen. In those with splenomegaly, up to 80–90% of the circulatory platelets are sequestered by the spleen.

Thrombocytopenia is a quantitative platelet disorder, where there is increased platelet destruction, decreased platelet production, or abnormal distribution and/or increased sequestration. These platelet abnormalities can be either inherited or acquired. The most common cause of thrombocytopenia is immunologic, where autoantibodies destroy existing platelets. These patients with immunologic cause of thrombocytopenia are best treated preoperatively with splenectomy, corticosteroids, or immunoglobulin.

In addition to the thrombocytopenias, there are adhesion defects, aggregation defects, and granular defects resulting in mucosal bleeding, surgical bleeding, or easy bruisability and needing platelet transfusion before any surgical procedure. That is why it is imperative that the platelets be evaluated before any surgery.

A single platelet concentrate usually yields an incremental rise in platelet levels of 10,000/μL/m^2. A platelet count should be obtained approximately 1 h after the appropriate platelet transfusion to confirm the desired estimate preoperatively. In general, a patient with a platelet count of 60,000–100,000/μL or greater can tolerate most routine surgeries. Considering that platelet survival postoperatively is affected by fever, infection, or bleeding, close monitoring of platelet levels followed by proper supplementation is essential.

It is imperative to recognize life-threatening causes of thrombocytopenia. These include drug-induced thrombocytopenia, thrombotic thrombocytopenic purpura, sepsis, disseminated intravascular coagulation (DIC), post-transfusion purpura, acute leukemia, and catastrophic antiphospholipid antibody syndrome. Examination of the blood smear is crucial for all patients with thrombocytopenia [2, 11].

22.8 Perioperative Management of Coagulation-Altering Therapy

Prophylactic and therapeutic use of coagulation-altering therapy has been increasing owing to the increase in prevalence of coronary artery disease, atrial fibrillation (AF), peripheral vascular disease, and other risk factors of the aging US population.

Before every invasive/surgical procedure, clinicians must assess the risk versus benefit of thrombosis associated with discontinuing any anticoagulation agent and balance that against the potential bleeding risk perioperatively. Therefore, deciding on patient-specific management plans such as holding, continuing, and bridging, anticoagulation therapy should usually be made in consultation with the prescribing physician and the oral health-care specialist performing the procedure, and then communicated directly to the patient.

Patients who are prescribed with anticoagulant medications are at different degrees of risk of a thrombotic event if the medications were to be discontinued. Patients who are at low thrombotic risk if the anticoagulant medication were discontinued are: aortic valve prosthesis without other thrombotic risk factors (like caged-ball or single tilting disk valve; atrial fibrillation; history of stroke, TIA, or other embolic event; left ventricular failure; and underlying hypercoagulable state, including cancer) or AF with low stroke risk or VTE >3 months previously. Patients within the low risk category have a risk of thrombosis of less than 5% if they are not anticoagulated. Patients who are at moderate thrombotic risk if the anticoagulant medication is discontinued are mitral or multiple prostheses or aortic prosthesis with risk factors for thrombosis or AF at high stroke risk or VTE within past 3 months. Patients with moderate and high thrombosis risk have a 5–10% and 10% annual risk of thrombosis or more, respectively.

Specific discussion pertaining to management of the maxillofacial surgery patient will be discussed later. However, generalizations pertaining to the medical management of these thrombotic risk categories are (1) low risk, anticoagulant can be stopped prior to surgery, and (2) high risk, if anticoagulant therapy is stopped, the patient should be "bridged" with heparin [12–14].

22.9 Adjunctive Measures

The best management of perioperative hemorrhage of maxillofacial surgeries is prevention. This includes proper preoperative patient assessment, knowledge of the various bleeding disorders, and the characterization of the correct methods of management.

Key preventive measures in patients with bleeding disorders include the following:

- Use hemostatic materials.
- Use lasers or electrocautery to reduce bleeding at the time of surgical intervention.
- Topical rinses, such as tranexamic acid, to inhibit fibrinolysis.
- Use various pressure dressings to the appropriate locations of the oral cavity.
- Avoid NSAIDS analgesics.
- Be cognizant that antibiotics (excluding a one-time dose for prophylaxis) may alter the effect of warfarin.

Conclusion

The perioperative management of patients with hematologic disorders or taking medications affecting hemostasis relies heavily on judicious history taking, physical examination and appropriate interpretation of blood tests, close collaboration between the surgeon, primary care physician, anesthesiologist, and hematologist is crucial for the safe management of patients undergoing maxillofacial surgery. For most dentoalveolar surgery, the patient's medications do not require modification. Local hemostatic measures should be used. For major oral and maxillofacial surgical procedures, the patient is managed in a manner comparable to other intermediate to high bleeding risk procedures.

References

1. World Health Organization. Nutritional anaemias: report of a WHO Scientific Group [meeting held in Geneva from 13 to 17 March 1967]. Geneva: World Health Organization, 1968
2. Lubin MF, Walker HK, Smith RB. Medical management of the surgical patient. 3rd ed. Philadelphia, PA: JB Lippincott; 1992.
3. Musallam KM, Tamim HM, Richards T, et al. Preoperative anaemia and postoperative outcomes in non-cardiac surgery: a retrospective cohort study. Lancet. 2011;378:1396–407.
4. Baron DM, Hochrieser H, Posch M, et al. Preoperative anaemia is associated with poor clinical outcome in non-cardiac surgery patients. Br J Anaesth. 2014;113:416–23.
5. Simon TL, et al. Practice parameter for the use of red blood cell transfusions: developed by the Red Blood Cell Administration Practice Guideline Development Task Force of the College of American Pathologists. Arch Pathol. 1998;122(2):130.
6. Carson JL, Carless PA, Hebert PC. Transfusion thresholds and other strategies for guiding allogeneic red blood cell transfusion. Cochrane Libr. 2012;4(1):CD002042.
7. Hoffman R, et al. Hematology: basic principles of practice. Philadelphia: Churchill Livingstone; 2005.
8. Nichols WL, et al. von Willebrand disease (VWD): evidence-based diagnosis and management guidelines, the National Heart, Lung, and Blood Institute (NHLBI) Expert Panel report (USA) 1. Haemophilia. 2008;14(2):171–232.
9. Berntorp E, Shapiro AD. Modern haemophilia care. Lancet. 2012;379(9824):1447–56.
10. Hayward CPM. Diagnostic evaluation of platelet function disorders. Blood Rev. 2011;25(4):169–73.
11. Arnold DM, Lim W. A rational approach to the diagnosis and management of thrombocytopenia in the hospitalized patient. Semin Hematol. 2011;48(4):251–8. WB Saunders.
12. Halaszynski TM. Administration of coagulation-altering therapy in the patient presenting for oral health and maxillofacial surgery. Oral Maxillofac Surg Clin North Am. 2016;28(4):443–60.
13. Kaboli P, Henderson MC, White RH. DVT prophylaxis and anticoagulation in the surgical patient. Med Clin North Am. 2003;87(1):77–110.
14. Ortel TL. Perioperative management of patients on chronic antithrombotic therapy. ASH Education Program Book. 2012;2012(1):529–35.

23 Oncologic Disorders and Maxillofacial Surgery

Victor A. Chang

Abstract

There has been tremendous progress in cancer treatment. Cancer patients are living longer with improved quality of life. It is likely that maxillofacial surgeons will encounter cancer patients in need of their expertise, whether their surgical intervention is an integral part of cancer treatment or for an unrelated issue. This chapter seeks to review major problems encountered in the perioperative setting by maxillofacial surgeons, including cancer treatment complications, pain management, and major psychiatric issues. In the later part of the chapter, some attention is devoted to the so-called immunotherapy that is revolutionizing cancer treatment. The chapter aims to remind the surgeon of the major problems encountered in cancer patients in the perioperative setting and offer some management guidance.

23.1 Introduction

The perioperative management of cancer patients can be complex. There are direct and indirect effects of cancer and side effects of cancer therapy. Their perioperative impact needs to be considered in maxillofacial surgery.

Preoperative evaluation of cancer patients should include an assessment of nutritional status, functional status, and symptom control, in addition to an assessment of general medical issues. The biology of the cancer and the after effects of any prior chemotherapy or radiation should be noted as well. The timing and purpose of the surgery can affect perioperative evaluation in cancer patients. Functional status over age should be considered in considering surgery [1].

23.2 Nutrition

Patients with cancer may become malnourished for many reasons. Eating and drinking may be impaired by pain, nausea, mucositis, or tumors involving the oropharynx or gastrointestinal tract. Metabolic disturbance may induce anorexia and weight loss [2–4].

V.A. Chang, M.D.
Yale University School of Medicine, New Haven, CT, USA
e-mail: vachang@hotmail.com

© Springer International Publishing AG 2018

E.M. Ferneini, J.D. Bennett (eds.), *Perioperative Assessment of the Maxillofacial Surgery Patient*, https://doi.org/10.1007/978-3-319-58868-1_23

Many studies have failed to show a survival benefit from preoperative nutritional intervention in cancer patients undergoing surgery, but some have found fewer operative complications and shorter length of hospital stay in severely malnourished patients receiving nutritional support prior to major surgery for the head and neck cancers [5].

23.3 Pain

Cancer patients often have severe pain and require medication for relief. Patients who have been receiving opioid analgesics can be expected to have some degree of tolerance and may require dose escalation in the postoperative period to attain adequate pain control. Many cancer patients are on long-acting forms of opioids and may require conversion to short-acting forms of narcotics in the perioperative period.

23.4 Cardiovascular Issues

23.4.1 Pericardial Disease

Cancer patients are at risk for malignant and nonmalignant pericardial disease. Metastases to the pericardium can cause effusions, tamponade, and constrictive pericarditis. Radiation treatment to the mediastinum can also cause constrictive pericarditis or effusions with tamponade. Pericarditis may occur months to years after radiation treatment [6].

Echocardiography should be performed if physical examination reveals findings consistent with tamponade or constriction (i.e., jugular venous distension, hypotension, narrowed pulse pressure, distant heart sounds, or excessive respiratory variation in blood pressure) or if electrocardiography (ECG) or imaging studies suggest a significant pericardial effusion [6].

Tamponade and constrictive pericarditis should be treated prior to surgery if possible, and patients with asymptomatic malignant pericardial effusions need to be monitored for the development of tamponade in the perioperative period [6].

23.4.2 Coronary Artery Disease and Conduction Disorder

Radiation therapy to fields that include the heart can lead to premature coronary heart disease and conduction disorder. Patients who have a history of thoracic radiation therapy should be assessed for heart disease as part of the preoperative history and exam and should have a preoperative ECG [6].

23.4.3 Cardiac Valvular Disease

Radiation therapy has also been associated with valvular heart disease, particularly of the mitral and aortic valves. Cardiac auscultation is an important part of the perioperative assessment for patients with a history of chest irradiation [6].

23.4.4 Cardiac Toxicity from Chemotherapy

Certain chemotherapy agents, particularly trastuzumab monoclonal antibody therapy and the anthracyclines (i.e., doxorubicin, daunorubicin, idarubicin, epirubicin, and mitoxantrone), cause significant cardiotoxicity. Dose-dependent cardiomyopathy and heart failure may occur in patients who have received cumulative doses of over 550 mg/m^2 of doxorubicin and 600 mg/m^2 of daunorubicin. Pre-existing heart disease, prior radiation therapy, and exposure to other potentially cardiotoxic chemotherapy agents (i.e., taxanes, trastuzumab) can lower the cumulative anthracycline dose threshold at which cardiomyopathy develops [7].

ECG abnormalities such as tachycardia, premature atrial or ventricular contractions, nonspecific *ST* and *T* wave changes, and low-voltage QRS complexes may be early signs of cardiotoxicity. They are insensitive indicators of cardiac dysfunction. Preoperative assessment of the left cardiac ventricular function, such as echocardiography, should be considered in patients who are at risk for cardiomyopathy, as they are at risk for heart failure [7].

Several chemotherapy drugs are associated with prolongation of the QT interval, particularly crizotinib, dasatinib, eribulin, and vascular endothelial growth factor inhibitors, including pazopanib, sorafenib, sunitinib, and vandetanib. These patients are at risk for potentially fatal arrhythmias [7].

23.5 Pulmonary Issues

Patients with tumors in or adjacent to the central airway are at risk for airway obstruction or superior vena cava (SVC) syndrome. Stridor, or any signs and symptoms of upper airway obstruction, should be assessed preoperatively by laryngoscopy [8].

The incidence of SVC syndrome due to thrombosis has risen due to increased use of intravascular devices, such as catheters and pacemakers. As much as 50 percent of nonmalignant cases of SVC syndrome are attributable to fibrosing mediastinitis, due to infection and radiation [8].

23.5.1 Cancer Treatment-Related Pulmonary Toxicity

Both chemotherapy and radiation can produce pulmonary toxicity that may be intensified when both are given concurrently.

Bleomycin is associated with pulmonary toxicity or pneumonitis in up to 10% of patients. Also, recent bleomycin treatment in the setting of receiving supplemental inhaled oxygen, such as during general anesthesia, may induce pulmonary toxicity several years after the chemotherapy treatment. For bleomycin-exposed patients who undergo subsequent surgery, supplemental oxygen during surgery should be carefully titrated, and intravenous fluids are administered sparingly to avoid volume overload and perioperative pulmonary edema. As with other preoperative patients who may have pulmonary disease, patients exposed to chest radiation therapy or chemotherapy should undergo a thorough history, review of systems, physical examination, and a preoperative chest radiograph. Pulmonary function testing and measurement of oxygen saturation may be appropriate for selected patients with abnormal examination findings or symptoms. Cancer patients at risk of postoperative pulmonary complications can benefit from special perioperative care [9].

23.5.2 Pleural Effusions

Cancer patients who have a pleural effusion that is large enough to be symptomatic may benefit from therapeutic thoracentesis prior to surgery [10].

23.6 Hematologic Issues

23.6.1 Hypercoagulability

Hypercoagulability is common in cancer patients, particularly those with advanced disease and primary brain tumors, and may be due to increased plasma levels of clotting factors, cytokines, procoagulants, or to increased release of tissue plasminogen activator [11]. Hypercoagulability, leading to arterial thrombosis, i.e., myocardial infarction or stroke as well as venous thrombosis such as deep vein thrombosis, is also a potential side effect of chemotherapy. Some of the drugs include bevacizumab anti-VEGF monoclonal antibody therapy and other drugs that target the vascular endothelial growth factor, thalidomide, lenalidomide, and combination chemotherapy with drugs including bleomycin, cisplatin, and vinblastine [12].

23.6.2 Neutropenia and Lymphopenia

Cancer patients who are myelosuppressed due to chemotherapy or hematologic malignancy are at increased risk of infection. The risk is higher with longer durations of neutropenia and lymphopenia [13].

Whenever possible, elective or non-emergent surgery should be postponed in neutropenic patients. Postoperative fever is common, and if it develops in the setting of neutropenia, aggressive diagnostic and therapeutic interventions are necessary. Neutropenic fever requires prompt administration of broad spectrum antimicrobials. Even when the neutropenia has resolved, cancer patients who received myelosuppressive chemotherapy remain relatively immunocompromised for a period of time [13].

Patients with lymphoma or hematologic cancer such as chronic lymphocytic leukemia have abnormal cellular and humoral-mediated immune responses due to defects in immune effector cells, and they are predisposed to infection, particularly if they are treated with purine analogs (e.g., fludarabine), chlorambucil, and alemtuzumab. These issues with immunity should be considered in the perioperative period [14].

23.6.3 Neutropenia

Neutropenia is usually defined as an absolute neutrophil count (ANC) <1500 cells/μL and severe neutropenia as an ANC <500 cells/μL or an ANC that is expected to decrease to <500 cells/μL over the next 48 h. The risk of clinically important infection rises as the neutrophil count falls below 500 cells/μL and is higher in those with a prolonged duration of neutropenia (>7 days). Fever in a neutropenic patient is usually defined as a single temperature ≥38.3 °C (101 °F) or a temperature ≥38 °C (100.4 °F) sustained over a 1-hour period [15].

After chemotherapy the absolute neutrophil count (ANC) decreases until it reaches its lowest point or nadir. The timing and depth of chemotherapy-induced nadirs vary based on patient factors and type of chemotherapy administered. In general the nadir occurs in 10–14 days. Granulocyte colony-stimulating factors (G-CSFs) may be considered and used in reducing the depth and duration of the nadir [15].

There is no established role for the use of G-CSFs in afebrile patients who have already developed severe neutropenia after chemotherapy. The lack of benefit from G-CSFs in this setting was illustrated in a controlled trial in which 138 afebrile outpatients with severe chemotherapy-induced neutropenia (absolute neutrophil count [ANC] ≤500/μL) were randomly assigned to G-CSF or placebo until the ANC recovered to at least 500/μL [16].

23.6.4 Neutropenia from Radiation Therapy

Granulocyte colony-stimulating factor (G-CSF; filgrastim) and pegfilgrastim (the pegylated formulation of G-CSF) are approved by the US Food and Drug Administration (FDA) for patients acutely exposed to myelosuppressive doses of radiation (i.e., >2 Gy). Daily injections of G-CSF are required until neutropenia improves. Owing to its prolonged half-life, pegfilgrastim should be administered as two doses of 6 μg/kg subcutaneously, separated by 1 week [17].

23.6.5 Thrombocytopenia

Thrombocytopenia in cancer patients occurs either as a result of the malignancy or from treatment. In general, a platelet count of at least 50,000/μL is adequate for most surgical procedures, but the specific procedure and the platelet function must also be considered. Consider postponing surgery until the platelet count has recovered if the thrombocytopenia is related to chemotherapy or radiation [18–20].

Medications that can interfere with platelet function (aspirin, clopidogrel, nonsteroidal anti-inflammatory drugs) should be discontinued long enough prior to surgery to allow for adequate recovery of platelet function. This period will depend upon the specific antiplatelet agent, the surgery, and the patient's other clinical conditions and medications [21].

23.6.6 Prophylactic Platelet Transfusion

Patients with leukemia, hematopoietic cell transplant (HCT), or those being treated with cytotoxic chemotherapy have a suppressed bone marrow that cannot produce adequate platelets. We use prophylactic transfusion in these settings. The thresholds suggested below apply to patients with thrombocytopenia who are afebrile and without active infection. If fever or sepsis is present, higher thresholds may be needed. In general, standard dose prophylactic transfusion is recommended at a threshold platelet count of 10,000/μL and transfusion for any bleeding greater than petechial bleeding [22, 23].

Patients with acute promyelocytic leukemia often have an associated coagulopathy that puts them at high risk for disseminated intravascular coagulation and bleeding. Prophylactic transfusion is recommended at a platelet count of 30,000–50,000/μL and treats any sign of bleeding, especially central nervous system bleeding, with immediate platelet transfusion [22, 23].

23.6.7 Anemia

Many factors may contribute to the development of anemia in the cancer patient. In determining which factors caused the anemia, it is important to correlate patients' clinical histories and physical exam findings with laboratory observations, realizing that there may be more than one contributing cause of the anemia [24].

As with anemias in general, three causes should be considered when assessing causes of anemia in patients with malignancies [25]:

Bleeding
Increased red blood cell (RBC) destruction or hemolysis
Decreased RBC production

One or more of the above three mechanisms may be responsible for the anemia. Some causes are specific for cancer patients [25]:

Direct bone marrow suppression by the cancer
Direct destruction of the RBC by the cancer
Effects of cancer treatment
Nutritional impairment with the cancer

23.6.8 Correction of Anemia

Iron supplementation—in surgical patients, intravenous iron—alone increased hemoglobin levels by 1–2 g in as little as 1 week, and a review of 14 studies reported a clinically and statistically significant increase in hemoglobin in patients treated with intravenous iron alone. Oral supplementation is an acceptable option in non-emergent or elective cases [26].

Results from randomized trials suggest preoperative recombinant human erythropoietin (rHuEPO) reduces risk of allogeneic transfusion [26].

While safety concerns have been raised about the use of rHuEPO, these risks were confined to repetitive use in cancer patients receiving chemotherapy. The FDA has issued a warning based on reports that erythropoiesis-stimulating agents are associated with serious cardiac and thrombovascular events and more rapid tumor progression with increased mortality in cancer patients [27].

However, there may be a role for preoperative rHuEPO to correct anemia in patients who would refuse allogeneic transfusion that are too anemic to qualify for autologous blood donation [28].

Preoperative transfusion may be required for patients who become unstable or who continue to bleed heavily before definitive therapy can be performed. The decision to transfuse should be based not only on hemoglobin level but also on individual patient characteristics and symptoms. In general, the different guidelines have recommended that transfusion is not indicated for hemoglobin >10 g/dL but the lower threshold varies from 6 to 8 g/dL. As a result, the 2016 AABB guidelines include the following recommendations for hemodynamically stable patients without active bleeding [28]:

- Hemoglobin <6 g/dL—transfusion recommended except in exceptional circumstances.
- Hemoglobin 6–7 g/dL—transfusion likely to be indicated.
- Hemoglobin 7–8 g/dL—transfusion may be appropriate in patients undergoing orthopedic surgery or cardiac surgery, and in those with

stable cardiovascular disease, after evaluating the patient's clinical status.

- Hemoglobin 8–10 g/dL—transfusion generally not indicated but should be considered for some populations (i.e., those with symptomatic anemia, ongoing bleeding, acute coronary syndrome with ischemia, and hematology/oncology patients with severe thrombocytopenia who are at risk of bleeding).
- Hemoglobin >10 g/dL—transfusion generally not indicated except in exceptional circumstances.

The guidelines emphasize that the decision to transfuse should not be based only on hemoglobin level but should incorporate individual patient characteristics and symptoms. Clinical judgment is critical in the decision to transfuse. To transfuse with RBCs above or below the specified hemoglobin threshold may be dictated by the clinical context. The decision not to transfuse with RBCs to a hemoglobin concentration below the recommended threshold is also a matter of clinical judgment [28].

23.7 Neurologic Issues

23.7.1 Paraneoplastic Syndromes

Paraneoplastic syndromes that affect neuromuscular function are relatively rare but are of particular concern in the perioperative period because treatment with anesthetic agents can exacerbate neuromuscular dysfunction, leading to respiratory failure or delayed extubation. Although a wide variety of tumor types may be responsible, many of these neuromuscular paraneoplastic syndromes arise in the setting of small cell lung cancer. Treatment of the cancer may mitigate these symptoms [29].

23.7.2 Screening for Brain Metastases

Routine imaging of the central nervous system is not mandatory in patients with cancer prior to surgery. However, radiographic imaging of the brain should be considered in the setting of unexplained symptoms referable to the central nervous system (CNS). Furthermore, if prophylactic anticoagulation is planned, radiographic screening for brain metastases, preferably with magnetic resonance imaging or MRI, should be done in those patients whose tumors have a propensity to spread to the CNS and spontaneously bleed, including melanoma, small cell lung cancer, choriocarcinoma, renal cell, breast, adenocarcinoma of the lung, or thyroid cancer. Cancer patients in general should be imaged if there are any symptoms suggesting brain metastasis, such as headaches, mental status changes, seizures, and other neurologic symptoms. The presence of untreated CNS metastases represents a relative contraindication to anticoagulation, and active intracranial bleeding is an absolute contraindication [30].

23.7.3 Stroke Risk in Patients Undergoing Neck Irradiation

Ischemic stroke can be a late complication of neck irradiation, with multiple factors contributing to this risk, including carotid artery stenosis, increased deposition of plaque, and pre-existing risk factors for cerebrovascular disease, such as smoking. A high index of suspicion for carotid artery disease in the perioperative setting should be maintained in patients who have received neck irradiation, particularly in conjunction with chemotherapy for head and neck cancer [31].

23.8 Endocrinopathy

23.8.1 Glucocorticoids

Many chemotherapy regimens include glucocorticoids, either as a therapeutic agent or as a component of premedication to prevent chemotherapy-induced nausea and vomiting or an infusion reaction. Glucocorticoids may unmask occult diabetes or exacerbate previously controlled blood sugar levels [32].

23.8.2 Adrenal Insufficiency

Adrenal insufficiency can occur in cancer patients as a result of adrenal suppression from chronic glucocorticoid treatment or, uncommonly, from metastatic disease to both adrenal glands. The presence or absence of adrenal suppression, and therefore the need for perioperative "stress-dose" glucocorticoid coverage, can often be anticipated from the dose and duration of the patient's glucocorticoid therapy [33].

The hypothalamic–pituitary–adrenal (HPA) axis suppression should be assumed to be present in patients taking prednisone at a dose greater than 20 mg/day for 3 weeks or more and in patients with a cushingoid appearance [33].

In general, patients who have taken any dose of glucocorticoids for less than 3 weeks or who have taken chronic alternate day therapy are unlikely to have a suppressed HPA axis and should continue on their usual dose of glucocorticoids perioperatively. Patients on intermediate doses of glucocorticoids should undergo testing, although many clinicians prefer empiric treatment with "stress-dose" glucocorticoids [33].

The so-called immunotherapy that is revolutionizing cancer treatment is well known for causing endocrinopathies including adrenal dysfunction. Please refer to the later section on immunotherapy side effects.

23.8.3 Hypothyroidism

Radiation therapy to the neck and chest can cause hypothyroidism [34].

Hypothyroidism may also complicate long-term treatment with the tyrosine kinase inhibitors *sunitinib* and less so with *sorafenib*. Because hypothyroidism is associated with poor surgical site healing, serum thyroid-stimulating hormone (TSH) and free T4 concentrations should be measured prior to surgery in patients who have received more than 10 Gy total dose to the neck or are receiving treatment with *sunitinib* or *sorafenib*. Patients found to be hypothyroid should receive supplemental thyroid hormone prior to surgery [35].

The so-called immunotherapy is well known for causing thyroid dysfunction. Please refer to the later section on immunotherapy side effects.

23.9 Electrolyte Imbalance

23.9.1 Hyponatremia

Preoperative hyponatremia can occur in cancer patients and may be attributed to paraneoplastic effects of the tumor or be caused by cancer treatments [36].

Preoperative hyponatremia can complicate perioperative management. In a cohort study of 964,263 adults undergoing major surgery at 200 hospitals over a 5-year period, a preoperative serum sodium concentration below 135 mmol/L was associated with significantly higher postoperative 30-day mortality (adjusted odds ratio [aOR] 1.44) and significantly higher rates of major adverse cardiac events (aOR 1.21), surgical site infection (aOR 1.24), and pneumonia (aOR 1.17), as well as a longer postoperative hospitalization, by a median of 1 day. Because the association was actually stronger for lower-risk surgeries and for younger patients and was independent of the time prior to surgery that the serum sodium was measured, hyponatremia was likely not the direct cause of postoperative complications but instead a marker for impaired fluid and electrolyte homeostasis associated with chronic conditions, such as chronic heart failure [37].

Therefore, the best approach to the patient with preoperative hyponatremia may be to identify the underlying related disorders, to avoid exacerbating the hyponatremia with hypotonic intravenous solutions, and to closely monitor and carefully manage the patient in the perioperative period [38].

23.9.2 Hypercalcemia

Hypercalcemia is a common complication of cancer, occurring in up to 15% of the patients. Therefore, a preoperative screening serum calcium measurement is often appropriate in cancer patients. If hypercalcemia is found, the patient's hydration should be optimized and calcium levels normalized prior to surgery, if possible [39].

Hypercalcemia is associated with a poor prognosis. The most common tumors that cause hypercalcemia are breast cancer, multiple myeloma, lymphoma, and squamous cell cancers [39].

There are three major mechanisms in malignant hypercalcemia [39]:

- Tumor secretion of parathyroid hormone-related protein (PTHrP)
- Osteolytic metastases with local release of cytokines
- Tumor production of 1,25-dihydroxyvitamin D

Hypercalcemia in patients with tumors secreting PTHrP is due to both increased bone resorption and distal renal tubular calcium reabsorption, whereas hypercalcemia in patients with osteolytic metastases is primarily due to increased bone resorption and release of calcium from the bone. In cancer patients with tumor production of 1,25-dihydroxyvitamin D, hypercalcemia is the result of a combination of increased intestinal calcium absorption and bone resorption [39].

The initial approach to determining the mechanism of hypercalcemia in the presence of a low-normal or low serum parathyroid hormone or PTH concentration (<20 pg/mL) includes measurement of PTHrP and vitamin D metabolites. If PTHrP and vitamin D metabolites are not elevated, another source for the hypercalcemia must be considered. Additional laboratory testing is warranted, such as serum and urine protein electrophoresis and serum free light chain assay, for possible multiple myeloma, TSH, and vitamin A [40].

Patients with hypercalcemia can present with few or no symptoms with mild chronic hypercalcemia to severe obtundation and coma. The degree of hypercalcemia, along with the rate of rise of serum calcium concentration, correlates with the symptoms and the severity and dictates the urgency of treatment intervention. Patients with a serum calcium concentration >14 mg/dL (3.5 mmol/L) require treatment, regardless of symptoms [40].

Patients with severe hypercalcemia, calcium >14 mg/dL (3.5 mmol/L), usually require aggressive therapy. Therapeutic intervention for severe hypercalcemia consists of three major approaches [41]:

- Volume expansion with isotonic saline at an initial rate of 200–300 mL/h that is then adjusted to maintain the urine output at 100–150 mL/h. In the absence of renal failure or heart failure, loop diuretic therapy to directly increase calcium excretion is not recommended, because of complication risks and the availability of drugs that inhibit bone resorption.
- Salmon calcitonin (4 international units/kg) can be given with repeat measurement of the serum calcium after several hours. If a hypocalcemic response is seen, then the patient is calcitonin sensitive and the calcitonin can be repeated every 6–12 h (4–8 international units/kg). Calcitonin may be used with a bisphosphonate in patients with severe or symptomatic hypercalcemia.
- Bisphosphonate administration with zoledronic acid (4 mg intravenously [IV] over 15 min) or pamidronate (60–90 mg IV over 2 h) can be given with isotonic hydration. Zoledronic acid is superior to pamidronate in reversing hypercalcemia related to malignancy.

The administration of calcitonin plus saline should result in substantial reduction in serum calcium concentrations within 12–48 h. The bisphosphonate will be effective by the second to fourth day, thereby maintaining control of the hypercalcemia. Rarely, more aggressive measures such as hemodialysis are necessary [41].

23.10 Side Effects of Chemotherapy

23.10.1 Hepatotoxicity

Several chemotherapy drugs are known for potential for hepatotoxicity. If there are signs or symptoms suggestive of hepatotoxicity, there is a need to check the prothrombin time as a test of adequate hepatic synthetic function prior to surgery [42].

Reactivation of viral hepatitis, especially hepatitis B virus, is a potential complication of myelosuppressive chemotherapy, particularly in patients receiving rituximab and ofatumumab. Patients who are positive for HBV surface antigen or for antibodies against HBV core antigen (anti-HBc) should have liver function tests done prior to surgery [43].

23.10.2 Nephrotoxicity

Many chemotherapy agents are potentially nephrotoxic, especially cisplatin. For all patients who have recently undergone chemotherapy, check serum blood urea nitrogen, creatinine, and electrolyte concentrations before surgery [44].

23.10.3 Wound Healing

Impaired wound healing is a complication of chemotherapy. It is notable for antiangiogenic agents targeting the vascular endothelial growth factor. Because of the long half-life of bevacizumab at 20 days, it is recommended that at least 28 days, but preferably 6–8 weeks, should have passed after a dose of bevacizumab before major surgery. Because of their shorter half-lives, it is suggested that orally active small molecular antiangiogenic tyrosine kinase inhibitors, including sunitinib, sorafenib, pazopanib, vandetanib, and cabozantinib, be stopped for at least 1 week before surgery and not reinitiated until adequate wound healing has occurred. For antiangiogenic tyrosine kinase inhibitors with a short half-life such as axitinib, it is suggested that drug stoppage occurs 48 h prior to surgery [45, 46].

More than 50% of cancer patients receive some form of radiation treatment, and despite improvements in radiation technique, poor wound healing is seen not infrequently. It is recommended to wait 3–6 weeks after radiation therapy before surgery or conversely to wait 3–4 weeks after surgery before starting radiation [47].

23.11 Side Effects of Immunotherapy

Checkpoint inhibitors, immunomodulatory antibodies that are used to enhance the immune system, have substantially improved the prognosis for patients with advanced melanoma as well as lung, bladder, and kidney cancers and lymphoma more recently. They are showing promise also in other types of malignancy, including GI and head and neck cancers. Inflammation of the pituitary, thyroid, or adrenal glands from checkpoint blockade often presents with nonspecific symptoms such as nausea, headache, fatigue, and vision changes [48].

The primary targets for checkpoint inhibition include [48]:

Programmed cell death 1 (PD-1) and PD-1 ligand (PD-L1) receptors—antibodies against PD-1 and PD-L1 have shown great promise in multiple malignancies. Nivolumab and pembrolizumab, both of which target PD-1, and atezolizumab, avelumab, and durvalumab, all of which target PD-L1, have been approved in multiple indications, including melanoma, renal cell carcinoma, non-small cell lung cancer, head and neck cancer, urothelial carcinoma, Hodgkin lymphoma, and Merkel cell carcinoma. Other indications are coming soon.

Cytotoxic T-lymphocyte-associated antigen 4 (CTLA-4)—ipilimumab, an anti-CTLA-4 antibody, is approved for use in patients with advanced melanoma. Another anti-CTLA-4 antibody, tremelimumab, will soon be available.

Checkpoint inhibition is associated with a unique spectrum of side effects referred to as immune-related adverse events. These include dermatologic, gastrointestinal, hepatic, endocrine, and other less common inflammatory events. They are believed to arise from general immunologic enhancement, and the use of immunosuppressive drugs including corticosteroids, tumor necrosis factor-alpha antagonists, mycophenolate mofetil, or other medications is often effective in ameliorating the events [49].

23.12 Immunizations Prior to Splenectomy

The spleen is the dominant site for the production of immunoglobulin M antibodies required for opsonizing encapsulated pathogens. Patients needing splenectomy should undergo preoperative immunization against *Streptococcus pneumoniae* (pneumococcus), *Neisseria meningitidis* (meningococcus), and *Haemophilus influenzae* type b. If vaccination was not possible prior to surgery, or unanticipated splenectomy was performed, the patient should be vaccinated postoperatively [50].

23.13 Anxiety and Depression

Cancer patients have a high rate of psychiatric comorbidity. Approximately one-half of the patients exhibit emotional difficulties. Common psychological problems in cancer patients include adjustment disorder, depression, anxiety, impoverished life satisfaction, or loss of self-esteem. Cancer patients most at risk for depression and other psychiatric illnesses are often those with advanced disease, a prior psychiatric history, poorly controlled pain, and other life stressors [51].

Anxiety, mood disorder, fatigue, and depression are common in head and neck cancer patients before and after treatment [52].

Body image reintegration and adjustment require compassion, patience, and encouragement from surrounding family and friends and treating physicians. Issues that can lead to social avoidance include physical limitations such as impaired speech and swallowing and concerns about one's appearance and disfigurement [53].

The National Comprehensive Cancer Network recommends routine screening of all cancer patients for psychological distress [54].

There are simple instruments to measure distress in cancer patients [55].

Please refer to the chapter on psychiatric disorders for management of anxiety and depression.

23.14 Delirium

Delirium is frequently seen in advanced cancer patients. It causes moderate to severe distress in both patient and caregivers. Delirium is an etiologically nonspecific, global, cerebral dysfunction, characterized by disturbances in the level of consciousness, attention, thinking, perception, memory, psychomotor behavior, emotion, and the sleep–wake cycle. Delirium can be due either to the direct effects of cancer on the central nervous system (CNS) or due to indirect CNS effects of the disease or related treatment. It is often multifactorial in origin. It is important to identify the cause of delirium in cancer patients since rapid and significant cognitive improvement can occur with treatment [56].

Early symptoms of delirium may be misdiagnosed as anxiety, anger, depression, psychosis, or unreasonable or uncooperative attitudes toward rehabilitative efforts or other treatments. The diagnosis should be considered in any patient with the acute onset of agitation, impaired cognitive function, altered attention span, or a fluctuating level of consciousness. A common error among medical and nursing staff is to conclude that a new psychiatric symptom is functional without completely ruling out all possible organic etiologies such as drug reaction or infection [57].

It can be difficult to differentiate delirium from dementia since they often share common clinical features such as disorientation and impaired memory, thinking, and judgment. Dementia can occur in relatively alert individuals with little or no clouding of consciousness. The temporal onset of symptoms in dementia is more insidious or chronically progressive, and the patient's sleep–wake cycle is generally intact. Patients with dementia have trouble with short- and long-term memory, impaired judgment and abstract thinking, and disturbance of higher cortical functions, such as aphasia and apraxia. Occasionally delirium is superimposed on an underlying dementia, particularly in the elderly, patients with AIDS, or cancer patients [58].

Conclusion

The perioperative management of cancer patients can be involved and challenging. The maxillofacial surgeon needs to consider the direct and indirect effects of the cancer and the side effects of cancer therapy. Their perioperative impact cannot be ignored for safe and effective patient management. By being mindful of the major problems encountered and related management, perioperative care of cancer patient is hopefully less daunting for the maxillofacial surgeon.

References

1. Ramesh HS, Pope D, Gennari R, Audisio RA. Optimising surgical management of elderly cancer patients. World J Surg Oncol. 2005;3:17.
2. Jain S, Palekar U, Shigli K, et al. Nutritional considerations for patients undergoing maxillofacial surgery—a literature review. Indian J Dent. 2014;5:52–5.
3. Teunissen SC, Wesker W, Kruitwagen C, et al. Symptom prevalence in patients with incurable cancer: a systematic review. J Pain Symptom Manage. 2007;34:94.
4. Davis MP, Dickerson D. Cachexia and anorexia: cancer's covert killer. Support Care Cancer. 2000;8:180.
5. Koretz RL, Avenell A, Lipman TO, et al. Does enteral nutrition affect clinical outcome? A systematic review of the randomized trials. Am J Gastroenterol. 2007;102:412.
6. Adams MJ, Hardenbergh PH, Constine LS, Lipshultz SE. Radiation-associated cardiovascular disease. Crit Rev Oncol Hematol. 2003;45:55.
7. Zamorano JL, Lancellotti P, Rodriguez Muñoz D, et al. ESC position paper on cancer treatments and cardiovascular toxicity developed under the auspices of the ESC Committee for Practice Guidelines: the task force for cancer treatments and cardiovascular toxicity of the European Society of Cardiology (ESC). Eur Heart J. 2016;37:2768.
8. Rice TW, Rodriguez RM, Light RW. The superior vena cava syndrome: clinical characteristics and evolving etiology. Medicine (Baltimore). 2006;85:37.
9. Klein DS, Wilds PR. Pulmonary toxicity of antineoplastic agents: anaesthetic and postoperative implications. Can Anaesth Soc J. 1983;30:399.
10. Heffner JE, Klein JS. Recent advances in the diagnosis and management of malignant pleural effusions. Mayo Clin Proc. 2008;83:235.
11. Young A, Chapman O, Connor C, et al. Thrombosis and cancer. Nat Rev Clin Oncol. 2012;9:437.
12. Lyman GH, Khorana AA, Kuderer NM, et al. Venous thromboembolism prophylaxis and treatment in patients with cancer: American Society of Clinical Oncology clinical practice guideline update. J Clin Oncol. 2013;31:2189.
13. Flowers CR, Seidenfeld J, Bow EJ, et al. Antimicrobial prophylaxis and outpatient management of fever and neutropenia in adults treated for malignancy: American Society of Clinical Oncology clinical practice guideline. J Clin Oncol. 2013;31:794.
14. Freifeld AG, Bow EJ, Sepkowitz KA, et al. Clinical practice guideline for the use of antimicrobial agents in neutropenic patients with cancer: 2010 update by the infectious diseases society of America. Clin Infect Dis. 2011;52:e56.
15. Crawford J, et al. Reduction by granulocyte colony-stimulating factor of fever and neutropenia induced by chemotherapy in patients with small-cell lung cancer. N Engl J Med. 1991;325:164–70.
16. Hartmann LC, Tschetter LK, Habermann TM, et al. Granulocyte colony-stimulating factor in severe chemotherapy-induced afebrile neutropenia. N Engl J Med. 1997;336:1776.
17. Smith TJ, Bohlke K, Lyman GH, et al. Recommendations for the use of WBC growth factors: American Society of Clinical Oncology Clinical Practice Guideline Update. J Clin Oncol. 2015;33:3199.
18. Wadhwa PD, Morrison VA. Infectious complications of chronic lymphocytic leukemia. Semin Oncol. 2006;33:240.
19. Chee YL, Crawford JC, Watson HG, Greaves M. Guidelines on the assessment of bleeding risk prior to surgery or invasive procedures. British Committee for Standards in Haematology. Br J Haematol. 2008;140:496.
20. Kumar A, Mhaskar R, Grossman BJ, et al. Platelet transfusion: a systematic review of the clinical evidence. Transfusion. 2015;55:1116.
21. Warner MA, Woodrum D, Hanson A, et al. Preprocedural platelet transfusion for patients with thrombocytopenia undergoing interventional radiology procedures is not associated with reduced bleeding complications. Transfusion. 2017;57:890.
22. Kaufman RM, Djulbegovic B, Gernsheimer T, et al. Platelet transfusion: a clinical practice guideline from the AABB. Ann Intern Med. 2015;162:205.
23. Schiffer CA, Anderson KC, Bennett CL, et al. Platelet transfusion for patients with cancer: clinical practice guidelines of the American Society of Clinical Oncology. J Clin Oncol. 2001;19:1519.
24. Macciò A, Madeddu C, Gramignano G, et al. The role of inflammation, iron, and nutritional status in cancer-related anemia: results of a large, prospective, observational study. Haematologica. 2015;100:124.

25. Tefferi A. Anemia in adults: a contemporary approach to diagnosis. Mayo Clin Proc. 2003;78:1274.
26. Shander A, Spence RK, Auerbach M. Can intravenous iron therapy meet the unmet needs created by the new restrictions on erythropoietic stimulating agents? Transfusion. 2010;50:719.
27. MedWatch Safety Alerts for Human Medical Products. http://www.fda.gov/medwatch/safety/2008/safety08.htm#ESA. Accessed 03 June 2008.
28. Carson JL, Guyatt G, Heddle NM, et al. Clinical practice guidelines from the aabb: red blood cell transfusion thresholds and storage. JAMA. 2016;316:2025.
29. Wirtz PW, Nijnuis MG, Sotodeh M, et al. The epidemiology of myasthenia gravis, Lambert-Eaton myasthenic syndrome and their associated tumours in the northern part of the province of South Holland. J Neurol. 2003;250:698.
30. Sperduto PW, Chao ST, Sneed PK, et al. Diagnosis-specific prognostic factors, indexes, and treatment outcomes for patients with newly diagnosed brain metastases: a multi-institutional analysis of 4,259 patients. Int J Radiat Oncol Biol Phys. 2010;77:655.
31. Scott AS, Parr LA, Johnstone PA. Risk of cerebrovascular events after neck and supraclavicular radiotherapy: a systematic review. Radiother Oncol. 2009;90:163.
32. Basch E, Prestrud AA, Hesketh PJ, et al. Antiemetics: American Society of Clinical Oncology clinical practice guideline update. J Clin Oncol. 2011;29:4189.
33. Salem M, Tainsh RE Jr, Bromberg J, et al. Perioperative glucocorticoid coverage. A reassessment 42 years after emergence of a problem. Ann Surg. 1994;219:416.
34. Tunio MA, Al Asiri M, Bayoumi Y, et al. Is thyroid gland an organ at risk in breast cancer patients treated with locoregional radiotherapy? Results of a pilot study. J Cancer Res Ther. 2015;11:684.
35. Hamnvik OP, Larsen PR, Marqusee E. Thyroid dysfunction from antineoplastic agents. J Natl Cancer Inst. 2011;103:1572.
36. Adrogué HJ, Madias NE. Hyponatremia. N Engl J Med. 2000;342:1581.
37. Leung AA, McAlister FA, Rogers SO Jr, et al. Preoperative hyponatremia and perioperative complications. Arch Intern Med. 2012;172:1474.
38. Vassalotti JA, DuPree E. Preoperative hyponatremia: an opportunity for intervention? Arch Intern Med. 2012;172:1482.
39. Stewart AF. Clinical practice. Hypercalcemia associated with cancer. N Engl J Med. 2005;352:373.
40. Bilezikian JP. Management of acute hypercalcemia. N Engl J Med. 1992;326:1196.
41. Maier JD, Levine SN. Hypercalcemia in the intensive care unit: a review of pathophysiology, diagnosis, and modern therapy. J Intensive Care Med. 2015;30:235.
42. Lee WM. Drug-induced hepatotoxicity. N Engl J Med. 1995;333:1118.
43. Voican CS, Mir O, Loulergue P, et al. Hepatitis B virus reactivation in patients with solid tumors receiving systemic anticancer treatment. Ann Oncol. 2016;27:2172.
44. Hensley ML, Hagerty KL, Kewalramani T, et al. American Society of Clinical Oncology 2008 clinical practice guideline update: use of chemotherapy and radiation therapy protectants. J Clin Oncol. 2009;27:127.
45. Erinjeri JP, Fong AJ, Kemeny NE, et al. Timing of administration of bevacizumab chemotherapy affects wound healing after chest wall port placement. Cancer. 2011;117:1296.
46. Harshman LC, RJ Y, Allen GI, et al. Surgical outcomes and complications associated with presurgical tyrosine kinase inhibition for advanced renal cell carcinoma (RCC). Urol Oncol. 2013;31:379.
47. Mendelsohn FA, Divino CM, Reis ED, Kerstein MD. Wound care after radiation therapy. Adv Skin Wound Care. 2002;15:216.
48. Naidoo J, Page DB, Li BT, et al. Toxicities of the anti-PD-1 and anti-PD-L1 immune checkpoint antibodies. Ann Oncol. 2015;26:2375.
49. Champiat S, Lambotte O, Barreau E, et al. Management of immune checkpoint blockade dysimmune toxicities: a collaborative position paper. Ann Oncol. 2016;27:559.
50. Rubin LG, Levin MJ, Ljungman P, et al. 2013 IDSA clinical practice guideline for vaccination of the immunocompromised host. Clin Infect Dis. 2013;58:e44.
51. Derogatis LR, Morrow GR, Fetting J, et al. The prevalence of psychiatric disorders among cancer patients. JAMA. 1983;249:751.
52. Veer V, Kia S, Papesch M. Anxiety and depression in head and neck out-patients. J Laryngol Otol. 2010;124:774.
53. Fingeret MC, Hutcheson KA, Jensen K, et al. Associations among speech, eating, and body image concerns for surgical patients with head and neck cancer. Head Neck. 2013;35:354.
54. National Comprehensive Cancer Network. Distress management. Clinical practice guidelines. J Natl Compr Canc Netw. 2003;1:344.
55. Jacobsen PB, Donovan KA, Trask PC, et al. Screening for psychologic distress in ambulatory cancer patients. Cancer. 2005;103:1494.
56. Bruera E, Bush SH, Willey J, et al. Impact of delirium and recall on the level of distress in patients with advanced cancer and their family caregivers. Cancer. 2009;115:2004.
57. Tuma R, DeAngelis LM. Altered mental status in patients with cancer. Arch Neurol. 2000;57:1727.
58. Inouye SK. Delirium in older persons. N Engl J Med. 2006;354(11):1157–65.

24 Substance Abuse and Maxillofacial Surgery

Thomas Hickey, Michael Kwakye,
and Pavan Tankha

Abstract

Acute and chronic substance abuse can adversely affect the perioperative course of maxillofacial surgery. Addictive substances modulate the brains reward pathways and manifest with altered behaviors. Substance use can affect all major organ systems, and identification of patients who are at risk will help minimize perioperative complications. Challenges include preoperative optimization, intraoperative management, and postoperative withdrawal treatment. Multimodal analgesia, with emphasis on regional and non-opioid medications, is recommended. Should postoperative withdrawal develop, prompt and effective treatment is warranted.

24.1 Medical Disease

In 2014, more than 21 million people over the age of 12 in the United States reported illicit or prescription drug misuse in the last year, with over 10% of the population reporting using an illicit drug within the past month [1]. Additionally, nearly 25% reported binge drinking within the last month [1]. The economic impact of substance misuse is more than $700 billion dollars a year when taking into account the costs of lost productivity, associated crime, and health-care costs [2, 3]. The cost in lives is the most staggering, as more than 183,000 people have died from prescription drug overdoses since 1999, with approximately 47,055 deaths in 2014 alone [4].

In the updated version of the American Psychiatric Association's *Diagnostic and Statistical Manual of Mental Disorders* (DSM-5), substance abuse and substance dependence were combined into substance use disorder (SUD). A SUD is defined as the recurrent use of drugs resulting in clinically significant impairment including poor health, disability, and/or problems of daily living (i.e., failure to meet demands at work, poor school attendance, or neglecting household tasks.) Diagnosing a SUD involves identifying two or more of the diagnostic criteria listed in the DSM-5 that occur within a 12-month period (Table 24.1).

T. Hickey, M.D. • P. Tankha, D.O. (✉)
Yale School of Medicine, New Haven, CT, USA

VA Connecticut Healthcare System,
West Haven, CT, USA
e-mail: Pavan.Tankha@va.gov

M. Kwakye, M.D.
Yale New Haven Hospital, New Haven, CT, USA

© Springer International Publishing AG 2018
E.M. Ferneini, J.D. Bennett (eds.), *Perioperative Assessment of the Maxillofacial Surgery Patient*,
https://doi.org/10.1007/978-3-319-58868-1_24

Table 24.1 Substance use disorder diagnostic criteria

A substance use disorder is characterized as a problematic pattern of substance use leading to clinically significant impairment or distress, as manifested by at least two of the abovementioned, occurring within a 12-month period	
Category	Criteria
Impaired control over substance use	1. The substance is often taken in larger amounts or over a longer period than was intended 2. There is a persistent desire or unsuccessful efforts to cut down or control substance use 3. A great deal of time is spent in activities necessary to obtain the substance, use the substance, or recover from its effects 4. Craving, or a strong desire or urge to use the substance
Social impairment	1. Recurrent substance use resulting in a failure to fulfill major role obligations at work, school, or home 2. Continued substance use despite having persistent or recurrent social or interpersonal problems caused or exacerbated by the effects of the substance 3. Important social, occupational, or recreational activities are given up or reduced because of substance use
Risky use of the substance	1. Recurrent substance use in situations in which it is physically hazardous 2. Substance use is continued, despite knowledge of having a persistent or recurrent physical or psychological problem that is likely to have been caused or exacerbated by the substance
Pharmacological	1. Tolerance, which is defined by a need for markedly increased amounts of the substance to achieve the desired effect or a markedly diminished effect with continued use of the same amount of the substance 2. Withdrawal symptoms

Source: *Diagnostic and Statistical Manual of Mental Disorders*, Fifth Edition

The DSM 5 does not classify addiction as a specific diagnosis, and the behavior aspects have been incorporated into the criteria for severe SUD. However, when referencing it, addiction refers to when a person is unable to control the urge/impulse to use drugs despite negative consequences; these changes are accompanied by changes in brain functioning as well. Physical dependence is seen when a substance taken on a regular basis (e.g., nicotine, antihypertensive) is suddenly stopped, manifesting with specific symptoms of withdrawal. Physical dependence can occur independent of or in conjunction with SUD, and this differentiation is important during the perioperative evaluation of patients.

24.1.1 Pathophysiology

The biopsychosocial basis of SUD is quite complex. Multiple neurobiological pathways within the brain including regions responsible for pleasurable effects, craving, and withdrawal are all thought to play a role. In addition, the initiation and continuation of substances include social cohesion, reduction or avoidance of negative emotions and social exclusion, and enhancement of feelings of joy or excitement [5]. A brief review of both normal and abnormal physiology can be helpful in conceptualizing these complex pathways.

The reward pathway of the brain, also known as the mesolimbic system, modulates the ability to feel pleasure but also motivates basic survival behavior (e.g., thirst, hunger, sex drive). It consists of the ventral tegmental area, which sends projections to the nucleus accumbens. The neurotransmitters that are responsible for signaling include glutamate (GLU), dopamine (DA), and gamma-aminobutyric acid (GABA) [6, 7]. Dopamine is thought to be the most important in addictive behavior with substances either directly or indirectly increasing its concentration in the reward pathway [6].

Initial exposure of an addictive substance powerfully activates the reward pathway, with a resultant increase in DA, and the euphoric effect is known as a “high.” With chronic use, less DA is released, and a greater amount of substance is required to generate a similar response (tolerance). There is also an anti-reward system involving the amygdala, which over time opposes the effects of the addictive substance eventually causing a dysphoric response [6]. Recurrent substance use can result in the reward center/anti-reward center balance favoring the latter, so the user is now taking the substance to avoid feelings of withdrawal rather than the pleasurable effects. With time, the prefrontal cortex, basal ganglia, and amygdala area are all affected, which manifests clinically as impulsive behavior and compulsivity [8].

While these addictive substances can alter multiple regions of the brain involved in memory, concentration, judgment, learning, behavior, and decision making, not all users develop severe substance use disorder. Ultimately, one's risk of abuse varies from person to person and is based on age, gender, genetic predisposition, age of initial exposure, and comorbid psychiatric disorders [9].

24.1.2 Prevalence

Substance abuse is now the number one cause of preventable illness and death in the United States. The following statistics from 2014, which include people aged 12 and older, will help put the magnitude of this problem into perspective [1]:

- An estimated 27 million people, or 10.2% of the population, misused illicit or prescription drugs. The percentage of people who were current illicit drug users has steadily trended upward since the early 2000s.
- 21.5 million people had substance use disorders in the past year, including 17 million people with alcohol use disorder and 7.1 million people with an illicit drug use disorder.
- Over one out of every four deaths in the United States (more than 500,000 deaths) is related to the abuse of tobacco, alcohol, or other drugs.
- More than half of Americans were current users of alcohol. Most were reported as moderate drinkers. Of the 176.6 million reported alcohol users, roughly 17 million had a diagnosis of alcohol use disorder.
- Roughly 4.2 million people, or 1.6% of the population, had a marijuana use disorder. This was similar to years during 2005–2013.
- 1.9 million people, or 0.7% of the population, had pain reliever use disorder. This was similar to years 2005–2013.
- An estimated 1.5 million people, or 0.6% of the population, used cocaine with approximately 354,000, or 0.2%, using crack. The percentage of people using cocaine and crack remained steady between 2009 and 2013, although the rate was lower in 2014 than the previous years.
- An estimated 1.6 million people used stimulants, which included 569,000 who were current methamphetamine users.
- Approximately 586,000 people had opioid use disorder (previously heroin use disorder) which represented 0.2% of the population. The percentage of people using opioids remained steady between 2011 and 2014.
- An estimated 330,000 people, or 0.1% of the population, were current nonmedical users of sedatives. The percentage of sedative drug users remained steady between 2002 and 2014.

24.1.3 Manifestations of Disease

While the neurological and behavioral effects of substance abuse are well known, it also impacts multiple organ systems simultaneously including cardiovascular, respiratory, hepatic, gastrointestinal, and immune. This subsequently increases the risk of perioperative complications, and a working knowledge of toxicity and treatments is essential.

24.1.3.1 Alcohol

Acute and chronic alcohol use can lead to significant medical complications affecting every organ system. Alcoholics are at increased risk for cirrhosis, gastrointestinal bleeding, pancreatitis, cardiomyopathy, trauma, cancers, nerve damage, anemia, and vitamin deficiencies (vitamin K, folate, B12) [10]. It can also lead to respiratory depression and increased risk of aspiration [11]. There is also evidence to suggest immunity is lowered and patients are at increased risk of infections in the lungs [12].

Chronic alcohol users can suffer from severe complications of withdrawal including seizures, blackout spells, tremors, tactile or auditory hallucinations, and, in the most severe cases, coma, delirium tremens, or death. As such, they may require medical intensive care management. Given these potential complications, a thorough alcohol history including frequency of usage and prior complications should be assessed prior to surgery.

24.1.3.2 Benzodiazepines

Benzodiazepines are prescribed for anxiety, panic attacks, insomnia, seizures, and alcohol withdrawal. They are most often administered orally. Acutely, abuse of benzodiazepines can manifest with slurred speech, incoordination, unsteady gait, nystagmus, stupor, or coma. Impairment of memory, specifically anterograde amnesia, is also a common manifestation of acute abuse.

Symptoms of withdrawal include sweating, insomnia, panic attacks, flu-like symptoms (muscle pain or weakness), visual problems, sensitivity to sound/light, and detachment from reality [13]. Patients who abuse this class of medications, with or without a prescription, who present with abrupt cessation are at increased risk of developing delirium in the postoperative setting and need to be monitored closely.

24.1.3.3 Cocaine

Cocaine is used as a local anesthetic for ear, nose, and throat surgeries where it is applied topically. When abused, the route of administration includes intranasal ("snorting"), smoking, or intravenous. Toxicity manifests as paranoia, anxiety, and psychosis. Vascular complications can include cerebral hemorrhage possibly resulting in stroke or coronary vasoconstriction possibly resulting in myocardial infarction. Snorting cocaine chronically can contribute to nosebleeds, difficulty swallowing, chronic inflammation, and irritation of the nasal septum [14]. Intravenous users are at increased risk of HIV and hepatitis C as well. Withdrawal symptoms are similar to other abused substances and include increasing anxiety, restlessness, sweating, and tremors.

24.1.3.4 Opioids

Prescribed opioids are most commonly seen in patients who are being treated for chronic pain. Depending on the medication, routes for administration include oral, sublingual, transmucosal, intravenous, subcutaneous, or intrathecal. Of note, many of the same routes can be utilized for abuse, but medications can also be crushed, then snorted, or injected. Newer drug formulations are "tamper resistant" making crushing and then abusing the medication much more difficult. Side effects include sedation, respiratory depression, nausea and vomiting, pruritis, and constipation. Symptoms of withdrawal, while unpleasant, are not life-threatening. Early symptoms include agitation, anxiety, muscle aches, insomnia, and sweating; late symptoms include nausea and vomiting, abdominal pain, diarrhea, dilated pupils, and goose bumps.

24.1.3.5 Heroin

Heroin, an opioid, was originally synthesized, and it was thought to be a more effective yet less addictive substitute to morphine. Those claims were very shortly dismissed, and the drug is currently an illicit substance with high addictive potential. It is most often abused via an intravenous or subcutaneous ("skin popping") route. Given the chemical similarity to morphine (heroin is diacetylmorphine), the acute and chronic effects are similar and are discussed above. As with any other drug of abuse that requires the skin to be penetrated, there is an increased risk of infection that includes the development of abscess, infection of the heart valves, HIV, and Hepatitis B and C. Of note, many additives found in street heroin consist of substances not readily dissolvable and may cause obstruction of blood vessels in the brain, lungs, kidney, and liver. Symptoms of withdrawal can start as soon as 6 h following the last dose and are essentially unchanged from withdrawal from other opioids.

24.1.3.6 Tobacco

Cigarette smoking is harmful to every organ in the body and is responsible for a quarter of all cancer-related deaths [15]. Smoking has been linked to over 90% of lung cancers, which is still the number one cancer responsible for overall deaths in men and women [16]. In addition, cigarettes contribute to cancers of the pharynx and larynx, esophagus, kidney, and bladder. Chronic respiratory conditions including bronchitis and emphysema and increased risk of ischemic cardiovascular events (e.g., stroke, myocardial infarction) are also associated with smoking. What is important to note is the increased likelihood of substance use disorder in smokers than nonsmokers, so further questioning regarding drugs of abuse should be made [17]. Symptoms of withdrawal include anger, irritability, increased appetite, or insomnia [18].

24.1.3.7 Cannabinoids

Marijuana use can develop into problem use like all of the substances mentioned beforehand. Studies have shown that marijuana use before the age of 18 results in adults who are 4–7 times more likely to develop marijuana use disorder than people who begin using it as adults [18]. Indeed, the percent of patients with marijuana use disorder ranges from 9% if use is started when an adult to as high as 17% if started before the age of 18 years old [19, 20]. Marijuana smoke is an irritant to the throat and lungs and can contribute to the development of a chronic cough. Irritation of the respiratory tract can lead to lung hyperinflation, increased airway resistance, and airway inflammation, which can impede adequate airway flow. Clinically, patients will present sedated, with red eyes, and often lack motivation and interest. Signs of withdrawal include nausea, vomiting, sweating, irritability, and depressed mood.

24.1.4 Anesthetic Risk

The anesthetic risk associated with substance use disorder is dependent on the substance, frequency and route of misuse, as well as any end-organ damage that may have occurred secondary to chronic use. Hence preoperative interview and identifying these factors beforehand are important. An example of this would be inducing anesthesia with ketamine in a patient who chronically abuses cocaine. If the patient has depleted stores of catecholamines, significant cardiac depression may occur at induction. Indeed, if an attempt to treat that hypotension/bradycardia is with ephedrine, another medication that relies on stored catecholamines, the results could be disastrous. In the sections below, we will discuss specifics with each medication class.

24.2 Preoperative Assessment

24.2.1 Workup

The importance of a thorough history cannot be overemphasized when it comes to SUD. Questions regarding current and past alcohol, tobacco, and drug use (not covered in the medication history) should be an integral part of the social history. Prefacing these questions with assurances of confidentiality, as well as the importance to the perioperative workup, can also put the patient at ease and ensure honest answers. Information regarding frequency of use, last use, and symptoms of withdrawal can also help guide management. While the majority of patients answer these questions honestly, certain subsets of patients at high risk or suspected of SUD (exhibiting signs of withdrawal, smell of alcohol, track marks visible on extremities, poor dentition) should receive further workup [21].

24.2.2 Laboratory Tests

Urine testing remains a reliable first step in assessing the presence of both prescription and illegal drugs the patient may be taking. The drugs that can be tested for include opioids, cocaine, marijuana, amphetamines, benzodiazepines, oxycodone, barbiturates, and methadone. Since this is a qualitative test, it simply indicates whether or not the drug is present, and not the amount or if any metabolites are present. One should also be aware that heroin use will result in a positive test for opioids, so if you suspect this is being abused, confirmatory testing of the sample should be carried out. While the sensitivity and specificity for these tests are high, they are not 100%, so confirmatory testing using gas chromatography/mass spectroscopy would then be indicated. It should be noted that if test results indicate acute or chronic use and the surgery is elective, consider postponing the procedure and refer the patient for substance abuse treatment.

24.2.3 Steps to Optimize the Patient

Patient optimization is dependent on whether the patient is actively abusing, on maintenance therapy, or in remission. Those patients with active SUD who present for elective surgery should be referred for treatment first. If they present for urgent or emergent surgery, identification of the abused drug should be made as quickly as possible with appropriate intraoperative and postoperative management as noted below.

Patients on maintenance therapy should be stratified into one of three groups based on the anticipated postsurgical pain: minimal, intermediate, and severe. For those in the minimal category undergoing elective surgery, opioid-sparing techniques (regional blockade) and non-opioid medications (NSAIDs, acetaminophen) should be discussed with the patient. Those in the intermediate and severe groups should have their maintenance medications weaned in the days and weeks leading up to elective surgery. Consultation with the prescribing provider may prove beneficial to ensure the chance of relapse is minimized. An effort to maximize non-opioid therapy with the judicious use of opioids postoperatively is advised. In the event of an urgent or emergent surgery where the maintenance medication cannot be weaned, higher doses of perioperative opioids will be required to achieve pain relief. Given the increased affinity to the mu receptor, fentanyl is often a good first choice.

24.2.4 Reasons to Cancel the Case

The decision to cancel the case will be based on a number of factors. Some institutions may have their own policies regarding this matter, and so the decision is made for you. However, if no guidelines exist at your practice, consider cancelation if the patient is exhibiting signs of clinical toxicity. Patient hemodynamics, behavior, and symptoms may be more indicative of potential perioperative complications than an asymptomatic patient with a positive urine toxicology. There is evidence in the literature that even when patients present with acute cocaine use, perioperative outcomes remain unchanged [22–24]. As previously discussed, should the case be urgent or emergent, then the guidelines set out below will be beneficial in guiding the patient through the perioperative period.

24.3 Intraoperative Management

24.3.1 Effect of Anesthesia on Disease

24.3.1.1 Alcohol

Acute alcohol ingestion causes sedation on a wide spectrum encompassing mildly impaired cognition to respiratory depression and death. As would be expected with a substance with a depressant effect, there is a decrease in overall anesthetic requirements. Chronic alcoholics develop tolerance and may require increased levels of anesthesia, though other end-organ damage (i.e., liver, kidneys) may change these requirements. In addition, because of the potential for increased levels of anesthesia, these patients may be at increased risk of awareness under anesthesia.

24.3.1.2 Benzodiazepine

When acute benzodiazepine intoxication is suspected, the reversal agent flumazenil can be administered. There are rarely significant intraoperative concerns associated with chronic benzodiazepines, other than possible increased anesthetic requirements. Postoperative withdrawal is characterized by anxiety, insomnia, tremors, and seizure. In order to minimize the risk of postoperative complications, these medications should be continued or tapered perioperatively.

24.3.1.3 Cocaine

Acute cocaine ingestion predisposes to arrhythmia, coronary artery vasospasm with myocardial ischemia, aortic dissection, QT prolongation, stroke, and seizure. The use of beta-blockers in acutely intoxicated patients has been discouraged given the possibility of hypertension in the setting of unopposed alpha adrenergic stimulation. In addition, hemodynamic changes (hyper- or hypotension) may occur secondary to catecholamine release or depletion and should be anticipated. For chronic, intranasal users, care should be taken as destruction of the nasal septum, and/or soft palate may make intubation or gastric tube placement dangerous.

24.3.1.4 Opioids

Chronic opioid use results in tolerance, which increases overall anesthetic requirements and predisposes to difficult-to-treat postoperative pain. A comprehensive approach utilizing multimodal analgesia should be employed, baseline/preoperative opioids should be maintained, and additional opioids should be prescribed for breakthrough pain. If opioids are withheld perioperatively, patients should be monitored for signs and symptoms of withdrawal. Opioid withdrawal is rarely life-threatening but very uncomfortable for the patient; symptoms and signs include craving, irritability, nausea, pain, anxiety, insomnia, tachycardia, diaphoresis, hypertension, pupillary dilation, and fever.

24.3.1.5 Heroin

Treatment is similar to patients on opioids (see above). In those who present with overdose, there is a potential for pulmonary edema or aspiration, so securing the airway takes special importance. Multimodal analgesia is recommended with close monitoring for uncontrolled pain.

24.3.1.6 Tobacco

There are no specific concerns regarding patients who smoke unless end-organ damage presents (COPD). However, patients who smoke do report more pain and may require higher doses of postoperative opioids [25].

24.3.1.7 Marijuana

Anesthetic concerns are similar to the standard respiratory concerns associated with smoking tobacco. Withdrawal symptoms are mild and do not require any special treatment. Patients may be using marijuana to treat chronic conditions such as pain, which may make perioperative pain management more challenging.

24.3.2 What Anesthetic Medications to Use and Not to Use?

Medications exclusively cleared by the liver should be used cautiously in alcoholics with cirrhosis and impaired hepatic function. Acetaminophen should also be used cautiously in this population given the risk for acute liver injury. There is a synergistic response to CNS depressants in those patients who use benzodiazepines, so slow titration to effect is recommended. In patients who abuse cocaine, there may be depleted catecholamine stores, so when administering medications such as ketamine or ephedrine as the desired response may not occur.

24.3.3 Potential Problems

Chronic alcoholism causes multi-system disease. These patients are more likely to have comorbid psychiatric disease, neurological disease associated with their nutritional deficiencies, cardiovascular disease including alcohol induced cardiomyopathy, hepatic disease as described below, and hematological disturbances including anemia. There is increased risk of gastrointestinal disease including esophagitis, gastritis, and pancreatitis.

Cirrhosis is a special category within alcoholism and can be particularly challenging. One scoring model for risk stratification is the MELD score, which ranges from 6 to 40 points and consists of serum bilirubin, serum creatinine, and INR; hyponatremia is another useful prognostic factor. Elective surgeries should be avoided in patients with MELD scores above 15. Mortality rates in cirrhotic patients undergoing common surgeries such as open cholecystectomy have been reported as high as 25% [26, 27]. Cirrhotic patients may present with the following morbidities, in addition to the aforementioned sequelae of chronic alcoholism:

Renal: susceptibility to acute kidney injury, hepatorenal syndrome, hyponatremia

Cardiovascular: systemic vasodilation, hypervolemia and hyperdynamic state, cardiomyopathy with reduced ejection fraction, portopulmonary hypertension

Hepatic disease: portal hypertension, ascites, varices, decreased metabolic function, hypoalbuminemia, decreased gluconeogenesis with increased risk of labile glucose, insulin resistance

Pulmonary: increased aspiration risk, hepatopulmonary syndrome, atelectasis and restrictive lung disease in setting of ascites, pleural effusions

Neurological: encephalopathy, cerebral edema, increased intracranial pressure

Hematologic: bleeding and thrombosis, pancytopenia

24.3.4 Monitoring

The standard American Society of Anesthesiology monitors should be applied, which include an oxygen analyzer, pulse oximeter, capnography, ECG monitoring, blood pressure measurement, and temperature. Given the type of surgery, patient comorbidities, and preoperative anesthesia concerns, additional monitors may be indicated.

24.3.5 What Depth of Anesthesia Is Appropriate?

The appropriate depth of anesthesia will vary with the type/length of procedure. However, given the increased tolerance to anesthesia with chronic substance use, it is likely more anesthesia will be required to maintain the appropriate depth.

24.3.6 Airway Management

If general anesthesia is required, emergent cases involving acutely intoxicated patients should be treated as full stomachs and undergo either awake endotracheal intubation or intubation using a rapid sequence intubation (RSI) technique. As noted earlier, caution is required in chronic, intranasal cocaine use as the nasal septum and soft palate may be compromised making intubation dangerous.

24.3.7 Fluid Management

If patients are arriving for scheduled, elective surgery and preoperative evaluation was not concerning, fluid management would be routine. However, if an acutely intoxicated patient presents and the case cannot be delayed or rescheduled, they may be hypovolemic and may require fluid resuscitation. Care must be taken as certain substance can predispose to cardiomyopathy, while others may compromise kidney function.

24.4 Postoperative Management

24.4.1 Airway Management

Patients should be extubated according to standard extubation criteria. Noninvasive positive-pressure ventilation may be useful in the recovery of obese patients or those with known obstructive sleep apnea; however, this ventilatory support requires cooperative patients. Aspiration precautions should be applied in the postoperative period.

24.4.2 Pain Management

Multimodal analgesia including NSAIDs and acetaminophen should be maintained for moderate, or greater, postoperative pain. The use of opioids should be used judiciously in all patients, but given the known history of substance use, these patients are at increased risk for abuse or relapse.

As such, emphasis on opioid-sparing regimens should be emphasized, but their pain should be addressed appropriately.

Note that an increasing subset of patients with substance use disorder are on opioid partial agonists such as buprenorphine and naltrexone. These medications have a mild analgesic effect but, more importantly, bind the opioid receptor so tightly that the analgesic effects of full opioid agonists (i.e., morphine, hydromorphone) are blocked. For this reason, if moderate, or greater, postoperative pain is anticipated, these medications should be discontinued for 72 h and in the case of IM naltrexone 30 days. Coordination of these changes is most often arranged by the prescriber. Note that patients who remain on these medications perioperatively may require very high doses of full agonist to achieve any effect, which together with the variable pharmacology of buprenorphine and naltrexone increases the risk of opioid-induced respiratory depression. For these reasons, these patients' respiratory status should be monitored closely postoperatively. Patients on methadone may have QT prolongation, and other medications that may prolong the QT interval should be administered judiciously.

24.5 Postoperative Complications

Withdrawal is the primary concern for substance use disorder in the postoperative period. Chronic alcohol withdrawal ranges from craving and irritability to seizure and life-threatening delirium tremens. Alcoholics in particular should be managed in a setting where they can be monitored aggressively for mental status changes, hyperthermia, tachycardia, dysrhythmia, hypo- and hypertension, seizure, and delirium tremens, which occurs 2–4 days after the last drink. Various measurement tools including the Clinical Institute Withdrawal Assessment (CIWA) scales exist to guide the assessment and management of alcohol withdrawal. Treatment of mild alcohol withdrawal is with benzodiazepines and beta-blockers, whereas severe symptoms may need supportive care in an ICU setting.

Benzodiazepine withdrawal can be treated in a two-step fashion. To combat symptoms of withdrawal, restarting the patient on the medication is most effective. However, to prevent future abuse, a taper plan, which must be closely monitored by the prescribing physician, can take effect and lasts 1 week to a month.

Tobacco and cannabinoid withdrawal can be treated with replacement products. There are various nicotine patch formulations that can be started postoperatively as well as THC replacements. Counseling regarding cessation should be offered to all patients.

Opioid and heroin withdrawal are treated symptomatically. As stated previously, withdrawal is not life-threatening but can be very uncomfortable for the patient. However, given the risk of nausea and vomiting following maxillofacial surgery, prompt identification and treatment of withdrawal is warranted.

Conclusions

Many patients with substance use disorder, sometimes as a direct result of abuse of these drugs, may require maxillofacial surgery. Identifying patients through a thorough history will allow the provider to optimize perioperative care and avoid potentially dangerous intraoperative and postoperative complications.

References

1. Results from the 2013 National Survey on Drug Use and Health: summary of national findings. Rockville, MD: Substance Abuse and Mental Health Services Administration, Center for Behavioral Health Statistics and Quality; 2013.
2. The health consequences of smoking—50 years of progress. Rockville, MD: Department of Health and Human Services; 2014.
3. Excessive drinking costs U.S. $223.5 billion. 2014. http://www.cdc.gov/features/alcoholconsumption. Accessed 17 Apr 2014.
4. Rudd RA, Seth P, David F, Scholl L. Increases in drug and opioid-involved overdose deaths—United States, 2010–2015. MMWR Morb Mortal Wkly Rep. 10.15585/mmwr.mm6550e1. ePub: 16 Dec 2016.
5. Cooper ML. Motivations for alcohol use among adolescents: development and validation of a four factor model. Psychol Assess. 1994;6:117–28.
6. Gardner EL. Brain reward mechanisms. In: Lowinson JH, Ruiz P, Millman RB, Langrod JG, editors.

Substance abuse: a comprehensive textbook. 4th ed. Philadelphia: Lippincott Williams & Wilkins; 2005. p. 48–97.
7. Koob GF. Drugs of abuse: anatomy, pharmacology and function of reward pathways. Trends Pharmacol Sci. 1992;13:177–84.
8. Goldstein RZ, Volkow ND. Dysfunction of the prefrontal cortex in addiction: neuroimaging findings and clinical implications. Nat Rev Neurosci. 2011;12:652–69.
9. Demers CH, Bogdan R, Agrawal A. The genetics, neurogenetics and pharmacogenetics of addiction. Curr Behav Neurosci Rep. 2014;1:33–44.
10. Stein M. Medical consequences of substance abuse. Psychiatr Clin North Am. 1999;22:351–70.
11. Langhan ML. Acute alcohol intoxication in adolescents: frequency of respiratory depression. J Emerg Med. 2013;44(6):1063–9. https://doi.org/10.1016/j.jemermed.2012.11.041. Epub 2013 Feb 26.
12. Nelson S, Kolls JK. Alcohol, host defence and society. Nat Rev. 2002;2:205–9.
13. The diagnostic and statistical manual of mental disorders. 5th ed. (DSM-5), American Psychiatric Association; 2013. Sedative, hypnotic, and anxiolytic intoxication, p. 556.
14. Guyuron B, Afrooz PN. Correction of cocaine-related nasal defects. Plast Reconstr Surg. 2008 Mar;121(3):1015–23.
15. Siegel RL, Jacobs EJ, Newton CC, Feskanich D, Freedman ND, Prentice RL, Jemal A. Deaths due to cigarette smoking for 12 smoking-related cancers in the United States. JAMA Intern Med. 2015;175(9):1574–6.
16. Centers for disease control and prevention website. https://www.cdc.gov/cancer/lung/basic_info/risk_factors.htm.
17. Lai S, Lai H, Page JB, McCoy CB. The association between cigarette smoking and drug abuse in the United States. J Addict Dis. 2000;19:11–24.
18. Howell LL, Kimmel HL. Monoamine transporters and psychostimulant addiction. Biochem Phamcol. 2008;75:196–217.
19. Lopez-Quintero C, Pérez de los Cobos J, Hasin DS, et al. Probability and predictors of transition from first use to dependence on nicotine, alcohol, cannabis, and cocaine: results of the National Epidemiologic Survey on Alcohol and Related Conditions (NESARC). Drug Alcohol Depend. 2011;115(1–2):120–30.
20. Anthony JC. The epidemiology of cannabis dependence. In: Roffman RA, Stephens RS, editors. Cannabis dependence: its nature, consequences and treatment. Cambridge, UK: Cambridge University Press; 2006. p. 58–105.
21. Brown J, Kranzier HR, Del Boca FK. Self-reports by alcohol and drug abuse inpatients: factors affecting reliability and validity. Br J Addict. 1992;87(7):1013–24.
22. Ryb GE, Cooper C. Outcomes of cocaine-positive trauma patients undergoing surgery on the first day after admission. J Trauma. 2008;65(4):809–12.
23. Hadjizacharia P, Green DJ, Plurad D, et al. Cocaine use in trauma: effect on injuries and outcomes. J Trauma. 2009;66(2):491–4.
24. Barash PG, Kopriva CJ, Langou R. Is cocaine a sympathetic stimulant during general anesthesia? JAMA. 1980;243(14):1437–9.
25. Zvolensky MJ, McMillan K, Gonzalez A, Asmundson GJ. Chronic pain and cigarette smoking and nicotine dependence among a representative sample of adults. Nicotine Tob Res. 2009;11:1407–14.
26. Ziser A, Plevak DJ, Wiesner RH, Rakela J, Offord KP, Brown DL. Morbidity and mortality in cirrhotic patients undergoing anesthesia and surgery. Anesthesiology. 1999;90:42–53.
27. Del Olmo JA, Flor-Lorente B, Flor-Civera B, Rodriguez F, Serra MA, Escudero A, et al. Risk factors for nonhepatic surgery in patients with cirrhosis. World J Surg. 2003;27:647–52.

25 Perioperative Management of the Tobacco User

Laura Romito

Abstract

Tobacco use remains a significant cause of morbidity and mortality and can produce myriad adverse effects on the oral and maxillofacial complex. As smoking negatively impacts both anesthetic management and healing and surgical outcomes, it is incumbent upon oral and maxillofacial surgeons to address tobacco use in the patients for whom they render care. This chapter will address nicotine addiction, systemic and oral consequences of tobacco use and environmental tobacco smoke, perioperative concerns, and the available, effective office-based tobacco interventions.

In 2004 and then again in 2012 with more instructive criteria, the Joint Commission established parameters for patient tobacco screening and smoking cessation counseling [1]. Considering its impact on society and the surgical patient, the time has arrived to more actively address this issue within our offices in a more credible manner to optimize surgical outcome and overall patient health. This chapter will address nicotine addiction, systemic and oral consequences, perioperative concerns, and available office-based tobacco interventions.

L. Romito, D.D.S., M.S., M.B.A.
Nicotine Dependence Program, Indiana University School of Dentistry, Indianapolis, IN, USA
e-mail: lromitoc@gmail.com

25.1 Tobacco Products and Their Harmful Constituents

Currently, there are several available forms of smoking tobacco, including cigarettes, cigars, and pipe tobacco, as well as less traditional forms such as hookah, bidis, and kreteks. Among US adults, cigarettes constitute by far the most popular form, followed by cigars, roll-your-own, and pipe tobacco [2].

25.2 Long-Term Systemic Consequences

The addictive properties of nicotine are due in part to its rapid uptake by the brain following inhalation. When smoking, high levels of nicotine enter the lungs and are quickly absorbed into the bloodstream. Nicotine reaches the brain in

© Springer International Publishing AG 2018

E.M. Ferneini, J.D. Bennett (eds.), *Perioperative Assessment of the Maxillofacial Surgery Patient*,
https://doi.org/10.1007/978-3-319-58868-1_25

about 10 s provoking pleasurable sensations and the craving for additional tobacco. Following inhalation, nicotine enters the circulation whereby the heart pumps it immediately to the brain and other body organs at elevated levels. It's these high concentrations delivered so rapidly that make nicotine highly addictive. Nicotine alters brain chemistry by increasing the quantity of nicotinic cholinergic receptors (nAChRs), which are triggered by cues that increase a user's desire to smoke. Binding of nicotine to receptors in the brain promotes the release of dopamine, norepinephrine, serotonin, beta-endorphins, acetylcholine, and vasopressin. The resulting CNS effects include a feeling of enhanced mood and cognition as well as appetite suppression [3]. Continued use of tobacco often results in the development of tolerance and physical dependence.

Although countless nicotinic receptors will be eliminated when a smoker stops using tobacco, the remaining receptors can be triggered by cues; this phenomenon is sometimes referred to as euphoric recall. Furthermore, when attempting to quit, smokers experience withdrawal symptoms such as such as anxiety, depression, craving, nervousness, and irritability. For many, these symptoms are most pronounced during the first several days of cessation and diminish over time [4]. However, the craving to smoke may still be experienced months or even years after quitting. This renders the ex-smoker highly susceptible to relapse of tobacco use [5, 6].

The effects of tobacco use are dose dependent, and adverse effects can be seen in every body system. Smoking causes lung cancer, emphysema, and chronic bronchitis by damaging the bronchial tubes and alveoli of the lungs and enabling tar and other tobacco chemicals to be deposited on lung tissue. Smoking is one of the major causes of peripheral vascular disease, cardiovascular disease, stroke, and aneurysm. Smoking has been linked to the formation of arterial plaque, elevated blood pressure, and reduced oxygen carrying capacity due to carbon monoxide levels. Recent studies have also shown that smoking may reduce memory and cognitive abilities long-term [7, 8].

Tobacco use has been associated with numerous cancers including lung, pancreas, oral, pharyngeal, bladder, kidney, uterus, and cervical cancer. Along with other lung carcinogens, tumor promoters, and cocarcinogens, tobacco smoke contains 4-(methylnitrosamino)-1-(3-pyridyl)-1-butanone (NNK) and polycyclic aromatic hydrocarbons (PAHs). The potential of NNK and PAHs to exercise their carcinogenic potential depends upon the balance of activating and detoxifying factors within the user's system; this balance differs among individuals and will result in differing levels of cancer risk. Although the smoker receives small doses of carcinogens with each use, through many years and/or high doses of smoking, the cumulative damage produced can be considerable [8, 9].

Smoking can modify the activity of many human hormones and has been implicated as a risk factor in endocrine disorders, for example, thyroid diseases, even affecting thyroid function of children exposed to environmental tobacco smoke (ETS). Smoking stimulates the release of adrenal gland hormones and several pituitary hormones, which may influence a number of body functions, for example, fertility and blood pressure through actions on prolactin, and antidiuretic hormone, respectively. Smoking has major effects on human reproductive potential and, in women, produces an antiestrogen effect. The activity of insulin is antagonized by smoking as is parathyroid hormone (PTH) and vitamin D. These changes make the smoker more susceptible to elevated blood glucose and lowered calcium absorption [10]. Tobacco use is now recognized as a causal factor for type II diabetes mellitus [8].

Tobacco use can contribute to infertility. Smoking during pregnancy increases a woman's risk of stillborn, premature delivery, miscarriage, and low birth weight babies. A pregnant woman who smokes more than 20 cigarettes per day increases the risk that her baby, should the offspring ever begin smoking, will become dependent on tobacco [11].

Although it does not generate many of the toxins found in burning tobacco, smokeless tobacco is not harmless. The adverse oral effects of smokeless tobacco are numerous and range from the benign stained dentition to severe periodontal disease to oral carcinoma. After being absorbed into circulation, the carcinogens and toxins in spit tobacco products may have a deleterious effect on various tissues. Smokeless tobacco affects the operation of CYP-450 enzymes which are integral to numerous body functions such as hormone synthesis and regulation and metabolism of toxins and medications. Animal studies have shown that smokeless tobacco also alters DNA in the lung, kidney, and liver [12]. However, smokeless tobacco's effects on these tissues in humans are less clear. Nonetheless, spit tobacco's effects on the human cardiovascular system have been demonstrated and are similar to smoking [13–16].

Environmental tobacco smoke (ETS), or secondhand smoke, remains an important public health issue. The Centers for Disease Control and Prevention (CDC) reported that from 2011 to 2012 approximately 58 million nonsmokers were exposed to secondhand smoke. Those most at risk for exposure to passive smoking were of low socioeconomic status, African-American, blue-collar, service, and construction workers. Overall, one in five children and seven of ten African-American children were exposed to ETS [17]. It is estimated that more than 41,000 deaths per year can be attributed to secondhand smoke—7,330 deaths from lung cancer and 33,950 deaths from heart disease [8]. Aside from these conditions, in nonsmokers ETS produces respiratory problems and diminished lung function. ETS exposure in babies and children increases their risk for sudden infant death syndrome, middle ear disease, acute and lower respiratory tract infections, and complicated asthma. Children exposed to ETS experience irritation of the upper respiratory tract which can significantly reduce lung function and increase frequency and severity of symptoms in asthmatic children [18].

In recent years, battery-powered electronic cigarettes (e-cigarettes), vaporizers, and other electronic nicotine delivery systems (ENDS) have skyrocketed in popularity and experienced sharp growth in online sales and through "vape shops," malls, and other local outlets [19]. Some ENDS resemble traditional smoking tobacco while others, such as the larger tank-style devices, do not; ENDS mimic smoking, but without the many of the toxicants and tobacco smoke carcinogens. Along with glycerin, propylene glycol, flavorings, and other ingredients, they contain liquid nicotine, which is vaporized upon inhalation and absorbed by the user's oral mucosa [20]. The CDC reported that in 2014, 12.6% of US adults had tried e-cigarettes, while nearly 4% were regular users. However, among children and teenagers, use of ENDS has grown dramatically and overtaken use of cigarettes: by 2015, e-cigarettes were currently used by 16% of high schoolers and 5.3% of middle school children [21–24].

As ENDS do not generate the myriad hazardous chemicals associated with combustible tobacco, they are viewed by some as a safer substitute for smoking, particularly for smokers who have been unsuccessful in quitting. Further, some contend that these devices may be useful as aids in smoking cessation [25]. However, there is much variability in the components of the products, and the long-term health effects of e-cigarettes are unknown [26].

While ENDS are potentially less harmful than traditional tobacco products [27], they emit aerosols which contain substances which may pose health risks [28–31]. The adverse effects of e-cigarette vapor on gingival epithelial cells may lead to dysregulated gingival cell function and result in oral disease [32]. As there is much variation among products, more studies are needed [33]. However, there have been dozens of reported cases of explosions of e-cigarettes which have resulted in serious injury, including injuries of the maxillofacial complex [34–36].

Secondhand exposure to e-cigarette vapor is also a concern, particularly on children. One review found that although the risks appear to be less than those from ETS from combustible tobacco, ENDS vapor has the potential to produce health harms [37].

In 2016, the US Food and Drug Administration (FDA) assumed regulatory control over all ENDS such as vaporizers, vape/hookah pens, and e-cigarettes. This rule, which allows the FDA to regulate the manufacture, importation, packaging, labeling, promotion, sale, and distribution of ENDS, has created a number of new requirements intended to improve safety and curtail use of the products by minors [21].

25.3 Effects on Anesthetic Management and Wound Healing

Smoking is associated with increased perioperative morbidity and mortality [38, 39]. It negatively impacts both anesthetic management and surgical outcomes. Smoking affects both the pulmonary and cardiovascular system. Smoking has both chronic and acute effects on both systems. The acute effects of smoking on the respiratory system result from an increase in carbon monoxide within the blood. This results in an increase in carboxyhemoglobin, which results in a decrease in tissue oxygenation as a result of both less oxygen being carried by hemoglobin and less oxygen being released to the peripheral tissues. The half-life of carboxyhemoglobin is 4 h. Counseling the patient to stop smoking for 24 h prior to surgery can therefore have a significant benefit in reversing the detrimental effect on tissue oxygenation, which is associated with carboxyhemoglobin. The benefit achieved from an overnight cessation in smoking for a morning procedure is more limited because the half-life of carboxyhemoglobin is prolonged during sleep [40].

The chronic effects on the respiratory system secondary to smoking include impaired mucociliary clearance, mucous hypersecretion, and ventilation-perfusion mismatch. This results in an increased incidence of airway irritability contributing to laryngospasm and airway obstruction. Children exposed to passive smoking have also been demonstrated to have a higher incidence of perioperative complications [41].

In 1989, an article was published in the Mayo Clinic Proceedings, which reported that smoking cessation within 8 weeks prior to a general anesthetic was associated with increased airway secretions and irritability [42]. This conclusion has been challenged, and other authors have demonstrated that smoking cessation is associated with reduced pulmonary complications after just 4 weeks and is not associated with an increased risk of pulmonary complications less than 4 weeks [43].

The effects of smoking on the cardiovascular system result both from the activation of the sympathoadrenergic system and arterial thromboembolism and coronary artery vasospasm resulting in a hypercoagulable state. Activation of the sympathoadrenergic system is attributed to the high concentration of nicotine in inhaled smoke resulting in increased peripheral resistance, heart rate and blood pressure. In the patient under general anesthesia, there is also a higher occurrence of ST depression, which correlates with elevated levels of expired carbon monoxide [44].

Tobacco smoke negatively affects wound and bone healing. There are multiple factors that contribute to the adverse effects secondary to smoking. Tobacco smoke contains multiple toxins including nicotine, carbon monoxide, and hydrogen cyanide. Carbon monoxide and hydrogen cyanide decrease tissue oxygenation. Nicotine activates the sympathoadrenergic system, which diminishes tissue perfusion. Nicotine can also contribute to an increase in bone matrix resorption, which can impair bone healing [45]. Smoking modulates the expression of selected genes (bone sialoprotein, osteocalcin, and type I collagen) modifying bone repair [46]. The hypercoagulable state associated with platelet aggregation contributes to wound necrosis. Tobacco also interferes with neutrophil function and suppresses the immune response.

Smoking contributes to adverse effects following dentoalveolar procedures, implant surgery, and major surgical procedures such as facial fracture repair and orthognathic surgery [47]. Smoking affects bone formation in extraction sites as well as increases the incidence of alveolar osteitis [48, 49]. Smoking also results in a higher rate of implant failures [50]. It also contributes to increased marginal bone loss and peri-implantitis in patients whose implants have osseointegrated and are deemed successful [51, 52].

25.4 Perioperative Smoking Cessation: Brief Interventions for Tobacco Dependence

Planned surgical procedures provide a useful occasion in which to address tobacco use and dependence and encourage tobacco cessation efforts. Smokers may not be aware of their increased surgery-associated risks so the perioperative period has been hailed as a teachable moment during which a patient may have increased motivation to quit when advised by their doctor [53, 54]. Although surgeons and anesthesiologists can play an active role in motivating patients to quit using tobacco prior to surgical procedures, this appears to be uncommon in clinical practice [55]. However, it has been demonstrated that perioperative tobacco interventions can have an impact on smoking cessation up to 1 year later [56–58]. A Cochrane review by Thomsen and colleagues on preoperative smoking cessation interventions concluded that combined behavioral and pharmacotherapeutic smoking interventions applied at least 4 weeks prior to surgery can reduce surgical complications and increase perioperative and long-term smoking cessation [59].

As tobacco use is an oral health problem and can adversely impact oral and maxillofacial surgical treatments, it is important that those involved in the provision of oral healthcare, including oral and maxillofacial surgeons, be actively involved in addressing tobacco use and dependence in those that they care for. Furthermore, with increasing evidence to support an oral-systemic health connection, tobacco dependence treatment by oral health providers reinforces the goals of integrated health promotion and holistic patient care. It has been shown that individuals who receive a clinician-provided tobacco intervention quit using tobacco at nearly twice the rate of those who do not receive clinician assistance [60]. For the past several decades, national medical and dental organizations have advocated for healthcare providers to become more actively engaged in providing tobacco interventions [8, 60–62]. Current scientific evidence indicates that behaviorally based tobacco interventions delivered by oral healthcare providers in an office-based or community setting and involving an oral exam may increase cessation rates among spit tobacco users and cigarette smokers [63].

Among US dentists, more than 90% of those in a national survey indicated that they ask about tobacco use, while 45% reported that they refer patients for pharmacotherapy and/or tobacco cessation counseling [64]. As clinicians in the oral surgical specialties may be even more likely to have smoking adversely affect their therapeutic outcomes, it is relevant for them to encourage and assist in tobacco interventions. A survey of practicing oral and maxillofacial surgeons by Crews et al. found that approximately 90% of respondents reported asking about and documenting tobacco use in the patient's medical record, 63% advised tobacco users to quit, and only 40% reported assessing patient interest in cutting down, quitting, or remaining tobacco abstinent; even fewer clinicians said that they provided assistance for patients' quit attempts or arranged for follow-up [65]. A similar survey of practicing periodontists found that while 92% believed that tobacco cessation was a responsibility of their profession, they reported low rates of comprehensive tobacco interventions in clinical practice. Oral health providers' perceived barriers to helping patients quit tobacco have been cited as low patient acceptance of treatment, lack of time, and lack of training [66].

Because tobacco dependence often requires repeated interventions and several attempts to achieve sustained abstinence from tobacco, tobacco dependence is considered a chronic disease [60]. In addition to physiological dependence on nicotine, there are sociocultural issues and psychological dependence factors that are interwoven to create a chain of addiction wherein each of the component factors must be addressed to achieve long-term abstinence from tobacco [67].

The US Public Health Service Clinical Practice Guideline *Treating Tobacco Use and Dependence* serves as the evidence-based guide to help clinicians address tobacco use and dependence in their patient populations. The

Guideline, which recommends that all healthcare providers deliver brief tobacco interventions, provides clinicians with both pharmacological and behavioral tobacco interventions that may be employed in the clinical setting. Brief interventions can be effective, save lives, and can often be performed in less than 3 min [60].

An approach to the brief intervention process with tobacco users described in the Guideline involves the "5As". This approach includes asking about tobacco use, advising tobacco users to quit, assessing their willingness to quit, assisting in their quit attempt, and arranging for follow-up to evaluate progress toward quitting. As part of the 5As, when obtaining the health history, all patients should be asked about their tobacco use. This can be facilitated by a question such as, "Have you used any form of tobacco within the past 30 days?" The clinician should ask about any and all tobacco use because oftentimes non-daily or social smokers do not define themselves as smokers [68]. The type(s) of tobacco used, frequency of use, and duration of use, that is, how many months/years the individual has been using tobacco, should then be documented in the patient record.

If a patient is identified as a current tobacco user, they should be advised to discontinue use, in a clear, strong, personalized manner that is directed toward their individual health assessment and risks. While the message should be very clear and personalized, it should also be encouraging, nonjudgmental, and respectful. Many smokers contemplate quitting and attempt, unsuccessfully, numerous times [69]. The clinician should display empathy when discussing tobacco use and dependence and share with tobacco users that even if they have attempted quitting previously without sustainable abstinence from tobacco, this is not unusual. In fact, recent research suggests that it may take up to 30 quit attempts to achieve long-term abstinence [70]. It is also important to have the tobacco user understand that tobacco use is an oral health problem and can affect treatment outcomes as well; hence, the appropriateness of your speaking to them about the topic. Oftentimes the "advise" message is linked to specific findings in the oral cavity such as leukoplakia, periodontal disease, or other conditions and in advance of dental treatments where outcomes would be improved by tobacco abstinence.

The clinician's communication style when discussing tobacco use and advising the user to quit is very important in order to increase motivation for quitting. Rather than simply telling the tobacco user to quit, the clinician should use a patient-centered approach and first ask permission to continue the conversation about tobacco. Asking permission to continue the conversation changes the tone of the communication from adversarial to inclusive and from parental to collegial. It leaves the patient in control [71, 72].

By using an "ask-tell-ask" technique, the clinician allows the patient to feel in control of the direction of the conversation. In the first step, the clinician asks the patient if they would like to know more. For example, in a patient who is pregnant yet continues to smoke, the provider might say one of these three examples in the ask step: What would you like to know about ….? Would it be OK with you if ….? Are you open to hearing about?

In the second "tell" step, the clinician gives the patient information in a neutral, nonjudgmental manner. This step may be made less judgmental by referencing the existing evidence for the information being shared (e.g., With regard to smoking and wound healing, the research has indicated ….)

Lastly, it is important to respectfully ask about the patient's understanding so that the conversation can move forward. Immediately following the final request of the patient to express their understanding and relevance of the cessation messages, the clinician should offer to help by saying, for example, "Now that you've learned this, what can I do to help?" Of course the tobacco user may or may not accept that offer; however, regardless of their response, the clinician should proceed with the "assess" of the 5As.

The clinician may assess the patient's willingness to quit by asking, for example, "Are you interested in quitting tobacco in the next 30 days?" If a patient indicates that they are willing, the clinician should offer to provide assistance. Above all, the clinician should express empathy and be encouraging to support the tobacco user's motivation and self-efficacy in quitting. The clinician should ask the patient to set a quit date within the next 2–5 weeks. Additionally, the clinician may assist the patient to identify family, friends, or coworkers who would be supportive in their quit attempt and discuss triggers for tobacco use and how to cope with these triggers and additional stresses after quitting. The patient should be informed about the available FDA-approved medications for smoking cessation, and the clinician may recommend or prescribe medications considering the effectiveness, cost, medical history, and patient preferences. The patient may also be provided with supplemental materials, information, and referral to other tobacco dependence treatment resources, including telephone counseling quit lines (e.g., 1-800-QUIT-NOW [1-800-784-8669], local health organizations/societies, hospital- or faith-based tobacco treatment counseling services, as well as online tobacco dependence treatment support (e.g., www.smokefree.gov and www.women.smokefree.gov) [73].

The last step of the 5As, arrange, includes arranging at follow-up contacts to assess progress for those who did make a quit attempt. At this time, the clinician and patient should discuss any difficulties the patient may have encountered in their quit attempt, what triggered them, and how they might be prevented in the future. If the patient is using pharmacotherapy for tobacco cessation, they should also discuss any adverse effects and the medication effectiveness and make medication adjustments if needed. The clinician should take the opportunity to discuss the patient's use of counseling and support during the quitting process and encourage continued abstinence. Clinicians employing this approach may utilize the CDT code D1320 (Tobacco Interventions for the Control and Prevention of Oral Disease) for office-based tobacco counseling.

25.5 Ask-Advise-Refer

For busy oral and maxillofacial surgery practices, the brief 5As intervention may be used in a condensed three-step format—as ask, advise, and refer. In this case, the assess, assist, and arrange steps of the intervention are performed by a referral source, not the oral health provider. When using the ask, advise, and refer approach, if the patient expresses a general interest in quitting tobacco or is open to receiving information on quitting, they are referred to a tobacco cessation expert resource for further information, assessment, and assistance in quitting when they are ready. Common referral sources include the state tobacco quit line (1-800-QUIT-NOW), the American Cancer Society, the American Lung Association, or local hospital, community, or faith-based tobacco dependence treatment counseling services. After documenting tobacco use and advising the patient to quit, a referral to tobacco dependence treatment resources may be given [60].

25.6 Motivational Interviewing and the 5Rs

For tobacco users who are not ready to make a quit attempt, the Guideline advocates using the "5Rs"to enhance patient motivation. These consist of the following: discussing with the patient the relevant reasons to quit, the risks associated with continued tobacco use, the rewards of cessation, and the roadblocks or barriers to quitting, as well as asking the patient permission to consider the issue again in the future (repetition) should the opportunity arise [60].

The clinician should tailor the communication so that the reasons for quitting tobacco are personal and relevant to the particular patient, speaking in terms of what they have shared with the clinician. Discussion of risks of continued tobacco use should be open and frank, however, not intended to invoke fear or scare tactics, as these are not successful in motivating individuals to quit tobacco [74]. Talk specifically about the risks identified in the clinical assessment and/or conversation with the patient. Be clear in the benefits of quitting to that particular individual; if the patient has included others in the reasons why they want to or should quit, the clinician can reinforce this as well. However, external motivators tend not to be long-term motivators. Clinicians can ask open-ended questions to facilitate patients' identification of barriers to making a quit attempt. Tobacco users will often share numerous reasons why the present is not a good time to quit tobacco However, if the clinician can enable nonjudgmental, empathetic dialogue on the issue, sometimes by just talking about it, patients will arrive at their own solutions to the stated barriers.

If the opportunity avails itself, revisiting the message at future interactions is important. For those who were unwilling to quit, at a follow-up visit, the clinician can assess their progress at cutting down smoking or willingness to quit. When these patients return for care, document tobacco use and reassess their interest in quitting. Oftentimes a tobacco user will not be open to a quit message today or will be contemplating quitting, but not quite ready to take the next step. However, by a subsequent visit, the patient may have changed their mind. Because it's impossible to predict which tobacco users will be ready to quit and when, reexamining the issue of quitting tobacco at follow-up appointments is essential.

25.7 Pharmacotherapeutic Aids

Because tobacco use and dependence is a chronic disease, it requires multiple treatment approaches including both behavioral and pharmacotherapeutic. All clinicians should inform tobacco users of the currently available safe and effective medications for facilitating tobacco cessation. Clinicians should encourage those interested in making a quit attempt to use one or a combination of these medications, as appropriate considering their medical history, age, pregnancy, and tobacco use level. Available FDA-approved pharmacotherapies for tobacco cessation include five forms of nicotine replacement therapy (NRT). NRT is available over-the-counter as the patch, gum, and lozenge. The nicotine inhaler and nasal spray are available as prescription products. Additionally, two non-nicotine-based medications are also available: bupropion and varenicline. With the exception of case-specific contraindications or with specific populations for which there is insufficient evidence of effectiveness (e.g., pregnant women, smokeless tobacco users, light smokers, and adolescents), for all of the aforementioned FDA-approved first-line medications, there is empirical evidence indicating safety and effectiveness for use in tobacco dependence treatment, and as such, they should be clinicians' first choice in recommending pharmacotherapy [60] (Table 25.1).

NRT nicotine is delivered at a slower rate than nicotine from smoking; peak plasma levels of NRT nicotine are also lower than would be obtained from smoking. NRT has been shown to improve quit rates by reducing cravings and other nicotine withdrawal symptoms by gradually reducing the amount of nicotine in the tobacco user's system. NRT has an excellent record of safety and is not an independent risk factor for acute myocardial events. There are only a few patients in which these products should be used with caution, including those who have experienced a myocardial infarction in the previous 2 weeks, serious arrhythmias, and unstable angina pectoris.

In December 2016, the FDA updated the drug safety communication regarding use of bupropion and varenicline medications for tobacco dependence treatment. After reviewing data from a recent large clinical trial, the FDA determined that the "risk of serious side effects on mood, behavior, or thinking with the stop-smoking medicines Chantix (varenicline) and Zyban (bupropion) is lower than previously suspected." Subsequently, the FDA removed the boxed warning for adverse mental health effects from varenicline and bupropion labeling. The FDA review also reconfirmed the utility of these medications as well as NRT in helping people quit smoking more effectively than placebo and recommended that all healthcare professionals counsel patients on quitting smoking and discuss the utility and the risks and benefits of the FDA-approved pharmacotherapy in facilitating sustained abstinence from tobacco [75].

The Guideline recommends that for patients making an attempt to quit tobacco and willing to use pharmacotherapy, clinicians should consider recommending certain combinations of these medications. These include the following three options: (1) long-term (>14 weeks) NRT patch

Table 25.1 Pharmacotherapy for treating tobacco use and dependence

Medication	Dosage	Duration of treatment	Coding	Cautions	Common adverse effects
NRT gum	1 piece q 1–2 h If < 24 cpd; 2 mg If > 24 cpd or smokeless tobacco: 4 mg	6–14 weeks >14 weeks	Usual duration Long duration	Adherence to dental work No food/drink during use	Oral soreness, hiccups, heartburn
NRT lozenge	2 mg: smoking > 30 min after waking 4 mg: if smoking < 30 min after waking Weeks 1–6: 1 q 1–2 h Weeks 7–9: 1 q 2–4 h Weeks 10–12: 1 q 4–8 h	6–14 weeks >14 weeks	Usual duration Long duration	No food/drink 15 min before or during use 1 lozenge at a time 20 lozenges per day maximum	Hiccups, heartburn, nausea, cough
NRT patch	Usual dose/day: 15 mg/16 h/day OR 21 mg/24 h/day High dose > 25 mg/day Use 1 patch/day If > 10 cpd: 21 mg for 4 weeks, then 14 mg for 2 weeks, then 7 mg for 2 weeks If < 10 cigs/day: 14 mg for 4 weeks, then 7 mg for 4 weeks	6–14 weeks >14 weeks	Usual duration Long duration	Not recommended for patients with severe eczema or psoriasis	Localized skin irritation where patch is placed; insomnia, vivid dreams
NRT nasal spray	1 dose = 1 squirt/nostril 1–2 doses/h 8–40 doses/day Do not inhale	3–6 months; taper at end >6 months taper at end	Usual duration Long duration	Not recommended for patients with severe asthma, bronchospasm, and reactive airway disease	Nasal irritation
NRT inhaler	6–16 cartridges/day	Up to 6 months; taper at end >6 months taper at end	Usual duration Long duration	No food/drink during use Keep stored > 40°F	Local mouth/throat irritation, cough, rhinitis
Bupropion SR	Days 1–3: 150 mg each morning Days 4-end 150 mg bid	Start 1–2 weeks before quit date Up to 14 weeks 14 weeks–6 months	Usual duration Long duration	Medication interactions Use of bupropion in other forms History of seizures History of eating disorders	Insomnia, nausea, dizziness, headache, xerostomia, constipation, weight loss, anxiety
Varenicline	Days 1–3: 0.5 mg each morning Days 4–7: 0.5 mg bid Day 8-end: 1 mg bid	Start 1 week before quit date Up to 14 weeks 14 weeks–6 months	Usual duration Long duration	Renal impairment Psychological disorders	Nausea, constipation, and gas Insomnia, vivid or unusual dreams

Adapted from Fiore MC, Jaén CR, Baker TB, et al. Treating tobacco use and dependence: 2008 update. Clinical Practice Guideline. Rockville, MD: U.S. Department of Health and Human Services. Public Health Service; 2008: 35–43

plus other ad libitum NRT (e.g., gum, lozenge, or spray), (2) NRT patch plus the nicotine inhaler, and (3) The NRT patch plus bupropion SR [60].

The Guideline also describes research which has assessed patients' use of NRT for helping to reduce smoking, rather than quitting tobacco entirely. In these cases, results indicated that there is an increased likelihood that the individuals will make a quit attempt and will be successful in quitting. Thus, clinicians' recommendations for NRT use surrounding treatment may also increase patients' motivation and success in quitting [60].

As a result of a body of new research evidence indicating that the use of OTC NRT prior to quitting tobacco is safe and may effectively increase abstinence rates, the FDA allowed for the labeling of these medications to change to remove the warnings prohibiting use of NRT products for individuals who are still smoking or using any other nicotine-containing product [76]. As with any medication, clinicians should encourage patients using tobacco cessation pharmacotherapy to contact them promptly to report any possible side effects that they notice from taking the medication.

25.8 Behavioral Therapy

Behavioral therapy is a proven method for tobacco dependence treatment. Practical counseling provides education and information on nicotine addiction, withdrawal symptoms, and other elements of the quitting process, along with developing coping skills on coping with cravings, individual tobacco triggers, and stress, as well as recognizing the triggers that might lead to relapse. Additionally, support and encouragement for tobacco abstinence as part of treatment also has been found to enhance success in quitting tobacco [60].

Tobacco dependence treatment counseling is often provided on an individual basis, or in groups by certified tobacco treatment specialists (CTTS), or other behavioral clinicians with special training in tobacco dependence treatment. Phone counseling via the national network of quit-line services, web and smartphone apps, and text-based counseling programs are also available. Current research strongly supports combining counseling with the use of pharmacotherapy as the combination is more effective in enhancing success in quitting tobacco than either counseling or pharmacotherapy alone. As such, patients should be encouraged to utilize both modalities when attempting to quit using tobacco [60].

25.9 Other Tobacco Cessation Aids

Currently, there is insufficient evidence to support the use of hypnosis, massage therapy, acupuncture, and similar methods to help quit tobacco. As healthcare providers are obligated to recommend evidence-based treatment protocols, patients should be encouraged to utilize the previously discussed behavioral and pharmacotherapeutic cessation aids. However, patients should not be discouraged from quit attempts and may be informed that although alternative methods are not proven to be effective in increasing cessation rates, they may be helpful on an individual basis, and the potential risks and benefits to the particular patient should be considered.

The cold turkey method of quitting tobacco is an inexpensive and feasible initial option for many people. The best candidates for this method may be those who are not heavy users and have a relatively low level of nicotine dependence. A recent study comparing gradual quitters to those quitting abruptly with a cold turkey approach found that at 1 month, 39% of the gradual quitters were nonsmokers, while 49% of those using the cold turkey approach were successful in quitting. Six months later, 22% of the abrupt quitters were still not smoking, while only 16% of the gradual quitters remained abstinent [77].

Tapering (Controlled Smoking, Harm Reduction) is the gradual reduction of tobacco consumed over time, typically by cutting down the number cigarettes and/or the amount of each cigarette smoked.

There are two methods for tapering: counting the number of cigarettes smoked and decreasing that number every day until it reaches zero, or postponing each cigarette until a predetermined length of time has passed between cigarettes. Tapering may be considered as a tool in tobacco cessation, particularly for those who desire to cut down the amount they use in preparation for a future quit attempt. Doing so puts the responsibility for taking action in quitting on the patient and may also make a smoother transition from levels of nicotine obtained through smoking with that obtained from NRT which may be used after quitting. However, it is important to remember that decreasing the number of cigarettes, for example, does not decrease the health risks. Smokers who taper cigarette use may compensate for the decrease in nicotine consumption by inhaling more deeply, occluding the filter vents on their cigarettes, or taking more frequent puffs. Another disadvantage of tapering is the ease at which a smoker can return to his/her previous level of tobacco use.

For patients currently using electronic cigarettes or other similar ENDS to quit smoking, clinicians should support the quit attempt and encourage quitting all traditional tobacco use in lieu of using the ENDS product exclusively. Then, the clinician should strongly recommend that the patient plan for quitting ENDS use by setting a quit date. For patients who have not tried to utilize ENDS, such as electronic cigarettes, to quit smoking, the clinician should encourage the use of the available, evidence-based, effective methods for tobacco dependence treatment and emphasize lack of scientific evidence for safety and efficacy of electronic cigarettes [78].

Conclusion

Oral and maxillofacial surgeons can, and should, play an essential role in helping their patients quit tobacco by increasing their motivation to make a quit attempt. Although the decision to be tobacco-free rests with the patient, oral and maxillofacial surgeons can facilitate the process by providing a rationale for quitting, advising patients to quit, assisting with the quit attempt, and supporting patient progress over time. As tobacco use poses substantial risks to oral and systemic health, all oral healthcare providers have a moral and professional responsibility to actively address tobacco use and dependence in their patient population.

References

1. Fiore MC, Goplerud E, Schroder SA. The Joint Commission's new tobaccos-cessation measure: will hospitals do the right thing? New England Journal of Medicine. 2012;366:1172–4.
2. U.S. Department of Health and Human Services. Smoked tobacco products. Washington, D.C. https://betobaccofree.hhs.gov/about-tobacco/Smoked-Tobacco-Products/index.html. Accessed 25 Feb 2017.
3. Zevin S, Gourlay SG, Benowitz NL. Clinical pharmacology of nicotine. Clin Dermatol. 1998;16(5):557–64.
4. Hughes JR. Effects of abstinence from tobacco: valid symptoms and time course. Nicotine Tob Res. 2007;9(3):315–27.
5. Pomerleau OF, Pomerleau CS, Mehringer AM, Snedecor SM, Cameron OG. Validation of retrospective reports of early experiences with smoking. Addict Behav. 2005;30(3):607–11.
6. Shiffman S, Kirchner TR. Cigarette-by-cigarette satisfaction during ad libitum smoking. J Abnorm Psychol. 2009;118(2):348–59. https://doi.org/10.1037/a0015620.
7. Sabia S, Elbaz A, Dugravot A, Head J, Shipley M, Hagger-Johnson G, Kivimaki M, Singh-Manoux A. Impact of smoking on cognitive decline in early old age: the Whitehall II cohort study. Arch Gen Psychiatry. 2012;69(6):627–35. https://doi.org/10.1001/archgenpsychiatry.2011.2016.
8. U.S. Department of Health and Human Services. The Health Consequences of Smoking—50 Years of Progress: A Report of the Surgeon General. Atlanta: U.S. Department of Health and Human Services, Centers for Disease Control and Prevention, National Center for Chronic Disease Prevention and Health Promotion, Office on Smoking and Health, 2014.
9. Hecht SS. Tobacco smoke carcinogens and lung cancer. J Natl Cancer Inst. 1999;91(14):1194–210.
10. Tweed JO, Hsia SH, Lutfy K, Friedman TC. The endocrine effects of nicotine and cigarette smoke. Trends Endocrinol Metab. 2012;23(7):334–42. https://doi.org/10.1016/j.tem.2012.03.006. Published online 2012 May 2.
11. MMWR women and smoking: a report of the surgeon general. 30 Aug 2002/51(RR12); pp. 1–30. https://www.cdc.gov/mmwr/preview/mmwrhtml/rr5112a4.htm.
12. Avti PK, Kumar S, Pathak CM, Vaiphei K, Khanduja KL. Smokeless tobacco impairs the antioxidant defense in liver, lung, and kidney of rats. Toxicol Sci. 2006;89(2):547–53; Epub 2005 Nov 9
13. Stepanov I, Villalta PW, Knezevich A, Jensen J, Hatsukami D. Hecht SS Analysis of 23 polycyclic aromatic hydrocarbons in smokeless tobacco by gas chromatography-mass spectrometry. Chem Res Toxicol. 2010;23(1):66–73. https://doi.org/10.1021/tx900281u.

14. Lawler TS, Stanfill SB, Zhang L, Ashley DL, Watson CH. Chemical characterization of domestic oral tobacco products: total nicotine, pH, unprotonated nicotine and tobacco-specific N-nitrosamines. Food Chem Toxicol. 2013;57:380–6. https://doi.org/10.1016/j.fct.2013.03.011. Epub 2013 Mar 19.
15. Avti PK, Vaiphei K, Pathak CM, Khanduja KL. Involvement of various molecular events in cellular injury induced by smokeless tobacco. Chem Res Toxicol. 2010;23(7):1163–74. https://doi.org/10.1021/tx900458x.
16. Hecht SS. Progress and challenges in selected areas of tobacco carcinogenesis. Chem Res Toxicol. 2008;21(1):160–71. Epub 2007 Dec 4
17. Centers for Disease Control and Prevention. Vital signs: disparities in nonsmokers' exposure to secondhand smoke—United States, 1999–2012. Morb Mortal Wkly Rep. 2015;64(4):103–8. [accessed 2017 Feb 21].
18. U.S. Department of Health and Human Services. The health consequences of involuntary exposure to tobacco smoke: a report of the Surgeon General. Atlanta: U.S. Department of Health and Human Services, Centers for Disease Control and Prevention, National Center for Chronic Disease Prevention and Health Promotion, Office on Smoking and Health; 2006. [accessed 2017 Feb 21].
19. Romito LM, Hurwich RA, Eckert GJ. A snapshot of the depiction of electronic cigarettes in YouTube videos. Am J Health Behav. 2015;39(6):823–31. https://doi.org/10.5993/AJHB.39.6.10.
20. The U.S. Food and Drug Administration. Tobacco products vaporizers, E-cigarettes, and other electronic nicotine delivery systems (ENDS). https://www.fda.gov/TobaccoProducts/Labeling/ProductsIngredientsComponents/ucm456610.htm.
21. Centers for Disease Control and Prevention. Tobacco use among middle and high school students—United States, 2011–2015. Morb Mortal Wkly Rep. 2016;65(14):361–7.
22. Centers for Disease Control and Prevention. Tobacco product use among middle and high school students—United States, 2011–2014. Morb Mortal Wkly Rep. 2015;64:381–5.
23. Villanti AC, Johnson AL, Ambrose BK, et al. Use of flavored tobacco products among U.S. youth and adults; findings from the first wave of the PATH Study (2013–2014). Am J Prev Med. 2017;53(2):139–51.
24. Schoenborn CA, Gindi RM. Electronic cigarette use among adults: United States, 2014. NCHS data brief, no. 217. Hyattsville, MD: National Center for Health Statistics; 2015.
25. Rom O, Pecorelli A, Valacchi G, Reznick AZ. Are E-cigarettes a safe and good alternative to cigarette smoking? Ann N Y Acad Sci. 2015;1340:65–74. https://doi.org/10.1111/nyas.12609. Epub 2014 Dec 31.
26. Rahman MA, Hann N, Wilson A, Worrall-Carter L. Electronic cigarettes: patterns of use, health effects, use in smoking cessation and regulatory issues. Tob Induc Dis. 2014;12:21.
27. Oh AY, Kacker A. Do electronic cigarettes impart a lower potential disease burden than conventional tobacco cigarettes? Review on E-cigarette vapor versus tobacco smoke. Laryngoscope. 2014;124(12):2702–6. https://doi.org/10.1002/lary.24750. Epub 2014 Oct 9.
28. Fernández E, Ballbè M, Sureda X, Fu M, Saltó E, Martínez-Sánchez JM. Particulate matter from electronic cigarettes and conventional cigarettes: a systematic review and observational study. Curr Environ Health Rep. 2015;2(4):423–9. https://doi.org/10.1007/s40572-015-0072-x.
29. Schober W, Szendrei K, Matzen W, Osiander-Fuchs H, Heitmann D, Schettgen T, Jörres RA, Fromme H. Use of electronic cigarettes (e-cigarettes) impairs indoor air quality and increases FeNO levels of e-cigarette consumers. Int J Hyg Environ Health. 2014;217(6):628–37. https://doi.org/10.1016/j.ijheh.2013.11.003. Epub 2013 Dec 6.
30. Leigh NJ, Lawton RI, Hershberger PA, Goniewicz ML. Flavourings significantly affect inhalation toxicity of aerosol generated from electronic nicotine delivery systems (ENDS). Tob Control. 2016;25(Suppl 2):ii81–7. https://doi.org/10.1136/tobaccocontrol-2016-053205. Epub 2016 Sep 15.
31. Kosmider L, Sobczak A, Prokopowicz A, Kurek J, Zaciera M, Knysak J, Smith D, Goniewicz ML. Cherry-flavoured electronic cigarettes expose users to the inhalation irritant, benzaldehyde. Thorax. 2016;71(4):376–7. https://doi.org/10.1136/thoraxjnl-2015-207895. Epub 2016 Jan 28.
32. Rouabhia M, Park HJ, Semlali A, Zakrzewski A, Chmielewski W, Chakir J. E-cigarette vapor induces an apoptotic response in human gingival epithelial cells through the caspase-3 pathway. J Cell Physiol. 2017;232(6):1539–47. https://doi.org/10.1002/jcp.25677. Epub 2016 Nov 30.
33. Callahan-Lyon P. Electronic cigarettes: human health effects. Tob Control. 2014;23(Suppl 2):ii36–40. https://doi.org/10.1136/tobaccocontrol-2013-051470.
34. Harrison R, Hicklin D Jr. Electronic cigarette explosions involving the oral cavity. J Am Dent Assoc. 2016;147(11):891–6. https://doi.org/10.1016/j.adaj.2016.03.018. Epub 2016 May 6.
35. Rogér JM, Abayon M, Elad S, Kolokythas A. Oral trauma and tooth avulsion following explosion of E-cigarette. J Oral Maxillofac Surg. 2016;74(6):1181–5. https://doi.org/10.1016/j.joms.2015.12.017. Epub 2016 Jan 7.
36. Brownson EG, Thompson CM, Goldsberry S, Chong HJ, Friedrich JB, Pham TN, Arbabi S, Carrougher GJ, Gibran NS. Explosion injuries from E-cigarettes. N Engl J Med. 2016;375(14):1400–2.
37. Hess IM, Lachireddy K, Capon A. A systematic review of the health risks from passive exposure to electronic cigarette vapour. Public Health Res Pract. 2016;26(2):pii: 2621617. 10.17061/phrp2621617.

38. Schmid M, Sood A, Campbel L, et al. Impact of smoking on perioperative outcomes after major surgery. Am J Surg. 2015;210:221–9.
39. Turan A, Mascha EJ, Roberman D, et al. Smoking and perioperative outcomes. Anesthesiology. 2011;114:837–46.
40. Munday IT, Desai PM, Marshall CA, Jones RM, Phillips ML, Rosen M. The effectiveness of pre-operative advice to stop smoking: a prospective controlled trial. Anaesthesia. 1993;48:816–8.
41. Jone DT, Bhattacharyya N. Passive smoke exposure as a risk factor for airway complications during outpatient pediatric procedures. Otolaryngol Head Neck Surg. 2006;135:12–6.
42. Warner DO, Offord KP, Warner ME, et al. Role of preoperative cessation of smoking and other factors in postoperative pulmonary complications: a blinded prospective study of coronary artery bypass patients. Mayo Clinic Proc. 1989;64:609–16.
43. Wong J, Lam DP, Abrishami A, et al. Short-term preoperative smoking cessation and postoperative complications: a systematic review and meta-analysis. Can J Anesth. 2012;9:268–79.
44. Woehlck HJ, Connolly LA, Cinguegrani MP, et al. Acute smoking increases ST depression in humans during general anesthesia. Anesth Analg. 1999;89:856.
45. Katono T, Kawato T, Tanabe N, et al. Nicotine treatment induces expression of matrix metalloproteinases in human osteoblastic Saos-2 cells. Acta Biochim Biophys Sin. 2006;38:874–82.
46. de Campos JM, Prati AJ, Cirano FR, et al. Smoking modulates gene expression of type 1 collagen, bone sialoprotein, and osteocalcin in human alveolar bone. J Oral Maxillofac Surg. 2015;73:2123–31.
47. Kuhlefelt M, Laine P, Suominen AL, et al. Smoking as a significant risk factor for infections after orthognathic surgery. J Oral Maxillofac Surg. 2012;70:1643–7.
48. Ozkan A, Bayar GR, Altug HA, et al. The effect of cigarette smoking on the healing of extraction sockets: an immunohistochemical study. J Craniofac Surg. 2014;25(4):e397–402. https://doi.org/10.1097/SCS.0b013e31829ae609.
49. Tarakji B, Saleh LA, Umair A, et al. Systemic review of dry socket: Aetiology, treatment, and prevention. J Clin Diagn Res. 2015;9(4):ZE10–3. https://doi.org/10.7860/JCDR/2015/12422.5840. Epub 2015 Apr 1.
50. Bain CA, Moy PK. The association between the failure of dental implants and cigarette smoking. Int J Oral Maxillofac Implants. 1993;8:609–15.
51. De la Rosa M, Rodriguez A, Sierra K, et al. Predictors of peri-implant bone loss during long-term maintenance of patients treated with 10-mm implants and single crown restorations. Int J Oral Maxillofac Implants. 2013;28:798–802.
52. Heitz-Mayfield LJ. Peri-implant diseases: diagnosis and risk indicators. J Clin Periodontol. 2008;35:292–304.
53. Webb AR, Robertson N. Sparrow M smokers know little of their increased surgical risks and may quit on surgical advice. ANZ J Surg. 2013;83(10):753–7. https://doi.org/10.1111/ans.12096. Epub 2013 Feb 17.
54. Wong J, Chung F. Peri-operative cessation of smoking: time for anaesthetists to act. Anaesthesia. 2015;70(8):902–6. https://doi.org/10.1111/anae.13183.
55. Zaballos M, Canal MI, Martínez R, Membrillo MJ, Gonzalez FJ, Orozco HD, Sanz FJ, Lopez-Gil M. Preoperative smoking cessation counseling activities of anesthesiologists: a cross-sectional study. BMC Anesthesiol. 2015;15:60. https://doi.org/10.1186/s12871-015-0036-6.
56. Webb AR, Robertson N, Sparrow M, Borland R, Leong S. Printed quit-pack sent to surgical patients at time of waiting list placement improved perioperative quitting. ANZ J Surg. 2014;84(9):660–4. https://doi.org/10.1111/ans.12519.
57. Wong J, Abrishami A, Yang Y, Zaki A, Friedman Z, Selby P, Chapman KR, Chung F. A perioperative smoking cessation intervention with varenicline: a double-blind, randomized, placebo-controlled trial. Anesthesiology. 2012;117(4):755–64.
58. Lee SM, Landry J, Jones PM, Buhrmann O, Morley-Forster P. Long-term quit rates after a perioperative smoking cessation randomized controlled trial. Anesth Analg. 2015;120(3):582–7. https://doi.org/10.1213/ANE.0000000000000555.
59. Thomsen T, Villebro N, Møller AM. Interventions for preoperative smoking cessation. Cochrane Database Syst Rev. 2014;3:CD002294. https://doi.org/10.1002/14651858.CD002294.pub4.
60. Fiore MC, Jaén CR, Baker TB, et al. Treating tobacco use and dependence: 2008 update. Clinical practice guideline. Rockville, MD: U.S. Department of Health and Human Services. Public Health Service; 2008. p. 35–43.
61. Academy of General Dentistry. Can tobacco products harm my mouth? 2008. http://www.agd.org/public/oralhealth/Default.asp?IssID=335&Topic=T&ArtID=3815#body. Accessed 18 Feb 2017.
62. American Dental Association. Summary of policy and recommendations regarding tobacco 1964-present. http://www.ada.org/2056.aspx.
63. Carr AB, Ebbert J. Interventions for tobacco cessation in the dental setting. Cochrane Database Syst Rev. 2012;6:CD005084.
64. Jannat-Khah DP, McNeely J, Pereyra MR, et al. Dentists' self-perceived role in offering tobacco cessation services: results from a nationally representative survey, United States, 2010–2011. Prev Chronic Dis. 2014;11:E196.
65. Crews KM, Sheffer CE, Payne TJ, Applegate BW, Martin A, Sutton T. A survey of oral and maxillofacial surgeons' tobacco-use-related knowledge, attitudes and intervention behaviors. J Am Dent Assoc. 2008;139:1643–51.

66. Patel A, Blanchard S, Christen A, Bandy R, Romito L. A survey of United States periodontists' knowledge, attitudes, and behaviors related to tobacco-cessation interventions. J Periodontol. 2011;82:367–76.
67. Christen AG. Tobacco cessation, the dental profession, and the role of dental education. J Dent Educ. 2001;65(4):368–74.
68. Levinson AH, Campo S, Gascoigne J, Jolly O, Zakharyan A, Tran ZV. Smoking, but not smokers: identity among college students who smoke cigarettes. Nicotine Tob Res. 2007;9(8):845–52.
69. Borland R, Partos TR, Yong HH, Cummings KM, Hyland A. How much unsuccessful quitting activity is going on among adult smokers? Data from the International Tobacco Control Four Country cohort survey. Addiction. 2012;107(3):673–82. https://doi.org/10.1111/j.1360-0443.2011.03685.x.
70. Chaiton M, Diemert L, Cohen JE, Bondy SJ, Selby P, Philipneri A, Schwartz R. Estimating the number of quit attempts it takes to quit smoking successfully in a longitudinal cohort of smokers. BMJ Open. 2016;6(6):e011045. https://doi.org/10.1136/bmjopen-2016-011045.
71. Vuckovic N, Polen MR, Hollis JF. The problem is getting us to stop. What teens say about smoking cessation. Prev Med. 2003;37(3):209–18.
72. Hahn SR. Patient-centered communication to assess and enhance patient adherence to glaucoma medication. Ophthalmology. 2009;116(11 Suppl):S37–42. https://doi.org/10.1016/j.ophtha.2009.06.023.
73. Fiore MC, Baker TB. Clinical practice. Treating smokers in the health care setting. N Engl J Med. 2011;365(13):1222–31.
74. Janine K, Cataldo JK, Petersen AB, Sheon N. Positive and instructive anti-smoking messages speak to older smokers: a focus group study. Tob Induc Dis. 2015;13:2. https://doi.org/10.1186/s12971-015-0027-x.
75. U.S. Food and Drug Administration. FDA drug safety communication: FDA revises description of mental health side effects of the stop-smoking medicines Chantix (varenicline) and Zyban (bupropion) to reflect clinical trial findings. https://www.fda.gov/Drugs/DrugSafety/ucm532221.htm.
76. U.S. Food and Drug Administration. Federal register. Modifications to labeling of nicotine replacement therapy products for over-the-counter human use. https://www.federalregister.gov/documents/2013/04/02/2013-07528/modifications-to-labeling-of-nicotine-replacement-therapy-products-for-over-the-counter-human-use.
77. Lindson-Hawley N, Banting M, West R, Michie S, Shinkins B, Aveyard P. Gradual versus abrupt smoking cessation: a randomized, controlled noninferiority trial. Ann Intern Med. 2016;164(9):585–92. doi:10.7326/M14-2805. Epub 2016 Mar 15.
78. Malas M, van der Tempel J, Schwartz R, Minichiello A, Lightfoot C, Noormohamed A, Andrews J, Zawertailo L, Ferrence R. Electronic cigarettes for smoking cessation: a systematic review. Nicotine Tob Res. 2016;18(10):1926–36. https://doi.org/10.1093/ntr/ntw119. Epub 2016 Apr 25.

Check for updates

Chronic Pain Management and Maxillofacial Surgery

26

Avni Gupta, Pavan Tankha, and Mahmood Ahmad

Abstract

Chronic pain is an increasingly common pathology that is encountered perioperatively. A disease process in itself, chronic pain affects the biological, psychological, and sociological domains with treatment that extends well beyond identifying a localized pain generator. Postoperative pain control is often challenging in this patient population, requiring identification of preoperative treatment regimens as well as making perioperative modifications to improve patient outcomes and patient satisfaction. With multidisciplinary planning, optimal postoperative pain control can be achieved while minimizing adverse effects.

26.1 Medical Disease

26.1.1 Pathophysiology

Pain is a symptom that serves an essential function: It warns us of harm from mechanical, thermal, or chemical insults to the body. Also, there is an unpleasant emotional response which also modifies our behavior for healing and avoiding similar injury in the future. Pain can be defined in numerous ways such as clinically into somatic or visceral, temporally into acute or chronic, or by pathology into cancer or non-cancer-related. Acute pain lasts less than 6 weeks and will remain until the pathological process resolves or healing is complete. Chronic pain, present for more than 6 weeks, transitions from a symptom to a disease entity and often lacks any identifiable pathology. It can be present after

A. Gupta, M.D.
Department of Psychiatry & Behavioral Medicine, University of Illinois-Peoria, Peoria, IL, USA

Millennium Pain Center, Unity Point Health-Methodist Hospital, Peoria, IL, USA
e-mail: agupta@millenniumpaincenter.com

P. Tankha, D.O. (✉)
Department of Anesthesiology, Yale School of Medicine, New Haven, CT, USA

Pain Management Section, VA Connecticut Healthcare System, West Haven, CT, USA
e-mail: Pavan.Tankha@va.gov

M. Ahmad, M.D.
Anesthesiology and Pain Medicine Specialist, Shaheed Zulfiqar Ali Bhutto Medical University, Islamabad, Pakistan

© Springer International Publishing AG 2018

E.M. Ferneini, J.D. Bennett (eds.), *Perioperative Assessment of the Maxillofacial Surgery Patient*,
https://doi.org/10.1007/978-3-319-58868-1_26

tissue healing has taken place and has many of the psychological overlays which are not present in acute pain. Before a discussion on chronic pain can begin, a brief overview of the normal pain physiology is necessary.

Peripheral nerves contain three distinct fibers: sensory, motor, and sympathetic postganglionic axons. The sensory afferents, whose cell bodies lie in the dorsal root ganglion (DRG), can be differentiated by diameter and myelination. The large myelinated A-beta fibers found in abundance in the skin are responsible for the sensations of mechano-proprioception (light touch, motion). Small myelinated A-delta fibers and small unmyelinated C-fibers, also known as primary afferent nociceptors, are responsible for conducting painful stimuli and are located throughout the skin and deeper somatic and visceral tissues. Pain from these two fiber types is also described as fast or slow pain which correlates with A-delta and C-fibers, respectively. Fast pain is an acute, sharp, or electric sensation. It is rare in the deeper visceral tissues. Slow pain is chronic, burning, and aching and can be felt both on the skin and in deeper tissues.

The physiology of pain can be broken down into four pathways: transduction, transmission, modulation, and perception. Transduction includes primary afferent nociceptors which are stimulated via chemical, mechanical, and thermal insult. The chemical substances include products of tissue destruction as well as released mediators during an inflammatory response including potassium ions, bradykinin, histamine, acetylcholine, serotonin, and acid [1]. Of note, two other products of inflammation, substance P and prostaglandins, do not directly stimulate peripheral nociceptors but rather sensitize the receptors [2]. Sensitization is a process whereby intense and prolonged stimulation of nociceptors will lower the pain threshold; this can occur peripherally or centrally. Also, neighboring receptors that may not be involved with the inciting injury can also be recruited during sensitization [3]. Ultimately, these pain mediators will cause the nociceptor to depolarize, carrying the signal into the DRG where proximal projections terminate on neurons in the dorsal horn of the spinal cord.

The dorsal horn is a fascinating intersection of the transduction, transmission, and modulation pathways. The afferent pain fibers terminate in the posterior aspect of the dorsal horn. Here they synapse with second-order neurons in the Rexed lamina and project contralaterally up the spinothalamic tract. A-delta fibers terminate in laminae I and V, and C-fibers in laminae II, VII, and VIII, located in the ventral horn, are also involved with painful cutaneous stimuli. The excitatory amino acids glutamate and aspartate activate second-order neurons. The dorsal horn is also the location of interneurons and opioid receptors which, via the modulation pathway, will inhibit pain transmission.

Transmission begins after transduction produces depolarization of sensory afferents. It then includes the excitation of second-order neurons in the dorsal horn which transmits afferent signals via the spinothalamic tract to third-order neurons in the contralateral thalamus. These third-order neurons subsequently terminate in two areas: (1) the somatosensory cortex, which helps discriminate the location and quality of the pain, and (2) the limbic system, which is responsible for the emotional and behavioral aspects of pain.

Modulation, also known as descending inhibition, plays an integral role in the brain's ability to regulate painful stimuli. There are numerous areas of the brain thought to be responsible for this which include the frontal cortex and hypothalamus. These two regions project to the periaqueductal gray (PAG) and rostral ventromedial medulla (RVM). The PAG and RVM have projections to laminae I, II, and V where they are thought to act on interneurons to inhibit pain transmission [1]. The transmitters responsible for this suppression of pain are endogenous endorphins, specifically enkephalin, at the level of the dorsal horn. Enkephalin release which works both presynaptically and postsynaptically in the dorsal horn inhibits primary afferent nociceptive signals. One additional way ascending signals can be suppressed is through stimulation of larger A-beta fibers. It is thought that stimulation of these fibers activates inhibitory interneurons, which suppress presynaptic transmission at the level of the dorsal horn [4].

While the prior three pathways give us an understanding of the somatosensory aspects of pain, it is the perception which allows us to understand the potent emotional and behavioral aspects of chronic pain. There are a number of emotions that are intimately linked with pain including anger or fear. Acutely, these emotions are also linked to physiologic changes in sympathetic activity, muscle contraction, and cortisol release [1]. There are also changes in the limbic system such that there is a heightened perception of pain [5]. Functional imaging of the brain has shown an overlap in areas of the brain where pain and emotion are processed [6]. Also, there are significant behavioral adaptations that take place after encountering painful stimuli. Acutely these are of benefit as they can be protective (guarding) and also alert others to distress (grimacing).

The pathophysiology of chronic pain is complex and is still incompletely understood. However, using the prior pain pathways as a guide, numerous changes occur peripherally as well as centrally that are implicated in its pathogenesis.

Pathology, as it relates to transduction, is thought to occur with injury to peripheral nerves. These injuries include the mechanical, thermal, and chemical injuries mentioned above but can also include inflammatory changes (i.e., post-herpetic neuralgia) or metabolic changes (diabetic peripheral neuropathy) [7]. When this injury occurs, there can either be increased sensitivity to adrenergic stimulation, or the fiber develops ectopic activity [7]. As such, otherwise innocuous stimuli will now cause pain or lead to sensitization of nociceptors in the area of injury. In the case of ectopic activity, it is thought voltage-gated sodium channels, which are otherwise inactive or not present, begin spontaneous firing primary afferent nociceptors resulting in abnormal nociceptive signals [7].

Changes at the dorsal horn include a process known as "windup" and are thought to play a central role in chronic pain [8]. Windup refers to the process by which C-fibers, through repetitive stimulation, enhance the responsiveness of wide dynamic range (WDR) neurons in the dorsal horn. This process is thought to be responsible for the remodeling of neurons in the dorsal horn known as central sensitization [8]. Clinically, a stimulus that would otherwise be innocuous, or even limit pain, such as touch, can now lead to allodynia.

Alterations with perception also play a role in chronic pain. One such thought is that chronic pain may be a learned behavior that initially begins with an inciting event (either painful or innocuous) [9]. The appropriate acute pain behaviors are then rewarded, causing reinforcement of pain behavior. Common reinforcements are family members taking care of the patient and keeping them in a sick role, financial compensation, medications, or emotions [9].

26.1.2 Prevalence

The estimates for chronic pain in the general population widely vary from 10% to 50% [10]. In a 2012 survey, it was estimated that 25.3 million Americans, or 11.2% of the population, experienced chronic pain. Another report estimated that nearly 100 million Americans suffer from chronic pain [11]. To put these numbers into perspective, it is estimated that 26 million Americans suffer from diabetes, 16 million from coronary heart disease, and 12 million from cancer. In another study, respondents were asked what effect pain had on their lives, and 77% reported feeling depressed, 86% responded difficulty with sleeping, and 59% stated the pain interfered with their enjoyment of life [12].

Reported rates of various types of pain include low back pain at 27%, headaches at 15%, cervical pain at 15%, and facial pain at 4%. Of note, those who reported low back pain are more likely than other types of pain to report limited activity, poor health, and psychologic distress [6].

This vast prevalence undoubtedly has economic implications as evidenced by reports that suggest chronic pain costs businesses hundreds of billions of dollars in lost productivity, the majority of which is a result of decreased work performance [13].

There are numerous risk factors that have been associated with the transition to chronic pain.

Modifiable risk factors include severe acute pain, psychiatric comorbidities (anxiety, depression, PTSD), smoking, increased body mass index, and malnutrition [14]. Non-modifiable risk factors include advanced age, female sex, lower socioeconomic status, a history of abuse, and ethnic or cultural predisposition.

26.1.3 Manifestations of Disease

The manifestations of chronic pain include those associated with the nociceptive features but also involve a significant psychological overlay. Depending on the degree of treatment the patient has received, symptoms range on a spectrum of unmanaged to well-managed pain; it should be noted that complete pain relief from chronic pain is often not a realistic expectation. Often the nociceptive aspects cannot be treated appropriately, and, as such, a greater degree of attention has been moved toward increasing functionality, irrespective of the level of pain so that patients can gain a greater sense of control over their pain and lives. A discussion of signs, symptoms, and treatments will help clarify these varied clinical presentations.

Symptomatically, chronic pain will manifest similarly to acute pain. Pain can vary from sharp and well localized to dull and poorly localized, or combinations of both may be present. A distinguishing feature with chronic pain is it can be constant even though there is no clear, identifiable cause. In some patients, intermittent pain may predominate, which can include hyperalgesia and allodynia, commonly seen in chronic pain conditions.

Psychologically, depression, anxiety, pain catastrophizing, fear avoidance, distraction, job satisfaction, and pain expectations have all been implicated in the development or as a consequence of chronic pain. Indeed, 27% of patients who present to the primary care provider meet the diagnostic criteria for depression [15], and the overall incidence of comorbid psychiatric disorders is two to three times higher than the general population [16, 17]. Patients with depression also report greater pain and increased disability [18]. In addition to depression and anxiety, substance abuse disorder is also seen at higher rates in chronic pain patients than the general population which may also lead to maladaptive pain behaviors [16, 17, 19].

Pain catastrophizing is an exaggerated focus on the pain and its possible negative consequences. It has been associated with greater pain and increased disability than those without it [20]. Patients' expectation for their pain can also be a strong factor to overcome. If patients believe the pain will cause disability, this may slowly hold true despite the actual degree of disability and even carry over to expected outcomes of treatment effects [21].

The biopsychosocial model of pain treatment is an essential aspect of chronic pain treatment. As has been elucidated in the previous discussion, chronic pain has its underpinnings in physiologic and psychologic changes, and as such simply targeting one aspect will unlikely be beneficial to the patient. This model of treatment acknowledges that treating both the biological and psychological aspects of pain using multidisciplinary treatments is indicated.

26.1.4 Anesthetic Risk

Chronic pain as a disease entity does not pose any specific anesthetic risks. However, the biopsychosocial aspects and treatment associated with it should be considered perioperatively. As will be discussed further in the chapter, patients in chronic pain may have limited physical function, and, as such, evaluating physical capacity can be difficult. Psychological comorbidities are also more prevalent and may pose a challenge with perioperative pain control. Finally, there are numerous classes of medications and implantable devices that need to be addressed before surgery to prevent possible withdrawal or neurological complications.

26.2 Preoperative Assessment

A preoperative assessment is an opportunity to develop a patient-centered, comprehensive perioperative plan utilizing appropriate resources for the complex pain patient. One of the major challenges with this particular patient population is the postoperative pain control [22]. Uncontrolled postoperative pain increases the risk of morbidity, reduces patient satisfaction, and can lead to chronic pain. Recognition of chronic pain is often the first step in establishing trust in the physician-patient relationship. The goal of preoperative evaluation is optimizing of pain regimen, planning of a multimodal perioperative analgesic plan, and setting up patient expectations which reduce patient anxiety related to surgery. Multimodal analgesia involves the combination of several pharmacological and non-pharmacological modalities with different mechanisms of action to improve analgesia through synergistic and additive effects while minimizing side effects of any one class of medication, especially opioids [23, 24]. A multidisciplinary team effort utilizing coordination and open communication between anesthesiologist, surgical team, chronic pain specialist, acute pain service, and nursing staff can result in the successful outcome and improved patient satisfaction [22]. Hence, ideally, these patients should be referred to an anesthesiologist well ahead of time of their scheduled surgery for preoperative evaluation. The guidelines published by Vickers et al. highlight the high-risk patients [25]:

1. Previous difficulty with adequate postoperative pain management
2. Long-term opioid therapy
3. At risk for neuropathic pain, including patients who will sustain nerve damage during surgery, e.g., thoracotomy or amputation
4. Have a chronic pain syndrome
5. Have significant anxiety over postoperative pain

The fundamentals are same for any preoperative assessment with a focus on a comprehensive evaluation of their chronic pain history. This includes a detailed history and physical exam pertinent to the cause of chronic pain, specific aggravating and relieving factors, functional impairment due to pain, current and past medications, therapies with response to treatment, associated psychological comorbidities, and history of chemical dependency.

Documentation of the underlying cause and mechanism of pain (e.g., nociceptive, neuropathic, mixed, oncological) will help direct multimodal treatment in the perioperative period. The aggravating factors, if known, in some patients such as those suffering from trigeminal neuralgia (e.g., by pressure on trigger zones, certain smells, cold) can be avoided in the perioperative period. Information on current and previous treatment, exact dosage, schedule, route of administration, prescriber, pharmacy, effectiveness, side effects, and the reason for discontinuation of drugs should be noted. The medication management for chronic pain may consist of opioids, anti-inflammatory, anticonvulsants, antidepressants, muscle relaxers, and adjunctive treatments as acupuncture, physical therapy, psychotherapy, transcutaneous electrical nerve stimulation, and herbal supplements. Further laboratory evaluation will depend on this interview and is discussed later in the chapter. Attention should be paid to identify and quantify any potential difficulties and existing medical conditions that may complicate analgesia to improve safety [26].

26.2.1 What to Do About Chronic Medications?

The general principle is to continue the preoperative pain regimen throughout the perioperative period unless there are reasons to hold medications for surgical reasons.

26.2.1.1 Opioids

An estimated 20% of patients presenting to physician offices with non-cancer pain or pain-related diagnoses (including acute and chronic pain) receive an opioid prescription [27]. Opioid-tolerant patients present multiple challenges with control of postoperative pain as well as increased medication toxicity ultimately leading to poor outcomes and increased hospital stay [28]. Increasing postoperative opioid doses are required due to tolerance. However, this can also sometimes lead to worsening of pain due to opioid-induced hyperalgesia and poses risks such as respiratory depression, sedation, and ileus [29]. Hence, incorporation of multimodal analgesia in the perioperative planning is of paramount importance to improve patient outcomes and is started 1–2 h before the surgery.

Many opioids are available for chronic pain patients, such as morphine, codeine, hydrocodone, hydromorphone, oxycodone, oxymorphone, buprenorphine, fentanyl, methadone, tapentadol, and tramadol. Oral opioids include immediate- and extended-release preparations. Also, subcutaneous, sublingual, transdermal, intrathecal routes are sometimes used. There should be minimal disruption of patient's usual daily regimen. This provides the basal analgesia for controlling their ongoing chronic pain and prevents an opioid debt along with possible withdrawal. If the patient does not take their AM opioid dose, its equivalent must be given on the morning of surgery or at induction.

For the majority of oral maxillofacial (OMF) surgeries, transdermal fentanyl patches can be continued throughout the perioperative period. However, caution should be taken to place them away from any area of intraoperative concern and away from the heating blanket application. Fentanyl absorption can be altered unpredictably depending on the type of surgery, amount of fluids administered intraoperatively, and skin temperature at the end of the procedure [30, 31]. In the event the fentanyl patch needs to be removed, it is recommended to administer an equianalgesic dose parentally [32].

Special situations, such as prolonged preoperative fasting prohibiting oral intake of patient's home medication regimen, warrant a similar approach. The total daily opioid consumption of the patient must be assessed. Cross-reference tables are available and can be used to determine the patient's baseline opioid level [33]. However, these tables are just a guide and do not take into account incomplete cross-tolerance. Hence, reducing the equianalgesic dose by 50% when moving from one opioid to another is strongly recommended [34, 35]. Opioid-tolerant patients undergoing major OMF surgery should be forewarned regarding the possibility of opioid rotation perioperatively as the benefits of incomplete cross-tolerance can be taken advantage of. It is, therefore, important to document the efficacy of previously trialed medications for pain relief and their side effects. Additional medications should be available to manage acute postoperative pain. This could mean two to four times of the morphine dose appropriate for an opioid-naive patient having the same procedure [36].

26.2.1.2 Antidepressants

Low-dose tricyclic antidepressants (TCAs) and serotonin and norepinephrine reuptake inhibitors (SNRIs) are commonly prescribed as first-line agents for several neuropathic conditions [37]. Cessation of antidepressants perioperatively has shown to increase symptoms of depression, delirium, and confusion [38]. However, one should be aware of the possibility of the rare phenomena of serotonin syndrome with drug interactions in the perioperative period in patients taking selective serotonin reuptake inhibitors (SSRIs) or SNRIs [39]. The risk increases with co-administration of drugs like tramadol or TCAs. Typical symptoms like tremor, agitation, myoclonus, hypertension, and hyperthermia may be masked under anesthesia and can first present postoperatively.

26.2.1.3 Anticonvulsants

Gabapentinoids are an important class of drugs for managing neuropathic pain [37]. Abrupt cessation of these drugs in the perioperative period can lead to seizures [40]. Continuation of these drugs in the perioperative period has shown to decrease postoperative pain and opioid requirements [41, 42]. Long-term use may, however, lead to hematological and biochemical abnormalities, and hence a full blood work including blood count and electrolytes is recommended [43].

26.2.1.4 Implantables

Advanced treatment options for chronic pain include implantable therapies such as neuromodulators as well as intrathecal pumps. Neuromodulation involves stimulation of targeted areas of the spinal cord (e.g., dorsal column, dorsal root ganglion) or a peripheral nerve field through implantable electrodes connected to a pulse generator. Of particular importance in OMF surgeries are peripheral nerve stimulators placed for refractory facial pain like trigeminal neuralgia, neuropathy, and atypical facial pain [44]. The electrodes are subcutaneously inserted into the painful area and tunneled to the generator. It is important to be aware of the presence of such a device and where the leads and generator exist. If needed, radiological confirmation of exact location can be ordered as the leads can interfere with the surgical field. Case reports of serious injuries including permanent neurological damage and even death are present due to heating of electrodes with diathermy, so bipolar electrocautery is recommended [45]. The current recommendations are to turn off the device before the surgery and keep it off until the patient is fully conscious and acute postoperative pain control is stabilized. Interrogation of the stimulator could be done in the postoperative period to ensure proper functioning [46]. Antibiotic prophylaxis is not routinely needed.

Special attention toward patients with intrathecal drug delivery systems is warranted. The system includes a subarachnoid catheter connected to a subcutaneous programmable pump infusing various combinations of drugs such as opioids, baclofen, ziconotide, and local anesthetics for the management of chronic pain. Careful attention toward the contents of the pump should be made as well as refill date of the pump to ensure there is enough medication for the perioperative period. The pump should be interrogated pre- and postoperative to ensure proper functioning [47]. Abrupt cessation of a baclofen pump can lead to life-threatening complications that can be refractory to treatment. It should be noted that the pump cannot be used to manage the postoperative pain but can be used to resume their baseline regimen. Since these patients can be quite opioid tolerant, multimodal analgesia should be used to manage the postoperative pain. Additional analgesia through oral, IV, or PCA should be available. Unlike spinal cord stimulation, the functioning of the pump is not affected by cautery. Antibiotic prophylaxis is not routinely needed for intrathecal pumps.

26.2.2 Steps to Optimize the Patient

The major challenge in the chronic pain patient is postoperative analgesia. Multimodal analgesia has been shown to reduce the postoperative opioid requirements, surgical complications, and hospital stay [48–51]. The specific selection of the drugs will vary based on specific patient and surgery. Acetaminophen (by mouth and IV), NSAIDs, COX-2 inhibitors, gabapentinoids (gabapentin and pregabalin), glucocorticoids, local anesthetics, IV infusions, NMDA-receptor antagonists (ketamine, magnesium), and α-2 agonists (clonidine and dexmedetomidine) have been found to be successful components of multimodal analgesia [52–62].

Various combinations of these agents are typically started 1 or 2 h before surgery and continued throughout the postoperative period. The combination of IV Tylenol, Celebrex, and pregabalin started before the surgery and continued around the clock which afterward has shown to decrease the opioid requirements [63]. A single dose of pregabalin and dexamethasone before rhinoplasty showed decreased postoperative opioid requirements [58].

Depression and anxiety should be screened for in the preoperative period, and appropriate referrals should be made for management of these conditions [64].

26.2.3 Lab Work/Work-Up

1. *Cardiovascular evaluation:* The evaluation of cardiac-pulmonary status is similar to any other patient undergoing similar surgery. However, patient's sufferings with chronic pain tend to have decreased functional status and impaired mobility due to pain. Methadone can interact with voltage-gated potassium channels in the myocardium, causing QT prolongation and

ventricular arrhythmias such as torsades de pointes [65]. A baseline EKG should be obtained in patients on methadone. The possibility of drug interactions with other drugs that also cause QT prolongation (e.g., ondansetron, promethazine, fluoxetine, quetiapine, or amitriptyline) should also be kept in mind.
2. Full blood count and comprehensive metabolic profile should be obtained on patients taking anticonvulsants.
3. *Urine drug screen:* Baseline urine drug screen may be useful to determine potential substance misuse, abuse, or diversion. See chapter on substance use disorder for more information.
4. Cervical spine X-rays with flexion and extension views should be considered in chronic pain patients suffering from neck pain or post-fusion to evaluate the stability of cervical spine for airway manipulation [66].

26.2.4 Why Cancel Surgery?

In the face of active, undiagnosed substance abuse, a joint decision between the surgeon and anesthesiologist should be made, weighing the risks of the abuse on both the patients' current health and surgical outcome.

26.3 Intraoperative Management

26.3.1 Effect of Anesthesia on Chronic Pain

There are no specific adverse effects related to anesthesia and chronic pain. In fact, there are studies to suggest, depending on the type of surgery and anesthetic utilized, they may reduce the likelihood of chronic pain or control pre-existing chronic pain [67, 68]. Ketamine, a NMDA-receptor antagonist, has been shown, when infused at sub-anesthetic doses, to improve postoperative pain control in patients [68]. It should be noted, however, that some of the medications the patient may be on preoperatively related to chronic pain may have an effect on the anesthetic (as discussed below).

26.3.2 What Anesthetics to Use and Not Use?

There are no specific contraindications to any anesthetic for patients with chronic pain. However, some medications the patient may be taking can alter the amount of volatile anesthetic required for the procedure. Specifically, patients on chronic opioids, TCAs, SSRIs, or SNRIs, will have increased requirement for volatile anesthetics. Conversely, patients who have been acutely exposed to opioids or patients on alpha-2 agonists, gabapentinoids (gabapentin, pregabalin), or calcium channel blockers will have decreased volatile anesthetic requirements.

If possible, adding a regional anesthetic to the procedure may also prove beneficial to the patient. Also, regional anesthetics are shown to be opioid sparing. Patients often have greater postoperative pain relief when the regional anesthetic is still functioning. However, skill in the procedures is required as there are numerous targets in the head and neck that if inadvertently injected into may cause serious neurological side effects.

26.3.3 Potential Problems

Barring any illicit drug use before surgery and ensuring proper medications have either been taken or replaced on the day of surgery, there are no specific concerns related to chronic pain and the intraoperative anesthetic technique. Assuming a proper multimodal plan has been instituted, there may be decreased anesthetic requirements intraoperatively for the patient, as well.

26.3.4 Monitoring

It is recommended that standard ASA monitors be placed and the patient is under proper supervision throughout the entire procedure. The need for invasive monitoring will be based on the surgical procedure, not pre-existing chronic pain.

26.3.5 What Depth of Anesthesia Is Appropriate?

The depth of anesthesia is related to the surgery being performed as well as other comorbidities that the patient may have. Concurrent pain and adjuvant medications may either increase or reduce the concentration of volatile anesthetic that is required.

26.3.6 Airway Management

Whether the airway needs to be secured via an endotracheal tube, laryngeal mask airway or nasal cannula is dependent on the scheduled surgery. Indeed, if a regional anesthetic is used without any sedation, there is no need for specific airway manipulation. However, there are no specific concerns with chronic pain and airway management assuming the pain is not being generated from a structure related to the airway.

26.3.7 Fluid Management

There are no specific concerns related to fluid management and chronic pain. As such, standard fluid guidelines associated with the scheduled surgery should be followed.

26.4 Postoperative Management

26.4.1 Airway Management

Airway management and extubation criteria are similar to any other patient undergoing similar surgery. However, opioid-tolerant patients should be carefully monitored for respiratory depression. Additional airway support may be needed in the postoperative period.

26.4.2 Pain Management

Postoperative pain management poses the biggest challenge in these patients [29, 69, 70]. Inadequate pain control is associated with myocardial ischemia, impaired pulmonary function, thromboembolism, ileus, impaired immune function, wound infection, anxiety, and reduced patient satisfaction [71]. In addition to increased hospital costs secondary to postoperative complications, hospital reimbursements are now linked to patient satisfaction scores [72].

Opioid-tolerant patient poses dual challenges of uncontrolled pain due to less response to exogenous opioids and increased complications associated with higher opioid doses. Increased doses of opioids may worsen the pain due to opioid-induced hyperalgesia [73]. Hence, the primary emphasis should be on an opioid-sparing approach through multimodal analgesia ideally started in the preoperative period.

A home regimen of opioids should be resumed, and additional analgesia should be available. Patients should restart their long-acting opioid medications as soon as possible in the postoperative period. In special situations of prolonged preoperative fasting, baseline opioid equivalent should be continued parentally. One of the approaches is to offer a patient-controlled analgesia (PCA) pump with a basal infusion and demand dosage. The basal infusion per hour is equating to the daily parental dose divided by 24 h [36]. Additional analgesia can be provided through demand dosage in the PCA which increases patient satisfaction and reduces anxiety [74, 75]. This could mean two to four times of the morphine dose appropriate for an opioid-naive patient having the same procedure [36]. As soon as the patient can take oral medications, the home regimen for long-acting opioids should be restarted and basal infusion should be stopped. Conversion from intravenous to oral opioids requires the expertise of the acute pain service led by anesthesiologists.

Long-term opioid use often begins with the treatment of acute pain. According to the new Centers for Disease Control (CDC) guidelines, when opioids are used for acute pain, clinicians should prescribe the lowest effective dose of immediate-release opioids and should prescribe no greater quantity than needed for the expected duration of pain severe enough to require opioids. Three days or less will often be sufficient; more than seven days will rarely be needed (recommendation category, A; evidence type, 4) [76]. In an opioid-tolerant patient, this could mean two to four times the dose for an opioid-naive patient [36]. The physician managing patient's chronic pain should be notified the possible need to adjust the dose and to schedule follow-up appointments after discharge.

Patients with a history of difficulty in management of postoperative pain, who live at a distance from the hospital, or otherwise pose a challenge requiring close monitoring in the perioperative period may benefit from planned hospital admission to manage complications postoperatively even for what may otherwise be considered routine outpatient procedures [77].

Postoperative nausea and vomiting may be challenging in these patients. Besides the risk factors involved in oral surgeries, increase in opioid requirements in chronic pain population due to opioid tolerance may increase the risk for postoperative nausea and vomiting. Hence, multiple agents such as 5-HT3 receptor antagonists, gastrokinetics, steroids, and butyrophenones are recommended for prophylaxis and treatment [66].

26.4.3 Postoperative Risks

Moreover, chronic opioid consumption is thought to induce some effects that are still poorly explained, e.g., delay in scar formation, increased complication rate, and increased risk of chronic pain. Absorption of transdermal fentanyl can be affected by postoperative fever [78]. And, as mentioned earlier, uncontrolled acute pain can be a cause for the development of chronic pain via windup and central sensitization.

26.5 Postoperative Complications

Postoperative complications can be related to one of two issues: poorly controlled postoperative pain or pharmacological withdrawal. As described above, chronic pain patients, especially those on preoperative opioids, will have increased requirements for pain control [36]. As such, unless their baseline opioid requirements are met with the addition of an appropriate multimodal pain plan, uncontrolled acute pain can result. This can affect multiple systems and can potentially cause issues with the surgical wound especially if strict hemodynamic parameters are required for proper healing. The effects of uncontrolled pain are varied and include tachycardia, hypertension, hypoxia, hypercarbia, decreased cough, nausea, vomiting, ileus, impaired wound healing, anxiety, anger, delirium, and urinary retention. Quickly addressing the uncontrolled pain is of the utmost importance.

The second issue to address is medication withdrawal. With appropriate preoperative education, the patient is made aware of which medications to take the morning of surgery. However, if these medications are not taken the day of surgery or not started postoperatively, the risk of withdrawal increases. These medications include opioids, benzodiazepines, and baclofen. While opioid and benzodiazepine withdrawal are unpleasant for the patient, baclofen withdrawal can be life-threatening with associated hallucinations and seizures that are potentially intractable to standard treatments. As such, restarting these medications, either orally, intravenously, or via a pre-existing intrathecal pump, is recommended as soon as possible after surgery. Also, sudden discontinuation of gabapentin may cause anxiety, insomnia, nausea, pain, and sweating. Patients with seizures may also experience increased seizure activity. Indeed, any unexpected changes postoperatively may warrant a close examination of preoperative medications or possible illicit substances.

Conclusions

While acute pain is indicative of potential tissue damage, chronic pain often lacks any identifiable pathology or treatment and is thought to represent "hurt, not harm." Also, pain is universally an unpleasant experience with associated negative emotions and behavioral modifications. It should then come as no surprise that chronic pain has a large psychological overlay and in the absence of harm can result in significant functional disability.

Chronic pain can be caused by varied, though often unknown, pathologies and can manifest anywhere along the pain pathway. The associated conditions include cancer, diabetes, back pain, headache, atypical facial pain, arthritis, temporomandibular joint pain, peripheral neuropathy, gastrointestinal disorders, pelvic pain, and numerous other conditions. The challenge in chronic pain management is some conditions are known to produce chronic nociceptive pain, neuropathic pain, or inflammatory pain, whereas others can be caused by minor injuries that result in central sensitization well after healing is complete. Appropriate treatment via the biopsychosocial model is recommended for the best possible pain management.

The perioperative considerations for the chronic pain patient include thorough discussions of postoperative pain relief plans as well as optimizing the patient before surgery. Care should be taken to assess the pain medications the patient is on as well as any implantable devices that may need to be turned off or identified preoperatively. Numerous intraoperative choices are available for the patient including regional anesthesia, intravenous infusions, or NMDA antagonists.

References

1. Hall JE, Guyton AC. Guyton and Hall textbook of medical physiology. Philadelphia, PA: Saunders Elsevier; 2011.
2. Sahbaie P, Shi X, Guo T-Z, et al. Role of substance *P* signaling in enhanced nociceptive sensitization and local cytokine production after incision. Pain. 2009;145(3):341–9. https://doi.org/10.1016/j.pain.2009.06.037.
3. Latremoliere A, Woolf CJ. Central sensitization: a generator of pain hypersensitivity by central neural plasticity. J Pain. 2009;10(9):895–926. https://doi.org/10.1016/j.jpain.2009.06.012.
4. Melzack R, Wall PD. Pain mechanisms: a new theory. Science. 1965;150(3699):971–9.
5. Ahmad AH, Zakaria R. Pain in times of stress. Malays J Med Sci. 2015;22(Spec Issue):52–61.
6. Wager T, Atlas L, Lindquist M, et al. An fMRI-based neurologic signature of physical pain. N Engl J Med. 2013;368:1388–97.
7. Costigan M, Scholz J, Woolf CJ. Neuropathic pain: a maladaptive response of the nervous system to damage. Annu Rev Neurosci. 2009;32:1–32. https://doi.org/10.1146/annurev.neuro.051508.135531.
8. Mendell LM. Constructing and deconstructing the gate theory of pain. Pain. 2014;155(2):210–6. https://doi.org/10.1016/j.pain.2013.12.010.
9. Tyrer SP. Learned pain behavior. Br Med J (Clin Res Ed). 1986;292(6512):1–2.
10. Johannes CB, Le TK ZX, Johnston JA, Dworkin RH. The prevalence of chronic pain in United States adults: results of an Internet-based survey. J Pain. 2010;11(11):1230–9. https://doi.org/10.1016/j.jpain.2010.07.002. Epub 25 Aug 2010.
11. Institute of Medicine of the National Academies Report. Relieving pain in America: a blueprint for transforming prevention, care, education, and research. Washington DC: The National Academies Press; 2011.
12. American Pain Foundation. Voices in Chronic Pain Survey. American Pain Society. 2006. http://www.painmed.org/files/facts-and-figureson-pain.pdf.
13. Stewart WF, Ricci JA, Chee E, Morganstein D, Lipton R. Lost productive time and cost due to common pain conditions in the US workforce. JAMA. 2003;290(18):2443–54. https://doi.org/10.1001/jama.290.18.2443.
14. Van Hecke O, Torrance N, Smith BH. Chronic pain epidemiology: where do lifestyle factors fit in? Br J Pain. 2013;7(4):209–17. https://doi.org/10.1177/2049463713493264.
15. Bair J, Robinson RL, Katon W, Kroenke K. Depression and pain comorbidity: a literature review. Arch Intern Med. 2003;163:2433–45.
16. Cheatle MD, Gallagher RM. Chronic pain and comorbid mood and substance use disorders: a biopsychosocial treatment approach. Curr Psychiatry Rep. 2006;8(5):371–6. https://doi.org/10.1007/s11920-006-0038-7.
17. Knaster P, Karlsson H, Estlander A, Kalso E. Psychiatric disorders as assessed with SCID in chronic pain patients: the anxiety disorders precede the onset of pain. Gen Hosp Psychiatry. 2012;34(1):46–52.
18. Arnow BA, Hunkeler EM, Blasey CM, Lee JDH, Constantino MJ, Fireman B, et al. Comorbid depression, chronic pain, and disability in primary care. Psychosom Med. 2006;68(2):262–8.
19. Polatin PB, Kinney RK, Gatchel RJ, Lillo E, Mayer TG. Psychiatric illness and chronic low-back pain. The mind and the spine: which goes first? Spine. 1993;18(1):66–71.
20. Quartana PJ, Campbell CM, et al. Expert review of neurotherapeutics. 2009;9(5):745–58.

21. Johansson AC, Linton SJ, et al. Disability and rehabilitation. 2010;32(7):521–9.
22. American Society of Anesthesiologists Task Force on Acute Pain Management. Practice guidelines for acute pain management in the perioperative setting: an updated report. Anesthesiology. 2004;100:1573–81.
23. Kehlet H, Dahl J. The value of "multimodal" or "balanced analgesia" in postoperative pain treatment. Anesth Analg. 1993;77:1048–56.
24. Langford R. Pain management today. What have we learned? Clin Rheumatol. 2006;25:S2–8.
25. Vickers A, Bali S, Baxter A, et al. Consensus statement on the anticipation and prevention of acute postoperative pain: multidisciplinary RADAR approach. Curr Med Res Opin. 2009;25:2557–69.
26. The Royal College of Anaesthetists and The British Pain Society. Pain management services good practice. London: The Royal College of Anaesthetists and The British Pain Society; 2003.
27. Daubresse M, Chang HY, Yu Y, et al. Ambulatory diagnosis and treatment of nonmalignant pain in the United States, 2000–2010. Med Care. 2013;51:870–8.
28. Armaghani S, Lee D. Bible Jet al. Increased preoperative narcotic use and its association with postoperative complications and length of stay in patients undergoing spine surgery. Clin Spine Surg. 2016;29:E93–8.
29. Carroll IR, Angst MS, Clark JD. Management of perioperative pain in patients chronically consuming opioids. Reg Anesth Pain Med. 2004;29:576–91.
30. Rose DK, Cohen MM, Yee DA. Changing the practice of pain management. Anesth Analg. 1997;84:764–72.
31. Frolich MA, Giannotti A, Modell JH. Opioid overdose in a patient using a fentanyl patch during treatment with a warming blanket. Anesth Analg. 2001;93:647–8.
32. Andreas K, Anne B, Christoph S. Perioperative management of the chronic pain patient. Best Pract Res Clin Anaesthesiol. 2005;19(1):59–76.
33. Joly V, Richebe P, Guignard B, et al. Remifentanil-induced postoperative hyperalgesia and its prevention with small-dose ketamine. Anesthesiology. 2005;103:147–55.
34. Lewis N, Williams J. Acute pain management in patients receiving opioids for chronic and cancer pain. Contin Educ Anaesth Crit Care Pain. 2005;5:127–9.
35. Hadi A, Morley-Forster P, Dain S, Horril K, Moulin D. Brief review: preoperative management of the patient with chronic non-cancer pain. Can J Anaesth. 2006;53:1190–9.
36. Richebe P, Beaulieu P. Perioperative pain management in the patient treated with opioids: continuing professional development. Can J Anesth. 2009;56:969–81.
37. Attal N, Cruccu G, Baron R, Haanpa M, Hansson P, Jensen TS, et al. EFNS guidelines: EFNS guidelines on the pharmacological treatment of neuropathic pain: 2010 revision. Eur J Neur. 2010;17:1113–23.
38. Kudoh A, Katagai H, Takazawa T. Antidepressant treatment for chronic depressed patients should not be discontinued prior to anaesthesia. Can J Anaesth. 2002;49:132–6.
39. Jones D, Story D. Serotonin syndrome and the anaesthetist. Anaesth Intensive Care. 2005;33:181–7.
40. Barrueto F, Green J, Howland MA, Hoffman RS, Nelson LS. Gabapentin withdrawal presenting as status epilepticus. Toxicol Clin Toxicol. 2002;40:925–8.
41. Ho K, Gan T, Habib A. Gabapentin and postoperative pain- a systematic review of randomized controlled trials. Pain. 2006;1(26):91–101.
42. Kong V, Irwin M. Gabapentin: a multimodal perioperative drug? Br J Anaesth. 2007;99:775–86.
43. Henry D, Lawson DH, Reavey P, Renfrew S. Hyponatraemia during carbamazepine treatment. BMJ. 1977;1:83–4.
44. Klein J, Sandi-Gahun S, Schackert G, Juratli TA. Peripheral nerve field stimulation for trigeminal neuralgia, trigeminal neuropathic pain, and persistent idiopathic facial pain. Cephalalgia. 2015;36(5): 445–53.
45. Witters DM, von Maitzahn G, Bassen HI. In vitro assessment of tissue heating near metallic medical implants by exposure to pulsed radio frequency diathermy. Phys Med Biol. 2003;48(291):9–28.
46. British Pain Society. Spinal cord stimulation for the management of pain: recommendations for best clinical practice. 2009. www.britishpainsociety.org/pub_professional.htm.
47. Grider J, Brown R, Colclough G. Perioperative management of patients with an intrathecal drug delivery system for chronic pain. Anaesth Anal. 2008;107:1393–6.
48. Michelson JD, Addante RA, Charlson MD. Multimodal analgesia therapy reduces length of hospitalization in patients undergoing fusions of the ankle and hindfoot. Foot Ankle Int. 2013;34:1526–34.
49. Larson DW, Lovely JK, Cima RR, et al. Outcomes after implementation of a multimodal standard care pathway for laparoscopic colorectal surgery. Br J Surg. 2014;101:1023–30.
50. Helander Erik M, Menard Bethany L, Harmon Chris M. Multimodal analgesia, current concepts, and acute pain considerations. Curr Pain Headache Rep. 2017;21(1):3.
51. Elia N, Lysakowski C, Tramer MR. Does multimodal analgesia with acetaminophen, nonsteroidal antiinflammatory drugs, or selective cyclooxygenase-2 inhibitors and patient-controlled analgesia morphine offer advantages over morphine alone? Anesthesiology. 2005;103:1296–304.
52. Hamidreza E, Reza T, Hamidreza K, et al. Evaluation of a single dose intravenous paracetamol for pain relief after maxillofacial surgery: a randomized clinical trial study. J Maxillofac Oral Surg. 2014;13(4):478–82.
53. Marković Aleksa B, Ljubomir T. Postoperative analgesia after lower third molar surgery: contribution of the use of long-acting local anesthetics, low-power laser, and diclofenac. Oral Surg Oral Med Oral Pathol Oral Radiol Endodontol. 2006;102(5):e4–8.
54. Takayuki A, Yoshihide O, Yusuke M. Analgesic efficacy of celecoxib in patients after oral surgery: special reference to time to onset of analgesia and

duration of analgesic effect. Oral Maxillofac Surg. 2016;20(3):265–71.
55. Hurley RW, Cohen SP, Williams KA, et al. The analgesic effects of perioperative gabapentin on postoperative pain: a meta-analysis. Reg Anesth Pain Med. 2006;31:237–47.
56. Wai CC, Shan CW, Yan LY, et al. A double-blind randomized crossover study to evaluate the timing of pregabalin for third molar surgery under local anesthesia. J Oral Maxillofac Surg. 2012;70(1):25–30.
57. Zhang J, Ho KY, Wang Y. Efficacy of pregabalin in acute postoperative pain: a meta-analysis. Br J Anaesth. 2011;106:454–62.
58. Demirhan A, Tekelioglu UY, Akkaya A. Effect of pregabalin and dexamethasone addition to multimodal analgesia on postoperative analgesia. Aesthetic Plast Surg. 2013;37(6):1100–6.
59. Rood JP, Coulthard P, Snowdon AT, et al. Safety and efficacy of levobupivacaine for postoperative pain relief after the surgical removal of impacted third molars: a comparison with lignocaine and adrenaline. Br J Oral Maxillofac Surg. 2002;40(6):491–6.
60. Sharif NM, Yates C. Bupivacaine as pre-emptive analgesia in third molar surgery: randomised controlled trial. Br J Oral Maxillofac Surg. 2006;44(6):501–3.
61. Daykin H. The efficacy and safety of intravenous lidocaine for analgesia in the older adult: a literature review. Br J Pain. 2017;11(1):23–31.
62. Albrecht E, Kirkham KR, Liu SS, Brull R. Perioperative intravenous administration of magnesium sulphate and postoperative pain: a meta-analysis. Anaesthesia. 2013;68(1):79–90.
63. Trabulsi EJ, Patel J, Viscusi ER, et al. Preemptive multimodal pain regimen reduces opioid analgesia for patients undergoing robotic-assisted laparoscopic radical nephrectomy. Urology. 2010;76:1122–4.
64. Szumita RP, Szumita PM, Just N. Understanding and managing patients with chronic pain. Oral Maxillofac Surg Clin North Am. 2010;22(4):481–94.
65. Krantz M, Lowery C, Martell B, et al. Effects of methadone on QT-interval dispersion. Pharmacotherapy. 2005;25:1523–9.
66. Krohner RG. Anesthetic considerations and techniques for oral and maxillofacial surgery. Int Anesthesiol Clin. 2003;41(3):67–89.
67. Ah-Reum C, Jae-Young K, Kyung-Hoon K, et al. The effects of anesthetics on chronic pain after breast cancer surgery. Anesth Analg. 2013;116(3):685–93.
68. Kaur S, Saroa R, Aggarwal S. Effect of intraoperative infusion of low-dose ketamine on management of postoperative analgesia. J Nat Sci Biol Med. 2015;6(2):378–82. https://doi.org/10.4103/0976-9668.160012.
69. de Leon-Casasola OA, Myers DP, Donaparthi S, et al. A comparison of postoperative epidural analgesia between patients with chronic cancer taking high doses of oral opioids versus opioid-naive patients. Anesth Analg. 1993;76:302–7.
70. Rapp SE, Ready LB, Nessly ML. Acute pain management in patients with prior opioid consumption: a case-controlled retrospective review. Pain. 1995;61:195–201.
71. Joshi GP, Ogunnaike BO. Consequences of inadequate postoperative pain relief and chronic persistent postoperative pain. Anesthesiol Clin North America. 2005;23:21–36.
72. Hospital Consumer Assessment of Healthcare Providers and Systems [HCAHPS]. https://www.cms.gov/medicare/quality-initiatives-patient-assessment-instruments/hospitalqualityinits/hospitalhcahps.html.
73. Chapman CR, Davis J, Donaldson GW, et al. Postoperative pain trajectories in chronic pain patients undergoing surgery: the effects of chronic opioid pharmacotherapy on acute pain. J Pain. 2011;12(12):1240–6.
74. Thomas V. Psychological characteristics and the effectiveness of patient-controlled analgesia. BJA. 1995;74:271–6.
75. Taylor N, Hall G, Salmon P. Is patient controlled analgesia controlled by the patient? Soc Sci Med. 1996;43(1):1137–43.
76. CDC guidelines for prescribing opioids for chronic pain. https://www.cdc.gov/drugoverdose/prescribing/guideline.html.
77. Brooks MR, Golianu B. Perioperative management in children with chronic pain. Paediatr Anaesth. 2016;26(8):794–806.
78. Ashburn M, Lazarre Ogden L, Zhang J, Love G, Basta S. The pharmacokinetics of transdermal fentanyl delivered with and without controlled heat. J Pain. 2003;4:291–7.

27 Perioperative Management of the HIV Patient

Lydia Aoun Barakat and Jacques Emile Mokhbat

Abstract

Human immunodeficiency virus (HIV) infection is a chronic condition and requires lifelong treatment. HIV-infected patients are living longer and have multiple comorbidities. In this chapter, we discuss the epidemiology, pathophysiology, clinical manifestations, and perioperative management specific to HIV-infected patients. We outline in detail the operative and anesthesia risk, drug-drug interaction, and antiretroviral therapy related to HIV management.

27.1 HIV Disease

27.1.1 Pathophysiology

Acquired immune deficiency syndrome (AIDS) was first described in 1981 [1]. In 1983, the retrovirus human immunodeficiency virus (HIV) was identified as the underlying infectious cause of AIDS. There are two subtypes of the virus, HIV-1 and HIV-2. HIV-1 is responsible of the vast majority of infections in the world and specifically in North America and Europe. HIV-2 is mainly prevalent in West Africa and appears to have similar but rather slower clinical course.

HIV infection is acquired through blood exposure, sexual intercourse, and perinatal transmission. Infectious virus can be recovered from blood, semen, and cervical or vaginal secretions.

After acquisition of HIV, the virus targets human T lymphocyte cells. The viral envelop protein (gp120) attaches to the CD4 complex of the host cell. Once HIV is inside the cell, it integrates its own genome into the host cell DNA. The viral genetic material is then transcribed into new RNA which eventually produces more infectious HIV viral particles that will ultimately leave one cell and infect other CD4 T cells. Figure 27.1 illustrates the life cycle of the HIV virus.

The replication of HIV triggers virus directed and immune killing of the CD4 T lymphocytes [2] which leads to a drop in the total pool of human T cells that ranges around 1400 cell/μL in

L.A. Barakat, M.D. (✉)
Section of Infectious Disease, Yale University School of Medicine, New Haven, CT, USA
e-mail: Lydia.barakat@yale.edu

J.E. Mokhbat, M.D.
Division of Infectious Diseases, Department of Medicine, Lebanese American University School of Medicine, Beirut, Lebanon
e-mail: Jacques.mokhbat@lau.edu.lb

© Springer International Publishing AG 2018
E.M. Ferneini, J.D. Bennett (eds.), *Perioperative Assessment of the Maxillofacial Surgery Patient*,
https://doi.org/10.1007/978-3-319-58868-1_27

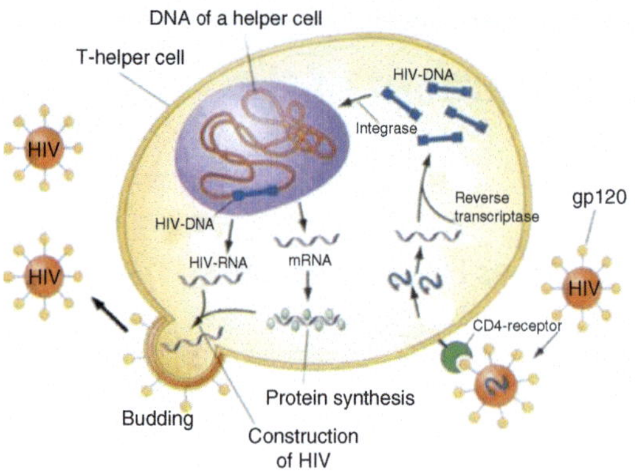

Fig. 27.1 HIV life cycle

a normal host [3]. The amount of circulating virus or HIV viral load is measured by the number of HIV RNA copies of the virus in 1 mL of plasma. In the absence of antiretroviral therapy (ART), the CD4 T cells decline is estimated at a rate of 4% per year per log copies/ml of HIV viral load and on average 50 cell/μL per year [4]. When the total CD4 count fall below 200 cell/μL or 14%, the patient is identified as having AIDS [2, 5, 6]. Figure 27.2 displays the natural history of HIV infection.

27.1.1.1 HIV Diagnosis

The case definition of HIV diagnosis includes a positive HIV antibody/antigen assay (fourth-generation enzyme-linked immunoassay) or a positive HIV viral load. The Western blot confirmatory test is no longer required. The fourth-generation EIA test identifies HIV-1 and HIV-2 virus within 2 weeks of infection [7].

27.1.2 HIV Prevalence

Worldwide, there are around 36.9 million people living with HIV infections as of June 2016; the majority are in Africa (Fig. 27.3). An estimated two million new infections were diagnosed in 2014 and 1.2 million people died from AIDS-related illnesses in 2015 globally. There are approximately 1.4 million HIV-infected individuals the United States of America with an estimated 55,000 new infections annually.

The vast majority of HIV infections are spread through sexual contact. In man, the highest rate of transmission is through men who have sex with men (MSM) contact and via heterosexual intercourse in women.

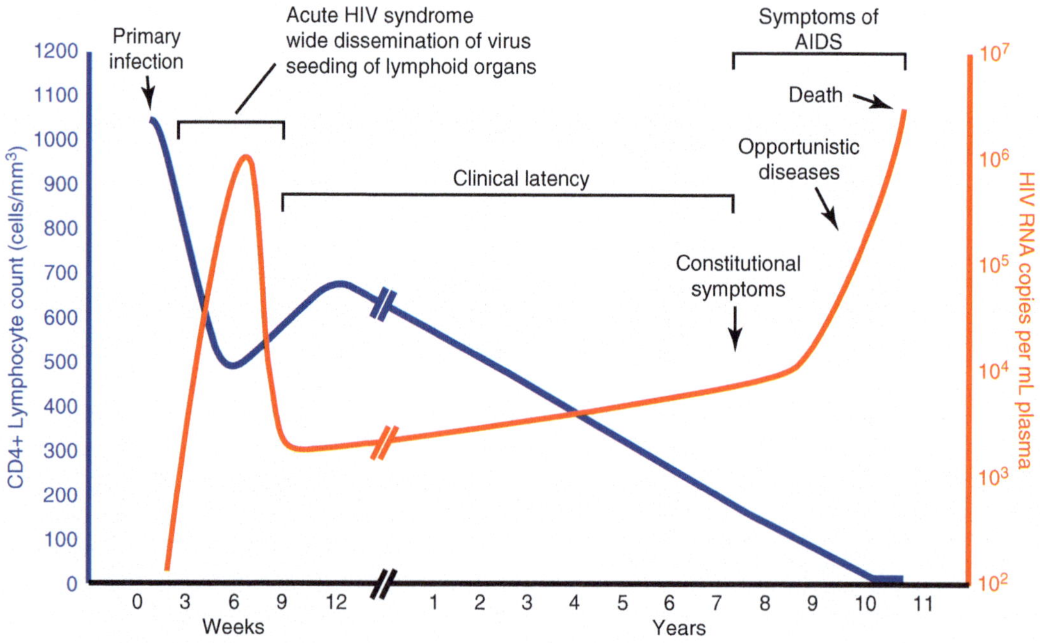

Fig. 27.2 The natural history of HIV infection

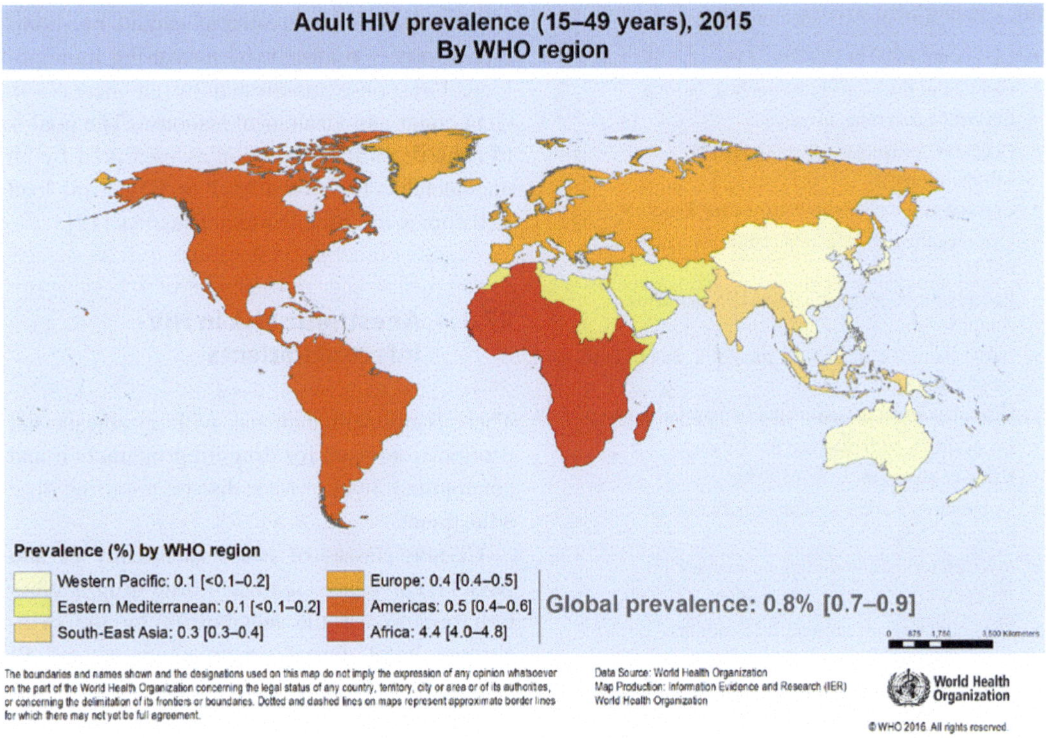

Fig. 27.3 The global HIV prevalence

27.1.3 Manifestations of HIV Disease

The median interval between HIV seroconversion and progression to AIDS has been estimated to be 8–10 years [2] as shown in Fig. 27.2. However, cases of elite controllers, long-term nonprogressors, and rapid progressors have been described [8, 9].

Prior the effective antiretroviral therapy (ART), the AIDS-associated illnesses and opportunistic infection infections were the principal cause of morbidity and mortality. However, with increased access to effective ART, the life expectancy of HIV-infected patients is almost similar to HIV-uninfected [10].

The Center for Disease Control and Prevention (CDC) HIV classification is the most widely used and included immunological criteria based on CD4 cell count and clinical criteria [7, 11].

Chronic HIV infection is divided into four stages.

Asymptomatic HIV infection: usually CD4 count >500 cell/μL. The patients are asymptomatic except for possible persistent generalized lymphadenopathy (PGL).

Symptomatic HIV infection: usually CD4 count 200–500 cell/μL. The patients are usually asymptomatic but can have occasionally thrush, vaginal candidiasis, hairy cell leukoplakia, herpes zoster, peripheral neuropathy, or idiopathic thrombocytopenic purpura.

AIDS: CD4 count <200 cell/μL or AIDS defining illness as outlined in Table 27.1.

Advanced AIDS: CD4 count <50 cell/μL with life expectancy of 12 month if not treated.

The introduction of highly active antiretroviral therapy (ART) in 1996 has tremendously impacted the natural history of HIV. The overall mortality, progression to AIDS, and opportunistic infection rates have decreased significantly [10]. Although there is no cure for HIV, patients are living longer and have a life expectancy almost similar to the HIV-uninfected population. As the patients are growing older, there is a potential increase in the need for surgeries including in the area of the ear, nose, and throat (ENT).

Table 27.1 List of AIDS defining illness

• CD4 count <200 or CD4% < 14%
• Candida of the esophagus, trachea, or lung
• Cervical carcinoma, invasive
• Coccidioidomycosis, disseminated or extrapulmonary
• Cryptosporidiosis, with diarrhea for 1 month
• Cytomegalovirus infection (not in liver, spleen, or LN)
• Encephalopathy due to HIV, AIDS dementia complex
• Herpes simplex, ulcer for 1 month or pneumonitis or esophagitis
• Histoplasmosis, disseminated or extrapulmonary
• Isosporiasis, with diarrhea for 1 month
• Kaposi's sarcoma
• Lymphoma, Burkitt's or immunoblastic or primary CNS
• Mycobacteriosis, including pulmonary TB
• *Pneumocystis carinii* pneumonia
• Pneumonia, recurrent within 12 months
• Progressive multifocal leukoencephalopathy
• Salmonella (non-typhoid) septicemia, recurrent
• Toxoplasmosis of the brain
• Wasting syndrome due to HIV

The US Department of Health and Human Services (DHHS) recommends that ART be initiated to all HIV-infected patients regardless of their CD4 T cell count and HIV viral load. There are five classes of ART. As of 2016, it is recommended to use three drug regimens [12]: two from the nucleoside reverse transcriptase inhibitor (NRTI) class and one from the nonnucleoside reverse transcriptase inhibitor (NNRTI), protease inhibitor (PI), or integrase inhibitor (INSTI) class. Many of the ART combination are currently available in single-tablet regimen (STR). Currently, there are six different ART available in STR:

- Atripla (tenofovir/emtricitabine/efavirenz)
- Complera (tenofovir/emtricitabine/rilpivirine)
- Stribild (tenofovir/emtricitabine/elvitegravir/cobicistat)
- Triumeq (abacavir/lamivudine/dolutegravir)
- Odefsey (tenofovir/alafenamide/emtricitabine/rilpivirine)
- Genvoya (tenofovir/alafenamide/emtricitabine/elvitegravir/cobicistat)

The response to treatment should be monitored every 3–6 months by measuring immunological response manifested by an increase in CD4 count and virological response. The goal is to achieve viral suppression as measured by an undetectable HIV viral load or HIV viral load <20 copies/mL by the available assays [12].

27.1.4 Anesthetic Risk in HIV-Infected Patients

There is no significant risk with anesthesia, but caution is advised for drug-drug interaction and concomitant liver or renal disease requiring dose adjustment.

Certain classes of ART, specifically PI and NNRTI, can cause significant drug-drug interaction because of the metabolism by the cytochrome P450. For example, efavirenz and PI increase the level of midazolam and triazolam and should not be coadministered [12, 13]. In-depth discussion about specific anesthetic is discussed in Sect. 27.3.

27.2 Preoperative Assessment of HIV-Infected Patient

27.2.1 Workup

Preoperative evaluation of the HIV-infected patient is similar to that of the general population. However, HIV-infected patient can have increased risk of comorbidities and polypharmacy [14–16].

In preparation for the surgery, the patient should complete a physical exam and routine baseline laboratory studies. These studies include complete blood count, creatinine, glucose, liver function test, albumin, prothrombin time, and partial thromboplastin time. Additionally a CD4 cell count and an HIV viral load should be repeated if results are unavailable in the past 3–6 months. HIV-infected patients are at higher risk for coronary artery disease [17], and certain ART are associated with QT prolongation such as atazanavir, a PI, and rilpivirine, an NNRTI [12]. Therefore, it is prudent to perform a careful cardiac risk assessment and obtain an electrocardiogram preoperatively.

In addition, the prevalence of underlying pulmonary disease is increased in HIV population in part due to high prevalence of smoking among HIV population [15, 18, 19]. A chest X-ray should be considered if no record available in the past 6–12 months and assess respiratory complications in the perioperative period.

27.2.2 Discuss Laboratory Tests and Anticipated Results and What Abnormal Results Indicate

Neutropenia is common in HIV-infected patients with severe immunosuppression or chronic liver disease. It is very unlikely to require G-CSF use to maintain an absolute neutrophil count >1000 cells/mm^3 [20].

Thrombocytopenia: One of the causes of thrombocytopenia is idiopathic thrombocytopenic purpura that can occur at any stage of HIV infection. It is prudent to consult with a hematologist prior to surgery for patient with platelet count <50,000/mm^3.

Abnormal liver function test: Elevated transaminases can be secondary to drug toxicity such as NRTI or statins. However, coinfection with hepatitis B or C can predispose the patient to increased bleeding risk due to coagulopathy or thrombocytopenia. Isolated hyperbilirubinemia can be associated with the protease inhibitor atazanavir and is reversible after discontinuation of the medication.

Abnormal renal function: There are many reasons for a decline in renal function. However, tenofovir is one of the NRTI that can be associated with nephrotoxicity and Fanconi's syndrome. A GFR <50 mL/min requires dose adjustment of the medication; therefore it has an impact on anesthesia dosing and selection.

Low albumin: It is associated with advanced liver disease; however, it can be a predictor of abnormal nutritional status, and it was shown to be associated with post-op complications.

CD4 count and HIV viral load results: Virological staging is important prior to surgery in order to discuss the risk and benefit with the patient. CD4 T cell count and HIV viral load should be ordered if not available in the past 3–6 months.

27.2.3 What to Do About Chronic Medications?

HIV-infected patients are on lifelong antiretroviral medications. ART should not be stopped and be safely continued perioperatively. ART can be held on the day of surgery if the patient is required to be in a "nothing per mouth" or "nil per os (NPO)" status. These medications should be resumed as soon as feasible, specifically in patient with hepatitis B coinfection. ART interruption for few days would not have a detrimental consequence on their potency and effectiveness. In this case, all ART should be stopped at the same time. If ART are being administered intermittently, viral resistance would emerge and will lead to multiple drug resistance. In special situations when the patient is unable to swallow pills, a liquid substitution is available to several ART drugs, or certain pills can be crushed [12], as summarized in Table 27.2.

Currently, there are no FDA-approved intravenous ART. It is advisable to consult with an HIV specialist to guide ART management.

Patients who have AIDS or low CD4 T cell count are required to take medications for prophylaxis against opportunistic infections. These medications can be held for several days or can be substituted with parenteral form when available. For example, trimethoprim-sulfamethoxazole (available intravenously) or atovaquone (liquid) is used to prevent *Pneumocystis jiroveci* pneumonia when CD4 count <200 cell/μL and toxoplasmosis for CD4 count <100 cell/μL. Azithromycin or clarithromycin (available intravenously) is used to prevent *Mycobacterium avium* complex (MAC) for CD4 count <50 cell/μL [21].

Table 27.2 List of antiretroviral agents and bioavailability

ART	Liquid	Soluble in water	Crushable
Zidovudine (AZT)	Yes	No	Yes
Lamivudine (3TC)	Yes	No	Yes
Abacavir	Yes	No	No
Tenofovir	Yes	Yes	Yes
Tenofovir alafenamide	No	Yes	Yes
Emtricitabine	Yes	Yes	Yes
Efavirenz	Yes	No	No
Rilpivirine	No	No	No
Nevirapine	Yes	Yes	Yes
Etravirine	No	Yes	Yes
Raltegravir	Yes	No	No
Elvitegravir	No	No	No
Dolutegravir	No	Yes	Yes
Lopinavir/ritonavir	Yes	No	No
Atazanavir	Yes	Yes	Yes
Darunavir	Yes	Yes	Yes

27.2.4 Steps to Optimize Patient: Pre-op Preparation

Several steps can be taken in order to optimize the patient status for surgery:

- Review patient surgical risk based on patient medical condition using the American Society of Anesthesiologists (ASA) score or American College of Surgeons.
- Evaluate the laboratory and imaging results with the patient and make appropriate referrals to specialists if needed.
- Emphasize the importance of ART and ensure HIV viral suppression.
- Discuss the risk of medication interruption, specifically ART with the patient and alternative options.
- Identify any medication allergies or active drug/alcohol use.
- Address advance directives and healthcare proxy prior to surgery to ensure that patient confidentiality regarding HIV status is protected in case of an emergency or adverse outcome.

27.2.5 What Should Cancel Surgery? Discuss Risk Factors

In the current ART era, patients living with HIV have good surgical outcomes. Neither CD4 count nor HIV viral load should be used as sole contributing factor to surgical risk or should be a factor to cancel surgery [22–24]. Some studies suggested that HIV-infected patients have higher rate postoperative complications or mortality compared to HIV-uninfected patients independent of CD4 cell count [25–27]. However, another retrospective matched study found the same complication rate in HIV-infected and HIV-uninfected patients except for pneumonia [28].

Certain studies suggested poorer surgical outcomes with low CD4 cell count, and others report better outcomes when patients are on ART and have a suppressed viral load [22, 26, 27, 29]. Thus, it is ideal for the patient to have an optimized ART management preoperatively by and HIV expert in order to achieve HIV suppression and lead to immune reconstitution prior to elective surgery.

Certain conditions that might contribute to delaying surgeries include but not limited to ongoing bacterial or fungal infection that is not controlled by antimicrobial agents, acute kidney injury from unclear or irreversible condition, acute decompensated liver cirrhosis that can impact dosing or selection of anesthesia, and coagulopathy due to liver disease or ITP that can cause potential risk for intra- or postoperative bleeding.

There are concerns among HIV-uninfected surgeon regarding HIV acquisition during surgery of an HIV-infected patient. Surgeons have the highest risk among healthcare workers for percutaneous blood exposure, approximately a dozen exposures per person-year [30]. In almost 30 years, there were 150 possible cases and 58 documented cases of occupationally acquired HIV infection, and none of them were surgeons. Additional information regarding occupational HIV transmission are available at the center of disease control and prevention website *www.cdc.gov*.

In case of high risk occupational HIV exposure, healthcare worker should report to their occupational health provider in order to receive timely ART for post-exposure prophylaxis [31].

27.3 Intraoperative Management

27.3.1 Effects of Anesthesia on Disease

Several studies have reported a decline in immune function with general anesthesia. Therefore, general anesthesia should be approached with caution in immunosuppressed individuals with HIV. This immunosuppression starts shortly upon induction within 15 min and may last up to 11 days postoperatively. In addition, putting a patient to sleep and intubation may be associated with increased risk of aspiration pneumonia and inhalation-associated respiratory infection. The longer the use of artificial ventilation, the higher the risk of ventilator-associated pneumonia [32].

Many anesthetic agents may have significant interactions with antiretroviral agents especially through cytochrome p450 induction. Antiretroviral agents should be given as close as possible to the anesthesia. However, they will have to be interrupted around surgery and possibly for prolonged period if the patient has to be kept fasting for long periods pre- or postoperatively. If interruption is of a very short duration (i.e., only the duration of surgery), this does not represent a major difficulty. Viral resistance is not likely to occur if all antiretroviral agents are interrupted simultaneously. In that case, the difference in half-lives of agents should be addressed with caution. For example, most NNRTIs have very prolonged half-lives, and if a triple combination containing an NNRTI, for example, efavirenz, is to be interrupted, this should be done gradually with modification of the regimen to a protease inhibitor-based combination for a period of 2 weeks prior to surgery. Eventually, antiretroviral agents will be administered via nasogastric feeding tubes. However, if interruption is anticipated to last longer, it is important to modify the regimen in a way that all drugs should have similar half-lives to avoid maintaining one of the drugs (e.g., efavirenz) having a persistent serum concentration alone, while the other drugs have already been excreted.

If antibiotics are used for primary or secondary prophylaxis (i.e., cotrimoxazole), these should be converted to parenteral forms to maintain the patient on them during the potential period of prolonged fasting [33–35].

What anesthetic medications to use or not to use: Several anesthetic agents may interact with the antiretroviral medications, particularly benzodiazepines, opioids, and nonsteroidal anti-inflammatory agents [36]. The main agents associated with such interactions are the boosted protease inhibitors leading to risks of over dosage [13]. The safest agents for induction should have limited cytochrome p450 metabolism, such as etomidate. However, there is no clear contraindication to the use of other induction agents such as propofol or thiopental. The latter may reduce plasma concentrations of protease inhibitors and should be avoided in case of a PI-based regimen. Desflurane has also minimal metabolism and may be safely used. As far as opioids, remifentanil and morphine are acceptable agents. Other opiates such as fentanyl and alfentanil may incur altered metabolism resulting in higher concentrations when used in individuals treated with PIs or in lower concentrations in patients treated with an NNRTI-based regimen and should best be avoided. However, doses may have to be increased especially in patients treated with NNRTIs and reduced in case of protease inhibitor-based regimen. Pethidine or meperidine is to be avoided because of accumulation of metabolites and the risk of seizures. Curarizing agents such as atracurium and cis-atracurium are generally safe. Whenever possible regional anesthesia or spinal or epidural anesthesia is preferable, unless contraindicated in case of coagulopathy or neuropathy or azotemia [37].

27.3.2 What Anesthetic Medications to Use and Not to Use?

General anesthesia may depress immunity [38]. Even in the pre-highly active antiretroviral therapy era, a study done in 343 HIV-infected individuals undergoing surgery under general anesthesia demonstrated that HIV does not increase postoperative complications or death [39]. In another case-controlled study of cesarean section in 45 HIV-infected women as compared to 450 seronegative women [40], it appeared that HIV-positive women are at higher risk of postoperative complications with statistically significant higher incidence of postoperative of mild anemia, fever, urinary tract infections, and pneumonia. These complications correlated with lower CD4 cell counts. Similar findings are also described in infected children as compared to uninfected ones in a study of surgical complications in pediatric population [41]. HIV-infected children had statistically significant higher complication rate (41.5%) and mortality rate (7.3%) as compared to uninfected children (5.7% and 0%, respectively). Even HIV-exposed children had higher rates of complications (23.5%) and mortality (5.2%). Spinal anesthesia: In a case-controlled study, elective cesarean section under spinal anesthesia in 44 pregnant women with HIV infection was not associated with intraoperative or postoperative complications as compared to 45 non-HIV-infected women [42]. However, infection through spinal anesthesia was found to be associated with worsening of HIV disease [37]. In a more recent study of 90 patients, 30 patients underwent spinal anesthesia [43]. None acquired a nervous system infection and patients tolerated such anesthesia well.

27.3.3 Potential Problems

The incidence of complications in general anesthesia is a little higher, but it has been shown that this form of anesthesia is reliable and safe irrespective of the disease state prior to surgery [44]. Some authors showed also that there was no difference between various anesthetic approaches in persons living with HIV [45]. An increased incidence of postoperative fever was demonstrated in an older study [46], but this correlated with the severity of the primary disease and the type of surgery.

1. Risk to the anesthesiologists and to the surgical team: Universal precautions have to adopt with any patient regardless of HIV serostatus or viral load [47]. The risk to the surgical team is lower when patients have undetectable viral load.
2. Organ dysfunction:
   (a) Hepatic insufficiency or alteration of function: Liver damage from antiretroviral agents or from hepatitis viruses coinfection should be taken in consideration. Precautions from hepatitis virus are similar to the universal precautions that would

prevent transmission of HIV or any other blood-borne pathogen. Liver function tests have to be taken in consideration prior to anesthesia and prior to administration of any drug for choice of agents and proper dosing.

(b) Renal dysfunction: HIV may induce a nephropathy which is best managed by antiretroviral agents. In addition, several drugs may alter kidney function, for example, tenofovir which may lead to proteinuria, increases in creatinine, and even severe Fanconi's syndrome. Renal function has to be fully evaluated in order to dose medications properly and avoid drugs that may alter blood levels of antiretroviral agents or which could be associated with increased renal toxicity [48].

(c) Lung: Preexisting pulmonary infection with hypoxemia will affect the decision to subject the patient to general anesthesia. Patients with HIV infection may be more predisposed to develop postoperative infections especially in advanced HIV infection with altered leukocyte functions and numbers. It is noteworthy that smoking is frequently reported in some vulnerable populations and this should be taken in consideration during administration of general anesthesia [19, 49].

(d) Hematologic disturbances: These may be either induced by the virus itself or because of some opportunistic infections (cytomegalovirus, infection, non-tuberculous mycobacterial infection, etc.) or a side effect of some antiretroviral agent (e.g., zidovudine) or agents used for treatment or prophylaxis of opportunistic infections (e.g., co-trimoxazole). Correction of anemia is essential prior to surgical procedure. HIV infection is also a classical cause of thrombocytopenia. Evaluation by a hematologist should be discussed prior to surgery. It is also necessary to monitor the leukocyte count and eventually administer G-CSF to increase the neutrophil count to more than $1000/mm^3$ prior to a surgical procedure [20, 50].

27.3.4 Monitoring

1. Colonization by resistant organisms: Individuals should be checked for colonization by resistant organisms. For example, persons who inject drugs tend to be more frequently colonized by methicillin-resistant *Staphylococcus aureus*. This will impact the choice of preoperative prophylactic antibiotics, requiring the administration of a glycopeptide instead of the usual cephalosporin [51].
2. Persons who inject drugs or who are self-administering substances of abuse would benefit from preparation with a period of abstinence or the administration of opiate substitution agents (methadone, buprenorphine, etc.) prior to anesthesia. A preoperative toxicology screen is indicated [52].
3. Persons living with HIV tend to have increased risk of allergic reactions to medications. This should be carefully investigated and monitored.

27.4 Postoperative Management

27.4.1 Pain Management

Administration of pain medications should take in consideration the history of substance abuse. Appropriate dosing should be adapted accordingly. Pain medications cannot be withdrawn because an individual is an opiate user.

27.4.2 Antiretroviral Agents

ART may have to be interrupted prior to anesthesia. Such therapeutic break should be of the shorted possible duration and should involve the whole regiment to avoid development of resistance [13]. It should be restarted as soon as possible postoperatively, as soon as gastrointestinal transit permits. It is preferable to avoid prolonged interruption of agents, and these could be administered as soon as oral intake is acceptable, as discussed in previous section.

27.5 Postoperative Complications

Fluid management should be adapted according to cardiac and renal function and to the potential for drug toxicity. Operated patients with HIV infection may be at increased risk of thromboembolic disease, and special care should be given for prevention [13].

27.5.1 Postoperative Infections

Most postoperative infections in persons living with HIV are similar to HIV-uninfected individuals. However, neutropenic and severely immunosuppressed patients may not mount the usual inflammatory response, and therefore diagnostic workup may have to rely mostly on clinical suspicion and microbiological diagnosis rather than on typical clinical or routine laboratory findings. The risk of hospital-acquired pathogens such as *Staphylococcus aureus, Pseudomonas aeruginosa,* and extended spectrum beta-lactamase-producing *Enterobacteriaceae* is increased especially in neutropenic patients particularly in the pre-ART era [53, 54].

27.5.2 Surgical Outcomes

With the increasing coverage with highly active antiretroviral therapy (HAART), most studies have reported low surgical risk. In a large study comparing surgical outcomes between HIV-infected individuals and HIV-uninfected control patients matched for age, gender, race, type of surgery, and various comorbidities including smoking (332 individuals in each group); the rate of postoperative infections was similar except for postoperative pneumonia and potential 12-month mortality (although the deaths were not thought linked to surgery). Among the HIV-infected individuals, those with a CD4 count of less than 50 cells/mm^3 had higher complication rate [28]. In another report of 25 patients infected with HIV with acceptable CD4 counts while on HAART and undergoing cardiac surgery primarily for infective endocarditis (56%), the outcome was excellent with a postoperative mortality rate of 4% (one patient), and 5 patients had severe postoperative complications [25].

Conclusion

During their lifetime, HIV-infected patients will potentially require surgical interventions including maxillofacial surgeries. Patients who are on ART and have HIV virologic suppression with elevated CD4 count have a surgical outcome comparable to those HIV-uninfected.

It is ideal for the surgical team to be aware of the potential surgical risk and complications for HIV-infected patient as detailed in this chapter. Effective communication with the HIV provider to assist in challenging perioperative management is recommended.

References

1. Centers for Disease Control (CDC). Pneumocystis pneumonia--Los Angeles. MMWR Morb Mortal Wkly Rep. 1981;30(21):250–2.
2. Lang W, Perkins H, Anderson RE, Royce R, Jewell N, Winkelstein W Jr. Patterns of T lymphocyte changes with human immunodeficiency virus infection: from seroconversion to the development of AIDS. J Acquir Immune Defic Syndr. 1989;2(1):63–9.
3. Henrard DR, Phillips JF, Muenz LR, et al. Natural history of HIV-1 cell-free viremia. JAMA. 1995;274(7):554–8.
4. Gottlieb GS, Sow PS, Hawes SE, et al. Equal plasma viral loads predict a similar rate of CD4+ T cell decline in human immunodeficiency virus (HIV) type 1- and HIV-2-infected individuals from Senegal, West Africa. J Infect Dis. 2002;185(7):905–14.
5. Touloumi G, Pantazis N, Pillay D, et al. Impact of HIV-1 subtype on CD4 count at HIV seroconversion, rate of decline, and viral load set point in European seroconverter cohorts. Clin Infect Dis. 2013;56(6):888–97.
6. Lodi S, Phillips A, Touloumi G, et al. Time from human immunodeficiency virus seroconversion to reaching CD4+ cell count thresholds <200, <350, and <500 cells/mm(3): assessment of need follow-

ing changes in treatment guidelines. Clin Infect Dis. 2011;53(8):817–25.
7. Centers for Disease Control and Prevention (CDC). Revised surveillance case definition for HIV infection--United States, 2014. MMWR Recomm Rep. 2014;63(RR-03):1–10.
8. Migueles SA, Connors M. Long-term nonprogressive disease among untreated HIV-infected individuals: clinical implications of understanding immune control of HIV. JAMA. 2010;304(2):194–201. https://doi.org/10.1001/jama.2010.1925.
9. Dinoso JB, Kim SY, Siliciano RF, Blankson JN. A comparison of viral loads between HIV-1-infected elite suppressors and individuals who receive suppressive highly active antiretroviral therapy. Clin Infect Dis. 2008;47(1):102–4.
10. Antiretroviral Therapy Cohort Collaboration. Life expectancy of individuals on combination antiretroviral therapy in high-income countries: a collaborative analysis of 14 cohort studies. Lancet. 2008;372(9635):293–9. https://doi.org/10.1016/S0140-6736(1008)61113-61117.
11. Osmond D, Chaisson R, Moss A, Bacchetti P, Krampf W. Lymphadenopathy in asymptomatic patients seropositive for HIV. N Engl J Med. 1987;317(4):246.
12. AIDSinfo DHHS HIV Treatment Guidelines 2016.pdf.
13. Bornard L, Blay M, Roger PM, Raucoules-Aime M, Carles M. Anaesthesia for HIV-infected patients. Ann Fr Anesth Reanim. 2011;30(6):501–11. https://doi.org/10.1016/j.annfar.2011.1003.1016.
14. Hasse B, Ledergerber B, Furrer H, et al. Morbidity and aging in HIV-infected persons: the Swiss HIV cohort study. Clin Infect Dis. 2011;53(11):1130–9.
15. Akgun KM, Tate JP, Oursler KK, et al. Association of chronic obstructive pulmonary disease with frailty measurements in HIV-infected and uninfected veterans. AIDS. 2016;30(14):2185–93. https://doi.org/10.1097/QAD.0000000000001162.
16. Ando M, Tsuchiya K, Nitta K. How to manage HIV-infected patients with chronic kidney disease in the HAART era. Clin Exp Nephrol. 2012;16(3):363–72. https://doi.org/10.1007/s10157-10012-10585-10157.
17. Goulet JL, Fultz SL, Rimland D, et al. Aging and infectious diseases: do patterns of comorbidity vary by HIV status, age, and HIV severity? Clin Infect Dis. 2007;45(12):1593–601. https://doi.org/10.1086/523577.
18. Mdodo R, Frazier EL, Dube SR, et al. Cigarette smoking prevalence among adults with HIV compared with the general adult population in the United States: cross-sectional surveys. Ann Intern Med. 2015;162(5):335–44. https://doi.org/10.7326/M7314-0954.
19. Niaura R, Shadel WG, Morrow K, Tashima K, Flanigan T, Abrams DB. Human immunodeficiency virus infection, AIDS, and smoking cessation: the time is now. Clin Infect Dis. 2000;31(3):808–12.
20. Kedzierska K, Rainbird MA, Lopez AF, Crowe SM. Effect of GM-CSF on HIV-1 replication in monocytes/macrophages in vivo and in vitro: a review. Vet Immunol Immunopathol. 1998;63(1-2):111–21.
21. AIDSinfo Guidelines for prevention and Treatment of Opportunistic Infections 2016.pdf.
22. King JT Jr, Perkal MF, Rosenthal RA, et al. Thirty-day postoperative mortality among individuals with HIV infection receiving antiretroviral therapy and procedure-matched, uninfected comparators. JAMA Surg. 2015;150(4):343–51.
23. Snir N, Wolfson TS, Schwarzkopf R, et al. Outcomes of total hip arthroplasty in human immunodeficiency virus-positive patients. J Arthroplast. 2014;29(1):157–61.
24. Cacala SR, Mafana E, Thomson SR, Smith A. Prevalence of HIV status and CD4 counts in a surgical cohort: their relationship to clinical outcome. Ann R Coll Surg Engl. 2006;88(1):46–51.
25. Filsoufi F, Salzberg SP, Harbou KT, Neibart E, Adams DH. Excellent outcomes of cardiac surgery in patients infected with HIV in the current era. Clin Infect Dis. 2006;43(4):532–6.
26. Guth AA, Hofstetter SR, Pachter HL. Human immunodeficiency virus and the trauma patient: factors influencing postoperative infectious complications. J Trauma. 1996;41(2):251–5; discussion 255–256
27. Guild GN, Moore TJ, Barnes W, Hermann C. CD4 count is associated with postoperative infection in patients with orthopaedic trauma who are HIV positive. Clin Orthop Relat Res. 2012;470(5):1507–12.
28. Horberg MA, Hurley LB, Klein DB, et al. Surgical outcomes in human immunodeficiency virus-infected patients in the era of highly active antiretroviral therapy. Arch Surg (Chicago, Ill: 1960). 2006;141(12):1238–45.
29. Snir N, Kaye ID, Klifto CS, et al. 10-year follow-up wear analysis of first-generation highly crosslinked polyethylene in primary total hip arthroplasty. J Arthroplast. 2014;29(3):630–3.
30. Joyce MP, Kuhar D, Brooks JT. Notes from the field: occupationally acquired HIV infection among health care workers – United States, 1985–2013. MMWR Morb Mortal Wkly Rep. 2015;63(53):1245–6.
31. Kuhar DT, Henderson DK, Struble KA, et al. Updated US public health service guidelines for the management of occupational exposures to human immunodeficiency virus and recommendations for postexposure prophylaxis. Infect Control Hosp Epidemiol. 2013;34(9):875–92.
32. Nelson L, Fried M, Stewart K. HIV-infected patients: the risks of surgery. J Perioper Pract. 2009;19(1):24–30.
33. Julg B, Goebel FD. Treatment interruption in HIV therapy: a SMART strategy? Infection. 2006;34(3):186–8.
34. King JR, Yogev R, Aldrovandi G, Chadwick E, Acosta EP. Pharmacokinetics of antiretrovirals administered to HIV-infected children via gastrostomy tube. HIV Clin Trials. 2004;5(5):288–93.
35. Soni N, Pozniak A. Continuing HIV therapy in the ICU. Crit Care. 2001;5(5):247–8.
36. Littlewood KE. The immunocompromised adult patient and surgery. Best Pract Res Clin Anaesthesiol. 2008;22(3):585–609.

37. Evron S, Glezerman M, Harow E, Sadan O, Ezri T. Human immunodeficiency virus: anesthetic and obstetric considerations. Anesth Analg. 2004;98(2):503–11.
38. Wyniecki A, Zetlaoui P, Bruyere M, Benhamou D. Bilateral catheter for continuous TAP block and postoperative pain relief after gynecologic surgery. Ann Fr Anesth Reanim. 2011;30(1):67–9.
39. Ayers J, Howton MJ, Layon AJ. Postoperative complications in patients with human immunodeficiency virus disease. Clinical data and a literature review. Chest. 1993;103(6):1800–7.
40. Ferrero S, Bentivoglio G. Post-operative complications after caesarean section in HIV-infected women. Arch Gynecol Obstet. 2003;268(4):268–73.
41. Karpelowsky JS, Millar AJ, van der Graaf N, van Bogerijen G, Zar HJ. Outcome of HIV-exposed uninfected children undergoing surgery. BMC Pediatr. 2011;11:69.
42. Avidan MS, Groves P, Blott M, et al. Low complication rate associated with cesarean section under spinal anesthesia for HIV-1-infected women on antiretroviral therapy. Anesthesiology. 2002;97(2):320–4.
43. Zhang WW, Wang YP, Wang YQ, Ji XM, Zhang MY. Effects of different anesthetic approaches on postoperative complications in HIV-infected patients. Genet Mol Res. 2015;14(3):9130–5.
44. Blair JM, Fagan JL, Frazier EL, et al. Behavioral and clinical characteristics of persons receiving medical care for HIV infection – medical monitoring project, United States, 2009. MMWR Suppl. 2014;63(5):1–22.
45. Rodriguez-Merchan EC. HIV and HCV coinfected haemophilia patients: what are the best options of orthopaedic treatment? Haemophilia. 2006;12(Suppl 3):90–101.
46. Bremerich DH, Ahr A, Buchner S, et al. Anesthetic regimen for HIV positive parturients undergoing elective cesarean section. Anaesthesist. 2003;52(12):1124–31.
47. Lee KG, Soni N. AIDS and anaesthesia. Anaesthesia. 1986;41(10):1011–6.
48. Gupta SK, Eustace JA, Winston JA, et al. Guidelines for the management of chronic kidney disease in HIV-infected patients: recommendations of the HIV medicine Association of the Infectious Diseases Society of America. Clin Infect Dis. 2005;40(11):1559–85. Epub 2005 Apr 1522
49. Tesoriero JM, Gieryic SM, Carrascal A, Lavigne HE. Smoking among HIV positive New Yorkers: prevalence, frequency, and opportunities for cessation. AIDS Behav. 2010;14(4):824–35.
50. Hoffman RM, Currier JS. Management of antiretroviral treatment-related complications. Infect Dis Clin N Am. 2007;21(1):103–32, ix
51. Diep BA, Chambers HF, Graber CJ, et al. Emergence of multidrug-resistant, community-associated, methicillin-resistant Staphylococcus aureus clone USA300 in men who have sex with men. Ann Intern Med. 2008;148(4):249–57.
52. Whetten K, Reif SS, Napravnik S, et al. Substance abuse and symptoms of mental illness among HIV-positive persons in the southeast. South Med J. 2005;98(1):9–14.
53. Witt DJ, Craven DE, McCabe WR. Bacterial infections in adult patients with the acquired immune deficiency syndrome (AIDS) and AIDS-related complex. Am J Med. 1987;82(5):900–6.
54. Shepp DH, Tang IT, Ramundo MB, Kaplan MK. Serious Pseudomonas aeruginosa infection in AIDS. J Acquir Immune Defic Syndr. 1994;7(8):823–31.

28 Psychiatric Disorders and Maxillofacial Surgery

Jayesh Kamath and Shakaib Khan

Abstract

Patients with psychiatric illnesses present a major challenge to the surgical teams due to high rates of medical and substance use comorbidities, complexity of psychotropic medical regimens increasing the risk of serious drug-drug interactions, and difficulties with patient-provider communications. Psychiatric patients fall under one of the three major categories: mood disorders, anxiety disorders, or psychotic disorders. Patients from each of these categories present with unique challenges due to their distinct symptomatology, cognitive status, and ability to understand and engage in informed consent.

Perioperative management of psychiatric patients should include a careful review of patient's psychiatric status, medical status, substance use comorbidities, and their psychotropic medication regimens for potential drug-drug interactions including interactions with anesthesia. Decisions related to high-risk psychotropic medications should be informed by risk-benefit ratio including risk of psychiatric relapse and/or withdrawal symptoms. Close monitoring of these patients is essential given the documented high mortality risk in psychiatric patients in the postoperative period compared to patients without psychiatric illness.

The present chapter provides an overview of psychiatric disorders, their epidemiology, pathophysiology, and manifestation of symptoms relevant to perioperative management. It then takes a more in-depth look at the preoperative, intraoperative, and postoperative care of psychiatric patients and provides recommendations for their care throughout the surgical period.

28.1 Introduction

In any given year, approximately one in five adults or about 18.5% of the US population experience psychiatric illness [1]. Out of the 43.8 million that experience mental illness, approximately ten mil-

J. Kamath, M.D., Ph.D. (✉)
Psychiatry and Immunology, Mood and Anxiety Program, University of Connecticut Health Center, Farmington, CT, USA
e-mail: jkamath@uchc.edu

S. Khan, M.D.
Department of Psychiatry, University of Connecticut Health Center, Farmington, CT, USA

© Springer International Publishing AG 2018
E.M. Ferneini, J.D. Bennett (eds.), *Perioperative Assessment of the Maxillofacial Surgery Patient*,
https://doi.org/10.1007/978-3-319-58868-1_28

lion carry diagnoses of serious mental illness (SMI) such as major depressive disorder, bipolar disorder, or schizophrenia [1]. It is highly likely that surgical teams encounter patients with psychiatric disorders in their day to day practice. It is important that surgical teams have adequate knowledge about the psychiatric illnesses; their impact on patient's emotional, cognitive, and other functioning; frequent medical comorbidities these patients present with; and the psychotropic medications including their pharmacokinetic and pharmacodynamics interactions with treatments used during perioperative management.

Psychiatric patients can present a major challenge to the surgical teams due to several factors. Patients with SMI, such as schizophrenia, are at increased risk of medical illnesses such as diabetes and cardiovascular illnesses due to their lifestyle and due to the side effects associated with their psychotropic medications, e.g., antipsychotic medications [2]. These medical comorbidities can present a major problem during the perioperative care. Evidence suggests higher-mortality risk in the postoperative period in patients with serious mental illness [3]. Surgical teams may be confronted with multiple other challenges with these patients, especially in patients with serious mental illness. Such challenges include problems with communication with these patients, concerns about patient's ability to give informed consent, high rates of substance use comorbidities, and potential for serious drug-drug interaction.

In the present chapter, we discuss major psychiatric illnesses, their epidemiology and pathophysiology, their diagnostic criteria, and critical aspects of communication with these patients relevant to their psychiatric illness. Subsequently, we delineate evidence-based perioperative assessment and management of these patients including management of their psychotropic medications, their potential interactions with anesthesia and other medications used during perioperative care, and strategies to improve postoperative outcomes.

28.2 Major Psychiatric Illness Categories

There are three major categories of psychiatric illnesses: mood disorders, psychotic disorders, and anxiety disorders. Following is a description of each of these categories, major psychiatric illnesses in each of these categories, and their epidemiology, pathophysiology, diagnostic criteria, and disease manifestations.

28.2.1 Mood Disorders

Mood disorders are the most prevalent disorders in psychiatry. These include unipolar depression and bipolar disorder. Communication with patients with mood disorders can be difficult due to several reasons depending on their mental status. Patients experiencing clinical state of depression may be slow to respond, have difficulties making decision, may have low frustration tolerance, and may have low tolerance for pain and discomfort, while patients in hypomanic/manic state of bipolar disorder may be disinhibited, overtalkative, unable to focus, easily distractible, and in extreme cases may get easily agitated.

28.2.1.1 Epidemiology

Unipolar Depression (Major Depressive Disorder)

Unipolar depression is the most prevalent mental health disorder with a lifetime prevalence of 17% and a 1-year prevalence of 6.7% [4]. The mean age of onset of unipolar depression is 40 years. The lifetime prevalence of unipolar depression is higher in women (17%) compared to men (9%) [5]. Prashant et al. suggest high rates of clinically relevant depression and anxiety in patients with disfiguring facial injuries. These rates were especially high in women. Depression and anxiety scores were high at the time of diagnosis and remained elevated at 1-month and at 6-month follow-ups [6].

28.2.1.2 Bipolar Disorder

Bipolar disorder usually starts earlier than depression with a mean age of onset of 30 years. Men are affected by mania more than women, whereas women have more depressive or mixed episodes. The lifetime prevalence of bipolar disorder ranges between 2 and 5%. The 1-year prevalence is 0.5–1.4% and is similar for men and women [4].

Both unipolar depression and bipolar disorder are frequently associated with comorbidities such as the anxiety disorders and substance use disorders [4]. Patients with mood disorders carry a high suicide risk. Men carry a higher risk and are more likely to die by suicide than women.

28.2.1.3 Pathophysiology

The pathophysiology of mood disorders is likely multifactorial. Most theories revolve around the monoamine hypothesis or the biogenic amine hypothesis which is the leading hypothesis at this time [7]. The biogenic amine hypothesis suggests dysregulation in three major neurotransmitter systems: serotonin, norepinephrine, and dopamine. Decrease in the levels of neurotransmitters has been linked to depression, while increase in their levels has been linked to symptoms of mania such as disinhibition [7]. Evidence suggests that other bodily systems such as the neurobehavioral system, endocrine system (e.g., hypothalamic-pituitary-adrenal axis), and immune system (e.g., pro-inflammatory cytokines) also play a major role in the pathophysiology of these disorders [8].

It should be noted that clinical depression or manic-like symptomatology can also be iatrogenic. Medications such as beta blockers and interferon treatments can cause depression, while steroids can lead to manic-like symptoms. Furthermore, certain medical conditions and substance use disorders can mimic symptoms of these disorders, e.g., encephalopathies, metabolic disorders, and use of certain illicit substances such as cocaine and ecstasy.

28.2.1.4 Manifestations of Disease

Patients with these disorders may present to the surgical team in depressed or hypomanic/manic state. Patients with mood symptomatology (depression or hypomania/mania) frequently present with comorbid anxiety, distractibility, and cognitive deficits as a result of their mood symptoms. Additionally, patients with atypical depression may present with hypersomnia, fatigue, lack of motivation, and cognitive slowing. I should also be noted that patients in a severe depressed or manic state may present with comorbid psychotic symptoms. All of these symptoms can seriously compromise patient's ability to engage in a meaningful conversation about their surgery, informed consent, and perioperative care. Table 28.1 describes the diagnostic criteria for major mood disorders according to the Diagnostic and Statistical Manual of Mental Disorders (DSM-5) [9].

28.2.2 Psychotic Disorders

Patients with psychotic disorders (also known as thought disorders) present with gross impairment of reality testing. The level of impairment depends on severity of symptoms at the specific point in time. Psychotic symptoms include positive symptoms such as hallucinations, paranoia, delusions, and symptoms indicating disruption in the form or organization of thinking. Psychotic disorders category include diagnoses such as schizophrenia, schizoaffective disorder, schizophreniform disorder, brief psychotic disorder, and delusional disorder.

28.2.2.1 Epidemiology

The prevalence of schizophrenia is approximately 1% with no difference in prevalence between men and women [4]. Onset is earlier in men with a peak age of onset being 10–25. There is a bimodal onset in women with 25–35 or after 40 years of age [4].

Table 28.1 Mood Disorders

Criteria* for major depressive disorder

1. Five (or more) of the following symptoms have been present during the same 2-week period and represent a change from previous functioning; at least one of the symptoms is either (1) depressed mood or (2) loss of interest or pleasure
   (a) Depressed mood most of the day, nearly every day, as indicated by either subjective report (e.g., feels sad, empty, hopeless) or observation made by others (e.g., appears tearful)
   (b) Markedly diminished interest or pleasure in all, or almost all, activities most of the day, nearly every day (as indicated by either subjective account or observation)
   (c) Significant weight loss when not dieting or weight gain (e.g., a change of more than 5% of body weight in a month) or decrease or increase in appetite nearly every day
   (d) Insomnia or hypersomnia nearly every day
   (e) Psychomotor agitation or retardation nearly every day (observable by others, not merely subjective feelings of restlessness or being slowed down)
   (f) Fatigue or loss of energy nearly every day
   (g) Feelings of worthlessness or excessive or inappropriate guilt (which may be delusional) nearly every day (not merely self-reproach or guilt about being sick)
   (h) Diminished ability to think or concentrate, or indecisiveness, nearly every day (either by subjective account or as observed by others)
   (i) Recurrent thoughts of death (not just fear of dying), recurrent suicidal ideation without a specific plan, or a suicide attempt or a specific plan for committing suicide
2. The symptoms cause clinically significant distress or impairment in social, occupational, or other important areas of functioning
3. The episode is not attributable to the physiological effects of a substance or another medical condition
4. The occurrence of the major depressive episode is not better explained by schizoaffective disorder, schizophrenia, schizophreniform disorder, delusional disorder, or other specified and unspecified schizophrenia spectrum and other psychotic disorders
5. There has never been a manic episode or a hypomanic episode

Criteria* for bipolar disorder

Manic episode

1. A distinct period of abnormally and persistently elevated, expansive, or irritable mood and abnormally and persistently increased activity or energy, lasting at least 1 week and present most of the day, nearly every day (or any duration if hospitalization is necessary)
2. During the period of mood disturbance and increased energy or activity, three (or more) of the following symptoms (four if the mood is only irritable) are present to a significant degree and represent a noticeable change from usual behavior:
   (a) Inflated self-esteem or grandiosity
   (b) Decreased need for sleep (e.g., feels rested after only 3 hours of sleep)
   (c) More talkative than usual or pressure to keep talking
   (d) Flight of ideas or subjective experience that thoughts are racing
   (e) Distractibility (i.e., attention too easily drawn to unimportant or irrelevant external stimuli), as reported or observed
   (f) Increase in goal-directed activity (either socially, at work or school, or sexually) or psychomotor agitation (i.e., purposeless non-goal-directed activity)
   (g) Excessive involvement in activities that have a high potential for painful consequences (e.g., engaging in unrestrained buying sprees, sexual indiscretions, or foolish business investments)
3. The mood disturbance is sufficiently severe to cause marked impairment in social or occupational functioning or to necessitate hospitalization to prevent harm to self or others, or there are psychotic features
4. The episode is not attributable to the physiological effects of a substance (e.g., a drug of abuse, a medication, other treatment) or another medical condition

Hypomanic episode

1. A distinct period of abnormally and persistently elevated, expansive, or irritable mood and abnormally and persistently increased activity or energy, lasting at least 4 consecutive days and present most of the day, nearly every day

Table 28.1 (continued)

2. During the period of mood disturbance and increased energy and activity, three (or more) of the following symptoms (four if the mood is only irritable) have persisted, represent a noticeable change from usual behavior, and have been present to a significant degree:
   (a) Inflated self-esteem or grandiosity
   (b) Decreased need for sleep (e.g., feels rested after only 3 h of sleep)
   (c) More talkative than usual or pressure to keep talking
   (d) Flight of ideas or subjective experience that thoughts are racing
   (e) Distractibility (i.e., attention too easily drawn to unimportant or irrelevant external stimuli), as reported or observed
   (f) Increase in goal-directed activity (either socially, at work or school, or sexually) or psychomotor agitation
   (g) Excessive involvement in activities that have a high potential for painful consequences (e.g., engaging in unrestrained buying sprees, sexual indiscretions, or foolish business investments)
3. The episode is associated with an unequivocal change in functioning that is uncharacteristic of the individual when not symptomatic
4. The disturbance in mood and the change in functioning are observable by others
5. The episode is not severe enough to cause marked impairment in social or occupational functioning or to necessitate hospitalization. If there are psychotic features, the episode is, by definition, manic
6. The episode is not attributable to the physiological effects of a substance (e.g., a drug of abuse, a medication, other treatment) or another medical condition

Major depressive episode

1. Five (or more) of the following symptoms have been present during the same 2-week period and represent a change from previous functioning; at least one of the symptoms is either (1) depressed mood or (2) loss of interest or pleasure
   (a) Depressed mood most of the day, nearly every day, as indicated by either subjective report (e.g., feels sad, empty, or hopeless) or observation made by others (e.g., appears tearful)
   (b) Markedly diminished interest or pleasure in all, or almost all, activities most of the day, nearly every day (as indicated by either subjective account or observation)
   (c) Weight loss when not dieting or weight gain (e.g., a change of more than 5% of body weight in a month) or decrease or increase in appetite nearly every day
   (d) Insomnia or hypersomnia nearly every day
   (e) Psychomotor agitation or retardation nearly every day (observable by others; not merely subjective feelings of restlessness or being slowed down)
   (f) Fatigue or loss of energy nearly every day
   (g) Feelings of worthlessness or excessive or inappropriate guilt (which may be delusional) nearly every day (not merely self-reproach or guilt about being sick)
   (h) Diminished ability to think or concentrate, or indecisiveness, nearly every day (either by subjective account or as observed by others)
   (i) Recurrent thoughts of death (not just fear of dying), recurrent suicidal ideation without a specific plan, or a suicide attempt or a specific plan for committing suicide
2. The symptoms cause clinically significant distress or impairment in social, occupational, or other important areas of functioning
3. The episode is not attributable to the physiological effects of a substance or another medical condition

Bipolar I disorder

1. Criteria have been met for at least one manic episode (criteria A–D under "manic episode" above)
2. The occurrence of the manic and major depressive episode(s) is not better explained by schizoaffective disorder, schizophrenia, schizophreniform disorder, delusional disorder, or other specified or unspecified schizophrenia spectrum and other psychotic disorder

Bipolar II disorder

1. Criteria have been met for at least one hypomanic episode (criteria A–F under "hypomanic episode" above) and at least one major depressive episode (criteria A–C under "major depressive episode" above)
2. There has never been a manic episode
3. The occurrence of the hypomanic episode(s) and major depressive episode(s) is not better explained by schizoaffective disorder, schizophrenia, schizophreniform disorder, delusional disorder, or other specified or unspecified schizophrenia spectrum and other psychotic disorder
4. The symptoms of depression or the unpredictability caused by frequent alternation between periods of depression and hypomania causes clinically significant distress or impairment in social, occupational, or other important areas of functioning

*According to the diagnostic and statistical manual of mental disorders (5th ed.); DSM–5; American Psychiatric Association, 2013

28.2.2.2 Pathophysiology

The dopamine biochemical hypothesis is the leading hypothesis for psychotic disorders [10]. It is believed that the positive symptoms (auditory or visual hallucinations, paranoia, delusions) are due to dysregulation of dopaminergic activity in the mesolimbic system and the negative symptoms (diminished emotional expression, avolition) are related to dopamine dysregulation in the mesocortical system. This hypothesis is based on the treatment response to neuroleptics which are known to be dopamine antagonists. It is also based on the fact that psychotic symptoms are caused by drugs like cocaine and amphetamines which are known to increase dopamine in the mesolimbic system.

Other systems and pathways have also been implicated in the pathophysiology of psychotic disorders [10]. These include dysregulation in the glutamatergic/serotonin pathways and disruptions in immune and endocrine systems [10]. Evidence also suggests that schizophrenia is a neurodevelopmental disorder with disturbances in early brain development [10].

28.2.2.3 Manifestations of Disease

Patient with these disorders may present with chronic psychotic symptoms, significant cognitive deficits, and comorbid depression/anxiety symptoms. They may be guarded and may have difficulty understanding the risks-benefits of the surgery raising concerns about the informed consent process. However, their ability to participate in the informed consent process depends on their mental status at the specific time point. Their ability to give the informed consent and participation in the perioperative care is mainly compromised by the disorganization and cognitive deficits associated with the illness. Substance use is also highly comorbid with these disorders and can have a significant negative impact on perioperative care. Table 28.2

Table 28.2 Psychotic Disorders

Criteria* for schizophrenia
1. Two (or more) of the following, each present for a significant portion of time during a 1-month period (or less if successfully treated). At least one of these must be (1), (2), or (3): (a) Delusions (b) Hallucinations (c) Disorganized speech (e.g., frequent derailment or incoherence) (d) Grossly disorganized or catatonic behavior (e) Negative symptoms (i.e., diminished emotional expression or avolition)
2. For a significant portion of the time since the onset of the disturbance, level of functioning in one or more major areas, such as work, interpersonal relations, or self-care, is markedly below the level achieved prior to the onset (or when the onset is in childhood or adolescence, there is failure to achieve expected level of interpersonal, academic, or occupational functioning)
3. Continuous signs of the disturbance persist for at least 6 months. This 6-month period must include at least 1 month of symptoms (or less if successfully treated) that meet criterion A (i.e., active-phase symptoms) and may include periods of prodromal or residual symptoms. During these prodromal or residual periods, the signs of the disturbance may be manifested by only negative symptoms or by two or more symptoms listed in criterion A present in an attenuated form (e.g., odd beliefs, unusual perceptual experiences)
4. Schizoaffective disorder and depressive or bipolar disorder with psychotic features have been ruled out because either (1) no major depressive or manic episodes have occurred concurrently with the active-phase symptoms or (2), if mood episodes have occurred during active-phase symptoms, they have been present for a minority of the total duration of the active and residual periods of the illness
5. The disturbance is not attributable to the physiological effects of a substance (e.g., a drug of abuse, a medication) or another medical condition
6. If there is a history of autism spectrum disorder or a communication disorder of childhood onset, the additional diagnosis of schizophrenia is made only if prominent delusions or hallucinations, in addition to the other required symptoms of schizophrenia, are also present for at least 1 month (or less if successfully treated)

Table 28.2 (continued)

Criteria* for schizoaffective disorder
1. An uninterrupted period of illness during which there is a major mood episode (major depressive or manic) concurrent with criterion A of schizophrenia Note: The major depressive episode must include criterion A1: depressed mood
2. Delusions or hallucinations for 2 or more weeks in the absence of a major mood episode (depressive or manic) during the lifetime duration of the illness
3. Symptoms that meet criteria for a major mood episode are present for the majority of the total duration of the active and residual portions of the illness
4. The disturbance is not attributable to the effects of a substance (e.g., a drug of abuse, a medication) or another medical condition

*According to the diagnostic and statistical manual of mental disorders (5th ed.); DSM–5; American Psychiatric Association, 2013

describes the diagnostic criteria for the two major psychotic disorders (schizophrenia and schizoaffective disorder) according to the Diagnostic and Statistical Manual of Mental Disorders (DSM-5) [9].

28.2.3 Anxiety Disorders

Anxiety is part of everyday life and can be a normal response to perceived danger or worry about a specific situation [11]. It involves activation of the sympathetic nervous system, specific areas in the brain, and certain other bodily systems, e.g., hypothalamic-pituitary-adrenal (HPA) axis [12]. The goal of such "fight or flight" activation is to enhance performance to address the specific situation or stressor. However, anxiety can become pathological if it becomes too intense, frequent, or persistent and negatively impacts performance drive and interferes with functioning and daily life. Such pathological anxiety is the basis of anxiety disorders [11]. The anxiety disorders encompass several acute and chronic disorders: generalized anxiety disorder, panic disorder, agoraphobia, obsessive compulsive disorder, and post-traumatic stress disorder.

28.2.3.1 Epidemiology

Anxiety disorders are some of the most common psychiatric disorders. Research shows that one in four people meet the diagnostic criteria for anxiety disorders [4]. There is a 12-month prevalence rate of 17.7%. Women are more likely to have an anxiety disorders as compared to men [4]. The prevalence of anxiety disorders decreases with higher socioeconomic status.

28.2.3.2 Pathophysiology

Evidence suggests that several central nervous system (CNS) structures, neurotransmitter systems, and neuroendocrine interactions play a critical role in the etiology and pathophysiology of anxiety disorders. The CNS structures known to play a major role in the pathophysiology of anxiety disorders include amygdala, thalamus, and hippocampus [13]. The three major neurotransmitter systems implicated in the pathophysiology of anxiety disorders include norepinephrine, gamma-aminobutyric acid (GABA), and serotonin [14]. Additionally, the autonomic nervous system plays an integral role in the anxiety response. Stimulation of the autonomic nervous system leads to cardiac, muscular, gastrointestinal, and respiratory symptoms, e.g., heart palpitations, dizziness, muscle tension, nausea, and difficulty breathing. Release of cortisol from the HPA axis, in response to perceived stress, also plays a critical role in the pathophysiology of anxiety disorders [12].

28.2.3.3 Manifestations of Disease

In order to make a diagnosis of an anxiety disorder, all medical diagnoses and substance use diagnoses must be ruled out. Table 28.3 describes the diagnostic criteria for the major anxiety disorders most relevant to surgery according to the Diagnostic and Statistical Manual of Mental Disorders (DSM-5) [9]. Patients with anxiety disorders can present a significant challenge to the surgical teams as they may be resistant to scheduling the surgery and may not show up for the

Table 28.3 Anxiety Disorders

Criteria* for generalized anxiety disorder

1. Excessive anxiety and worry (apprehensive expectation), occurring more days than not for at least 6 months, about a number of events or activities (such as work or school performance)
2. The individual finds it difficult to control the worry
3. The anxiety and worry are associated with three (or more) of the following six symptoms (with at least some symptoms having been present for more days than not for the past 6 months):
   (a) Restlessness or feeling keyed up or on edge
   (b) Being easily fatigued
   (c) Difficulty concentrating or mind going blank
   (d) Irritability
   (e) Muscle tension
   (f) Sleep disturbance (difficulty falling or staying asleep or restless, unsatisfying sleep)
4. The anxiety, worry, or physical symptoms cause clinically significant distress or impairment in social, occupational, or other important areas of functioning
5. The disturbance is not attributable to the physiological effects of a substance (e.g., a drug of abuse, a medication) or another medical condition (e.g., hyperthyroidism)
6. The disturbance is not better explained by another mental disorder

Criteria* for panic disorder

1. Recurrent unexpected panic attacks. A panic attack is an abrupt surge of intense fear or intense discomfort that reaches a peak within minutes and during which time four (or more) of the following symptoms occur:
   Note: The abrupt surge can occur from a calm state or an anxious state
   (a) Palpitations, pounding heart, or accelerated heart rate
   (b) Sweating
   (c) Trembling or shaking
   (d) Sensations of shortness of breath or smothering
   (e) Feelings of choking
   (f) Chest pain or discomfort
   (g) Nausea or abdominal distress
   (h) Feeling dizzy, unsteady, light headed, or faint
   (i) Chills or heat sensations
   (j) Paresthesias (numbness or tingling sensations)
   (k) Derealization (feelings of unreality) or depersonalization (being detached from oneself)
   (l) Fear of losing control or "going crazy"
   (m) Fear of dying

   At least one of the attacks has been followed by 1 month (or more) of one or both of the following:
   (a) Persistent concern or worry about additional panic attacks or their consequences (e.g., losing control, having a heart attack, "going crazy")
   (b) A significant maladaptive change in behavior related to the attacks (e.g., behaviors designed to avoid having panic attacks, such as avoidance of exercise or unfamiliar situations)
2. The disturbance is not attributable to the physiological effects of a substance (e.g., a drug of abuse, a medication) or another medical condition (e.g., hyperthyroidism, cardiopulmonary disorders)
3. The disturbance is not better explained by another mental disorder

Criteria* for agoraphobia

1. Marked fear or anxiety about two (or more) of the following five situations:
   (a) Using public transportation (e.g., automobiles, buses, trains, ships, planes)
   (b) Being in open spaces (e.g., parking lots, marketplaces, bridges)
   (c) Being in enclosed places (e.g., shops, theaters, cinemas)
   (d) Standing in line or being in a crowd
   (e) Being outside of the home alone
2. The individual fears or avoids these situations because of thoughts that escape might be difficult or help might not be available in the event of developing panic-like symptoms or other incapacitating or embarrassing symptoms (e.g., fear of falling in the elderly, fear of incontinence)
3. The agoraphobic situations almost always provoke fear or anxiety
4. The agoraphobic situations are actively avoided, require the presence of a companion, or are endured with intense fear or anxiety
5. The fear or anxiety is out of proportion to the actual danger posed by the agoraphobic situations and to the sociocultural context

Table 28.3 (continued)

6. The fear, anxiety, or avoidance is persistent, typically lasting for 6 months or more
7. The fear, anxiety, or avoidance causes clinically significant distress or impairment in social, occupational, or other important areas of functioning
8. If another medical condition (e.g., inflammatory bowel disease, Parkinson's disease) is present, the fear, anxiety, or avoidance is clearly excessive
9. The fear, anxiety, or avoidance is not better explained by the symptoms of another mental disorder

*According to the diagnostic and statistical manual of mental disorders (5th ed.); DSM–5; American Psychiatric Association, 2013

scheduled surgery due to high anxiety levels. Management of these patients throughout the perioperative period can also be a significant challenge and frequently requires close collaboration with psychiatric providers to manage their anxiety symptoms. Their management is further complicated by the interactions of antianxiety medications with anesthesia and medications used during the perioperative period.

28.3 Factors Affecting Perioperative Management of Psychiatric Patients

28.3.1 Psychiatric Status

Psychiatric status during perioperative period can have a significant impact on surgical outcomes. Adogwa et al. found that the preoperative Zung depression scale scores predicted patient satisfaction independent of surgical effectiveness in patients undergoing lumbar surgery [15].

All patients with current or past psychiatric illness should undergo careful assessment of their psychiatric symptomatology with two primary objectives. First objective is to assess their decision-making ability, including ability to participate in the informed consent process, in the context of their psychiatric stability and impact of other factors, e.g., their psychotropic medications. Psychiatric symptoms may play a critical role, but the most important factor in patients' decision-making ability is their cognitive status. Ghormley et al. investigated correlation between neuropsychological impairment and informed consent in patients with depression. They concluded that no generalization can be made in patients with depression. Their findings suggest that the surgical team can address the issue of informed consent by devoting more attention and effort [16]. They concluded that it is possible and important to protect the rights and autonomy of this vulnerable patient population. Howe et al. evaluated the ability to give informed consent in acutely psychotic patients with schizophrenia [17]. Notably, they found that the inability to give informed consent in these patients was dependent on patients' cognitive deficits and not simply the product of their diagnosis or psychiatric symptoms. They recommended that patients be evaluated at a symptom level. Patients with psychiatric illnesses, both acute and chronic, need more support and time spent on informed consent procedures.

The other objective of the psychiatric assessment is to determine patients' ability to engage in perioperative management and especially in postoperative rehabilitation and recovery as their psychiatric symptomatology can play a crucial role in their ability to engage in certain aspects of their care.

An important factor affecting perioperative management of psychiatric patients involves hopelessness and suicidality, comorbid with several psychiatric illnesses. Certain patients undergoing surgery, such as patients with head and neck cancer, may carry higher risk of suicide compared to the general population [18]. Suicidality and completed suicides have been associated with specific risk factors. These include being white, male gender, age older than 45 years, being unemployed, living alone, poor social supports, current mental illness, or history of one including substance abuse and having a family history of suicide [19]. Patients that express no further desire to live, have developed a suicide plan, have secured a lethal device, and have made a previous attempt are at a higher risk and require immediate intervention. Patients who have had cosmetic procedure such as blepharoplasty, coronal brow lift, rhinoplasty, and rhytidectomy are reported to have higher suicide rates than the general population [20].

Surgical teams should err on the side of caution and be mindful of signs and symptoms of suicidality throughout perioperative management. Certain measures can be taken once patients at high risk are identified. Such measures include a staff member staying with the patient until further arrangements can be made, inviting a family member if available to be with the patient, and removing all medications, surgical instruments, needles, scissors, and scalpels which can be used to inflict self-harm.

28.3.2 Medical Comorbidities

Patients with psychiatric illness, especially patients with SMI such as schizophrenia, frequently have multiple medical comorbidities due to their lifestyle (e.g., diet, smoking) and as a consequence of their psychotropic medications [2]. Their medical comorbidities include disorders such as cardiovascular and respiratory illnesses, diabetes, and metabolic syndrome [2]. Due to these comorbidities, they carry a higher risk of morbidity and mortality compared to the general population. Additionally, due to their physical morbidity, they have diminished functional capacity of organs (e.g., liver, kidney) which is critical for metabolism of drugs used during the perioperative period. This reduced functional capacity of organs can increase the risk of delirium and other behavioral problems during surgery and in the postoperative period.

28.3.3 Substance Use Comorbidities

Patients with serious mental illnesses (such as schizophrenia and bipolar disorder) commonly have comorbid substance use disorders [21]. Such substance use disorders may include disorders involving legal substances such as alcohol; illicit drugs such as cocaine, heroin, and club/designer drugs (e.g., ecstasy); and illegally obtained prescription medications such as stimulants, opioids, and benzodiazepines. These substance use disorders are not reported, or extent of the addiction is underreported by patients during the preoperative evaluation. This increases the risk of withdrawal and delirium during the perioperative period. Withdrawal from certain substances/medication, specifically alcohol, benzodiazepines, and barbiturates, can significantly increase the risk of mortality during the perioperative management.

28.3.4 Management of Psychotropic Medications

Psychotropic medication regimens of psychiatric patients can be simple or very complex depending on the patients' diagnosis and severity of their illness. There are five major psychotropic medication classes: antidepressants, antianxiety medications, antipsychotic medications, mood stabilizers, and hypnotics. There are several subclasses within each medication class based on the underlying mechanism of action. These psychotropic medications can have a significant impact on surgical outcomes due to their direct effects on various organs and systems due to certain indirect effects via drug-drug interactions, e.g., with drugs used for anesthesia or with other medications used in perioperative care. Table 28.4 delineates major psychotropic medication classes and medications, their effects/interactions relative to perioperative care, and critical aspects of their management during the perioperative period.

Following is a description of clinically relevant and potentially serious effects and interactions of these medications and management of these medications from a risk-benefit perspective. It is important to note that there are very few clinical studies evaluating these effects and interactions in patients undergoing maxillofacial

Table 28.4 Perioperative management of psychotropic medications

Medication class or medication	Relevant effects, interactions, and need for psychiatric consultation	Need to discontinue* and withdrawal risks
SSRIs[a]	Risk of gastrointestinal bleeding, risk of hyponatremia and serotonin syndrome Interactions: increased bleeding risk with NSAIDs, aspirin. Risk of serotonin syndrome with other serotonergic medications (e.g., tramadol). Effects on P450 system medication dependent Psychiatric consultation: on as needed basis	No* Risk of withdrawal and serotonin discontinuation syndrome with abrupt discontinuation If discontinued, taper essential
SNRIs[b]	Risk of hypertension and other cardiac issues. Risk of gastrointestinal bleeding, risk of hyponatremia and serotonin syndrome Interactions: increased cardiovascular risks with medications known to cause cardiovascular issues. Increased bleeding risk with NSAIDs, aspirin. Risk of serotonin syndrome with other serotonergic medications. Effects on P450 system medication dependent Psychiatric consultation: on as needed basis	No* Risk of serotonin discontinuation syndrome with abrupt discontinuation If discontinued, taper essential
NDRI[c]: bupropion	Dose-dependent seizure risk in patients with history of seizure disorder and in patients with electrolyte abnormalities (e.g., in patients with bulimia nervosa), insomnia, risk of weight loss Interactions: effects on P450 system primarily 2D6 inhibition. Increased seizure risk with medications known to reduce seizure threshold Psychiatric consultation: on as needed basis	No* If discontinued, usually no risk of withdrawal symptoms but taper recommended
Atypical antidepressant: mirtazapine	Sedation, dizziness. risk of hepatotoxicity and neutropenia. Decreased elimination in elderly. Weight gain risk with long-term use Interactions: increased sedation and dizziness risk in patients with similar effects (e.g., narcotic pain medications Psychiatric consultation: on as needed basis	No* If discontinued, usually no risk of withdrawal symptoms but taper recommended
Atypical antidepressant: trazodone	Sedation. Risk of orthostatic hypotension, dizziness, and priapism (rare) Interactions: increased sedation and orthostasis risks in patients with similar effects (e.g., opioids, antihypertensives) Psychiatric consultation: on as needed basis	No* If discontinued, usually no risk of withdrawal symptoms but taper recommended

(continued)

Table 28.4 (continued)

Medication class or medication	Relevant effects, interactions, and need for psychiatric consultation	Need to discontinue* and withdrawal risks
TCAs[d]	High risk of cardiotoxicity and neurotoxicity. Risk of seizures. Risk of weight gain and anticholinergic effects such as dry mouth, orthostatic hypotension, dizziness, and sedation. If continued: EKG and medication levels (when indicated) are recommended	Discontinuation recommended* Risk of cholinergic rebound and/or serotonin discontinuation depending on medications If discontinued, taper essential in most cases
	Interactions: hyper or hypotension when combined with certain medications (e.g., sympathicomimetics). Risk of seizures with enflurane. Effects on P450 system medication dependent	
	Psychiatric consultation: strongly recommended	
MAOIs[e]	Risks of serotonin syndrome and hypertensive crisis. Risk of orthostatic hypotension, dizziness, and anticholinergic side effects	Discontinuation recommended* Discontinuation: 2–4 week window recommended and taper essential
	If continued: psychiatric and pharmacy consultation strongly recommended	Risk of hypertension and/or serotonin discontinuation syndrome
	Interactions: multiple drug-drug interactions including risk of serotonin syndrome and hypertensive crisis when combined with certain medications (e.g., epinephrine)	
	Psychiatric and pharmacy consultation: strongly recommended	
Antipsychotic medications (except clozapine)	Agranulocytosis, cardiovascular effects including cardiac conduction change (QTc prolongation), hypotension, seizure risk, anticholinergic effects. Risk of neuroleptic malignant syndrome. Additionally first-generation antipsychotic medications (e.g., haloperidol) associated with extrapyramidal symptoms and second-generation antipsychotic medications (e.g., quetiapine) associated with metabolic syndrome, diabetes, weight gain, and hyperlipidemia	No* Risk of cholinergic rebound with certain medications If discontinued, taper recommended
	Interactions—increased sedation, cardiovascular and cerebrovascular risks, and seizure risk when combined with certain perioperative medications. Effects on P450 system medication dependent	
	Psychiatric consultation: recommended	

Table 28.4 (continued)

Medication class or medication	Relevant effects, interactions, and need for psychiatric consultation	Need to discontinue* and withdrawal risks
Clozapine	Severe agranulocytosis with infection risk, cardiovascular effects including cardiac conduction change, hypotension, seizure risk, anticholinergic effects. Risk of neuroleptic malignant syndrome. Weight gain, metabolic syndrome, diabetes, hyperlipidemia If continued: EKG is recommended	Discontinuation recommended* Risk of cholinergic rebound Taper recommended
	Interactions—increased sedation, agranulocytosis, cardiovascular and cerebrovascular risks, and seizure risk when combined with certain perioperative medications	
	Psychiatric and pharmacy consultation: strongly recommended	
Lithium[f]	Effects on kidneys and thyroid, cardiovascular effects including arrhythmias, seizure risk, central nervous system effects If continued, EKG and lithium levels is recommended	Discontinuation- recommended* If discontinued, usually no risk of withdrawal symptoms but taper recommended
	Interaction—with NSAIDs, diuretics, ACE-inhibitors (nephrotoxicity and increased lithium levels), increased sedation when combined with certain perioperative medications	
	Psychiatric and pharmacy consultation: strongly recommended	
Anticonvulsants[g] (mood stabilizers)	Hepatotoxicity, decreased blood counts especially platelet counts, hyponatremia, lipid changes, sedation, central nervous system effects	No* If discontinued, usually no risk of withdrawal symptoms but taper recommended
	Interactions—increased risk of sedation, hyponatremia, and decreased platelet count when combined with certain perioperative medications. Inhibitory or inducing effects on P450 enzymes depending on medication	
	Psychiatric consultation: recommended	
Benzodiazepines and hypnotics	Central nervous system (CNS) effects including sedative and cognitive effects. Risk of tolerance and abuse	No* Risk of serious withdrawal (including seizure risk) with abrupt discontinuation If discontinued, taper essential
	Interactions—increased risk of sedation and other CNS effects in combination with certain perioperative medications with similar effects (e.g., narcotic pain medications)	
	Psychiatric consultation: on as needed basis	

[a]Selective serotonin reuptake inhibitor, [b]serotonin-norepinephrine reuptake inhibitor, [c]norepinephrine-dopamine reuptake inhibitor, [d]tricyclic antidepressant (see text for details), [e]monoamine-oxidase inhibitor (see text for details). [f]See text for details, [g]medications such as valproate, carbamazepine

*Consider risk-benefit on a case-by-case basis: Considerations include medication role in psychiatric stability, risk of withdrawal symptoms, and risk of psychiatric relapse if discontinued

surgeries. The following description is based on known effects of these medications combined with evidence from studies conducted in other relevant patient populations, e.g., in patients with medical comorbidities or patients undergoing other surgeries.

28.3.4.1 Bleeding Risk

Antidepressants such as the specific serotonin reuptake inhibitors (SSRIs) and serotonin-norepinephrine reuptake inhibitors (SNRIs), tricyclic antidepressants (TCAs), monoamine oxidase inhibitors (MAOIs), and certain mood stabilizers (valproate and carbamazepine) are known to increase the risk of bleeding [22, 23]. The mechanism is not completely understood, but for serotonergic medications, it is believed to be related to reduction of serotonin receptors on platelet surface and reduction in platelet affinity [22]. Increased bleeding risk with valproate and carbamazepine is believed to be due to decreased platelet count and inhibition of platelet aggregation by these medications [23]. The risk of bleeding can increase substantially when these medications are combined with non-steroid anti-inflammatory agents (NSAIDs) and aspirin, medications known to contribute to bleeding risk [24].

28.3.4.2 Hemodynamic Instability

Certain antipsychotic medications are known to cause hypotension, partially due to their antagonistic effects on alpha-adrenergic receptors (e.g., chlorpromazine) [25]. Antipsychotic medications have also been associated with sudden death due to prolongation of the QTc interval and torsades des pointes (e.g., thioridazine) [26]. These cardiovascular effects of these medications can have serious interactions with anesthesia. Minor cardiovascular effects such as postural hypotension and tachycardia are also common in patients receiving these medications [27]. Some patients with schizophrenia continued on their antipsychotic medications in the perioperative period may experience profound hypotension and other hemodynamic issues during and after anesthesia induction [28]. However, it should be noted that cardiovascular effects of antipsychotic medications are variable and depend on the specific medications under consideration. The newer (atypical) antipsychotic medications have fewer issues with hemodynamic stability compared to the older (typical) medications [26]. Therefore, individualized preoperative assessment should be conducted based on known cardiovascular effects of the antipsychotic medication patients are receiving in the context of other risk factors such as pre-existing medical comorbidities and known anesthesia-related risk factors (e.g., age, use of antihypertensive medications). Postural hypotension can increase the risk of syncope and injury due to falls in the postoperative period [29].

Certain antidepressants, specifically SNRIs, are known to increase blood pressure and cause other cardiovascular effects due to their noradrenergic effects. These effects vary depending on the medications and are usually dose-dependent increasing with the dose.

28.3.4.3 Thermoregulation and Neuroleptic Malignant Syndrome (NMS)

Antipsychotic medications are known to affect hypothalamic temperature regulation due to dopamine blockade [30]. Hypothermia can be an important factor increasing postoperative morbidity and mortality in patients receiving antipsychotic medications [31]. NMS, a syndrome characterized by acute increases in body temperature, muscle rigidity, and autonomic nervous system instability, has been associated with use of antipsychotic medications. Among patients exposed to antipsychotic medications, prevalence of NMS ranges from 0.02 to 2.4% [32]. It remains unclear if there is a connection between NMS and malignant hyperthermia associated with anesthesia and what anesthetic precautions should be taken in patients with history of NMS.

28.3.4.4 Pain Sensitivity

Evidence suggests impairment of pain sensitivity in patients with schizophrenia [33]. Postoperative pain scores and analgesic consumption are significantly less in these patients compared to the general population [34]. This pain insensitivity may be related to N-methyl-D-aspartate (NMDA) receptor hypofunction and may also be due to analgesic effects of antipsychotic medications [35, 36]. This pain insensitivity can increase the risk of postoperative complications due to delay in diagnosis and treatment and can also increase risk of postoperative confusion [33].

On the contrary, pain sensitivity and perception may be heightened in patients with mood and anxiety disorders [37]. Adequate treatment of these disorders is critical for appropriate management of pain in these patients.

28.3.4.5 Paralytic Ileus

The anticholinergic and noradrenergic effects of antipsychotic medication can contribute to increased risk of paralytic ileus [38]. This is primarily a problem in patients undergoing abdominal surgery but can be an issue with other surgeries. Impairment of pain sensitivity due to antipsychotic medications can further complicate ileus due to delay in diagnosis and treatment.

28.3.4.6 Interaction with Other Medications

Psychotropic medications can complicate perioperative management due to their direct or indirect interaction with other medications. These interactions may include pharmacokinetic or pharmacodynamics interactions as follows:

Vasoconstrictors: Vasoconstrictors when administered in presence of certain antidepressants (e.g., TCAs) may increase the risk of hypertensive reaction and other sympathomimetic effects [39]. However, clinical relevance of this interaction remains unclear [40].

Paracetamol: Medications such as carbamazepine can cause induction of cytochrome (CYP) 1A2. This can increase the metabolism of paracetamol reducing its efficacy and potentially increasing hepatotoxicity due to accumulation of its metabolites [41]. Similarly, metabolism of TCAs can be slowed down by paracetamol increasing risk of toxicity due to higher TCA levels [42].

Non-steroid anti-inflammatory drugs (NSAIDs): As noted earlier, NSAIDs when co-administered with serotonergic medications can increase risk of bleeding. NSAIDs can also cause other drug-drug interactions, e.g., increase in valproate levels by displacing it from protein binding and by inhibiting its metabolism [23]. The most clinically relevant interaction NSAIDs have is with lithium. NSAIDs can increase lithium levels due to reduced clearance of lithium [43]. Rising lithium levels are seen in about 5–10 days after initiation of NSAID. Lithium toxicity involves ataxia and confusion and can cause permanent renal damage. It can be potentially fatal. More frequent monitoring of serum lithium levels is strongly recommended in patients receiving NSAIDs [44].

Antibiotics and antifungals: Similar to NSAIDs, tetracyclines and metronidazole can reduce renal clearance of lithium increasing risk of lithium toxicity [45]. Ciprofloxacin and macrolide antibiotics such as erythromycin inhibit isoenzymes CYP 3A4 and CYP 1A2. This can lead to increased levels of certain TCAs and SSRIs metabolized by these isoenzymes increasing risk of toxicity [46]. Antifungals such as ketoconazole, fluconazole, and terbinafine are potent inhibitors of the CYP 3A4 isoenzyme. This inhibition can increase levels of medications such as TCAs, carbamazepine, and trazodone increasing risk of toxicity due to these high levels [46, 47]. Fluconazole, when co-administered with valproate, can increase risk of bleeding due to enhanced inhibition of platelet aggregation [48].

Benzodiazepines: Concurrent administration of sedating medications such as TCAs, opioid analgesics with benzodiazepines, can be potentially problematic, especially in the elderly [49]. It can increase risk of sedation, confusion, and in some cases delirium. The benzodiazepines with longer half-lives (e.g., diazepam) can be more problematic than the ones with shorter half-lives such as the lorazepam.

28.3.4.7 Critical Psychotropic Medications

Following are medication/medication classes that may need to be discontinued or managed with continuous psychiatric/pharmacy consultation during the perioperative care. Decision to continue or discontinue these medications during perioperative period should be made considering risk-benefit on a case-by-case basis [50]. Factors affecting the risk-benefit ratio include medication role in psychiatric stability, risk of withdrawal symptoms, and risk of psychiatric relapse if discontinued.

TCAs (Tricyclic Antidepressants)

TCAs work by inhibiting presynaptic uptake of norepinephrine and serotonin. They also affect histaminergic and cholinergic systems leading to wide range of side effects. They include medications such as amitriptyline, imipramine, desipramine, doxepin, nortriptyline, and others.

TCAs can potentiate the effect of intraoperative anticholinergic medications and those that cross the blood-brain barrier. Increased availability of postsynaptic norepinephrine can lead to exaggerated blood pressure response to indirect acting vasopressors [39, 51]. If TCAs are continued, pancuronium-, ketamine-, meperidine-, and epinephrine-containing solutions should be avoided [51]. Chronic therapy with TCAs can reduce cardiac catecholamines. This can lead to decreased myocardial contractility potentiating the cardiac depressant effect of anesthetic agents [51]. Dysrhythmias can occur secondary to slowing of sodium channel electrical conduction. Seizures have been documented with amitriptyline and enflurane [52].

Monoamine Oxidase Inhibitors (MAOIs)

MAOIs are primarily to treat treatment-resistant depression. They exert their therapeutic effect by inhibition of the monoamine oxidase enzyme in the breakdown of norepinephrine and serotonin, thereby increasing their circulating concentration.

There exist multiple interactions between anesthetics and MAOIs [53]. Indirect-acting sympathomimetics may precipitate potentially fatal hypertensive crisis in combination with MAOIs. Direct-acting sympathomimetics may have an enhanced effect due to receptor hypersensitivity, and doses should be titrated appropriately. Pancuronium should be avoided as it releases stored noradrenaline. Two different reactions can occur with MAOIs and opioids [54]. Type I (excitatory) reactions occur with pethidine and dextromethorphan, both of which inhibit serotonin uptake. This can lead to serotonin syndrome which is life threatening. Type II (depressive) reaction are rare and are thought to be due to MOAI inhibition of hepatic enzymes resulting in enhanced effects of all opioids.

Propofol and etomidate can be used safely with MAOIs. Opioids like morphine, fentanyl, alfentanyl, and remifentanil can all be safely used. Benzodiazepines, inhalational anesthetic agents, anticholinergic drugs, and non-steroidal anti-inflammatory drugs can be used safely in patients taking MAOIs.

There should be a careful review of risks-benefits of stopping the MAOI prior to elective surgery with the involvement of the anesthesiologist, psychiatrist, and patient [53]. This review is particularly important because these medications are used primarily in patients with treatment-refractory depression, and discontinuation of these medications can cause significant psychiatric instability [55]. If decision is made to discontinue MAOIs, they should be tapered down and then stopped with adequate supervision. A two- to four-week window is recommended between stopping of these medications and scheduling of surgery and/or use of agents with potential interactions with these medications.

Lithium

Lithium is used primarily in the treatment of bipolar disorder [56]. It is also used as an adjunctive treatment in patients with treatment-refractory depression and psychotic disorders with affective component. Lithium has shown benefit in decreasing suicidal behaviors [56]. It has a narrow therapeutic index. Its side effects include gastrointestinal symptoms and central nervous system and cardiac effects [57]. Toxicity is usually related to its plasma levels of 1.5 mmol/L but might occur at lower levels. Lithium toxicity can occur with the use of NSAIDs due to nephrotoxic effects of these medications [57]. Lithium can also increase the duration of neuromuscular-blocking agents like pancuronium and succinylcholine making reversibility difficult. Similar to MAOIs, continuation or discontinuation of lithium prior to elective surgery should include a careful review of risks-benefits with the involvement of anesthesiologist, psychiatrist, and patient [50]. Patients responding to lithium treatment are generally stable on this medication for years and sometimes decades. Discontinuation of lithium in these patients can lead to significant exacerbation of their psychiatric illness.

Clozapine

Clozapine is an atypical antipsychotic medication. It is frequently used in the management of treatment-refractory psychosis [58]. It is highly effective, and its discontinuation can cause significant psychiatric instability including rapid onset psychosis. Clozapine carries risk of multiple side effects and drug-drug interactions [59]. Its major side effects include agranulocytosis, cardiac toxicity, and other cardiovascular side effects, e.g., hypotension, weight gain, increased risk of diabetes, metabolic syndrome, hyperlipidemia, sedation, hyperthermia, and lowering of seizure threshold [59]. Clozapine can be continued during the perioperative period with careful monitoring of cardiovascular, blood counts and avoiding or minimizing use of medications with potentially serious interactions with clozapine [50]. Psychiatric and pharmacy consultation during and throughout perioperative period is strongly recommended in management of all patients receiving clozapine [50]. Input of these services as well as patient input is essential if discontinuation of clozapine is considered during perioperative period.

28.4 Preoperative, Intraoperative, and Postoperative Management

28.4.1 Preoperative Management

Preoperative assessment includes evaluation of psychiatric and medical status. Psychiatric evaluation includes assessment of current mood, anxiety, psychotic symptoms, as well as use of substances. Assessment of suicidality and cognitive status are essential aspects of patient evaluations. As noted earlier, cognitive and psychiatric status may affect patients' ability to give informed consent. It is important to gather past psychiatric/substance use history and history of past suicidal ideation and/or attempts. Assessment of past history should include questions about patients' vulnerability to stressful situations, i.e., exacerbation of symptoms when under stress. Evaluation of medical status should include assessment of medical comorbidities frequently encountered in these patients, e.g., cardiovascular illness, diabetes, and metabolic syndrome related to antipsychotic medications.

Assessment of patients' psychotropic medication regimen should include impact of these medications on critical organs/systems (e.g., liver, kidney) and their pharmacodynamics and pharmacokinetic interactions with other medications. Feasibility of their usual route of administration should be considered in the context of requirements of preoperative fasting and other restrictions related to anesthesiological procedures. Some surgeries are followed by placement of gastric tubes. Potential impact on bioavailability of medications is an important consideration in dosing changes when medications are delivered via gastric tubes. In rare cases, medications need to be delivered via alternate routes, e.g., intravenous or intramuscular. In such case, availability of alternate formulations of their medications or similar medications needs to be explored. In extremely rare cases, certain medications have to be discontinued due to their potentially serious interactions with anesthesia or other aspects of perioperative management (e.g., MAOIs with certain types of anesthesia).

Discontinuation of psychotropic medications is associated with risk of withdrawal symptoms and/or relapse of psychiatric symptoms [50]. Serotonergic medications (SSRIs and SNRIs) if discontinued abruptly can lead to serotonin discontinuation syndrome [60]. This syndrome is characterized by dysphoric mood, anxiety, insomnia, headaches, dizziness, confusion, agitation, sensory disturbances (such as paresthesia), autonomic instability, and in rare cases seizures. Similarly, abrupt discontinuation of benzodiazepines is also associated with withdrawal symptoms with risk of heightened anxiety, tremors, agitation, autonomic instability, and risk of seizures [61]. Discontinuation of these medications can also lead to relapse of mood, anxiety, and psychotic symptoms depending on the medication and the indication it is used for [50]. Furthermore, replacing the current medication with similar medication, even from the same class, may lead to instability and worsening of psychiatric status as there can be subtle differences between medications belonging to the same class. Any discontinuation and/or substitution of psychotropic medication in a psychiatrically stable patient should be done in consultation with psychiatric services and should include careful consideration of risks and benefits [50].

Preoperative laboratory evaluation should include assessment of critical organs/systems known to be affected by patients' psychotropic medications and lifestyle as a result of serious mental illness, e.g., kidney and thyroid function in patients receiving lithium, liver function in patients receiving antipsychotic medications, and labs related to metabolic syndrome in patients receiving antipsychotic medications. Generally, laboratory evaluation should include assessment of kidney, liver, thyroid, blood counts, and lipid levels. Laboratory evaluations should also include assessment of medication levels when indicated, e.g., lithium, valproate, carbamazepine, and TCA levels. These baseline levels are critical for intra- and postoperative management of patients, especially if patients start experiencing exacerbation of psychiatric symptoms during these periods or experience side effects due to increased levels. Assessment of cardiac status, especially in patients receiving antipsychotic medication, is important. An electrocardiogram to assess QTc prolongation should be included in these patients.

28.4.1.1 What Should Cancel Surgery

Risk of suicide should be a strong consideration for canceling a surgery. Components of suicide assessment include evaluation of risk factors, patient's mental state, social context, and nonverbal signs of extreme distress or depression such as agitation or excessive slowing, poor eye contact [62]. Hopelessness is a powerful predictor of suicidal ideation and completed suicides [62]. History past suicidal ideation and/or attempts is another critical factor. Friedlander et al. conducted a comprehensive review of literature focusing on suicide risk in patients undergoing oral and maxillofacial surgery [19]. They recommend using well-established risk factors (the SAD PERSONS pneumonic) to identify patients at high risk of suicide [19]. Certain suicide screening tools such as the Beck Hopelessness Scale, the Suicide Intent Scale, and the Columbia-Suicide Severity Rating Scale are used to screen for suicide risk in the general population and in patients with mental illness [63]. It is important to note that patients with head and neck cancer which may include patients scheduled for maxillofacial surgery carry significantly higher risk of suicide [64].

The inability of giving informed consent should also be a strong consideration for canceling surgery [65]. A patient must be able to do four things to make a competent decision: express a treatment choice, appreciate the personal consequences of their choice, make a rational decision concerning treatment, and understand the treatment and its risks and benefits.

28.4.2 Intraoperative Management

Use of general vs. regional anesthesia in patients with psychiatric patients remains controversial and should be decided on a case-by-case basis considering surgical needs, patient risk factors, and interactions of psychotropic medications with proposed anesthesia [66]. As noted earlier, major risks as a result of interactions with psychotropic medications include hemodynamic instability, cardiac conduction changes, effects on thermoregulation, malignant hyperthermia, and effects on mental status in case of postoperative metabolic instability. Airway management can be complicated in patients receiving certain psychotropic medications and/or in patients with substance use disorders [67]. Sedation and other factors may increase risk of aspiration, aspiration pneumonia, and lung injury including risk of acute respiratory distress syndrome [67]. Care should be taken during intubation or placement of nasogastric/orogastric tube in patients with known history on intranasal substance use disorders (e.g., cocaine) as chronic intranasal substance use has been associated with septal destruction and soft palate necrosis [67].

28.4.3 Postoperative Management

Postoperative management of psychiatric patients is complicated by both medical and psychiatric factors. A major concern, especially in patients with SMI such as schizophrenia, is high mortality risk. Sudden death is about five times more frequent in these patients compared to the general population [68]. High mortality risk in these patients has been associated with cardiac arrhythmias such as QTc prolongation; respiratory arrest due to cardiac and respiratory complications; aspiration due to excessive sedation, agitated delirium, heat stroke, and NMS; and complications due to paralytic ileus [69–71]. Risk of postoperative confusion is very high in these patients compared to the general population [72]. Postoperative confusion in these patients has been correlated with increased cortisol, norepinephrine, and interleukin-6 (IL-6) levels and appears to be independent of type of anesthesia used [72, 73]. High rates of delirium have also been reported in patients with serious mental illness such as patients with depression and schizophrenia [74]. Evidence indicates that preoperative discontinuation of psychiatric medications may increase risk of postoperative delirium in these patients [75]. Treatment of postoperative confusion or delirium includes both behavioral and pharmacologic measures. Keeping the patient in an environment where they will not be overstimulated is important. Pharmacological management primarily includes treatment with antipsychotic medications and avoiding benzodiazepines.

Patients with psychiatric illness may carry a higher risk of postoperative water intoxication. This may be due to abnormal secretion of vasopressin, aldosterone, and atrial natriuretic peptide during anesthesia [75]. These abnormal secretions may be due to heightened surgical stress in these patients compared to patients without mental illness and may also be related to effects of chronic administration of antipsychotic medications [75]. Patients with history of psychiatric illness also carry a higher risk of local and systemic infections [76]. This includes delayed wound healing, wound infections, and risk of pneumonia. This may be due to immune and pituitary-adrenal dysregulation related to antipsychotic medications [77].

Pain management during postoperative period can be complicated in psychiatric patients due to impairment of pain responsiveness. As noted earlier, patients with mood and anxiety disorders report more pain locations and higher severity of pain compared to patients without these disorders [78]. They report higher number of locations and severity of pain even after remission of depression/anxiety symptoms, and they are also at higher risk for chronic pain [78]. On the other hand, patients with psychotic/thought disorders such as schizophrenia report less pain compared to the general patient population due to pain insensitivity [33]. Evidence suggests that their postoperative pain scores are significantly lower than control patients and their analgesic consumption is also about 60% lower than control patients [34]. Postoperative pain is an important risk factor for postoperative confusion, and inadequate pain relief in these patients can increase the risk of postoperative confusion.

It is important to closely monitor patients' psychiatric status in the postoperative period. The stress of surgery can cause exacerbation of psychiatric symptoms. Multiple other factors (e.g., discontinuation of psychotropic medications in the preoperative period) can contribute to psychiatric exacerbation. Patients with history of substance use may experience withdrawal symptoms in the postoperative period. Similarly patients may also experience withdrawal symptoms if certain psychotropic medications were discontinued abruptly (e.g., SSRIs or benzodiazepines) in the pre- or intraoperative period.

Conclusion

Psychiatric problems are common, and maxillofacial surgical teams frequently encounter these patients in their practices. Perioperative management of these patients can be challenging due to their multiple psychiatric, medical, and substance use comorbidities. Their management is further complicated by factors related to their psychotropic medication regimens, drug-drug interactions, issues related to informed consent, patient-provider communication difficulties, and risk of suicidality. Evidence suggests high risk of morbidity and mortality in these patients during preoperative period. Surgical teams should be aware of specific issues and risks in the management of these patients.

References

1. National Institute of Mental Health Web Site. https://www.nimh.nih.gov/health/statistics/prevalence/any-mental-illness-ami-among-us-adults.shtml.
2. Meyer JM, Stahl SM. The metabolic syndrome and schizophrenia. Acta Psychiatr Scand. 2009;119(1):4–14.
3. Kudoh A. Perioperative management for chronic schizophrenic patients. Anesth Analg. 2005;101(6):1867–72.
4. Kessler RC, Chiu WT, Demler O, Merikangas KR, Walters EE. Prevalence, severity, and comorbidity of 12-month DSM-IV disorders in the National Comorbidity Survey Replication. Arch Gen Psychiatry. 2005;62(6):617–27.
5. Hasin DS, Goodwin RD, Stinson FS, Grant BF. Epidemiology of major depressive disorder: results from the national epidemiologic survey on alcoholism and related conditions. Arch Gen Psychiatry. 2005;62(10):1097–106.
6. Prashanth NT, Raghuveer HP, Kumar D, Shobha ES, Rangan V, Rao TS. A comparative study of post-traumatic stress disorder, anxiety, depression and change in sexual functioning of patients with facial injuries and patients with extremity injuries. J Contemp Dent Pract. 2015;16(11):884–92.
7. Hillhouse TM, Porter JH. A brief history of the development of antidepressant drugs: from monoamines to glutamate. Exp Clin Psychopharmacol. 2015;23(1):1–21.
8. Müller N, Schwarz MJ. The immune-mediated alteration of serotonin and glutamate: towards an integrated view of depression. Mol Psychiatry. 2007;12(11):988–1000.
9. American Psychiatric Association. The diagnostic and statistical manual of mental disorders: DSM–5. 5th ed. Washington; London: American Psychiatric Association; 2013.
10. Howes OD, McCutcheon R, Owen MJ, Murray RM. The role of genes, stress, and dopamine in the development of schizophrenia. Biol Psychiatry. 2017;81(1):9–20.
11. McTeague LM, Lang PJ. The anxiety spectrum and the reflex physiology of defense: from circumscribed fear to broad distress. Depress Anxiety. 2012;29(4):264–81.
12. Furtado M, Katzman MA. Neuroinflammatory pathways in anxiety, posttraumatic stress, and obsessive compulsive disorders. Psychiatry Res. 2015;229(1–2):37–48.
13. Marek R, Strobel C, Bredy TW, Sah P. The amygdala and medial prefrontal cortex: partners in the fear circuit. J Physiol. 2013;591(10):2381–91.
14. Murrough JW, Yaqubi S, Sayed S, Charney DS. Emerging drugs for the treatment of anxiety. Expert Opin Emerg Drugs. 2015;20(3):393–406.
15. Adogwa O, Parker SL, Shau DN, Mendenhall SK, Bydon A, Cheng JS, Asher AL, McGirt MJ. Preoperative Zung depression scale predicts patient satisfaction independent of the extent of improvement after revision lumbar surgery. Spine J. 2013;13(5):501–6.
16. Ghormley C, Basso M, Candlis P, Combs D. Neuropsychological impairment corresponds with poor understanding of informed consent disclosures in persons diagnosed with major depression. Psychiatry Res. 2011;187(1–2):106–12.
17. Howe V, Foister K, Jenkins K, Skene L, Copolov D, Keks N. Competence to give informed consent in acute psychosis is associated with symptoms rather than diagnosis. Schizophr Res. 2005;77(2–3):211–4.
18. Lydiatt WM, Moran J, Burke WJ. A review of depression in the head and neck cancer patient. Clin Adv Hematol Oncol. 2009;7(6):397–403.
19. Friedlander AH, Rosenbluth SC, Rubin RT. The adult suicide-prone patient: a review of the medical literature and implications for oral and maxillofacial surgeons. J Oral Maxillofac Surg. 2012;70(5):1253–60.
20. Witte TK, Didie ER, Menard W, Phillips KA. The relationship between body dysmorphic disorder behaviors and the acquired capability for suicide. Suicide Life Threat Behav. 2012;42(3):318–31.
21. Lipari RN, Hedden SL, Hughes A. Substance use and mental health estimates from the 2013 National Survey on drug use and health: overview of findings. The CBHSQ Report. Rockville, MD: Substance Abuse and Mental Health Services Administration (US); 2013.
22. Serebruany VL. Selective serotonin reuptake inhibitors and increased bleeding risk: are we missing something? Am J Med. 2006;119(2):113–6.
23. Reisner L, Pettengill CA. The use of anticonvulsants in orofacial pain. Oral Surg Oral Med Oral Pathol Oral Radiol Endod. 2001;91(1):2–7.

24. Hersh EV, Pinto A, Moore PA. Adverse drug interactions involving common prescription and over-the-counter analgesic agents. Clin Ther. 2007;29(Suppl):2477–97.
25. Leung JY, Barr AM, Procyshyn RM, Honer WG, Pang CC. Cardiovascular side-effects of antipsychotic drugs: the role of the autonomic nervous system. Pharmacol Ther. 2012;135(2):113–22.
26. Glassman AH, Bigger JT Jr. Antipsychotic drugs: prolonged QTc interval, torsade de pointes, and sudden death. Am J Psychiatry. 2001;158(11):1774–82.
27. Buckley NA, Sanders P. Cardiovascular adverse effects of antipsychotic drugs. Drug Saf. 2000;23(3):215–28.
28. Kudoh A, Katagai H, Takase H, Takazawa T. Effect of preoperative discontinuation of antipsychotics in schizophrenic patients on outcome during and after anaesthesia. Eur J Anaesthesiol. 2004;21(5):414–6.
29. Ray WA, Griffin MR, Schaffner W, Baugh DK, Melton LJ 3rd. Psychotropic drug use and the risk of hip fracture. N Engl J Med. 1987;316(7):363–9.
30. Young DM. Risk factors for hypothermia in psychiatric patients. Ann Clin Psychiatry. 1996;8(2):93–7.
31. Kramer MR, Vandijk J, Rosin AJ. Mortality in elderly patients with thermoregulatory failure. Arch Intern Med. 1989;149(7):1521–3.
32. Casey DE. Side effect profiles of new antipsychotic agents. J Clin Psychiatry. 1996;57(Suppl 11):40–5.
33. Dworkin RH. Pain insensitivity in schizophrenia: a neglected phenomenon and some implications. Schizophr Bull. 1994;20(2):235–48.
34. Kudoh A, Ishihara H, Matsuki A. Current perception thresholds and postoperative pain in schizophrenic patients. Reg Anesth Pain Med. 2000;25(5):475–9.
35. Olney JW, Farber NB. Glutamate receptor dysfunction and schizophrenia. Arch Gen Psychiatry. 1995;52(12):998–1007.
36. Patt RB, Proper G, Reddy S. The neuroleptics as adjuvant analgesics. J Pain Symptom Manag. 1994;9(7):446–53.
37. Ghoneim MM, O'Hara MW. Depression and postoperative complications: an overview. BMC Surg. 2016;16:5.
38. Kudoh A, Ishihara H, Matsuki A. Pituitary-adrenal and parasympathetic function in chronic schizophrenic patients with postoperative ileus or hypotension. Neuropsychobiology. 1999;39(3):125–30.
39. Yagiela JA. Adverse drug interactions in dental practice: interactions associated with vasoconstrictors. Part V of a series. J Am Dent Assoc. 1999;130(5):701–9.
40. Gómez-Moreno G, Guardia J, Cutando A, Calvo-Guirado JL. Pharmacological interactions of vasoconstrictors. Med Oral Patol Oral Cir Bucal. 2009;14(1):E20–7.
41. Becker DE. Psychotropic drugs: implications for dental practice. Anesth Prog. 2008;55(3):89–99.
42. Little JW. Dental implications of mood disorders. Gen Dent. 2004;52(5):442–50.
43. Phelan KM, Mosholder AD, Lu S. Lithium interaction with the cyclooxygenase 2 inhibitors rofecoxib and celecoxib and other nonsteroidal anti-inflammatory drugs. J Clin Psychiatry. 2003;64(11):1328–34.
44. Clark DB. Dental care for the patient with bipolar disorder. J Can Dent Assoc. 2003;69(1):20–4.
45. Hersh EV. Adverse drug interactions in dental practice: interactions involving antibiotics. Part II of a series. J Am Dent Assoc. 1999;130(2):236–51.
46. Hersh EV, Moore PA. Adverse drug interactions in dentistry. Periodontol. 2008;46:109–42.
47. van der Kuy PH, Hooymans PM. Nortriptyline intoxication induced by terbinafine. BMJ. 1998;316(7129):441.
48. Hupp WS. Seizure disorders. Oral Surg Oral Med Oral Pathol Oral Radiol Endod. 2001;92(6):59.
49. Turner LN, Balasubramaniam R, Hersh EV, Stoopler ET. Drug therapy in Alzheimer disease: an update for the oral health care provider. Oral Surg Oral Med Oral Pathol Oral Radiol Endod. 2008;106(4):467–76.
50. Huyse FJ, Touw DJ, van Schijndel RS, de Lange JJ, Slaets JP. Psychotropic drugs and the perioperative period: a proposal for a guideline in elective surgery. Psychosomatics. 2006;47(1):8–22.
51. Hansen D, Föhring U, Eyrich K. Long-term antidepressive medication-- an increased anesthetic risk? Anaesthesist. 1990;39(4):205–10.
52. Sprague DH, Wolf S. Enflurane seizures in patients taking amitriptyline. Anesth Analg. 1982;61(1):67–8.
53. Krings-Ernst I, Ulrich S, Adli M. Antidepressant treatment with MAO-inhibitors during general and regional anesthesia: a review and case report of spinal anesthesia for lower extremity surgery without discontinuation of tranylcypromine. Int J Clin Pharmacol Ther. 2013;51(10):763–70.
54. Gillman PK. Monoamine oxidase inhibitors, opioid analgesics and serotonin toxicity. Br J Anaesth. 2005 Oct;95(4):434–41.
55. Shulman KI, Herrmann N, Walker SE. Current place of monoamine oxidase inhibitors in the treatment of depression. CNS Drugs. 2013;27(10):789–97.
56. Müller-Oerlinghausen B, Berghöfer A, Ahrens B. The anti-suicidal and mortality-reducing effect of lithium prophylaxis: consequences for guidelines in clinical psychiatry. Can J Psychiatr. 2003;48(7):433–9.
57. Gitlin M. Lithium side effects and toxicity: prevalence and management strategies. Int J Bipolar Disord. 2016;4(1):27.
58. Iqbal MM, Rahman A, Husain Z, Mahmud SZ, Ryan WG, Feldman JM. Clozapine: a clinical review of adverse effects and management. Ann Clin Psychiatry. 2003;15(1):33–48.
59. Lundblad W, Azzam PN, Gopalan P, Ross CA. Medical management of patients on clozapine: a guide for internists. J Hosp Med. 2015;10(8):537–43.
60. Bingham K, Hawa R, Sockalingam S. SSRI discontinuation syndrome following bariatric surgery: a case report and focused literature review. Psychosomatics. 2014;55(6):692–7.
61. Lader M, Kyriacou A. Withdrawing benzodiazepines in patients with anxiety disorders. Curr Psychiatry Rep. 2016;18(1):8.

62. Morriss R, Kapur N, Byng R. Assessing risk of suicide or self-harm in adults. BMJ. 2013;347:f4572.
63. Bolton JM, Gunnell D, Turecki G. Suicide risk assessment and intervention in people with mental illness. BMJ. 2015;351:h4978.
64. Misono S, Weiss NS, Fann JR, Redman M, Yueh B. Incidence of suicide in persons with cancer. J Clin Oncol. 2008;26(29):4731–8.
65. Brown S, Greenwood M, Meechan JG. General medicine and surgery for dental practitioners. Part 5--psychiatry. Br Dent J. 2010;209(1):11–6.
66. Attri JP, Bala N, Chatrath V. Psychiatric patient and anaesthesia. Indian J Anaesth. 2012;56(1):8–13.
67. Moran S, Isa J, Steinemann S. Perioperative management in the patient with substance abuse. Surg Clin North Am. 2015;95(2):417–28.
68. Ruschena D, Mullen PE, Burgess P, Cordner SM, Barry-Walsh J, Drummer OH, Palmer S, Browne C, Wallace C. Sudden death in psychiatric patients. Br J Psychiatry. 1998;172:331–6.
69. Haddad PM, Anderson IM. Antipsychotic-related QTc prolongation, torsade de pointes and sudden death. Drugs. 2002;62(11):1649–71.
70. Laposata EA, Hale P Jr, Poklis A. Evaluation of sudden death in psychiatric patients with special reference to phenothiazine therapy: forensic pathology. J Forensic Sci. 1988;33(2):432–40.
71. Tueth MJ. Emergencies caused by side effects of psychiatric medications. Am J Emerg Med. 1994;12(2):212–6.
72. Kudoh A, Takahira Y, Katagai H, Takazawa T. Schizophrenic patients who develop postoperative confusion have an increased norepinephrine and cortisol response to surgery. Neuropsychobiology. 2002;46(1):7–12.
73. Kudoh A, Takase H, Takahira Y, Katagai H, Takazawa T. Postoperative confusion in schizophrenic patients is affected by interleukin-6. J Clin Anesth. 2003;15(6):455–62.
74. Copeland LA, Zeber JE, Pugh MJ, Mortensen EM, Restrepo MI, Lawrence VA. Postoperative complications in the seriously mentally ill: a systematic review of the literature. Ann Surg. 2008;248(1):31–8.
75. Kudoh A, Kudo M, Ishihara H, Matsuki A. Increased plasma vasopressin and atrial natriuretic peptide in chronic schizophrenic patients during abdominal surgery. Neuropsychobiology. 1998;37(4):169–74.
76. Felker B, Yazel JJ, Short D. Mortality and medical comorbidity among psychiatric patients: a review. Psychiatr Serv. 1996;47(12):1356–63.
77. Kudoh A, Sakai T, Ishihara H, Matsuki A. Plasma cytokine response to surgical stress in schizophrenic patients. Clin Exp Immunol. 2001;125(1):89–93.
78. Gerrits MM, van Marwijk HW, van Oppen P, van der Horst H, Penninx BW. Longitudinal association between pain, and depression and anxiety over four years. J Psychosom Res. 2015;78(1):64–70.

Perioperative Management of Pregnant & Postpartum Patients

29

Sarah T. Araji, Georges Yared, Deena Elkafrawi, and Tony G. Zreik

Abstract

Oral and maxillofacial surgery is rarely indicated in the pregnant patient. However, when such is indicated, the surgeon must be cognizant of the many physiologic changes that occur in the gravida female. This chapter will review the physiologic changes associated with pregnancy and the post-partum period as well as the perioperative anesthetic and surgical management. The chapter will also review considerations regarding the lactating mothers.

29.1 Medical Disease

29.1.1 Pathophysiology

Pregnancy is a period in a female patient's life notable for many physiological changes of various systems including the cardiovascular, respiratory, musculoskeletal, gastrointestinal, and hematological systems. As a result, many pregnant patients commonly complain of nausea and vomiting, nasal congestion, alteration in taste, food cravings, hyperventilation and shortness of breath, and fatigue. When operating on a pregnant patient, one must consider the well-being of both the mother and fetus. Below we will outline the various physiological changes in a pregnant female by system and how to manage them appropriately.

29.1.1.1 Cardiovascular System

Various changes occur in the hemodynamic and cardiovascular systems of gravid females. Cardiac output will increase in the first trimester, plateaus in the second trimester and minimally increases in the third trimester. Cardiac output increases 30–50% during pregnancy, due to a 20–30% increase in heart rate and a 20–50% increase in stroke volume [1]. Increased stroke volume due to an increase in left ventricular mass and total blood volume by 25–52% during gestation is most likely responsible for the early increase in cardiac output [1].

S.T. Araji, M.D.
PGY3 Obstetrics and Gynecology, Saint Joseph's Regional Medical Center, Paterson, NJ, USA

G. Yared, M.D. • T.G. Zreik, M.D., M.B.A. (✉)
Department of OB/GYN, Lebanese American University School of Medicine, Beirut, Lebanon
e-mail: tgzreik@lau.edu.lb

D. Elkafrawi, B.A.
St. George's University School of Medicine, True Blue, Grenada

© Springer International Publishing AG 2018
E.M. Ferneini, J.D. Bennett (eds.), *Perioperative Assessment of the Maxillofacial Surgery Patient*,
https://doi.org/10.1007/978-3-319-58868-1_29

Table 29.1 Dosing recommendations for lactating mothers

Drug	Dosage	Notes
Oxycodone/acetaminophen	5–10 mg by mouth every 4–6 h as needed for pain	Not to exceed 30–40 mg per 24 h
Hydrocodone	5–10 mg by mouth every 6 h as needed for pain	Not to exceed 30 mg per 24 h
Oral morphine sulfate	5–15 mg by mouth every 6 h as needed for pain	Correct dosage can be influenced by a number of factors
Ibuprofen	800 mg by mouth three times daily as needed for pain for 10 days	Should be taken with food

The above mentioned dosages are recommended both for mothers who have just delivered and for mothers who have had surgery when their baby is a little older

A decrease in blood pressure and cardiac output may occur while a gravid patient is in a supine position during the second and third trimester. This is due to decreased venous return to the heart secondary to compression of the inferior vena cava by the gravid uterus; ultimately a 14% reduction in cardiac output may result [1, 2]. Decrease in blood pressure occurs due to compression of the descending aorta, hence decreasing blood flow to the common iliac arteries. Supine hypotension syndrome characterized by hypotension, bradycardia, and syncope in the supine position may be noted; initially an increase in heart rate and blood pressure will occur and then a decrease. Even if a pregnant patient is asymptomatic in the supine position, a notable decrease in uteroplacental perfusion may occur. *Therefore, placing the patient in a 5–15% tilt on her left side can relieve supine hypotension; if not relieved, a full left lateral position may be needed* [1–3].

29.1.1.2 Hematological System

Total blood volume during pregnancy increases by 25–52%, and red blood cell mass increases 20% over non-gravid values by end of the third trimester [1]. As a result, physiological anemia of pregnancy is maximal by approximately 30–32 weeks of gestation. The purpose of these hematological changes is to protect the mother from volume depletion secondary to excessive peripartum hemorrhage. Additionally, this may reduce the chances of a thrombotic event from occurring. Studies have shown that a maternal hematocrit between 30 and 38% is protective against maternal and intrauterine thrombotic events [1]. Gestation increases leukocyte count leading to physiological leukocytosis of pregnancy. Leukocytes increase by 5000 to 10,000 cells secondary to increased circulation of catecholamines and cortisol leading to demargination of mature leukocytes from the endothelial lining of the vascular system [1–3] (Table 29.1).

Pregnant females are at five times increased risk of thromboembolic events in comparison to nonpregnant patients given the hypercoagulable state of pregnancy [1–3]. All coagulation factors are increased during pregnancy, except factors XI and XIII, which are decreased. Moreover, thrombin-mediated fibrin generation increases throughout pregnancy [1].

Anticoagulation is essential for the treatment of established PE and DVT and prophylaxis against venous thromboembolism in women with a history of thromboembolic disease. *Heparin is the anticoagulant of choice during pregnancy; given its large molecular size, it does not cross the placenta unlike Coumadin which poses a fetal risk* [1]. Heparin has a high-affinity binding sequence to antithrombin III, which undergoes a conformational change that increases its ability to inactivate coagulation factors Ia, Xa, and IXa. A retrospective study of 100 consecutive pregnancies where heparin was used showed that the rate of adverse fetal and neonatal outcomes was similar to that in normal pregnancies [1]. One major concern when using heparin in pregnant patients is heparin-induced thrombocytopenia (HIT). HIT is due to heparin-dependent IgG antiplatelet antibodies which lead to serotonin-induced platelet aggregation; it occurs 5–15 days after the start of heparin therapy; HIT substantially increases the risk of a thromboembolic event. Heparin-induced osteoporosis is a concern during pregnancy; while fractures during pregnancy are rare, they occur mainly in the pelvic region with no maxillofacial fractures reported [1].

Low-molecular-weight heparin (LMWH) is preferred over unfractionated heparin because of its longer half-life and less protein binding affinity, making the dose response more predictable [1]. Additionally, LMWH was found to be more effective than unfractionated heparin in preventing recurrence of clot and less likely to cause major bleeding due to its minimal effects on platelets and vascular permeability [1].

Acute thromboembolism during pregnancy necessitates intravenous anticoagulation for 5–10 days, followed every 8–12 h by subcutaneous injections to prolong the partial thromboplastin time at least to 1.5 times control throughout the dosing interval [1]. The current regimen for gravid women at risk for DVT includes 5000 U heparin twice a day in the first trimester, 7500 U twice a day in the second trimester, and 10,000 U twice a day in the third trimester [1]. For gravid patients with a history of a previous thromboembolic event, heparin 5000 U is recommended every 12 h or heparin adjusted to level of 0.1–0.2 IU/mL or clinical surveillance with periodic surveillance ultrasonography or Coumadin prophylaxis postpartum for 4–6 weeks; sequential pneumatic compression devices can be used concurrently [1].

29.1.1.3 Respiratory System

Changes in the nasal and upper airway mucosa are to be expected during pregnancy. The mucosa will become more engorged and edematous. Approximately 30% of gravid patients experience symptoms of rhinitis during pregnancy. These changes are likely secondary to the direct effects of estrogen and indirect effects of increased blood volumes. Rhinitis of pregnancy commences in the beginning of the second trimester and gradually increases in severity until delivery; symptoms will resolve 48 hours after delivery [1–3].

Pulmonary changes manifesting in the gravid patient include hyperventilation which begins in the first trimester and increases up to 42% in late pregnancy [1]. Hyperventilation may be secondary to increased maternal oxygen demands or lessened residual capacity of the lungs. Several factors play into the mechanism of action of hyperventilation—progesterone acts as a respiratory stimulant [1–3]. Additionally, a resting arterial carbon dioxide tension below 30 mmHg accompanied with increased renal bicarbonate excretion is a contributing factor. Twenty-five percent of supine gravid women present with moderate hypoxemia which improves significantly when shifted to the sitting position. Hence, gravid patients are expected to have mild respiratory alkalosis (pH 7.40–7.46) and blood gas parameters (serum bicarbonate between 18 and 22 mEq/L) that are altered by maternal position [1]. Therefore, using non-gravid ventilatory patterns may result in respiratory acidosis in the fetus and in the mother.

Dyspnea is a common complaint in pregnant women—approximately 50% will have symptoms by 19 weeks of gestation, which increases to 75% by 31 weeks. The dyspnea may occur by the hormonal changes to the mucosa of the respiratory tract. However, it may be simply that women who complain of dyspnea are more aware of increased ventilation of pregnancy [1–3].

From an anatomic standpoint, the diaphragm is displaced upward approximately 4 cm in a gravid patient; this is compensated for by an increase in the transverse diameter of the thorax and chest circumference, increasing vital capacity by 40% [1]. Functional residual capacity is reduced by 15–20% secondary to diaphragmatic displacement [1]. Additionally, oxygen consumption increases by 15% in a gravid patient. *Therefore, oxygen reserves are lowered, hence increasing hypoxia during periods of hypoventilation. As a result, inspired oxygen concentrations should be obtained before periods of apnea.*

29.1.1.4 Gastrointestinal System

Several changes occur in the gastrointestinal system during pregnancy. Gallbladder emptying time increases during pregnancy, impacting patient's digestion and increases risk of gallstone formation. Alterations of hepatic function in a gravid patient include increased production of hormone-binding globulin and decreased albumin, impacting the pharmacokinetics of certain medications. Also of significance is the elevation of liver-dependent clotting factors, such as fibrinogen, and the liver's production of alkaline phosphatase, which can be elevated to a level two to four times that of the non-gravid women. Gastrointestinal changes during pregnancy are secondary to displacement of the stomach onto the spleen and liver by the growing uterus, leading to an increase in intragastric pressure. Additionally, increased amounts of progesterone during pregnancy inhibit motilin production leading to decreased lower esophageal sphincter tone. Hence, pyrosis (heartburn) occurs in 70% of all pregnant women; additionally doubling of gastric time occurs in comparison to non-gravid females [2, 3].

Given the elevated gastric pressure, lowered esophageal sphincter tone, and slowed gastric emptying in gravid patients, there is an increase in episodes of gastric reflux and regurgitation. Preventing aspiration of gastric contents during surgery on a gravid patient is a serious concern. Maternal death occurred in 10–25% of reported cases of aspiration; the more acidic the aspirate, the higher the risk. Antacid therapy was first proposed in 1946 to decrease morbidity from gastric aspiration. Particulate antacids (magnesium and aluminum hydroxide) were in use until 1979 when it was revealed that they did not prevent pulmonary edema and impaired oxygenation after aspiration [1]. More studies have shown that sodium citrate (30 mL) and Bicitra (citric acid and sodium citrate) (30 mL) are effective in buffering gastric contents to a pH greater than 2.5 in 88% of obstetric patients [1]. Research on the efficacy of H2 antagonist cimetidine and ranitidine was shown to decrease the pH of gastric secretions [1]. *No published studies show with hard evidence that antacids or histamine antagonists decrease maternal mortality from pulmonary aspiration* [1].

29.1.2 Anesthetic Risk

Studies of outcomes in large numbers of pregnant women who underwent surgery suggest no increase in congenital abnormalities but a great risk of spontanous abortion, growth restriction, and low birth weight. These studies revealed that complications resulted from the surgical procedure itself or the primary disease rather than exposure to anesthesia [4].

29.1.2.1 Local Anesthetics

Pregnancy increases nerve sensitivity to local anesthetics. A study conducted on pregnant and non-pregnant animal models noted the time required for 50% depression of action potential of A, B, and C vagal fibers after applying bupivacaine [1]. The onset time for conduction of blockade in each type of nerve fibers was significantly faster in gravid as opposed to non-gravid animals. Initial findings suggested a slowing of nerve conduction velocity in humans as pregnancy progresses [1, 4].

Local anesthetics cross the placental barrier freely, hence making fetal toxicity a concern. Several amide type agents are bound alpha acid glycoprotein; pregnancy reduces alpha acid glycoprotein levels, hence increasing free local anesthetic plasma concentration [1, 4]. This increases the risk for toxic reactions specifically with bupivacaine. *Generally, the direct effects of local anesthesia on the neonate are minimal, even at higher doses* [1]. Administration of benzocaine, procaine and tetracaine, and lidocaine during pregnancy did not result in an increased rate of fetal malformations according to The Collaborative Perinatal Project [1].

Traditionally, when local anesthetic is administered in oral and maxillofacial surgery, it is dispensed in 1:100,000 epinephrine concentration [1, 4]. This is an issue of concern in gravid patients because accidental intravascular injection of 15 μg epinephrine can cause vasoconstriction of the uterine artery and decrease uterine blood flow [1]. Studies on animal models revealed that this decrease in uterine blood flow is only transient [1].

29.1.2.2 General Anesthetics

When administering general anesthesia to a pregnant patient, there are three primary concerns: maintaining fetal oxygenation, avoidance of teratogenic agents, and prevention of premature labor. Fetal oxygenation is maintained by normal maternal $PaCo_2$, PaO_2, uterine vascular resistance, and maternal blood pressure. General anesthesia in a gravid patient can lead to rapid onset of hypoxemia; this can be averted by short-term administration of high levels of oxygen without risk to the fetus; studies have shown that with a maternal PaO_2 of 600 mm Hg, the fetal PaO_2 does not rise above 50–60 mm Hg [1, 4]. Therefore, there is no risk of premature closure of the ductus arteriosus secondary to increased maternal oxygen content.

Intraoperatively, maternal hypotension secondary to administration of inhaled agents can lead to fetal hypoxia. Therefore, general anesthetics should be sufficient to accommodate surgical stress without decreasing maternal blood pressure. If maternal hypotension does occur, treatment should include intravenous fluid administration, repositioning patient to the lateral position, decreasing anesthetic concentration, and using an indirect acting vasoconstriction like ephedrine to avoid uterine vasoconstriction.

Nitrous oxide is an inhaled general anesthetic agent commonly used in oral and maxillofacial surgery. The teratogenic potential of nitrous oxide lies in its ability to inactivate methionine synthetase which is responsible for converting homocysteine and methyltetrahydrofolate to methionine and tetrahydrofolate; methionine is imperative for DNA synthesis. Several studies regarding the impact of chronic exposure to nitrous oxide were conducted. A study following female dental assistants found that working with non-scavenged nitrous oxide for 3 or more hours per week increased risk of spontaneous abortion. Scavenging and ventilation methods may reduce this concern [1].

29.2 Preoperative Assessment

As is the case with any surgical patient, a thorough medical and surgical history must be sought. Documenting chronic illnesses, allergies, medications, and the reason behind seeking the procedure must be sought. Illnesses that may cause physiological decompensation during surgery such as angina, seizure disorders, or asthma must be noted. A preanesthetic evaluation should also be conducted as part of the preoperative workup. Laboratory testing and imaging should only be performed if they would offer any valuable clinical information. Additionally, conditions that affect the postoperative phase such as diabetes, for instance, must be addressed. Generally speaking, in gravid patients all elective procedures such as orthognathic and cosmetic should be postponed until postpartum. If pregnancy is suspected in a female patient, no oral surgical intervention should be conducted unless emergent. Documentation of a patient's pregnancy status by her primary care provider or obstetrician should be obtained before commencing treatment [1–3, 5].

29.2.1 Workup

29.2.1.1 Imaging

Imaging is imperative for many dental and oral surgical procedures; however, using radiography in a pregnant patient requires several precautions, and their usage should be kept to a minimum. *Animal and human studies revealed that more than 10 cGy total exposure to radiation or more than 5 cGy during the first trimester is related to intrauterine growth retardation and congenital fetal abnormalities. Therefore, radiography is discouraged during the first trimester* [1, 2]. However, it is important to note that a full-mouth radiographic examination exposes 0.0001 cGy, and an orthopantomogram delivers 0.008 cGy. Therefore, a minimal use of dental radiographs after the first trimester is acceptable for pregnant patients. In general, head and neck films using a lead shield pose minimum risk to the mother and fetus [1–3, 5].

CT is useful in determining deep-seated infections and is the modality of choice in viewing lateral pharyngeal infections. CT doses are higher in comparison to plain radiography but lower than multiple slices for polytomography. MRI may be an alternative to CT when considering fetal irradiation. MRI has greater soft tissue sensitivity compared with CTF2′ and therefore may help even more in difficult cases of infection. MRI uses magnetic field-assisted nuclear alignment in creating images and provides no ionizing radiation. However, the risks of fetal exposure to strong magnetic fields are not known [1–3].

29.2.1.2 OB/Gyn and Maternal-Fetal Medicine Consultation

It is imperative to obtain an obstetrics/gynecology consultation early for maternal-fetal monitoring and ultrasonography. A maternal-fetal medicine specialist is recommended particularly when a pregnant patient also has a concomitant complication of pregnancy (i.e., gestational diabetes, multiple gestation, preeclampsia, or an abnormality of the uteroplacental unit) [5].

29.2.2 Discuss Laboratory Tests and Anticipated Results and What Abnormal Results Indicate

- It is recommended to obtain a baseline platelet count, fibrinogen levels, partial thrombin time, partial thromboplastin time, and fibrinogen degradation product analysis to monitor for later signs of maternal coagulopathy [5].
- Serum chemistry → Mild respiratory alkalosis (pH 7.40–7.46) is expected in pregnant females. Additionally, serum bicarbonate values are between 18 and 22 mEq/L during pregnancy [1, 5, 6].
- Hemoglobin/hematocrit → Physiological anemia of pregnancy is expected. Here are acceptable H/H values per trimester. *First trimester (0–13 weeks)*, 11/33; *second trimester (14–26 weeks)*, 10.5/32; *third trimester (27–40 weeks)*, 11/33 [1–3, 5].
- Pulmonary function tests → Primarily done in patients with a history of asthma, COPD, or scoliosis regardless of pregnancy state [5].
- Chest radiograph → Traditionally done for non-gravid patients with history of smoking, COPD, and recent URI.
- ECG → Conducted in patients with cardiac disease, advance age, or respiratory diseases regardless of gestational status. [5, 6]

29.2.3 Steps to Optimize Patient: Preop Preparation

29.2.3.1 Nutrition and Hydration

There are increased nutritional and vitamin requirements in pregnancy that need to be accounted for during treatment of the pregnant patient. Maternal nutrition is of outmost importance during the third trimester since the fetus is accumulating glycogen and brown fat stores for postpartum survival. Maternal fluid requirements are also increased with gravid patients requiring an additional 30 mL per day. The surgeon needs to be aware of the initial demands of increased nutrition and fluids in the patient with a maxillofacial infection, along with the compounded demands of pregnancy. In the non-gravid patient, sensible and insensible fluid losses increase from 300 to 325 mL per degree centigrade of fever. Additionally, caloric requirements increase by 5–8% per degree of fever [1]. Gravid patients who need enteral feedings during a severe maxillofacial infection may not be able to tolerate the oral route due to hyperemesis gravidarum or intestinal malabsorptive problems. Parenteral nutrition may need to be considered in these cases. Appropriate consultation is crucial for complicated nutritional needs and situations [1–3, 6].

29.2.3.2 Empirical Antibiotics

Penicillins and cephalosporins are safe to use in gravid patients [1–3, 7]. On the other hand, tetracyclines and fluoroquinolones are to be avoided during pregnancy. Tetracyclines are known to cause discoloration of teeth. Fluoroquinolones have been shown to cause irreversible arthropathy. Like penicillins, clindamycin does cross the placenta, and there are no first trimester concerns with its use. However, caution should be exercised in the use of metronidazole in the pregnant patient, especially in the first trimester. Mutagenicity occurs in rodents but has thus far not been shown in humans [1, 7]. Antibiotics in the management of a gravid patient are discussed in further details in the postoperative complications section.

29.2.4 What Should Cancel Surgery? Discuss Risk Factors

Current guidelines suggest that pregnant patients should never be denied indicated surgery, regardless of trimester. However, it is recommended that all elective surgeries be postponed until postpartum [5]. Additionally, non-urgent surgeries should be done in the second trimester when preterm contractions and spontaneous abortions are least likely [5]. Any abnormal fetal tracing noted on monitoring or abnormal fetal heart rate should be grounds to cancel the procedure [5]. Additionally, if the mother is not physiologically stable for any reason, the procedure should be terminated.

29.3 Intraoperative Management

It is imperative to inform the patient's obstetric care providers of the surgery and involve them in the decision-making process. If the provider is not available at the institution where the surgery will be performed, another obstetrician must be involved. In general, if fetal monitoring will be used, the surgery should be conducted at a facility with neonatal and pediatric services. Additionally, the institution should have an obstetric care provider with cesarean delivery privileges available. Lastly, an individual should be available to interpret fetal heart rate patterns. Below are some factors to consider during intraoperative management of a gravid patient [2, 3, 5].

29.3.1 Effect of Anesthesia on Pregnancy

When administering general anesthesia to a pregnant patient, there are three primary concerns: maintaining fetal oxygenation, avoidance of teratogenic agents, and prevention of premature labor. Fetal oxygenation is maintained by normal maternal $PaCo_2$, PaO_2, uterine vascular resistance, and maternal blood pressure [1, 4]. General anesthesia in a gravid patient can lead to rapid onset of hypoxemia; this can be averted by short-term administration of high levels of oxygen without risk to the fetus; studies have shown that with a maternal PaO_2 of 600 mm Hg, the fetal PaO_2 does not rise above 50–60 mm Hg. Therefore, there is no risk of premature closure of the ductus arteriosus secondary to increased maternal oxygen content.

Intraoperatively, maternal hypotension secondary to administration of inhaled agents can lead to fetal hypoxia. Therefore, general anesthetics should be sufficient to accommodate surgical stress without decreasing maternal blood pressure. If maternal hypotension does occur, treatment includes intravenous fluid administration, repositioning patient to the lateral position, decreasing anesthetic concentration, and using an indirect acting vasoconstriction like ephedrine to avoid uterine vasoconstriction [1, 4].

Nitrous oxide is an inhaled general anesthetic agent commonly used in oral and maxillofacial surgery. The teratogenic potential of nitrous oxide lies in its ability to inactivate methionine synthetase which is responsible for converting homocysteine and methyltetrahydrofolate to methionine and tetrahydrofolate; methionine is imperative for DNA synthesis. Several studies regarding the impact of chronic exposure to nitrous oxide were conducted. A study following female dental assistants found that working with non-scavenged nitrous oxide for 3 or more hours per week increased risk of spontaneous abortion. Scavenging and ventilation methods may reduce this concern [1, 4].

29.3.2 What Anesthetic Medications to Use and Not to Use?

Generally speaking, no currently used anesthetic agents have been shown to have any teratogenic effects in humans when using standard concentrations at any gestational age. Lidocaine and other common local anesthetics as stated earlier are not associated with fetal malformations [1, 4]. However, there is a higher potential for local anesthetic toxicity secondary to an overdose to occur during pregnancy given the increased vascular volume and permeability. Controversy arises with the use of vasoconstrictors (i.e., epinephrine) given that it may lead to uteroplacental vasoconstriction with subsequent fetal hypoxia if administered intravascularly [1, 4]. Ultimately, the use of epinephrine is acceptable given that caution is used not to administer it intravascularly. Usage of nitrous oxide is also controversial considering its ability to inhibit methionine synthetase as mentioned above.

However, it is agreed upon that using nitrous oxide in a gravid patient is acceptable as long as it is less than 50% of the inhalant, with the other part being oxygen [1, 4]. Additionally, the patient must be given supplemental vitamins to replace methionine as a precaution [1].

29.3.3 Potential Problems

29.3.3.1 Maternal Hypotension

As stated earlier, *maternal hypotension* secondary to administration of inhaled agents can lead to fetal hypoxia. If maternal hypotension does occur, treatment includes intravenous fluid administration, repositioning patient to the lateral position, decreasing anesthetic concentration, and using an indirect acting vasoconstriction like ephedrine to avoid uterine vasoconstriction [1, 4].

29.3.3.2 Aspiration During Anesthetic Induction

As stated earlier there is an increased risk of aspiration in a gravid patient secondary to multiple gastrointestinal changes. To alleviate this risk, several regimens have been recommended. Cimetidine or ranitidine combined with metoclopramide can reduce gastric volume to less than 25 mL. Manchikanti suggests a regimen for emergency surgical patients of intravenous administration of either cimetidine (5 mg/kg) or ranitidine (1 mg/kg) with metoclopramide (0.2–0.3 mg/kg) given that sufficient time is available [1]. The addition of a nonparticulate antacid could buttress safety if given 10–30 min before induction [1]. In cases of loss of consciousness or where laryngeal reflexes are compromised, cricoid pressure (Sellick's maneuver) and rapid tracheal intubation are recommended [2, 3].

29.3.4 Monitoring

Fetal monitoring is of utmost importance while performing nonobstetric surgery on a pregnant patient. General guidelines for fetal monitoring entail the following:

- In a previable fetus (i.e., a fetus between 20 0/7 and 25 6/7 weeks of gestation), confirming fetal heart rate by a Doppler before and after the procedure is sufficient [5].
- If the fetus is considered viable, at minimum, electronic fetal heart rate and contraction monitoring must be performed before and after the procedure to confirm fetal viability and absence of contractions [5].
- Intraoperative electronic fetal monitoring is appropriate given all the following apply:
  - Fetus is viable.
  - Placing an intraoperative electronic fetal monitoring is physically possible.
  - A provider with obstetric surgery privileges is willing and available to intervene during the procedure if fetal complications arise.
  - The patient has given informed consent to an emergency cesarean delivery.
  - The nature of the procedure to be performed provides safe interruption or alteration to perform an emergency delivery.

In certain situations intraoperative fetal monitoring may be needed for previable fetuses to facilitate positioning or oxygenation interventions [5].

29.3.5 What Depth of Anesthesia Is Appropriate?

Thiopental and propofol induction agents commonly used during anesthesia are relatively safe in gravid patients. During pregnancy thiopental requires approximately 35% of the average dose used in non-gravid patients, and its half-life is prolonged. Sensitivity of propofol during pregnancy is not yet known; however, it is an effective induction agent during pregnancy with a more rapid recovery period than thiopental and unchanged half-life during pregnancy. The minimum alveolar concentration (MAC) of halogenated volatile anesthetics is decreased by 20–40%; their induction rates are increased during pregnancy [1, 4]. High doses of halogenated anesthetics with MAC greater than 2.0 potentially lead to maternal hypotension and in return fetal hypoxia. Low-to-moderate doses of MAC (0.5–1.0), supplemented with intravenous narcotics such as fentanyl in doses of 50–100 pg, are shown to have no deleterious effects on the fetus or placenta [1, 4]. Commonly known halogenated agents such as halothane, isoflurane, enflurane, and desflurane are all considered safe during pregnancy assuming they are used in appropriate doses [1, 4]. Furthermore, no data indicates the teratogenic potential of halogenated agents [1].

29.3.6 Airway Management

As in non-gravid patients, airway assessment entails an evaluation of tongue mobility, floor of mouth swelling, deviation of the uvula, and lateral pharyngeal swelling. Endotracheal intubation using a 6.5 mm endotracheal or a surgical airway is established before commencing the procedure [4]. Airway management by a face mask, a laryngeal mask, or tracheal intubation may not be feasible during pregnancy secondary to increased anteroposterior chest wall diameter, breast enlargement, laryngeal edema, and weight gain affecting soft tissues of the neck [2–4]. With the increased risk of airway obstruction in gravid patients, it is imperative not to oversedate them; they are safely intubated either by blind nasal intubation or fiber optic-assisted intubation while seated and awake. The patient should be adequately preoxygenated because it is especially important to avoid maternal hypoxia [4].

29.4 Postoperative Management

29.4.1 Pain Management

29.4.1.1 Opioids

These agents include morphine-like agonists (e.g., morphine, hydromorphone, hydrocodone, codeine, and oxycodone), meperidine-like agonists, and synthetic opioid analogues (e.g., tramadol). Reproductive studies describing the use of narcotic analgesics in human pregnancies are limited, and there are no prospective, comparative studies. However, these drugs have been used in therapeutic doses by pregnant women for many years and have not been linked to elevated risk of major or minor malformations. The Collaborative Perinatal Project identified 448 morphine exposures at various stages of pregnancy and found no evidence of increased teratogenic effects [8].

Codeine is associated with fetal toxicity below maternal toxic doses in mice and hamster models leading to decreased fetal body weight. Codeine did not lead to any increases in structural changes in mice. In humans, no effects of maternal codeine intake during pregnancy were observed on infant survival or congenital malformations rate; however, the association with acute cesarean delivery and postpartum hemorrhage may justify a certain level of caution when administering codeine toward the end of pregnancy [9].

Meperidine and morphine are both safe when administered for anesthesia and analgesia for short periods of time. Chronic use has been shown to cause fetal growth retardation and neonatal withdrawal [1].

Nonsteroidal anti-inflammatory drugs (NSAIDs) inhibit prostaglandin synthesis which could potentially lead to premature closure of the fetal ductus arteriosus, inducing fetal pulmonary hypertension and fetal bleeding tendencies. *Therefore, pregnant women are discouraged from using analgesic doses of aspirin and other NSAIDs and encouraged to use acetaminophen instead* [1]. Studies have shown bleeding tendencies in infants whose mothers had ingested 5–10 g of aspirin 5 days before delivery; bleeding tendencies did not occur if the aspirin was consumed 6 days before delivery. A plethora of cases documented closure of ductus arteriosus secondary to the usage of indomethacin for tocolysis purposes. It is important to note that ibuprofen, the most widely used NSAID, had no published reports linking its use with congenital defects. *Cyclooxygenase (COX-2) inhibitors (celecoxib and rofecoxib) are to be avoided in pregnancy based on animal studies* [1].

29.5 Postoperative Complications

29.5.1 Infections

Postoperative maxillofacial infection in a gravid patient must be addressed immediately. Pregnant patients are more likely to develop infections for various reasons [10]. As stated earlier, hormonal changes make the mucosa in pregnant women dry, hence allowing chronic gingivitis to easily develop. Moreover, there is a mild immunosuppression which takes place during pregnancy. Management of mild infections entails incision/drainage under a local anesthetic followed by antibiotic coverage. Gravid patients must be treated aggressively to reduce the risk of infection to the fascial spaces. In cases of fascial spaces infections, airway assessment (if in doubt intubate), imaging (CT scan), and adequate incision and drainage in the operating room must be done. Empirical penicillin therapy is appropriate until culture/sensitivity results are available. Severe infections may require management in the operating room using general anesthesia with IV antibiotics and incision and drainage.

Choosing the appropriate antibiotic to treat infections in a gravid patient is of utmost importance given the teratogenic potential of certain classes of antibiotics. In general, studies have shown that there is no increase in congenital anomalies after exposure to penicillin in the first trimester. *Penicillin is the antibiotic of choice for treatment of oral infections in pregnant patients.* In cases of gravid patients with allergies to penicillin, certain macrolides such as erythromycin and clindamycin are used extensively; all macrolides are classified as class B, with the exception of clarithromycin which is class C by the FDA. Quinolones are associated with irreversible arthropathy and cartilage erosion in fetuses of multiple animal species. Hence, fluoroquinolones are not recommended to treat oral infections in gravid patients. Tetracyclines are to be avoided in pregnant patients and children up to 12 years old, given their risk of permanent dental staining.

Metronidazole, an antianaerobic antibiotic previously thought to be carcinogenic, is now justified for serious oral and maxillofacial infections in gravid patients. A study conducted on 17,000 fetuses exposed to metronidazole in the first trimester revealed no increase in rate of congenital anomalies. Another analysis revealed no increase in teratogenic risk with the use of metronidazole.

29.5.2 Deep Venous Thrombosis (DVT) and Pulmonary Embolism (PE)

In non-gravid surgical patients, DVT is a serious concern given the lack of mobility in the postoperative phase. However, as discussed earlier, decreased venous flow and increased levels of certain clotting factors during pregnancy further increase the chances of thromboembolism. As far as DVT/PE prophylaxis, it is advised that the supine position be avoided, if possible, and support stockings, a pneumatic compression device, or subcutaneous prophylactic heparin be applied. As mentioned previously, *the current regimen for subcutaneous heparin application is 5000 U twice a day in the first trimester, 7500 U twice a day in the second trimester, and 10,000 U twice a day in the third trimester. For gravid patients with a history of a previous thromboembolic event, heparin 5000 U is recommended every 12 h or heparin adjusted to level of 0.1–0.2 IU/mL or clinical surveillance with periodic surveillance ultrasonography or Coumadin prophylaxis postpartum for 4–6 weeks. Sequential pneumatic compression devices can be used concurrently* [1].

Pulmonary embolism is a leading cause of maternal mortality. Correct diagnosis of DVT and instituting heparin treatment decreased the incidence of PE by 320%, hence leading to a decrease in maternal mortality by almost 18-fold. Symptoms of DVT include pain, tenderness, swelling, edema, changes of limb color, a palpable cord, a positive Homan's sign, and a positive Lowenberg test (pain occuring distal to a blood pressure cuff rapidly inflated to 180 mm Hg) [2, 3]. Clinical diagnosis of DVT is difficult; in many cases, PE may occur in the absence of clinical symptoms. The first step in confirming the diagnosis of DVT is conducting real-time ultrasonographic imaging, using duplex Doppler as well as continuous wave Doppler, which provides valuable information. However, in pregnancy the iliac vessels are very hard to image due to pressure from the gravid uterus on the inferior vena cava. Therefore, venography is the diagnostic mainstay of DVT in pregnancy. Radiation exposure to the fetus is believed to be 0.0314 rad for unilateral venography, including fluoroscopy and spot films without an abdominal shield. This is below the minimum level of radiation exposure considered teratogenic [2, 3].

29.5.3 Pulmonary Edema and Adult Respiratory Distress Syndrome

The cardiorespiratory and hematologic alterations of pregnancy, as mentioned earlier, place the patient at a higher risk for developing pulmonary edema and adult respiratory distress syndrome (ARDS). Noncardiogenic pulmonary edema has multiple etiologies in a pregnant patient including aspiration, pneumonia, sepsis, blood transfusion reactions, amniotic fluid embolus syndrome, and disseminated intravascular coagulation. Clinical symptoms of pulmonary edema include tachypnea, dyspnea, tachycardia, wet rales, cardiomegaly, hypoxemia, and infiltrates on the chest radiograph. Pulmonary edema is an obstetric emergency which necessitates immediate treatment. The purpose of therapy regardless of the mechanism of pulmonary edema is to alleviate symptoms, maintain systemic arterial oxygenation, and decrease the total pressure causing liquid filtration. Initial treatment of pulmonary edema entails elevating the head of the patient's bed 45 degrees to decrease venous return to the lungs and improve breathing [2]. Supplemental oxygen should be administered to maintain maternal PaO_2 in excess of 60 mm Hg; this is imperative for maintenance of uteroplacental perfusion. Sufficient fetal oxygenation will occur if the maternal hemoglobin is greater than 10 g/dL and the maternal PaO_2 is greater than 60 mm Hg. Morphine sulfate decreases left atrial pressures, maternal catecholamines, and anxiety [1–3]. A furosemide dose of 20–40 mg intravenously will promote fluid removal in patients with pulmonary edema; however, providers should be aware that a large initial dose can produce marked maternal hypotension [1]. Ventilatory support and intubation are imperative in patients unresponsive to clinical measures and have PaO_2 less than 60 mm Hg or $PaCO_2$ greater than 45 mm Hg on room air or PaO_2 less than 70 mm Hg and a $PaCO_2$ greater than 55 mm Hg on 40% venti-mask. Positive end-expiratory pressure (PEEP) improves maternal oxygenation, decreases venous return, and counteracts pulmonary hydrostatic pressure. Continuous electronic fetal heart rate monitoring is recommended, and, if possible, delivery should be avoided until the pregnant woman has been stabilized [2, 3]. The mortality rate is 50%–90% in ARDS regardless of maximum treatment. Therapy for ARDS is supportive. The gravid patient requires adequate fluid to maintain intravascular volume to support blood pressure and to preserve renal function. The pulmonary artery catheter is a usual part of monitoring of pregnant women with ARDS; mechanical ventilation is crucial in supportive care for patients with ARDS. PEEP is useful for opening collapsed alveoli disease in ARDS. The goal of the therapy in ARDS is to use fractional inspired oxygen of less than 0.5 atm to maintain a SaO_2 of greater than 90% or a PaO_2 of greater than 60 mm Hg to prevent oxygen toxicity. Most clinicians recommend a PEEP level of 15–20 mm Hg to minimize FiO_2 and maintain a PaO_2 greater than 60 mm Hg [2, 3].

29.6 Maxillofacial and Oral Surgery Management in Postpartum Patients

Management of postpartum patients does not vary much from management of non-gravid patients. Special attention must be paid to the choice of anesthesia and analgesia if the mother is breastfeeding given the ability of some analgesia and anesthetic agents to pass through breast milk. Any elective surgery can be performed immediately postpartum especially that most elective cases will be delayed during a low-risk pregnancy until the postpartum period to avoid the risks on the mother and child [11]. However, any high-risk condition complicating the pregnancy must be taken into consideration in the postpartum period too before proceeding with surgery such as hypercoagulable state, hypertension, HELLP syndrome, and eclampsia; in these cases elective surgery should be delayed for at least a period of 12 weeks [12].

29.6.1 Postpartum Anesthesia

Drugs used for anesthetic induction such as propofol, midazolam, etomidate, or thiopental are present in the milk compartment only minimally since they have extraordinarily brief plasma distribution phases (only minutes); therefore, their transport to milk is low to nil. Literature is scant regarding the use of anesthetic gases in breastfeeding mothers. However, they also have brief plasma distribution phases, and their levels in breast milk are likely nil. A recent series of case reports suggests that xenon maintenance after propofol induction is allowed for breastfeeding immediately after surgery. The use of ketamine in breastfeeding mothers has not been reported. Local anesthetics are poorly absorbed orally, as such they should be safe in postpartum breastfeeding mothers. Milk levels of bupivacaine and ropivacaine are exceedingly low [13].

29.6.2 Postpartum Analgesics

29.6.2.1 Non-opioid Analgesics

Non-opioid analgesics should generally be the first choice for pain management in breastfeeding postpartum women since they do not impact maternal or infant consciousness. *Acetaminophen/paracetamol and ibuprofen are safe and effective for analgesia in postpartum mothers* [13]. Ketorolac is commonly used for postpartum analgesia, especially after cesarean section, despite a Food and Drug Administration black box warning against its use in breastfeeding women; studies have shown that ketorolac levels are low in breast milk after oral administration; however, the study did not take into consideration levels after parenteral administration [13]. Cyclooxygenase-2 inhibitors such as celecoxib may have some theoretical advantages if maternal bleeding is a concern; this must be balanced with higher cost and potential cardiovascular risks, which are minimal with short-term use in healthy young women [13]. Naproxen passage into milk is low, but gastrointestinal disturbances have been found in some infants following prolonged therapy. Therefore, short-term use (1 week) is probably safe [13].

29.6.2.2 Opioid Analgesics

Morphine is considered an ideal analgesic for breastfeeding mothers because of its limited transport to milk and poor oral bioavailability in infants. On the other hand, levels of meperidine/pethidine into breastmilk are low (1.7–3.5% of maternal weight-adjusted 550 dose). However, meperidine/pethidine and its metabolite (normeperidine) are associated with dose-related neonatal sedation; presence in milk and neonatal sedation have been present for up to 36 hours after a single dose [13]. *Therefore, they should be avoided in postpartum analgesia.* Infants of mothers who have been exposed to repeated doses of meperidine/pethidine should be closely monitored for sedation, cyanosis, bradycardia, and possibly seizures. Hydrocodone has been used frequently in breastfeeding mothers; there are some cases of neonatal sedation that have been documented, but these are rare and usually dose related. Doses of hydrocodone in breastfeeding mothers should be kept at the minimum necessary to control pain; it is important to note that frequent dosing throughout the day may lead to sedative effects in the breastfed infant [13].

The American Academy of Pediatrics recommends that other agents are preferred over codeine during breastfeeding [13]. Both the European Medicine Agency and the UK's Medicines and Healthcare Products Regulatory Agency recommend that codeine not be used in nursing mothers. Several small series suggest that codeine may be contributory to episodes of apnea, bradycardia, and cyanosis in the first week of life [13]. In addition, the reported neonatal death of a breastfed infant due to respiratory depression following the use of codeine in a mother who was found to be a CYP450 2D6 ultrarapid metabolizer (wherein levels of morphine following the use of codeine may be significantly elevated) suggests that the use of codeine in breastfeeding mothers should be monitored closely [13].

Oxycodone is not significantly safer for the rare mother who is a rapid metabolizer, as it is also a substrate for CYP2D6. A recent retrospective study showed that one in five breastfed infants with mothers medicated with oxycodone experienced central nervous system depression. The strong concordance between maternal and infant symptoms may be used to identify babies at higher risk. It is important to follow these infants carefully for drowsiness [14].

Accordingly, it is best to provide pain control with nonnarcotic analgesics; and if codeine-containing drugs are to be prescribed, it is recommended that maternal intake of oral codeine be limited to 4 days at a low dose with close infant monitoring. If the baby shows signs of increased sleepiness, difficult breastfeeding, breathing difficulties, or floppiness, medical care should be sought immediately [15, 16].

Conclusion

Perioperative management of the pregnant, postpartum, and lactating patient requires appropriate assessment and modification in delivered care. Proper knowledge and understanding of the situation allows the surgeon to optimize care of both patient and child during the perioperative period. Consultation with the patient's obstetrician or pediatrician may be indicated.

References

1. Dellinger TM, Mark Livingston H. Pregnancy: physiologic changes and considerations for dental patients. Dent Clin N Am. 2006;50(4):677–97.
2. Flynn TR, Susarla SM. Oral and maxillofacial surgery for the pregnant patient. Oral Maxillofac Surg Clin North Am. 2007;19(2):207–21.
3. Turner M, Aziz SR. Management of the pregnant oral and maxillofacial surgery patient. J Oral Maxillofac Surg. 2002;60(12):1479–88.
4. Walton NKD, Melachuri VK. Anaesthesia for non-obstetric surgery during pregnancy. Cont Educ Anaesth Crit Care Pain. 2006;6:83–5.
5. American College of Obstetricians and Gynecologists. Committee opinion no. 474: nonobstetric surgery during pregnancy. Obstet Gynecol. 2011;117:420–1.
6. Petranker S, Nikoyan L, Ogle OE. Preoperative evaluation of the surgical patient. Dent Clin North Am. 2012;56(1):163–81.
7. Steinberg BJ, et al. Oral health and dental care during pregnancy. Dent Clin N Am. 2013;57(2):195–210.
8. Heinonen OP, Slone D, Shapiro S. Birth defects and drugs in pregnancy. Littleton, MA: Publishing Sciences Group; 1977.
9. Nezvalová-Henriksen K, Spigset O, Nordeng H. Effects of codeine on pregnancy outcome: results from a large population-based cohort study. Eur J Clin Pharmacol. 2011;67(12):1253–1261. Published online 2011 Jun 9. https://doi.org/10.1007/s00228-011-1069-5.
10. Lawrenz DR, Whitley BD, Helfrick JF. Considerations in the management of maxillofacial infections in the pregnant patient. J Oral Maxillofac Surg. 1996;54(4):474–85.
11. Banu K, Srikanth G. Ludwig's angina in postpartum patient. J Maxillofac Oral Surg. 2014;13:208.
12. Jamadarkhana S, Law R. Seizures in the early postpartum period: a diagnostic dilemma. Indian J Anaesth. 2012;56(2):183.
13. Montgomery A, Hale TW, Academy of Breastfeeding Medicine. ABM clinical protocol# 15: analgesia and anesthesia for the breastfeeding mother, revised 2012. Breastfeed Med. 2012;7(6):547–53.
14. Sachs HC, the American Academy of Pediatrics committee on Drugs. The transfer of drugs and therapeutics into human breast milk: an update on selected topics. Pediatrics. 2013;132:e796–809. PMID: 23979084
15. United States National Library of Medicine. Toxnet. Toxicology data network. http://toxnet.nlm.nih.gov/cgi-bin/sis/htmlgen?LACT. Accessed 2013.
16. Therapeutic Goods Administration. Codeine use in children and ultra-rapid metabolisers. Pharmacovigilance and special access branch safety review. https://www.tga.gov.au/sites/default/files/codeine-use-children-and-ultra-rapid-metabolisers.pdf. Accessed Oct 2015.

Check for updates

Perioperative Management of Head and Neck Burns

30

Roselle E. Crombie and Amit Sood

Abstract

Burn injury is a devastating, life changing event that can forever change a patient's life. The injury can involve significant trauma, associated injuries, disfigurement, and psychological consequences. Care of this special patient population requires a multispecialty approach. This chapter will discuss the pathophysiology as well as burn classification. There will be a focused discussion on the surgical and supportive management of these complex patients.

30.1 Introduction

Burn injury is a devastating, life-changing event that can forever change a patient's life. The injury can involve significant trauma, associated injuries, disfigurement, and psychological consequences. Care of this special patient population is fraught with unique challenges in the initial phase as well as the long-term stable phase due to the injuries and ongoing scar contractures.

R.E. Crombie, M.D. (✉)
General Surgery, Hyperbaric Medicine, Surgical Critical Care, Bridgeport Hospital, Bridgeport, CT, USA
e-mail: Roselle.Crombie@bpthosp.org

A. Sood, D.M.D., M.D.
Division of Oral and Maxillofacial Surgery, School of Dental Medicine, University of Connecticut, Farmington, CT, USA

30.2 Burn Classification

Burn injury has been classified based on depth of the burn, and a basic understanding of the mechanisms and severity of burns can be extremely helpful in managing the care. These classifications apply to all burns, but given the relative thinness of the skin in regions of the head and neck, it is important to understand all types of burn degrees given that a relatively small amount of energy can denote a quicker deeper burn.

First-degree burn involves the most superficial injury to the epidermis of the skin. It is characterized by redness, pain, and is akin to the sunburn that many of us have experienced in our childhood. Burns to this depth are well tolerated and heal with virtually no scar in the time period for regular skin regeneration [1–3].

Second-degree burn involves injury to the epidermis and some portion of the next deeper layer of the skin, the dermis. The dermis houses the

© Springer International Publishing AG 2018

E.M. Ferneini, J.D. Bennett (eds.), *Perioperative Assessment of the Maxillofacial Surgery Patient*,
https://doi.org/10.1007/978-3-319-58868-1_30

key rete ridges of the skin which serve as the germinal centers for skin cells and the immune cells of the skin called the Langerhans cells. Here you can find the ever important hair follicle which is a specialized skin organ. Not only does the hair follicle produce its keratin outgrowth which is key to homeostasis, but it also houses the sweat glands that are responsible for maintaining the skin environment and health. Second-degree burn injury can have significant challenges depending on how deep into the dermis it falls [1–3]. Generally, the injuries are divided into superficial partial thickness (superficial second-degree burns) and deep partial thickness (deep second-degree burns). The former is more favorable as many of the dermal elements are preserved, so the ability to regenerate with minimal scar is attained [1–3]. The latter is more devastating and has similar characteristics to the third-degree burn (discussed below). Damage to the deeper layer of the dermis requires some thought into its management given its delayed ability to heal and wound closure is done mostly by scar formation [1–3].

Third-degree burn and beyond are among the most devastating of all the burn depths (Fig. 30.1). In this injury, there is no remnant of the dermis or regenerative elements of the skin present. Given the intense heat that causes this injury, there is often damage to the underlying subcutaneous fat noted with thrombosed vessels. Repair of this injury not only involves debridement down to healthy fat with brisk bleeding but will also require some type of skin graft for wound closure. Depending on the location of the third-degree burns particularly those with little underlying subcutaneous fat over muscle fascia, joints, or exposed cartilage, these areas may require grafting with dermal substitutes to facilitate underlying function and movement [1, 3].

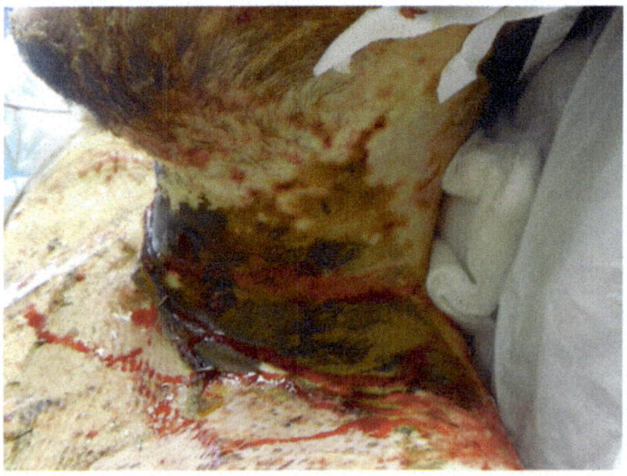

Fig. 30.1 Third-degree neck burn

Fourth-degree burn typically involves deeper tendon and bone. Given the tremendous destruction in this situation, debridement to healthy remnant of bone or complete resection of the tissue is often what is required. Complex reconstruction by plastic surgery is likely to be of help at this depth of burn [1, 3].

Severity of burns is graded both in the depth of burns (first, second, third, and fourth) as well as the total body surface area (TBSA) of burns. TBSA is measured to only include second-degree burn and deeper [1, 4, 5].

30.3 Airway Management

Diagnosing inhalation damage without delay is crucial in the prognosis of patients who have been exposed to fire or smoke. The initial assessment of the airway should consider the total body surface area injured, patient's age, past medical history, level of consciousness, and time since injury. The physical exam should include assessing the patient for the presence of facial burns, carbonaceous sputum, soot in mouth/nose/larynx, wheezing, and use of accessory muscles as these findings are suggestive of inhalational injury [1, 2, 6–9]. Fiber optic bronchoscopy is often employed to directly visualize the upper airway and is considered gold standard by some authors. A fiber optic bronchoscopy can be falsely negative if performed within the first several hours after injury, and therefore repeat bronchoscopy needs to be performed 24–48 h after injury [10–13]. Endotracheal intubation should be performed at the first signs of laryngeal injury as any delay could lead to significant laryngeal edema which will make intubation extremely difficult, possibly leading to emergent cricothyrotomy or tracheostomy. Another benefit of early intubation is the ability to place a larger diameter endotracheal tube prior to the development of airway edema. A larger ETT decreases airway pressures and allows for improved pulmonary hygiene. In the case of mild inhalation injury in which ETT placement is not indicated, the use of racemic epinephrine can be used to bronchodilate the upper airway and decrease stridor and potentially avoid an advanced airway [1, 7, 9–11, 14, 15].

Carbon monoxide is a toxic gas that can complicate the management of patients with burn injuries and smoke inhalation. Carbon monoxide is produced by the partial combustion of carbon-containing compounds such as wood, paper, coal, charcoal, methane, butane, propane, and petroleum products. It is a colorless and odorless gas and therefore difficult for individuals to detect. Carbon monoxide binds to hemoglobin to form carboxyhemoglobin and has an affinity for hemoglobin over 200 times that of oxygen [1, 6, 7, 10]. It also impairs mitochondrial function and causes brain injury through oxidative free radicals and inflammation. The central nervous system and cardiovascular system are most susceptible to carbon monoxide poisoning due to their sensitivity to hypoxia. To diagnose carbon monoxide poisoning, arterial COHb levels using a co-oximeter must be obtained. The partial pressure of oxygen (PaO_2) in arterial blood does not change in CO poisoning and therefore cannot be utilized for a diagnosis [1, 2, 6, 8–10]. Treatment of CO poisoning is 100% oxygen administered via nonrebreather mask or endotracheal tube until the COHb level is below 5–10%. There is controversy over the use of hyperbaric oxygen therapy to treat CO poisoning and to prevent delayed neurocognitive syndrome that presents 2–28 days postexposure; however the studies are inconclusive [1, 16].

Thermal or chemical injury to the airway causes the ciliary epithelium to become detached from its underlying basal membrane [1, 7]. The complement cascade is initiated which in turn leads to histamine release and subsequent development of oxygen free radicals [8, 17]. Oxygen free radicals can induce cells to undergo apoptosis but also can lead to recruitment of leukocytes to the affected region. This recruitment results in vasodilation and increased permeability and causes further influx of monocytes, macrophages, and polymorphonuclear neutrophils all which produces significant edema and damage to lung tissue which disrupts gas exchange [1, 7, 17]. Due to this significant edema and cellular damage, finding the right type of mechanical ventilation can be challenging. New studies have shown volume diffuse respirations (VDR) to be superior to both pressure control ventilation (PCV) and synchronized intermittent mechanical ventilation (SIMV) when concerning severe burn patients in both pediatric and adult populations. VDR is a high-frequency time-cycled pressure ventilator that can ventilate and oxygenate all while promoting airway secretion removal. VDR provides ventilation at lower peak airway pressures than those of SIMV and PCV [15, 16, 18, 19].

30.4 Fluid Management

Managing fluid resuscitation after burn injury is imperative 24–48 h after injury [6, 7]. Determining the appropriate fluid replacement by using standard formulas and algorithms is necessary to prevent under resuscitation which could lead to hemodynamic compromise but also to avoid over-resuscitation which could cause abdominal compartment syndrome which carries a high mortality rate. Due to these serious complications, hourly attention to urine output and hemodynamics are necessary [20–22].

To determine the amount and rate of fluid needed, it is first necessary to determine the total body surface area (TBSA) of the burn. The "rule of nines" in some studies has shown to overestimate volume resuscitation by as much as twofold, so alternative methods can be employed such as the Lund-Browder chart or "rule of hands," in which the patient's own hand represents 1% TBSA [20, 22, 23]. Lactate ringers are typically used because they are resuscitative fluid, given their ability to largely remain intravascular. The consensus from the American Burn Association is that anywhere from 2 to 4 mL*kg*TBSA should be given [3, 20, 22, 23]. This formula determines the total resuscitation for the first 24 h in which half is given over the first 8 h and the remaining over the next 16 h. For example, a 90-kg male with 30%TBSA will require a total of 10,800 mL (using Parkland formula) over 24 h of lactate ringers with 5400 mL given over the first 8 h and the remaining 5400 mL given over the last 16 h [20, 22, 23]. For pediatric, patients weighing less than 40 kg, the modified Brooke formula is 3 mL*kg*TBSA. Once the first 24 h of resuscitation have been provided, it is important to monitor and titrate fluid resuscitation. The most reliable measure of adequate resuscitation is urine output which should be 30–50 mL/h in adults and 0.5–1 mL/kg/h in pediatric population [20, 22–24].

In order to facilitate delivery of fluids, two large-bore intravenous catheters (18 gauge) should be placed, ideally in the antecubital fossa bilaterally, in the field or in the trauma bay. If intravenous access cannot be gained, intraosseous access must be sought. Once the patient arrives to the hospital, trained professionals should obtain central venous access. A central line is a tube that is passed through a vein and terminates in the thoracic portion of the vena cava (superior or inferior) [2, 7, 10]. Central venous access has several uses such as it allows monitoring of central venous pressure, pulmonary artery pressure, and pulmonary capillary wedge pressure. It can be used to deliver large amounts of fluid or blood products rapidly, deliver medications that affect the heart, and receive kidney dialysis for those patients with kidney failure [2, 3, 7, 10]. A central line can be placed via the neck (internal jugular vein), chest (subclavian or axillary vein), and groin (femoral vein). A Foley urethral catheter should be placed to obtain accurate hourly urine output to assess appropriate fluid resuscitation. Basic hemodynamic monitors should also be applied, either in the field or in the trauma bay such as pulse oximeter, EKG leads, and blood pressure cuff. If blood pressure cuff cannot be used, an arterial line should be obtained through the radial artery to give up-to-date blood pressure readings [2, 3, 7, 10].

30.5 Management of Neck Burns

Management of the burn patient may occur in phases. The surgeon may take the patient to surgery multiple times depending on the location and depth of burns as well as other physiologic demands [4, 5].

The 24–48-h resuscitation of a large burn (>20 TBSA) will illustrate how the tissues can change dramatically in this time period. When managing a large burn, the time point of maximal anasarca in the tissues is around the 48-h mark. Concurrently, it is also important to understand that it may take 48–72 h for the second-degree burn to declare itself as to whether it will be able to repair itself without surgical intervention or if it will convert to a deeper third-degree burn [1, 4, 7]. Given these two factors, with the exception of an emergent tracheostomy, there is no need to do immediate surgical intervention. The advantage in expectant management is allowing the wound to heal or fully declare itself and then have a true understanding of what clearly needs grafting versus what will be able to heal (Fig. 30.2). Although, in different areas of the body, allowing the second-degree burn to heal is prudent management, this may not be the best course of management in the neck region. Recall that healing of the skin is done by a combination of laying down scar as well as contracture. At the basic cell level, the key player is the fibroblast which lays down type I and type III collagen in combination with the elastin fibers that through a very complex process close the wound. Depending on how large the area of the neck burned, allowing the wound to scar down exclusively can have devastating functional and cosmetic consequences [1, 4, 7].

The neck region is truly a complex joint which needs for full range of motion. Key basic functions include eating, talking, breathing, etc. Some individuals depending on the flexibility of their neck joints can often achieve greater than 180 degrees of range of rotational motion from shoulder to shoulder, 0–180 degrees of forward flexion, and similar ranges for flexion. The goal as the surgeon

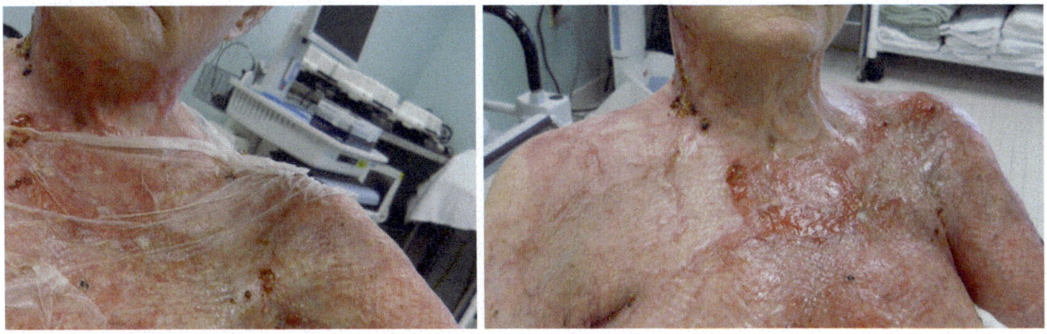

Fig. 30.2 Note scar band contractures at the neck in sections allowed to heal and at adjacent graft seams

is to help the patient achieve their maximal pre-injury range of motion functionally. Initial care of the patient should involve (after the C-spine has been cleared) an evaluation of the complete range of motion. If the initial exam is done closer to the 48-h mark in the large-burn patient, this may not be accurate based on the amount of swelling [1, 2, 7]. Additionally, the role of occupational therapy (OT) intervention immediately can be very helpful to maintain as much range of motion as possible. The therapy team should be involved as soon as possible to manage the areas of tightness due to the burn on the patient.

Deciding whether and when to operate on a neck burn is complex. Some scenarios are clear-cut where others are more based on the surgeon's judgment. The decision to operate should include the depth of the burn, cosmetics, and the surgeon's evaluation of the range of motion. In one scenario, if the initial evaluation demonstrates third- or fourth-degree burn, then the patient clearly needs excision and grafting [4, 5, 25]. If after the 48–72-h time point, the hallmarks of the second-degree burn (blanching, pain) are gone and replaced with a deeper second-degree or non-compliant third-degree tissue, then the surgeon should consider excision and grafting. If the surgeon recognizes pink well-perfused areas in the burn wounds, then it is possible that the neck will heal with a reasonable functional and cosmetic result. Also note that variegated areas of burns with intermixed first-, second-, and third-degree burns may have a reasonable result with expectant management if the third-degree burns are surrounded by mostly areas of first- and second-degree burns [4, 5, 25].

30.6 Burn Excision

30.6.1 Timing

If the patient needs operative intervention, there are a few things to consider and discuss. Timing of the excision should be done when the patient is through the initial resuscitation and much more stable. Given how sick some of these patients can be, it is in general not ideal to head to surgery if they are still on vasopressors. Perfusion to the skin organ should be considered seriously given that the depth of the excision will depend on what the surgeon sees in the operating room (OR) [4, 6, 7, 10].

30.6.2 Positioning

The surgeon should consider that he/she may need to excise the neck in multiple phases depending on the location and health of the wound bed. Ideally, the surgeon can start with the patient in the supine position but know that he/she will not have access to the posterior neck and may have limited access to the lateral neck. The patient should be placed on a beanbag for lateral positioning in the OR if the surgeon is planning on excision of a lateral burn. Axillary rolls are needed for the patient and plan on the operating surgeon to be present for the intubation so you can guide anesthesia as to where the ET tube should lie.

30.6.3 Consent for Operation

Because most of the intraoperative decision to excise, depth of excision, and type of grafting depend on what the surgeon sees with the patient anesthetized, it is prudent to include in the consent excision, grafting, and mention both a temporary graft and autograft in terms of wound coverage. Temporary grafts include both xenograft and allograft. It is important to note that a xenograft (different species) is derived from porcine dermis where an allograft (homograft or same species) is derived from donated cadaver skin. Xenograft is used more for a biologic dressing placed over superficial second-degree burns. Allograft is often used as a bridge to autograft (skin taken from the patient) to allow the wound bed to heal and grow granulation tissue (Fig. 30.3). Explaining all possibilities to patients is important for their understanding as well as highlighting any allergy or religious contraindications they may have to any of these options. Additionally, given the fact that amount of bleeding is considered in the operative management of burns, it is important not to underestimate the amount of blood loss with burns in a typical operation. Type and cross for surgery is best to have on hand prior to entering the operating room [4, 5].

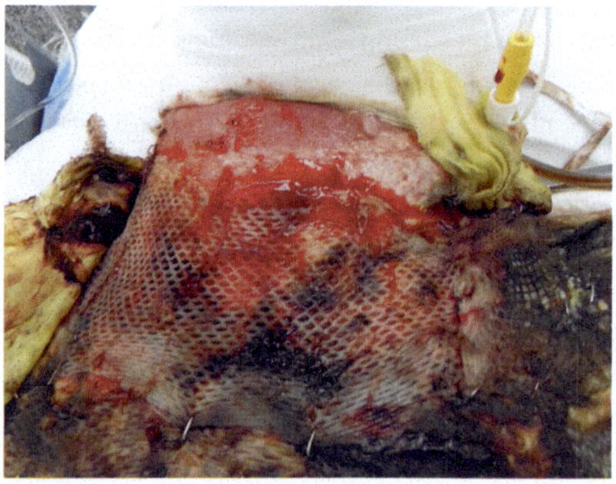

Fig. 30.3 Acute burn of the neck with allograft applied

30.6.4 Excision

After the patient is anesthetized and properly positioned, burn excision proceeds with multiple different tools. The goal is to get to a depth of punctate bleeding signifying healthy wound bed that can either repair if there is still some reticular dermis or is ready for autografting. In a superficial first- or second-degree burn, lap sponges, Dobie sponge (similar to a sterile dish sponge), or periosteal elevators can be used to debride away the overlying fibrin crust or superficial eschar. If superficial debridement reveals a healthy bleeding bed with punctate bleeding, then there is no need to excise to a greater depth. On the contrary, if the wound bed still appears pale, then deeper excision is necessary [4, 5].

Second- and third-degree burns are usually approached with a Weck or Goulian blade. This blade was designed to have tangential excision along to dermis to preserve as much reticular dermis as possible. Starting with a light pass of the blade is always wise with the goal also to get down to punctate bleeding. If only some bleeding is noted, it either needs to be excised further or the surgeon may consider placing temporary allograft to allow the area to heal and excise at a later date [4, 5]. The finer points of surgical decision-making come with experience, but maximal preservation of dermis is a key goal. Even with a thin-layer dermis, patients will have better range of motion and less contracture in the long run.

If the surgeon encounters a third-degree burn, then he/she can consider two options for excision. Initially excising with the Weck blade is one way to prove the depth. Another way to excise is to consider fascial excision through the eschar once the depth of viable tissues is confirmed. In the neck, there is often very little subcutaneous fat, and instead the surgeon will encounter the thin platysma muscle [4, 5, 25]. If possible, the platysma must be saved. Given the thinness of the neck and very thin subcutaneous tissue, even in a not so deep burn, the surgeon can find himself/herself faced with the underlying superficial veins and structures exposed down to the deeper muscles before healthy tissue is actually encountered. Thrombosed vessels denote a deeper burn warranting more excision either at the time or a later date when some of the bed has healed. In this scenario, consider only temporary graft with allograft at the time of first excision so the bed is allowed to heal [2, 4, 5].

30.7 Grafting

Decision for wound coverage at the time of surgery depends on many factors. Patient perfusion and factors should always trump the surgeon's decision. If it is the initial burn excision of the neck and the surgeon encounters a superficial burn with minimal excision, consider xenograft as a temporary biologic dressing. This is to be applied in the scenario where the surgeon believes that the dermis will heal on its own with minimal damage. The purpose of the xenograft is to cover the wound as well as help with patient comfort by covering exposed injured nerves.

If during debridement punctate bleeding is present and the surgeon is deeper into the dermis, he/she can consider an autograft. As alluded to earlier, even though there is reticular dermis that is healthy and able to repair, if the repair included scar and non-complaint epidermis and dermis, the neck is one of the areas where the surgeon should seriously consider an autograft (patient's own skin). In fact, autografting allows for wound closure with less contracture and scarring and when done properly can give the patient an excellent cosmetic result [4, 5]. Similar to what will be discussed for the face in the next section, the neck should be approached anteriorly with sheet grafting instead of the meshed graft for maximal cosmesis and least amount of scarring. Small drainage holes can be made through the graft with an 11-blade in order to accommodate fibrin exudate that may interfere with graft take [4, 5].

If the debridement reveals that there is a suboptimal underlying wound bed with minimally acceptable bleeding, then the surgeon should consider allograft as a bridge to autograft. Allograft in this case serves as the matrix for the cells to grow to as they repair the wound bed. Allowing the bed to heal for 5–7 days may enable growth of granulation tissue and allow preservation of some of the underlying wound bed. Plan for the next operating room trip to be within the next week is prudent. Depending on multiple factors, burn excision may take several trips to the operating room before the wound bed is ready for autografting [4, 5].

30.8 Underlying Factors Affecting Burn Healing

In the overall management of burn wounds, it would be remiss not to mention some key factors affecting the success of your wound closure. These can be classified into overall body physiology and innate skin characteristics.

The surgeon ideally wants to select a time when the wound has declared itself but not waited too long that the patient is placed at considerable risk of infection. Part of this depends on patient factors and part on the wound factors. Patients at risk for wound failure include diabetics, patients with peripheral vascular disease, and those in immunosuppressed states. Additionally, the surgeon should not underestimate the role of basic nutrition in wound healing [4, 5]. The ultimate measure of total body nutrition is still up for debate among many experts, but in general, patients with poor albumin stores and prealbumin measurements in the single digits should be approached with caution when considering autograft. Additionally, patients with a larger TBSA have a much higher metabolic demand on their system vs. a less than 10% TBSA burn only involving the neck. Conservative approaches to autografting should be followed in the larger burns. Lastly, patients requiring full anticoagulation can be tough to manage. By nature burn excision can be exsanguinating. This combined with any clot that may form under the autograft can risk complete autograft failure. It can be helpful to place these patients on a heparin drip in order to better precisely control the amount of anticoagulation around surgical procedures [3].

When discussing wound bed factors affecting burn healing, several things must be considered. First of all, the age and compliance of the skin have a lot to do with how quickly the wound will close. The extremes of age (infant/toddlers and geriatric) burns tend to need more delicate techniques for closure. Both have thinner dermal elements, and although the youngsters have more capacity to heal with quicker dividing cells, the dermal elements and overall considerations in depth of grafts are much closer to the elderly. For example, the standard depth of skin grafts is 12/1000th of an inch, but in the extremes of age, the surgeon may have to consider 8–10/1000th or a thinner graft for donor. Another element to consider is whether the wound bed has any signs of infection. On average, it can take as quick as 5 days to colonize a third-degree wound bed with significant bacteria. On the head and neck, this can be devastating given its proximity to key airway, ocular structures not to mention the implications on the fascial planes in the neck as high-risk areas [4, 5, 25]. If there is any concern at any point even within the early phases of burn resuscitation, expedient excision of devitalized infected tissue should be done with application of temporary graft. The role of the head and neck surgeon in this scenario is key as there are numerous key structures if injury warrants deeper excision. Lastly, bleeding and shear under an autograft need to be addressed. The neck is a mobile, very vascularized area. Complete hemostasis of the wound bed should be achieved in the operating room. Additionally, application of the graft using multiple modalities to limit autograft movement should be used [4, 5].

30.9 Management of Facial Burns

Facial burns are among the most devastating injury to the human body. Much of how we communicate and define each other and ourselves as self is hidden in the face. Additionally, as it houses key structures as the eyes, nose, and mouth, the face protects other key parts to our respiratory and digestive systems.

In the initial management of facial burns, consider first intubation and/or tracheotomy. Most burn injuries that produce facial burns also include significant airway trauma. Always attend to the airway first [1, 2].

Tracheostomy in a burn patient can be fraught with significant challenges. In the acute burn phase, the edema and anasarca can interfere with the normal locations of anatomical landmarks. Similarly, in the post burn, individual with thickened scar and distortions of landmarks can also be challenging. Palpation of the thyroid and cricoid cartilage landmarks can be virtually impossible. When setting up for the procedure, it is important to approach it in the way the surgeon normally does it (percutaneous or open) but have both modalities available. Also consider doing the procedure with an anesthesiologist or other qualified provider available as managing the neck can be as challenging as managing the airway. Ultrasound could be a helpful tool: familiarity with the appearance of the trachea versus vessels in a normal neck can be helpful when trying to identify the location of structures [6, 7, 9, 10, 15]

If the burn involves the eyes, it is important to have a proper evaluation of the eyes: pupillary reflex, cornea examination, fluorescein test, and vision test if possible. Keeping the eyes hydrated and clean is imperative in burn care. Ophthalmic bacitracin and vigilant care by the nurses can avoid painful, devastating corneal ulcers. One very important test is the eye tenotomy test. With severe burns to the face, there can be an ocular compartment syndrome due to the noncompliance of the tissues. If this is missed, blindness will occur. The pressure in the eye should be measured initially and then noted at regular intervals [4, 25]. In the event that the ocular pressure is elevated and the patient is still in your edematous stage, it is reasonable to consider performing a lateral canthotomy in order to release the pressure [4, 25].

Burn reconstruction of the face should be taken on last in the overall reconstruction. Over excision or too early excision risks significant subtle contour changes that can have devastating consequences. Working in conjunction with a facial or plastic surgeon who is familiar with burn reconstruction is imperative. Basic tenets for facial reconstruction were first documented by a surgeon in the 1950s named Gonzalez-Ulloa [4, 5, 25]. He realized that the face should be divided into separate esthetic units and hence reconstructed in full pieces as such. Burn surgeons today utilize this technique in order to accomplish this in a methodical way. Similar to reconstructing large pieces of a car, hiding the seams of these aesthetic units where natural

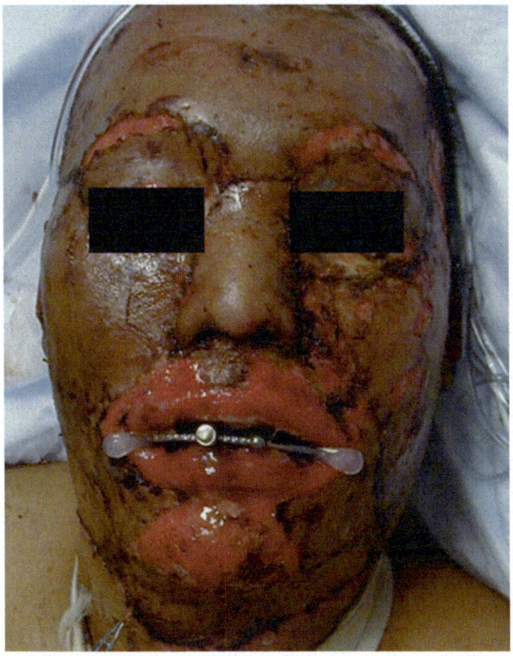

Fig. 30.4 Facial reconstruction done with aesthetic units of the face (early postoperative). Note the oral commissure splint to prevent contracture

folds/skin lines would normally fall will allow for the best cosmetic result. Depending on the defects of the underlying structure of the face, it may require certain contour adjustments or soft tissue flaps to occur prior to the overall skin grafts. Faces are reconstructed often with a combination of full-thickness grafts and thinner split-thickness skin grafts depending on the defect [4, 5]. Similar to the neck region, it is not uncommon to do this portion of the reconstruction in phases. As the skin heals and contractures occur, particularly around the ocular region, this is often the first esthetic unit to be addressed to help with preserving eyelid closer to prevent ocular desiccation. Oral splints are placed early even before surgery to prevent significant oral commissure contracture [4, 5] (Fig. 30.4).

Conclusion

In summary, burns of the head and neck pose significant challenges to the provider given the devastating loss of anatomy, landmarks, and essential structures that can be injured. Additionally, the potential danger of airway issues and injury to such organs as the eyes, nose, and oral structures can create problems for the provider. If the surgeon keeps certain principles in mind, you can safely manage simple problems in the acute burn prior to transfer to a verified burn center. Knowledge of the injury mechanism dynamic clinical status of the patient in the acute burn phase is important in the initial management, transfer of care, and definitive management of these patients.

References

1. Cancio LC. Airway management and smoke inhalation injury in the burn patient. Clin Plast Surg. 2009;36(4):555–67.
2. Traber DL, Pollard V. Pathophysiology of burn injury. In: Herdon DN, editor. Total burn care. London: WB Saunders; 1996. p. 175–83.
3. Nebraska Burn Institute Advisory Board. Initial assessment and management. In: Advanced burn life sup- port course: provider's manual. 2nd ed. Lincoln, NE: Nebraska Burn Institute; 1990. p. 8–9.
4. Neale HW, Billmire DA, Carey JP. Reconstruction following head and neck burns. Clin Plast Surg. 1986;13:119–36.
5. McCauley RL, Barret JP. Electrical injuries. In: Erickson E, editor. Plastic surgery; indications, operations and outcomes. St. Louis: Mosby, Inc; 2000. p. 375–87.
6. Ennis JL, Chung KK, Renz EM, et al. Joint Theater trauma system implementation of burn resuscitation guidelines improves outcomes in severely burned military casualties. J Trauma. 2008;64(Suppl 2):S146–51.
7. Sen S, Greenhalgh D, Palmieri T. Review of burn injury research for the year 2009. J Burn Care Res. 2010;31(6):836–48.
8. Lee-Chiong TL Jr. Smoke inhalation injury: when to suspect and how to treat. Postgrad Med. 1999;105(2):55–62.
9. Clark WR. Smoke inhalation: diagnosis and treatment. World J Surg. 1992;16(1):24–9.
10. Pham TN, Cancio LC, Gibran NS. American burn association practice guidelines: burn shock resuscitation. J Burn Care Res. 2008;29(1):257–66.
11. Easley RB, Segeleon JE, Haun SE, et al. Prospective study of airway management of children requiring endotracheal intubation before admission to a pediatric intensive care unit. Crit Care Med. 2000;28(6):2058–63.
12. Muehlberger T, Kunar D, Munster A, et al. Efficacy of fiberoptic laryngoscopy in the diagnosis of inhalation injuries. Arch Otolaryngol Head Neck Surg. 1998;124:1003–7.

13. Chou SH, Lin SD, Chuang HY, et al. Fiber-optic bronchoscopic classification of inhalation injury: prediction of acute lung injury. Surg Endosc. 2004;18(9):1377.
14. Lange M, Hamahata A, Traber DL, et al. Preclinical evaluation of epinephrine nebulization to reduce airway hyperemia and improve oxygenation after smoke inhalation injury. Crit Care Med. 2011;39(4):718–24.
15. Branson RD, Durbin CG. Invasive mechanical ventilation in adults: implementation, management, weaning and follow-up. Respir Care. 2002;47(3):247–8.
16. Fitzpatrick JC, Cioffi WG. Ventilatory support following burns and smoke inhalation injury. Respir Care Clin N Am. 1996;3(1):21–49.
17. Mayo D, Merrel P. Inhalation injury in the burn patient. Crit Care Nurs North Am. 2004;16(1):27–38.
18. Shimazu T, Yukioka T, Ikeuchi H, et al. Ventilation-perfusion alterations after smoke inhalation injury in an ovine model. J Appl Physiol (1985). 1996;81(5):2250–9.
19. Chung KK, Wolf SE, Renz EM, et al. High-frequency percussive ventilation and low tidal volume ventilation in burns: a randomized controlled trial. Crit Care Med. 2010;38(10):1970–7.
20. Goodwin CW, Dorethy J, Lam V, et al. Randomized trial of efficacy of crystalloid and colloid resuscitation on hemodynamic response and lung water following thermal injury. Ann Surg. 1983;197(5):520–31.
21. Reiss E, Stirman JA, Artz CP, et al. Fluid and electrolyte balance in burns. JAMA. 1953;152:1309–13.
22. Blumetti J, Hunt JL, Arnoldo BD, et al. The Parkland formula under fire: is the criticism justified? J Burn Care Res. 2008;29(1):180–6.
23. Ivy ME, Atweh NA, Palmer J, et al. Intra-abdominal hypertension and abdominal compartment syndrome in burn patients. J Trauma. 2000;49(3):387–91.
24. Markell KW, Renz EM, White CE, et al. Abdominal complications after severe burns. J Am Coll Surg. 2009;208(5):940–7.
25. Warpeha RL. Resurfacing the burned face. Clin Plast Surg. 1981;8:255–7.

Part 3

Perioperative, Pharmacological, and Supportive Management of the Surgical Patient

31 Treatment Planning and Perioperative Management of the Dental Implant Patient

Michael S. Block

Abstract

This chapter focuses on state-of-the-art methods to utilize preoperative planning to enhance implant therapy for our patients. The preoperative patient examination requires specific data to be obtained, including physical examination, radiographic examination, and photographic documentation. The final restorative plan must be visualized to provide the necessary information to place implants accurately. These visualization tools can then be matched with navigation methods for precise treatment. Navigation methods are discussed and illustrated in depth.

31.1 Introduction

The primary goal for implant placement is achieving high accuracy and precision. Surgeons should avoid placing implants with a wide variance from an ideal position. Repetitive accuracy and precision of placement result in a small standard deviation from a virtual planned position. All implants should be placed accurately with repeated precision.

The surgeon must have a clearly defined plan which is based on the anticipated final restoration. Based on the final restorative plan, the location of the implants can be precisely planned and placed.

Utilization of traditional stone models and wax-ups of the planned restoration involves laboratory support and a variety of guide stents. Digital and navigational technology has been reduced to practice for everyday use with high efficiency and improved accuracy. This chapter will outline several algorithms to guide clinicians to use technology to more accurately and precisely place implants in ideal restorative positions, based on perioperative planning and orchestration.

31.2 Perioperative Data Collection

Whether the patient is referred or comes into the office without a referral, the initial interview is similar. The patient is asked what they would like to achieve at the end of the treatment. They may desire function, esthetics, elimination of pain, or reestablishing their dentition to ideal health. Based on these desires, the clinician assembles diagnostic materials for treatment planning.

M.S. Block, D.M.D.
Private Practice, Metairie, LA, USA
e-mail: drblock@cdrnola.com

© Springer International Publishing AG 2018

E.M. Ferneini, J.D. Bennett (eds.), *Perioperative Assessment of the Maxillofacial Surgery Patient*,
https://doi.org/10.1007/978-3-319-58868-1_31

The exam should include evaluation of joint function, status of teeth including which are missing or non-restorable, soft tissue examination to eliminate coincident pathology, and esthetic evaluation of the patient.

31.2.1 Establishing the Planned Gingival Margin

The central incisor is used as the reference for positioning the anterior teeth. The incisive edge should be approximately 2–3 mm below the lip at rest, with the mouth slightly opened. The length of the central incisor ranges from 10 to 11 mm depending on facial profile. Longer faces will have longer teeth. Once the incisor edge is determined and the length of the central incisor is identified, the facial gingival margin can be located. The implant will need to be 3–4 mm superior to that vertical reference [1].

31.2.2 Cone Beam Scanning

The patient will need a cone beam scan taken to be used for perioperative assessment. For the patient who will have one or more teeth replaced, a clip with fiducials is placed prior to the cone beam scan for dynamic navigation planning. If available the scan can be taken with a restorative plan in place. In the edentulous patient, an initial scan is taken without a plan in place in order to assess bone availability, with the understanding that an additional scan may be necessary if navigation is planned for implant placement.

The cone beam is read thoroughly to assess airway, nasal septal deformity, sinus pathology, neck pathology, or other problems not previously identified.

31.2.3 Standardized Photographs

Each patient should have a standardized set of photographs taken. This can be used for communication to the patient and colleagues illustrating the pretreatment status of the patient. These photographs can also be used to create digital imaged plans and used to compare to the final result.

The following is included in a suggested series:

1. Incisor show at rest with the lips slightly apart and relaxed. The patient's central incisor show at rest is documented.
2. Smile line. With the patient expressing an animated smile, a photograph is taken to demonstrate the incisor show. This is especially important in the patient who starts treatment with gingival recession or for those patients who have short clinical crowns and may be candidates for crown lengthening at the incisor edge of the gingival margin.
3. Frontal, lateral, and full occlusal photographs are taken with retractors. Another important but often forgotten photograph is a lateral view of the anterior teeth in occlusion showing ridge relationships and lip posture.
4. A video of the patient talking and laughing is often useful for esthetic planning.

31.3 Methods to Visualize the Final Restorative Plan on Digital Plans for Navigated Implant Placement

Current case planning should include virtual placement of teeth to understand exactly what surgical adjunctive hard and soft tissue procedures are necessary to place implants in the desired locations. By loading the data from a cone beam scan into appropriate software, the clinician can identify implant position based on the restorative plan. The digital method eliminates several lab procedures which many dentists cannot perform. The restorative dentist may have to pay additional fees for plans made by a laboratory technician. Surgical plans or guides will need to be fabricated to accurately place implants based on analog or digital preoperative plans. The patient benefits from less invasive surgery and a more accurate implant placement when navigation is used [2, 3].

31.3.1 Use of Radiopaque Tooth Replicas

Models are made and teeth are set in the ideal position. The setup can use denture teeth or wax. The model with the setup is duplicated and a vacuum form made. The setup is removed from the model leaving the edentulous space. A radiopaque material is placed into the vacuum form and pressed onto the model. Barium sulfate is inexpensive and easily used. The barium sulfate powder is dissolved in monomer and then acrylic powder added. The resultant duplication of the setup is now in a radiopaque form. Holes are drilled into the occlusal of the planned teeth replicas simulating implant axis emergence. The patient is then scanned with this radiopaque plan in place. For dynamic navigation, the implants are placed virtually with their axes emerging from the holes (Fig. 31.1—use Takia).

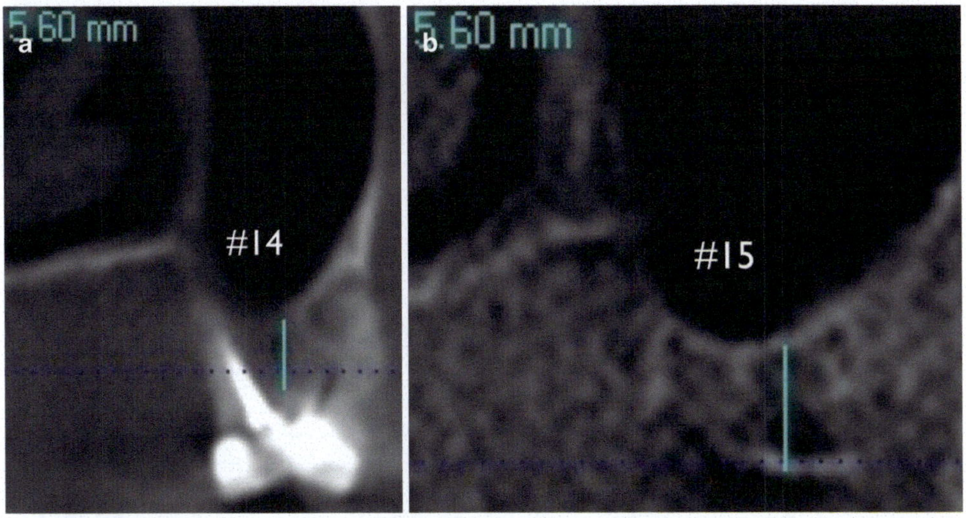

Fig. 31.1 (**a**) Maxillary left first molar with 5.6 mm of vertical bone present in the furcation. Tooth planned for removal with eventual implant placement. (**b**) Maxillary edentulous left second molar location. Note 5 mm of vertical bone present. Treatment planned for implant placement. (**c**) Surgical procedure included sulcular incisions with crestal extension and vertical release. The first molar tooth was removed. A Piezosurgery crosscut bit was used to create osteotomies connecting the three sockets. (**d**) The mobilized furcation bone was gently tapped and elevated approximately 5–6 mm to gain vertical dimension. Graft was then placed into the socket and elevated portion of the molar site. A crestal approach was also used in the second molar region and grafted to gain additional vertical bone dimension. (**e**) These cross sections from the 4-month postoperative cone beam scan show 10–11 mm of bone present in the first and second molar regions. (**f**) Prior to scanning the patient for the final navigation planning, denture teeth were set on models in proper occlusion. The setup was duplicated and a vacuum form made. The molars were recreated in radiopaque resin within the vacuum form. Holes were then drilled in the desire implant emergence location. The patient had a cone beam scan taken with the radiopaque teeth in her mouth with a clip with fiducials on the right side of her maxilla. Planning by Dr. Greg Guerra. (**g**) This image is from the navigation planning screen. A virtual implant is placed and aligned to emerge within the predrilled holes in the template. At the time of surgery, the radiopaque guide will not be in the mouth because the navigation system has the virtual tooth in the correct position and the implant is placed fully guided. (**h**) Implant is accurately and precisely positioned in the first molar location. (**i**) After 4 months for implant integration, custom abutments were fabricated and placed into the implants. (**j**) Final crowns in place (**k**) 1-year follow-up radiographs showing excellent bone levels

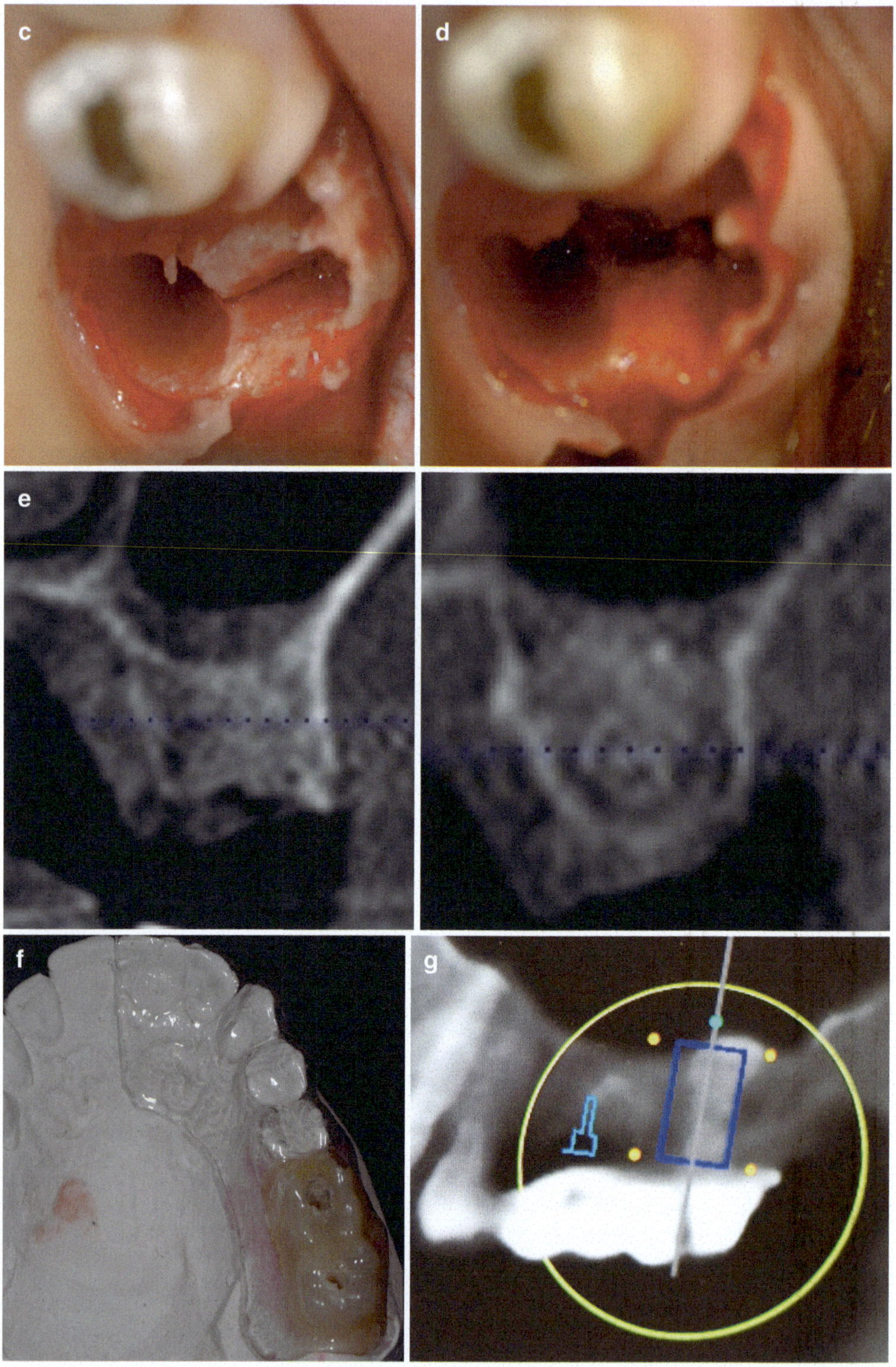

Fig. 31.1 (continued)

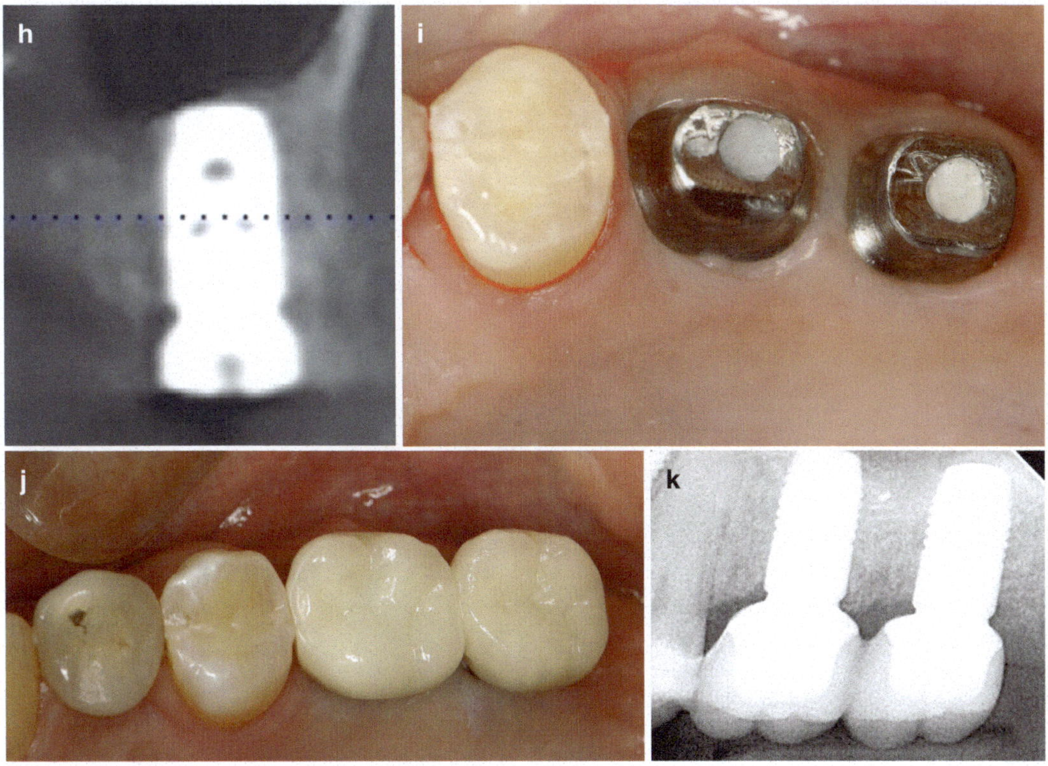

Fig. 31.1 (continued)

31.3.2 Use of .stl Files to Superimpose on Cone Beam Scans

Models are made and sent articulated to a lab. The lab creates a setup of the planned restoration. The plan is then scanned in the lab creating an output .stl file. The .stl file is securely sent to the clinician who is using the planning software. The .stl file is superimposed on the patient's cone beam scan for planning. This method is useful for dynamic or static guides. The planned image is outlined on cross-section views allowing for virtual implant placement taking into consideration the cervical margin, labial contour, incisive edge position, or fossae of the planned restoration (Fig. 31.2—Ellensworth).

31.3.3 Use of Virtual Tooth Position on Planning Software

Planning software that utilizes cone beam files usually has the features built-in that allow for placing virtual crowns on the images. For missing single teeth, the virtual crown feature eliminates the need for an analog setup. The tooth to be replaced can be easily visualized aligning with the adjacent teeth (Fig. 31.3—virtual tooth setup—use lateral case).

If a patient has teeth in place but they are not in the planned position, adjustments can be made using virtual tooth setup. For example, a patient will have their anterior dentition removed and implants placed. The physical evaluation of the patient identifies the need to

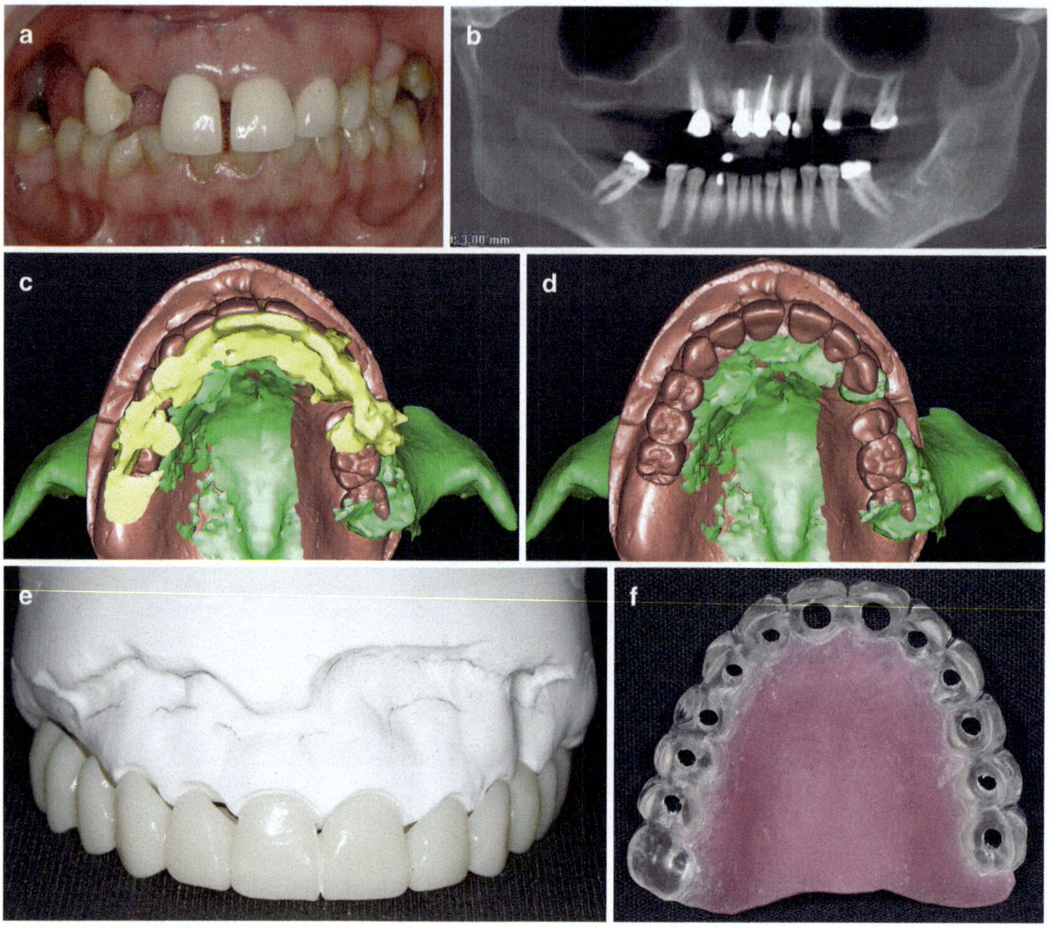

Fig. 31.2 (**a**) This patient presents with a goal of having teeth that allow to smile. Her maxillary teeth are malposed, have secondary decay, and are not esthetically satisfactory. (**b**) Reconstructed panoramic image from an initial cone beam scan shows bone present from canine to first molar locations, malposition and non-restorable teeth in her maxilla. (**c**) For this patient models were sent to the lab (Lars Hanson, CDT) where a wax-up of the final teeth positions was completed. The wax-up was scanned to create an .stl output file. The .stl file was electronically sent to the surgeon. This image is an occlusal view of the original teeth in yellow, with the .stl image of the plan superimposed on the cone beam scan (Simplant, Dentsply, Waltham Mass). This shows the necessary compensations to be made to accurately and precisely position implants using navigation. (**d**) This occlusal view shows the plan with the original teeth removed from the image. Note how clear the images are and can be used for final planning of implant size and positioning. (**e**) From the accepted plan, a milled resin provisional is fabricated in the laboratory for placement at the time of implant placement. There is no flange nor pink gingiva substitutes planned for this patient. (**f**) This drill guide is also made to verify implant position at the time of surgery. The palatal portion allows for accurate seating of the guide. (**g**) This image is from the navigation screen (X-Nav, Lacombe, PA). The .stl output file has been superimposed on the imported cone beam scan. Using the superimposed plan as a guide, implants are then virtually positioned in an ideal prosthetic position. (**h**) This view shows the vertical alignment of the planned implants. Note the angulation of the posterior right molar implant which provides information on the necessary angulated abutment that will be needed at the time of surgery. (**i**) This view shows the implant intended positions and their alignment to match the planned placement of the crowns. Note that the implant positions do not match the patient's natural teeth positioned because the planned corrected for the malposition of the teeth. (**j**) The implants were placed using dynamic navigation and the provisional converted. Note the anterior teeth are created with embrasures to allow for tissue ingrowth. (**k**) Occlusal view of the provisional. (**l**) Three months post implant placement showing an esthetic result satisfactory to the patient. She will have an all-ceramic full arch restoration milled as the final prosthesis

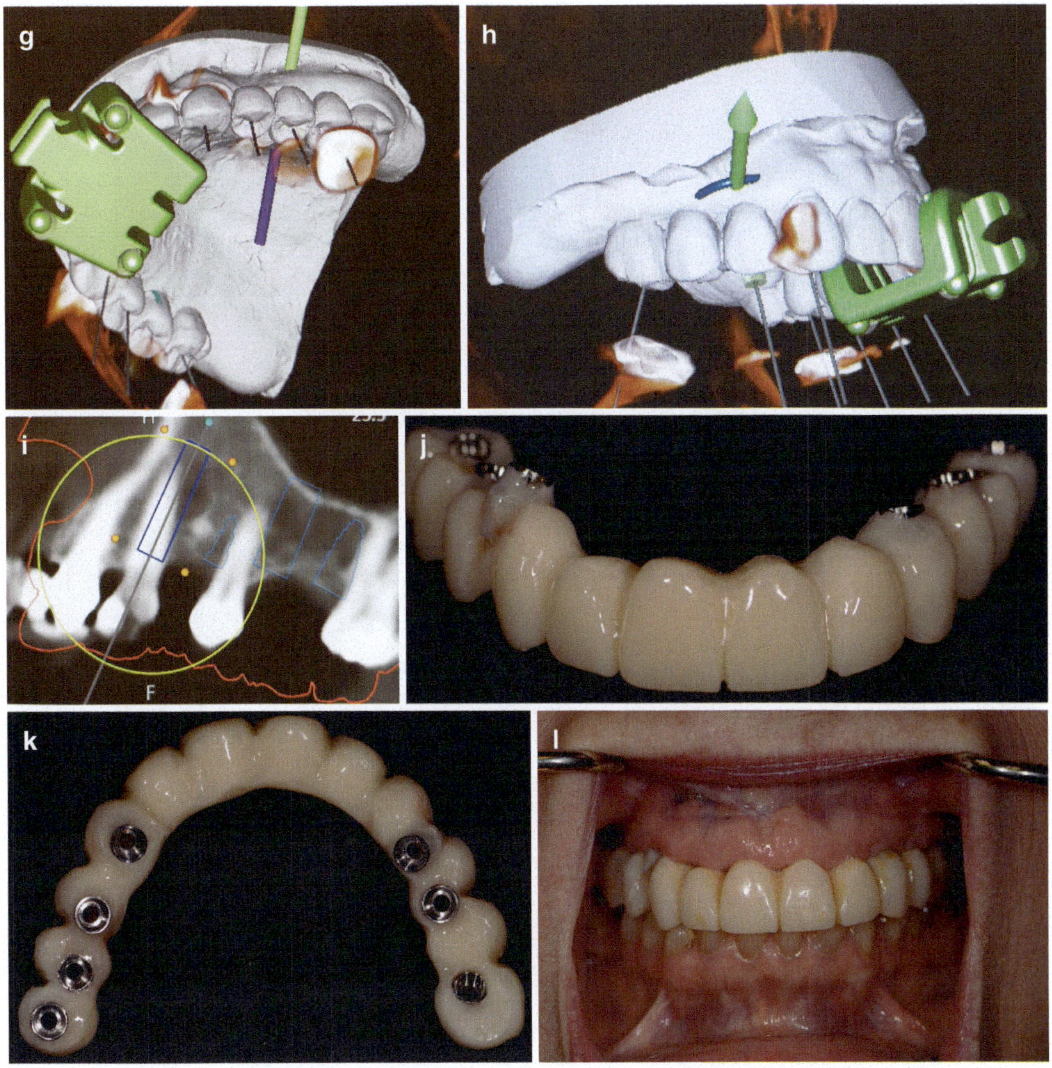

Fig. 31.2 (continued)

move the incisor edge inferiorly for improved incisor show and may need to change angulation to avoid excessive protrusion. These parameters are noted in the initial evaluation and with consultation with the restorative dentist. The virtual tooth placement over the existing teeth corrects their malposition. The corrected, virtual plan is now used to plan implant position. This will result in correct placement of the implant in the anterior-posterior position with angulation to plan for screw retention if desired (Fig. 31.4).

For a full arch maxillary case, preoperative models are made and articulated. A setup is performed in the laboratory. The setup is scanned and an .stl file is electronically sent to the surgeon. The surgeon takes the .stl file of the planned setup and superimposes in onto the cone beam file to position implants. Often these patients have significant dental malposition with spacing

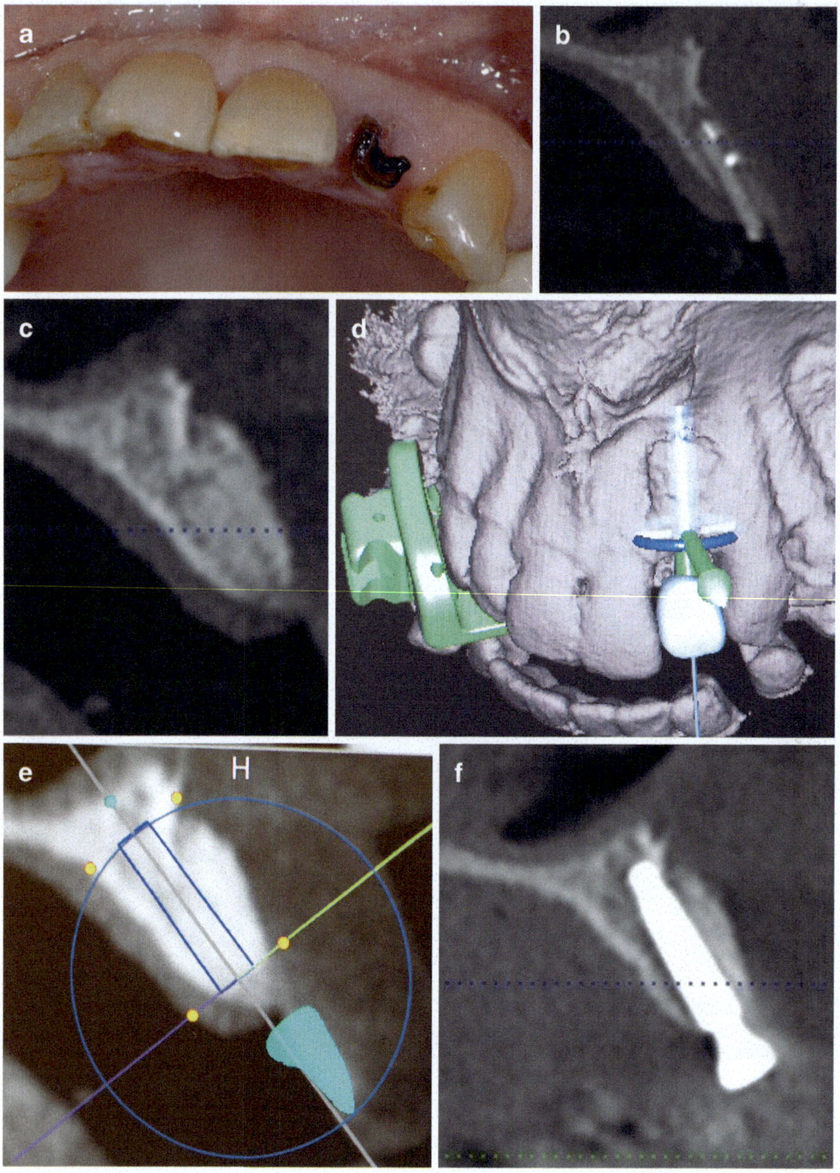

Fig. 31.3 (**a**) This 75-year-old male who presented with a desire to have an implant placed in the left lateral incisor location. The tooth is fractured with loss of labial bone. (**b**) A cone beam scan was taken with a fiducial clip on the right maxillary teeth. This cross-section image from the cone beam shows lack of bone and the obvious need for a graft to restore ridge width. At the time of tooth removal, a flap was elevated and the tooth removed. Allograft was placed into site confluent with the adjacent bone. A 2 mm layer of xenograft was placed to prevent severe resorptive changes since sintered xenograft will minimally resorb. (**c**) A second scan with the original fiducial containing clip was taken after 4 months. This image shows the restored ridge form. (**d**) The digital file from the second cone beam scan was imported into navigation computer. A virtual lateral incisor crown was positioned, followed by placement of a virtual implant emerging according to the virtual crown placement. (**e**) This cross-section image from the navigation screen shows the virtual implant position with at least 2 mm of graft labial to the implant with the implant emerging in the position agreed to by the restorative dentist. He plans to place a cemented crown. (**f**) Navigation was used to place the implant. The incision did include a small palatal flap with no labial reflection to protect the graft. A mesh analysis was performed confirming less than 1° of divergence from the virtual plan. (**g**) This is a 2-year follow-up radiograph showing the maintenance of bone around the implant. (**h**) This is a 2-year follow-up of the crown with an adequate band of keratinized gingiva which allows for tissue health long term

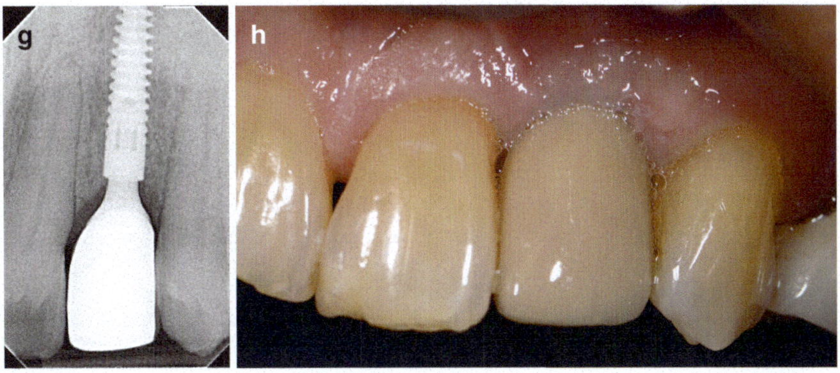

Fig. 31.3 (continued)

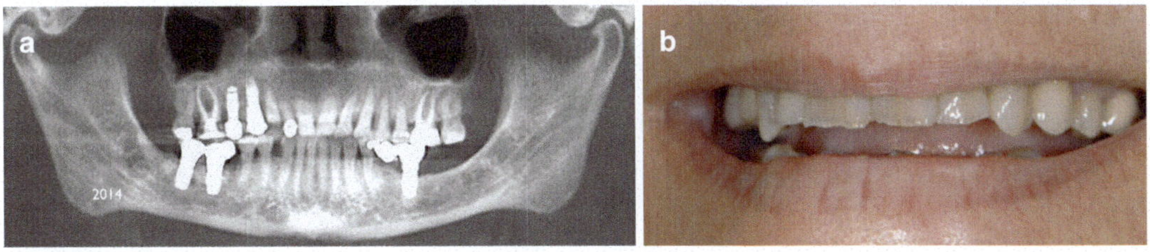

Fig. 31.4 (**a**) This woman has a long-standing history of mobile anterior maxillary teeth. Her desire is to have teeth that do not move when she chews and to have teeth that are more esthetic in appearance. (**b**) At smile she shows 4 mm of clinical crown. At rest she shows −1 mm of tooth. (**c**) Her anterior maxillary teeth are not symmetric. The crown of the central incisors measures 8.5 mm in height. Her occlusion shows attrition and is in need of vertical readjustment. (**d**) This image is from planning software (Simplant, Dentsply Implants, Waltham, Mass). The cone beam scan was imported into the software program. The patient's original teeth split from the underlying bone to simulate their removal by a simple click of an icon. Virtual teeth were placed using the natural teeth as references. The virtual teeth added 2.5 mm to the incisor height, maintaining her gingival margin position. (**e**) This image is the planned virtual teeth in position with removal of the patient's natural teeth. This allows the treatment team to visualize the final restoration. With this clarity implant positions can be determined and a surgical plan finalized. The laboratory technician (Michael Bellerino, Metairie La) then created a wax-up following the virtual plan and fabricated a transitional removable appliance for the patient to wear while the implants integrated. (**f**) This occlusal view shows the planned position of four implants. The implants can be placed along the palatal aspect of each extraction site. A drill guide was fabricated to insure proper vertical positioning of the implants. (**g**) At the time of surgery, sulcular incisions were made and the gingiva conservatively elevated. No vertical incisions were made. The teeth were removed with the aid of a periotome, preserving bone. Implants were placed into the palatal slope of the extractions sites. A surgical guide stent was used to confirm accurate positioning. The guide stent, fabricated based on the pretreatment planning, had vertical references made to ensure that the implants were appropriately submerged. The gaps between the implants and the intact labial bone were grafted with xenograft. The sockets were also grafted with xenograft. Short healing abutments were placed to avoid trauma from the removable provisional prosthesis. (**h**) Postoperative panoramic reconstruction from the cone beam showing implant placement positioned as planned. (**i**) After 4 months for integration, the short healing abutments were replaced with longer abutments for ease of use by the restorative dentist (Dr. Randall Green, Metairie, LA). (**j**) Implant level impressions were taken, abutments chosen, and a screw-retained milled provisional made. The design was based on the pretreatment virtual planning. Note the gentle emergence of the provisional with minimal ridge lap. This is a maintainable prosthetic plan. (**k**) The added length of the incisors is satisfactory to the patient. (**l**) Frontal view showing symmetry and a highly esthetic restoration of six anterior teeth. Note no pink gingival substitutes were used. (**m**) The occlusal view shows the screw retention sites as planned. (**n**) One-year follow-up radiographs showing well-maintained bone levels. The patient has decided to use the milled provisional as her final restoration. If it fractures, it can be remilled using the digital file used to fabricate the provisional

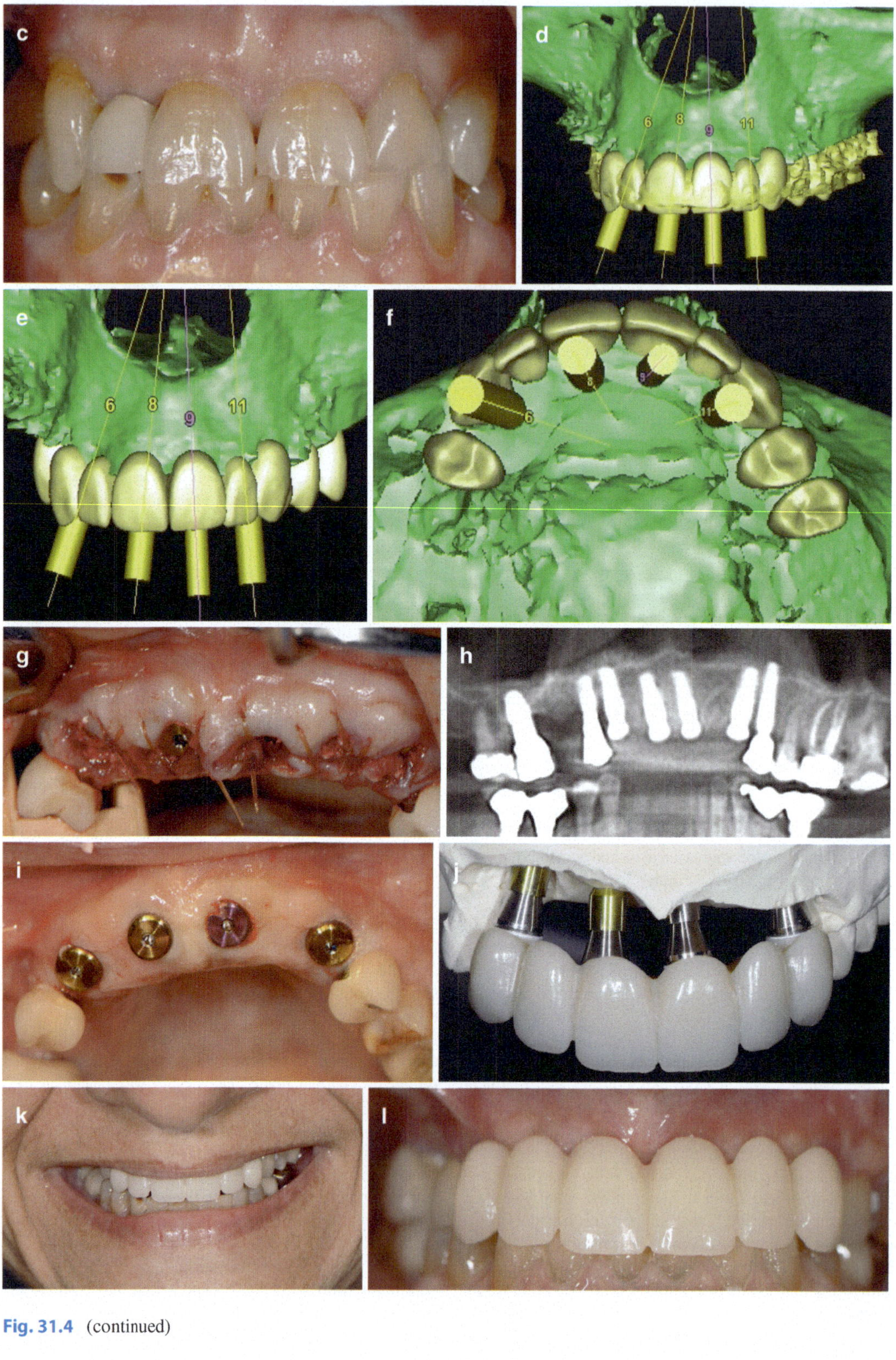

Fig. 31.4 (continued)

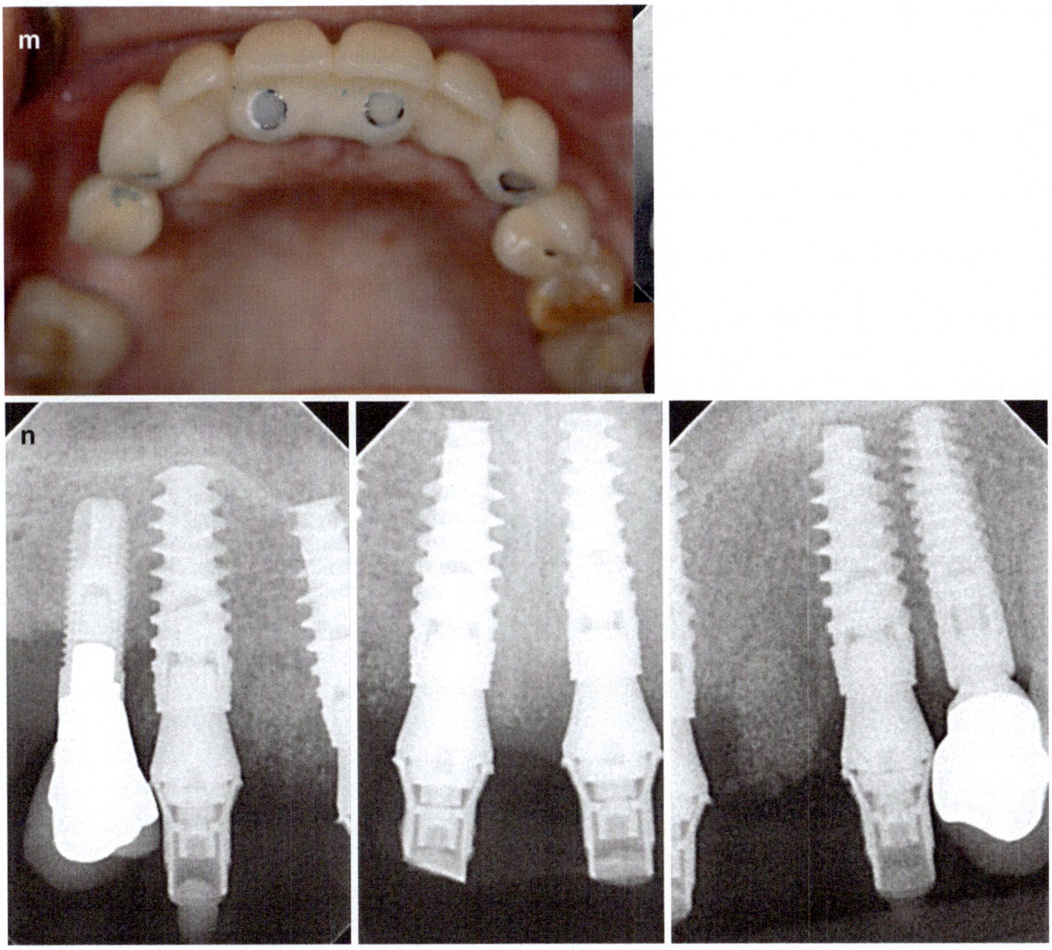

Fig. 31.4 (continued)

issues, so the planned setup will allow precise implant placement with the final restoration guiding the surgery (Fig. 31.2).

31.4 Static or Dynamic Navigation

Navigated surgery uses a guidance system to more accurately and precisely perform a given surgical procedure. For placement of dental implants, two navigation methods are available. A *static* navigation guide uses a manufactured acrylic stent with cylinders in place to guide implant placement. The specific implant system, length, width, depth, and angulation are determined on a computer. Once chosen the implant placement is rigid and cannot easily be changed at the time of surgery.

Dynamic navigation uses a GPS-like method real time. The implant image is placed onto a radiographic image of the patient, within the navigation computer. A patient tracking array is secured to the patient's jaw. The handpiece for site preparation also has a tracking array on it. Light is emitted from an overhead light source.

Its reflection from the patient tracking array and the handpiece is captured by high-definition cameras, resulting in a three-dimensional view and guidance for implant placement. The surgeon can change the plan at any time during the procedure, resulting in great flexibility.

Why should the clinician consider static or dynamic navigation? Navigation can result in accurate depth control and should decrease the chance of damage to the inferior alveolar nerve. Navigation allows for flapless or limited flap elevation resulting in less patient postoperative morbidity. Navigation with virtual implant placement provides accurate spacing and angulation of implants compared to freehand approaches. Virtual implant planning and navigated placement can ensure appropriate implant angulation and depth for esthetic situations. The use of virtual implant planning and subsequent navigation allows prosthetic/surgical collaboration with precise planning and accurate orchestration of the plan to achieve a high level of patient-specific results. There are limitations with both static and dynamic navigation systems, as discussed below.

31.4.1 Static Guides

A static system uses computerized tomography (CT)-generated stents, with metal tubes and a surgical system which uses specific drills and sleeves to prepare and subsequently place implants using the guide stent (Fig. 31.5). Implant position is dependent on the stent without the ability to change implant position. Static is meant to be consistent with predetermined implant position without real-time visualization of the implant preparation site as it is being developed. No intraoperative position changes can be made with a static system unless the use of the stent is abandoned during the surgical procedure.

To fabricate a CT-generated surgical guide for static navigation, a cone beam CT scan (CBCT) is taken with the prosthetic plan in the mouth as an imaging guide. The fabrication of the imaging guide requires pre-scan lab work, as well as time to transmit data or stone models. There will be a time delay between scan- and guide-directed surgeries, since the guides are manufactured by a company often in another location. There may be additional costs to the team and hence added cost to the patient. In-house printing of guide stents may improve on the time and cost considerations using static guides.

The CBCT DICOM data must be entered into the planning software. One disadvantage for the use of digital software is that it requires training to use the software. Clinicians may not proficiently learn the software and may decide to use a third party to plan the case. After the team finalizes the plan, the plan is uploaded to the stent manufacturer. A model or an optical scan of the arch is needed to fabricate a guide that seats accurately on the teeth. This requires impressions, pouring stone, and trimming the model and adds time and costs to the static guide method. The stent manufacturer will evaluate the uploaded scan and determine if it meets quality control parameters. The clinician may need to repeat the process if the static guide does not seat accurately on the teeth or tissues. There can be 2 weeks between upload and delivery of the guide stent. At this point the surgery can be performed. The cost for static guides will differ between manufacturers. The required preoperative procedures and added costs, combined with the clinician's reluctance to gain proficiency with the planning software, create a workflow barrier for the use of a static CT-generated guide. Therefore static guides are often reserved for "special" cases.

When using a static guide, the surgeon will require the use of a specific surgical kit for the implant system chosen for the patient. The implant

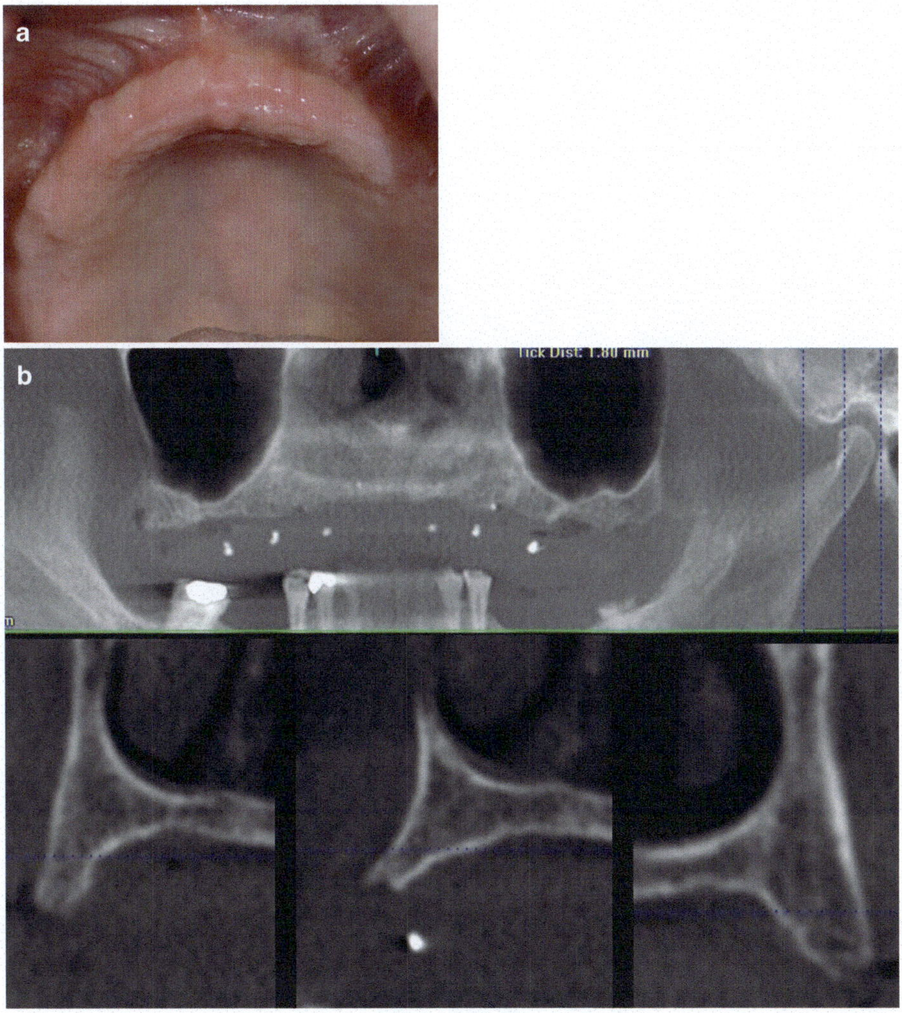

Fig. 31.5 (**a**) A patient edentulous in the maxilla for 10 years desires a set of teeth that do not have to be removed. He has funds for the implants placement and prosthetics but not for additional costs of an immediate fixed provisional. (**b**) A new denture was fabricated and used with fiducials for dual scan protocols. These images demonstrate adequate bone for a fixed provisional. (**c**) For a static guide, the image of the new denture was superimposed on the bone using planning software. Six implants are positioned within the bone. The anterior four can be paralleled to use straight emergence abutments. The posterior implants will require 30° angle correction abutments. (**d**) The view of the planned prosthesis with the implants. (**e**) The planning positioned the implants within the crowns of the teeth in order to minimize flange and allow for a prosthesis made of ceramics if the patient found this option financially acceptable. (**f**) This occlusal view shows the planned position of the implants to allow for a screw-retained prosthesis. (**g**) The planning software designs the surgical guide stent. This allows the surgeon to view its design prior to manufacture. (**h**) This is the surgical guide stent fabricated by the dual scan virtual method. (**i**) These views show implant analogs mounted to the cylinders within the guide stent. Stone can be poured to provide a presurgical model for additional planning or provisional prosthesis conversion. (**j**) This is a stone model made from the implant analogs placed into the guide stent. This is available preoperatively to allow the restorative dentist visible confirmation of the plan. This model can be used to choose abutments, trim retentive coping, and convert a provisional prior to the surgical procedure. (**k**) This photo shows the surgical guide stent in position with the implants placed and pins securing the stent to the maxilla. (**l**) Implants have been placed and cover screws placed. This allows the patient to wear his denture during the healing period with minimal pressure placed on the implants. (**m**) Reconstructed panoramic image showing implants placed as planned. (**n**) This is the zirconia prosthesis immediately after milling. (**o**) Final prosthesis with staining for esthetics (laboratory work by Mr. Renzo Cassellini). (**p**) Occlusal view showing metal inserts to allow for metal-to-metal contact when screw retaining the prosthesis. (**q**) Occlusal view of prosthesis in mouth. (**r**) Photo showing appropriate soft tissue support and tooth show. (**s**) Frontal view of prosthesis in place with space for maintenance (Restorative dentist is Dr. Laurie Glaser)

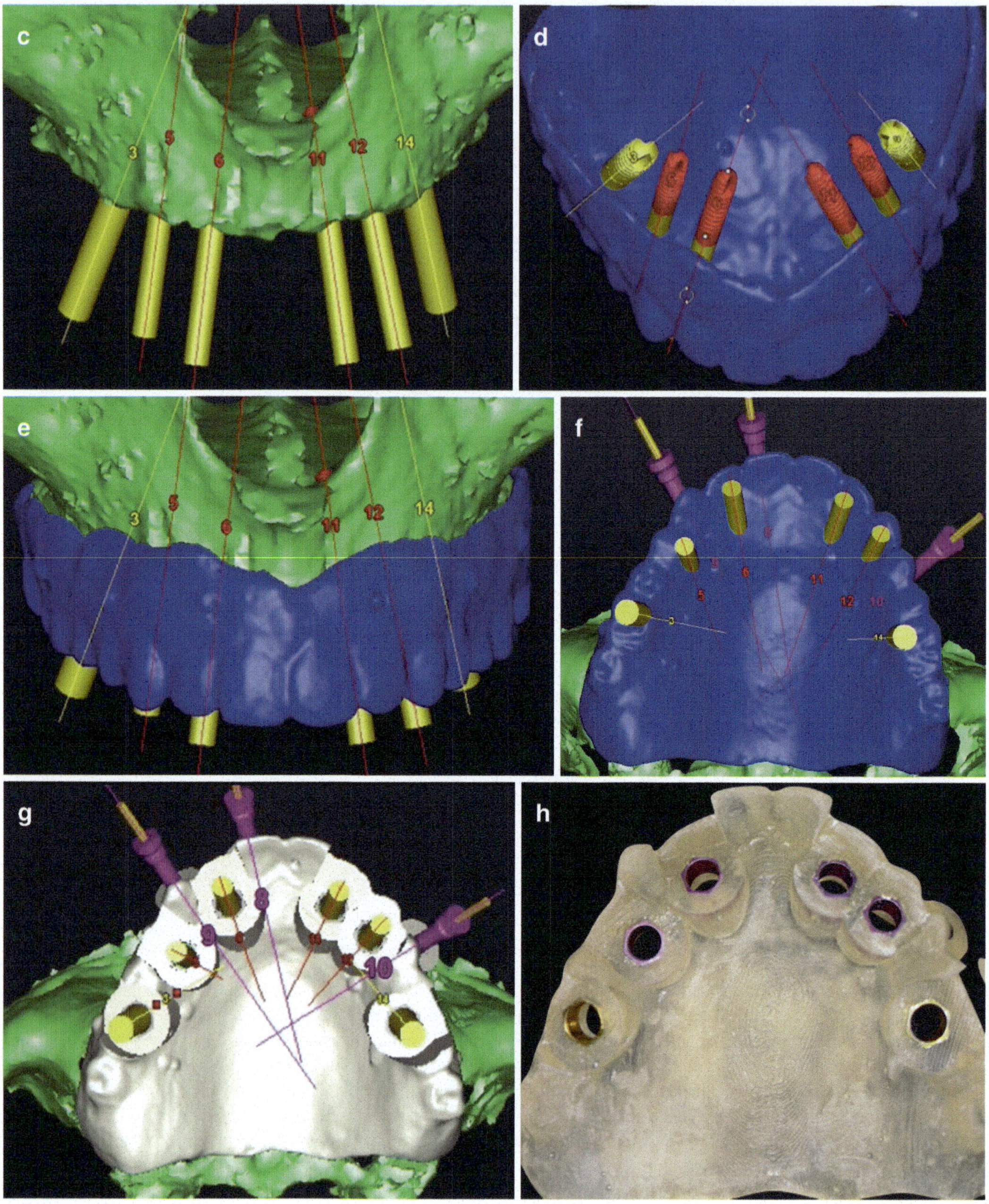

Fig. 31.5 (continued)

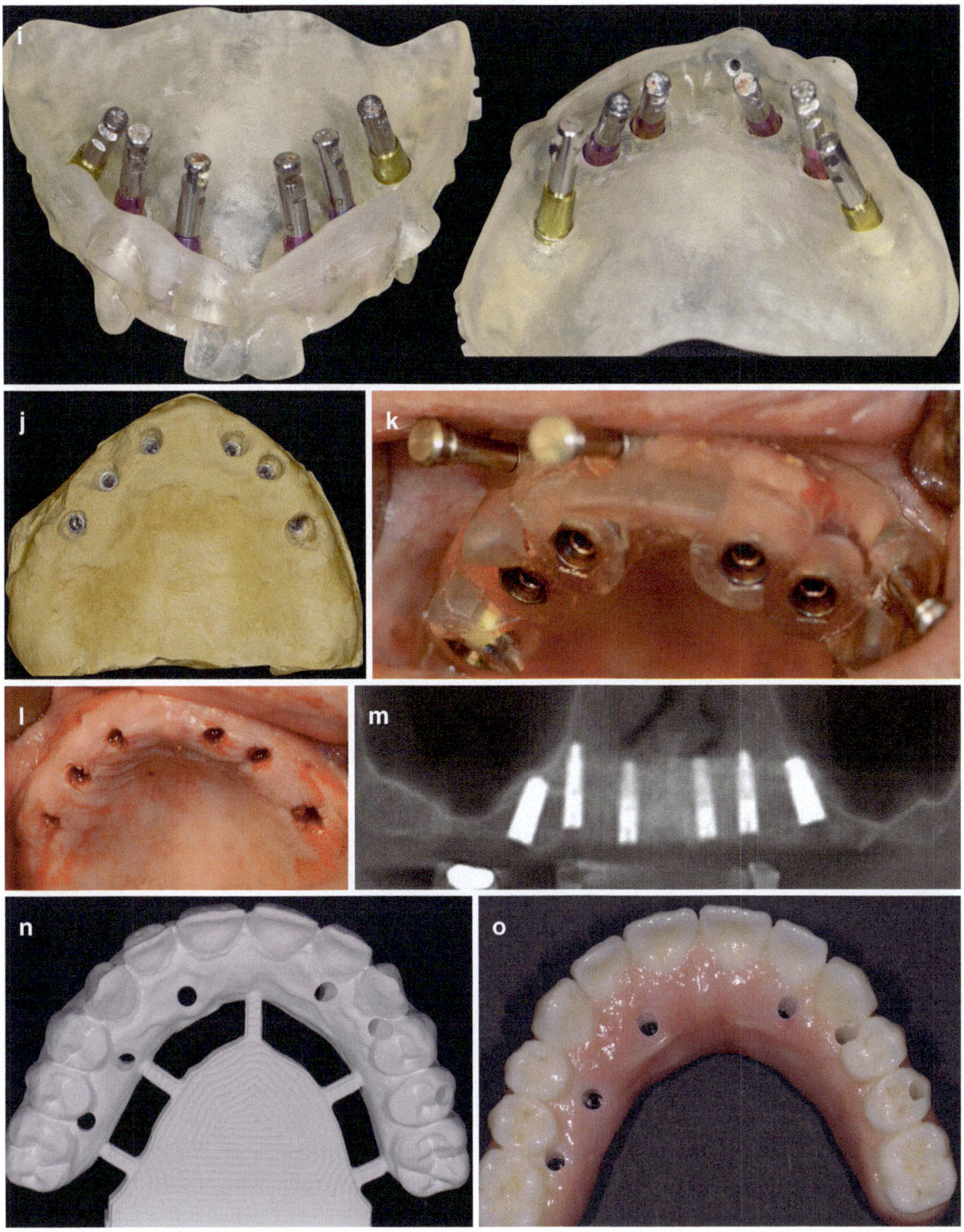

Fig. 31.5 (continued)

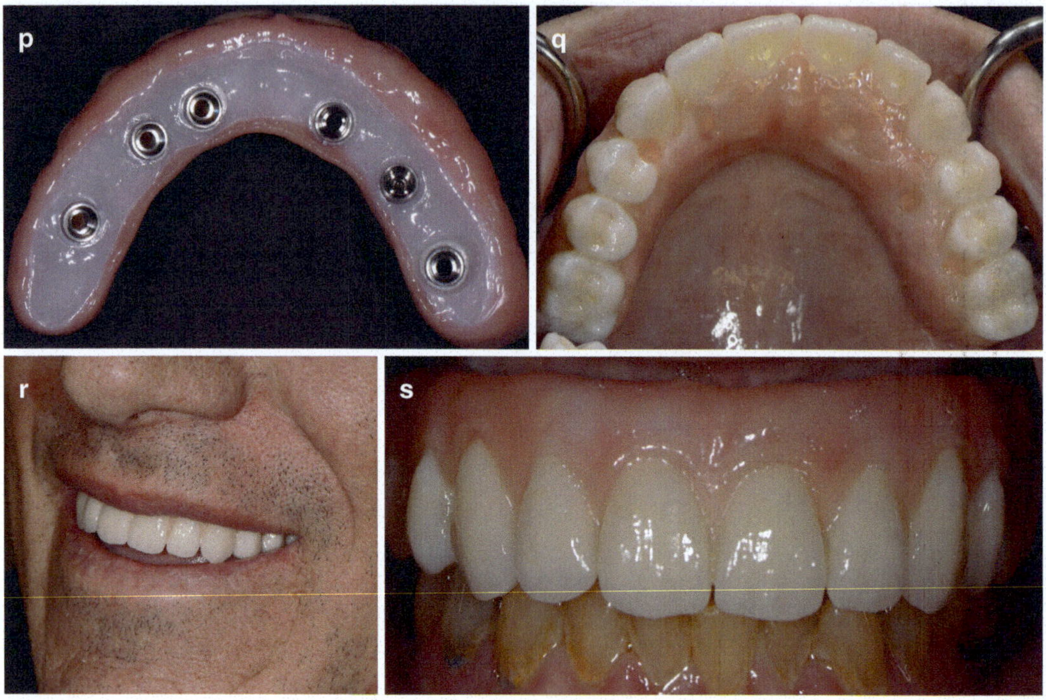

Fig. 31.5 (continued)

choice cannot be easily changed once the guide stent has been fabricated. During surgery, the implant placement position cannot be changed unless the surgeon abandons the use of the guide stent. The use of the static guide stent also limits the ability to irrigate the drill during the process since access is limited to the bone, with the potential for increased heat production [4].

The use of static guides is difficult when the patient has limited mouth opening or for placement in the second molar regions. This problem is most evident in the posterior region of the mouth or in selected patients who have limited interocclusal opening, such as scleroderma patients.

The advantages of using a static guide stent are the accurate implant placement, the use of flapless approach, the ability to use the guide stent to preoperatively fabricate fixed provisional restorations, and in general less invasive surgery which results in less patient morbidity.

31.4.2 Dynamic Navigation

Presently available dynamic navigation systems for dental implant placement use passive tracking arrays to track the patient and the handpiece and to display images onto a monitor [5, 6]. Passive systems reflect light emitted from a light source back to high-definition cameras.

Most dynamic navigation systems require the use of fiducials securely attached to the patient's arch during the CBCT (Fig. 31.6). The fiducials, typically three in a triangular pattern, are within a clip-type device that allows for the connection of an extraoral tracking array. A similar array is on the handpiece. At the time of surgery, the patient tracking array and the handpiece's array must be within line of site to the overhead cameras, with no interferences (Fig. 31.7).

During the preparation of the implant site, the normal drill sequence is used. The surgeon uses the navigation screen to guide drilling with mini-

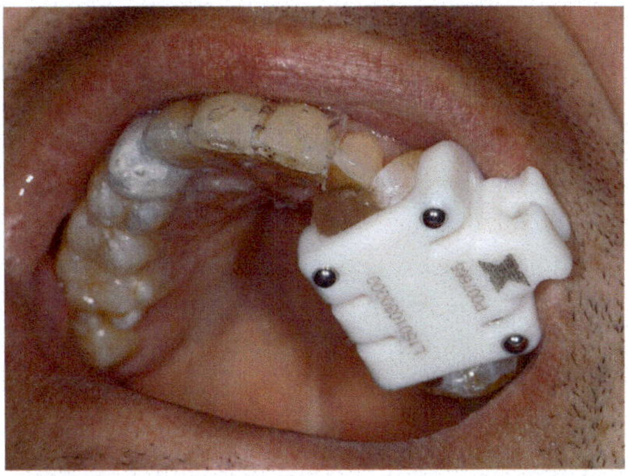

Fig. 31.6 This photo shows a barium sulfate radiopaque maxillary right premolar within a vacuum form, which is on the teeth on the right quadrant. The clip, which has three fiducials, is custom molded to fit onto the teeth in the left quadrant. The cone beam scan is then taken with cotton rolls in place to open the bite to allow for a clear registration of the fiducials

mal direct visualization of the drill in the patient's mouth [7–15].

The workflow for dynamic navigation can be simplified to use this method for 90% of implant patients who have at least three teeth adjacent to each other in the arch. The clip with fiducials is placed, the scan is taken, the digital data is transferred to the navigation computer, and the implant is planned. This usually takes less than 30 minutes to accomplish and is ideally performed after the patient's initial visit. Instrument calibration is unique for each navigation system and is performed by surgical staff prior to the patient entering the surgical room. The time for administration of anesthesia is the same as freehand approaches. The extent of flap reflection is less with navigation. The time for implant placement using freehand compared to navigation is approximately

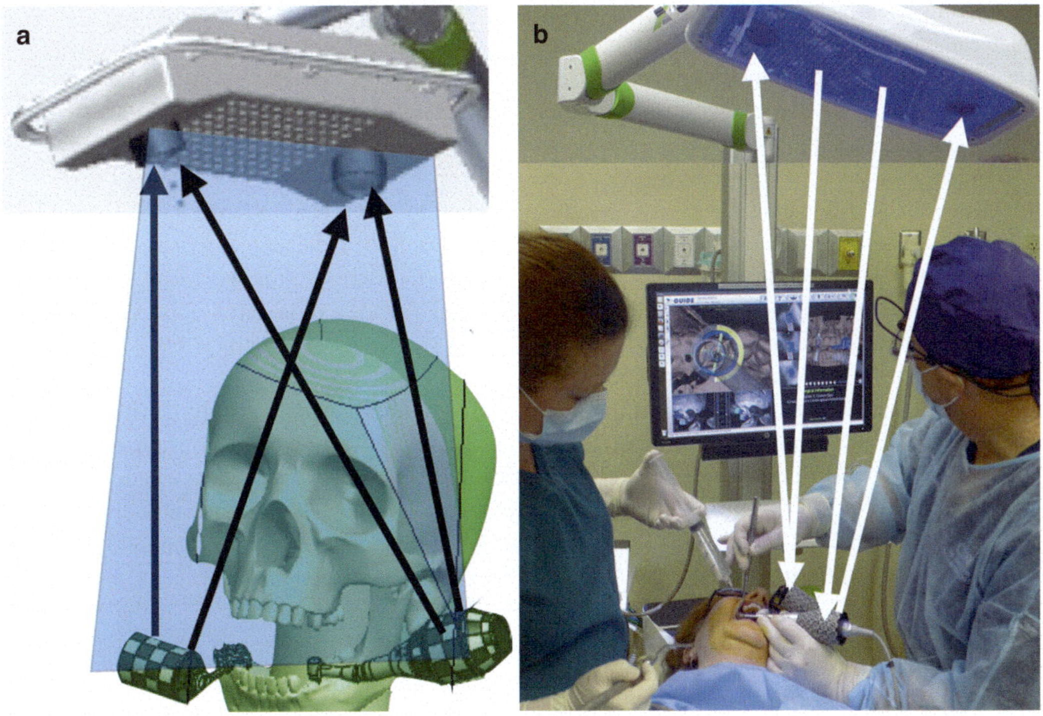

Fig. 31.7 (**a**) A diagrammatic depiction of the navigation system setup. A source light projects light to the patient. A patient tracking array is attached to the clip used to take the cone beam scan. The implant handpiece also has a tracking array. These arrays reflect the light back to the overhead panel. Two high-definition cameras received the reflection, and the system then depicts a three-dimensional view onto the screen. (**b**) Setup for actual surgery. Note the overhead light panel sends the light to the arrays which is then reflected back to the overhead panel. A clear line of sight is necessary

the same. The early experience with the system may add time, but after 15 cases the author has found that the dynamic navigation adds only 2–5 min to the case.

The surgeon positions the patient and arrays for direct line of sight to the overhead cameras. The drills are oriented following the three-dimensional images on the screen, which includes depth. The surgical assistant focuses on irrigation, retraction, and suctioning as usual. The implant can be placed fully or partially guided or by hand depending on clinician preference.

The advantages of the dynamic navigation method is accuracy [16–19], less invasive flap reflection compared to freehand approaches, less trauma to the surgeon since posture is improved with less back and neck bending, and the ability to change implant size, system, and location during the surgical procedure. In a patient who has difficulty in opening or in a second molar site which can be difficult to access, dynamic navigation allows implant placement relying on the navigation screen to guide the drills without direct visualization in the mouth.

There is a variable learning curve to develop proficiency using a dynamic navigation system. The medical literature reports between 15 and 125 case experiences depending on the procedure and the use of surgical simulators prior to the clinician developing proficiency with new surgical procedures [20, 21]. Dynamic navigation requires a team approach. Both the surgeon and the first assistant must learn to work together for efficient use of a dynamic navigation system.

31.5 Accuracy Considerations

31.5.1 Static CT-Generated Guides

What is the accuracy of static navigation systems? Static guide stents result in more accurate implant placement and depth control compared to the freehand procedure or model-based nonrestricted guides [9–12]. Mucosa-supported guides have mean deviations ranging from 1.6 mm at the implant apex to 1.4 mm at the shoulder, with angulation deviations ranging from 2.5 to 4.75 degrees from the virtual plan. More than half of the implants placed with static guides are placed more superficially than planned [22, 23]. In two meta-analyses [24, 25] with static guides, there was a mean deviation of 1.04 mm (up to 4.5 mm) at the entry point, 1.4 mm (up to 3.75 mm) deviation at the implant's apex, and angulation error less than 5°. Analyses using freehand methods were model based [24, 25]. CT-generated static-guided methods had less deviation from the virtual plan compared to model-based freehand methods [24–32].

There is also a difference in accuracy between clinicians. Some clinicians are more accurate with CT-guided implant placement than others, regarding the positions of the apex, depth, and angle. When inexperienced surgeons were supervised by experienced surgeons, there was no significant difference between inexperienced or experienced surgeons regarding implant placement accuracy when using CT-generated stents [33].

31.5.2 Dynamic Navigation System Accuracy

Studies by Chiu [16], Kramer [17], Brief [23], and Casap [19] indicate that dynamic navigation systems have entry error approximating 0.4 mm and angular deviation error approximating 4°. Model studies report accuracy that is superior to clinical trials.

This author has been involved with an ongoing IRB-approved prospective evaluation on the accuracy of one dynamic navigation system (X-Nav, Lansdale, Pa). The results of 120 consecutive patients are referenced [3]. Three hypotheses were evaluated [3].

Hypothesis 1: The accuracy of the evaluated dynamic navigation system is similar to the accuracy reported in patients using static CT-generated guides.

As seen in the adjacent table, there is similar accuracy comparing dynamic to static navigation. In the meta-analyses, it is very difficult to identify a standard deviation comparing multiple references, so the standard deviation is not included in the table. Readers can review each study within the meta-analysis if desired.

Hypothesis 2: The accuracy of the evaluated dynamic navigation system is similar to freehand implant placement.

Freehand data: 20 patients had clips placed onto their teeth, and a virtual navigation plan was made. However, due to regulatory restraints, the dynamic navigation system was not used. These 20 patients had their implants placed freehand. Routine preoperative and immediate postoperative CBCT scans were mesh analyzed to provide freehand data [3].

As seen in the adjacent table, there is a difference between freehand and navigation. In every study evaluated, it is obvious that the freehand approach is not as accurate or precise compared to navigation, whether dynamic or static.

Hypothesis 3: After 20 cases, there are minimal accuracy differences between surgeons.

Navigation surgery is known to have a learning curve associated with it. The learning curve of cardiothoracic and vascular surgical procedures has been summarized in a total of 48 studies. Based on operating time, the learning curve for coronary artery bypass surgery ranged between 15 and 100 cases; for endoscopic vessel harvesting and other cardiac vessel surgery, between 7 and 35 cases; for valvular surgery, which included repair and replacement, between 20 and 135 cases; for video-assisted thoracoscopic surgery, between 15 and 35 cases; for vascular neurosurgical procedures, between 100 and 500 cases, based on complications; for endovascular vessel repairs, between 5 and 40 cases; and for ablation procedures, between 25 and 60 cases. They concluded that the learning curves for cardiothoracic and vascular procedures varied depending on the procedure and the level of experience of the clinician.

Simulation of dynamic navigation has been used to decrease the learning curve for clinicians performing colonoscopy. Simulators improved training of novice endoscopists. In a study involving colonoscopy procedures, the mean cecal intubation time decreased from a baseline of 9.50 to 2.20 min at completion of the training. Colonic insertion depth improved from 29.4 to 63.7 cm. The learning effect of simulator training ceased after 60 colonoscopies. This study demonstrates the rationale for intensive simulator training in the early learning curve of novices performing colonoscopy. It is recommended for all clinicians using a dynamic navigation system to have training on manikins, mentoring with over-the-shoulder observation, and if possible hands-on mentoring when performing the initial case surgeries.

As previously reported [3], the repeated measure ANOVA showed a significant difference in accuracy between case experiences (0–30 surgeries, and 0–20 vs. 21–40) for both platform deviation ($P = 0.001$, $P = 0.025$) and apical deviation ($P = 0.008$, $P = 0.005$). It showed no difference in accuracy between case experiences for angular deviation ($P = 0.548$, $P = 0.131$). There was no significant difference in accuracy between surgeons for any of the three deviations ($P = 0.619$, $P = 0.274$, $P = 0.176$).

The accuracy data did demonstrate a learning curve for the surgeons. As seen in Fig. 31.8, the accuracy for cases 1–10, 11–20, 21–30, and 31–40 were slightly different. It appears that after 20 cases, minimal differences were noted [2, 3] (Table 31.1).

31.6 Indications for Each Method

There are clinical situations that either method is advantageous over the freehand method. The choice of static or dynamic navigation will depend on the clinician's preference and experience. Either navigation method can be used for:

1. Flapless approaches: A site that has had previous ridge augmentation and the clinician wants to avoid disturbing the superficial part of the graft with flap elevation.
2. Placement of adjacent implants requiring accurate spacing between implants and adjacent teeth. This ensures appropriate spacing of the implants from the teeth and provides accuracy in maintaining appropriate space between implants.
3. The need for accurate implant angulation which is especially important in the esthetic zone and for screw-retained prostheses.

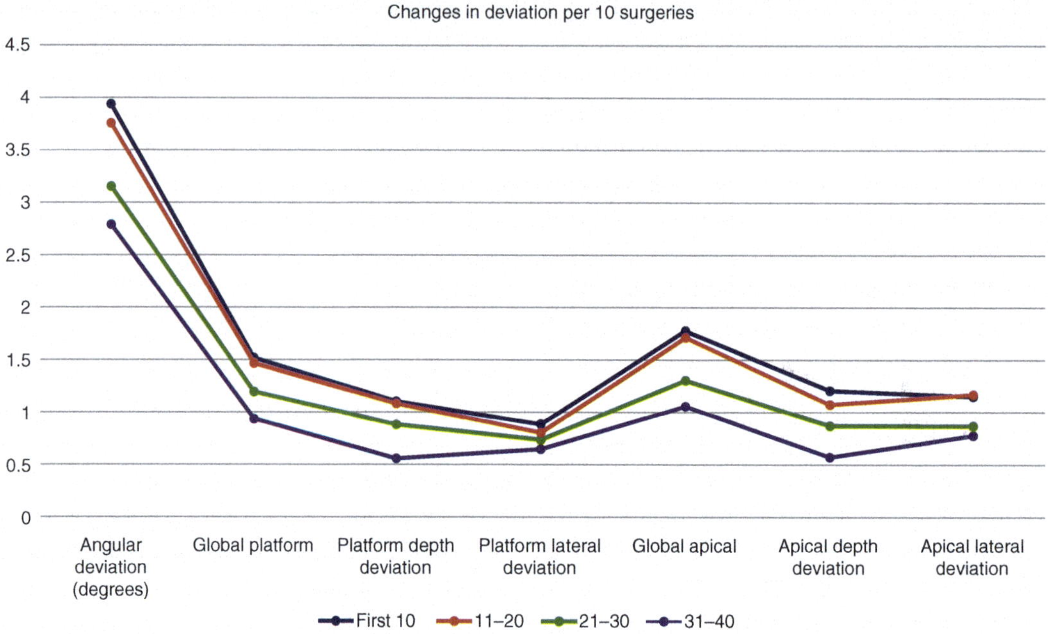

Fig. 31.8 Graphic depiction of learning curve

Table 31.1 Comparison of accuracy between implant placement methods

	Angular deviation (degrees)	Platform deviation (mm)	Apical deviation (mm)
Dynamic navigation [3]	3.15 ± 2.1	1.2 ± 0.5	0.88 ± 0.5
Static navigation [25]	3.89 ± ?	1.12 ± ?	1.39 ± ?
Freehand [3]	7.69 ± 4.9	1.67 ± 0.4	2.21 ± 0.99

4. Control of depth placement:
   (a) To avoid nerve trauma
   (b) To place the preparation osteotomy adjacent to the sinus floor, when elevating the sinus floor through the implant preparation site
   (c) To intentionally engage the floor of the sinus or nasal floor for bicortical implant stability

A CT-generated static guide is recommended for edentulous cases. Dynamic navigation requires registration of the jaw to the navigation system which is currently not evidence based on intrabony fiducials. For the edentulous case, a static CT-generated guide is used when:

1. A flapless method is desired.
2. The CT-generated guide can be used to preoperatively fabricate a provisional prosthesis on models generated from the static guide itself.
3. The clinician desires the use of a bone reduction guide to accurately provide space for the planned prosthesis.
4. Implant placement is critical for a planned full arch fixed crown and bridge-type prosthesis.

Dynamic navigation is indicated when the surgeon plans:

1. Placement of implants in cases with limited mouth opening
2. Placement of implant on the same day the CBCT is taken
3. Placement of implants in difficult access locations such as the second molar
4. Placement of implants when direct visualization is difficult
5. Placement of implant in tight interdental spaces when static guides cannot be used due to tube size

6. Placement of implants adjacent to natural teeth in situations where static guide tubes interfere with ideal implant placement

Additional considerations for dynamic navigation:

What are the common reasons for error when placing dental implants? The presence of asymmetric density in bone can result in deviation of the implant position. Dense bone will deflect drills while creating osteotomies and implants when they are delivered. For example, this occurs when placing an implant immediately into a mandibular molar extraction site, when placing an implant after removing an anterior incisor, or when placing an implant early after grafting lost facial cortical bone with the lateral portion of the graft being softer than the lingual or palatal bone. When the surgeon recognizes these phenomena, the position of the implant drills can be compensated. This problem is present with or without the use of guided surgery; however, using dynamic navigation the deflection can be visualized on the monitor.

A surgeon will have either right- or left-handed dominance. The position of the arrays will be affected by the surgeon's dominant hand. For a left-handed surgeon, placement of the arrays on the right side of the arch allows for less interference with the direct line of sight to the patient-mounted arrays. The position of the patient reclined or sitting will affect the ability of the cameras to track the drill array, which in general should be parallel to the overhead camera. Each surgeon will need to practice different positions with the camera behind, over, or in front of the patient and get comfortable.

Working at high magnification allows the surgeon to acquire new skills. The surgeon has the ability to visualize implant placement within a "sphere of accuracy." The sphere of accuracy is affected by the surgeon's ability to hold the instrumentation, the rigidity of the instrumentation, the resolution of the CT, and the inaccuracy of the tracking system itself. Dynamic systems presented have graphics that show a 1 mm sphere of accuracy. When drill extensions are used, the inaccuracy compounded by these flexible components can be visualized.

The surgeon must learn to trust the navigation system and their own presurgical planning. This will require a slower approach in the early stages as the surgeon confirms implant positioning after each drill is used.

Conclusion

Accuracy and precision are required for implant placement. The use of planning prior to implant placement will provide patients with care that they should expect on a routine basis. The material presented in this chapter has been reduced to everyday practice and can be implemented by all clinicians.

References

1. Block MS. Esthetic anterior implant restorations: surgical techniques for optimal results. In: Color atlas of dental implant surgery. 4th ed. St Louis, MI: Elsevier; 2015. p. 365–419.
2. Block MS, Emery RW. Static or dynamic navigation for implant placement-choosing the method of guidance. J Oral Maxillofac Surg. 2016;74(2):269–77.
3. Block MS, Emery RW, Lank K, Ryan J. Implant placement accuracy using dynamic navigation. Int J Oral Maxillofac Implants. 2017;32(1):92–9.
4. dos Santos PL, Queiroz TP, Margonar R, de Souza Carvalho AC, Betoni W Jr, Rezende RR, dos Santos PH, Garcia IR Jr. Evaluation of bone heating, drill deformation, and drill roughness after implant osteotomy: guided surgery and classic drilling procedure. Int J Oral Maxillofac Implants. 2014;29:51–8.
5. Nijmeh AD, Goodger NM, Hawkes D, Edwards PJ, McGurk M. Image-guided navigation in oral and maxillofacial surgery. Br J Oral Maxillofac Surg. 2005;43:294–302.
6. Bouchard C, Magil JC, Nikonovskiy V, Byl M, Murphy BA, Kaban LB, Troulis MJ. Osteomark: a surgical navigation system for oral and maxillofacial surgery. Int J Oral Maxillofac Surg. 2012;41:265–70.
7. Strong EB, Rafii A, Holhweg-Majert B, Fuller SC, Metzger MC. Comparison of 3 optical navigation systems for computer-aided maxillofacial surgery. Arch Otolaryngol Head Neck Surg. 2008;134:1080–4.
8. Casap N, Wexler A, Eliashar R. Computerized navigation for surgery of the lower jaw: comparison of 2 navigation systems. J Oral Maxillofac Surg. 2008;66:1467–75.
9. Poeschl PW, et al. Comparison of cone-beam and conventional multislice computed tomography for image-guided dental implant planning. Clin Oral Investig. 2013;17:317–24.

10. Ewers R, et al. Basic research and 12 years of clinical experience in computer-assisted navigation technology: a review. Int J Oral Maxillofac Surg. 2005;34:1–8.
11. Wittwer G, Adeyemo WL, Schicho K, Birkfellner W, Enislidis G. Prospective randomized clinical comparison of 2 dental implant navigation systems. Int J Oral Maxillofac Implants. 2007;22:785–90.
12. Wanschitz F, et al. Evaluation of accuracy of computer-aided intraoperative positioning of endosseous oral implants in the edentulous mandible. Clin Oral Implants Res. 2002;13:59–64.
13. Lueth TC, Wenger T, Rautenberg A, Deppe H. RoboDent and the change of needs in computer aided dental implantology during the past ten years. In: 2011 IEEE International Conference on Robotics and Automation (ICRA). Shanghai, China: IEEE; 2011. p. 1–4.
14. Casap N, Laviv AW. Computerized navigation for immediate loading of dental implants with a prefabricated metal frame: a feasibility study. J Oral Maxillofac Surg. 2011;69:512–9.
15. Siessegger M, et al. Use of an image-guided navigation system in dental implant surgery in anatomically complex operation sites. J Craniomaxillofac Surg. 2001;29:276–81.
16. Chiu WK, Luk WK, Cheung LK. Three-dimensional accuracy of implant placement in a computer-assisted navigation system. J Oral Maxillofac Implants. 2006;21:465–70.
17. Kramer F-J, Baethge C, Swennen G, Rosahl S. Navigated vs. conventional implant insertion for maxillary single tooth replacement. Clin Oral Implants Res. 2005;16:60–8.
18. Brief J, Edinger D, Hassfeld S, Eggers G. Accuracy of image-guided implantology. Clin Oral Implants Res. 2005;16:495–501.
19. Casap N, Wexler A, Persky N, Schneider A, Lustmann J. Navigation surgery for dental implants: assessment of accuracy of the image guided implantology system. J Oral Maxillofac Surg. 2004;62:116–9.
20. Arora KS, Khan N, Abboudi H, Khan MS, Dasgupta P, Ahmed K. Learning curves for cardiothoracic and vascular surgical procedures – a systematic review. Postgrad Med. 2015;127:202–14.
21. Koch AD, Ekkelenkamp VE, Haringsma J, Schoon EJ, de Man RA, Kuipers EJ. Simulated colonoscopy training leads to improved performance during patient-based assessment. Gastrointest Endosc. 2015;81:630–6.
22. Hultin M, Svensson KG, Trulsson M. Clinical advantages of computer-guided implant placement: a systematic review. Clin Oral Implants Res. 2012;23(Suppl 6):124–35.
23. Wittwer G, Adeyemo WL, Wagner A, Enislidis G. Computer-guided flapless placement and immediate loading of four conical screw-type implants in the edentulous mandible. Clin Oral Implants Res. 2007;18:534–9.
24. Tahmaseb A, Wismeijer D, Coucke W, Derksen W. Computer technology application in surgical implant dentistry: a systemic review. Int J Oral Maxillofac Implants. 2014;29(Suppl):25–42.
25. Jung RE, Schneider D, Ganeles J, Wismeijer D, Zwahlen M, Hammerle CHF, Tahmaseb A. Computer technology applications in surgical implant dentistry: a systemic review. Int J Oral Maxillofac Implants. 2009;24(suppl):92–109.
26. Vercruyssen M, Cox C, Coucke W, Naert I, Jacobs R, Quirynen M. A randomized clinical trial comparing guided implant surgery (bone- or mucosa-supported) with mental navigation or the use of a pilot-drill template. J Clin Periodontol. 2014;41:717–23.
27. Park JM, Kim SM, Kim MJ, Lee JH, Kim MJ. An assessment of template-guided implant surgery in terms of accuracy and related factors. J Adv Prosthodont. 2013;5:440–7.
28. Pettersson A, Kero T, Söderberg R, Näsström K. Accuracy of virtually planned and CAD/CAM-guided implant surgery on plastic models. J Prosthet Dent. 2014;112:1472–8.
29. Di Giacomo GA, da Silva JV, da Silva AM, Paschoal GH, Cury PR, Szarf G. Accuracy and complications of computer-designed selective laser sintering surgical guides for flapless dental implant placement and immediate definitive prosthesis installation. J Periodontol. 2012;83(4):410–9.
30. Ersoy AE, Turkyilmaz I, Ozan O, McGlumphy EA. Reliability of implant placement with stereolithographic surgical guides generated from computed tomography: clinical data from 94 implants. J Periodontol. 2008;79(8):1339–45.
31. Ozan O, Turkyilmaz I, Ersoy AE, McGlumphy EA, Rosenstiel SF. Clinical accuracy of 3 different types of computed tomography-derived stereolithographic surgical guides in implant placement. J Oral Maxillofac Surg. 2009;67(2):394–401.
32. Valente F, Schiroli G, Sbrenna A. Accuracy of computer-aided oral implant surgery: a clinical and radiographic study. Int J Oral Maxillofac Implants. 2009;24(2):234–42.
33. Van de Wiele G, Teughels W, Vercruyssen M, Coucke W, Temmerman A, Quirynen M. The accuracy of guided surgery via mucosa-supported stereolithographic surgical templates in the hands of surgeons with little experience. Clin Oral Implants Res. 2015;26(12):1489–94. https://doi.org/10.1111/clr.12494. [Epub ahead of print].

32 Navigational Surgery and Computer Assisted Treatment Planning

Akashdeep Villing and Jasjit Dillon

Abstract

The maxillofacial region presents a distinctive challenge with respect to surgical approaches and complex anatomy. The area has unique functional and esthetic requirements, making surgical precision mandatory. In recent years, a trend toward dynamic imaging modalities to help improve the accuracy of maxillofacial reconstruction has developed (Haflfeld et al. Int J Oral Maxillofac Surg 24:111–9, 1995). CT-guided navigation surgery allows the operator to link previously acquired imaging with clinical findings in the operating room (Haflfeld et al. Int J Oral Maxillofac Surg 24:111–9, 1995). This enables a live three-dimensional (3D) map of the patient's anatomy in relation to the surgical site. This utility aids in reducing surgical error and is an area of great interest in the head and neck region. This chapter will review the applications of navigation in maxillofacial surgery.

32.1 Introduction

The maxillofacial region presents a unique challenge with respect to surgical approaches and complex anatomy. The area has unique functional and esthetic requirements, making surgical precision mandatory. Traditional modes of imaging have been utilized to help reconstruct maxillofacial defects for several decades. The progression from plain films to computed tomography (CT) and magnetic resonance imaging (MRI) as adjuncts to clinical findings for treating injuries and pathology in the head and neck region has been well documented [1]. In recent years, a trend toward dynamic imaging modalities to help improve the accuracy of maxillofacial reconstruction has developed [1]. CT-guided navigational surgery enables the surgeon to link previously acquired imaging with clinical findings in the operating room [1], allowing for a live three-dimensional (3D) map of the patient's

A. Villing, D.M.D.
Department of Oral and Maxillofacial Surgery, University of Washington, Seattle, WA, USA

J. Dillon, DDS, MBBS, FDSRCS, FACS (✉)
Department of Oral and Maxillofacial Surgery, Harborview Medical Center, University of Washington, Seattle, WA, USA
e-mail: dillonj5@uw.edu

© Springer International Publishing AG 2018
E.M. Ferneini, J.D. Bennett (eds.), *Perioperative Assessment of the Maxillofacial Surgery Patient*,
https://doi.org/10.1007/978-3-319-58868-1_32

anatomy in relation to the surgical site of concern. Furthermore, this enables dynamic tracking to ensure appropriate positioning of surgical instruments and implants used for reconstruction. This utility of dynamic imaging to aid in reducing surgical error is an area of great interest in the head and neck region. This chapter will review the applications of navigation in maxillofacial surgery.

32.2 History

Surgical approaches in the head and neck region often make it challenging to accurately visualize the entire injury when approaching a surgical correction [1]. For years surgeons have had to rely primarily on experience and peripheral confirmation including occlusion or subjective analysis of symmetry when confirming final trauma reductions or secondary revisions. These techniques rely heavily on imaging for preoperative assessment and surgical planning, not only for appropriate and efficient time allotment but also for outcome predictability in the operating room (OR). However, there is a constant desire for improvement. In recent years, pre-surgical virtual planning options which improve surgical accuracy, outcomes, and, in training institutions, resident education have become popularized. Virtual planning allows an infinite number of surgical options to be assessed on a computer using specialized software now available from multiple companies. With computer-aided software becoming more and more sophisticated, including CAD/CAM (computer-aided design/computer-aided manufacturing), increasingly, the utility of navigational planning in maxillofacial reconstruction has become more prominent. This transition may be done with or without presurgical virtual planning. Intraoperative navigation systems were initially limited as the early "Digital Imaging and Communications in Medicine" (DICOM) datasets did not allow for dynamic movements or alterations in position during CT scanning, making the assessment of symmetry challenging [1]. As CAD/CAM developed, manipulation of CT datasets was more easily achievable [1]. This allowed surgeons to examine multiple planes and mirror image the face for symmetry, in addition to allowing for virtual planning of osteotomies and movements. The utility remained limited until the integration of integrative stereolithographic models [1] enabling physical models of the facial skeleton to be used as templates actively in the operating room [1]; these models allowed for static navigation. However, it was not until intraoperative dynamic navigation was utilized could live/real-time updates on hard and soft tissue adjustments be achieved. The addition of CAD/CAM and surgical navigation systems have allowed surgeons to more accurately address challenges unique to the maxillofacial region in the planning phase, arming them with more information prior to entering the operating room. Navigation effectively enables real-time live assessment of planned treatment, providing increased accuracy in obtaining the desired outcome. It should be noted that intraoperative navigation while a newer technology in the world of maxillofacial surgery has been used for several years in other surgical specialties, notably otolaryngology and neurosurgery.

Although stereolithographic models may not always be indicated, the intraoperative accuracy and ease of utility have expanded the use of surgical navigation into the realms of trauma, orthognathic surgery, implantology, and pathology.

32.3 Programs

Several available CAD/CAM programs exist to allow for surgical planning and navigation. Although an extensive discussion of each individual system is outside the scope of this chapter, an overview of software applications is appropriate in understanding the utility of different systems. Irrespective of which software is utilized, the key to effectiveness is the ability to import DICOM data and perform virtual manipulation in the operating room [1]. The DICOM format is used in most current CT scanners, CAD/CAM software, and surgical navigation systems.

Currently, the two main craniofacial navigation systems used in the United States are manufactured by Stryker® (Kalamazoo, MI USA) and Brainlab® (Munich, Germany). While Medtronic is also available, it is currently only for neurosurgical and ENT (skull base) cases. The readers are encouraged to review the literature in case this changes. For the purposes of this chapter, further detailed information regarding the two craniofacial systems and setup will be discussed with focus on the Stryker system as this is most familiar to the senior author. Readers are encouraged to educate themselves on the systems available within their medical centers.

The Stryker Cranial Navigation system (iNtellectCranial®, CranialMap® [2.0–3.0]) can be used as a real-time guide during reconstructive surgery assessing the defect site but also using the mirrored, uninvolved/healthy side of a patient to reconstruct the defect side [2]. iNtellectCranial is older software but has mirroring capacity. CranialMap 2.0 while newer could not mirror. Most recently the Food and Drug Administration approved CranialMap 3.0 which is the most superior with mirroring capacity. Using the software, a patient CT according to the company protocol is obtained. It must contain all the relevant images of the healthy side and the side to be reconstructed. This CT is then uploaded into the software and reviewed. If satisfactory the bone window cuts are used to mirror the dataset. This is done by adding the patient's information as CT01 (corresponding to the ORIGINAL image set). This CT dataset is then reselected and intentionally the orientations are switched from left to right in the coronal views to obtain the mirror imaging. This is then saved as CT02. Once the two new image sets are available, the planning software automatically produces the fully automatic image correlation dialog [2] by superimposing the two images. Since most human heads are fairly symmetrical, the correlation will be quite accurate. It is usually red (mirrored imaging) over green (original dataset). Skull segmentation is then performed first on the original image (CT01/the non-mirrored skull), followed by segmentation of the mirrored (area to be reconstructed skull/CT02). To guide during surgery, the patient is registered to the original dataset (CT01) [2] In the OR, the Stryker Navigation System accomplishes registration to the software and planned simulation using an auto-registration mask, along with traditional point-to-point registration. The software automatically detects the mask's LED positions as high density points on the intra-op scan and then during registration, software matches LEDs affixed to the patient. For the Stryker system, the mask is positioned on the upper nasal bridge with the central LED on the deepest point between the eyes [3]. The lowest LED along the midline is placed on the nose tip. The mask is approximated as close as possible to bony structures [3]. When applying the lower parts of the side sections, the central LED is placed near the edge of the orbital cavity (Fig. 32.1). The upper section is applied such that the lower LEDs are approximated near the eyebrows [3]. This system's built-in software will respond to the activation of the mask by starting the mask registration workflow [3]. At this stage the surgeon can ensure that the mask is within the working space of the camera. Registration is confirmed by the following color-coded indications: light green, visible; red, not visible; and gray, defective [3]. Utilization of known anatomical landmarks further confirms registration. Oftentimes in panfacial cases, the mask will be in the surgical field. To circumvent this, at this stage the operator can transfer registration of the mask to a skull post tracker which is screwed onto usually the parietal bone. Either way, the surgeon can then confirm registration is accurate by touching known anatomic landmarks. The senior author uses the maxillary incisor teeth edges and the medial canthi. It should be noted that imaging for registration must be current. Any facial swelling that has occurred post-injury must have resolved or the result will be an inaccurate face mask registration with a large error noted during registration conformation. The senior author recommends to obtain a CT scan per Stryker protocol within 24 h (idea)—1 week of surgery. Depending upon the case, the surgeon must then decide if the registration is accurate and what degree of error is acceptable. Normally within 1 mm is acceptable for non-dental implant cases. If the registration appears inaccurate, addi-

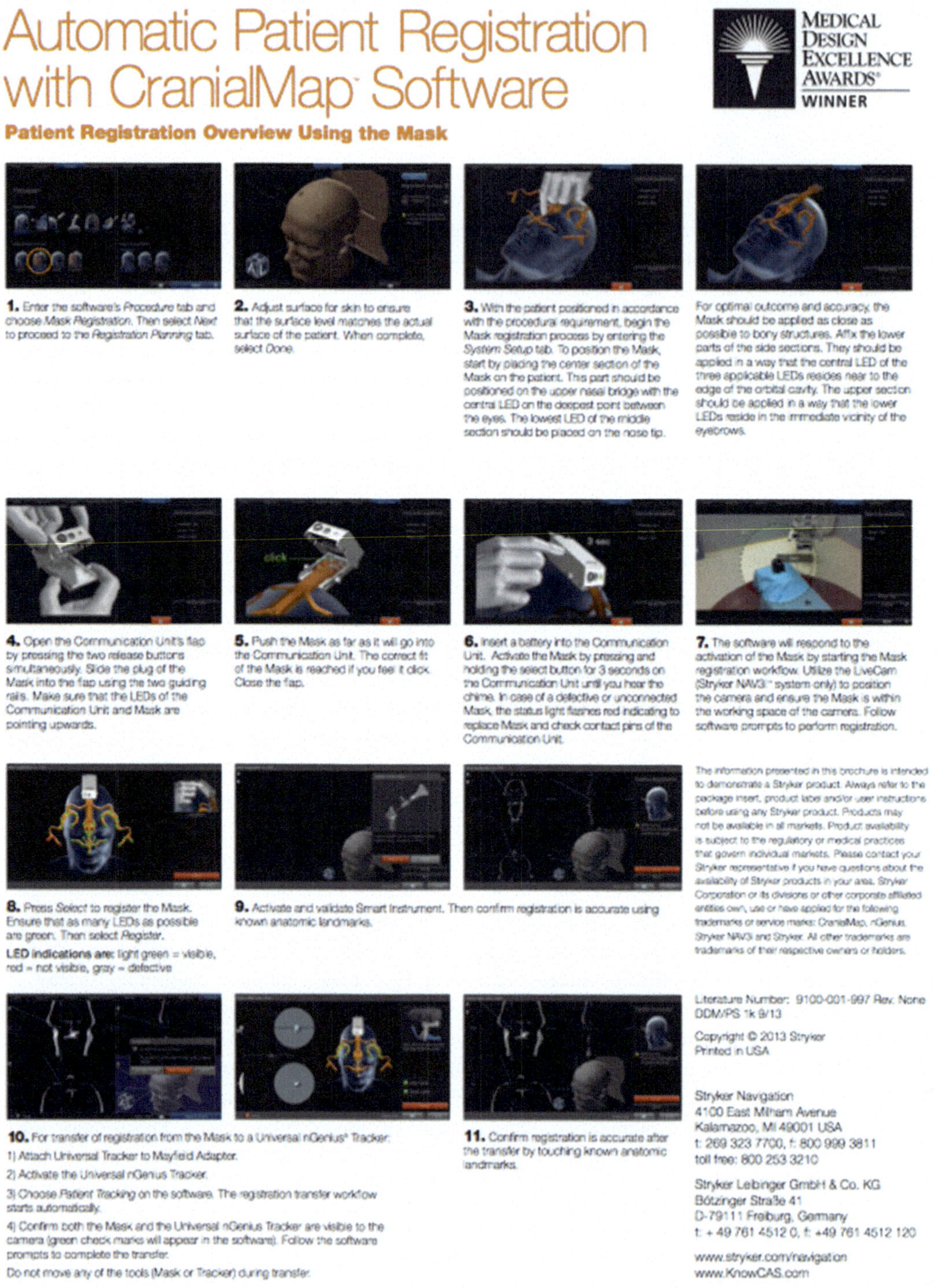
Automatic Patient Registration with CranialMap™ Software

MEDICAL DESIGN EXCELLENCE AWARDS® WINNER

Patient Registration Overview Using the Mask

1. Enter the software's *Procedure* tab and choose *Mask Registration*. Then select *Next* to proceed to the *Registration Planning* tab.

2. Adjust surface for skin to ensure that the surface level matches the actual surface of the patient. When complete, select *Done*.

3. With the patient positioned in accordance with the procedural requirement, begin the Mask registration process by entering the *System Setup* tab. To position the Mask, start by placing the center section of the Mask on the patient. This part should be positioned on the upper nasal bridge with the central LED on the deepest point between the eyes. The lowest LED of the middle section should be placed on the nose tip.

For optimal outcome and accuracy, the Mask should be applied as close as possible to bony structures. Affix the lower parts of the side sections. They should be applied in a way that the central LED of the three applicable LEDs resides near to the edge of the orbital cavity. The upper section should be applied in a way that the lower LEDs reside in the immediate vicinity of the eyebrows.

4. Open the Communication Unit's flap by pressing the two release buttons simultaneously. Slide the plug of the Mask into the flap using the two guiding rails. Make sure that the LEDs of the Communication Unit and Mask are pointing upwards.

5. Push the Mask as far as it will go into the Communication Unit. The correct fit of the Mask is reached if you feel it click. Close the flap.

6. Insert a battery into the Communication Unit. Activate the Mask by pressing and holding the select button for 3 seconds on the Communication Unit until you hear the chime. In case of a defective or unconnected Mask, the status light flashes red indicating to replace Mask and check contact pins of the Communication Unit.

7. The software will respond to the activation of the Mask by starting the Mask registration workflow. Utilize the LiveCam (Stryker NAV3i™ system only) to position the camera and ensure the Mask is within the working space of the camera. Follow software prompts to perform registration.

8. Press *Select* to register the Mask. Ensure that as many LEDs as possible are green. Then select *Register*.

LED indications are: light green = visible, red = not visible, gray = defective

9. Activate and validate Smart Instrument. Then confirm registration is accurate using known anatomic landmarks.

The information presented in this brochure is intended to demonstrate a Stryker product. Always refer to the package insert, product label and/or user instructions before using any Stryker product. Products may not be available in all markets. Product availability is subject to the regulatory or medical practices that govern individual markets. Please contact your Stryker representative if you have questions about the availability of Stryker products in your area. Stryker Corporation or its divisions or other corporate affiliated entities own, use or have applied for the following trademarks or service marks: CranialMap, nGenius, Stryker NAV3i and Stryker. All other trademarks are trademarks of their respective owners or holders.

10. For transfer of registration from the Mask to a Universal nGenius® Tracker:

1) Attach Universal Tracker to Mayfield Adapter.

2) Activate the Universal nGenius Tracker.

3) Choose *Patient Tracking* on the software. The registration transfer workflow starts automatically.

4) Confirm both the Mask and the Universal nGenius Tracker are visible to the camera (green check marks will appear in the software). Follow the software prompts to complete the transfer.

Do not move any of the tools (Mask or Tracker) during transfer.

11. Confirm registration is accurate after the transfer by touching known anatomic landmarks.

Literature Number: 9100-001-997 Rev. None
DDM/PS 1k 9/13

Copyright © 2013 Stryker
Printed in USA

Stryker Navigation
4100 East Milham Avenue
Kalamazoo, MI 49001 USA
t: 269 323 7700, f: 800 999 3811
toll free: 800 253 3210

Stryker Leibinger GmbH & Co. KG
Bötzinger Straße 41
D-79111 Freiburg, Germany
t: + 49 761 4512 0, f: +49 761 4512 120

www.stryker.com/navigation
www.KnowCAS.com

Fig. 32.1 Stryker navigation mask application protocol

tional surface registration can be done to enhance accuracy.

Brainlab (Munich, Germany) offers a different technique for referencing patients to the system. Surface matching with touch-based pointers or a laser touch pointer allows for a quicker registration process. Both devices register CT and MR images without headsets or markers, and as a result, registration scans can be avoided, leading to a reduction in the costs associated with navigation surgery. Using a universal instrument holder, the surgeon can then target preplanned trajectories. This feature allows continuous feedback intraoperatively. In addition to the above features, Brainlab Cranial is also compatible with most neurosurgery microscopes. Utilizing markers attached to the microscope allows for positional tracking for the microsurgeon. Heads-up display improves ergonomic position orientation while operating with the microscope. Multiple other systems are utilized worldwide with similar registration processes as described for Stryker and Brainlab. As navigation surgery evolves, the registration process will likely continue to be streamlined to allow for reduced setup time.

32.4 Applications

32.4.1 Trauma

32.4.1.1 Orbital Reconstruction

Orbital reconstruction presents a unique challenge to maxillofacial surgeons due to the complexity of the anatomy of this region. Even the "best" results can be humbling. Surgical approaches have required creativity to avoid anatomically crucial structures including muscles, nerves for vision and extraocular movement, vasculature, and the globe itself. Functional and esthetic requirements are paramount during orbital surgery, and particular attention must be paid to maintaining periorbital esthetics, baseline visual acuity, and extraocular movement [4]. Errors are unforgiving and secondary reconstruction is fraught with challenges and increased risk—the greatest being loss of vision. Functional and esthetic deficits in this region are poorly tolerated and can be caused iatrogenically when reducing fractures or correcting pathological deformities. Restoring the three-dimensional form and function of both the orbital frame and orbital volume is the goal of complex orbital reconstruction [4]. Postsurgical enophthalmos and diplopia remain frequent complications in part due to errors in orbital reconstruction and soft tissue manipulation [5]. In trauma cases, post-traumatic edema and scarring add to the complexity, leading to increasingly challenging access and poor visualization of fracture segments [5]. Combining computer-assisted preoperative planning using stereolithographic models with intraoperative navigation has aimed to aid the surgeon in providing more predictable outcomes for patients. Utilizing virtual correction by mirroring the anatomy of the unaffected side to the affected side has allowed for accurate reproduction of bony contours and globe projection [5]. In cases where alloplastic materials are utilized to replace or repair defects, stereolithographic models allow for presurgical manipulation of plates and intraoperative real-time navigation based on the models and navigation markers. With the advent of 3D printing, custom implants are now being made in real time. Case 1 is an example of a simple large orbital blowout fracture, where preoperative planning and intraoperative surgical navigation was utilized to aid in accurate orbital reconstruction (Figs. 32.2, 32.3, 32.4, and 32.5). Since the fracture continued to the posterior ledge, navigation enabled assess-

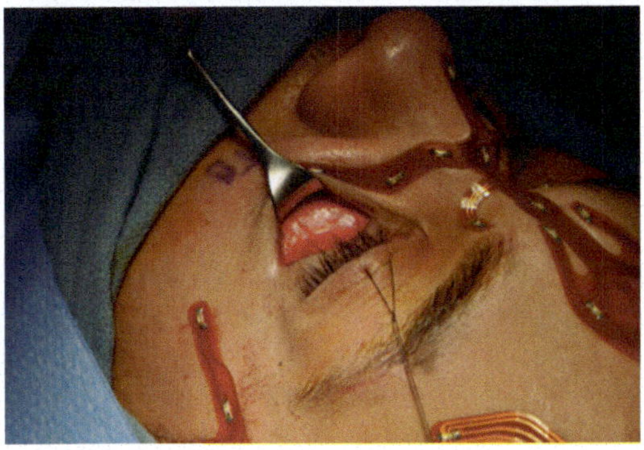

Fig. 32.2 Large orbital blowout fracture with navigation mask in place

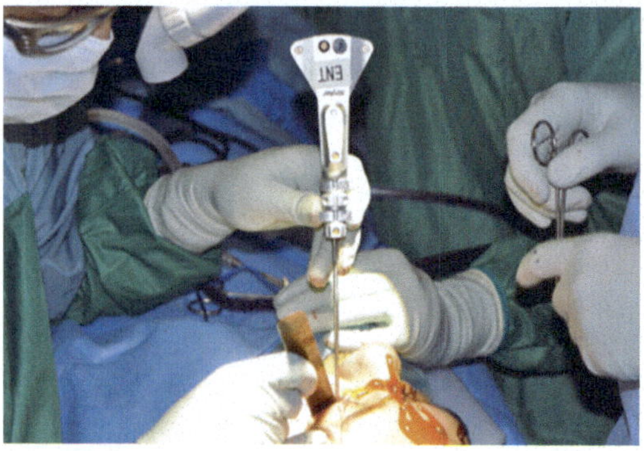

Fig. 32.3 Intraoperative photo utilizing navigation for orbital fracture

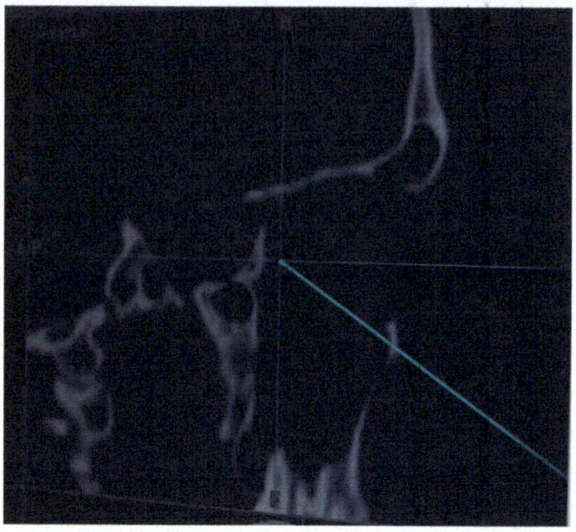

Fig. 32.4 Intraoperative real-time movements on CT

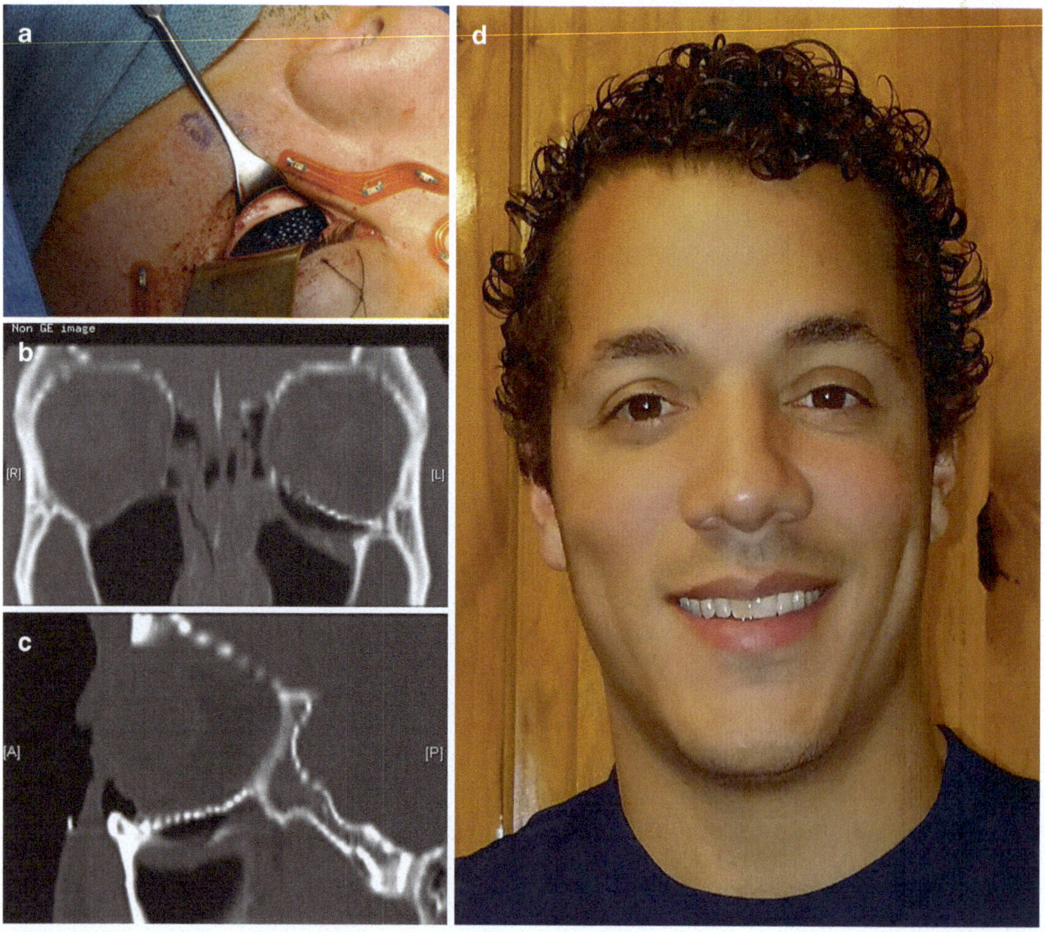

Fig. 32.5 Orbital floor following repair and hardware placement. (**a**) Intraoperative clinical photo showing navigation set up. (**b**) Intraoperative CT coronal bone window. (**c**) Intraoperative CT sagittal bone window (**d**) Post-operative clinical photo

ment of the optic canal and posterior as well as medial and lateral placement of the implant following surgical correction (Figs. 32.2, 32.3, 32.4, and 32.5b). Intraoperative CT imaging confirmed satisfactory implant placement.

32.4.1.2 Panfacial Fractures

Panfacial fractures are uniquely challenging for the craniomaxillofacial surgeon as key landmarks and references may be lost. Surgical access, distorted anatomy, and multiple fractured bone segments with hard and soft tissue losses may compound treatment planning complexity. CT imaging becomes increasingly important, as each individual fracture must be assessed in detail to fully plan for reconstruction. Surgical planning with the assistance of intraoperative navigation helps to reduce postoperative complications [6].

An example of this is a 52-year-old woman who was involved in high-speed MVC and sustained multiple craniomaxillofacial injuries including multiple facial lacerations, right NOE type III fracture, frontal sinus fracture, four-wall orbital fractures, right ZOMC fracture, and a subarachnoid hemorrhage (Fig. 32.6). Due to the intracranial injury, maxillofacial reconstruction was delayed after neurosurgery has repaired the cranial base fracture. Navigation was used to reduce the maxillofacial fractures which were further challenged by the frontal bandeau being repositioned posteriorly secondary to neurosurgical correction and the orbit having a significantly comminuted four-wall defect (Fig. 32.7). At 8-month follow-up, asymmetry was noted due to right infraorbital depression and scar tissue. A preoperative CT using Stryker protocol software displays posterior and lateral disposition of zygoma and lateral displacement of lateral orbital wall with increased orbital volume (Figs. 32.8 and 32.9). Using the CT, 3D models were fabricated for preoperative planning (Fig. 32.10). After clinical and radiographic review and computer simulation, the areas of concern were focused on posterolateral position of the orbitozygomatic complex, right lateral canthus dystopia. The surgical plan was for hardware removal, reosteotomy and anterior repositioning of zygoma, reosteotomy of orbit walls and rim, and medial repositioning of lateral wall to improve orbital volume using navigation and mirror imag-

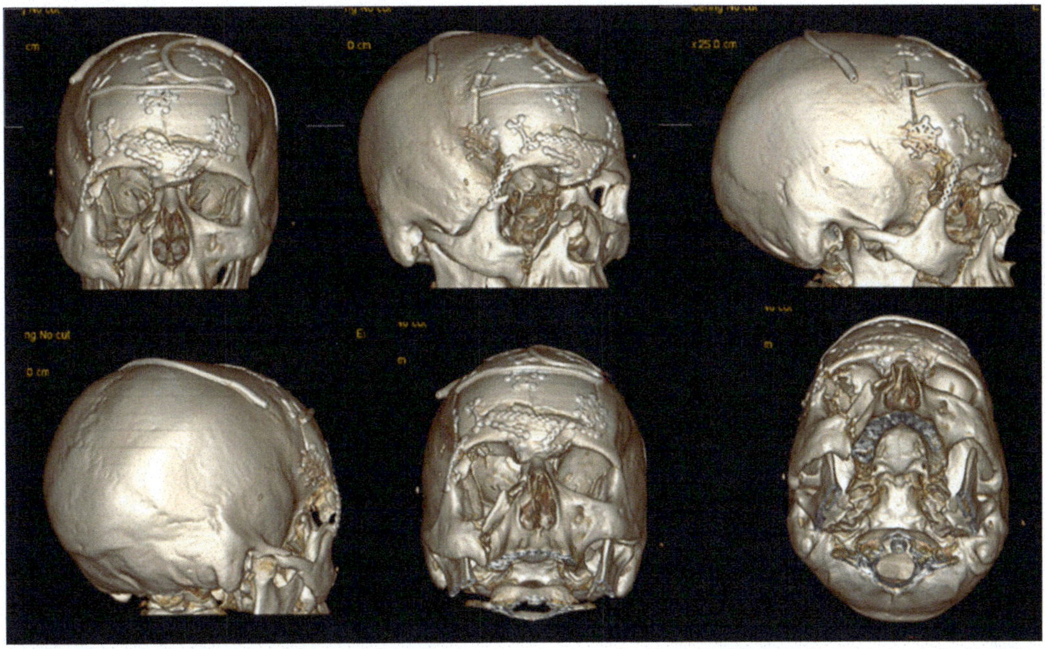

Fig. 32.6 3D CT reconstruction showing multiple facial lacerations, right NOE type III fracture, frontal sinus fracture, four-wall orbital fractures, right ZOMC fracture

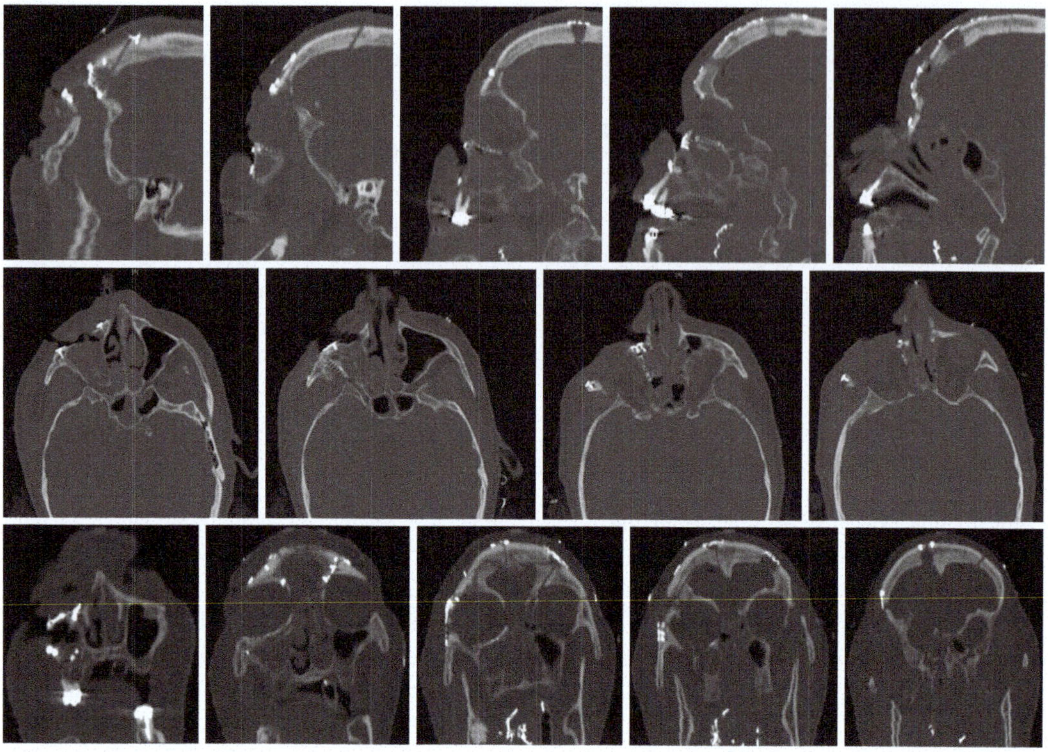

Fig. 32.7 CT showing multiple facial lacerations, right NOE type III fracture, frontal sinus fracture, four-wall orbital fractures, right ZOMC fracture

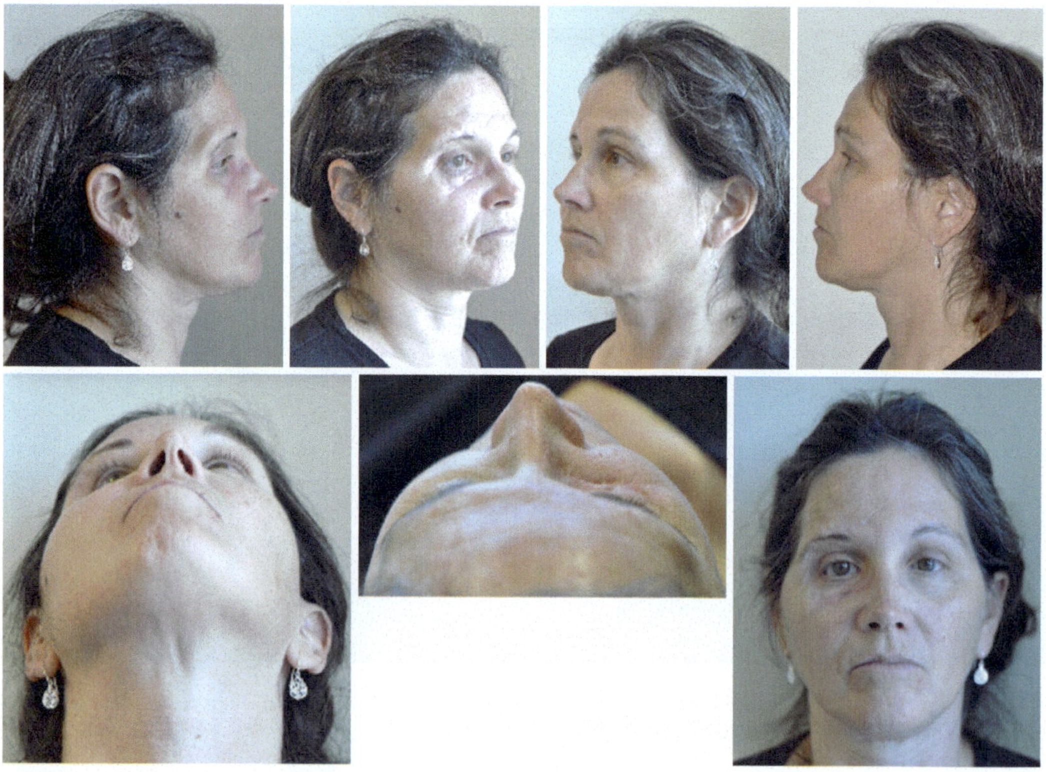

Fig. 32.8 Post-initial maxillofacial surgery. Pre-revision facial views

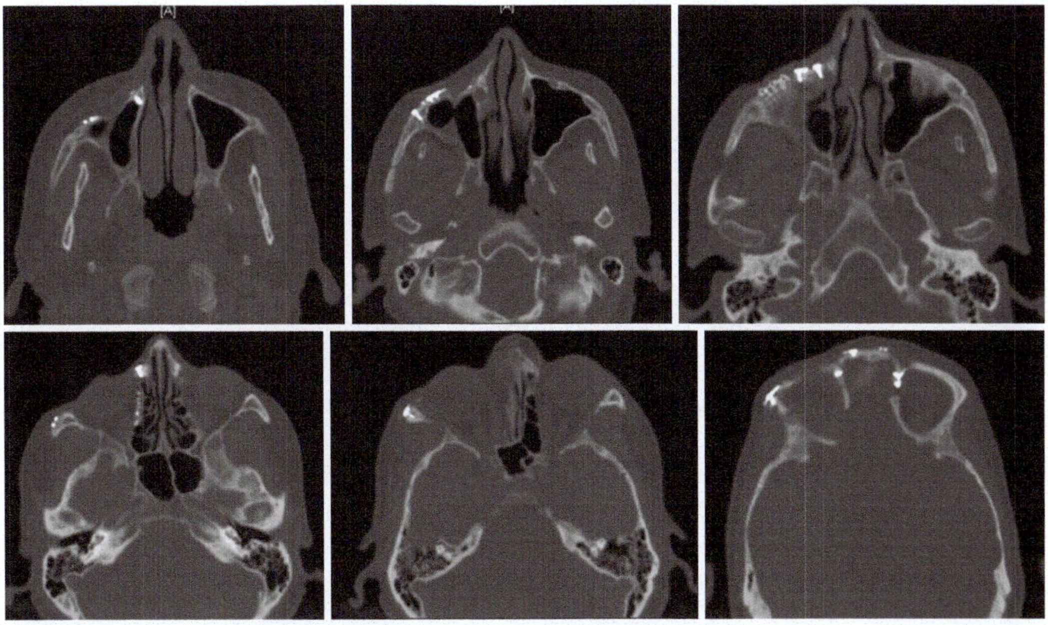

Fig. 32.9 CT showing positioning of hardware—pre-revision CT scan. Post-initial surgery

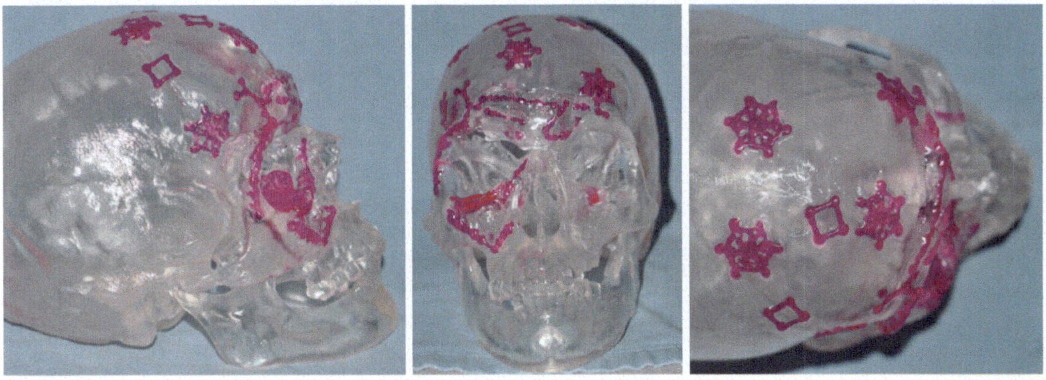

Fig. 32.10 3D models were fabricated for preoperative planning

ing. A Stryker navigation mask was placed, and registration was performed to confirm accuracy. Navigation allowed evaluation of the plan in detail with regard to important anatomic features on the patient's craniofacial skeleton (Figs. 32.11 and 32.12). The zygomaticomaxillary complex was advanced using navigation, until it superimposed onto the preoperative surgically planned position (Fig. 32.12). An intraoperative CT scan was obtained, showing that the reconstructed position corresponded with the surgical plan (Figs. 32.13 and 32.14). Figure 32.14a is

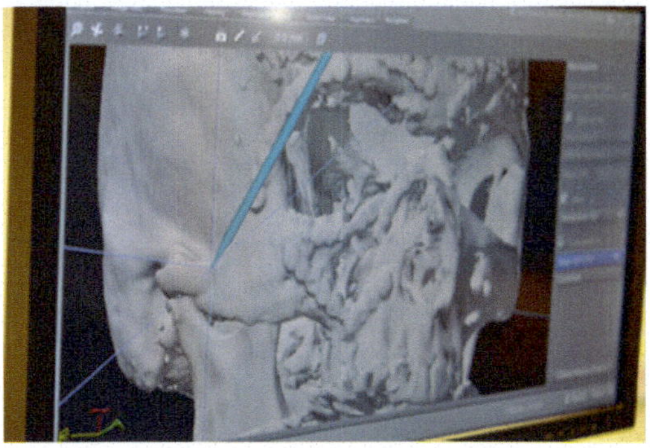

Fig. 32.11 Intraoperative navigation

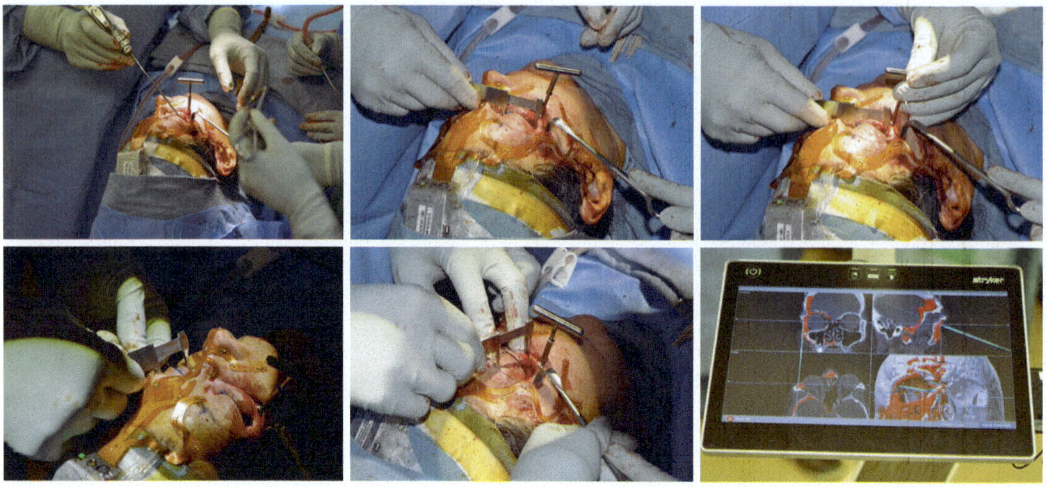

Fig. 32.12 Clinical photo showing the utilization of intraoperative navigation

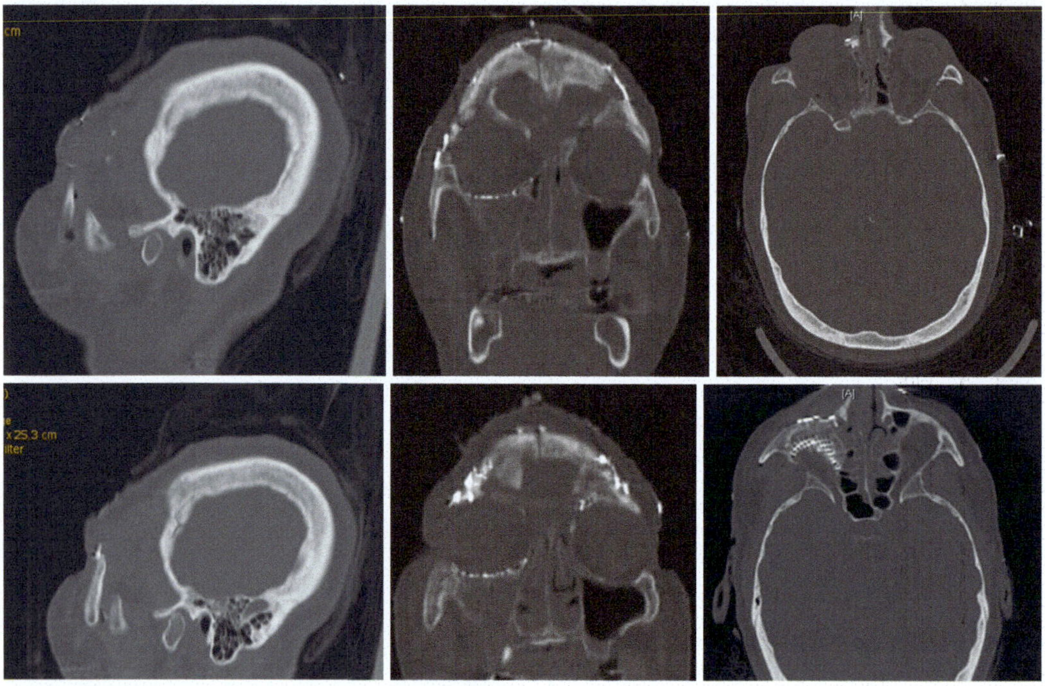

Fig. 32.13 Intraoperative CT scan

comparison of a current and preoperative (postprimary maxillofacial surgery) facial views with improved enophthalmos; however, further soft tissue revision is required and is in progress.

Current technology does not afford ease of use of navigation in mandibular trauma due to movement secondary to the condyles. However, the senior author has used it in difficult condylar fractures when the proximal segment has been very medially displaced. The technique requires the mandible being closed to replicate the preoperative CT scan or avoid error.

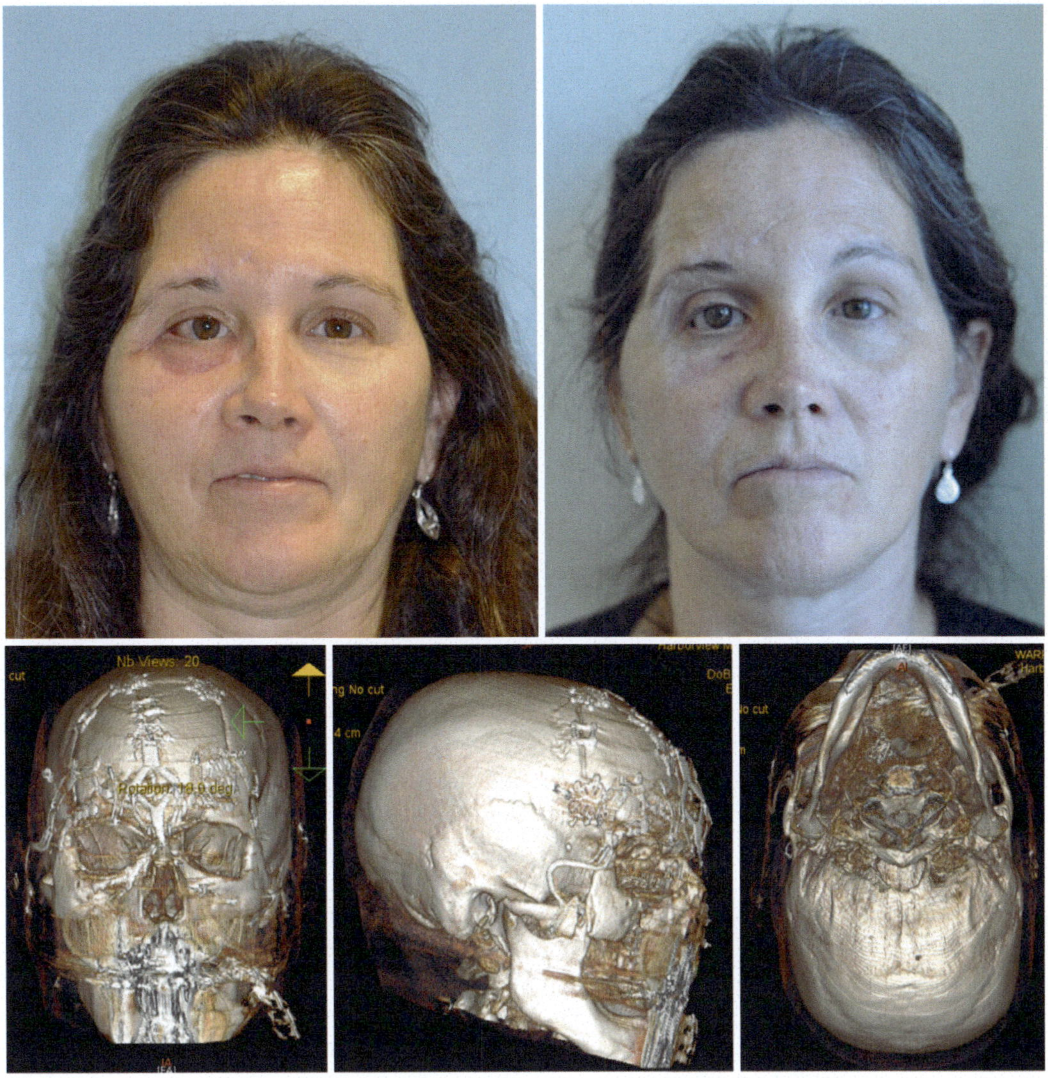

Fig. 32.14 3D reconstruction following treatment. (**a**) Pre- and post-revision facial views

32.4.2 Implantology (Please Refer to Dr. Block's Chapter, Figs. 32.15 and 32.16)

32.4.3 Orthognathic

Orthognathic surgery is entirely dependent upon preoperative planning to achieve ideal results. Frequent dialogue between the surgeon and the orthodontist allows for ideal function and esthetics. Computer planning with stereolithographic models in conjunction with machine-generated splints helps correlate presurgical planning with intraoperative outcomes [5]. Furthermore, navigation with intraoperative markers helps predictably allow for three-dimensional movement. Combining intraoperative navigation with the two commonly used systems for virtual surgical planning (VSP) of orthognathic cases, DePuy Synthes® (West Chester, PA USA) and KLS Martin ® (Jacksonville, FL USA) to name a few companies, has allowed for increased

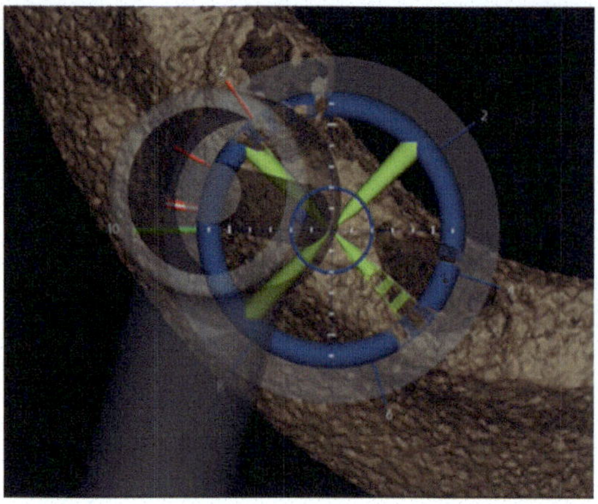

Fig. 32.15 X-Nav technology live implant placement showing desired implant positioning

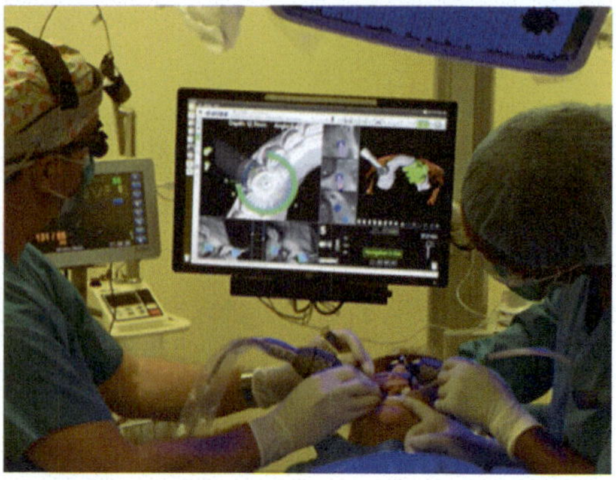

Fig. 32.16 Intraoperative photo showing the utilization of intraoperative navigation for implant placement

accuracy in orthognathic surgery. For both systems a full set of records are required, including standard orthognathic clinical images, updated panoramic image, lateral cephalometric X-ray, CT Face without contrast with three-dimensional (3D) reconstruction, updated casts with existing occlusal records, and simulated occlusal records of the final occlusal positioning. Once received by the parent company, an online planning session is undertaken by the surgeon and the software team, at which time movements are simulated. Prior to entering the OR, the surgeon now simulates movements to the ideal result. Based on this planning session, surgical stents are milled and sent to the surgeon. For double-jaw cases, both intermediate and final splints are provided. This allows for significant reduction in lab time by eliminating the manual steps of model surgery and splint fabrication. Once in the OR, the surgeon uses the simulated movements as a guide and inserts the splints to confirm movements. These movements can be combined with intraoperative navigation to further enhance the predictability of the surgically planned movements.

32.4.4 Pathology

32.4.4.1 Benign Pathology

Navigation surgery can also be utilized in the treatment of benign and malignant pathology guiding extirpation of lesion while preserving local critical anatomy or limiting the surgical approach to a more conservative one. The following case is an example where navigation allowed the location and removal of a displaced tooth and associated keratocystic odontogenic tumor. Preoperative imaging and intraoperative navigation allowed predictable access to the tooth (Figs. 32.17, 32.18, and 32.19). The position of the tooth posed a challenge, as the proximity to the orbit increased risk of iatrogenic injury or further displacement during the removal attempt. Utilization of intraoperative navigation allowed removal without further damage to adjacent

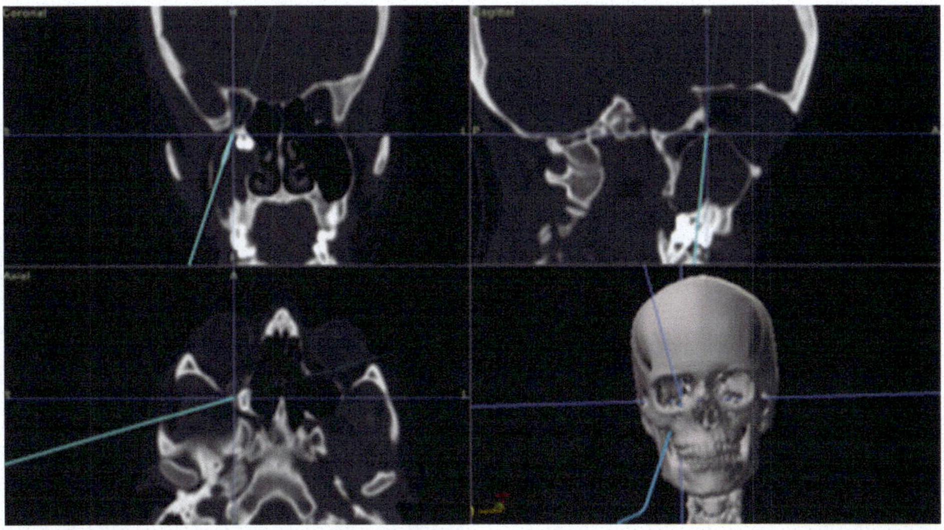

Fig. 32.17 Preoperative imaging showing displaced tooth

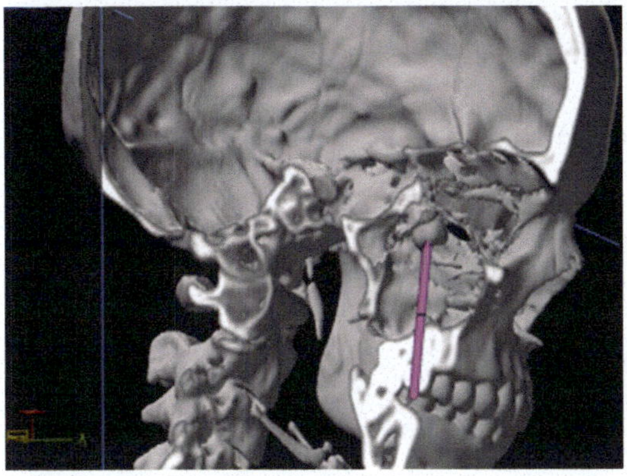

Fig. 32.18 Intraoperative planning for removal of displaced tooth

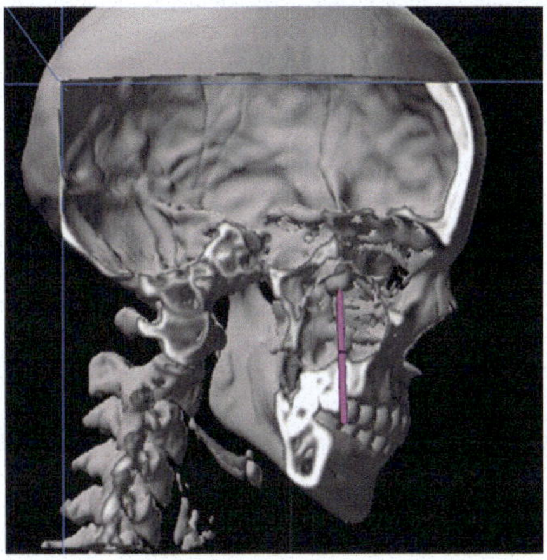

Fig. 32.19 Intraoperative planning for removal of displaced tooth

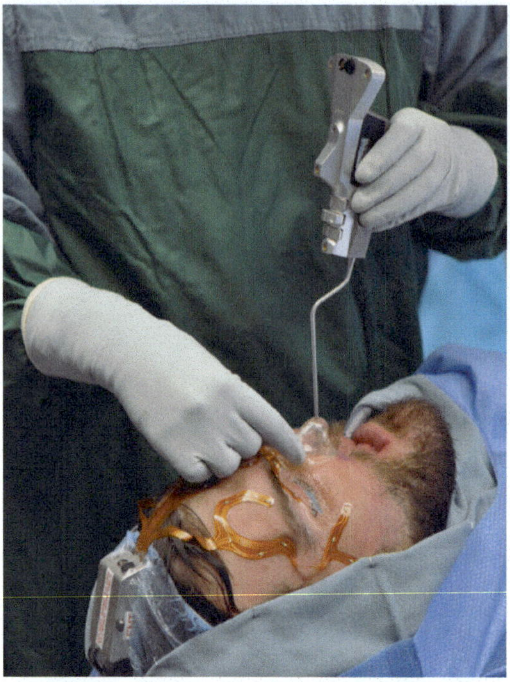

Fig. 32.20 Navigation registration for implant case

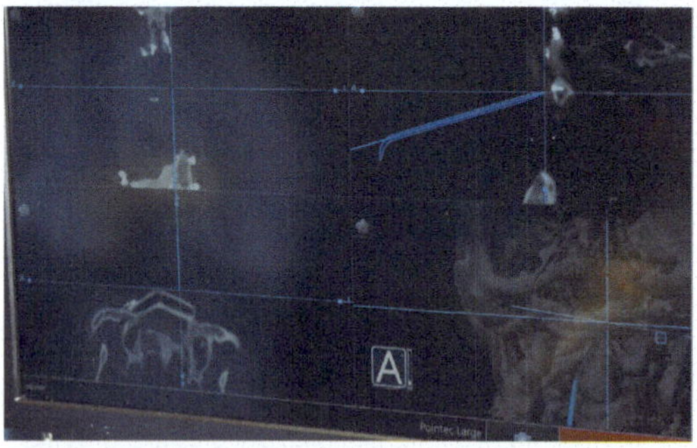

Fig. 32.21 Live CT navigation

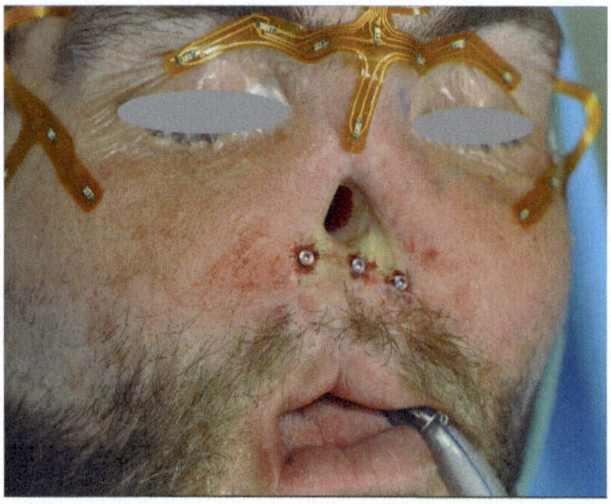

Fig. 32.22 Patient status post-trans-facial implant placement

anatomy (Figs. 32.20, 32.21, and 32.22) via a small intraoral posterior tuberosity window.

In a second case highlighting the benefits of intraoperative navigation in the treatment of benign maxillofacial pathology, intraoperative

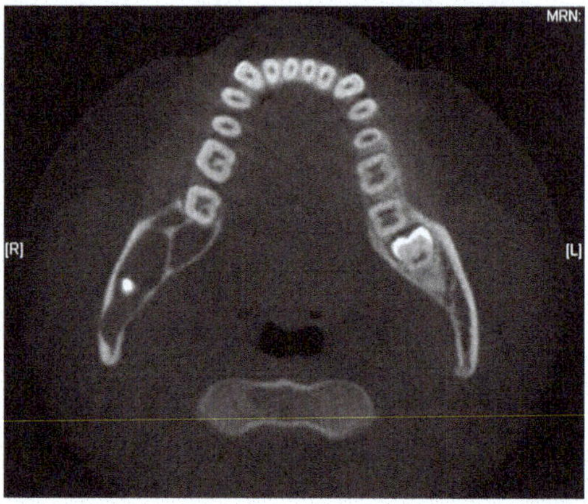

Fig. 32.23 Preoperative CT with axial cut showing recurrent KCOT

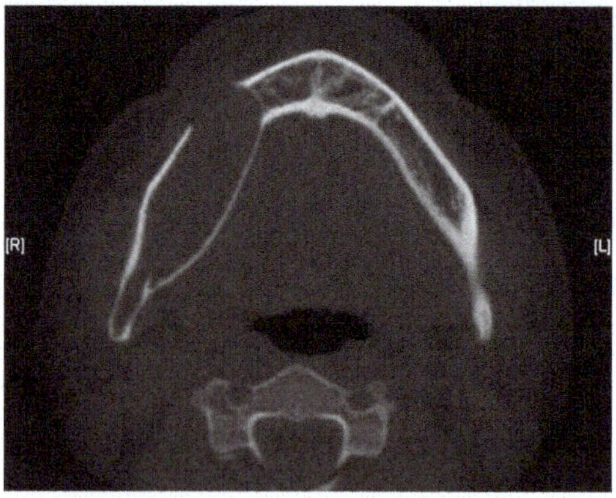

Fig. 32.24 Preoperative CT with axial cut showing recurrent KCOT

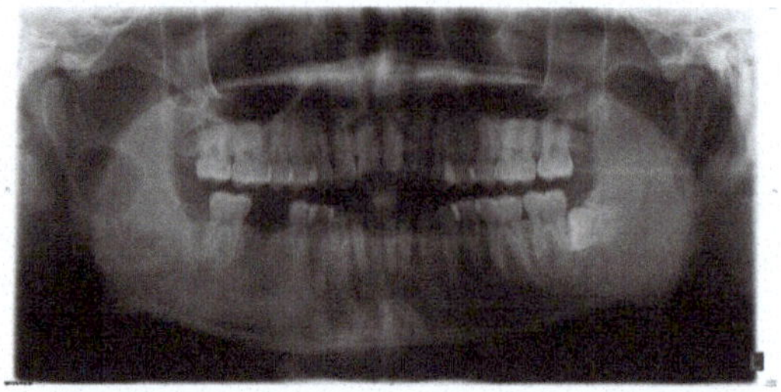

Fig. 32.25 Preoperative panoramic image showing recurrent right-sided KCOT

navigation was utilized in the treatment of a recurrent keratocystic odontogenic tumor/ odontogenic keratocyst. The patient was a 27 year old male who had previously bene treated at an outside facility with enucleation, curettage and Carnoy's solution (Figs. 32.23, 32.24, and 32.25). The patient had neurosensory changes notably initial anesthesia of the inferior alveolar nerve (IAN) with gradual return of sensation over 6–9 months. He was referred due to a recurrence/residual tumor in the ramus and wanted a conservative approach with

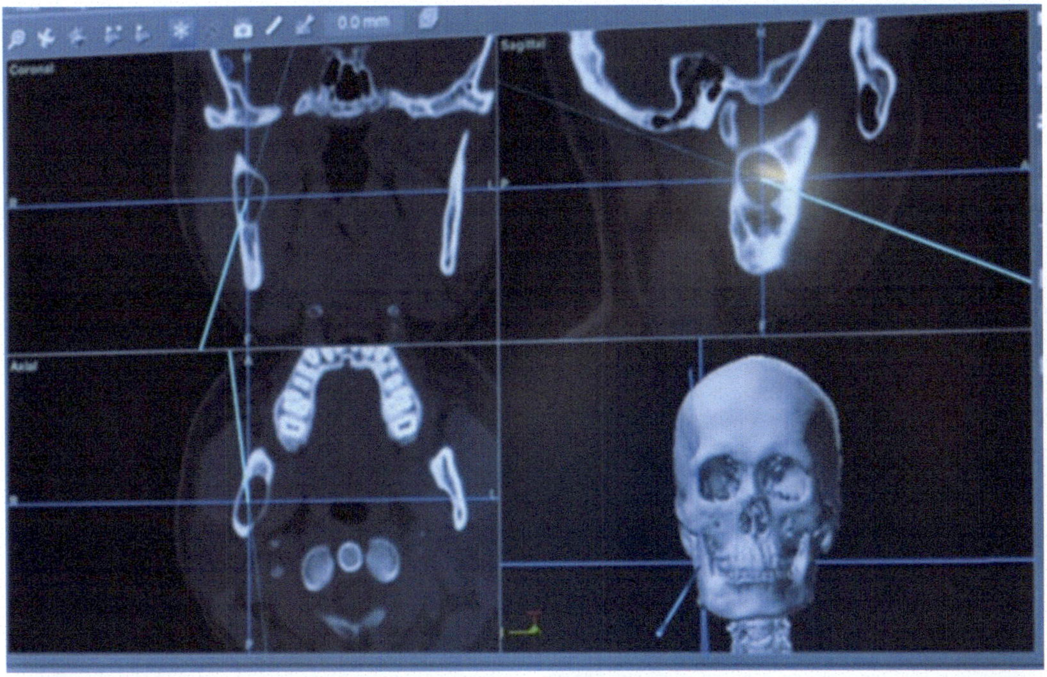

Fig. 32.26 Preoperative CT with coronal cut showing recurrent KCOT

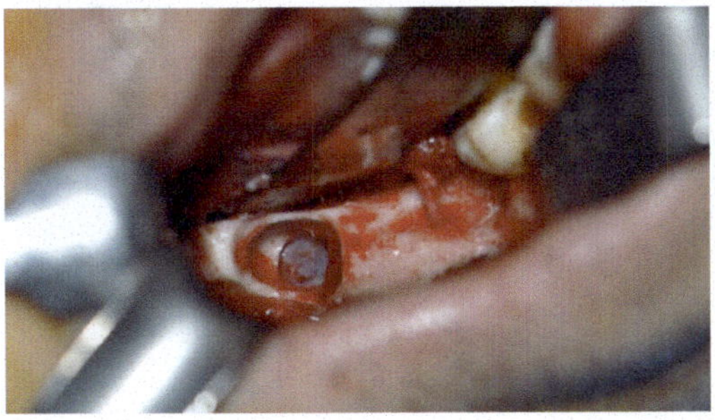

Fig. 32.27 Intraoperative image showing navigation

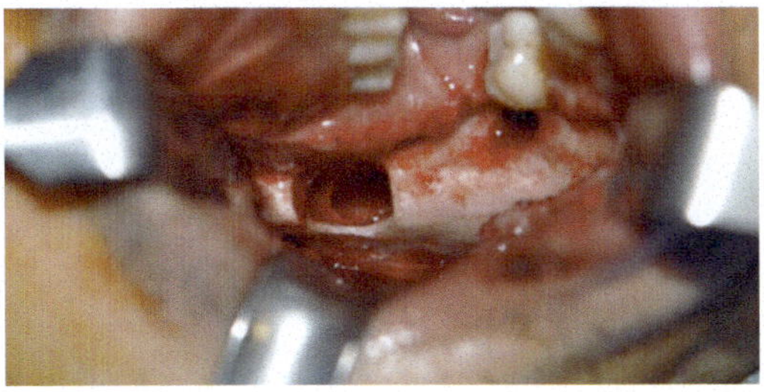

Fig. 32.28 Intraoperative image showing surgical exposure of lesion

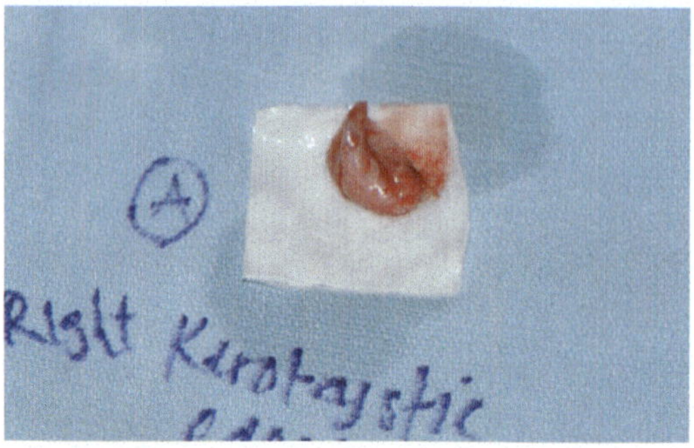

Fig. 32.29 Intraoperative image showing site post removal

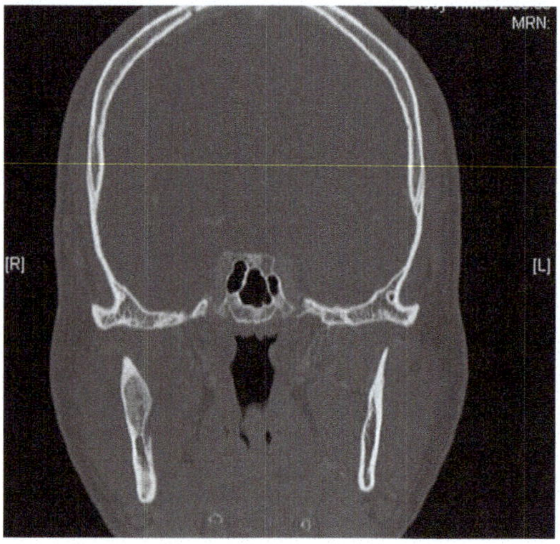

Fig. 32.30 Right-sided KCOT following excision

minimal risk to the IAN. Navigation was used to identify the position of the inferior alveolar nerve in relation to the tumor precisely and to confirm adequate removal (Figs. 32.26, 32.27, 32.28, 32.29, and 32.30). On follow-up there was no neurosensory deficit. Six months later the site has bony filling (Fig. 32.30).

32.4.4.2 Temporomandibular Joint

The temporomandibular joint (TMJ) region provides another unique challenge to the craniomaxillofacial surgeon. Facial nerve branches, the parotid gland, and muscle attachments greatly limit surgical approaches [7]. Combining stereolithographic models and intraoperative CT-based navigation can help improve the overall outcomes of TMJ surgery [8]. When treating TMJ ankylosis, it is critical that all the bone is removed, and medially where risks of catastrophic bleeding exist, some bone may be left due to limited access, direct visualization, and vasculature. Navigation can guide the surgeon to the area of the bone medially, avoiding the great vessels but

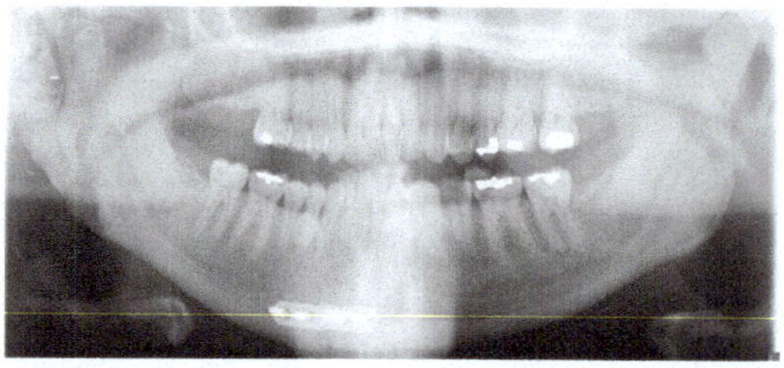

Fig. 32.31 Preoperative panoramic image showing right-sided TMJ ankylosis

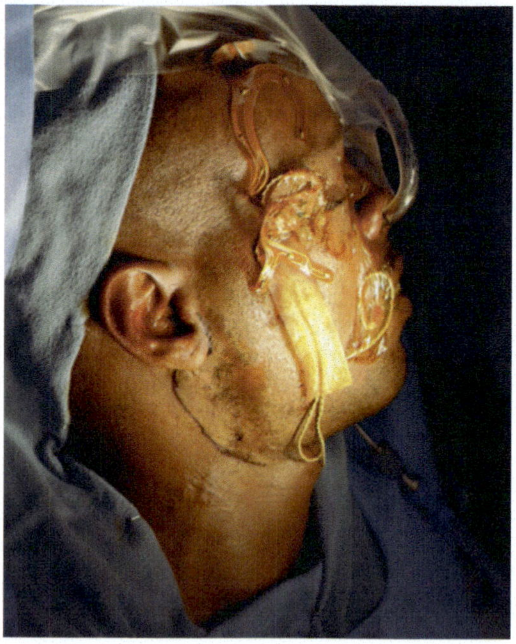

Fig. 32.32 Intraoperative image showing planned incision

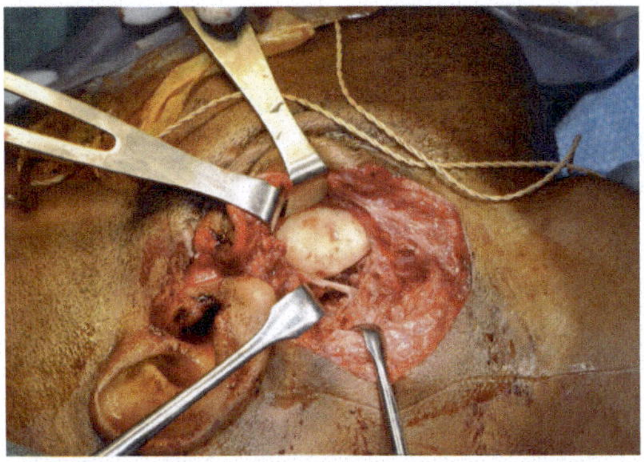

Fig. 32.33 Intraoperative image showing anatomically displaced cervicofacial trunk of cranial nerve VII

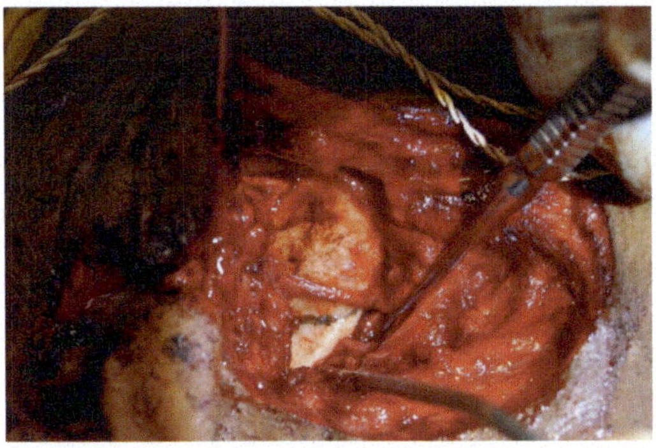

Fig. 32.34 Intraoperative image showing cervicofacial trunk of cranial nerve VII with planned osteotomy

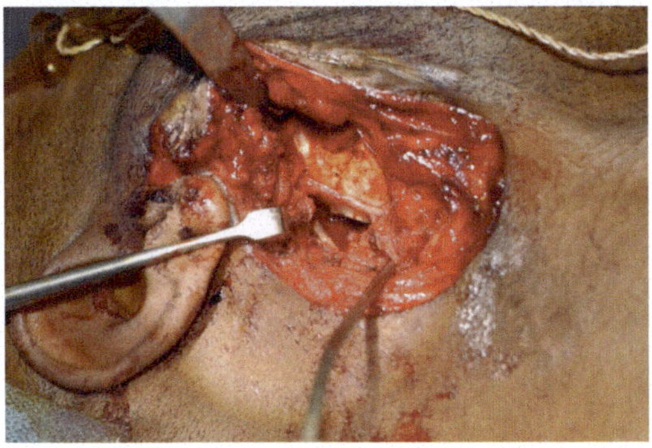

Fig. 32.35 Osteotomy with nerve intact

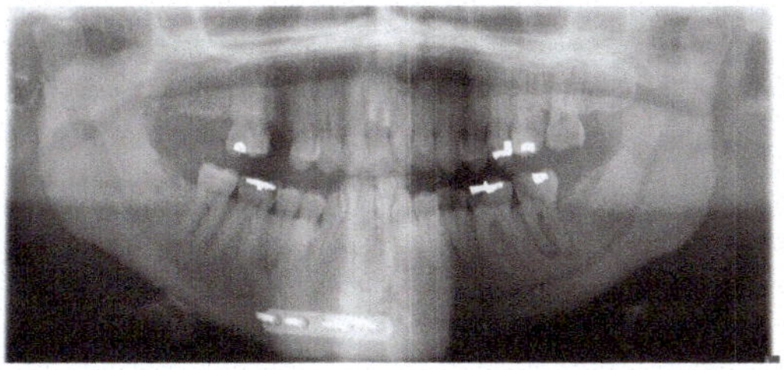

Fig. 32.36 Postoperative panoramic image following removal of bony ankylosis with remodeling

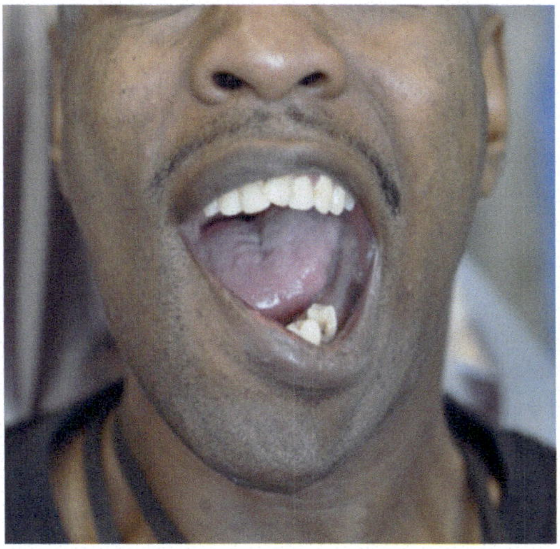

Fig. 32.37 Postoperative image showing improved maximal incisal opening 3 years postoperatively

still achieving the desired result. Navigation was used in the case of a 27-year-old male otherwise healthy status post motor vehicle accident 3 years prior presenting with ankylosis and facial nerve injury. His initial House-Brackmann score was 3/6, and he was clinically unable to open more than 7 mm. Imaging revealed ankylosis of the ramus to the mastoid process in close approximation to the facial nerve trunk. Intraoperative navigation, facial nerve monitoring, and a stereolithographic model were used to remove the bony ankylosis while preserving and maintaining the integrity of the facial nerve (Figs. 32.31, 32.32, 32.33, 32.34, 32.35, 32.36, and 32.37).

Conclusion

Surgery in the maxillofacial region provides unique challenges that require precision and accuracy. Minor deviations from the ideal surgical outcome are tolerated poorly by patients from both a functional and esthetic perspective. The use of navigation to improve surgical outcomes has become increasingly evident. Complex cases can be approached with increased confidence with respect to the end result. Navigation surgery is not a substitute for clinical expertise but an adjunct to guiding treatment and improving outcomes. In maxillofacial training institutions, navigation allows additional education benefits as the surgery can be visualized on screen and allows trainees to experience an enhanced learning platform. Maxillofacial surgeons are presented with challenging surgical situations regularly, the aid of virtual surgical planning, and navigation help guide treatment intraoperatively.

Conflict of Interest Nothing to disclose.

References

1. Haflfeld S, Mfihling J, ZO'ller J. Intraoperative navigation in oral and maxillo- facial surgery. Int J Oral Maxillofac Surg. 1995;24:111–9. 9 Munksgaard
2. Lin H, Lo L. Three-dimensional computer-assisted surgical simulation and intraoperative navigation in orthognathic surgery: a literature review. J Formos Med Assoc. 2015;114:300–7.
3. Stryker. Patient Registration Mask. Literature Number: 9100-001-997 Rev. None 9/13 Copyright © 2013 Stryker Printed in USA.
4. Markiewicz MR, et al. Reliability of intraoperative navigation in restoring normal orbital dimensions. J Oral Maxillofac Surg. 2011;2011(69):2833–40.
5. Bell RB, Markiewicz MR. Computer-assisted planning, stereolithographic modeling, and intraoperative navigation for complex orbital reconstruction: a descriptive study in a preliminary cohort. J Oral Maxillofac Surg. 2009;67:2559–70.
6. Zhang S, et al. Navigation-guided correction of midfacial post-traumatic deformities (Shanghai experience with 40 cases). J Oral Maxillofac Surg. 2012;2012(70): 1426–33.
7. Eggers G, Mühling J, Marmulla R. Image-to-patient registration techniques in head surgery. Int J Oral Maxillofac Surg. 2006;35:1081–95.
8. Wagner A, Undt G, Watzinger F, et al. Principles of computer- assisted arthroscopy of the temporomandibular joint with optoelectronic tracking technology. Oral Surg Oral Med Oral Pathol Oral Radiol Endod. 2001;92:30.

Perioperative Management of Temporomandibular Joint and Myofascial Pain

33

Gary F. Bouloux

Abstract

Current evidence suggests that arthrocentesis without the instillation of hyaluronic acid or corticosteroid remains an effective treatment for many patients with temporomandibular joint pain. The treatments for bruxism and myofascial pain have less evidence to support or refute commonly employed management strategies. The use of an occlusal splint, muscle relaxants, and occasionally botulinum toxin appears to be reasonable choices for bruxism. Myofascial pain may also benefit from the same treatments although jaw exercises, heat, spray and stretch, transcutaneous electrical nerve stimulation, dry needling, trigger point injections (TrP) with local anesthesia, tricyclic antidepressants, and neuromodulators may be equally effective. Supplemental analgesics should also be employed to reduce pain and improve quality of life, while the use of opioids is generally not supported.

33.1 Introduction

The management of patients with facial and head pain remains very challenging given the multitude of possible diagnoses, challenges in making the correct diagnosis, and varying treatment options. The choice of treatment is often guided more by physician preference and experience than science. However, whenever possible, decision-making should be based on scientific research. It is important to stratify the research based on the quality of the research methodology to ensure that one appreciates the different levels of evidence that are possible as well as the validity of the conclusions that are drawn from such research. The purpose of this chapter is to discuss several currently relevant topics and treatments as well as provide a scientific basis for treatment choices. Arthrocentesis for the treatment of temporomandibular joint pain and limited function is well documented. The potential benefit of the intra-articular instillation of adjunct medications remains controversial. Similarly, the management of myofascial pain, tension headache, and

G.F. Bouloux, M.D., D.D.S., M.D.Sc.
Division of Oral and Maxillofacial Surgery, Department of Surgery, Emory University School of Medicine, Atlanta, GA, USA
e-mail: gfboulo@emory.edu

© Springer International Publishing AG 2018

E.M. Ferneini, J.D. Bennett (eds.), *Perioperative Assessment of the Maxillofacial Surgery Patient*,
https://doi.org/10.1007/978-3-319-58868-1_33

bruxism varies considerably with little evidence to really support or refute many of the treatments. It remains clinically important to reduce pain and suffering in patients using evidence-based treatments and be mindful of the increasing societal problem with opioid addiction and abuse. This chapter will attempt to address these topics and provide a rationale to optimize treatment and patient outcomes.

33.2 Arthrocentesis

The usefulness of arthrocentesis in the management of temporomandibular joint (TMJ) arthralgia, internal derangement, and closed lock has been well documented [1]. Success rates vary in part as a result of the heterogeneous nature of TMJ pain and the potential for additional sources of pain in the head and neck region [2–12]. The concentration of inflammatory mediators within the joint appears to have some correlation with severity of pain [13–18]. There is significant variation in the volume of irrigation used during arthrocentesis although 200 ml has been shown to remove inflammatory cytokines and a majority of degraded joint proteins [19]. Despite this fact, the therapeutic outcome following arthrocentesis is influenced by both the initial concentration of inflammatory mediators within the joint and the degree to which they are reduced [20–22]. Nitzan has further shown that a "stuck disk" may also play a role in joint pain and closed lock with arthrocentesis able to increase intra-articular pressure effectively releasing the disk to improve both pain and range of motion (ROM) [1, 2, 7, 23–26].

Various medications have been injected into the joint after arthrocentesis in an attempt to further reduce pain and improve ROM. The most common medications injected include hyaluronic acid (HA), corticosteroid (CS), local anesthetics, and opioids. Hyaluronic acid and CS are known to reduce inflammation as a result of the anti-inflammatory properties of both agents. Opioids readily bind to μ receptors within the joint and are thought to reduce nociception and decrease both peripheral and central sensitization.

Hyaluronic acid (HA) has been shown to reduce reactive oxygen species, cytokine production, vascular permeability, and polymorph migration resulting in reduced inflammation and increased joint translation [27, 28]. Corticosteroids are synthetic drugs that play a key role in carbohydrate, fat, and protein metabolism as well as modulating the immune system. The overall effect is suppression of inflammation within the temporomandibular joint [29–33]. Local anesthetics such as lidocaine, bupivacaine, and carbocaine have also been used during arthrocentesis. They provide immediate anesthesia to allow the procedure to be performed but may also be additionally injected at the completion of the procedure. They effectively bind to sodium channels of the sensory nerves within the joint to provide anesthesia and analgesia of varying durations. Opioids are typically used to modulate pain through binding of opioid receptors in the central nervous system and spinal cord. This typically requires oral, intramuscular, or parenteral administration. The use of intra-articular opioids such as morphine, tramadol, and buprenorphine within the TMJ has been reported with a reduction in short- and long-term pain [34–37].

The challenge in assessing the benefit of injecting HA, CS, local anesthesia, or opioid after arthrocentesis is largely the result of a lack of double-blind randomized clinical trials and the failure to compare to a control group receiving only arthrocentesis. A recent double-blind randomized multicenter clinical trial compared arthrocentesis alone to arthrocentesis with HA and arthrocentesis with CS. A total of 102 subjects completed the study with the authors finding a clinically significant reduction in pain and an improvement in ROM for all three groups at both 1 and 3 months. There was no difference between the groups for pain reduction or ROM at either time point. This would suggest that arthrocentesis alone is sufficient to treat intra-articular TMJ pain and consideration should be given to avoiding additional medications unless new clinical trials establish superiority over arthrocentesis alone [38].

33.3 Bruxism

Bruxism is classically defined as repetitive jaw muscle activity resulting in jaw clenching and grinding. The activity can occur during sleep or while awake suggesting the existence of two similar but separate entities: sleep bruxism and awake bruxism [39]. Sleep bruxism appears to have an association with obstructive sleep apnea with both resulting in sleep arousals although the relationship between the two remains unclear [40]. There appears to be a genetic predisposition to the development of bruxism based on concordance rates among twin siblings [41]. Children as well as adults can be affected by bruxism [42]. Multiple potential causes exist for the development of bruxism including stress, personality traits, genetic factors, obstructive sleep apnea, medications, illicit drugs, tobacco, alcohol, caffeine, cerebral palsy, autism, and trauma. The net result appears to be an increase in the release of central neurotransmitters with a corresponding increase in muscle activity. The diagnosis of bruxism can be challenging, and generally speaking there should be a positive history of clenching and facial pain combined with a clinical examination revealing myofascial pain. The likelihood of making a correct diagnosis is further increased with the use of electromyography (EMG) or polysomnography (PSG) which can objectively quantitate muscle activity. Potential consequences of bruxism include the development of temporomandibular joint dysfunction (TMD) with myofascial pain more common than intra-articular pain and internal derangement. Damage to the teeth and periodontium is also possible in the face of bruxism.

The mainstay of treatment for bruxism involves the use of splints, behavioral modification, and the use of medications [39, 43]. The use of occlusal splints to treat bruxism remains somewhat controversial. The benefit of splints in mitigating the damage to teeth seems unequivocal, but whether splints actually reduce bruxism is less clear. Some studies report reduced muscle activity with splints as measured with EMG (nocturnal and during wakefulness) and PSG. Other studies report reduced facial pain on awakening and use this as an indirect barometer of success. The type of occlusal splint seems less important with various studies showing the benefit of a hard flat plane splint, nociceptive trigeminal inhibitor (NTI), and a mandibular advancement device (MAD). Support for soft occlusal splints, simple shell splints, and occlusal adjustment is lacking.

The use of behavioral modification has also been shown to reduce bruxism whether nocturnal or during wakefulness. Biofeedback remains the most popular technique with patients. While awake, patients can be trained to control their jaw muscle activity through auditory or visual feedback from a surface EMG. For sleep bruxism, auditory, electrical, vibratory, and even taste stimuli can be used for feedback. These techniques are time-consuming and not readily available.

Pharmacological management of bruxism remains popular despite little evidence. The number of studies evaluating the efficacy of pharmacological drugs is limited with most reporting on very small sample sizes. Additionally the primary end point differs between studies making comparisons almost impossible. Muscle relaxants, benzodiazepines, tricyclic antidepressants, dopaminergic drugs, clonidine, propranolol, and botulinum toxin have all been advocated although only a few have been subject to randomized clinical trials (Table 33.1).

Table 33.1 Medications evaluated in RCTs for the management of bruxism

Drug	Dose	Results
Amitriptyline	25 mg	No change in EMG activity
Levodopa	100 mg	Reduced muscle activity on PSG
Bromocriptine	7.5 mg	No change in muscle activity on PSG
Propanolol	120 mg	No change in muscle activity on PSG
Clonidine	0.3 mg	Reduced muscle activity on PSG
Botulinum toxin A	50–100 mouse units	No change in muscle activity on PSG Reduced strength of contraction on PSG

Table 33.2 Common medications for the management of sleep bruxism

Drug	Dose
Amitriptyline	10–25 mg PO QHS
Baclofen	10–20 mg PO QHS
Tizanidine	2–4 mg PO QHS
Cyclobenzaprine	5–10 mg PO QHS
Methocarbamol	1000 mg PO QHS
Metaxalone	400–800 mg PO QHS
Carisoprodol	250–350 mg PO QHS
Clonazepam	0.25–1 mg PO QHS
Temazepam	15–30 mg PO QHS
Botulinum toxin A	100–200 units IM every 3–6 months

Despite the lack of evidence to support the use of medication in the management of sleep bruxism, the use of pharmacological agents remains popular in addition to occlusal splints. Medications that may be considered to help manage bruxism are listed (Table 33.2).

For nocturnal bruxism medications should be taken shortly before sleep is anticipated. These medications can also be used to manage awake bruxism, but with the exception of baclofen and botulinum toxin, they tend to produce variable degrees of sedation and therefore tend to not be well tolerated during wakefulness. One additional treatment for sleep bruxism that has some evidence to support it is contingent electrical stimulation. In principle, a low-level electrical stimulation is applied to inhibit the muscles when they become active during sleep bruxism. Despite the evidence supporting this modality, patient compliance remains a challenge.

33.4 Myofascial Pain Dysfunction and Headache

Myofascial pain dysfunction refers to pain in the masticatory muscles, tendons, and ligaments that is worse with jaw function or parafunction. The diagnostic criteria axis I diagnoses include local myalgia, myalgia, myofascial pain, and myofascial pain with referral [44]. Myofascial pain is characterized by the presence of latent or active trigger points (TrPs) within the muscles [45]. Active TrPs produce spontaneous pain with activity, while latent TrPs produce pain with palpation. Trigger points are thought to represent focal areas of ectopic activity and are associated with increased focal muscle metabolism and an altered biochemical milieu. The source of pain appears to be the decreased oxygen tension in hyperactive muscle fibers with the production of K^+, prostaglandins, histamine, and kinins. Peripheral sensitization quickly develops followed by central sensitization, neuroplasticity, and increased receptor fields [46]. Social, behavioral, and psychological factors are known to be associated with MPD.

The diagnosis of MPD is facilitated by a thorough history and examination following the diagnostic criteria for temporomandibular disorders [47]. Palpation of the masticatory muscles is achieved in a systematic manner. Three temporal areas should be palpated with 2 lbs. pressure (Fig. 33.1). They should also be palpated independently (Fig. 33.2).

The masseter muscle should also be palpated in three areas with similar pressure (Fig. 33.3). Again the three areas should be palpated independently (Fig. 33.4).

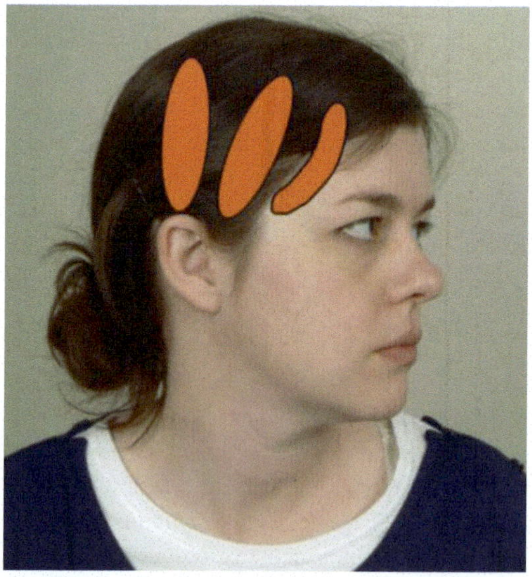

Fig. 33.1 Temporal areas. Adapted from diagnostic criteria temporomandibular disorders. Clinical examination protocol. Ohrbach R, Gonzalez Y, List T, Michelotti A, Schiffman E. Version Jan 6 2014

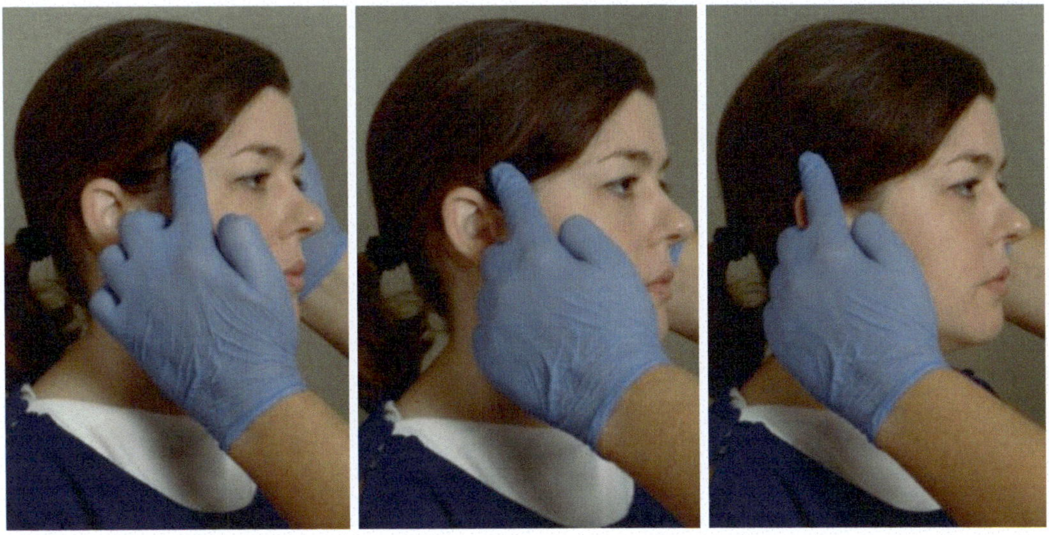

Fig. 33.2 Anterior, middle, and posterior palpation. Adapted from diagnostic criteria temporomandibular disorders. Clinical examination protocol. Ohrbach R, Gonzalez Y, List T, Michelotti A, Schiffman E. Version Jan 6 2014

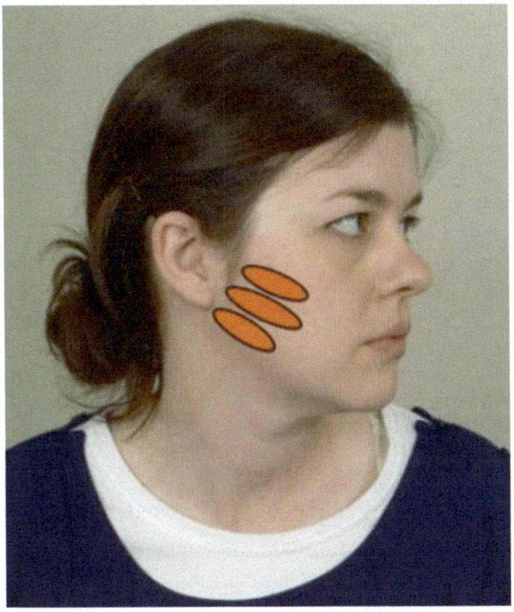

Fig. 33.3 Masseter areas. Adapted from diagnostic criteria temporomandibular disorders. Clinical examination protocol. Ohrbach R, Gonzalez Y, List T, Michelotti A, Schiffman E. Version Jan 6 2014

Treatment for MPD includes passive and active jaw exercises, heat, spray and stretch, transcutaneous electrical nerve stimulation, occlusal splints, dry needling, TrP injections with local anesthesia, tricyclic antidepressants, muscle relaxants, and neuromodulators.

Myofascial pain and fibromyalgia are distinct entities, and the pathophysiology of pain is likely to be different. Despite this, there is some evidence that treatment modalities which are considered appropriate for fibromyalgia may be beneficial for MPD.

An elegant way to compare the results of different studies with inconsistent methodologies and outcome measures is to calculate the number of patients needed to treat (NNT) to see a clinical reduction in pain which for most patients is a reduction of 30%. The smaller the NNT, the better the medication in producing the desired result. Nonsteroidal anti-inflammatory drugs, cognitive-based therapy, gabapentinoids, tricyclic antidepressants, and selective serotonin norepinephrine reuptake inhibitors have all been shown to be of benefit in some patients [48] (Table 33.3).

Myofascial pain often presents with headache as a component. Whether this represents MPD with referral or the coexistence of two entities is not always clear. The treatment approach for chronic daily headaches and migraine is different. The latter can often be aborted or attenuated with the use of triptans and caffeine-based analgesics when infrequent. Chronic daily headaches,

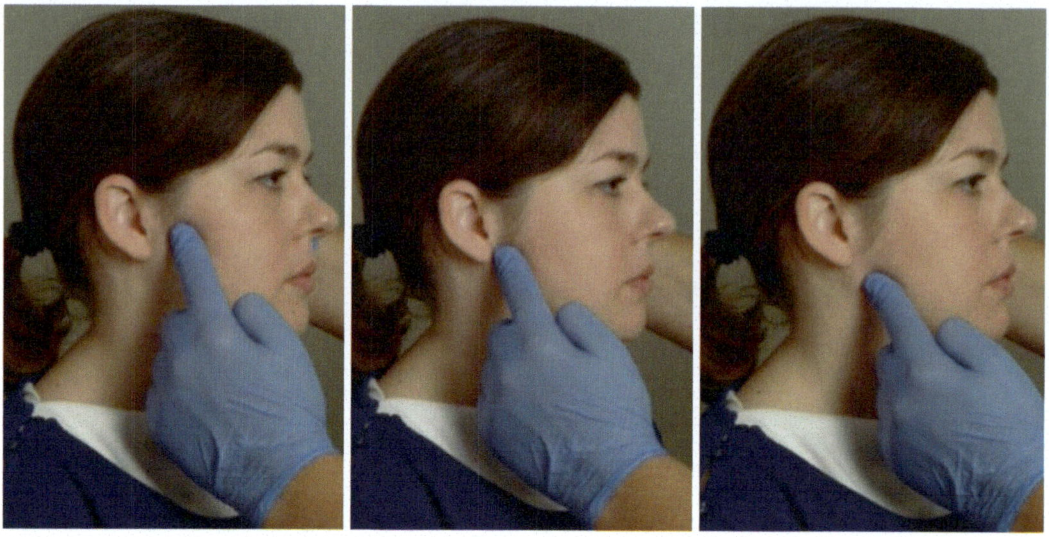

Fig. 33.4 Superior, middle, and inferior palpation. Adapted from diagnostic criteria temporomandibular disorders. Clinical examination protocol. Ohrbach R, Gonzalez Y, List T, Michelotti A, Schiffman E. Version Jan 6 2014

Table 33.3 Fibromyalgia and MPD

Evidence-based fibromyalgia/myofascial pain treatments	
Treatments	Numbers needed to treat
1. Gabapentinoids (Pregabalin)	13
2. TCA (Amitriptyline)	4.9
3. SNRI (Duloxetine)	10.0
4. Cognitive behavior therapy	Not available
5. Opioid therapy	Not available

Adapted from: Clark G, Padilla M, Dionne R. Medication treatment efficacy and chronic orofacial pain. Oral and Maxillofacial Surg Clin N Am. 2016; 28, 409

Table 33.4 Chronic daily headache

Evidence-based chronic daily headache treatments	
Treatments	Numbers needed to treat
1. Long-acting NSAID (Naproxen)	Not available
2. β-Blocker (Propranolol)	1.5
3. TCA (Amitriptyline)	3.2
4. AED (Valproate)	3.0–4.0
5. AED (Topiramate)	4.0
6. NMDA blocker (Memantine)	Not available
7. Opioids	Not available

Adapted from: Clark G, Padilla M, Dionne R. Medication treatment efficacy and chronic orofacial pain. Oral and Maxillofacial Surg Clin N Am. 2016; 28, 409

including migraine, require a different approach to help prevent headache development. Several medications have been suggested as potentially beneficial although the NNT cannot be adequately established for some drugs (Table 33.4).

Botulinum toxin A is approved by the FDA for the treatment of chronic headaches. Silberstein provides an excellent review on the use of botulinum toxin A for headache disorders [49]. The use of botulinum toxin for MPD is strictly off label, and the evidence to support its use for MPD remains somewhat inconclusive [50–54].

Botulinum toxin exists as seven antigenically different neurotoxin forms (A–G) all with similar structure. Only two forms are FDA approved to clinical use, botulinum toxin A and botulinum toxin B. The toxin binds to cholinergic receptors and the neuromuscular junction, autonomic ganglia, and postganglionic nerve endings. Once internalized it binds to a group of SNARE proteins and prevents fusion of the synaptic vesicles with the axon membrane effectively preventing the release of acetylcholine and impulse transmission. Botulinum toxin is indicated for the treatment of spasticity, non-dystonic muscle disorders, focal dystonias, strabismus, smooth muscle hyperactivity, sialorrhea, rhinitis, hyperhidrosis, and chronic pain. It is the latter that has resulted in the increasing use for chronic headache, tension headache, migraine, and myofascial pain. Proposed mechanisms of reducing pain include muscle relaxation as well as reduced levels of substance P, calcitonin gene-related peptide, and glutamate [55].

The reconstituted toxin can be administered in standardized locations within muscles, or it can be directed at specific painful sites (Fig. 33.5). The dose of botulinum toxin A for headache and migraine varies from 25 to 100 units. Beneficial effects of the drug are seen from 2 weeks to several months after injection and may last up to 12 months. Repeat injections are generally required for continued benefit although with this comes the potential for developing neutralizing antibodies in a small number of individuals.

The treatment of myofascial pain dysfunction requires the administration of botulinum toxin into the masseter and temporalis muscles. Occasionally the medial or lateral pterygoid muscle is also targeted. Doses typically vary from 100 to 300 units. The use of electromyographic (EMG) guidance is not required unless the pterygoid muscles are being injected. Short-term

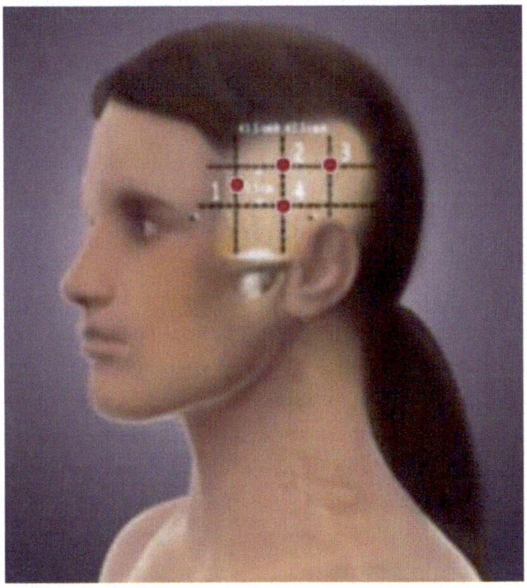

Fig. 33.5 Temporalis injection sites for headache. Adapted from Silberstein S; The use of botulinum toxin in the management of headache disorder. Semin Neurol; 2016, 36, 92

improvement in pain has been reported by some authors, while others have no difference when compared to placebo. Direct comparisons between studies is challenging given the heterogenous nature of headache and myofascial pain and the lack of consistency in the clinical examination used to identify subjects.

33.5 Supplemental Analgesia

The use of paracetamol and nonsteroidal anti-inflammatory drugs (NSAIDs) remains the mainstay of managing pain of mild or moderate quality. When pain is severe, the use of opioid medication alone or in combination with paracetamol or NSAIDs is warranted. The mechanism of action for both drugs appears to be through inhibition of cyclooxygenase pathway and the generation of prostaglandins. As with all medications, the potential side effects of these medications must be considered [56]. Paracetamol is the safest of the analgesics but can be associated with an allergic response in some individuals as well as liver failure when excessively consumed or in patients with pre-existing liver disease. Nonsteroidal anti-inflammatory drugs may be associated with gastritis, peptic ulcer disease, and acute kidney injury. Opioids have the potential for sedation, hypotension, nausea and emesis, constipation, and urinary retention as well as the potential for addiction and adverse drug-related behavior. Additionally the excessive consumption of opioids is associated with respiratory depression and death. In an attempt to overcome these issues, the surgeon may consider several other medication classes that may provide analgesia or reduce the dose of acetaminophen, NSAIDs, or opioids needed to provide adequate pain relief.

Reducing the need for opioids in the postsurgical patient remains a priority given the potential side effects. A reduction in the need for opioids has been shown for acetaminophen, NSAIDs, and selective Cox 2 inhibitors with a mean reduction in morphine use of 6.3, 10.2, and 10.9 mg, respectively, in the first 24 h after surgery [57]. Given the general safety profile of these medications, consideration should be given in using them for minor and major oral and maxillofacial surgery procedures. The potential to further reduce postoperative pain with the use of gabapentinoids may also be considered [58]. The mechanisms of action remain largely unknown although an increase in gamma-aminobutyric acid (GABA), the binding of calcium ion channels, and interaction with N-methyl-D-aspartate (NMDA) receptors have all been suggested. Side effects which include sedation, visual disturbances, and dizziness have been described, but the clinical significance remains less clear. The mean reduction in morphine use exceeds 13 mg during the first 24 h with gabapentin. A single preoperative dose of gabapentin is what is usually required with a dose ranging from 600 to 1200 mg depending in part on the type of surgery. Additionally, the reduction in morphine dose appears to result in a significant reduction in nausea, emesis, and urinary retention. The effect of pregabalin is a little more modest with a mean reduction in morphine dose of 8.8 mg for pregabalin doses less than 300 mg per day and a mean reduction of 13.4 mg morphine for pregabalin doses greater than 300 mg per day [57].

One new opioid that is associated with fewer side effects and adverse events is tapentadol. It has a novel mechanism of action that involves traditional mu-receptor binding in the central nervous system as well as inhibiting the reuptake of norepinephrine [59]. The immediate release formulation has been shown to compare favorably with traditional opioids for pain relief although whether this holds true for all surgery types including oral and maxillofacial surgery remains unclear.

Several non-systemic interventions also have the potential to reduce acute postoperative pain. Long-acting local anesthetics (LA) such as bupivacaine have been shown to reduce postoperative pain and increase the time to rescue medication when compared to shorter-acting local anesthetics such as lidocaine. The favorable toxicity profile and ease of administration for longer-acting LA make them a simple choice for most patients. The recent development of a liposomal bupivacaine formulation has further increased the opportunity to reduce postoperative pain. Exparel[1] provides extended local anesthesia as a result of the liposomal formulation which ensures that the bupivacaine is released slowly from the site of deposition to provide long-acting analgesia. It has been shown to reduce opioid consumption for certain types of surgery; although this seems to have considerable potential for oral and maxillofacial surgery, further studies are needed. The use of liposomal bupivacaine may eliminate traditional methods to continuously deliver local anesthesia regionally through the use of devices such as the ON-Q[2] without the risks related to the placement and removal of indwelling catheters.

The management of chronic pain remains a challenge for all practitioners given the excessive use of opioids and the potential for adverse events (AE) and adverse drug-related behavior (ADRB). Temporomandibular joint dysfunction and its treatment can result in chronic pain states that require long-term management. The use of transcutaneous electrical nerve stimulation (TENS), lidocaine patches, capsaicin, and iontophoresis with NSAID gels may be of benefit in some patients while reducing the need for systemic analgesics and neuromodulating drugs. As with acute postoperative pain, paracetamol, NSAIDs, and selective Cox 2 inhibitors should be considered first. When these drugs fail, the use of opioids may be considered. The efficacy of opioids in chronic cancer pain is generally well established although not without problems in some patients related to a lack of effect of a need to discontinue due to side effects. The use of opioids in chronic non-cancer pain such as TMD remains controversial. The use of long-acting opioids and drugs such as tapentadol should however be considered although further studies are clearly needed. Consideration should be given to the use of adjunct medications including gabapentin, pregabalin, tricyclic antidepressants, and serotonin norepinephrine reuptake inhibitors in these patients. The complexity of these patients with respect to peripheral and central sensitization, somatization, genetic polymorphisms, and

[1] Pacira Pharmaceuticals, San Diego, Ca

[2]™ Halyard Health, Irvine, CA

coping mechanisms generally ensures that they be managed by a dedicated pain specialist who can also monitor for AE and ADRB.

Conclusion

Arthrocentesis remains a simple and efficacious treatment for temporomandibular joint pain and limited opening. The instillation of hyaluronic acid or corticosteroid after the procedure appears to offer no advantage and should be discontinued in the majority of patients without a specific indication (e.g., inflammatory arthropathy). The treatments for bruxism continue to lack strong support suggesting that the most conservative approach appears to be the most reasonable until new evidence is available. Occlusal splints, select muscle relaxants, and botulinum toxin remain the best choices. The ideal management of myofascial pain and headache continues to require a multimodal approach that should also include occlusal splints, physical therapy, and the judicious use of gabapentinoids, tricyclic antidepressants, SNRI medications, propranolol, or botulinum toxin. Opioids have little to offer our patients, and it behooves the physician to exhaust all forms of supplemental analgesia to reduce pain, improve quality of life, and minimize adverse events such as opioid addiction and abuse.

References

1. Al-Belasy FA, Dolwick MF. Arthrocentesis for the treatment of temporomandibular joint closed lock: a review article. Int J Oral Maxillofac Surg. 2007;36:773–82.
2. Frost DE, Kendell BD, Part II. The use of arthrocentesis for treatment of temporomandibular joint disorders. J Oral Maxillofac Surg. 1999;57:583–7.
3. Onder ME, Tuz HH, Kocyigit D, Kisnisci RS. Long-term results of arthrocentesis in degenerative temporomandibular disorders. Oral Surg Oral Med Oral Pathol Oral Radiol Endod. 2009;107:e1–5.
4. Wiesend M, Kanehl S, Esser E. Arthrocentesis--a highly efficient therapy for acute TMJ arthropathy. Mund Kiefer Gesichtschir. 2006;10:341–6.
5. Brennan PA, Ilankovan V. Arthrocentesis for temporomandibular joint pain dysfunction syndrome. J Oral Maxillofac Surg. 2006;64:949–51.
6. Emshoff R. Clinical factors affecting the outcome of arthrocentesis and hydraulic distension of the temporomandibular joint. Oral Surg Oral Med Oral Pathol Oral Radiol Endod. 2005;100:409–14.
7. Emshoff R, Rudisch A. Determining predictor variables for treatment outcomes of arthrocentesis and hydraulic distention of the temporomandibular joint. J Oral Maxillofac Surg. 2004;62:816–23.
8. Emshoff R, Rudisch A, Bosch R, Strobl H. Prognostic indicators of the outcome of arthrocentesis: a short-term follow-up study. Oral Surg Oral Med Oral Pathol Oral Radiol Endod. 2003;96:12–8.
9. Alpaslan C, Dolwick MF, Heft MW. Five-year retrospective evaluation of temporomandibular joint arthrocentesis. Int J Oral Maxillofac Surg. 2003;32:263–7.
10. Spallaccia F, Rivaroli A, Cascone P. Temporomandibular joint arthrocentesis: long-term results. Bull Group Int Rech Sci Stomatol Odontol. 2000;42:31–7.
11. Nishimura M, Segami N, Kaneyama K, Suzuki T. Prognostic factors in arthrocentesis of the temporomandibular joint: evaluation of 100 patients with internal derangement. J Oral Maxillofac Surg. 2001;59:874–7. discussion 8
12. Carvajal WA, Laskin DM. Long-term evaluation of arthrocentesis for the treatment of internal derangements of the temporomandibular joint. J Oral Maxillofac Surg. 2000;58:852–5. discussion 6–7
13. Milam SB, Schmitz JP. Molecular biology of temporomandibular joint disorders: proposed mechanisms of disease. J Oral Maxillofac Surg. 1995;53:1448–54.
14. Milam SB, Zardeneta G, Schmitz JP. Oxidative stress and degenerative temporomandibular joint disease: a proposed hypothesis. J Oral Maxillofac Surg. 1998;56:214–23.
15. Zardeneta G, Milam SB, Lee T, Schmitz JP. Detection and preliminary characterization of matrix metalloproteinase activity in temporomandibular joint lavage fluid. Int J Oral Maxillofac Surg. 1998;27:397–403.
16. Zardeneta G, Milam SB, Schmitz JP. Presence of denatured hemoglobin deposits in diseased temporomandibular joints. J Oral Maxillofac Surg. 1997;55:1242–8. discussion 9
17. Zardeneta G, Milam SB, Schmitz JP. Elution of proteins by continuous temporomandibular joint arthrocentesis. J Oral Maxillofac Surg. 1997;55:709–16. discussion 16–7
18. Bouloux GF. Temporomandibular joint pain and synovial fluid analysis: a review of the literature. J Oral Maxillofac Surg. 2009;67:2497–504.
19. Kaneyama K, Segami N, Nishimura M, Sato J, Fujimura K, Yoshimura H. The ideal lavage volume for removing bradykinin, interleukin-6, and protein from the temporomandibular joint by arthrocentesis. J Oral Maxillofac Surg. 2004;62:657–61.
20. Kaneyama K, Segami N, Sato J, Fujimura K, Nagao T, Yoshimura H. Prognostic factors in arthrocentesis of the temporomandibular joint: comparison of bradykinin, leukotriene B4, prostaglandin E2, and substance P level in synovial fluid between success-

ful and unsuccessful cases. J Oral Maxillofac Surg. 2007;65:242–7.
21. Nishimura M, Segami N, Kaneyama K, Sato J, Fujimura K. Comparison of cytokine level in synovial fluid between successful and unsuccessful cases in arthrocentesis of the temporomandibular joint. J Oral Maxillofac Surg. 2004;62:284–7. discussion 7–8
22. Emshoff R, Puffer P, Strobl H, Gassner R. Effect of temporomandibular joint arthrocentesis on synovial fluid mediator level of tumor necrosis factor-alpha: implications for treatment outcome. Int J Oral Maxillofac Surg. 2000;29:176–82.
23. Nitzan DW. Rationale and indications for arthrocentesis of the temporomandibular joint. Alpha Omegan. 2003;96:57–63.
24. Nitzan DW. Arthrocentesis--incentives for using this minimally invasive approach for temporomandibular disorders. Oral Maxillofac Surg Clin North Am. 2006;18:311–28. vi
25. Nitzan DW, Dolwick MF, Martinez GA. Temporomandibular joint arthrocentesis: a simplified treatment for severe, limited mouth opening. J Oral Maxillofac Surg. 1991;49:1163–7. discussion 8–70
26. Nitzan DW, Samson B, Better H. Long-term outcome of arthrocentesis for sudden-onset, persistent, severe closed lock of the temporomandibular joint. J Oral Maxillofac Surg. 1997;55:151–7. discussion 7–8
27. Alpaslan C, Bilgihan A, Alpaslan GH, Guner B, Ozgur Yis M, Erbas D. Effect of arthrocentesis and sodium hyaluronate injection on nitrite, nitrate, and thiobarbituric acid-reactive substance levels in the synovial fluid. Oral Surg Oral Med Oral Pathol Oral Radiol Endod. 2000;89:686–90.
28. Shi Z, Guo C, Awad M. Hyaluronate for temporomandibular joint disorders. Cochrane Database Syst Rev. 2003;1:CD002970.
29. Shi ZD, Yang F, Zhang JY, Shi B. Randomized controlled trial of sodium hyaluronate for degenerative disorders of the temporomandibular joint. Zhongguo Xiu Fu Chong Jian Wai Ke Za Zhi. 2002;16:11–5.
30. Manfredini D, Rancitelli D, Ferronato G, Guarda-Nardini L. Arthrocentesis with or without additional drugs in temporomandibular joint inflammatory-degenerative disease: comparison of six treatment protocols*. J Oral Rehabil. 2012;39:245–51.
31. Huddleston Slater JJ, Vos LM, Stroy LP, Stegenga B. Randomized trial on the effectiveness of dexamethasone in TMJ arthrocentesis. J Dent Res. 2012;91:173–8.
32. Giraddi GB, Siddaraju A, Kumar A, Jain T. Comparison between betamethasone and sodium hyaluronate combination with betamethasone alone after arthrocentesis in the treatment of internal derangement of TMJ-using single puncture technique: a preliminary study. J Maxillofac Oral Surg. 2015;14:403–9.
33. Giraddi GB, Siddaraju A, Kumar B, Singh C. Internal derangement of temporomandibular joint: an evaluation of effect of corticosteroid injection compared with injection of sodium hyaluronate after arthrocentesis. J Maxillofac Oral Surg. 2012;11:258–63.
34. Kunjur J, Anand R, Brennan PA, Ilankovan V. An audit of 405 temporomandibular joint arthrocentesis with intra-articular morphine infusion. Br J Oral Maxillofac Surg. 2003;41:29–31.
35. Sipahi A, Satilmis T, Basa S. Comparative study in patients with symptomatic internal derangements of the temporomandibular joint: analgesic outcomes of arthrocentesis with or without intra-articular morphine and tramadol. Br J Oral Maxillofac Surg. 2015;53:316–20.
36. Ziegler CM, Wiechnik J, Muhling J. Analgesic effects of intra-articular morphine in patients with temporomandibular joint disorders: a prospective, double-blind, placebo-controlled clinical trial. J Oral Maxillofac Surg. 2010;68:622–7.
37. Prager TM, Mischkowski RA, Zoller JE. Effect of intra-articular administration of buprenorphine after arthrocentesis of the temporomandibular joint: a pilot study. Quintessence Int. 2007;38:e484–9.
38. Bouloux GF, Chou J, Krishnan D, Aghaloo T, Kahenasa N, Smith J, Giankopoulos H. Are hyaluronic acid or corticosteroid superior to lactated ringers in the short-term reduction of temporomandibular joint pain after arthrocentesis? J Oral Maxillofac Surg. 2017;75(1):52–62.
39. Lobbezoo F, van der Zaag J, van Selms MK, Hamburger HL, Naeije M. Principles for the management of bruxism. J Oral Rehabil. 2008;35:509–23.
40. Manfredini D, Guarda-Nardini L, Marchese-Ragona R, Lobbezoo F. Theories on possible temporal relationships between sleep bruxism and obstructive sleep apnea events. An expert opinion. Sleep Breath. 2015;19:1459–65.
41. Lobbezoo F, Visscher CM, Ahlberg J, Manfredini D. Bruxism and genetics: a review of the literature. J Oral Rehabil. 2014;41:709–14.
42. Manfredini D, Restrepo C, Diaz-Serrano K, Winocur E, Lobbezoo F. Prevalence of sleep bruxism in children: a systematic review of the literature. J Oral Rehabil. 2013;40:631–42.
43. Guaita M, Hogl B. Current treatments of bruxism. Curr Treat Options Neurol. 2016;18:10.
44. Schiffman E, Ohrbach R. Executive summary of the diagnostic criteria for temporomandibular disorders for clinical and research applications. J Am Dent Assoc. 2016;147:438–45.
45. Dommerholt J, Grieve R, Layton M, Hooks T. An evidence-informed review of the current myofascial pain literature--January 2015. J Bodyw Mov Ther. 2015;19:126–37.
46. Fricton J. Myofascial pain: mechanisms to management. Oral Maxillofac Surg Clin North Am. 2016;28:289–311.
47. Schiffman E, Ohrbach R, Truelove E, et al. Diagnostic criteria for temporomandibular disorders (DC/TMD) for clinical and research applications: recommendations of the international RDC/TMD consortium net-

work* and orofacial pain special interest group†. J Oral Facial Pain Headache. 2014;28:6–27.
48. Clark GT, Padilla M, Dionne R. Medication treatment efficacy and chronic orofacial pain. Oral Maxillofac Surg Clin North Am. 2016;28:409–21.
49. Silberstein SD. The use of botulinum toxin in the management of headache disorders. Semin Neurol. 2016;36:92–8.
50. Chen YW, Chiu YW, Chen CY, Chuang SK. Botulinum toxin therapy for temporomandibular joint disorders: a systematic review of randomized controlled trials. Int J Oral Maxillofac Surg. 2015;44:1018–26.
51. Soares A, Andriolo RB, Atallah AN, da Silva EM. Botulinum toxin for myofascial pain syndromes in adults. Cochrane Database Syst Rev. 2014;7:CD007533.
52. Ernberg M, Hedenberg-Magnusson B, List T, Svensson P. Efficacy of botulinum toxin type a for treatment of persistent myofascial TMD pain: a randomized, controlled, double-blind multicenter study. Pain. 2011;152:1988–96.
53. Canadian Agency for Drugs and Technologies in Health. Botulinum toxin A for myofascial pain syndrome: a review of the clinical effectiveness. Ottawa, ON: Canadian Agency for Drugs and Technologies in Health; 2014.
54. Sidebottom AJ, Patel AA, Amin J. Botulinum injection for the management of myofascial pain in the masticatory muscles. A prospective outcome study. Br J Oral Maxillofac Surg. 2013;51:199–205.
55. Patil S, Willett O, Thompkins T, et al. Botulinum toxin: pharmacology and therapeutic roles in pain states. Curr Pain Headache Rep. 2016;20:15.
56. Mathiesen O, Wetterslev J, Kontinen VK, et al. Adverse effects of perioperative paracetamol, NSAIDs, glucocorticoids, gabapentinoids and their combinations: a topical review. Acta Anaesthesiol Scand. 2014;58:1182–98.
57. Dahl JB, Nielsen RV, Wetterslev J, et al. Postoperative analgesic effects of paracetamol, NSAIDs, glucocorticoids, gabapentinoids and their combinations: a topical review. Acta Anaesthesiol Scand. 2014;58:1165–81.
58. Chang CY, Challa CK, Shah J, Eloy JD. Gabapentin in acute postoperative pain management. Biomed Res Int. 2014;2014:631756.
59. Argoff CE. Recent management advances in acute postoperative pain. Pain Pract. 2014;14:477–87.

Facial Cosmetic Surgery

34

LisaMarie Di Pasquale, Mohammad Banki,
and Elie M. Ferneini

Abstract

Facial cosmetic surgery is becoming popular in our society. In order to provide the most predictable surgical procedure, it is imperative for the surgeon to be able to define elements of facial aesthetics as well as the signs of an aging face. The surgeon must able to objectively and systematically analyze facial features preoperatively in order to correctly identify areas of concern and to arrive at an appropriate treatment plan for each patient. This chapter will review how to properly work up the facial cosmetic surgery patient. Clinical assessment and evaluation will be reviewed.

34.1 Introduction

Surgical correction of the aging face is an evolving art form. For over 200 years, facial cosmetic surgery has been researched and discussed in the literature. In the late nineteenth century, many surgeons were offering reconstructive procedures; however, few were writing about cosmetic improvements to an aging face. In the early twentieth century, many surgeons made very significant contributions to the field of cosmetic surgery, including Miller, Kolle, Bettman, and Booth through detailed reporting of face-lifting operations, eyelid surgery, and correction of the double chin [1].

Over the past two decades, however, numerous aesthetic techniques have been described to improve the results of facial rejuvenation. The current life expectancy in North America is now nearly 70 and approaching 80 years old [2]. Life

L. Di Pasquale, D.D.S., M.D. (✉)
Division of Oral and Maxillofacial Surgery, School of Dental Medicine, University of Connecticut, Farmington, CT, USA

M. Banki, M.D., D.M.D., F.A.C.S.
Artistic Contours, Warwick, RI, USA

Department of Surgery, Warren Alpert Medical School of Brown University, Providence, RI, USA

Division of Oral and Maxillofacial Surgery, University of Connecticut, Farmington, CT, USA

E.M. Ferneini, M.D., D.M.D., M.H.S., F.A.C.S. (✉)
Beau Visage Med Spa/Greater Waterbury OMS, Cheshire, CT, USA

Division of Oral and Maxillofacial Surgery, University of Connecticut, Farmington, CT, USA
e-mail: eferneini@yahoo.com

© Springer International Publishing AG 2018

E.M. Ferneini, J.D. Bennett (eds.), *Perioperative Assessment of the Maxillofacial Surgery Patient*,
https://doi.org/10.1007/978-3-319-58868-1_34

expectancy is increasing, and the aging population is generally healthier than the previous generation. The public has extreme interest for procedures that are new, have little to no recovery time, and produce a noticeable difference. These social demands are evidenced in the development of technologies and techniques directed at accomplishing this intervention [3]. Safe and effective surgical techniques with reduced downtime and long-lasting natural appearing results have emerged [4]. These minimally invasive facial rejuvenation procedures include the use of neuromuscular blocking agents and injectable fillers that offer temporary, low morbidity approach for the correction of many age-related abnormalities. The advantages include less swelling, no incisions, and minimal downtime to allow the patient to engage in regular activities as soon as the injection is completed [3]. As such, technical advances in minimally invasive cosmetic procedures have made facial rejuvenation increasingly more popular and widely available [4].

Successful cosmetic surgery relies both on the surgeon's ability to tend to the patient's operative wishes and attractively complete the operation and also the ability to appropriately select surgical candidates. The true goal of any plastic surgery procedure is to satisfy the cosmetic surgery patient [5]. Traditionally, these patients are increasingly educated consumers who have extensive sought data with which to make informed decisions [6]. Facial cosmetic surgery seeks to improve and refresh the appearance of the face without any signs of obvious surgical intervention after the healing is complete [4]. Understandably, the desires of the patient must be balanced with the treatment requirements of the surgeon. These requirements are critical in determining the advantages of one technique over the other [7, 8].

Facial aesthetic surgery is an elective process that aims to improve the appearance of the patient. The assessment of patient experiences, preferences, and perceptions in aesthetic surgery is especially necessary because patient satisfaction is the predominant factor in determining success. A thorough consultation with the patient including a complete history, a focused physical examination, and a consideration of psychological and psychosocial factors will lead to the highest possible chance of patient satisfaction and a good outcome. It is important to understand what specific goals the patient hopes to achieve and whether there are anatomic, medical, and psychological barriers that would hinder these desired aesthetic objectives [2]. Rejuvenation techniques include improving the overall health of the patient and their skin, in addition to using adjunctive surgical procedures to enhance beauty [4]. Thus, any medical comorbidities that would put the patient at increased risk for a complication or suboptimal result should be considered relative or absolute contraindications. Absolute contraindications are those that prevent adequate healing and lead to significantly increased risks [2]. Once a mutual agreement between the surgeon and the patient has been reached, it is then up to the surgeon's intimate understanding of facial anatomy, as well as the physiology of the aging process to produce the desired result.

34.2 Patient Selection

34.2.1 Patient Interview

The goal of maxillofacial cosmetic surgeons is to accurately identify areas where a patient's appearance may be modified for the desired outcome. One of the keys to achieving patient satisfaction, as well as a good surgical result, is proper patient analysis and selection [2]. Cosmetic surgeons must perform a systematic and thorough aesthetic evaluation to accurately diagnose and satisfy a patient's desires [9]. It is equally important to know when to operate as well as how to operate [10].

The process of connection with a prospective patient begins as soon as the patient enters the office. Office staff should be warm, courteous, and well informed for the patient. The reception area and the waiting room should be comfortable and welcoming [11]. The patients may receive calls from the office staff or a welcome letter sent in the mail prior to the consultation regarding what to expect. Pre-consultation medical forms, health questionnaires, and detailed patient packets may be sent. This useful information may include postoperative instructions, morbidity of procedures, complications of cosmetic surgery, and anticipated recovery time for various procedures [10]. This can save the surgeon time and offer understanding into the patient relationship. Once the patient has met the staff and the patient coordinator, other records, photographs, and vital signs may be taken.

The initial meeting between the oral and maxillofacial surgeon and patient is a complex interaction. The consultation should be an open discussion that involves two-way discussion and decision-making. During this time, the patient evaluates the surgeon, deciding whether to be operated on by that surgeon. Simultaneously, it is the responsibility of the facial cosmetic surgeon to thoroughly analyze the patient anatomically, medically, and psychologically to be able to discuss all of the options that may serve the patient's desired aesthetic goals [2, 10].

The history is of utmost importance with cosmetic surgery patients [2]. Most of the time, the patient will present with stated objectives such as bothersome aspects of their facial appearance or other specific concerns. During this time, it is not uncommon for patients to seek the opinion of the surgeon or request the surgeon to make recommendations regarding other procedures that would help the patient achieve their goals [10]. Photographs, computer imaging, or pictures of the surgeon's other cases can aid in the discussion with the patient. It may be helpful to include various stages of healing in the postoperative course to help the patient understand the natural history of the surgery [11]. Adequate time should be given to each patient to allow for all questions and concerns to be addressed.

34.2.2 Patient Selection

During the initial consultation, the surgeon must perform a careful evaluation of the patient's psychological, emotional, and physical profile. The evaluation process of determining which patient is a good psychological candidate is very complex and often is influenced by many factors. Sufficient time in the consultation allows the relationship between the patient and the surgeon to deepen, so the surgeon can understand the position and perspective of the patient and insight into their true motivation for having cosmetic surgery. Cosmetic surgery patients desire change and usually request surgery. Additionally, surgeons usually want to perform cosmetic surgery. Care must be taken by both the patient and the surgeon to avoid the erroneously thinking that great surgical result may make a psychologically imperfect patient contented [5]. For these reasons, careful communication during the initial consultation is essential in establishing a healthy surgeon-patient relationship. Helpful topics to address include:

1. The patient's initial desire for surgery and changes anticipated
2. Why the patient feels this time is appropriate for surgery
3. Available support of friends and family
4. The financial implications of the surgery
5. The patient's ability to tolerate the postsurgical course [12]

The consultation provides the surgeon a chance to educate the prospective patient. A realistic portrayal of what can and cannot be achieved must be explained to the patient. The conversation must include the morbidities and possible complications of surgery, as well as discussion of predictable suboptimal outcomes, as unfavorable results may rarely be predicted. It is imperative that the patient gains a firm knowledge of the anticipated postoperative course, realistic expectations, and an understanding of his/her responsibility to partake in adequate postoperative care. The time spent in patient education will allow for less overall misunderstanding, increased patient compliance, and improved patient-doctor rapport. If unrealistic expectations cannot be eradicated with patient education, the patient may not be a good fit for cosmetic surgery [11].

The surgeon must elicit a medical history from the patient. Prior medical issues, current overall medical health, discussion of the physical and mental stress of cosmetic surgery, and compliance issues should be reviewed.

A complete list of oral and topical medications including herbal and health supplements must be specifically asked from the patient. The surgeon should be wary of relevant medications and herbal medications that have blood-thinning properties, such as listed in Table 34.1 [2].

A thorough surgical history should be obtained, including previous facial cosmetic surgery. Many cosmetic procedures require extreme persistence and attentive care by patients in the postoperative period. A lack of compliance can significantly affect the outcome of a cosmetic procedure greatly. Thus, every effort must be made by the surgeon to ascertain the degree of compliance that patients might have before choosing the type and extent of cosmetic surgery appropriately [12]. Attention should be given to patient's anger or remorse over previous cosmetic procedures.

34.2.3 Psychiatric Considerations

During the interview about medical history, the surgeon must also be evaluating issues such as poor self-image, possible personality disorders, and body dysmorphic disorder (BDD) [5]. The surgeon must identify characteristics that may predispose the patient toward postoperative dissatisfaction with the surgical result [5, 12]. Studies have shown that the best indication for facial cosmetic surgery was a lack of self-confidence associated with a desire for social interaction in relation to a specific physical blemish [13]. This is an important distinction because if the surgeon believes that the patient has overall poor self-image and is generally an unhappy person, surgery is highly unlikely to create personal happiness for such a patient. An unhealthy motivation for surgery and poor self-image combine to make a patient who often is psychologically unfit for cosmetic surgery. Patients who have poor self-image often have unattainable expectations and have an accentuated dissatisfaction with the surgi-

Table 34.1 Medications and herbal health supplements to stop prior to surgery

	Relevance	When to Stop
Medication		
NSAIDs (nonexhaustive list)	Inhibit platelet synthesis	2 weeks prior to surgery
Aspirin, ibuprofen, naproxen, meloxicam, celecoxib	Vitamin K antagonist (clotting cascade)	1 week prior to surgery
Warfarin (Coumadin)	Inhibit platelet synthesis	1 week prior to surgery
Clopidogrel (Plavix)	Inhibits platelet aggregation	1 week prior to surgery
Alcohol	Inhibit platelet synthesis	1 week prior to surgery
Systemic steroids	Inhibits platelet aggregation	1 week prior to surgery
Isotretinoin	May inhibit wound healing	6 weeks prior to surgery
	May inhibit wound healing	6 months to 1 year prior to surgery
Herbal/Hearth Supplement		
Natural foods high in salicylate	Inhibit platelet synthesis	2 weeks prior to surgery
Curry, cayenne pepper, ginger, paprika, thyme, cinnamon, dill, oregano, turmeric, licorice, peppermint, raisins, cherries, cranberries, oranges, prunes, grapes, strawberries, chewing gum, honey, wine, cider, vinegar		
Vitamin E		
Fish oil/omega-3 fatty acids	Vitamin K antagonist (clotting cascade)	1 week prior to surgery
Gingko biloba	Inhibit platelet synthesis	2 weeks prior to surgery
St. Johns wort	Inhibits platelet aggregation	1 week prior to surgery
Garlic	Possible inhibitor platelet synthesis	1 week prior to surgery

cal result. Interestingly, in the 1960s, Edgerton and colleagues found that the following characteristics were associated with poor outcomes: male sex, seeking surgery at the request of another, unrealistic expectations, clinical depression, and surgery in a period of marital problems [9].

It is important for the surgeon to be aware of the patient's psychological profile preoperatively and to communicate concerns and potential issues with the patient during the consultation. Certain patients are predisposed to unhappiness and dissatisfaction. These patients, who may be psychologically unstable for surgery, include very difficult and exacting patients, those dissatisfied with the work of other surgeons despite good outcomes, the obsessive patient, the depressed patient, the narcissistic patient, and the patient with body dysmorphic disorder.

The difficult patient is a patient that challenges the surgeon's judgment, patient management, and surgical skills. They are often a stress on the surgeon and entire staff. Preoperatively, these patients may conceptualize their problems as much higher severity than what is reasonable [14]. In such consultations, surgeons must be aware that with any surgical intervention, they may bear this patient's dissatisfaction [12].

Cosmetic surgery patients tend to be more depressed than the average population. During the consultation, depressed patients may appear or express sadness, irritability, and hopelessness. Cosmetic surgery is statistically ineffective as a treatment of this disorder [14]. If a certain event or factor is contributing to the depression, it may be best to advise the patient to wait for the event to settle first and reconsider the request later in order to improve patient's self-confidence [13]. Another common personality disorder encountered by cosmetic surgeons is narcissistic personality disorder. These patients possess a grandiose sense of self and inflated sense of self-importance. In a surgical consultation, they are likely to present their ideals and demand treatment.

Various methods exist for dissuading the psychologically unfit patient from surgery. Firstly, the importance of spending enough time discussing all potential outcomes and implications with patients before cosmetic surgery cannot be stressed enough. It always must be stressed to patients that although perfection is the goal, a realistic approach should be taken, noting possible risks, suboptimal outcomes, and complications [12]. Scheduling a second or third consultation to rediscuss issues may prove very beneficial with certain patients. This allows time for patients to collect their thoughts and understand their motivations. If the second consultation reveals more challenging patient behavior, the extra time is warranted, and a decision to not offer surgery is acceptable. Once the surgeon determines that the patient is not a good surgical candidate, it is important to explain the situation directly and offer reasonable alternatives. Minimally invasive services, such as injection of botulinum toxin or facial fillers, are reversible and may fit to serve the patient's needs. This also allows the surgeon to care for the patient and observe how the patient engages in the post-procedure course [5]. When dealing with challenging patients, it is important to remember, the most common source of dissatisfaction can be traced back to inadequate pre- and perioperative counseling [12]. Building rapport with these patients is important. The approaches may be individualized for each patient, but facial cosmetic surgeons must master dealing with patients in these categories (Fig. 34.1).

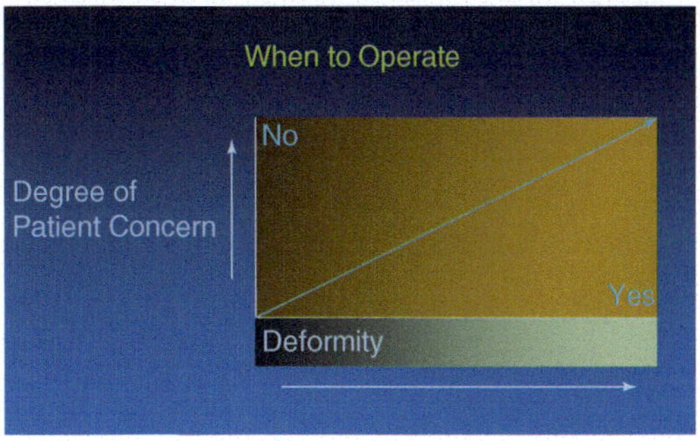

Fig. 34.1 Graph showing when to operate on a cosmetic patient [2]

34.3 Pre-op Evaluation of the Aging Face

A thorough mastery of facial anatomy and aesthetics is a requisite for all facial cosmetic surgeons. Perception of beauty will vary between surgeons and will be different for each patient. Care is taken to view each face with an objective analysis. While facial analysis should take into account sex, age, and racial differences, beauty is harmony, and this is a universal concept that typically transcends genders, ages, and ethnicities [2, 11]. Generally, all patients who present for aesthetic facial surgery desire an improved and more youthful appearance. As surgical techniques have evolved, a better understanding of facial anatomy and the aging process has also progressed. Thus, a basic fundament to obtaining consistent results in facial cosmetic surgery is an understanding of the changes that occur to an aging face. The surgeon must have a thorough knowledge of the anatomy of the head and neck while incorporating current concepts of beauty accordingly.

34.3.1 Anatomic Landmarks

Facial analysis is dependent on both soft tissue and skeletal, cephalometric anatomic landmarks. Soft tissue reference points are skeletal reference points defined by cephalometric analysis and are listed in Table 34.2 [15] (Figs. 34.2 and 34.3).

The Frankfort horizontal plane is the horizontal line from the external auditory canal to the inferior aspect of the infraorbital rim measured while the patient is in natural head position with the head parallel to the floor. It is the standard reference point for patient positioning in clinical records [15].

34.3.2 Facial Proportions

Facial proportions have long been established in historical texts. These provide a definition and guide for the facial cosmetic surgeon. When performing facial analysis, it is helpful to think of three components: the bony facial skeleton, the soft tissues, and the skin. All three components are discussed with the patient preoperatively in relation to different procedural options [2]. This

Table 34.2 Skeletal and soft tissue landmarks

Soft Tissue Anatomic Landmarks	Cephalometric Reference Points
Trichion (Tr): Anterior hairline in the midline	(S) Sella: The midpoint of the hypophysial fossa
Glabella (G): Most prominent point of the forehead on profile	(Or) Orbitale: The most inferior point on the infraorbital rim
Nasion (N): The deepest depression at the root of the nose; typically corresponds to the nasofrontal suture	(P) Porion: The most superior point on the external auditory meatus
Radix: Root of the nose, a region and not a point; part of an unbroken curve that begins at the superior orbital ridge and continues along the lateral nasal wall	(Cd) Condylion: The most superior point on the head of the mandibular condole
Rhinion (R): Soft-tissue correlate of the osseocartilaginous junction on the nasal dorsum	(Ar) Articulate: The point of intersection of the posterior margin of the ascending mandibular ramus and the margin of the cranial base
Sellion: Osseocartilaginous junction on the nasal dorsum	(ANS) Anterior nasal spine
Supratip: Point cephalic to the tip	(PNS) Posterior nasal spine
Tip (T): Ideally, the most anterior projection of the nose on profile	(A) Point A, subspinale: The deepest point in the concavity of the premaxilla
Subnasale (Sn): Junction of columella and upper lip	(Pr) Prosthion: The lowest most anterior point on the alveolar portion of the premaxilla
Labrale superius (Ls): Vermilion border of upper lip	
Stomion (S): Central portion of interlabial gap	(Id) Infradentale: The highest most anterior point on the alveolar portion of the mandible
Stomion superius: Lowest point of upper lip vermilion	
Stomion inferius: Highest point of lower lip vermilion	(B) Point B, supramentale: The most posterior point in the outer contour of the mandibular alveolar process
Labrale inferius (Li): Vermilion border of lower lip	

Table 34.2 (continued)

Soft Tissue Anatomic Landmarks	Cephalometric Reference Points
Mentolabial sulcus (Si): Most posterior point between lower lip and chin	(Pg) Pogonion: Most anterior point on the bony chin in the midline
Pogonion (Pg): Most anterior midline soft-tissue point of chin	(Gn) Gnathion: A point between the most anterior (Pg) and inferior (Me) point on the chin
Menton (Me): Most inferior soft-tissue point on chin	(Me) Menton: The lowest point on the mandible
Cervical point (C): The innermost point between the submental area and the neck	(Go) Gonion: The midpoint at the angle of the mandible

will point out the limitations of various procedures possible and modify patient expectations. Additionally, it is important to include the patient in this discussion with thoughtful reassurance that nearly all faces have some degree of disproportionate measure [2].

The initial assessment of the face evaluates symmetry. The face can be divided into facial units vertically and then horizontally (Figs. 34.4 and 34.5). Facial height is commonly assessed by one of two methods. The first method, the Da Vinci method, divides the face into equal horizontal thirds. Measurements are made, so the upper third extends from the trichion to the glabella, the middle third from the glabella to the subnasale, and the lower third from the subnasale to the menton [2, 11]. The lower facial third can be further subdivided into thirds from the subnasale to the stomion, the stomion to mentolabial sulcus, and then onto the menton [11]. Another method for measuring facial height excludes the upper facial third due to the variable position of the hairline and considers only the middle and lower third of the face [11, 15]. Measurements in this method are made from the nasion, not glabella, to the subnasale and from the subnasale to the menton. This method divides the face such that the midface represents 43% of the height, with the lower face representing 57% [2, 15]. Facial width is evaluated by dividing the face into equal fifths. These vertical fifths are based on the lateral projection of the helix to the lateral canthus, lateral canthus to the medial canthus, and intercanthal distance and so on to the contralateral side [11]. Thus, the width of each eye and the intercanthal distance each consumes a respective vertical fifth [15].

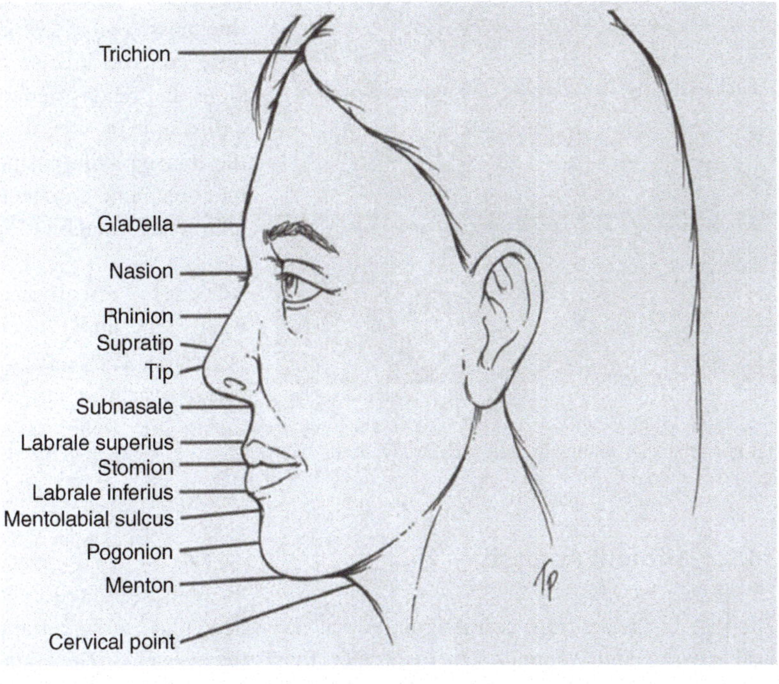

Fig. 34.2 Cephalometric analysis: soft tissue anatomic landmarks [15]

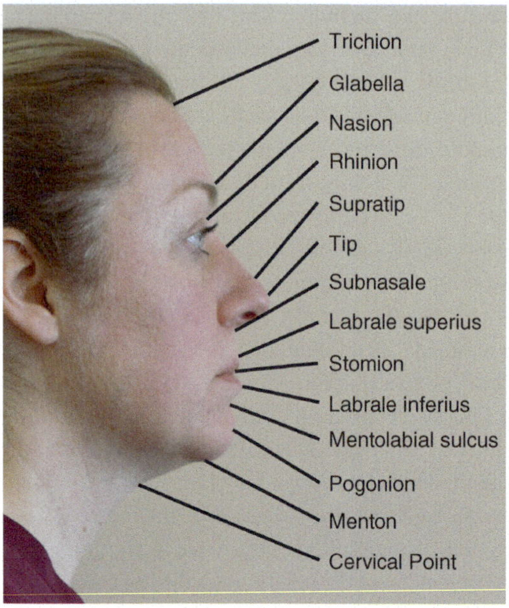

Fig. 34.3 Right profile view detailing anatomic landmarks

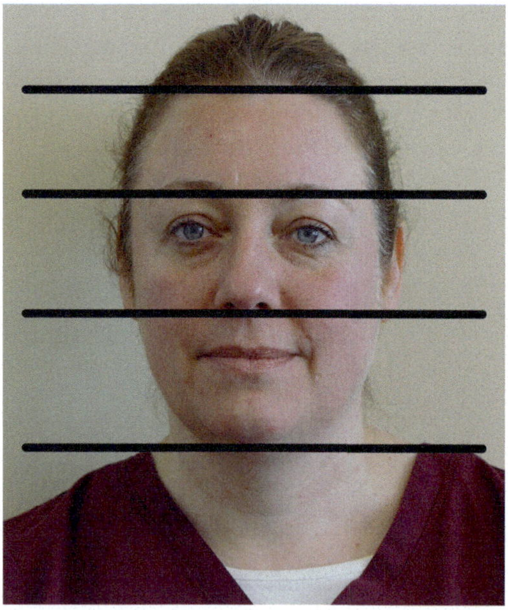

Fig. 34.4 Front view: *horizontal lines* passing through hairline, glabella, subnasale, and menton divide the face into equal thirds

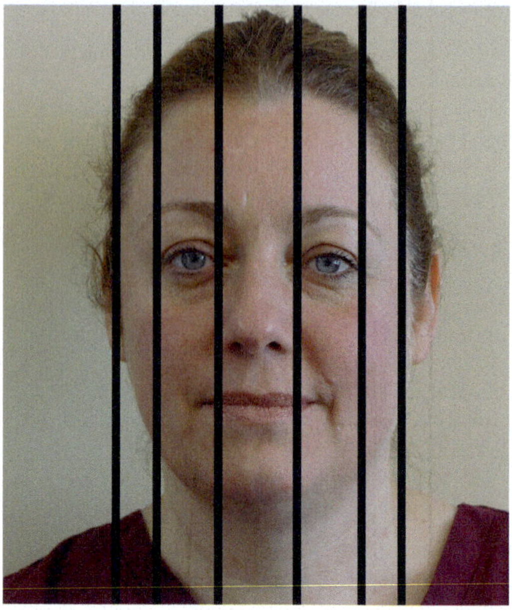

Fig. 34.5 Front view: *vertical lines* dividing the face into five equal zones, each measuring width of palpebral fissure. Distances are equal from helix to lateral canthus, from lateral canthus to medial canthus, and between the two medial canthi

34.3.3 Subunit Analysis

The face is divided into aesthetic units that are further divided into subunits. The major units that are classically defined for facial analysis include the forehead, eyes, nose, lips, chin, ears, and neck. The units and subunits are based on skin thickness, color, texture, and underlying structural contour. Precise planning of surgical incisions and reconstruction requires analysis of the entire unit or subunit. Incisions should parallel the relaxed skin tension lines and lie within the unit or subunit borders to result in the most favorable scar formation [15].

34.3.3.1 Forehead/Bones/Hair

Firstly, the bony structure of the face must be evaluated. The bony structure provides the foundation over which the soft tissues are draped and dictate the final aesthetic result [11]. Thinner angular faces typically have more prominent bone structure and fare better with cosmetic surgery results [11].

The eyes and upper face should be viewed in the context of the forehead and cheeks. The forehead plays an important role in the appearance of the eyes [11]. The boundaries of the forehead are from the hairline (trichion) to the glabella and make up the upper third of the face. The anterior hairline is usually 7.5–9.5 cm from the glabella [11]. The contour of the forehead should have a gentle convexity. The nasofrontal angle is the angle created by an intersection of lines tangent to glabella-nasion and tangent to the nasal dorsum. The average measurement of this angle is 115–135° [15].

34.3.3.2 Eyes

The boundaries of the orbits span the border between the upper and middle facial thirds. As previously discussed, the width of one eye from the medial to lateral canthus, as well as the intercanthal distance, should each measure one fifth of the total facial width [15]. Average intercanthal distance is approximately 30 mm [11]. In general, the eye should be almond shaped, with the lateral canthus approximately 2–4 mm superior to the medial canthus with the eyes open. The highest point of the upper eyelid at the medial limbus and the lowest point of the lower eyelid is at the lateral limbus [2]. The horizontal width of the palpebral fissure should measure 25–30 mm, and its vertical height should measure 10 mm [2].

An ideal eyebrow shape has a gentle curvature that begins medially and tapers laterally (Fig. 34.6) [2]. In male patients, brows are at the level of the supraorbital rim, whereas in females, the brow lies 1 cm above the supraorbital rim, with a peak just above the lateral limbus [11]. The medial extent of the brow terminates at a vertical line that passes through the lateral nasal ala and the medial canthus [15]. In women, the highest point of the eyebrow arc is in line with the lateral limbus. Medial and lateral brow should end in the same horizontal plane, with the lateral taper of the brow ending at a point on a line drawn from the nasal ala through the lateral canthus of the eye [2]. The distance between the upper lid lash line and the inferior aspect of the brow should be 25 mm at the midpupillary line [2]. Brow ptosis can account for dermatochalasis. Often blepharoplasty must occur in conjunction with correction of ptotic brows [11].

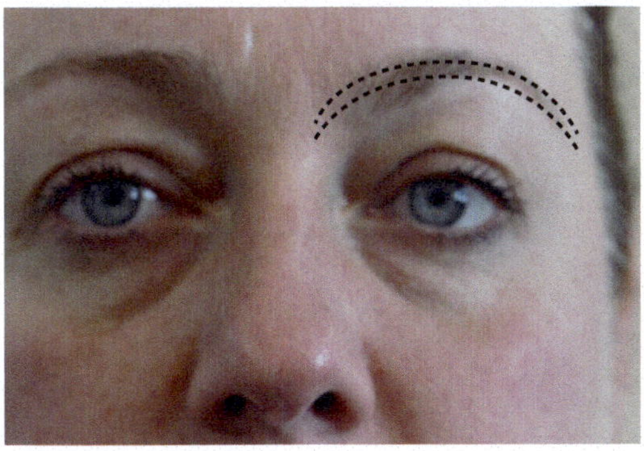

Fig. 34.6 Ideal brow shape with a gentle curvature that begins medially and tapers laterally

The upper lid crease is the anatomical line created by the insertion of the levator aponeurosis and orbital septum into the orbicularis oculi and dermis [15]. The supratarsal crease is evaluated by lifting the brow and asking the patient to look down. Distance from the upper lid margin to the crease is 8–11 mm in women and 6–9 mm in men [11]. Any measurement greater than this may be related to levator aponeurosis disinsertion. The upper eyelid normally covers a small portion (2 mm) of the iris and limbus but not the pupil. Blepharoptosis is measured using marginal reflex distance (MRD)-1 for the upper lid and MRD-2 for the lower lid. This is measured from the corneal light reflex to the eyelid margin in the midpupillary line. Reference range is 4.0–4.5 mm in the upper eyelid and 5.0–5.5 mm in the lower eyelid. Ptosis may cause values below these normal ranges, while values above these measurements may be from eyelid retraction or levator disinsertion [11]. The lower eyelid is within 1 to 2 mm of the iris on neutral gaze [15].

Orbital complex preoperative examination should include a visual acuity test, extraocular motion, and assessment for xerophthalmia [11]. The quality and excess of the skin, pseudoherniation and excess orbital fat, position of supratarsal crease, blepharoptosis, and lid retraction should be evaluated. Orbital fat pseudoherniation is more common in the nasal compartment superiorly and is possible in all three compartments inferiorly. This may be evaluated with gentle ballottement of the globe to highlight the weakened orbital septum and allow excess fat to bulge out [11]. Snap test is used to measure eyelid laxity. This test is performed by pulling the lower lid downward and outward and allowing it to snap back into rest position. In a normal test, the lower lid should return quickly and fully into a position contacting the globe; otherwise, eyelid laxity is present. Also, the lower lid is closely associated with the cheek. Settling and descending of the malar fat pad is common with age [11]. As this happens, the infraorbital rim becomes more exposed, and the delineation between the lower lid and the cheek is more obvious. This causes a double convexity deformity. Often this will be addressed with elevation of the cheek fat pad in addition to fat augmentation or transposition [11].

34.3.3.3 Nose

Nasal anatomy is highly variable, and aesthetic ideals should be viewed in relation to the individual patient's facial anatomy and desires. The nose should occupy the middle third of facial length (Fig. 34.7) [10]. Certain ideal nasofacial and intranasal relationships are essential in evaluating a nose. The three most important measures of nasal aesthetics are nasal length, tip projection, and rotation.

The nose is positioned in the middle third of the face, starting at the nasion, in line with the superior palpebral fold, and extending down the face to the end at the soft tissue point subnasale. The nose is so cosmetically prominent in the midface; it forms very significant and well-defined relationships with surrounding facial structures. Powell and Humphreys classically described the ideal values of these anatomic relationships [2]. They defined the relationships between the nasofrontal angle, nasolabial angle, nasofacial angle, and nasomental angle. The nasofrontal angle, as previously described, is the angle created by the intersection of lines tangent to the glabella-nasion and to the nasal dorsum. The average measurement of this angle is 115–135°. The nasolabial angle is the angle between the columella and the upper lip (Fig. 34.8). This angle should measure 95–110° in women and 90–95° in men [15]. The nasofacial angle is a measure of the angle created by a line tangent to the nasal dorsum intersecting a vertical line from the glabella to pogonion. The ideal nasofacial angle ranges from 30 to 40°. The nasomental angle describes the angle between lines tangent to the nasal dorsum intersecting with a vertical line from the nasal tip to the pogonion. The range of this angle is from 120 to 132°. Of all the stated

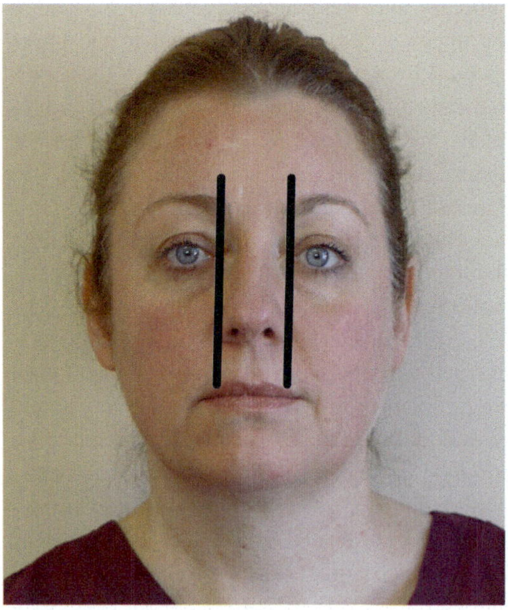

Fig. 34.7 Nasal landmarks: *Vertical line* drawn through lateral nasal tip passes through medial canthi

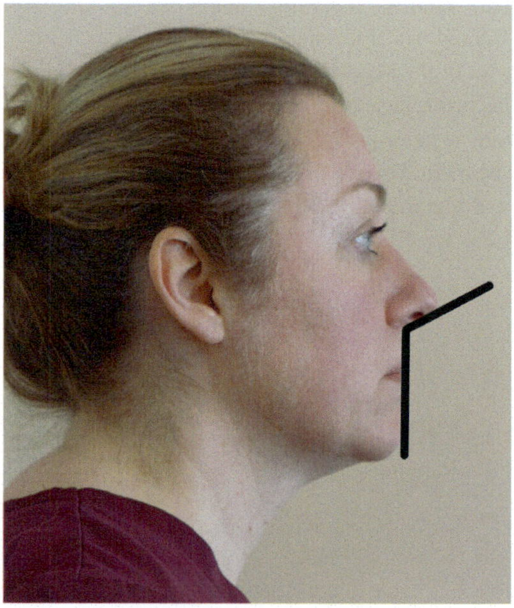

Fig. 34.8 Nasolabial angle is the angle between the columella and the upper lip

angles, the nasomental angle is the most inconsistent between individuals, as it is heavily influenced by variable lip and chin anatomy.

Nasal rotation and tip projection must be discussed in the cosmetic nasal analysis. Tip rotation is generally measured on an arc that is centered at anatomic landmark porion or the external auditory canal. Tip rotation increases along the superior aspect of the arc and decreases along the inferior portion. Ideal nasal tip projection described by Simons includes the upper lip, stating that the ratio of the upper lip should be equal to the base length of the nose in a 1:1 ratio [16]. Simons method is unique in that it incorporates the length of the upper lip into the measurement. Another method attributed to Goode uses a triangle to represent nasal tip projection. One side of the triangle is formed from a line vertical from the nasion through the alar groove, the second a perpendicular line going from the alar groove to the nasal tip, and the third a line tangent to the nasal dorsum through the nasion that completes the triangle [16]. The ratio derived by comparing the length of the perpendicular line (alar groove to the nasal tip) with that of the nasal length (nasion to the tip) should be 0.55–0.60 [15]. On lateral view, columellar show of 3–5 mm is acceptable and expected. From the basal view, the nose should be triangular in shape and divided into three equivalent units [15] (Fig. 34.9).

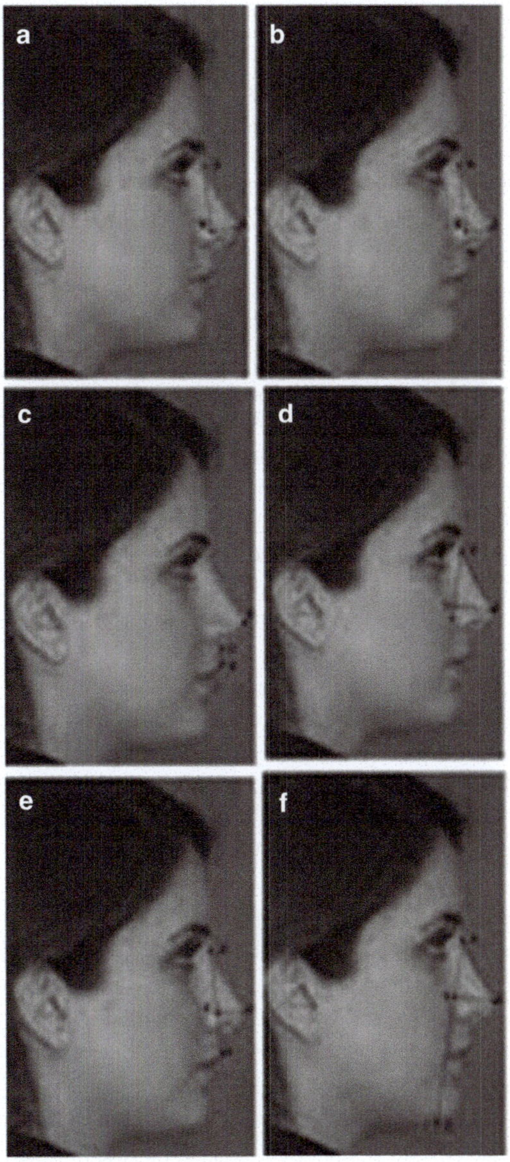

Fig. 34.9 Each of the six nasal tip projection ratios as defined by Baum (**a**), Powell (**b**), Simons (**c**), Goode (**d**), Crumley 1 (**e**), and Crumley 2 (**f**) [16]

34.3.3.4 Ears

The width of the ear is approximately one half its length. The superior aspect of the ear lies at the level of the eyebrow, whereas its inferior aspect is at the level of the nasal ala. Thus, the proportionate length of the ear should approximately that of the nose measured from the nasion to the subnasale. The ear lies between two parallel, horizontal lines: one drawn through the eyebrow superiorly and the nasal ala inferiorly. The ear protrudes from the skull at an angle of approximately 20–30°, which usually translates into a measurement of 15–25 mm from the helix to the mastoid skin [2, 15]. The long axis of the ear should be parallel to the long axis of the nasal dorsum.

34.3.3.5 Lips

With aging, several significant changes occur to the lips. The upper lip lengthens, the cupid's bow becomes flatter, and the white roll also becomes less defined causing blunting of the philtrum. Additionally, the commissures may turn down and the overall fullness of the lips is decreased. For assessment of lip projection, a line is drawn from the subnasale to pogonion. The upper lip should lie 3.5 mm anterior to the line and the lower lip around 2.2 mm anterior to the line. In the elderly, changes in dentition and loss of alveolar height can lead to decreased projection of the lips [11]. The upper lip should be approximately half the height of the lower lip, forming a ratio of approximately 1:2 [2].

The boundaries of the lip are entirely within the lower one third of the face. The upper lip is measured from the subnasale to a reference point called stomion superius. Likewise, the lower lip is measured from the stomion inferius to the menton [15]. An alternative method for determining horizontal placement of the lips is using the ideal nasomental angle. The lips should fall just behind this line at a distance of 4 mm for the upper lip and 2 mm for the lower lip [15].

34.3.3.6 Chin

A careful analysis of the chin is required to adequately analyze the nose or the neck, as the chin is a foundation unit in the lower facial third. The boundaries of the chin lie in the lower third of the face and can be measured from the mentolabial crease to the menton [2]. With aging, the mandibular alveolus and body tend to resorb leading to altered lower facial height. Chin and cheek augmentation may be necessary to achieve a certain result. Many patients simply will not be able to get their desired jaw definition without chin augmentation or genioplasty. The Gonzales-Ulloa method gives a measurement for where the ideal chin position (or pogonion soft tissue landmark) should rest. A vertical line is drawn from the nasion to the pogonion perpendicular to the Frankfort horizontal, and the pogonion landmark should approach or just touch this line [15]. If it does not, the patient must be evaluated for microgenia, micrognathia, or retrognathia. An alternative method for analyzing chin position has already been described in the lip section, where the mentolabial sulcus lies approximately 4 mm behind this line [15]. Additionally, the malar fat pads tend to atrophy causing a hollowed appearance with age. A facelift procedure alone will not correct this deformity, and malar augmentation procedures should be discussed with appropriate patients. Also, the position of the hyoid bone will greatly affect the cervicomental angle. A high hyoid bone provides greatest amount of contour and definition between the chin and the neck. [11].

34.3.3.7 Neck

The neck should be well defined from the mandible with a smooth jaw-neck line. Ideally the cervicomental angle, measured as the angle between a line from the glabella to pogonion intersecting with a line tangent from the menton to the cervical point, where the cervical point is defined as the innermost point between the submentum and neck [2, 15]. The ideal cervicomental angle is acute and should be 80–95°. The relationship between the chin and the neck is very important. When evaluating chin position, attention should be given to the cervicomental angle, as an obtuse angle may cause the appearance of poor chin projection [15].

34.3.3.8 Skin

During cosmetic surgery, consideration should also be given to skin quality. Rhytids, texture, pigmentation, elasticity, presence of subcutaneous fat, and other factors of the aging face may not be treated best with surgery, and other cosmetic procedures may be indicated to get the optimal outcome. This should be discussed with the patient preoperatively to mitigate expectations for the outcome from a surgical procedure [11]. Skin type can be classified using Fitzpatrick's description for pigmentation, whereas solar damage and rhytids can be described with Glogau's photoaging classification. Of most importance in skin examination is the evaluation of rhytids. Hyperdynamic facial lines are specifically those lines caused by facial expressions and related to facial muscle contraction, such as forehead furrows, crow's feet, or smile lines [2]. Static wrinkles are lines that are present when not forming facial expressions. They are natural to aging as a result of loss of skin structure and decreased volume of collagen, elastic, and hyaluronic acid (Table 34.3, Box 34.1) [15].

Table 34.3 Fitzpatrick classification

Fitzpatrick classification of Sun-reactive skin type		
Skin type	Skin color	Characteristics
I	White	Always burns, never tans
II	White	Usually burns, tans with difficulty
III	White	Sometimes burns, sometimes tans
IV	White	Rarely burns, tans with ease
V	Brown	Very rarely burns, tans very easily
VI	Black	Never burns, always tans

Box 34.1: Glogau classification

Glogau photoaging classification
Type I: No keratoses, few wrinkles, age 20–30, rarely wears makeup
Type II: Early lentigenes, wrinkles on animation, age 30–40, sometimes wears makeup
Type III: Advanced photoaging, wrinkles present at rest, age 50–60, always wears makeup
Type IV: Severe photoaging, severe wrinkling, age 60–70, makeup has minimal benefit

34.4 Clinical Evaluation/Assessment

34.4.1 Preoperative Medical Assessment

Facial cosmetic surgery is an elective process, and no elective procedures are worth an unfavorable outcome such as death. Proper preoperative assessment includes picking appropriate patients for the given procedure. Many patients undergoing cosmetic procedures are elderly and may have many medical comorbidities. Most patients will do well with proper medical, anesthetic, and surgical management; however, some patients are clearly not suitable surgical candidates [17]. Any medical conditions that could possibly lead to an increased risk for a complication should be considered. As discussed, the preoperative assessment will include a complete medical and surgical history. Conditions that are considered absolute contraindications are those that would increase surgical risks and affect healing leading to a suboptimal result. Such illnesses include uncontrolled diabetes, hypertension, end-stage renal or hepatic disease, autoimmune or connective tissue disorders, bleeding disorders, or other chronic illnesses.

The appropriate laboratory workup should be guided by the patient's age and medical comorbidities. All patients should obtain at least a complete blood count. Any patient with metabolic syndromes, such as diabetes, should have a hemoglobin A1C level checked. Patients with liver disease should obtain hepatic and coagulation panels. If a history of renal disease is noted, an electrolyte profile should be obtained. Additionally, patients and the surgeon should include the patient's primary care physician in the decision to proceed with elective surgery, particularly if the primary care doctor is managing medical comorbidities.

Some patients will require preoperative risk stratification from their primary care physicians or medical specialists pertinent to their medical conditions. For example, patients who have controlled hypertension or diabetes are most often cleared by a primary care physician from a medical standpoint and generally fare well [17]. Patients with cardiopulmonary problems present more of a risk. If a patient has cardiopulmonary history or is over the age of 40, a chest x-ray and electrocardiogram should be obtained [2]. If a patient has a history of angina or coronary artery disease, preoperative work by a cardiologist is warranted. If the patient is to undergo a cardiac CT or a stress test, pertinent information for the surgeon to know includes valvular function, ventricular function, the status of the coronary artery system, and any identified arrhythmias. Patients who have significant lung disease must undergo pulmonary consultation and related tests, such as pulmonary function tests [17].

A smoker undergoing facial cosmetic surgery incurs a major risk of postoperative complications [18]. Smokers present well-known surgical risks, specifically with wound healing, as well as many anesthesia risks. Anesthetically, they have increased secretions, more reactive airways, decreased lung capacity, and oxygenation problems. All in all, a smoker is 1.38 times more likely to die on the operating table than a nonsmoker [19, 20]. After surgery, they are more at risk for tissue necrosis and delayed healing [17]. Notably, two studies showed heightened risk of cutaneous necrosis in patients having undergone a cervical-facial lift (odds ratio of 4.6 [18] and 12.4 [21]). Another study found a correlation between smoking and hematoma formation [22]. Active smoking may contribute to hematoma formation due to bronchial hyperreactivity and increased secretions leading to excess coughing and therefore increased pressure [20]. Laser surgery may also be contraindicated in smoking patients [17].

Deep vein thrombosis (DVT) or resultant pulmonary embolus is a problem that may occur in longer operations. Combining multiple facial cosmetic procedures can lead to prolonged immobilization of a patient under general anesthesia. Obese patients, medically compromised patients, and patients on hormonal therapy including oral contraceptive pills may have an increase in the incidence of DVT. Pneumatic compression devices and compression hose should be used on all patients when appropriate.

Facial cosmetic surgery in patients receiving antiplatelet or anticoagulant therapy is debated. These medications are typically given to patients with valvular heart disease, prosthetic valves, atrial fibrillation, or history of a stroke. Surgeons typically discontinue the use of aspirin and vitamin K antagonists (warfarin) perioperatively. A balance must be obtained between surgical bleeding risk and exposing high-risk patients to thromboembolic complications. Traditionally, patients on anticoagulant therapy may be bridged from their warfarin therapy with heparin or low molecular weight heparin in the perioperative period [23].

In recent years, new oral anticoagulants have been developed with evidence of equivalent benefit and improved safety profile. These drugs are beneficial in that they do not require regular lab monitoring or routine dose adjusting. However, little evidence exists for their use, particularly with reversing their effects in the perioperative period [24].

The first of such novel oral anticoagulants are the factor Xa inhibitors, rivaroxaban, apixaban, and edoxaban. This class of anticoagulants blocks the function of factor Xa in the conversion of prothrombin to thrombin (factor II). As mentioned, these drugs do not require routine monitoring. Elimination profiles of these drugs are both hepatic and renal, with some interactions among drugs that are also dependent on hepatic CYP3A4 metabolism. Direct thrombin inhibitors, such as dabigatran, block thrombin from converting fibrinogen into fibrin. The direct thrombin inhibitors rely predominantly upon renal clearance [24].

For elective surgery, factor Xa and factor II inhibitors have predictable clearance times, provided normal renal function. This allows for the drug to be stopped at a certain time preoperatively and a concomitant decrease in anticoagulant effect observed, depending on the time of the last dose of the drug [24]. Once appropriate, the drugs may be restarted, and the patient is quickly brought back into the therapeutic window. Many groups have set forth recommendations for when to stop these novel drugs preoperatively. Cessation of the factor Xa inhibitors for 24 h before low bleeding risk procedures and at least 48 h before for high bleeding risk procedures is advised [24]. Attention must be given to patients with impaired renal function, as these patients will take longer to clear the anticoagulant effect of the drug. For patients with impaired renal function, a longer period of cessation (up to 96 h) is recommended. If postoperative bleeding is controlled, re-dosing of the thrombin or factor X inhibitors may start almost immediately within 24 h. If the surgical procedure is higher risk for postoperative bleeding, a period of 48–72 h is recommended prior to restarting the anticoagulation.

Unfortunately, no specific reversal agent exists for these anticoagulants. In emergent situations, the degree of anticoagulation can be measured using the activated partial thromboplastin time (APTT), prothrombin time (PT), or anti-factor Xa assays. Qualitative measurement of thrombin inhibitors may be assessed by certain tests that directly measure thrombin times, but these are not widely available [24]. Packed red blood cells or fresh frozen plasma transfusions can be given to aid in reversal of the anticoagulant effect. The use of prothrombin complex concentrate has been studied to reverse the anticoagulant effects of the novel oral agents; however, there is very little data to support the practice.

Conclusion

Finally, this chapter summarizes the preoperative management of the facial cosmetic surgery patient. Knowledge of surgical anatomy, a systematic preoperative assessment, and a detailed surgical plan allow for optimal patient outcomes.

References

1. Sykes PJ. The origins and personalities of facial cosmetic surgery. Ann Plast Surg. 2010;65(2):118–22.
2. Karimi K, Adamson P. Patient analysis and selection in aging face surgery. Facial Plast Surg. 2011;27(1):5–15. Web
3. Fedok F. Advances in minimally invasive facial rejuvenation. Curr Opin Otolaryngol Head Neck Surg. 2008;16(4):359–68.
4. Jo C, Bagheri SC. Facial cosmetic surgery. Clin Rev Oral Maxillofac Surg. 2008;303–34. Web.
5. Sykes JM. Patient selection in facial plastic surgery. Facial Plast Surg Clin North Am. 2008;16(2):173–6. Web
6. Kosowski TR, Mccarthy C, Reavey PL, Scott AM, Wilkins EG, Cano SJ, Klassen AF, Carr N, Cordeiro PG, Pusic AL. A systematic review of patient-reported outcome measures after facial cosmetic surgery and/or nonsurgical facial rejuvenation. Plast Reconstr Surg. 2009;123(6):1819–27. Web
7. Ghali GE, Lustig JH. Complications associated with facial cosmetic surgery. Oral Maxillofac Surg Clin North Am. 2003;15(2):265–83. Web
8. Ferneini E, Gady J, Nuveen E. Complications associated with facial soft-tissue fillers. Am J Cosmet Surg. 2014;31(4):238–42. Web
9. Ghali GE, Harris CM. Cosmetic surgery considerations in the female patient. Oral Maxillofac Surg Clin North Am. 2007;19(2):235–44. Web
10. Willett JM. Facial plastic surgery. Stamford, CT: Appleton & Lange; 1997. Print
11. Truswell W. Surgical facial rejuvenation: a road map to safe and reliable outcomes. New York: Thieme Medical; 2009. Print
12. Frodel JL. Dealing with the difficult trauma and reconstructive surgery patient. Facial Plast Surg Clin North Am. 2008;16(2):225–31. Web
13. Meningaud J-P, Benadiba L, Servant J-M, Herve C, Bertrand J-C, Pelicier Y. Depression, anxiety and quality of life: outcome 9 months after facial cosmetic surgery. J Cranio-Maxillofac Surg. 2003;31(1):46–50. Web
14. Chatham D. Avoiding and correcting complications in facial plastic surgery: patient selection. Facial Plast Surg. 2012;28(3):253–9. Web
15. Zimbler MS, Ham J. Aesthetic facial analysis. In: Cummings head and neck surgery. St. Louis: Mosby; 2015.
16. Devcic Z, Rayikanti BA, Hevia JP, Popenko NA, Karimi K, Wong BJF. Nasal tip projection and facial attractiveness. Laryngoscope. 2011;121(7):1388–94. Web
17. Niamtu J. Complications in facelift surgery and their prevention. Oral Maxillofac Surg Clin North Am. 2009;21(1):59–80. Web
18. Riefkohl R, Wolfe JA, Cox EB, Mccarty KS. Association between cutaneous occlusive vascular disease, cigarette smoking, and skin slough after Rhytidectomy. Plast Reconstr Surg. 1986;77(4):592–5. Web
19. Pluvy L, Panouillères M, Garrido I, Pauchot J, Saboye J, Chavoin JP, Tropet Y, Grolleau JL, Chaput B. Smoking and plastic surgery, part II. Clinical implications: a systematic review with meta-analysis. Ann Chir Plast Esthet. 2015;60(1):e15–49.
20. Turan A, Mascha EJ, Roberman D, Turner PL, You J, Kurz A, Sessler DI, Saager L. Smoking and perioperative outcomes. Anesthesiology. 2011;114(4):837–46. Web
21. Rees TD, Liverett DM, Guy CL. The effect of cigarette smoking on skin-flap survival in the face lift patient. Plast Reconstr Surg. 1984;73(6):911–5. Web
22. Grover R, Jones BM, Waterhouse N. The prevention of haematoma following Rhytidectomy: a review of 1078 consecutive facelifts. Br J Plast Surg. 2001;54(6):481–6. Web
23. Alcalay J. Cutaneous surgery in patients receiving warfarin therapy. Dermatol Surg. 2001;27(8):756–8. Web
24. Munson CF, Reid AJ. Novel oral anticoagulants in plastic surgery. J Plast Reconstr Aesthet Surg. 2016;69(5):585–93. Web

35 Peri-operative Management of the Orthognathic Surgery Patient

Christian A. Moore and Bernard J. Costello

Abstract

Orthognathic surgery exists as one of the cornerstones for correcting dentofacial deformities. While these surgical procedures are reliable and safe, proper preoperative evaluation is essential for optimal patient outcomes. Surgical planning and data collection have evolved to provide more optimal patient care with the adoption of virtual surgical planning. Proper patient management requires intense attention to detail during preoperative evaluation and planning, as well as an in-depth understanding of anatomy and physiology both intraoperatively and postoperatively in order to prevent any potential complications.

35.1 Introduction

Orthognathic surgery has been performed since the early 1900s but has become significantly more refined with rigid fixation and more recently, virtual surgical planning. Pioneers like Obwegeser and Bell more clearly defined and improved techniques that have expanded the realm of possibility from a surgical standpoint. Many others have created modifications and improvements to expand the versatility and applicability of orthognathic surgery procedures, but many of the same principles of perioperative planning and management remain.

Treatment of facial disproportion and dental misalignment through the combination of orthodontic and surgical approaches can confer striking changes both aesthetically and functionally. A complete understanding of the patient's motivations for pursuing surgery must be understood, and patient expectations must be managed appropriately. An understanding of the limitations of different techniques is essential to achieving desired outcomes. Presurgical planning is generally a long process, but the long-term

C.A. Moore, D.M.D., M.D (✉)
Department of Oral and Maxillofacial Surgery, University of Pittsburgh, Pittsburgh, PA, USA
e-mail: mooreca3@upmc.edu

B.J. Costello, D.M.D., M.D., F.A.C.S.
Faculty Affairs, University of Pittsburgh School of Dental Medicine, Pittsburgh, PA, USA

Department of Oral and Maxillofacial Surgery, University of Pittsburgh, Pittsburgh, PA, USA

Department of Otolaryngology, University of Pittsburgh, Pittsburgh, PA, USA
e-mail: bjc1@pitt.edu; costbj@upmc.edu

© Springer International Publishing AG 2018
E.M. Ferneini, J.D. Bennett (eds.), *Perioperative Assessment of the Maxillofacial Surgery Patient*,
https://doi.org/10.1007/978-3-319-58868-1_35

outcomes particularly from a psychosocial standpoint can be dramatic [1]. Orthognathic surgery also has a role in the management of obstructive sleep apnea (OSA), a problem estimated to impact between 27 and 43% of women and men in this country, respectively [2]. When properly planned and executed, skeletal manipulation can effectively improve sleep quality and quality of life for patients with a potentially life-threatening disease process [3]. These patients, however, present a unique perioperative management challenge.

The most important principles in preoperative planning for orthognathic surgery are obtaining a proper preoperative diagnosis and the development of a tailored approach to every patient. A thorough medical and surgical history and physical exam are important to patient health and safety. Preoperative workup should be performed in a similar fashion for each patient and should assess all aspects of dental and skeletal deformity in a uniform, routine way. It is important, however, to address the patient's aesthetic concerns in order to develop a reasonable plan that achieves the goals of both the patient and the surgeon. Virtual surgical planning has further revolutionized the preoperative planning, allowing three-dimensional manipulation of jaw and dental segments and decreasing sources of error inherent in the more traditional model surgery approach.

This section will address the perioperative assessment of the orthognathic surgical patient including the process of virtual surgical planning. Despite proper planning, difficulties can occur during orthognathic surgical procedures. While a large body of literature exists on the technical aspects of performing orthognathic surgery, this chapter will discuss the preoperative evaluation and treatment of orthognathic surgery patients in the perioperative setting. It will also address the role of VSP in surgical planning. It will also address the perioperative surgical management of the OSA patient.

35.2 Orthognathic Surgery: The Preoperative Examination

The preoperative examination should first be focused on the problems perceived by the patient. Classical studies have shown that most patients who seek surgical treatment are motivated by aesthetics [4], but more recent studies indicate that the majority of patients actually seek improved occlusion and masticatory function [5]. Addressing the aesthetic and/or functional concerns should be the primary goal of the surgeon.

Because orthognathic surgery can reliably improve facial proportion and aesthetics, surgeons should be cautious of patients that show signs of body dysmorphic disorder (BDD). BDD is a condition estimated to have a prevalence of 1–2% in the US population [6], and performing surgery may not be appropriate. While orthognathic surgery can be aesthetically beneficial to many patients, understanding surgical limitations is crucial. Predicting and managing patients' expectations can better help the surgeon plan appropriate surgical intervention.

The physical exam should be completed but with the majority of its focus on the head and neck to help formulate a surgical plan. Besides the typical data collected on exam that relates to the reconstructive procedures, a number of other areas will be helpful in assessing patients for this type of surgery that have a less direct relationship to surgical outcome. A thorough head and neck exam will be helpful in planning the patient's anesthetic. Facial asymmetry, TMJ range of motion, neck mobility, and thyromental distance are important to help assess the potential difficulty of endotracheal intubation. Often, signs of systemic illness can be present on head and neck exam. A patient with glossitis or conjunctival pallor should prompt the surgeon to investigate the possibility of anemia. Scleral icterus and jaundice of the buccal mucosa are often some of the first signs of hepatic dysfunction. The patient's neck thickness and respiratory patterns can be signals of obstructive sleep apnea or pulmonary disease processes. Endocrinopathies, though rare, can precipitate anesthetic complexities. If any suspicion exists for diabetes, adrenal insufficiency, or thyroid disorder, care may be provided in consultation with the patient's primary care physicians or specialists. Other disorders, such as immunodeficiency or blood dyscrasias, may have a direct impact on the surgical procedures themselves or the potential healing after the procedures.

A dedicated TMJ exam should be performed prior to undertaking orthognathic surgery. Many patients will present citing temporomandibular joint, pain in the muscles of mastication, or head and neck pain symptoms as a reason for seeking surgery. It is possible that orthognathic surgery could provide some relief of temporomandibular joint symptoms, but most of the data is conflicting and does not have a clear cause and effect relationship. As such, in the authors' opinion, there is no predictive evidence that orthognathic surgical procedures improve symptoms [7].

Recently, an increased focus on the perioperative outcomes of obstructive sleep apnea (OSA) patients has become the focus of a large body of interest [8]. While these patients may be presenting for surgical consultation as a result of failed other treatments, current recommendations support the proper identification of these patients as they are at higher risk of perioperative complications. Though there is not currently evidence to support the delay of surgeries as a result of diagnosed or suspected OSA, screening questionnaires in the preoperative appointment may prompt referral to primary care providers for workup of comorbid conditions such as obesity hypoventilation syndrome, pulmonary hypertension, and resting hypoxemia. At times, a number of additive comorbidities such as symptoms of airway obstruction, obesity, polydipsia, and polyuria in a patient without proper routine medical evaluations may prompt the need for a more extensive workup. Thorough preoperative evaluations with appropriate triggers can help prevent adverse outcomes by coming up with appropriate risk stratification of patients with potential comorbidities.

35.3 Permissive Hypotension in Orthognathic Surgery

Hypotensive anesthesia, first introduced by Schaberg in 1976 [9], is a well-established hemostatic strategy in maxillofacial surgery [10–12], and preoperative assessment should address whether the patient is able to tolerate this permissive hypotension. Blood pressure goals, especially during certain portions of craniofacial osteotomies such as maxillary downfracture, should include a mean arterial pressure (MAP) 30% less than the patient's usual MAP with a minimum goal of 50 mmHg in healthy patients that can tolerate this change without affecting perfusion pressures significantly [13]. Additionally, the systolic blood pressure is held to less than 100 mmHg if possible. A number of studies [10, 14] have reported up to 45% reduction in intraoperative blood loss when effective hypotensive anesthesia is implemented.

Significant intraoperative blood loss which is not easily controlled by surgical maneuvers can occur during orthognathic surgery. Due to the rich vascularity of the head and neck and the relative inaccessibility of certain vessels in the associated area, surgical bleeds can be brisk, and hemoglobin levels can reach transfusion thresholds relatively quickly if blood loss is not easily controlled. Studies have shown reduced blood loss when utilizing permissive hypotension [15, 16], and recent trauma studies indicate that permissive hypotension may be an effective method of resuscitating patients while controlling blood loss [17, 18]. Anesthesiologists and anesthetists that may be unfamiliar with these techniques may have concerns utilizing hypotensive anesthesia due to the risk of hypoperfusion of vital organs [19–22].

Various targets for intraoperative mean arterial pressure (MAP) have been proposed, but the patient's age, general health status, and preexisting medical comorbidities must be taken into consideration [10, 23–25]. The normal range of cerebral autoregulation exists at cerebral perfusion pressures between 50 and 150 mmHg [26], and the protective autoregulatory response is lost when MAPs deviate significantly from this range (Fig. 35.1).

Though the definition of "elderly" is vague, a MAP of 80 mmHg is considered to be a safe, effective blood pressure goal for older patients [27], and this data seems to be supported by recent trauma literature suggesting that permissive hypotension appears to be a potential management strategy in elderly trauma patients [28].

Potential complications of hypotensive anesthesia include cerebral, cardiovascular, renal, hepatic, and dermatologic effects and are related to hypoperfusion injury. Cerebral damage and neurological deficit [23, 29], stroke [30], dysrhythmia [31], and cardiac arrest [32] have all been reported as complications of deliberate hypotension. Though urine output has been shown to decrease during deliberate hypotension, it quickly returns to normal at the cessation of anesthesia [33, 34]. These studies also suggest that perioperative creatinine levels respond unpredictably. Hepatic impairment from induced hypotension is rare and appears to be minimal and transient [35]. Skin necrosis of the nasal tip [36] as well as alopecia [37] have been reported following vascular interruption though these complications tend to be more related to pressure necrosis than systemic hypoperfusion injury. Conceivably these complications could be induced by prolonged hypotension, and care should be exercised to ensure that adequate padding and positioning are utilized to prevent unnecessary pressure on the face, head, and other pressure areas.

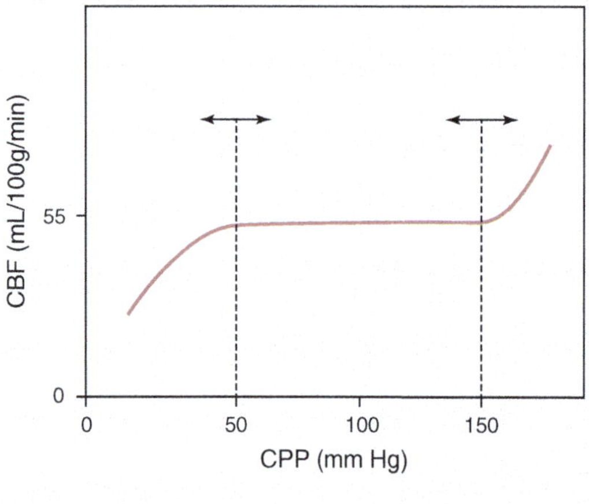

Fig. 35.1 Classic cerebral autoregulation curve. Cerebral autoregulation maintains a relatively constant rate of cerebral blood flow (CBF) across a wide range of cerebral perfusion pressure (CPP), as shown (plateau). The normal pressure limits of autoregulation (*vertical broken lines*) may be shifted to the left or right in certain conditions (*arrows*) and impaired or abolished in others (see text for details). Note the respective relatively steep rise and fall in CBF as CPP changes above and below the normal limits of autoregulation. Reprinted with permission from: Burrows, Anthony M.; Brown, Desmond A.; Klaas, James P.; Khurana, Vini G.; Benarroch, Eduardo E.; Meyer, Fredric B.. Published January 1, 2017. Pages 3012–3039. e11 © 2017

When utilizing hypotensive anesthetic techniques, continuous monitoring of vital signs must be performed throughout the procedure. Standard monitoring in the form of pulse oximetry, EKG, blood pressure, end tidal CO_2, temperature, and urine output should be utilized to assess patient status. Continuous blood pressure monitoring in the form of an arterial line is a safe and effective method of monitoring hypotension and eliminates the concern over the intermittent nature of noninvasive blood pressure monitoring. Arterial access also facilitates easy access for arterial blood gas analysis if complications arise. In older or more medically compromised patients, this monitoring should be utilized. Most orthognathic surgery patients are young, healthy individuals capable of tolerating longer periods of deliberate hypotension, and thus, hypotensive anesthesia is considered to be an effective procedure for orthognathic procedures [12]. Patients with a history of cardiovascular disease, hypertension, or other disorders that do not tolerate altered blood pressure are not typically candidates for this technique. As such blood products may be a consideration as the risk for volume loss and bleeding may be increased.

35.4 Virtual Surgical Planning

With the progress that has been made in advanced imaging and computer-aided surgery, we have improved the accuracy and efficiency of orthognathic surgery in terms of preoperative planning and intraoperative management. In addition to more efficient workup and decreased potential sources of error in treatment planning, virtual surgical planning (VSP) also provides other benefits. CT scanning allows the surgeon to visualize anatomic structures such as the inferior alveolar nerve and enables osteotomies to be planned that avoid these structures. Cutting jigs and custom fixation can be fabricated for increased precision and a decreased operative time. Custom printed cutting guides in conjunction with custom plating have provided the opportunity for "splintless" surgery in some applications. In addition, the CT reconstruction allows the surgeon to interact with the entire facial skeleton in three dimensions to gain a better appreciation for the implications of seemingly minute changes in the maxillomandibular complex. This improves the fit of bony segments and often decreases the need for extensive mitering prior to fixation. A better appreciation of the effect of three-dimensional repositioning of segments also improves the ability to judge improvements in symmetry in complex cases. Though the final surgical outcome still requires accurate and meticulous technique, VSP affords the surgeon the opportunity to create a precise surgical plan and has tremendous benefit when visualizing treatment planning complex movements.

The data collection process for VSP is very similar to that of traditional model-based surgical planning. As in traditional orthognathic planning, establishing a reproducible bite in centric relation is essential for surgical success and can be achieved with the aid of a wax bite registration. For planning purposes, a radiopaque marker is imbedded within the palatal portion of this bite registration. Because lip position plays such a large role in facial analysis, any excess wax must be trimmed from the labial and buccal aspects to prevent any lip posturing and any distortion of the facial soft tissue.

Once the patient's occlusion has been recorded, the patient's natural head position must next be established. This can be difficult but can often be achieved by having the patient pick a spot at eye level in front of them at a distance of 10–15 ft away. Photographs should be taken with the patient in this position that demonstrate the patient in repose and full smile from the frontal and lateral views which will be used during the VSP session to properly orient the scanned images [38].

Once the natural head position is established, the patient's head position is adjusted; markers are placed on the face to help further delineate the horizontal and vertical reference lines. These lines are established with the aid of a laser level and are helpful in cases of asymmetry. In the method used by the authors, the fiducial markers are placed at approximately the nasofrontal junction, menton, and the locations of the infraorbital nerves bilaterally. Establishing these points in the natural head position aids in positioning the patient's scan for virtual planning.

Soft tissue analysis of the face and head must be performed from an anterior and lateral view. Though cephalometric norms are used for treatment planning, each patient must be treated on an individual basis, and treatment is not wholly based on narrow views of limited numerical data. It is possible that patients could have cephalometric analysis that falls within the normal range but could still have large discrepancies causing poor occlusion and facial profile [39]. Ultimately, the changes orthognathic procedures produce are a result of changing the bony support of the facial soft tissues, and a judgment is made based on the expected draping of those soft tissues.

A medical grade or cone-beam CT scan of the patient's maxillofacial skeleton is next obtained with the patient's CR bite registration in place. Due to beam scatter from orthodontic appliances and restorations, CT imaging of the teeth and occlusal relationships is not accurate enough for planning purposes. One solution is to obtain die stone models of the patient's upper and lower arches and scan them with a cone-beam CT. Individual models of the upper and lower arches as well as the arches in occlusion are scanned, and this data is merged with CT data from the patient to create digital imaging and communication in medicine (DICOM) images of the patient's skeletal structure which is used to plan osteotomies and movement of bony segments.

Intraoral scanners are increasingly being adopted by dentists for obtaining digital impressions for crown and bridge restorations and for orthodontics. Surgeons are beginning to investigate this technology to obtain digital dental models to merge with CT data to provide accurate representation for virtual treatment planning [40]. Though data suggest that intraoral scanners produce an accurate representation of the dental arches and occlusion, more substantial studies are still needed to validate this method of data collection.

Once scanning data is obtained, it is then used to combine data sets with the CT imaging and render a complete merged image that can be manipulated virtually with the planned osteotomies. Two to three weeks prior to the scheduled surgery date, the final surgical plan is developed remotely via teleconference with the aid of biomedical engineers who can manipulate the images of the skeleton to precisely define the locations of osteotomies and planned skeletal movements.

One of the most useful aspects of virtual surgical planning is the ability to confirm the accuracy of data collection prior to the time of surgery. A key early step in virtual planning is confirmation of the accuracy of the merged CT scan and scanned dental images, ensuring that occlusal relationships, condylar position, midlines, and head position accurately reflect the patient. Next, maxillary osteotomies are simulated, and the treatment of any cant or midline issues is addressed. Anteroposterior and vertical changes in the position of the maxilla should be based on central incisor position [41]. The intermediate surgical splint can be generated once all maxillary movements are planned.

Once the final plan is established, occlusal splints are fabricated as well as osteotomy cutting guides if desired (Fig. 35.2).

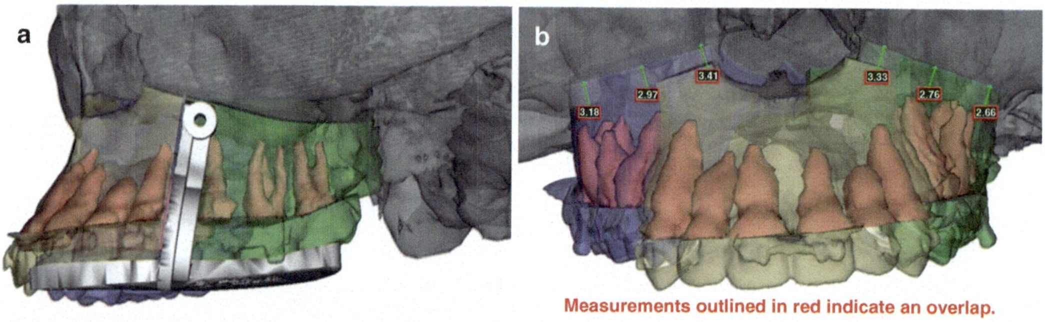

c

Point	Name	Anterior/Posterior	Left/Right	Up/Down
ANS	Anterior Nasal Spine	3.06mm Anterior	1.53mm Right	0.23mm Up
A	A Point	2.73mm Anterior	1.26mm Right	0.23mm Up
ISU1	Midline of Upper Incisor	2.02mm Anterior	0.59mm Right	0.00
U3L	Upper Left Canine	1.90mm Anterior	0.70mm Right	0.96mm Up
U6L	Upper Left Anterior Molar (mesiobuccal cusp)	1.63mm Anterior	0.43mm Right	3.27mm Up
U3R	Upper Right Canine	2.16mm Anterior	0.67mm Right	0.22mm Down
U6R	Upper Right Anterior Molar (mesiobuccal cusp)	2.21mm Anterior	0.68mm Right	3.64mm Up
ISL1	Midline of Lower Incisor	3.02mm Anterior	0.21mm Right	5.26mm Up
L6L	Upper Left Anterior Molar (mesiobuccal cusp)	2.74mm Anterior	0.14mm Right	3.58mm Up
L6R	Upper Right Anterior Molar (mesiobuccal cusp)	2.72mm Anterior	0.13mm Right	3.44mm Up
B	B Point	4.26mm Anterior	0.17mm Right	4.42mm Up
Pog.	Pogonion	5.28mm Anterior	0.17mm Right	4.40mm Up

Fig. 35.2 Generated surgical plan. (**a**) Simulated cutting guide for interdental osteotomy. (**b**) Simulated differential multi-piece maxillary impaction with cant and midline correction. (**c**) Planned surgical movements. Photo credit: Dr. Bernard J. Costello D.M.D., M.D

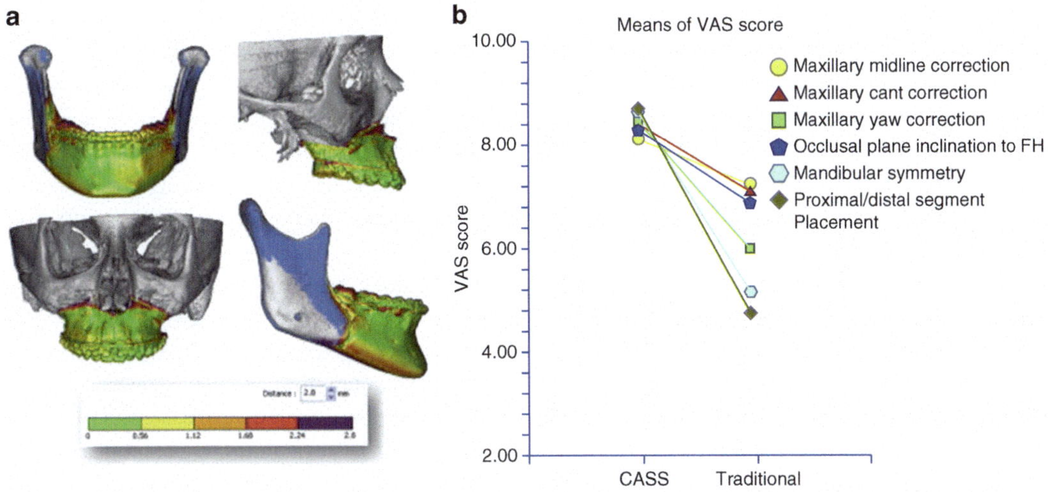

Fig. 35.3 (**a**) Superimposition of the CASS to postoperative CT scan via fixed reference points has been used to quantify the accuracy of the repositioned maxilla and mandible. (**b**) Improved outcomes for CASS compared with traditional model surgery. Reprinted with permission from Xia JJ, Shevchenko L, Gateno J, et al. Outcome study of computer-aided surgical simulation in the treatment of patients with craniomaxillofacial deformities. J Oral Maxillofac Surg 2011;69(7):2014–24

Full size replicas of the patient's skeleton can also be fabricated. These models are helpful both for the surgeon to identify anatomical boundaries and for helping the patient to understand the procedure. A detailed, precise list of planned movements is also generated by the software, effectively replacing the arduous task of planning complex movements using stone casts and model block measurements.

A benefit of this process is that treatment planning is often performed through teleconference, enabling the surgeon, orthodontist, and virtual technician to collaborate in the planning from any location with internet capabilities. More importantly, manipulation of the digital images allows the surgeon to assess the effects of movements of the maxillomandibular complex in relation to other structures of the maxillofacial skeleton. CASS can also help identify the need for potential endonasal surgery at the time of orthognathic surgery, such as turbinate reduction. Similarly, simulated mandibular movements can help the surgeon determine the degree of chin projection.

VSP is fast becoming a standard of care for orthognathic surgical treatment planning, especially in complicated cases of facial asymmetry [43]. Outcome studies have shown that VSP is able to achieve favorable, accurate results when compared with traditional model surgery [42–45] and can be helpful in visualizing a surgical plan (Fig. 35.3).

Utilizing this technique affords a more streamlined preoperative workup and more completely allows the surgeons to see the skeletal implications of movements of the maxillomandibular complex. VSP also allows the surgeon to proceed to the operating room with confidence in their surgical plan and the ability to anticipate and plan for potential intraoperative difficulties.

35.5 Surgical and Perioperative Management Challenges

Though orthognathic surgery is generally accepted to be the standard of care for management of dentofacial deformities, the procedure is not without complications. Short-term procedural and medical complication rates have been quoted at 5.4% nationally [46]. Preoperative evaluation should identify any medical comorbidities that increase the risk of complications, and attention must be paid to meticulous surgical technique to decrease the likelihood of surgical complications.

Delayed hemorrhage after maxillary surgery has been reported to occur anywhere from postoperative day zero through nine [47]. Maxillary impaction often involves the need for inferior turbinectomy which necessitates violating the nasal mucosa. Postoperative nasal bleeds are common after maxillary surgery, especially when concomitant endonasal surgery is performed. These bleeds, however, should be small volume, self-limited, and unilateral. They often respond to pressure and/or anterior packing. The presence of a high-volume bilateral bleed is much more concerning for large vessel injury and should be evaluated as quickly as possible.

The vessels most commonly implicated are the internal maxillary and descending palatine arteries, as well as the pterygoid venous plexus. If maxillomandibular fixation is present, it should be removed immediately. Provided that the patient is hemodynamically stable, immediate interventions include suction, visualization, local anesthetic (with vasoconstrictor) injection, and both anterior and posterior nasal packing. If the bleed is minor, these interventions along with bed rest for 3–5 days will likely be enough to stop the bleed. If bleeding is refractory to these interventions, endoscopic evaluation, surgical reexploration, or possible angiogram and embolization may be necessary. As with acute intraoperative bleeds, carotid ligation may be necessary in emergencies.

Post-extubation laryngospasm is a concern for all patients and is one of the most common causes of airway obstruction [48]. Management of post-extubation laryngospasm or obstruction may begin by providing airway support, supplemental oxygen, and positive pressure ventilation through bag-mask ventilation. This may be a difficult task in orthognathic surgery patients. Though not commonly used for orthognathic surgery, maxillomandibular fixation could interfere with airway management, and the more commonly utilized rigid internal fixation could become dislodged or fail secondary to airway management techniques. Hardware dislodgement is of secondary importance to the airway stability but may require further surgical procedures after the patient is stabilized.

If positive pressure ventilation is unable to break the laryngospasm, a paralytic is administered either intravenously or intramuscularly to allow the laryngeal muscles to relax and the spasm to break. During the period when the patient is paralyzed, airway management should be maintained either with bag-mask ventilation or placement of an airway device such as an LMA. Positive-pressure breaths through a facial mask could potentially introduce air and subcutaneous emphysema in orthognathic surgery patients, so supraglottic airway devices may be preferred in this situation.

Following laryngospasm, a potential complication is negative pressure pulmonary edema (NPPE). NPPE occurs in the setting of markedly negative intrathoracic pressure following an inspiratory effort against a closed or obstructed glottis. Muscular young males are predisposed to this condition [49] due to their ability to generate high intrathoracic pressure [50]. Signs of NPPE include pink, frothy sputum, bibasilar crackles on lung auscultation, and bilateral hazy interstitial opacity on chest x-ray. It is important to recognize the clinical signs and treat this condition quickly and aggressively. Any secretions should be suctioned from the patient's oropharynx, and the patient may need to be re-intubated to institute positive pressure ventilation. Occasionally re-intubation can be difficult so the provider should be prepared to perform an emergent cricothyroidotomy, tracheostomy, jet ventilation, or other support techniques.

After the airway is secured and positive pressure ventilation is instituted, pulmonary edema usually resolves in 24–48 h [51]. Lung-protective ventilation strategies such as maintaining low tidal volumes and plateau pressures help in decreasing the degree of acute insult to the lungs [52]. Diuretics may also be necessary to facilitate the off-loading of the transudated pulmonary fluid.

The use of corticosteroids in surgical patients is widely advocated for their ability to reduce swelling, pain, and postoperative nausea and vomiting (PONV). No major morbidity or impact has been clearly demonstrated with the use of steroids following single low-dose usage [53] which is why dexamethasone is used widely as prophylaxis for PONV. Long-term use of steroids, however, has been associated with adverse effects such as hyperglycemia, wound infections, delayed wound healing, gastric ulcers, and avascular necrosis [54–56]. Short-term corticosteroid use in orthognathic surgery has been shown to decrease postoperative analgesic and antiemetic use and appears to be a safe, effective practice [57]. Numerous studies have demonstrated a benefit to preoperative steroid administration, but there is little evidence to support an ideal therapeutic postoperative dose or dosing regimen. Intravenous doses of methylprednisolone greater than or equal to 85 mg appear to produce a significant decrease in edema [58]. Similarly, prednisolone has been shown to improve recovery of neurosensory impairment following orthognathic surgery [59] and betamethasone treatment regimens appear to be effective in decreasing edema and pain [60].

Antibiotic prophylaxis for prevention of surgical site infection in orthognathic surgery has been shown to be beneficial in decreasing operative site morbidity in orthognathic surgery [61]. The exact antibiotic choice and whether subsequent postoperative doses of antibiotic are warranted, however, is less clear. The surgical site in orthognathic surgery is considered "clean contaminated" and has a potential infection rate as high as 10–15% [62]. In the present era of resistant organisms, it is imperative that antibiotics be chosen practically. Additionally, the risk of side effects such as allergy and toxic reactions further supports limiting antibiotic use to only that which is necessary. Coverage should include gram-positive and anaerobic organisms; gram-negative coverage is less clear. Literature looking at head and neck surgery supports the use of ampicillin or clindamycin as appropriate antibiotic choices [63]. The duration of treatment remains vague but data favors long-term (greater than 24 h) antibiotic coverage after orthognathic procedures [64].

The nonsteroidal anti-inflammatory drug ketorolac is a frequently utilized adjunctive analgesic used in the management of postoperative pain. Unfortunately, despite its analgesic effect, the use of ketorolac is associated with increased risk of postoperative hemorrhage [65]. Ketorolac is also associated with a transient reduction in renal function [66], and with the fluid restriction and intraoperative hypotension often utilized during orthognathic surgery, a theoretical risk of renal failure exists. More recent data specifically suggest that the use of ketorolac is associated with increased risk of bleeding after tonsillectomy in adults [67] and possibly in children as well [68]. No specific data regarding ketorolac use in orthognathic surgery exists, but because of the close anatomic proximity of surgical sites, this data could conceivably be extrapolated to orthognathic surgery as well. Small studies indicate that diclofenac is an effective agent for controlling postoperative pain [69, 70] though bleeding complications where not specifically addressed. Unfortunately, strong evidence does not exist to conclusively support or refute the use of NSAIDs for management of postoperative pain following orthognathic surgery, but the theoretical risk of postoperative hemorrhage and renal dysfunction may be sufficient to preclude their use. Intravenous acetaminophen can also be a suitable substitute in some patients.

35.6 Orthognathic Surgery as a Treatment for Obstructive Sleep Apnea

As mentioned previously, it is important to get a proper history from patients seeking orthognathic surgery for OSA. Typically, elective orthognathic surgery is performed on healthy patients, and orthognathic surgery is deferred in patients with a physical status of III or greater. Many sleep apnea patients carry other diagnoses, and it is important to address and optimize these conditions prior to undergoing any operation. In general, OSA patients are older, have more comorbidities, and experience more complications than patients having orthognathic surgery for dentofacial deformities, often at a younger age [71].

The pathophysiology of OSA largely relates to inspiratory airway pressures that overwhelm muscular forces opposing airway collapse. The genioglossus muscle is activated at the same time as the inspiratory muscles of respiration to maintain patency of the airway, and in OSA patients, the activation of this muscle is depressed [72]. Loss of airway tone leads to episodes of apnea and hypopnea, and the severity of OSA is graded based on the number of these episodes occurring per hour of sleep. OSA is considered mild if the AHI is in the 5–15 range, moderate if between 15 and 30, and severe if over 30 [73]. The intermittent hypoxia and frequent nighttime arousals increase systemic sympathetic activation and oxidative stress which is thought to contribute to development of endothelial dysfunction, increased platelet aggregation, coronary artery disease, heart failure, stroke, and metabolic syndrome [74]. Hypoxia is also known to cause pulmonary vascular remodeling ultimately resulting in pulmonary hypertension and right ventricular hypertrophy [75].

Identification of these patients can help guide postoperative management [3]. Benzodiazepines and other respiratory depressants should be avoided in the perioperative period due to their propensity toward sedation and impaired airway function. After surgery, OSA patients should receive supplemental oxygen titrated to achieve an O_2 saturation the same as the patient's preoperative room air baseline. Positive airway pressure using noninvasive ventilation can be problematic in patients who have undergone orthognathic surgery. Air emphysema can occur if the device forces air into the surrounding tissues through fresh incisions. This can vary based upon the type of device used and the exact location of the incisions.

Monitoring should be determined on a case by case basis and should be decided based on the degree of oxygen supplementation required. The amount of opioid medication needed for adequate analgesia is a careful consideration. Generally, decreased amounts of opioids are preferred, and other medications that do not depress respiration are typically better choices in the setting of surgery involving the upper airway. Most patients who undergo orthognathic surgery will have anesthesia or dense paresthesia which, while uncomfortable, aides in pain control. Adjunct non-opioid medications such as dexmedetomidine, acetaminophen, long-lasting local anesthetics, and occasionally NSAIDs can all be effective in a multimodal analgesic strategy. Pregabalin and gabapentin have also been suggested as possible adjunctive pain medications but do carry a risk of sedation [76].

While considerably rare, patients with OSA are also predisposed to aspiration, ARDS, pulmonary embolism, arrhythmias, myocardial infarction, delirium, unplanned ICU admissions, and prolonged hospitalizations [39]. Because of this increased risk, it may be prudent to consider admission to an ICU for at least the first postoperative night for close monitoring. OSA appears to worsen after surgery starting from the first postoperative night and peaking between postoperative nights three and four [77]. Fluid and electrolyte balance should be managed actively in these patients. OSA patients are more prone to a process known as rostral fluid redistribution further increasing the risk of airway edema and obstruction [78]. Airway remodeling is a slow process, and with edema, recent surgical insult, and possible sedative effects of pain medications, these patients are at increased risk of postoperative complications. In patients with a higher risk for pulmonary and/or obstructive complications, it may also be advantageous to perform an elective tracheostomy prior maxillomandibular advancement to help ensure a secure airway in the postoperative period.

On examination, these patients may show good facial proportion, which is considerably different than those who undergo orthognathic surgery for growth discrepancies and malocclusions. Maxillomandibular advancement should be carefully planned in order to optimize aesthetics, prevent excessive incisor show and excessive protrusion of the lower facial third. Patients that are obese and have a thick soft tissue drape can tolerate larger movements with less noticeable effects on overall aesthetics.

Imaging in these patients may demonstrate decreased upper airway space on lateral cephalogram or CT, but it is important to remember that these imaging modalities are static; they are performed on awake patients with adequate airway tone and are not always captured in the supine position. A predictor of OSA is the mandibular plane to hyoid (MPH) distance as measured on lateral cephalometric radiographs. The tip of the hyoid bone is considered the end of the upper airway. And the distance from the mandibular plane to the tip of the hyoid effectively is a measure of the distance of the upper airway. Patients with OSA often have a lower-set hyoid bone which may contribute to soft tissue laxity and collapse [79]. Observed apnea and/or hypopnea episodes on polysomnography are the current gold standard for diagnosis of OSA [80]. Patients who are likely to benefit from maxillomandibular advancement as opposed to soft tissue surgery are those with true anteroposterior collapse of the airway and decreased airway space. This collapse is often able to be visualized on sleep endoscopy. Additional functional assessment of the airway via drug-induced sleep endoscopy (DISE) can also be helpful for diagnosis, airway phenotyping, and surgical treatment planning [81]. Customizing the surgical treatment plan based on the locations of airway obstruction can allow the team to target the etiology more effectively.

Orthognathic surgery for patients with OSA has undergone significant philosophical change over the past 20 years. Current research is focusing on the patient phenotype most likely to benefit from orthognathic surgery versus other surgical options. Alternatives to maxillomandibular advancement primarily involve soft tissue rather than bony surgery and include UPPP, hyoid suspension, epiglottoplasty, and more recently, implantation of a hypoglossal nerve stimulator. These soft tissue techniques were traditionally unreliable cures of the disease process, but newer implantable neurostimulation devices have been shown to be very effective in clinical trials [82].

Conclusions

Orthognathic surgery is a reliable way of producing dramatic improvements in facial proportion and occlusion but is not without risk. Bleeding, post-anesthetic complications, infection, swelling, and pain are all possible and must be anticipated. Orthognathic surgery for obstructive sleep apnea patients further increases the possibility of perioperative complications. Virtual surgical planning has revolutionized preoperative planning to streamline workup and improve efficiency and outcomes. Though orthognathic surgery has evolved since its inception, the central tenet remains that ideal outcomes are achieved with thorough and complete preoperative planning.

References

1. Soh CL, et al. Quality of life assessment in patients with dentofacial deformity undergoing orthognathic surgery—a systematic review. Int J Oral Maxillofac Surg. 2013;42:974–80.
2. Heinzer R, et al. Prevalence of sleep-disordered breathing in the general population: the HypnoLaus study. Lancet Respir Med. 2015;3:310–8.
3. Hsieh Y-J, Liao Y-F. Effects of maxillomandibular advancement on the upper airway and surrounding structures in patients with obstructive sleep apnoea: a systematic review. Br J Oral Maxillofac Surg. 2013;51:834–40.
4. Laufer D, Glick D, Gutman D, Sharon A. Patient motivation and response to surgical correction of prognathism. Oral Surg Oral Med Oral Pathol. 1976;41:309–13.
5. Proothi M, Drew SJ, Sachs SA. Motivating factors for patients undergoing orthognathic surgery evaluation. J Oral Maxillofac Surg. 2010;68:1555–9.
6. Chung KC, Pushman AG, Bellfi LT. A systematic review of ethical principles in the plastic surgery literature. Plast Reconstr Surg. 2009;124:1711–8.
7. Abrahamsson C, Ekberg EC, Henrikson T, Bondemark L. Alterations of temporomandibular disorders before and after orthognathic surgery. Angle Orthod. 2007;77:729–34.
8. Chung F, et al. Society of anesthesia and sleep medicine guideline on preoperative screening and assessment of patients with obstructive sleep apnea. Anesth Analg. 2016;123:452–73.
9. Schaberg SJ, Kelly JF, Terry BC, Posner MA, Anderson EF. Blood loss and hypotensive anesthesia in oral-facial corrective surgery. J Oral Surg. 1976;34(2):147–56.
10. Praveen K, et al. Hypotensive anaesthesia and blood loss in orthognathic surgery: a clinical study. Br J Oral Maxillofac Surg. 2001;39:138–40.
11. Chen CM, et al. Assessment of the related factors of blood loss and blood ingredients among patients under hypotensive anesthesia in orthognathic surgery. J Craniofac Surg. 2011;22:1594–7.
12. Choi WS, Samman N. Risks and benefits of deliberate hypotension in anaesthesia: a systematic review. Int J Oral Maxillofac Surg. 2008;37:687–703.
13. Rodrigo C. Induced hypotension during anesthesia with special reference to orthognathic surgery. Anesth Prog. 1995;42:41–58.

14. Shaberg SJ, Kelly JF, Terry BC, Posner MA, Anderson EF. Blood loss and hypotensive anesthesia in oral-facial corrective surgery. J Oral Surg. 1976;34:147–56.
15. Dolman RM, Bentley KC, Head TW, et al. The effect of hypotensive anesthesia on blood loss and operative time during Le Fort l osteotomies. J Oral Maxillofac Surg. 2000;58:834–9. [discussion 840]
16. Sollevi A. Hypotensive anesthesia and blood loss. Acta Anaesthesiol Scand Suppl. 1988;89:39–43.
17. Rodgrigues R, Carmona MJ, Junior JO. Bleeding and damage control surgery. Curr Opin Anaesthesiol. 2016;29:229–33.
18. Carrick MM, Leonard J, Slone DS, Mains CW, Bar-Or D. Hypotensive resuscitation among trauma patients. Biomed Res Int. 2016;2016:8901938., 8 Pages. https://doi.org/10.1155/2016/8901938.
19. Birch AA, Boyce WH. Changing renal blood flow following sodium nitroprusside in patients undergoing nephrolithotomy. Anesth Analg. 1977;56:102–9.
20. Nishimura S, Suzuki A, Hatazawa J, et al. Cerebral blood-flow responses to induced hypotension and to CO_2 inhalation in patients with major cerebral artery occlusive disease: a positron-emission tomography study. Neuroradiology. 1999;41:73–9.
21. Pasch T, Huk W. Cerebral complications following induced hypotension. Eur J Anaesthesiol. 1986;3:299–312.
22. Zayas VM, Blumenfeld JD, Bading B, et al. Adrenergic regulation of renin secretion and renal hemodynamics during deliberate hypotension in humans. Am J Phys. 1993;265:686–92.
23. Fromme GA, MacKenzie RA, Gould AB Jr, et al. Controlled hypotension for orthognathic surgery. Anesth Analg. 1986;65:683–6.
24. Ervens J, Marks C, Hechler M, et al. Effect of induced hypotensive anaesthesia vs isovolaemic haemodilution on blood loss and transfusion requirements in orthognathic surgery: a prospective, single-blinded, randomized, controlled clinical study. Int J Oral Maxillofac Surg. 2010;39:1168–74.
25. Kim NY, Yoo YC, Chun DH, et al. The effects of oral atenolol or enalapril premedication on blood loss and hypotensive anesthesia in orthognathic surgery. Yonsei Med J. 2015;56:1114–21.
26. Dagal A, Lam A. Cerebral autoregulation and anesthesia. Curr Opin Anaesthesiol. 2009;22:547–52.
27. Lin S, et al. Effects of hypotensive anesthesia on reducing intraoperative blood loss, duration of operation, and quality of surgical field during orthognathic surgery: a systematic review and meta-analysis of randomized controlled trials. J Oral Maxillofac Surg. 2017;75(1):73–86. https://doi.org/10.1016/j.joms.2016.07.012. pii: S0278-2391(16)30616-4, [Epub ahead of print]
28. Bridges LC, Waibel BH, Newell MA. Permissive hypotension: potentially harmful in the elderly? A national trauma data bank analysis. Am Surg. 2015;81:770–7.
29. Jones TH, Chiappa KH, et al. EEG monitoring for induced hypotension for surgery of intracranial aneurysms. Stroke. 1979;10(3):292–4.
30. Kim JS, Seok BK, Shin HE, et al. Perioperative stroke in the brain and spinal cord following an induced hypotension. Yonsei Med J. 2003;44:143–5.
31. Finegan BA, Clanachan AS. Clinical experience with adenosine for controlled hypotension during cerebral aneurysm surgery. Anesth Analg. 1987;66:229–34.
32. McLeod ME, et al. Anaesthetic management of arteriovenous malformations of the vein of Galen. Can Anaesth Soc J. 1982;29:307–12.
33. Goto F, Otani E, Kato S, Fujita T. Prostaglandin E1 as a hypotensive drug during general anaesthesia. Anaesthesia. 1982;37:530–5.
34. Toivonen J, Kaukinen S, Oikkonen M, Hannelin M. Effects of deliberate hypotension induced by labetalol on renal function. Eur J Anaesthesiol. 1991;8: 13–20.
35. Fukusaki M, et al. Effects of controlled hypotension with sevoflurane anaesthesia on hepatic function of surgical patients. Eur J Anaesthesiol. 1999;16:111–6.
36. Benvenuti D. Necrosis of the nasal tip. Plast Reconstr Surg. 1995;96:223–4.
37. Khalaf H, Negmi H, Hassan G, Al-Sebayel M. Postoperative alopecia areata: is pressure-induced ischemia the only cause to blame? Transplant Proc. 2004;36:2158–9.
38. Bobek SL, Farrell BB, Farrell BB, et al. Simplified protocol of virtual surgical planning for orthognathic surgery. J Oral Maxillofac Surg. 2012;70(9 Suppl 2):e68–9.
39. Garber DA, Salama H, Salama MA. Multidisciplinary cases: lessons learned. Paper presented at: 24th Annual Meeting of the American Academy of Esthetic Dentistry; Whistler, British Columbia, Canada, 6 Aug 1999.
40. De Waard O, et al. A novel method for fusion of intraoral scans and cone-beam computed tomography scans for orthognathic surgery planning. J Cranio-Maxillofac Surg. 2016;44:160–6.
41. Farrell B, Franco P, Tucker M. Virtual surgical planning in orthognathic surgery. Oral Maxillofac Surg Clin N Am. 2014;26:459–73.
42. Zhang N, et al. Accuracy of virtual surgical planning in two-jaw orthognathic surgery: comparison of planned and actual results. Oral Surg Oral Med Oral Pathol Oral Radiol. 2016;122:143–51.
43. Bobek S, et al. Virtual surgical planning for orthognathic surgery using digital data transfer and an intraoral fiducial marker: the Charlotte method. J Oral Maxillofac Surg. 2015;73:1143–58.
44. Xia J, Sheychenko L, Gateno J, et al. Outcome of computer-aided surgical simulation in the treatment of patient with craniomaxillofacial deformities. J Oral Maxillofac Surg. 2011;69:2014–24.
45. Hsu S, Gateno J, Bell R, et al. Accuracy of a computer-aided surgical simulation protocol for orthognathic surgery: a prospective multicenter study. J Oral Maxillofac Surg. 2013;71:128–42.

46. Berlin NL, Tuggle CT, Steinbacher DM. Improved short-term outcomes following orthognathic surgery are associated with high-volume centers. Plast Reconstr Surg. 2016;138:273e–81e.
47. Tiner BD, Van Sickels JE, Schmitz JP. Life threatening, delayed hemorrhage after Le Fort I osteotomy requiring surgical inter-vention: report of two cases. J Oral Maxillofac Surg. 1997;55:91–3.
48. Mamie C, Habre W, Delhumeau C, Argiroffo CB, Morabia A. Incidence and risk factors of perioperative respiratory adverse events in children undergoing elective surgery. Pediatr Anesth. 2004;14:218–24.
49. Deepika K, et al. Negative pressure pulmonary edema after acute upper airway obstruction. J Clin Anesth. 1997;9:403–8.
50. Udeshi A, et al. Postobstructive pulmonary edema. J Crit Care. 2010;25:538.e1–5.
51. Fremont RD, Kallet RH, Matthay MA, Ware LB. Postobstructive pulmonary edema: a case for hydrostatic mechanisms. Chest. 2007;131:1742–6.
52. Bhattacharya M, Kallet RH, Ware LB, Matthay MA. Negative-pressure pulmonary Edema. Chest. 2016;150:927–33.
53. Ho CM, Wu HL, Ho ST, Wang JJ. Dexamethasone prevents postoperative nausea and vomiting: benefit versus risk. Acta Anaesthesiol Taiwanica. 2011;49:100–4.
54. Guillot B. Glucocorticoid-induced cutaneous adverse events. Rev Med Interne. 2013;34:310–4.
55. Stanbury RM, Graham EM. Systemic corticosteroid therapy – side effects and their management. Br J Ophthalmol. 1998;82:704–8.
56. Wicke C, Halliday B, Allen D, et al. Effects of steroids and retinoids on wound healing. Arch Surg. 2000;135:1265–70.
57. Chegini S, Dhariwal DK. Review of evidence for the use of steroids in orthognathic surgery. Br J Oral Maxillofac Surg. 2012;50:97–101.
58. Dan AE, Thygesen TH, Pinholt EM. Corticosteroid administration in oral and orthognathic surgery: a systematic review of the literature and meta-analysis. J Oral Maxillofac Surg. 2010;68:2207–20.
59. Seo K, Tanaka Y, Terumitsu M, Someya G. Efficacy of steroid treatment for sensory impairment after orthognathic surgery. J Oral Maxillofac Surg. 2004;62:1193–7.
60. Widar F, Kashani H, Alsén B, Dahlin C, Rasmusson L. The effects of steroids in preventing facial oedema, pain, and neurosensory disturbances after bilateral sagittal split osteotomy: a randomized controlled trial. Int J Oral Maxillofac Surg. 2015;44:252–8.
61. Oomens M, Verlinden C, Goey Y, Forouzanfar T. Prescribing antibiotic prophylaxis in orthognathic surgery: a systematic review. Int J Oral Maxillofac Surg. 2014;43:725–31.
62. Zijderveld SA, Smeele LE, Kostense PJ, Tuinzing DB. Preoperative antibiotic prophylaxis in orthognathic surgery: a randomized, double-blind, and placebo-controlled clinical study. J Oral Maxillofac Surg. 1999;57(12):1403–6. [discussion 1406-7]
63. Johnson JT, Kachman K, Wagner RL, Myers EN. Comparison of ampicillin/sulbactam versus clindamycin in the prevention of infection in patients undergoing head and neck surgery. Head Neck. 1997;19(5):367–71.
64. Brignardello-Petersen R, Carrasco-Labra A, Araya I, Yanine N, Cordova Jara L, Villanueva J. Antibiotic prophylaxis for preventing infectious complications in orthognathic surgery. Cochrane Database Syst Rev. 2015;1:CD010266. https://doi.org/10.1002/14651858.CD010266.pub2.
65. Bailey R, Sinha C, Burgess LP. Ketorolac tromethamine and hemorrhage in tonsillectomy: a prospective, randomized, double-blind study. Laryngoscope. 1997;107:166–9.
66. Lee A, Cooper MG, Craig JC, Knight JF, Keneally JP. Effects of nonsteroidal anti-inflammatory drugs on postoperative renal function in adults with normal renal function. Cochrane Database Syst Rev. 2007;2:CD002765. https://doi.org/10.1002/14651858.CD002765.pub3.
67. Chan DK, Parikh SR. Perioperative ketorolac increases post-tonsillectomy hemorrhage in adults but not children. Laryngoscope. 2014;124:1789–93.
68. Lewis SR, Nicholson A, Cardwell ME, Siviter G, Smith AF. Nonsteroidal anti-inflammatory drugs and perioperative bleeding in paediatric tonsillectomy. Cochrane Database Syst Rev. 2013;7:CD003591. https://doi.org/10.1002/14651858.CD003591.pub3.
69. Öncül AMT, et al. Postoperative analgesia in orthognathic surgery patients: diclofenac sodium or paracetamol? Br J Oral Maxillofac Surg. 2011;49:138–41.
70. Tuzuner AM, et al. Preoperatıve diclofenac sodium and tramadol for pain relief after bimaxillary osteotomy. J Oral Maxillofac Surg. 2007;65:2453–8.
71. Passeri LA, et al. Morbidity and mortality rates after maxillomandibular advancement for treatment of obstructive sleep apnea. J Oral Maxillofac Surg. 2016;74:2033–43.
72. Faßbender P, Herbstreit F, Eikermann M, Teschler H, Peters J. Obstructive sleep apnea – a perioperative risk factor. Dtsch Arztebl Int. 2016;113:463–9.
73. American Academy of Sleep Medicine Task Force. Sleep-related breathing disorders in adults: recommendations for syndrome definition and measurement techniques in clinical research. The report of an American academy of sleep medicine task force. Sleep. 1999;22:667–89.
74. Ayas NT, Taylor CM, Laher I. Cardiovascular consequences of obstructive sleep apnea. Curr Opin Cardiol. 2016;31:599–605.
75. Sajkov D, et al. Obstructive sleep apnea and pulmonary hypertension. Prog Cardiovasc Dis. 2009;51:363–70.
76. Ahiskalioglu A, et al. Effects of a single-dose of preemptive pregabalin on postoperative pain and opioid consumption after double-jaw surgery: a randomized controlled trial. J Oral Maxillofac Surg. 2016;74:53.e1–7.

77. Lam T. Is perioperative fluid and salt balance a contributing factor in postoperative worsening of obstructive sleep apnea? Anesth Analg. 2016;122:1335–9.
78. White LH, Bradley TD. Role of nocturnal rostral fluid shift in the pathogenesis of obstructive and central sleep apnoea. J Physiol. 2013;591:1179–93.
79. Renata RL, et al. A cephalometric comparison of patients with the sleep apnea/hypopnea syndrome and their siblings. Sleep. 2005;28:315–20.
80. Berry RB, et al. Rules for scoring respiratory events in sleep: update of the 2007 AASM manual for the scoring of sleep and associated events. Deliberations of the sleep apnea definitions task force of the American academy of sleep medicine. J Clin Sleep Med. 2012;8:597–619.
81. Soose RJ. Novel surgical approaches for the treatment of obstructive sleep apnea. Sleep Med Clin. 2016;11:189–202.
82. Strollo PJ, et al. Upper-airway stimulation for obstructive sleep apnea. N Engl J Med. 2014;370:139–49.

36 Craniofacial Surgery

Jennifer E. Woerner and G.E. Ghali

Abstract

This chapter focuses on the perioperative assessment of the craniofacial patient, along with common craniofacial procedures. The preoperative data collection requires the use of multiple radiographic modalities, physical examination, and basic laboratory work. Vigilant intraoperative management of these patients is necessary due to the increased risk of blood loss during craniofacial procedures and the plethora of possible comorbidities that can be found in this population. Utilizing a mixture of these tools allows for better planning to ensure patient safety, excellent surgical outcomes, and an uneventful postoperative course.

36.1 Introduction

This chapter will focus on the nonsyndromic and syndromic forms of craniosynostosis and the preoperative data collection, roles of vital craniofacial team members during the assessment, methods for evaluation, basic surgical procedures, anesthetic management, and common complications for surgical procedures requiring a transcranial approach.

J.E. Woerner, D.M.D., M.D., F.A.C.S. (✉)
G.E. Ghali, DDS, MD, FACS, FRCS(Ed)
Louisiana State University Health Sciences Center-Shreveport, Shreveport, LA, USA
e-mail: jwoern@lsuhsc.edu

36.2 Classification

The cranial vault is made up of six major sutures. The coronal and lambdoid sutures are paired, and the metopic and sagittal are single sutures. There are also several minor sutures and two major fontanelles, designated as anterior and posterior. The patency of cranial sutures serves two functions: (1) to allow deformation of the head to facilitate vaginal delivery during childbirth and (2) to allow for expansion of the skull during periods of rapid brain and orbital growth [1, 2]. The brain, and therefore the cranial vault, grows very rapidly during the first year of life then steadily tapers off to a slow rate. By 2.5 years of age, 80–85% of brain and skull growth is complete [2]. Craniosynostosis is defined as the premature fusion of one or more cranial sutures [3]. This is most commonly an in utero event during fetal

© Springer International Publishing AG 2018

E.M. Ferneini, J.D. Bennett (eds.), *Perioperative Assessment of the Maxillofacial Surgery Patient*,
https://doi.org/10.1007/978-3-319-58868-1_36

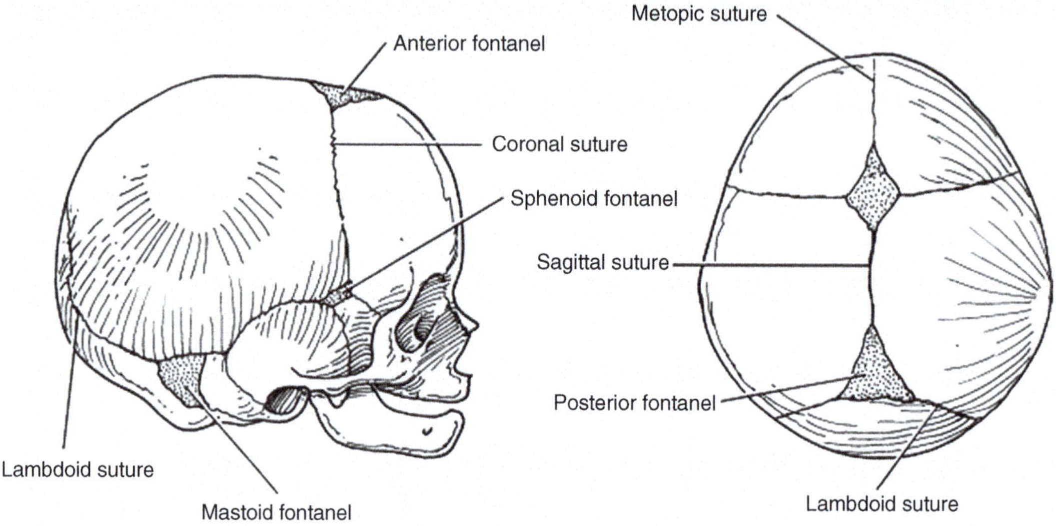

Fig. 36.1 Lateral and superior view of infant skull diagramming the sutures and fontanelles [1]

development. First defined by Virchow in 1851, there is restriction of growth perpendicular to the fused suture with compensatory growth at the sutures that remain patent [4]. This battle between restricted and compensatory growth results in a characteristically abnormal head shape depending on the suture(s) that are fused (Fig. 36.1).

36.2.1 Nonsyndromic Craniosynostosis

Nonsyndromic craniosynostosis occurs in 1 in 2000 live births and is not associated with other deformities or conditions [5, 6]. Approximately 90% of nonsyndromic craniosynostosis cases are random occurrences with the deformity limited to the skull and orbits [1, 2].

36.2.2 Syndromic Craniosynostosis

Syndromic craniosynostosis occurs in 1 in 20,000 live births and can be associated with a vast array of clinical findings, which often include hearing loss, midface hypoplasia, digital anomalies, and skeletal anomalies. There are now upwards of 180 identifiable syndromes that can be associated with craniosynostosis, though most are extremely uncommon [7]. Syndromic forms only represent about 15% of the total craniosynostosis cases [5, 6]. The most common gene mutations associated with syndromic craniosynostosis involve fibroblast growth factor receptors (FGFR-1, FGFR-2, or FGFR-3). Defects in FGFR cause an increase in bone deposition resulting in premature fusion of the cranial sutures. The most common syndromes associated with FGFR mutations that result in craniosynostosis are Apert, Crouzon, Pfeiffer, Muenke, and Saethre-Chotzen [2, 7].

36.3 Comorbidities Associated with Craniosynostosis

36.3.1 Intracranial Hypertension and Restriction of Cranial Vault Growth

One question that has plagued the craniofacial world relates to, "What value should be considered normal intracranial pressure (ICP)?" This has been debated since first described by Renier and his colleagues in 1982, but the "Paris" range for ICP is generally accepted, defining a normal ICP as <10 mmHg, borderline as 11–15 mmHg, and intracranial hypertension as >15 mmHg [8].

Previous studies have demonstrated a 13–14% incidence of intracranial hypertension with single-suture stenosis and up to a 42% incidence in children with multisuture stenosis [9, 10]. Increased intracranial pressure, if left untreated for extended periods of time, has been associated with lower developmental (DQ) and intelligence quotients (IQ) [11]. Clinical symptoms that may elucidate the practitioner to the possibility of intracranial hypertension include headaches, irritability, nausea and vomiting, difficulty sleeping, and possible developmental delay [12, 13]. On physical exam, findings such as tense, widely patent unaffected cranial sutures, bulging fontanelles, or engorged scalp veins may also be an indication of intracranial hypertension. Radiographic signs of intracranial hypertension may include cortical thinning or a lückenschädel (hammered metal) appearance of the inner table of the skull [14, 15]. If any clinical or radiographic exam findings suggest elevated ICP, the child should be evaluated by a pediatric ophthalmologist for a funduscopic exam to investigate for papilledema [16]. Although it is important to realize that papilledema and radiographic signs of increased ICP are necessary elements of the craniosynostosis workup, they are usually late findings or may not even be present if the intracranial hypertension has increased gradually [3, 16].

It is important to note that actual signs of intracranial hypertension are often late findings that occur after the age of one. These symptoms often present gradually and in infants, who have limited verbal communication, making them challenging to detect [17]. Another important factor may be the age of the patient when diagnosed with craniosynostosis. Arnaud, Renier, and Marchac found that ~20% of children presenting after the age of one presented with intracranial hypertension versus only 2% of patients presenting before 1 year of age [11]. Since most children with craniosynostosis are diagnosed before the age of 1, it may not be possible to predict who may develop intracranial hypertension if left untreated.

Considering the difficulty in diagnosing intracranial hypertension and the deleterious effects it can have on brain growth and development, there has been a modest amount of research published on measuring intracranial volume using noninvasive means such as computed tomography (CT) scans or magnetic resonance imaging (MRI). Most of the literature agrees there is little restriction of intracranial volume due to synostosis in patients over 6 months of age, with the exception of multiple suture synostoses [18]. This challenges the idea that craniosynostosis leads to inhibited volumetric growth of the cranium and an eventual increase in intracranial pressure due to restricted volume. Other factors that may be responsible for hypertension include intracranial venous congestion, hydrocephalus, and upper airway obstruction, all of which are more common in syndromic patients with craniosynostosis [18–21].

36.3.2 Hydrocephalus

Hydrocephalus may occur independently, but is not commonly associated with single-suture fusion. It is thought that hydrocephalus can affect 5–10% of patients with craniosynostosis. In patients with nonsyndromic forms of craniosynostosis, Cinalli and colleagues found that "dilation of the cerebral ventricles occurs with the same frequency as that observed in the normal population." In comparison, ~12% of children with syndromic forms of craniosynostosis developed hydrocephalus. The syndromes most commonly associated with hydrocephalus include Apert and Crouzon, and the presentation of hydrocephalus as either an early or late finding is thought to be dependent on the pattern in which the sutures fuse, along with the presence of jugular foramen stenosis. In addition, children with a kleeblattschädel deformity are at significant risk for hydrocephalus along with hindbrain herniation [22].

If a child suffers from craniosynostosis and hydrocephalus, one must consider the proper timing of ventriculoperitoneal (VP) shunt placement. Some surgeons prefer placement of a VP shunt following total cranial vault remodeling to prevent inadequate support of the bony segments due to drainage of the cerebrospinal fluid [23]. Children with moderate to severe forms of hydrocephalus or decreased compliance may require VP shunt placement prior to total cranial vault remodeling. Ultimately, the decision of when to place a VP shunt is left up to the judgment of the neurosurgeon after considering all neurologic findings.

36.3.3 Visual Acuity and Ocular Motility

Visual impairment related to craniosynostosis may include atrophy of the optic nerve, strabismus, ocular motility disorders, or direct trauma to the globe. Increased ICP may translate into clinically evident papilledema or disk edema. If left untreated, this may lead to optic atrophy resulting in complete or partial blindness. Stavrou and colleagues found that prognosis of visual acuity following cranial vault surgery was dependent on the preoperative insult and deficit. In their study, children with papilledema had improvement in their symptoms with vault expansion, but none of the patients suffering from optic nerve atrophy regained function [24].

In cases of unilateral coronal craniosynostosis, divergent or convergent non-paralytic strabismus may occur due to either orbital dystopia or abnormalities of the ocular muscles themselves. Vertical strabismus is very common and present in 37–50% of these patients. Abnormal ocular movements are present in 67% of patients with metopic craniosynostosis, possibly due to the ocular deformity [25]. Some forms of craniosynostosis may involve orbital hypertelorism and may lead to compromised visual acuity and restricted binocular vision. Forms of craniosynostosis causing restriction of forehead growth or recession of the supraorbital rims (unilateral coronal synostosis, Crouzon syndrome, and Apert syndrome) may cause an apparent exotropia requiring correction. Without correction, it places the patient at risk for corneal exposure and direct ocular trauma [26]. Of interest, new onset strabismus has been noted in 17–46% of patients that underwent fronto-orbital advancement but only resolved when present preoperatively in 3.4% [27, 28].

Proper evaluation of a child with synostosis by a pediatric ophthalmologist is important. Many of these impairments in ocular motility are easily correctable with surgery, and intervention can prevent long-term visual compromise.

36.3.4 Neuropsychiatric Disorders

The data differentiating whether or not children with single-suture craniosynostosis have higher rates of long-term cognitive, behavioral, or speech-related disorders is controversial. The recent data trending toward cognitive and/or behavioral disorders in children with single-suture craniosynostosis has found that these deficits may not be evident early on but often develop over early childhood [29–33]. It appears that many of these children suffer both delays in both mental and psychomotor development [34]. Several explanations include possible intracranial hypertension that goes unrecognized, an organic abnormality of the brain related to the specific synostosed suture, obstruction of cerebral blood flow, or alteration in CSF dynamics [29, 32]. Numerous studies have shown that cranial vault surgery may improve psychomotor function, but may not reverse the mental developmental delays that have already occurred. There is some evidence to show that surgery may prevent continued decline of mental function in these patients [34, 35].

Future studies utilizing larger patient populations improved long-term follow-up, and appropriate controls are necessary in order to stratify the risk of mental and psychomotor delays. It is important for children with single-suture craniosynostosis to have close follow-up, and it may be prudent for them to be routinely screened for cognitive, behavioral, and speech-related disorders by a qualified child psychologist.

36.4 Preoperative Data Collection

36.4.1 Patient History

The most critical data collected during the preoperative period is obtained from the history and physical examination. The basic data should include a thorough medical history, previous surgeries, family history, medication profile, allergies, and issues with previous anesthetics for the patient or their family. The standard of care, according to the American Cleft Palate and Craniofacial Association, for children suffering from craniosynostosis includes a multidisciplinary team approach [36, 37].

This well-organized craniofacial team should include audiology, craniofacial surgery, genetics, neurology, neurosurgery, ophthalmology, orthodontics, pediatrics, pediatric anesthesiology, pediatric critical care, psychology, and social work [36, 37]. The idea of the team approach was developed in response to the failures that commonly occurred when various aspects of care were not coordinated and when the relationships among coexisting problems were not known. The members work together in order to diagnose not only the conditions but any related deformities or symptomatology [38].

Most children with nonsyndromic craniosynostosis are healthy and require only basic preoperative laboratory evaluations. Syndromic patients, on the other hand, can have a wide variety of associated anomalies not limited to congenital heart defects, midface hypoplasia with resultant airway abnormalities, and limb abnormalities. Children at risk for cardiac abnormalities should undergo evaluation by a pediatric cardiologist. Approximately half of all children with Apert, Crouzon, or Pfeiffer syndrome suffer from obstructive sleep apnea. These children may benefit from a thorough airway evaluation or sleep study preoperatively, as they may be at an increased risk for obstruction during the postoperative period [39]. This thorough, multidisciplinary approach should allow the surgical team and anesthesiologist to prepare for any possible intraoperative complications or obstacles preventing a speedy recovery.

36.4.2 Physical Examination

In nonsyndromic craniosynostosis, there are very characteristic head shapes determined by the suture(s) involved. The overall head shape and position and symmetry of the ears should be inspected. Next, the head circumference should be measured and plotted on the appropriate growth curve. Restricted head growth or a patient that has fallen off the growth should be investigated for an organic cause. One cause of restricted head growth may be craniosynostosis, and this is more common when multiple sutures are involved. During physical examination, the skull should be palpated for patency of both the anterior and posterior fontanelle, along with all suture lines. The posterior fontanelle typically closes by 6 months of age and the anterior fontanelle by 12 months [40]. Premature closure of the fontanelle may be one clue that there is premature closure of one or more sutures. Normal fontanelles should feel soft and flat. Bulging and/or tense fontanelles may be an indication of increased intracranial pressure. Following palpation of the anterior and posterior fontanelle, all suture lines should be palpated for patency and ridging. Patent sutures should demonstrate a small amount of mobility of the cranial bones along the suture line. Both the bony orbit and projection of the globes should be examined. When viewing the skull from the superior aspect, the superior bony orbits should have adequate projection to protect the globe of the eye. Any exorbitism should be noted. If there are any indications of possible intracranial hypertension such as multiple suture synostoses, bulging fontanelles, engorged scalp veins, or widened unaffected cranial sutures, one should pursue an ophthalmology consult for a visual exam to examine for papilledema and consider other adjuncts to monitoring ICP [13, 16, 40].

36.4.3 Imaging

Surgeons may rely on conventional skull radiographs or CT scans with 3D reconstruction. Conventional skull radiographs should include skull films and lateral cephalograms. These films are inexpensive, expose the infant to a limited amount of radiation, and are easily accessible. Most cases of craniosynostosis can be easily identified on plain skull films. Normal or patent cranial sutures manifest as a radiolucent line. The absence of this finding in the normal anatomic position of a suture may suggest craniosynostosis [3].

CT scans are commonly used and allow for visualization of not only the stenosed suture but also the brain and ventricle anatomy. The definition of these elements and bony facial structures on high-resolution CT images with or without three-dimensional reconstruction is unmatched by other imaging techniques. CT scans are often an excellent aid to help describe head shape and suture abnormalities to families. In the postoperative period, a CT scan can be a valuable tool to

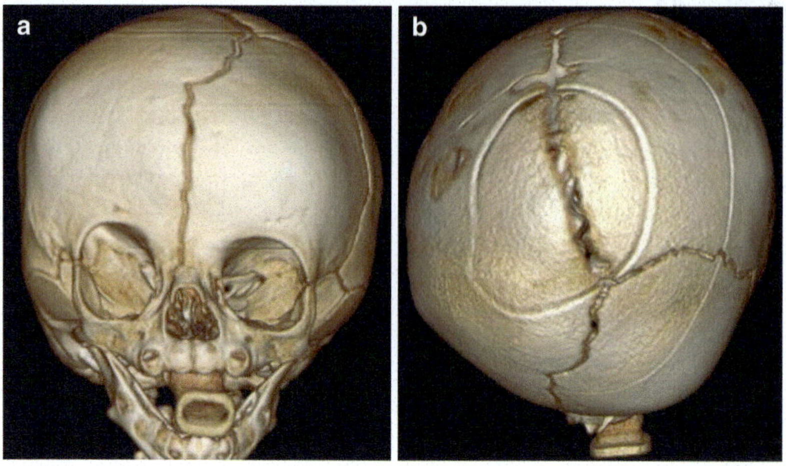

Fig. 36.2 (**a**) Frontal view of CT with 3D reconstruction and synostosis of the right coronal suture. (**b**) Superior view of CT with 3D reconstruction and synostosis of the right coronal suture

assess cranial expansion, supraorbital advancement, possible intracranial bleeds, and hydrocephalus, as well as a teaching tool for training surgeons and families (Fig. 36.2).

Due to increasing concerns over radiation exposure in children, along with the need for sedation to perform CT scans on many children, there has been some effort to explore high-resolution ultrasound (US) as a method in evaluating the patency of cranial sutures. Numerous studies have shown US to be a reliable method of determining patency of cranial sutures in children with abnormal head shapes [43–45]. It is possible for craniosynostosis to be identified as early as the third trimester of pregnancy on prenatal US. One limitation of US is that cranial suture patency is difficult to assess in children greater than 1 year of age due to the narrowing of the sutures and thickening of the skull bones [44].

36.4.4 Virtual Surgical Planning

Virtual surgical planning is rapidly gaining popularity within many facets of head and neck surgery, from orthognathic surgery to distraction osteogenesis, temporomandibular joint reconstruction, trauma reconstruction, and guides for resection and free tissue transfer [46–49]. These virtual plans are devised through computer-aided design and modeling (CAD/CAM). One drawback to traditional techniques in total cranial vault reconstruction is that the widening and advancement of the fronto-orbital bandeau, along with overall skull size and shape, is somewhat subjective. In other words, the surgeon, based on the appearance of the vault, determines the size, shape, and advancement of the fronto-orbital bandeau. Though craniofacial surgeons have been able to visualize deformities of the skull and face in the pediatric population since the mid-1990s, they were not been able to employ the CAD/CAM technology or 3D printing to aid in normalizing skull shape due to a lack of normative models [50, 51]. In 2011, Saber and colleagues closed that gap by extracting computed tomography (CT) data from 103 normocephalic individuals aged 8–12 months. They then used that data to make averaged, age-appropriate, normative three-dimensional (3D) models for the shape and size of the skull and supraorbital region [51]. This data can then be used to create stereolithic models for study and design standardized, age-appropriate templates for fronto-orbital bandeau reconstruction or 3D-printed patient-specific cutting guides and reconstruction templates for total cranial vault remodeling (TCVR) (Fig. 36.3) [47, 52, 53].

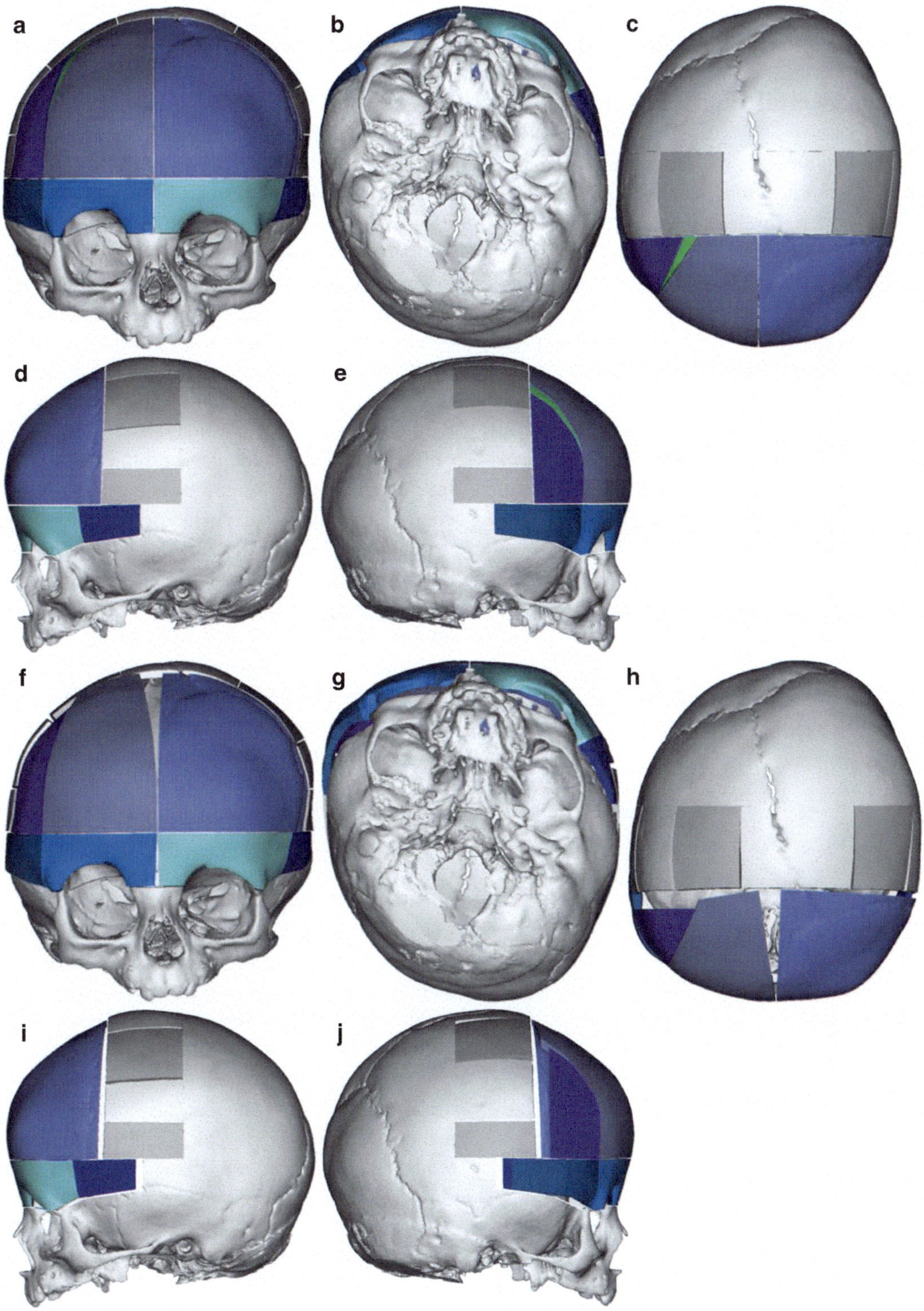

Fig 36.3 (**a**, **b**, **c**, **d**, and **e**) Frontal, inferior, superior, and lateral views of VSP planning for unilateral coronal synostosis. (**f**, **g**, **h**, **i**, and **j**) Frontal, inferior, superior, and lateral views of planned reshaping for unilateral coronal synostosis

36.5 Management of Craniosynostosis

36.5.1 Sagittal Synostosis

Sagittal synostosis is the most common form of craniosynostosis. It represents ~50% of all craniosynostosis cases in the United States and has an overall prevalence of 1 in 5000 live births [3, 23]. Sagittal synostosis is four times more common in males, and only 2% are considered familial [2, 3]. Sagittal synostosis is rarely associated with intracranial hypertension [14]. Clinical features include ridging of the sagittal suture, elongation of the skull in the anteroposterior dimension, and biparietotemporal narrowing and possible premature closure of the anterior fontanelle [2]. The term for this cranial vault deformity is "scaphocephaly" meaning "boat shaped." Usually, the midface and anterior cranial vault sutures are not affected (Fig. 36.4).

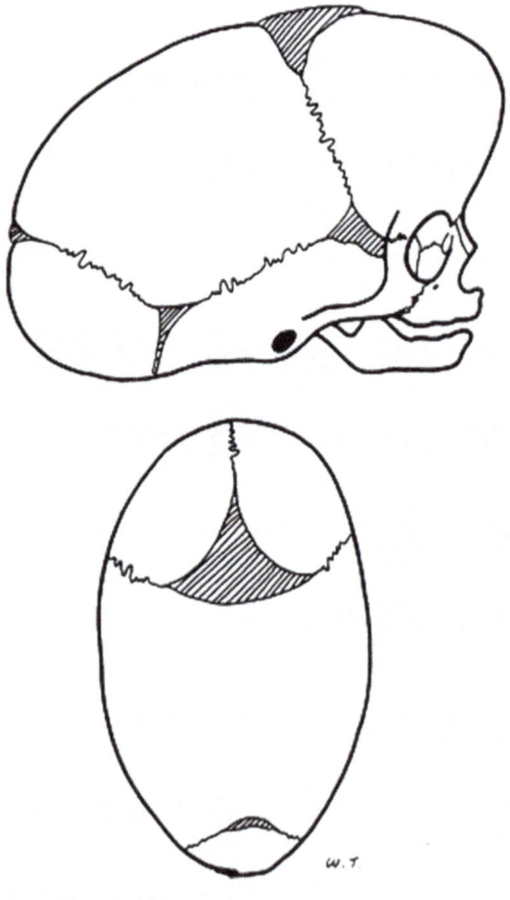

Fig. 36.4 Lateral and superior view of sagittal synostosis [14]

36.5.2 Unilateral Coronal Synostosis

Unilateral coronal synostosis is the second most common form of craniosynostosis. It represents ~20% of all craniosynostosis cases in the United States and occurs in 1 in 10,000 children [14, 23]. Two thirds of unilateral coronal synostosis cases occur in females, and ~10% are familial [2]. Clinical features include ridging or obliteration of the affected coronal suture, flattening of the frontal bone on the ipsilateral side, recession of the supraorbital and lateral orbital rim on the ipsilateral side, and significant bossing of the contralateral forehead [14]. These deformities result in nasal deviation and constriction, hypoplasia of the zygomatic arch, and a "harlequin eye deformity" on the affected side. This "harlequin eye deformity" is created by an orbital dystopia due to posterior and superior displacement of the bony orbit [2]. The term used to describe unilateral synostosis is "anterior plagiocephaly." One should rule out infant molding or positional plagiocephaly. One distinguishing difference is when the skull is viewed from the superior aspect, unilateral synostosis has an overall trapezoidal appearance, whereas positional plagiocephaly has a parallelogram shape. In anterior plagiocephaly, the anterior skull base is also affected resulting in absence of the frontoethmoidal, frontospheniodal, and sphenoethmoidal sutures [1]. This results in a continued long-term deformity in many patients, even following cranial vault remodeling with removal of the affected suture. This can also create future mandibular deviation and facial asymmetry requiring later correction (Fig. 36.5).

36.5.3 Bilateral Coronal Synostosis

Bilateral coronal synostosis is the most common syndrome-associated craniosynostosis and represents ~20% of the isolated craniosynostosis cases in the United States. It is also the most common cranial vault suture synostosis pattern associated

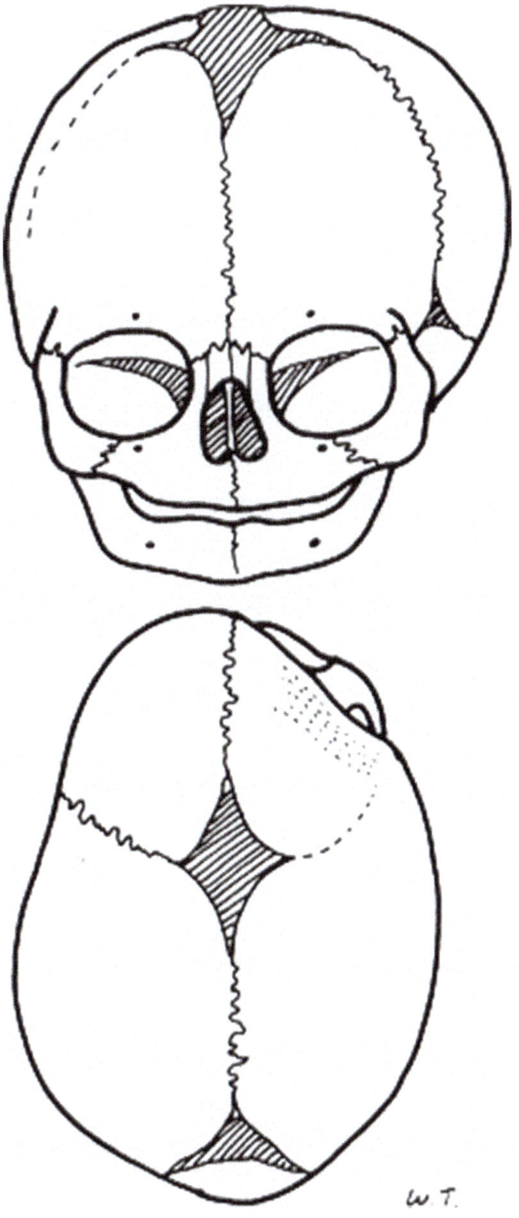

Fig. 36.5 Frontal and superior view of unilateral coronal synostosis [14]

with Apert, Crouzon, and Pfeiffer syndromes. The term nonsyndromic is used to describe bilateral coronal synostosis without midface deficiency or other known associated malformations [3, 14, 41]. Nonsyndromic bilateral coronal synostosis is more common in females by a ratio of 2:1 and is associated with advanced paternal age. It is believed that ~14% of nonsyndromic cases are familial [41]. Clinical features include recession of the frontoparietal region, posterior and superior displacement of the supraorbital rims and eyebrows, and widened palpebral fissures. Much like unilateral coronal synostosis, the lesser wing of the sphenoid is displaced superiorly resulting in bilateral "harlequin eyes" [41]. In addition to the recessed supraorbital bones and "harlequin eyes," the forehead appears to be lower, and there is sagittal shortening of the skull [3, 41]. The term for this cranial vault deformity is "brachycephaly." The upper orbits and anterior cranial base are short in the anteroposterior dimension and wide transversely. The overlying cranial vault is high in the superior-inferior dimension, with anterior bulging of the upper forehead that results from compensatory growth of the patent metopic suture (Fig. 36.6) [3, 41].

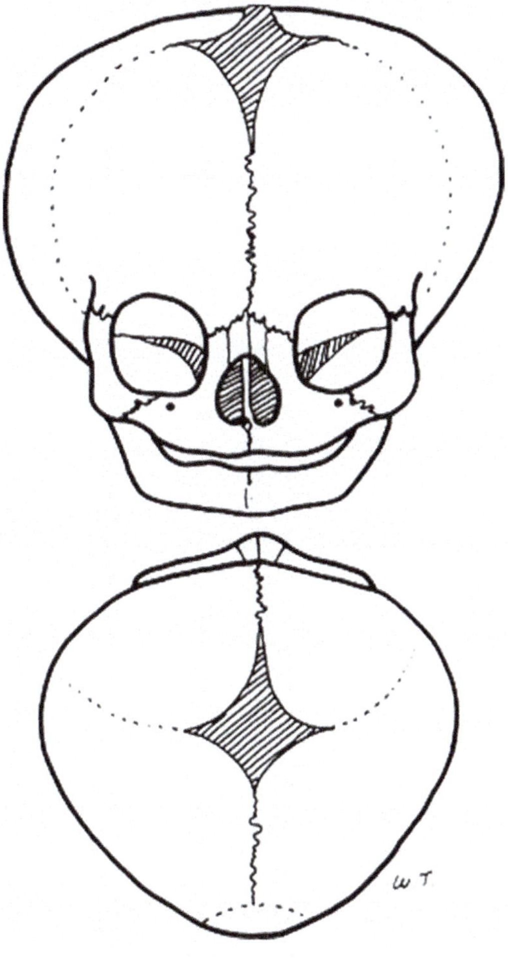

Fig. 36.6 Frontal and superior view of bilateral coronal synostosis [14]

36.5.4 Metopic Synostosis

Metopic synostosis accounts for ~10% of the isolated craniosynostosis cases in the United States and occurs in 1:15,000 children [1, 14]. This condition is more common in males, and ~5% of cases are familial. It is believed that up to 1/3 of metopic cases may be syndromic; therefore, genetic evaluation is warranted in children presenting with other congenital malformations [2]. Clinical features include ridging of the metopic suture, posteriorly sloped forehead, bitemporal narrowing, posteroinferior recession of the lateral orbital rims, associated hypotelorism, and often overcompensated growth of the posterior cranial vault. The decrease in bitemporal width and constriction of the forehead result in abnormal shape and decreased volume of the anterior cranial vault. This results in an overall triangular shape to the skull and is termed "trigonocephaly" (Fig. 36.7).

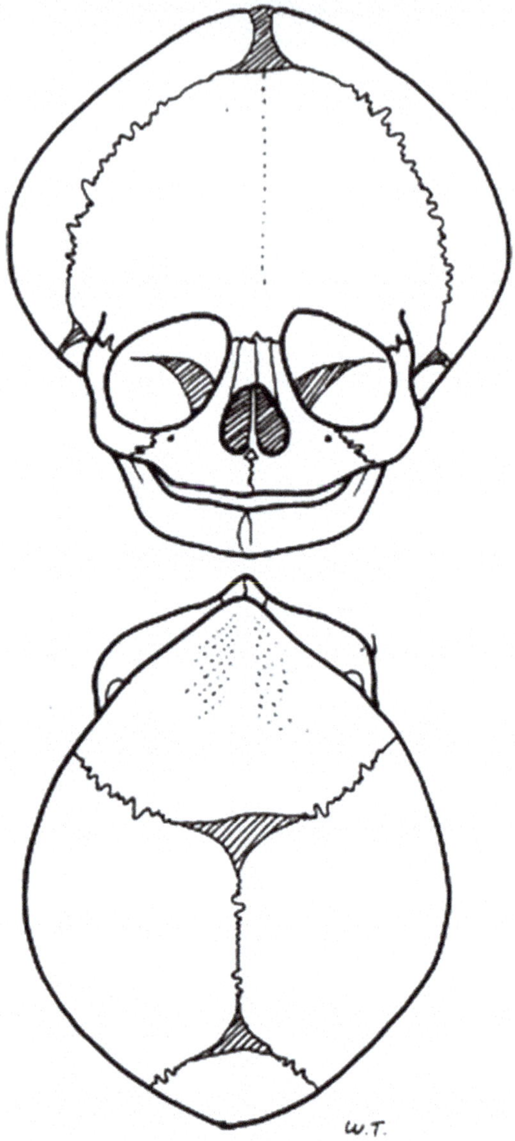

Fig. 36.7 Frontal and superior view of metopic synostosis [14]

36.5.5 Unilateral Lambdoid Synostosis

Unilateral lambdoid synostosis accounts for ~3% of isolated craniosynostosis cases in the United States and occurs in 1:150,000 live births [1, 3]. Clinical features include ridging or obliteration of the affected lambdoid, retrusion of the ipsilateral parieto-occipital region, retrusion of the forehead on the ipsilateral side, and superior-posterior displacement of the ipsilateral ear. The term for this cranial vault deformity is "posterior plagiocephaly." Lambdoid synostosis is extremely rare, and when suspected, a noncontrast CT scan of the head should be performed for diagnosis. Of critical importance is ruling out posterior positional plagiocephaly. With positional (or deformational) plagiocephaly, the head takes on a parallelogram shape in comparison to the trapezoidal shape encountered in lambdoid synostosis. In positional plagiocephaly, there is flattening of the contralateral forehead and anterior displacement of the ipsilateral ear. It is important to ensure proper diagnosis, as lambdoid synostosis is treated through surgical reconstruction and positional plagiocephaly is treated with conservative management such as "tummy time" or cranial remodeling orthosis (Fig. 36.8) [1, 3].

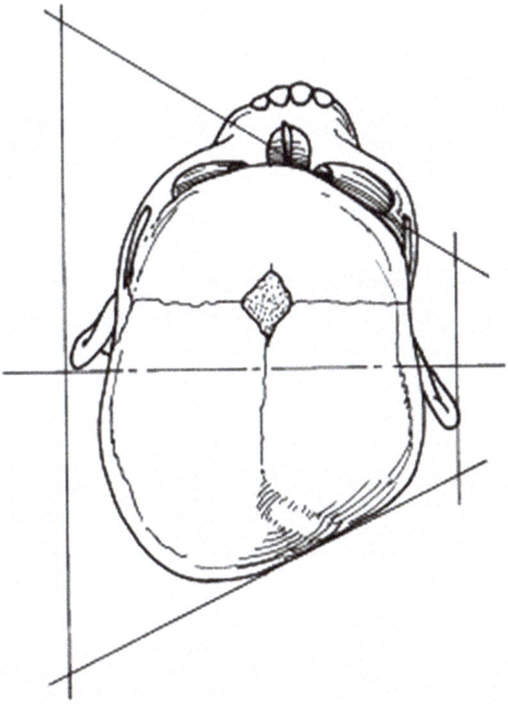

Fig. 36.8 Typical head shape associated with lambdoid synostosis [42]

36.6 Intraoperative Considerations

36.6.1 Laboratory Studies

Though cranial vault remodeling has been shown to be safe, it is still an invasive procedure for such a young infant [54, 55]. Basic laboratory tests should be obtained to include hemoglobin, hematocrit, platelet count, type and screen, and coagulation studies [56]. These laboratory values can then assist in monitoring fluid and electrolyte abnormalities and can serve as trigger levels for the implementation of transfusion protocols. The presenting authors often use blood gas samples drawn from the arterial line to vigilantly monitor for possible acidosis and the need for transfusion once all osteotomies are complete. At this point, a majority of the blood loss has occurred making it an appropriate time to address any fluid, electrolyte, hemoglobin, or coagulation abnormalities.

36.6.2 Airway Management

Airway evaluation should be performed on all craniofacial patients to help plan the safest anesthetic technique. It is important to investigate whether the child has undergone previous anesthetics and if they had any difficulty with the anesthesia. Children born with craniofacial syndromes, such as Apert and Crouzon, may present with severe midface hypoplasia that can make mask ventilation, intubation, or extubation challenging. These children may benefit from airway maneuvers and oropharyngeal or nasopharyngeal airways during mask ventilation. If intubation is expected to be challenging, one may consider the use of direct laryngoscopy with a video laryngoscope or fiber-optic intubation. Following intubation, it is necessary to check for equal bilateral breath sounds once the patient is appropriately positioned. It is also essential to ensure the endotracheal tube is not at risk of being kinked or moved because it is not easily accessible once the procedure begins [39]. At the author's institution, the patient is intubated orally utilizing a reinforced endotracheal tube that is secured through the chin to the periosteum of the mandibular symphysis with a silk suture. The position of the tube and proper ventilation are then rechecked prior to sterile preparation and draping.

36.6.3 Monitoring

Standard monitoring according to the American Society of Anesthesiologists should be employed. This includes end tidal CO_2 monitored continuously through capnography, capnometry, or mass spectroscopy. Blood oxygenation should be monitored continuously as well through pulse oximetry. In craniofacial surgery cases, it is necessary to place an arterial line to continuously monitor blood pressure and detect hypotension [39, 56, 57].

In young patients, it is vital to monitor the patient's core temperature. Children undergoing craniofacial procedures are at an increased risk for hypothermia due to the surface area of a child's head, administration of intravenous fluids, and blood loss. Hypothermia can impair coagulation and increase bleeding. In order to prevent hypothermia, the operating room should be kept warm, while the patient is being positioned and undergoing induction of anesthesia [56–58]. Once the patient is prepped and draped, active warming should occur. At the author's institution, a core-temperature Foley catheter is placed to monitor closely for hypothermia, and a forced air convection blanket is used during the surgical procedure.

36.6.4 Transfusion Protocol

To be safe, teams should be prepared to transfuse if necessary. Actual transfusion protocols, along with the use of erythropoietin and cell salvage, are controversial and often institution dependent [59]. Numerous studies have shown that children undergoing craniofacial surgery can lose, on average, anywhere from 21 to 65% of estimated blood volume [60]. At the author's institution, the average blood loss for craniosynostosis repair was 42.7%; therefore, all patients are typed and cross-matched for blood products, and families are given the opportunity to be direct donors, if possible [61]. Transfusion is begun at the time of incision to coincide with a majority of blood loss. Blood loss is most common during two periods: (1) at initial scalp incision and flap reflection and (2) during skull osteotomies [59]. It is vital that communication occur between the surgeon and the anesthesia team because children at this age and weight can easily become under-resuscitated [56, 58, 59]. In order to minimize the amount of blood to be transfused and the number of exposures from different donors, institutional transfusion protocols should be implemented. These protocols are often dictated either by hemodynamic parameters, such as arterial blood pressure, during times of blood loss or laboratory values such as hemoglobin/hematocrit (H/H), prothrombin time/partial thromboplastin time (PT/PTT), and platelet count during times of hemodynamic stability [56, 59].

36.7 Surgical Technique

36.7.1 Timing of Repair

Although the timing of craniosynostosis repair remains controversial and individualized, the presenting authors prefer early surgical repair between the ages of 4 and 8 months. Early surgical repair allows for rapid frontal lobe growth which supports forehead and supraorbital ridge advancement. At this age, the cranium is highly malleable and, therefore, easier to contour. Also, during this period of rapid growth, residual bony defects heal more rapidly [1, 62].

36.7.2 Overview of Technique

Once the patient is positioned, the hair is parted or the head is shaved. A coronal incision is drawn out with a marking pen, and local anesthetic is injected subcutaneously. Following sterile prepping and draping of the patient, a coronal incision is created through skin, subcutaneous tissue, galea, temporalis muscle bilaterally, and the periosteum. The temporalis muscles are incised and remain attached to the coronal flaps during dissection. Pre- or postauricular extension can be utilized if necessary. Care is taken to prevent entrance into the anterior or posterior fontanelles and possible violation of the sagittal sinus. The coronal flap is then reflected in a subperiosteal fashion to expose the cranial vault. In cases where a supraorbital bandeau is necessary, the supraorbital rims, superior half of the orbit, nasofrontal suture, and the zygomaticofrontal sutures are exposed. Once complete, the flaps are secured with surgical stays to facilitate surgical site exposure. Next, the osteotomy designs are drawn onto the skull using either a marking pen or sterile pencil. A bifrontal craniotomy is then performed by the pediatric neurosurgeon to provide access for additional craniofacial osteotomies. The skeletal segments are reshaped and replaced into position and stabilized using resorbable plates and screws. These plates, which are composed of polylactic and polyglycolic acid, are completely resorbed by hydrolysis within 9–14 months while maintaining tensile strength for initial stabilization [63–65]. As a result, growth restrictions are minimized, as is the potential for transcranial migration.

36.7.2.1 Sagittal Synostosis

- Premature closure of the sagittal suture often requires total cranial vault reshaping in the prone position.
- Following access, the synostotic suture is removed utilizing the Midas Rex. Barrel staves are made in the parietal, temporal, and frontal bones. The skull is then widened using the Tessier benders in the biparietal dimension and reduced in the anterior-posterior (AP) dimension.
- If it is determined that the posterior vault is prominent, it can be set anteriorly and/or rotated during the cranial vault reshaping to reduce the AP dimension of the skull. This bony segment can then be secured in place with resorbable plates and screws (Fig. 36.9).

36.7.2.2 Unilateral Coronal Synostosis

- Patient is positioned supine, and a coronal flap is elevated as previously described.
- Bilateral subperiosteal reflection extends to the periorbital and zygomaticotemporal regions anteriorly while maintaining the attachment of the medial canthal tendons. Posteriorly, the scalp flap is reflected midway between the coronal and lambdoid sutures. Markings for the bifrontal craniotomy and fronto-orbital bar/bandeau are indicated.
- Bifrontal craniotomy using the Midas Rex drill is used to develop a 1.5 cm bandeau.
- Retraction of the frontal and temporal lobes of the brain facilitates superior orbital and temporal osteotomies. Bilateral tongue-in-groove (tenon) extensions are developed via a reciprocating saw to the level of pterion.
- Intracranial retraction of frontal lobes, as well as intraorbital retraction of the periorbita, is necessary to achieve the anterior skull base osteotomy. The level of the lateral orbital rim osteotomy is at the zygomaticofrontal suture. The bandeau is transected from the root of the nose at or above the nasofrontal suture.
- The bandeau is adjusted bilaterally via removal of wedges from the recessed side and scoring of the over-projected side. Bending the recessed side and straightening the over-projected side allow for recontouring of the bandeau.
- Barrel-staving osteotomies are placed in the parietal and/or temporal bones as needed for reshaping.
- Resorbable plates and screws are utilized for stabilization of the bandeau and forehead (Fig. 36.10).

36.7.2.3 Bilateral Coronal Synostosis

- Surgical positioning, approach, and osteotomy design is similar to that previously described for repair of a unilateral coronal synostosis. Bilateral osteotomies are indicated to achieve proper advancement and contour.
- Following osteotomies, reshaping, and fixation of the bandeau and forehead is completed with resorbable plates and screws (Fig. 36.11).

36.7.2.4 Metopic Synostosis

- Surgical positioning, approach, and initial osteotomy design is similar to that previously described for uni- or bilateral coronal synostosis.
- Osteotomies of the anterior cranial vault and superior orbital rims with creation of an orbital

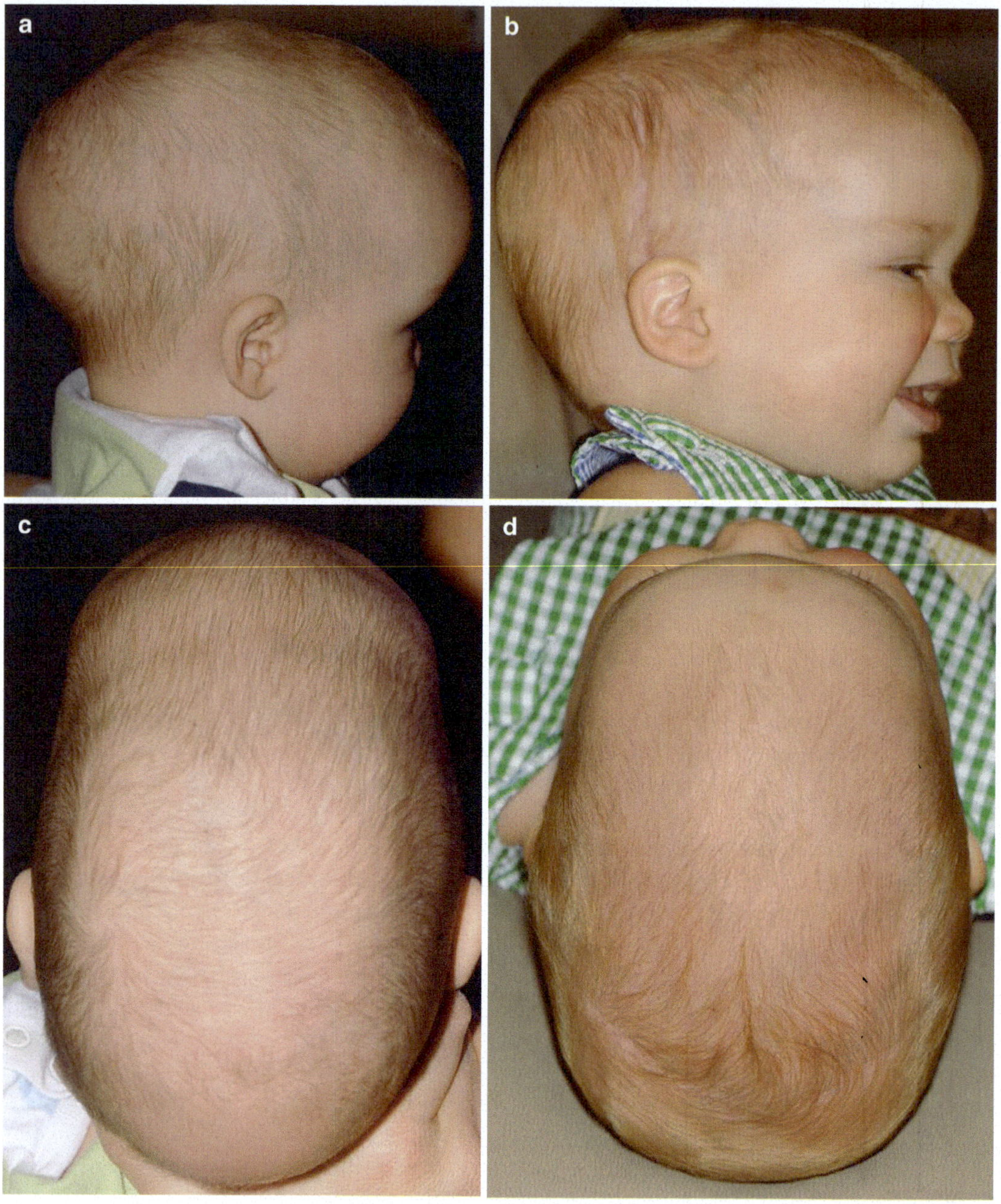

Fig. 36.9 (**a**, **b**) Pre- and postoperative lateral view of sagittal synostosis correction. (**c**, **d**) Pre- and postoperative superior view of sagittal synostosis correction. (**e**) Intraoperative view of coronal incision. (**f**) Markings for removal of sagittal suture and barrel staves. (**g**) Following osteotomy and biparietal expansion. (**h**) Markings for removal of posterior vault and barrel staves. (**i**) Inset and rotation of posterior vault with resorbable plate and screw fixation

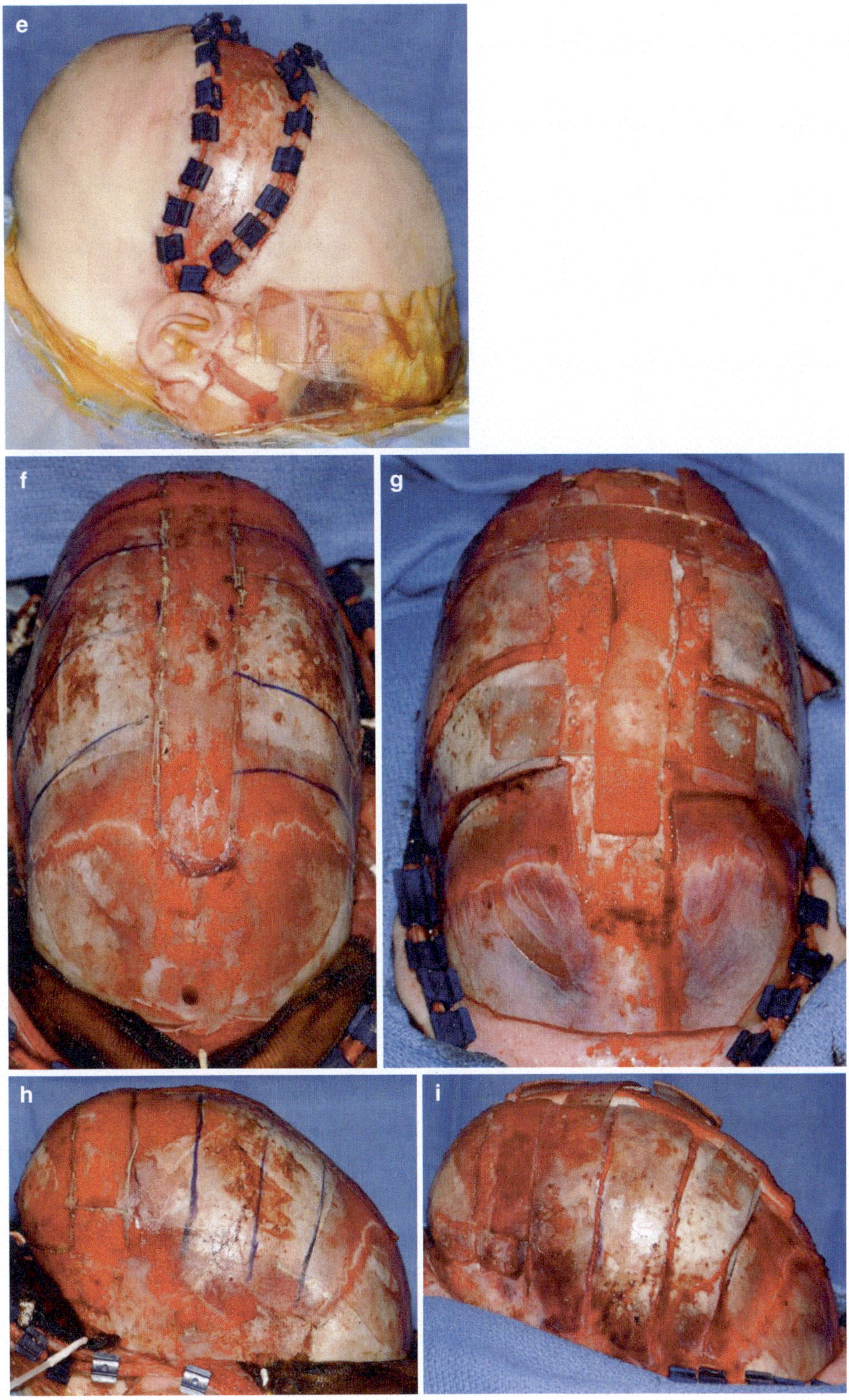

Fig. 36.9 (continued)

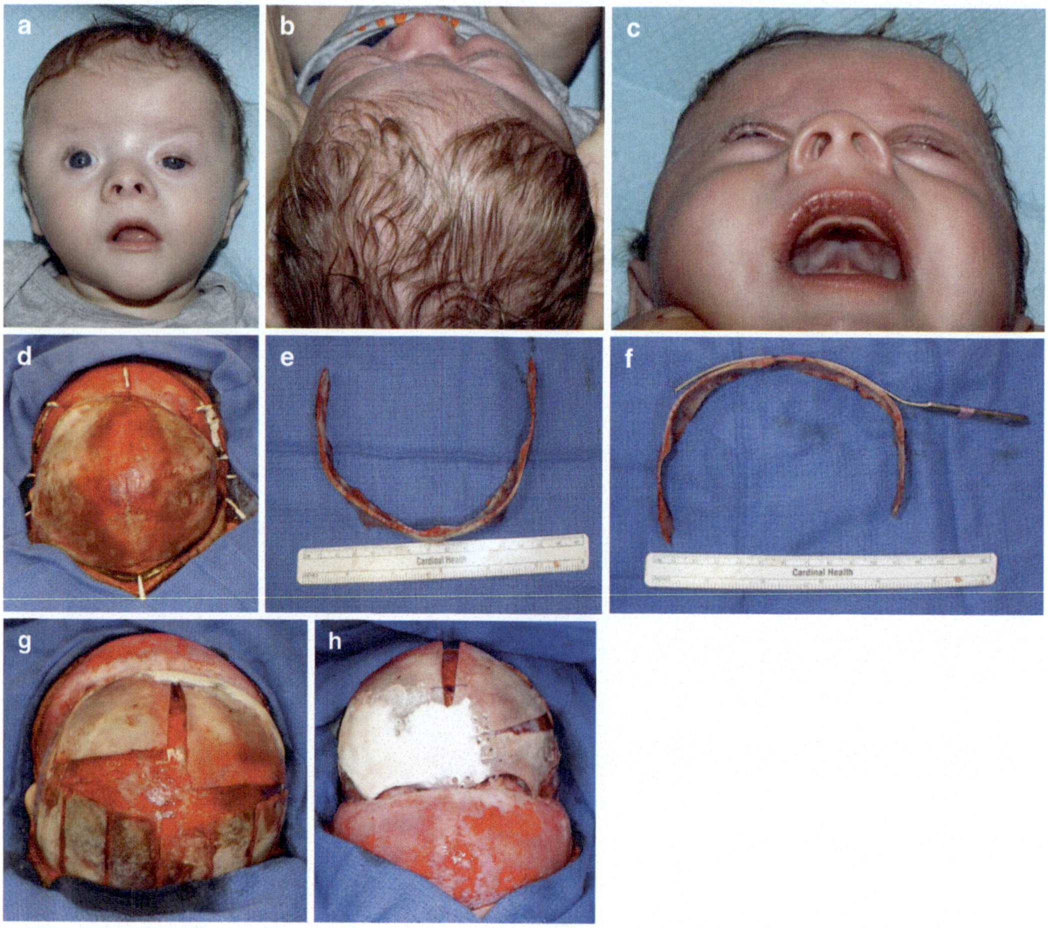

Fig. 36.10 (**a**) Frontal view of child with right unilateral synostosis. (**b**) Superior view of child with right unilateral synostosis. (**c**) Inferior view of child with right unilateral synostosis. (**d**) Intraoperative superior view of right unilateral synostosis. (**e**) Superior view of orbital bandeau showing recession of right supraorbital region. (**f**) Superior view of recontoured orbital bandeau with Marchac Bar to show contour. (**g**) Superior view showing expansion of vault with barrel staves and securing of frontal bones with resorbable plates and screws. (**h**) Frontal view of reshaped unilateral coronal synostosis and additional contouring with calcium phosphate cement

bandeau are necessary for adequate and advancement and reshaping.

- If true hypotelorism is present, the bandeau can be split at the midline and an autogenous cranial bone graft placed between the segments.
- The orbital bandeau can then be secured to the parietal bone with resorbable plates and screws extending from the tenon extensions. Evaluating the advancement of the bandeau for symmetry and expansion is done by retracting the frontal lobes and assessing the length of the gap between the anterior cranial fossa and the bandeau both laterally and at the orbits.
- Barrel staving is often needed bilaterally to widen the temporal and parietal bones prior to fixation of the frontal bones (Fig. 36.12).

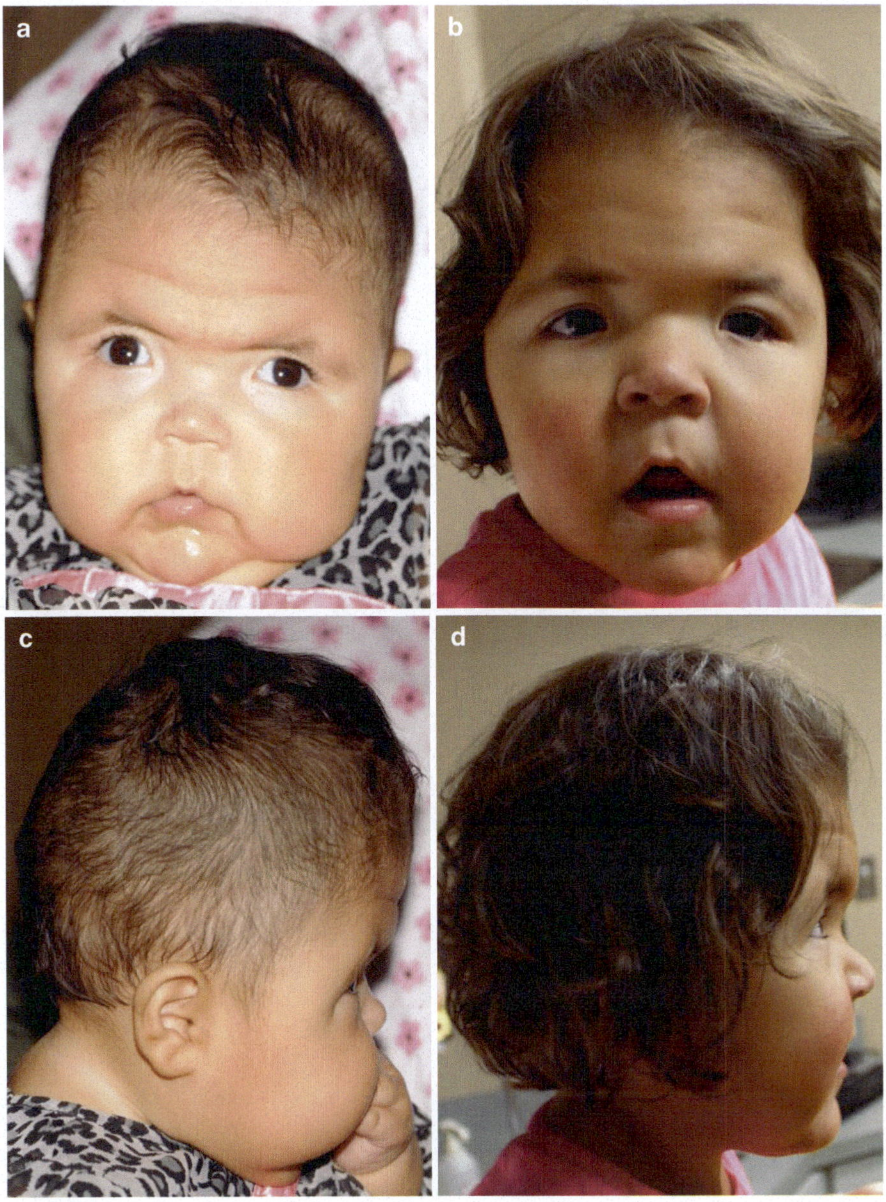

Fig. 36.11 (**a**, **b**) Pre- and postoperative frontal view of child with bilateral coronal synostosis. (**c**, **d**) Pre- and postoperative lateral view of child with bilateral coronal synostosis. (**e**) Superior view following removal of anterior cranial vault and supraorbital bandeau and expansion of barrel staves. (**f**) Lateral view of complete reconstruction showing advancement of frontal bones and supraorbital bandeau with resorbable plate and screw fixation

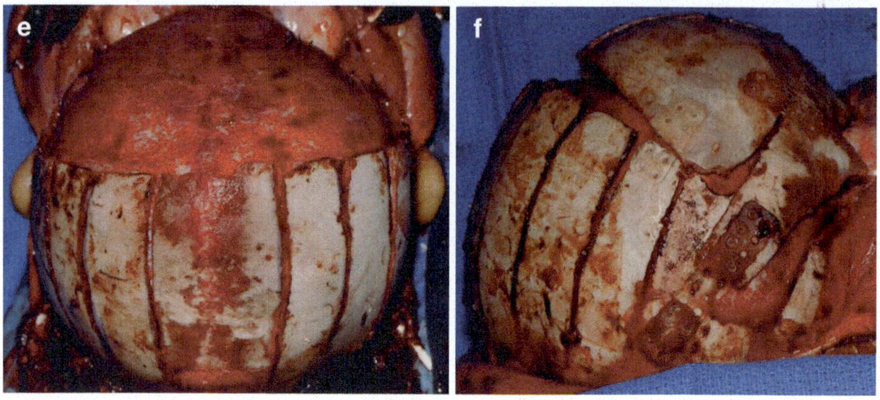

Fig. 36.11 (continued)

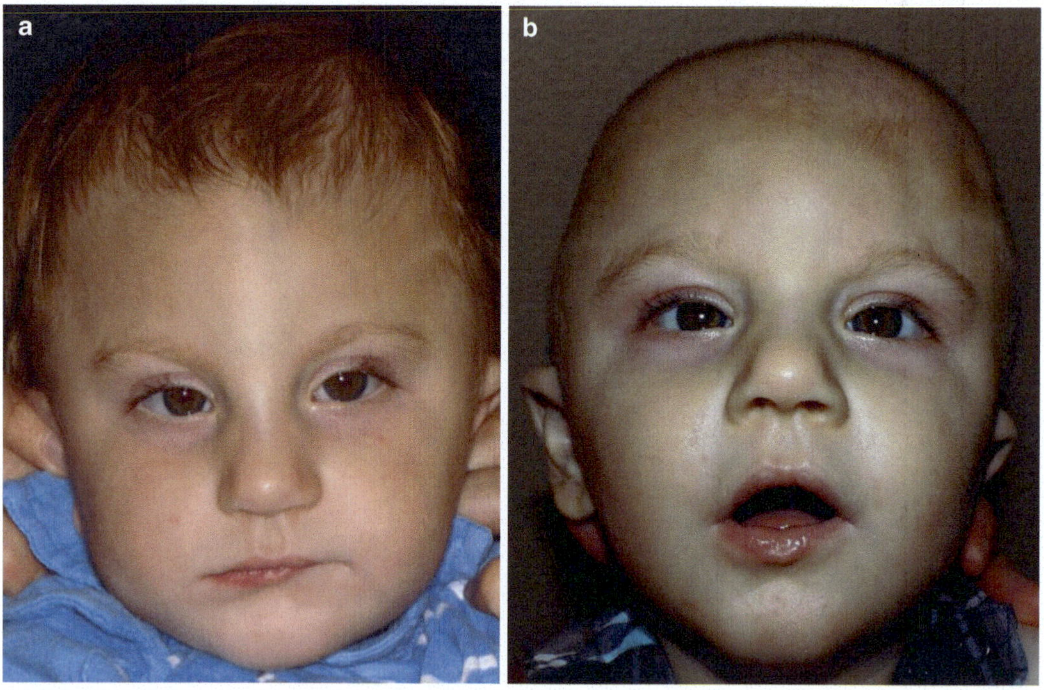

Fig. 36.12 (**a**, **b**) Pre- and postoperative frontal view of child with metopic synostosis. (**c**, **d**) Pre- and postoperative superior view of child with metopic synostosis. (**e**) Markings for removal of metopic suture, frontal bones, and barrel staves. (**f**) Superior view following removal of anterior cranial vault and supraorbital bandeau and expansion at barrel staves. (**g**) Superior view of frontal bones and supraorbital bandeau prior to reshaping. (**h**, **i**) Superior and frontal view of orbital bandeau following reshaping and placement of resorbable plates and screws. (**j**) Frontal/superior view of supraorbital bandeau fixated into place following reshaping. (**k**) Superior view of supraorbital bandeau fixated into place following reshaping with retraction of the frontal lobe to assess distance and symmetry of advancement. (**l**, **m**) Lateral and frontal view following complete reconstruction

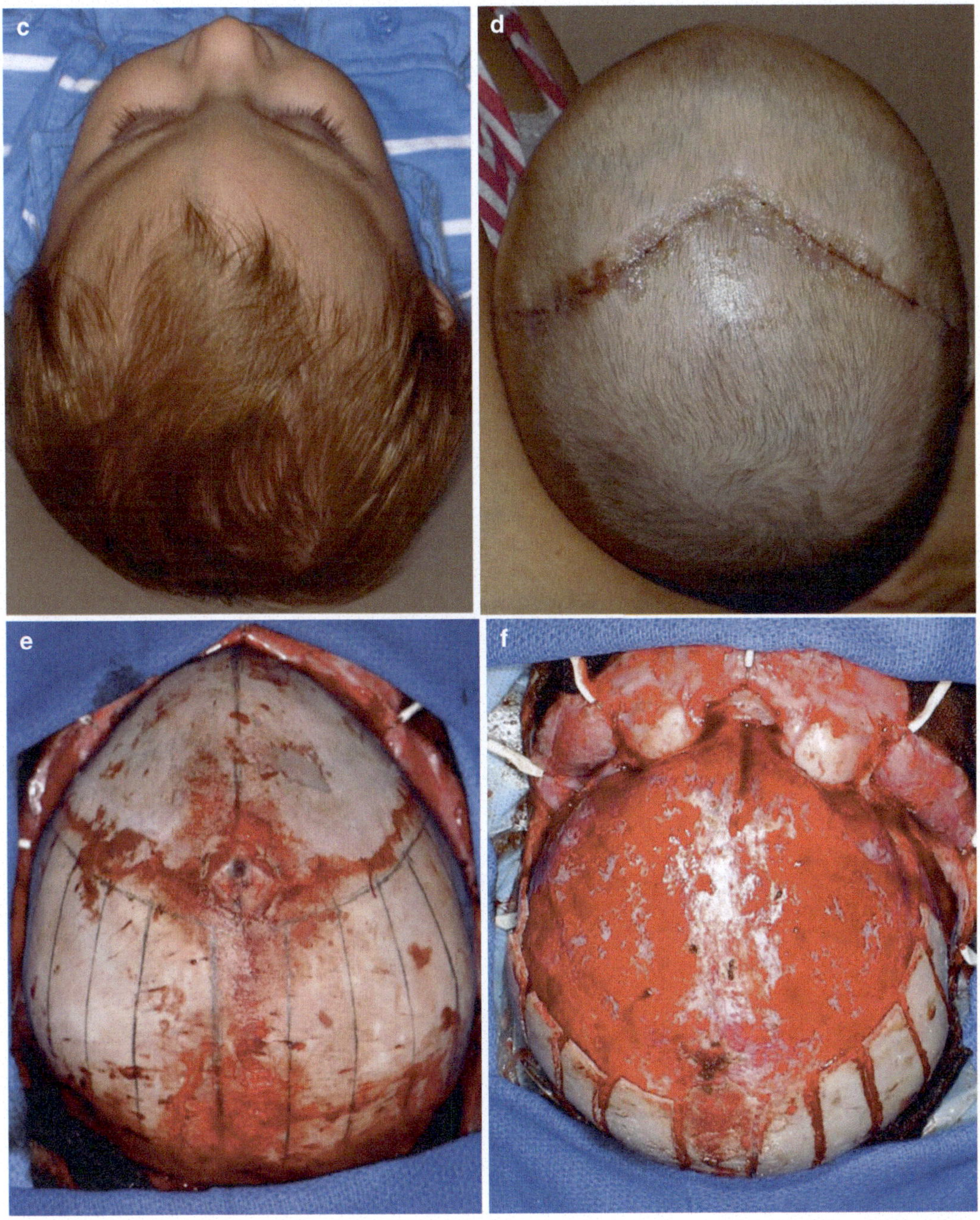

Fig. 36.12 (continued)

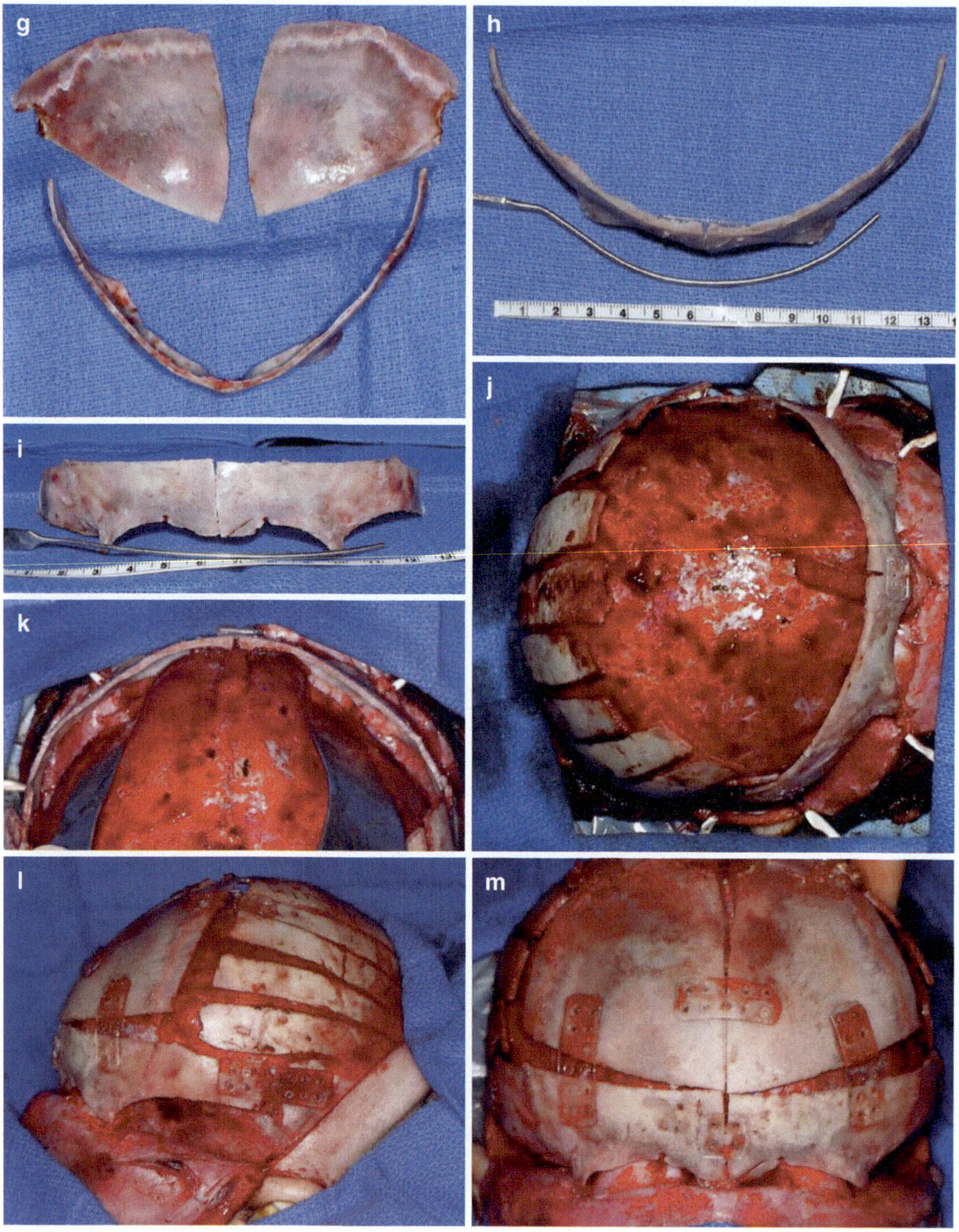

Fig. 36.12 (continued)

36.7.2.5 Unilateral Lambdoid Synostosis

- Surgical positioning, approach, and initial osteotomy design is similar to that previously described for sagittal synostosis in the prone position.
- The posterior cranial vault is then removed and reshaped to create a natural form.

36.8 Postoperative Care

Once the vault reshaping is completed, the authors advocate placement of a flap Jackson-Pratt (JP) drain in the subperiosteal plane that exits directly behind the ear and is attached to bulb suction. The periosteum and temporalis muscles are then closed with a 3-0 Vicryl sutures. The subcutaneous layer is then approximated with 4-0 Vicryl sutures in an interrupted fashion. The skin is then closed with skin adhesive such as cyanoacrylate. Following closure, a light head wrap is placed using Kerlix and Coban wrap. Once the patient is turned back over to anesthesia, the authors advocate transferring the patient to the pediatric intensive care unit while still intubated. A CT scan of the head is then obtained at 6–8 h postoperatively to check for possible subdural hemorrhage, possible hydrocephalus, and to confirm position of cranial vault reshaping. Once the postoperative CT scan is reviewed and shows no abnormalities, the patient can be extubated. A majority of the patients at the authors' institution spend 1–2 days in the PICU and 1–2 days on the pediatric floor. The average length of stay is 3 days. Once the patient is tolerating per os (po), voiding normally, a majority of the periorbital swelling is decreased, and the drain is removed; the patient may be discharged home.

36.9 Complications

Craniosynostosis repair is a safe and reliable procedure considering the invasiveness. Nguyen and colleagues utilized the Agency for Healthcare Research and Quality (AHRQ), Healthcare Cost and Utilization Project (HCUP), and Kids' Inpatient Database (KID) for 1997, 2000, 2003, and 2006 in order to look at the complication rates associated with cranial vault remodeling. They identified 3426 patients undergoing craniosynostosis repair, and a majority of these procedures (98%) were performed in teaching centers in urban areas. They found a mortality rate of less than 1% nationwide and an overall complication rate of 10% across all age groups. The mean hospital stay was 4.2 days, and the two most common complications were hematoma/hemorrhage and airway/respiratory failure [60].

At the authors' institution, a similar study was conducted on 100 consecutive craniosynostosis repairs showing good long-term results with a low complication rate. Out of 100 patients, most of the complications were mild and included two hematomas, two wound infections, one subgaleal abscess, six dural tears, three patients requiring reoperation for residual deformity, four cases requiring coronal scar revision, and one sagittal sinus bleed. Out of the 100 cases, there was 1 intraoperative death due to intraoperative pacemaker failure and was unrelated to the actual craniosynostosis repair. The most common complications associated with craniosynostosis repair during the operative, early postoperative, and late postoperative periods are listed in Table 36.1. Below we will discuss some of the rare yet most severe intraoperative complications encountered during transcranial procedures.

The most serious intraoperative complications to occur during a transcranial approach include venous air embolism, hemorrhage, dural tears, and death, though all of these are exceedingly rare. Venous air embolism occurs when diploic channels are exposed during cranial vault osteotomies. Air can then enter through these channels and into venous circulation till it reaches the right atrium. In approximately 35% of the population, a patent foramen ovale can also exist. If a patient has a patent foramen ovale, and a venous air embolism occurs, pulmonary hypertension and increased right atrial pressure can result, therefore creating a right to left shunt. Air can then pass directly into the coronary or cerebral circulation and possibly cause profound hypotension and, in rare cases, cardiovascular collapse [66,

Table 36.1 Most common complications

Intraoperative	Early postoperative	Late postoperative
Excessive blood loss	Bleeding	Incisional alopecia
Subdural hematoma	Hematoma	Hypertrophic scarring
Cerebrospinal fluid loss	Corneal abrasion	Skull and orbital irregularities
Anesthetic complications	Stitch abscess	Diplopia, strabismus
Periorbital injury	Cerebrospinal fluid leak	Sterile abscess secondary to plate hydrolysis
Death	Volume and electrolyte disturbances (SIADH/CSW syndromes)	
	Infection/meningitis	
	Loss of vision	
	Airway obstruction	
	Death	

67]. Symptomatic venous air embolism is a rare occurrence. Meyer et al. reported life-threatening air emboli in 2.6%, and the Royal Children's Hospital in Melbourne, Australia, reported only four cases of symptomatic air emboli in over 1000 transcranial cases [68]. If venous air embolism is suspected, the head of the bed should be lowered below the heart, bone wax should be used to control bleeding from diploic channels, the surgical site should be irrigated, the patient should be placed on 100% oxygen, and surgery should be ceased until resolution of symptoms. In severe cases, air can be removed through the central venous catheters. If cardiac collapse ensues, the patient can undergo closed cardiac massage to force air into the pulmonary circulation or open massage with possible aspiration of intracardiac air [66, 68].

Hemorrhage during these lengthy procedures was discussed previously in regard to blood transfusion protocols. It is important to remember that blood loss begins with scalp incision and, from then on, continues as constant ooze. Blood loss can also increase during bone osteotomies. The best way to manage blood loss is by prevention and continuous monitoring of losses for replacement [66]. At the authors' institution, meticulous attention is paid to blood loss prevention by the use of local anesthetic, reverse Trendelenburg, warming protocols to maintain normothermia, cauterizing bleeding areas along the coronal flap, use of bone wax on emissary veins when necessary, local measures to prevent bleeding from the dura, and operating room efficiency to reduce surgical time. One of the most worrisome sources of hemorrhage can be from the dural venous sinuses. This is more common in syndromic patients or those with severely dysplastic cranial deformities. Dural venous sinus tears are usually managed with local repair or maintaining pressure on the tear with delayed vascular repair [60, 61, 66].

Tearing of the dura during surgical dissection or craniotomy has been reported in 5–60% of cases [69–72]. Like dural venous sinus tears, lacerations of the dura occur more often in syndromic children or those with severely dysplastic cranial deformities due to the difficulty of dissection. Most often, these dural lacerations are easily repaired by primary closure. If the dural lacerations are large in size or challenging to close, a patch or use of a sealant such as fibrin glue may be necessary [66, 73].

Transcranial procedures have been proven to be safe and effective, but are not without risk. Most importantly, one must be able to recognize and address complications quickly when they do arise.

Conclusion

Craniofacial surgery has been evolving since the 1960s. It first began with detailed description of transcranial surgical techniques. In the present day, technology is evolving at a rapid pace to allow better assessment through imaging techniques and improved surgical planning utilizing 3D planning and the construction of surgical guides. In many cases, these advances have helped to improve accuracy, reduce operative times, and aid in the prediction of possible complications. Though craniofacial surgery is relatively safe, it is not without the risk of significant morbidity and mortality. Further investigation is necessary in order to advance the specialty, reduce risks, and help prevent sequela.

References

1. Ruiz RL, Ritter AM, Turvey TA, Costello BJ, Ricalde P. Nonsyndromic craniosynostosis: diagnosis and contemporary surgical management. Oral Maxillofac Surg Clin North Am. 2004;16(4):447–63.
2. Kirmi O, Lo SJ, Johnson D, Anslow P. Craniosynostosis: a radiological and surgical perspective. Semin Ultrasound CT MR. 2009;30(6): 492–512.
3. Ghali GE, Sinn DP. Nonsyndromic craniosynostosis. In: Miloro M, Ghali GE, Larsen PE, Waite P, editors. Peterson's principles of oral and maxillofacial surgery, vol. 2. 2nd ed. Ontario: BC Decker; 2004. p. 887–900.
4. Virchow R. Uber den cretinismus, nametlich in Franken, under uber pathologische. Schdelformen Verk Phys Med Gessellsch Wurxburg. 1851;2(2):230–71.
5. Singer S, Bower C, Southall P, et al. Craniosynostosis in Western Australia, 1980–1994. Am J Med Genet. 1999;83(5):382–7.
6. Boyadjiev S, International Craniosynostosis Consortium. Genetic analysis of non-syndromic craniosynostosis. Orthod Craniofac Res. 2007;10(3):129–37.
7. Agochukwu NB, Solomon BD, Muenke M. Hearing loss in syndromic craniosynostoses: otologic manifestations and clinical findings. Int J Pediatr Otorhinolaryngol. 2014;78(12):2037–47.
8. Renier D, Sainte-Rose C, Marchac D, Hirsch J-F. Intracranial pressure in craniostenosis. J Neurosurg. 1982;57(3):370–7.
9. Marchac D, Renier D. Treatment of craniosynostosis in infancy. Clin Plast Surg. 1987;14.(0094–1298 (Print):61–72.
10. Renier D, Lajeunie E, Arnaud E, Marchac D. Management of craniosynostoses. (0256-7040 (Print). Childs Nerv Syst. 2000;16(10–11):645–58.
11. Arnaud E, Renier D, Marchac D. Prognosis for mental function in scaphocephaly. J Neurosurg. 1995;83(3):476–9.
12. Ghali GE, Banker AR. Nonsyndromic craniosynostosis. In: Miloro G, Larsen W, editors. Peterson's principles of oral and maxillofacial surgery, vol. 2. 3rd ed. Shelton, CT: People's Medical Publishing House; 2012. p. 979–94.
13. Baird LC, Gonda D, Cohen SR, et al. Craniofacial reconstruction as a treatment for elevated intracranial pressure. Childs Nerv Syst. 2012;28(3):411–8.
14. Ghali GE, Sinn DP, Tantipasawasin S. Management of nonsyndromic craniosynostosis. Atlas Oral Maxillofac Surg Clin North Am. 2002;10(1):1–41.
15. Badve CA, K MM, Iyer RS, Ishak GE, Khanna PC. Craniosynostosis: imaging review and primer on computed tomography. Pediatr Radiol. 2013;43(6):728–42.
16. Cohen SR, Persing JA. Intracranial pressure in single-suture craniosynostosis. Cleft Palate Craniofac J. 1998;35(3):194–6.
17. Turvey TA Ruiz RL. Craniosynostosis and craniofacial dysostosis. In: Fonseca RJ, Stephen B Baker Wolford LM, ed. Oral and maxillofacial surgery. Philadelphia: WB Saunders; 2000:195–220.
18. Sgouros S. Skull vault growth in craniosynostosis. Childs Nerv Syst. 2005;21(10):861–70.
19. Hayward R. Venous hypertension and craniosynostosis. Childs Nerv Syst. 2005;21(10):880–8.
20. Gault DT, Renier D, Marchac D, Ackland FM, Jones BM. Intracranial volume in children with craniosynostosis. J Craniofac Surg. 1990;1(1):1–3.
21. Gault DT, Renier D, Marchac D, Jones BM. Intracranial pressure and intracranial volume in children with craniosynostosis. Plast Reconstr Surg. 1992;90(3):377–81. 0032-1052 (Print)
22. Cinalli G, Sainte-Rose C, Kollar EM, et al. Hydrocephalus and craniosynostosis. J Neurosurg. 1998;88(2):209–14.
23. Pattisapu JV, Gegg CA, Olavarria G, Johnson KK, Ruiz RL, Costello BJ. Craniosynostosis: diagnosis and surgical management. Atlas Oral Maxillofac Surg Clin North Am. 2010;18(2):77–91.
24. Stavrou P, Sgouros S, Willshaw HE, Goldin JH, Hockley AD, Wake MJC. Visual failure caused by raised intracranial pressure in craniosynostosis. Childs Nerv Syst. 1997;13(2):64–7.
25. Baranello G, Vasco G, Ricci D, Mercuri E. Visual function in nonsyndromic craniosynostosis: past, present, and future. Childs Nerv Syst. 2007;23(12):1461–5.
26. Posnick JC. Anterior plagiocephaly: unilateral coronal synostosis and skull molding. In: Posnick JC, editor. Craniofacial and maxillofacial surgery in children and young adults, vol. 1. First ed. Philadelphia: W.B. Saunders Company; 2000. p. 128.
27. Samra F, Paliga JT, Tahiri Y, et al. The prevalence of strabismus in unilateral coronal synostosis. Childs Nerv Syst. 2015;31(4):589–96.
28. Gosain AK, Steele MA, McCarthy JG, Thorne CH. A prospective study of the relationship between strabismus and head posture in patients with frontal plagiocephaly. Plast Reconstr Surg. 1996;97(5):881–91.
29. Becker DB, Petersen JD, Kane AA, Cradock MM, Pilgram TK, Marsh JL. Speech, cognitive, and behavioral outcomes in nonsyndromic craniosynostosis. Plast Reconstr Surg. 2005;116(2):400–7. 1529-4242 (Electronic)

30. Kapp-Simon KA. Mental development and learning disorders in children with single suture craniosynostosis. Cleft Palate Craniofac J. 1998;35(3):197–203.
31. Kapp-Simon KA, Leroux B, Cunningham M, Speltz ML. Multisite study of infants with single-suture craniosynostosis: preliminary report of presurgery development. Cleft Palate Craniofac J. 2005;42(4):377–84.
32. Chieffo D, Tamburrini G, Massimi L, et al. Long-term neuropsychological development in single-suture craniosynostosis treated early. J Neurosurg Pediatr. 2010;5(3):232–7.
33. Kapp-Simon KA, Collett BR, Barr-Schinzel MA, et al. Behavioral adjustment of toddler and preschool-aged children with single-suture craniosynostosis. Plast Reconstr Surg. 2012;130(3):635–47.
34. Da Costa AC, Anderson VA, Holmes AD, et al. Longitudinal study of the neurodevelopmental characteristics of treated and untreated nonsyndromic craniosynostosis in infancy. Childs Nerv Syst. 2013;29(6):985–95.
35. Warschausky S, Angobaldo J, Kewman D, Buchman S, Muraszko KM, Azengart A. Early development of infants with untreated metopic craniosynostosis. Plast Reconstr Surg. 2005;115(6):1518–23. 1529-4242 (Electronic)
36. Association ACPA. Parameters for the evaluation and treatment of patients with cleft lip/palate or other craniofacial anomalie. Chapel Hill, NC: American Cleft Palate-Craniofacial Association; 2009.
37. McCarthy JG, Warren SM, Bernstein J, et al. Parameters of care for craniosynostosis. Cleft Palate Craniofac J. 2011;49(S1):1S–24S.
38. Ghali GE, Woerner JE, Dashow JE. Surgical management of craniosynostosis, vol. 2. 3rd ed. USA: Elsevier; 2017.
39. Thomas K, Hughes C, Johnson D, Das S. Anesthesia for surgery related to craniosynostosis: a review. Part 1. Paediatr Anaesth. 2012;22(11):1033–41. 1460-9592 (Electronic)
40. Kliegman R, Nelson WE. Nelson textbook of pediatrics. Philadelphia, PA: Elsevier/Saunders; 2011.
41. Posnick JC. Brachycephaly: bilateral coronal synostosis without midface deficiency. In: Posnick JC, editor. Craniofacial and maxillofacial surgery in children and young adults, vol. 1. First ed. Philadelphia: W.B. Saunders Company; 2000. p. 249–68.
42. Caccamese J, Costello BJ, Ruiz RL, Ritter AM. Positional plagiocephaly: evaluation and management. Oral Maxillofac Surg Clin. 2004;16(4):439–46.
43. Rozovsky K, Udjus K, Wilson N, Barrowman NJ, Simanovsky N, Miller E. Cranial ultrasound as a first-line imaging examination for craniosynostosis. Pediatrics. 2016;137:e20152230. 1098-4275 (Electronic)
44. Regelsberger J, Delling G, Helmke K, Tsokos M, Kammler G, Kränzlein H, Westphal M. Ultrasound in the diagnosis of craniosynostosis. J Craniofac Surg. 2006;17(4):623–5. 1049-2275 (Print)
45. Krimmel M, Will B, Wolff M, Kluba S, et al. Value of high-resolution ultrasound in the differential diagnosis of scaphocephaly and occipital plagiocephaly. Int J Oral Maxillofac Surg. 2012;41(7):797–800. 1399-0020 (Electronic)
46. Steinbacher DM. Three-dimensional analysis and surgical planning in craniomaxillofacial surgery. J Oral Maxillofac Surg. 2015;73(12 Suppl):S40–56. 1531-5053 (Electronic)
47. Chim H, Wetjen N, Mardini S. Virtual surgical planning in craniofacial surgery. Semin Plast Surg. 2014;28(3):150–8. 1535-2188 (Print)
48. Tahiri Y, Taylor JA. In support of using computer-aided design and modeling for periorbital osteotomies. J Craniofac Surg. 2015;26(1):100–3. 1536-3732 (Electronic)
49. Xia JJ, Gateno J, Teichgraeber JF. Three-dimensional computer-aided surgical simulation for maxillofacial surgery. Atlas Oral Maxillofac Surg Clin North Am. 2005;13(1):25–39.
50. Vander Sloten J, Degryse K, Gobin R, Van der Perre G, Mommaerts MY. Interactive simulation of cranial surgery in a computer aided design environment. J Cranio-Maxillofac Surg. 1996;24(2):122–9.
51. Saber NR, Phillips J, Looi T, et al. Generation of normative pediatric skull models for use in cranial vault remodeling procedures. Childs Nerv Syst. 2012;28(3):405–10.
52. Seruya M, Borsuk DE, Khalifian S, Carson BS, Dalesio NM, Dorafshar AH. Computer-aided design and manufacturing in craniosynostosis surgery. J Craniofac Surg. 2013;24(4):1100–5. 1536-3732 (Electronic)
53. Soleman J, Thieringer F, Beinemann J, Kunz C, Guzman R. Computer-assisted virtual planning and surgical template fabrication for frontoorbital advancement. Neurosurg Focus. 2015;38(5):E5. 1092-0684 (Electronic)
54. Ghali GE, Zakhary G. Craniosynostosis: esthetic protocol in open technique. Ann Maxillofac Surg. 2013;3(1):62–5. 2231-0746 (Print)
55. Esparza J, Hinojosa J. Complications in the surgical treatment of craniosynostosis and craniofacial syndromes: apropos of 306 transcranial procedures. Childs Nerv Syst. 2008;24(12):1421–30. 1433-0350 (Electronic)
56. Koh JL, Gries H. Perioperative management of pediatric patients with craniosynostosis. Anesthesiol Clin. 2007;25(3):465–81. 1932-2275 (Print)
57. Anesthesiologists ASo. Standards for basic anesthetic monitoring. In: Anesthesiologists ASo, editor. 2015. http://www.asahq.org2015:4.
58. Stricker PA, Fiadjoe JE. Anesthesia for craniofacial surgery in infancy. Anesthesiol Clin. 2014;32(1):215–35. 1932-2275 (Print)
59. Hughes C, Thomas K, Johnson D, Das S. Anesthesia for surgery related to craniosynostosis: a review. Part 2. Paediatr Anaesth. 2013;23(1):22–7. 1460-9592 (Electronic)

60. Nguyen C, Hernandez-Boussard T, Khosla RK, Curtin CM. A national study on craniosynostosis surgical repair. Cleft Palate Craniofac J. 2012;50(5):555–60.
61. Zakhary GM, Montes DM, Woerner JE, Notarianni C, Ghali GE. Surgical correction of craniosynostosis. A review of 100 cases. J Craniomaxillofac Surg. 2014;42(8):1684–91. 1878-4119 (Electronic)
62. McCarthy JG, Epstein F, Sadove M, et al. Early surgery for craniofacial synostosis: an 8-year experience. Plast Reconstr Surg. 1989;73:521–33.
63. Cohen SR, Holmes RE, Meltzer HS, Nakaji P. Immediate cranial vault reconstruction with bioresorbable plates following endoscopically assisted sagittal synostectomy. J Craniofac Surg. 2002;13(4):578–82. discussion 583-574
64. Pietrzak WS, Kumar M, Eppley BL. The influence of temperature on the degradation rate of LactoSorb copolymer. J Craniofac Surg. 2003;14(2):176–83.
65. Ahmad N, Lyles J, Panchal J, Deschamps-Braly J. Outcomes and complications based on experience with resorbable plates in pediatric craniosynostosis patients. J Craniofac Surg. 2008;19(3):855–60.
66. Greensmith AL, Meara JG, Holmes AD, Lo P. Complications related to cranial vault surgery. Oral Maxillofac Surg Clin North Am. 2004;16(4):465–73.
67. Phillips RJ, Mulliken JB. Venous air embolism during a craniofacial procedure. Plast Reconstr Surg. 1988;82:155–9.
68. Meyer P, Renier D, Arnaud E, Jarreau MM, et al. Blood loss during repair of craniosynostosis. Br J Anaesth. 1993;71:854–7.
69. Poole MD. Complications in craniofacial surgery. Br J Plast Surg. 1988;41:608–13.
70. David DJ, Cooter RD. Craniofacial infection in 10 years of transcranial surgery. Plast Reconstr Surg. 1987;80:213–23. 0032-1052 (Print)
71. Munro IR, Sabatier RE. An analysis of 12 years of craniomaxillofacial surgery in Toronto. Plast Reconstr Surg. 1985;76:29.
72. Marchac D, Renier D. Complications. In: Marchac D, Renier D, editors. Craniofacial surgery for craniosynostosis. Boston: Little, Brown and Company; 1982.
73. Marchac D, Renier D. Fibrin glue in craniofacial surgery. J Craniofac Surg. 1990;1(1):32–4. 1049-2275 (Print)

Microvascular Flap Management During Maxillofacial Surgery

37

Roderick Youngdo Kim and Brent Benson Ward

Abstract

The need for oral and maxillofacial surgeons to replace and reconstruct defects of the head and neck is common. Trauma, pathology, and congenital etiologies may all lead to the necessity of pedicled or free vascularized flaps. These procedures are a growing part of the specialty and have become important skills in the armamentarium of many maxillofacial surgeons. Although there is plenty of literature in the method of harvest and the usage of each flap, the day-to-day care of these flaps and the perioperative considerations have not been as frequently outlined. In this chapter, we will discuss perioperative management of patients with flap reconstruction.

37.1 Introduction

The need for oral and maxillofacial surgeons to replace and reconstruct defects of the head and neck is common. Trauma, pathology, and congenital etiologies may all lead to the necessity of pedicled or free vascularized flaps. These procedures are a growing part of the specialty and have become important skills in the armamentarium of many maxillofacial surgeons. Although there is plenty of literature in the method of harvest and the usage of each flap, the day-to-day care of these flaps and the perioperative considerations have not been as frequently outlined. In this chapter, we will discuss perioperative management of patients with flap reconstruction.

37.2 Preoperative Assessment

As with any new patient visit, our initial meeting with the patient follows the typical history and physical exam. A medical history is important to establish the fitness of the patient who

R.Y. Kim (✉)
Former Resident, University of Michigan Oral and Maxillofacial Surgery, Current Fellow, Head and Neck Oncologic and Microvascular Reconstructive Surgery, John Peter Smith Hospital, Baylor Scott & White, Fort Worth, Texas, TX, USA
e-mail: Rodkim@umich.edu

B.B. Ward, M.D., D.D.S.
Department of Surgery, Section of Oral and Maxillofacial Surgery, University of Michigan, Ann Arbor, MI, USA
e-mail: Bward@med.umich.edu

© Springer International Publishing AG 2018
E.M. Ferneini, J.D. Bennett (eds.), *Perioperative Assessment of the Maxillofacial Surgery Patient*,
https://doi.org/10.1007/978-3-319-58868-1_37

will undergo a major surgery. Review of systems including functional assessments is particularly important, both as a way to optimize each patient's health prior to the surgery and as an indicator of the overall health of the patient. Indications of conditions that lead to atherosclerosis and claudication should be elicited, given the importance of vasculature associated with flaps.

Previous surgical history is also of importance when considering harvest of a flap. For example, relative contraindications for a pectoralis myocutaneous flap include if the patient has had recent subclavian cannulation, chest wall surgery, and axillary dissection, as it is generally considered that the muscle and vasculature are compromised. Total joint replacements of the shoulder, hips, or knees should be elicited for considering scapula, deep circumflex iliac artery, and fibula free flap, to avoid violation and contamination of the total joint prosthesis.

It is crucial to speak with patients regarding the extent of their surgery, including their perioperative expectations. A discussion regarding the "normal" recovery is important to make sure that the patient does not have unrealistic expectation of both esthetic and functional outcomes, as well as the donor site morbidity associated with the procedure. Furthermore, despite our best efforts, the disease itself may yield some permanent dysfunction in cases of advanced tumors, for example, and frank and clear conversations are important. In addition, many patients are unaware of the need for adjunctive procedures in addition to resection and reconstruction, such as extractions, blood transfusion, feeding tube placement/gastric tube placement and tracheostomy. It is also important to discuss with the patient the possibility of salvage flaps and additional indicated procedures. The number of additional preoperative visits, needed studies, length of hospital stay, and anticipated follow-up regimen are also important discussions for setting expectations. It is sometimes beneficial to have a preoperative appointment after the initial visit to discuss many of these points further and reassure that the appropriate preoperative studies are completed. Adjunctive staff can also speak with the patient over the phone to discuss any remaining questions prior to the surgery date and save time in clinic. Having a clear idea of their perioperative course reassures the patient and also allows for the recruitment of appropriate support beyond the hospital if needed. It is important to understand family or other support dynamics, as many patients undergoing these surgeries will need adjunctive treatments, for example, radiation/chemotherapy, in the postoperative setting.

An important aspect of the patient's social history is their occupation, which may on occasion have bearing on the flap choice. Considerations should be given for patients who use their hands or wrist frequently for their occupation when using radial forearm free flap, for which one of the complications include contracture. Their dominant hand should also be noted and preferably the contralateral arm used. Furthermore, while healing, they will not be able to perform jobs that necessitate exposure or frequently cleansing of the hands and wrist, especially while wearing the volar splint to allow the skin graft to take. For lower extremity flaps, consideration may be given to the ability to drive postoperatively: using the left leg leads to less potential for long-term disruption. For scapula free flaps, it would be of concern if the patient has an occupation that requires heavy usage of their shoulder, such as hairdresser or waiter. These examples are given as it is possible for surgeons focusing on the defect and the ideal reconstructive option to lose sight of the overall goal of return to optimal function in the most rapid fashion possible.

Finally, physical exam to verify the suitability of flap should be done in the clinic. One commonly described test is the Allen's test [1] for the radial forearm flap. After elevating the hand above the heart, the surgeon occludes the radial and ulnar arteries, while the patient mechanically exsanguinates the hand by opening and closing the hand. When the hand is pale, the surgeon continues to occlude the artery planned for harvest, whether it is the radial or ulnar. Typically, if the capillary refill of the hand is <12 s, it is considered safe to harvest the artery, and the palmar arch from the opposing artery is adequate for hand perfusion. Flap thickness is also reviewed for adequate bulk and tissue availability for the defect. For defects where the forearm flap may be too small, an anterolateral thigh (ALT) flap may be considered. However, in obese patients and females with preferential adipose tissue deposition, the ALT flap may be too bulky; therefore, other flaps such as parascapular fasciocutaneous flap should be considered.

37.3 Studies and Preoperative Review

For most pedicled or free flaps for oral and maxillofacial surgeons, preoperative imaging is not necessary. Computed tomography angiography (CTA) for free fibula flap is the most routine study to evaluate for normal three-vessel runoff: the peroneal, anterior, and posterior tibial arteries. Vessels are also verified for reconstitution at the feet. Furthermore, the peroneal take off from the posterior tibial artery can be checked and is useful for planning the reconstruction, such as the availability of the pedicle length (Fig. 37.1). CTA to assess the neck vessels is indicated in the previously operated neck where the question of recipient targets exists.

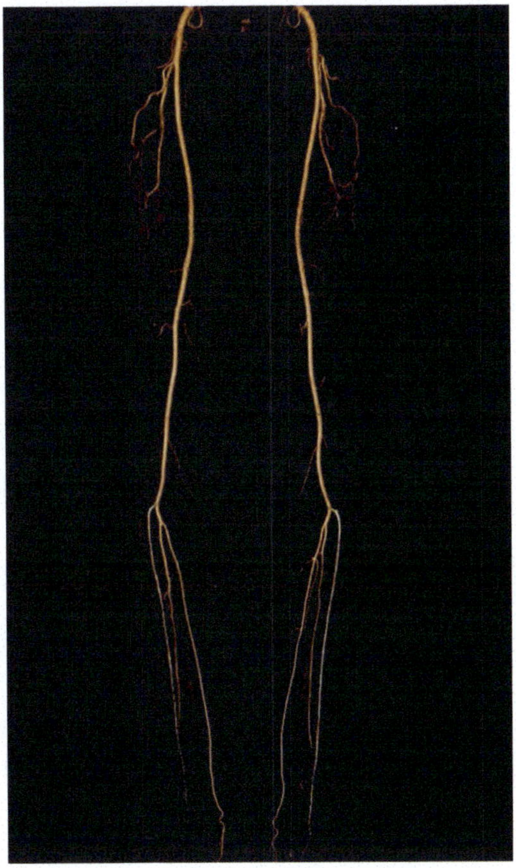

Fig. 37.1 CTA showing bilateral three-vessel runoff with normal take off of the peroneal vessels from posterior tibial artery

Recently there is a large push for preoperative health optimization, known as prehabilitation [2], which optimizes the health of the patient as much as possible prior to surgery. This includes emphasis toward increasing activity, pulmonary rehabilitation and smoking cessation, diet optimization, relaxation techniques, and information that provides support and education for the patient. Initial data in multiple randomized controlled trials show promise in improving patient outcomes and morbidity [3].

37.3.1 3D Planning

With the advent of 3D surgery planning, CT scans are now taken for diagnosis but also for medical modeling in bony reconstruction. Previously, stereolithographic (SLA) models were used to aid in plate bending and surgical planning. More recently, it is common for patients to undergo a CT of the scapula or hip in addition to the fibula for patient-specific custom cutting guides (Fig. 37.2). Furthermore, virtual surgical planning with engineers also allows planning of tumor margins. This has the advantage of 3D view and orientation. With the tumor margins expressed in 3D (Fig. 37.3), ideal tumor margins can be reviewed, and this allows resection without having to sacrifice significant amounts of uninvolved tissue. Furthermore, reconstruction planning can also be done simultaneously in a patient-specific way with the specific flap of choice. 3D planning allows for a more guided reconstruction and saves operating room time by providing custom surgical cutting guides for the resection as well as for reconstruction.

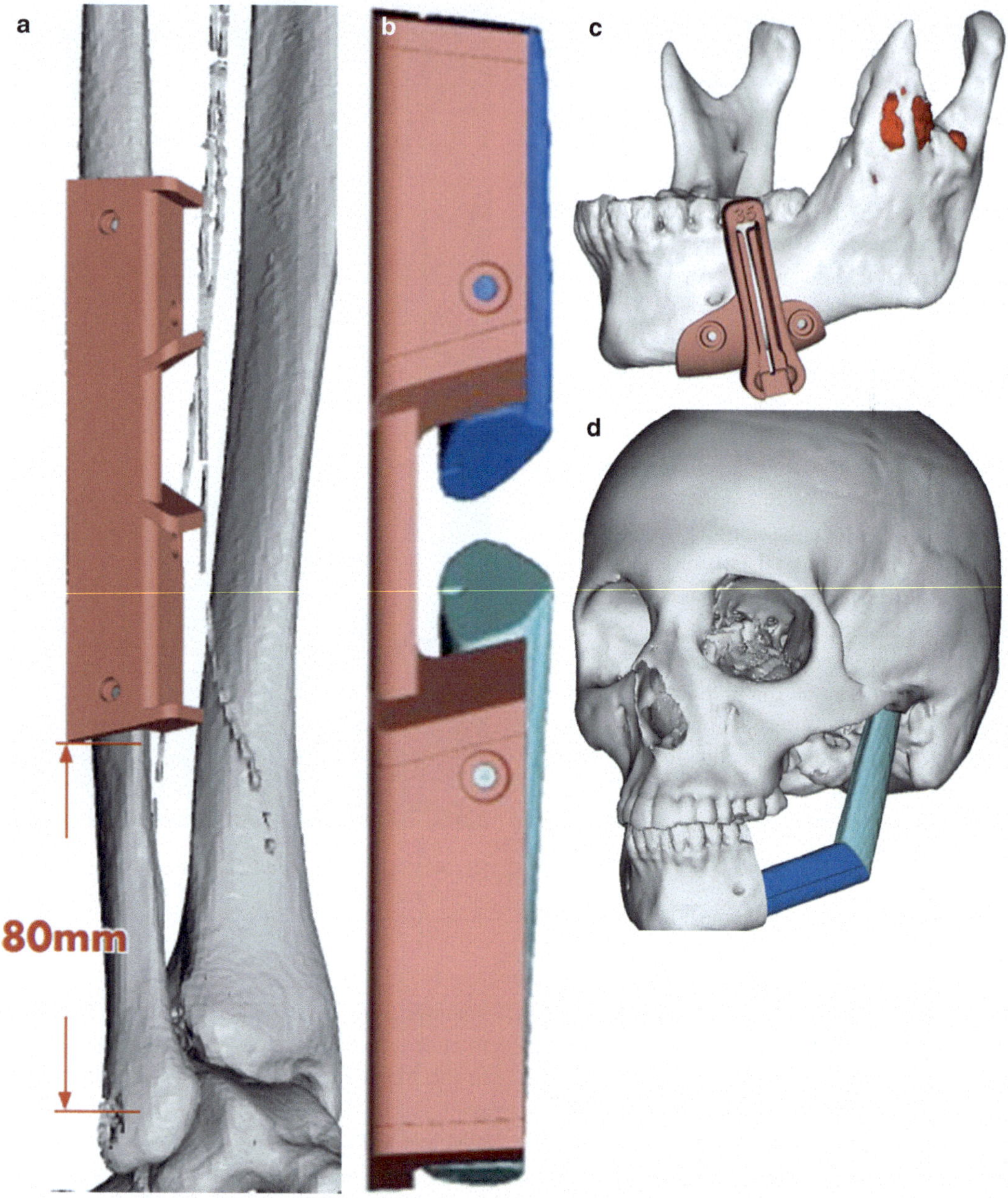

Fig. 37.2 Custom fibula cutting guide (**a**, **b**) and mandibular resection guide (**c**) from virtual surgical planning. Final planned mandibular reconstruction (**d**) (3D Systems Healthcare, Littleton, CO)

37.3.2 Preoperative Holding

The most important consideration in the preoperative holding environment is line access. It is very important to make sure that the patient does not receive an IV or arterial line on a site where surgery is planned. Overall, the extremity planned for flap is marked and not to be touched by anyone except for the surgical team.

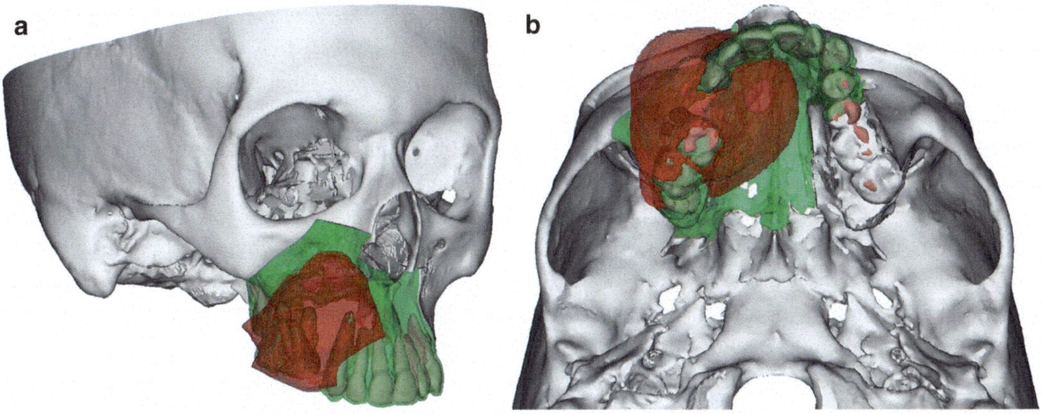

Fig. 37.3 Tumor represented in 3D with red and 1 cm margins planned for resection in green. (**a**) ¾ view. (**b**) Worm's eye view (3D Systems Healthcare, Littleton, CO)

37.4 Intraoperative Assessment

37.4.1 Anesthesia Care

During the initial phase of the surgery, long-acting muscle relaxants are not recommended, and this is clearly communicated with the anesthesiologists. Whether for vessel exploration in the neck or surgical margins nearing the facial nerve, the option to stimulate and evaluate nerve function is important and can be hampered by long-term muscle relaxants.

Additionally, it is important to have good communication with the anesthesia colleagues about fluids, pressors, and intraoperative medications management. There is a significant number of anecdotal recommendations but many with limited evidence for intraoperative care of vascularized free flap patients. For example, it is generally considered not ideal to use pressors during free tissue transfer surgery as this may lead to arterial insufficiency. Some advocate heparin usage, and in addition to preoperative 5000 units subcutaneously, surgeons utilize 500–1000 units intravenously prior to vessel separation. Blood transfusion for intraoperative anemia is also recommended to theoretically increase oxygen-carrying capacity and improve oxygenation of the flap [4]. There have also been recommendations for utilization of volume expanders such as colloids. However, there is belief that colloids can also lead to increased flap failure, perhaps due to increased bleeding risk [5].

Pattani et al. performed a literature review of intraoperative factors leading to free flap failure in head and neck reconstruction. In their study reviewing available flap failure literature, they noted factors that do show evidence in negative flap outcome. These include >7 L of intraoperative fluids, patients with significant medical comorbidity, and prolonged operative time of greater than 10 h. However, they saw no significant evidence in pressors, colloid usage, or avoiding hypotension in flap failure [6]. Some of these findings were further supported by Ettinger et al., who studied intraoperative fluid management, type of volume expanders, as well as other anesthesia care [7]. In this study, they saw significantly increased risk of any complications, when total fluids were greater than 5.5 L and when using colloids. Interestingly, there was no significant difference in odds ratio when colloids were stratified into individual types. Furthermore, they noted no significant increase in risk of any complication with pressor usage, although when separated by type of pressor, ephedrine had significantly increased risk. Lastly, usage of packed red blood cells (pRBC) also increased risk of any complication with flaps. However, when stratified to major versus minor complication, usage of fluids greater than 7 L and usage of pRBC were factors that remained statistically significant, while colloid usage had no significantly increased risk.

For transfusion, several authors have demonstrated that low preoperative hemoglobin levels can lead to adverse flap outcomes, typically when hemoglobin is <10 g/dL [8, 9]. However, Pattani et al. agreed with the previous literature that due to the fear of increased blood viscosity with pRBC, there is minimal support for correction of mild to moderate anemia [6]. Furthermore, multiple authors in head and neck reconstruction have noted that greater than three units of blood compared to non-transfused patient increased risk of negative outcomes including death [10, 11]. The reported threshold for transfusion of hgb <8 or hct <24 is based on critical care literature with outcome of death [12, 13], and there is paucity of data for transfusion criteria for flap survival. Notable head and neck threshold comes from Rosmiller et al., who reported that hct <25 for transfusion criteria did not negatively affect free flap outcome [14]. Therefore, this is a topic that requires further clarification through sound research. However, it is reasonable to consider transfusion at hct of 24, given the data currently shows no difference with flap outcomes with hct <25 but does show increased risk of death with hct <24.

Finally, in terms of heparin usage, Khouri et al. have noted no significant evidence in decreased thromboembolic risk for the flap when intraoperative heparin was used as luminal irrigation solution. However, they did note lower incidence of postoperative thrombosis when subcutaneous heparin was used [15]. A recent study by Lighthall et al. showed a significantly increased complication rate when thromboprophylaxis regimen was used compared with no postoperative anticoagulation [16]. However, they noted a higher flap salvage rate when the combination of aspirin with heparin/low molecular heparin or heparin drip was used. Therefore, the literature in this topic is controversial, and ultimately patient safety should be considered before flap survival. Bahl et al. from the University of Michigan studied chemoprophylaxis for venous thromboembolism (VTE) for head and neck surgery patients [17]. Specifically, for microvascular free tissue reconstruction patients, they noted that these patients had higher Caprini risk score, a score to determine VTE risk [18]. Furthermore, in patients who did not receive chemoprophylaxis, there were significantly higher incidences of VTE for all Caprini scores, compared to those who received chemoprophylaxis. Given that VTE can lead to pulmonary embolism and death and that microvascular tissue transfer patients have higher Caprini score, chemoprophylaxis should be administered, but therapeutic anticoagulation is likely unnecessary.

Based on these findings and more, the current recommendations are to minimize fluids to less than 7 L; colloids can be used but mostly albumin, while hydroxyethyl starch is rarely used. Use meticulous surgical techniques to minimize the need for packed red blood cells, but also transfuse if hct <24. Finally, preoperative subcutaneous heparin is recommended, but not routine intravenous heparin, and based on their Caprini risk score, patients should receive postoperative chemoprophylaxis to prevent VTE.

37.4.2 Harvest

A tourniquet is usually placed sterilely with limb protection sleeves underneath. Depending on the site, pressure is elevated from 250 to 350 mmHg. The site should be evaluated to make sure inadvertent placement of soft tissue is not pinched in the tourniquet. There are some data that shows the tourniquet time >120 min can lead to injury to soft tissue, nerve, and ischemic injuries [19]. Therefore, it is generally recommended to let down the tourniquet once every 2 h, for 15 min or longer.

After harvest of the flap is complete, whether pedicled or free, the tissue is wrapped in moist gauze, and the pedicle is kept moist. For osseous flaps, some surgeons perform the osteotomy, while the pedicle is intact. This allows ample time without compromise of the flap. However, there are some limitations of freedom, and inadvertent traction can cause damage of the pedicle.

Due to these limitations, many prefer to complete these tasks on the "back table" after dividing the pedicle. Regardless, prior to division, the tourniquet is deflated to allow for reperfusion, verify vascularity, and achieve hemostasis.

37.4.3 Microvascular

Typically, a partial or full inset of the flap is achieved prior to anastomosis. This allows improved stability of the pedicle's final location to verify that the inset does not lead to poor arc of rotation or kinking of the pedicle. The vessels are cleaned and are prepared at both ends of the anastomosis. An additional consideration is the need or desire to perform the anastomosis of two veins where this option exists. Two-vein anastomosis has been debated in terms of benefit for flap survival. While it makes intuitive sense that having a backup vein in case one fails would be beneficial, controversy to this approach exists [20]. Chen et al. were able to show significant decrease of take-backs for both vascular and venous insufficiency when using two-vessel anastomosis with minimal increase in operative time [21]. Opponents argue that a second anastomosis reduces blood flow, and animal models have shown stasis-induced thrombosis during microvascular repair [22–24]. It is true in the authors' experience that second vein anastomosis can lead intraoperative first vein thrombosis in some patients. Recent data from Heidekrueger et al., in a study of lower extremity reconstruction, did not note any significant difference in one- versus two-vein anastomosis, but they encouraged two-vein anastomosis when easily feasible [25]. Two-vein anastomosis can be considered for select patients or based on the surgeon's preference where concerns of venous compromise exist, and it does not lead to stasis or sluggish flow intraoperatively.

The use of indwelling venous Dopplers is a consideration for all flaps but especially in the buried flap patient. There are two main versions of the internal Doppler: Cook-Swartz Doppler probe (Cook Medical, Bloomington, IN) and GEM Flow Coupler (Synovis, Birmingham, AL). Cook-Schwartz Dopplers are small probes attached to silastic sheath and secured around the vein with Ligaclip, distal to the anastomosis (Fig. 37.4). GEM Flow Couplers are similar to traditional venous coupler, but the Doppler probe is attached to the coupler. These Dopplers are connected to an amplifier and continuously monitored by the nursing staff. Typically, the lines are secured with Tegaderm (3 M, Two Harbors, MN) to decrease the area that is exposed and can be inadvertently removed (Fig. 37.5).

Cook-Swartz venous Doppler has demonstrated in multiple studies to be a reliable measurement of flap status and improves salvage rate of compromised flaps [26]. Furthermore, a recent study comparing the Cook-Swartz and the Flow coupler found a low rate of false positivity and virtually no false-negative Doppler signal. There

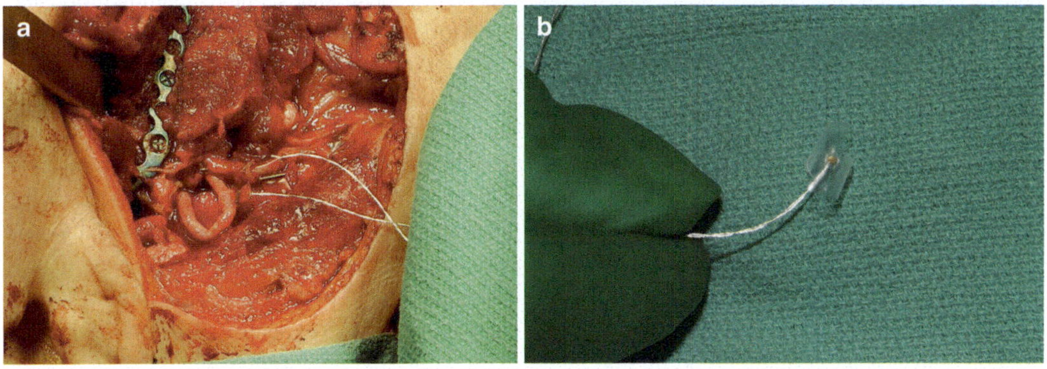

Fig. 37.4 (**a**) Cook-Swartz Doppler probe (Cook Medical, Bloomington, IN) secured with Ligaclip in both arterial and venous anastomoses (Photo Courtesy of Dr. Payam Afzali, University of Michigan). (**b**) Cook internal Doppler probe

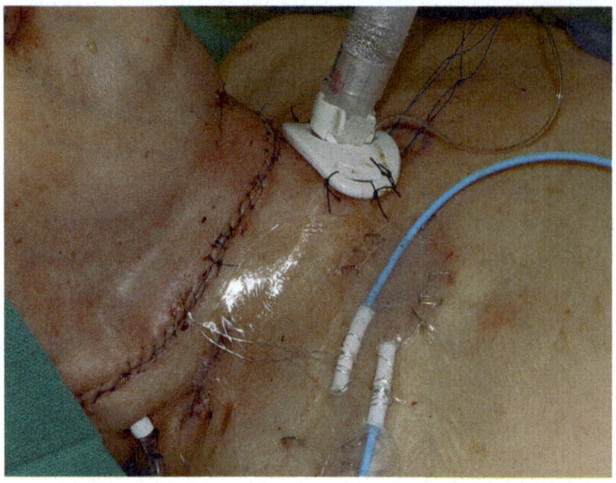

Fig. 37.5 Internal Doppler lines are secured with Tegaderm (3 M, Two Harbors, MN)

was no statistically significant superior device, and one major perceived benefit of the Flow coupler was that it does not involve a separate procedure to place the Doppler [27]. While there is some perceived increased operating time and learning curve when using the Cook-Swartz Doppler, this was not statistically significant. However, high cost associated with indwelling Dopplers should be considered especially when noting occasional failure or malfunction of the device, as well as not infreuqent iatrogenic detachment of the probe wire [28]. Given their significantly improved salvage rate and zero false-negative signals, the indwelling venous coupler may be routinely considered and particularly indicated for higher risk flaps and buried flaps.

37.5 Immediate Postoperative Assessment

Eighty to ninety percent of flap failure occurs in the first 48 h postoperatively, with 90% of arterial thrombosis occurring within 24 h, while venous congestion is the most common etiology of flap compromise [29–31]. Therefore, the flaps are monitored frequently and carefully, especially in this immediate postoperative time. If no cutaneous component is harvested with perforator, then only a venous internal Doppler is used and listened continuously. If there is any significant decrease in the sound, then further investigation may be required. For flaps with a visible and Dopplerable skin paddle, a superficial suture marking in the area noted intraoperatively as a strong signal can be helpful. Flaps are generally checked hourly for the first 24–48 h. Internal Dopplers may be dislodged easily and lead to "false-positive alarms." Once the internal Doppler is down, alternative methods of assessing flap viability may be required. External Doppler can also be useful if the sites of the pedicle have been appropriately marked and if no other vessels are in the area to confuse the signal. However, all these methods are in addition to clinical examination of flap color, the presence of capillary refill, and temperature that give indication of viability. Color should be slightly pinker to the donor site given the initial loss of sympathetic tone of the vasculature [32]. Capillary refill should be less than 2–3 s. If very rapid, this may be a sign of pending arterial insufficiency secondary to narrowing of the lumen leading to increased flow.

If there is difficulty with Doppler monitoring or any concerns of poor perfusion, such as pallor of the skin paddle, then pinprick with a needle can confirm the presence or lack of vascularity and is generally considered to be the most reliable method to verify that the flap is perfused [33]. Visual inspection for venous congestion is important given that pinprick of the flap will still lead to bleeding in the early onset. Delays in clinical signs are also concerning, given some report up to 5–6-h difference between the flap compromise and clinical signs [34, 35] (Fig. 37.6). Therefore, vigilant clinical examination and monitoring is crucial.

Surgeons must have a low threshold to return to the OR for vessel exploration and possible thrombectomy and thrombolysis. In general, with pedicled flaps, returning to the OR for exploration is limited to concerns of compression at the pedicle secondary to hematoma or limited tunnel dissection for the pedicle. Therefore, patient optimization including blood transfusion as necessary is typically indicated. However, for free flaps, most likely, etiology includes the anastomotic compromise. Therefore, exploration and verification of the anastomotic patency are

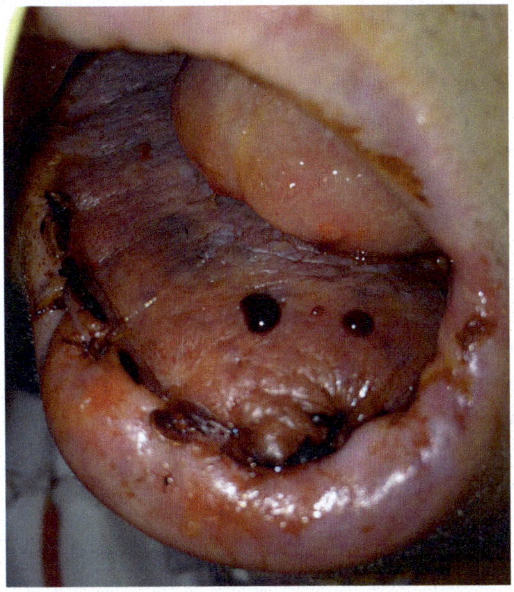

Fig. 37.6 Congested skin paddle of fibula free flap on postoperative day 1, with dark venous blood at the locations of pinprick test

pursued. Successful flap salvage has been reported at approximately 80% for thrombectomy of venous clot [30, 31]. Typical medications used in flap salvage include tissue plasminogen activator (tPA), heparin, topical nitroglycerine, and leeches. Heparin potentiates the activity of antithrombin III, thus deactivates clotting factors, and also has direct vasodilatory property [36]. tPAs are enzymes that catalyze the conversion of plasminogen to plasmin, a major enzyme for clot breakdown. Leeches produce hirudin, a selective thrombin inhibitor and vasodilator, while removing local blood directly [37]. They are most commonly used for bridge therapy to surgical revision while sometimes used to allow time for new venous channels to develop [38, 39]. Lastly, topical nitroglycerine is used for both arterial and venous congestion and works by topical absorption, conversion to nitric oxide radicals, and creating venous and arterial vasodilation [40].

Typical intraoperative vessel irrigation, in conjunction with mechanical thrombectomy, is done with heparinized saline and tPA. Any nidus for a clot such as a kink in the vessel or suboptimal suture placement is revised. For pedicled flap venous congestion, typical salvage medications include leeches and topical nitroglycerine. Nitroglycerine paste is applied every 4–6 h in a thin application [40, 41]. Although data exists in mastectomy flaps [42], no head and neck data exists for flap salvage using nitroglycerine paste. It is also prudent to relieve any signs of compression, whether anatomic or by fluid accumulation, such as seroma or hematoma formation. All these therapies allow decompression of the venous congestion, although they do not replace early and appropriate clinical recognition and return for definitive treatment in the operating room. It is important to keep in mind that each time the surgical wound is opened, there is a higher incidence of infection and skin flap compromise [43].

37.5.1 New Techniques for Monitoring Flaps

There are multiple ways to monitor the flaps that are coming into the scene. In addition to conventional handheld acoustic and implantable Dopplers, near-infrared spectroscopy, color duplex ultrasonography, and laser Doppler flowmetry are being introduced. Near-infrared spectroscopy, commercially known as Vioptix (Vioptix, Fremont, CA, USA) is a probe that is secured externally to the skin paddle and delivers near-infrared light to the tissue underneath. This light is selectively absorbed by hemoglobin and, similar to pulse oximetery, measures oxygen content [44]. Near-infrared spectroscopy has shown promise in detecting earlier flap compromise [45] and has higher reliability in detecting a threatened flap [46]. There is also an app on your mobile device for distant monitoring.

Color duplex ultrasonography is a noninvasive monitor that uses ultrasound to visualize the vessels. Benefit of this technique includes accuracy, speed, and noninvasiveness [47, 48]. Color is used to distinguish flow and their velocities [49]. These are typically done by monitors and ultrasound readily available in hospitals. This involves a trained technician and radiologist interpretation [49]. Furthermore, these monitors are not specifically designed for head and neck reconstruction and may be difficult to monitor deep buried flaps.

Lastly, laser Doppler flowmetry uses a laser light that is produced, and the backscattered light is collected from the area in question. This scatter is used to determine the frequency shift, which is proportional to the number and velocity of the red blood cells in the field [50]. Therefore, this is an indirect measurement of vascularity and flow. This is also a noninvasive monitor and currently uses multiple types of probes that can be applied to skin, muscle, and internal structures [49]. They can monitor areas at depth up to 8 mm deep and therefore can measure areas that are buried. These and many novel ways of accurately monitoring and recognizing early flap compromise are being studied and introduced. However, their accuracy and reliability are continuing to be studied.

37.6 Postoperative Assessment

Generally, after 48 h, there are fewer complications associated with the flap, and we begin to optimize the patient for the anticipated discharge from the hospital. This is a complex interplay between multiple disciplines. A way to ensure this intricate postoperative assessment is optimized, and interdisciplinary care is coordinated is with the usage of care pathways. Care pathways clearly outline duties and medical and surgical recovery milestones that the patients are expected to meet in a normal postoperative course. They include but are not limited to pain management, feeding advancement, physical therapy regimen, occupational therapy, mobility limitation and regimen, flap care frequency, tracheostomy care, and drain care. It allows the surgeon and the rest of the team to ensure no steps are skipped, acts as a checklist for discharge optimization and allows coordination of multidisciplinary care in an efficient manner. Recently, Yetzer et al. also described the significant difference in average length of stay and discharge within 7 days for patients who underwent head and neck reconstruction with free flaps while utilizing a care pathway [51]. Furthermore, there are some new data showing that care pathways significantly decrease the rates of major complications [52].

For the airway, patients are typically intubated nasally or a tracheostomy was performed. Based on their cuff leak test and exceeding the extubation criteria based on parameters such as negative inspiratory force and rapid shallow breath index, most patients that are kept intubated postoperatively are extubated on postoperative day 1 or 2. If tracheostomy is performed, most patients are able to wean from the ventilator as soon as their general anesthetic wears off and are on tracheostomy mask on postoperative day 0 or 1. Typically, downsizing or early removal occurs prior to discharge, so patients can usually begin speaking with a Passy-Muir (Passy-Muir Inc. Irvine, CA) one-way valve or from tracheostomy removal. In cancer patients with large flaps, the tracheostomy tube generally remains until definitive adjuvant therapy is determined. Depending on the location of the planned adjuvant radiation therapy, tracheostomy may be kept in during the duration of therapy, as significant airway edema, fibrosis, and stenosis may occur [53]. It is important to note that a metal Jackson is reserved for patients who will not receive radiation therapy, as significant scatter may occur with the metal Jackson. For patients with benign lesions, they can have their tracheostomy tube plugged for 24–48 h without airway issues; then, they can be decannulated.

Nutrition consultation is done on postoperative day 1, and tube-feeding regimen based on needed caloric intake is recommended. Some flexibility such as volume and type of feeds are available as necessary. Typical cases to alter feeding regimen include lactose intolerance, nausea secondary to volume of feeds, and chyle leak. With minimal chyle leak, typically <600 mL per day, low-fat tube feeds may provide enough slowing of the flow, allowing spontaneous closure of the chylous fistula [54].

For flap checks, as described previously, it is checked often in the immediate postoperative period. Practices vary but careful monitoring for the first 48 h is especially critical. Although a significant portion of our focus is given to the flap, the donor site is also checked multiple times a day. They are checked for swelling, graft evaluation, and neurovascular evaluation. To prevent unnecessary alarms, it is important to discuss with the whole team what is considered normal postoperative edema or surgical anatomy. With pectoralis myocutaneous flaps, a neck hematoma may have similarity with the muscle tunneled under the neck. Facial edema can be quiet striking and may worsen for the first 48–72 h and most likely does not represent infection, hematoma, or seroma.

In terms of donor site splints, multiple modalities ensure optimal recovery and prevent complications. Scapula free flap patients can be equipped with a sling to stabilize the arm and reminded not to perform extreme range of motion in the immediate postoperative period. Radial forearm free flap patients are equipped with volar splints that hyperextends their wrist. This allows stabilization of the wrist to allow the typical full or partial thickness skin graft to heal without risking shear force associated with flexing and extending the wrist. In the fibula free flap donor site, if a skin paddle is taken and a split thickness skin graft is placed on the donor site, there is a bolster dressing which stays in place for 5 days postoperatively. They are also equipped with L'nard boots while in bed, which stabilizes their foot in a neutral position to prevent foot drop and pneumatic below-knee boot while ambulating. Following a predetermined protocol, nursing staff as well as physical and occupational therapists achieve early ambulation and return to function. Physical and occupational therapists begin working with patients typically on postoperative day 2. They also help instruct the patients of their limitations until full recovery while preventing long-term limitations and instruct in methods to perform daily duties in perhaps different ways until full recovery. Lastly, physical and occupational therapists determine immediate discharge destination, home versus rehabilitation facility.

It is common for patients to be discharged to an extended care facility. Patients in this setting are able to receive higher level of wound care and other nursing care such as pulmonary hygiene, which may be difficult for patient's caregivers.

Most patients, until surgical and wound stabilization, have frequent clinic follow-ups. Typical delayed signs of compromised flap is wound breakdown. The periphery of the wound may also give the look of vascular congestion and will declare itself. At this juncture, usually conservative intervention at these wound edges with gauze packing is recommended. Delayed donor site complications can include hematoma, seroma formation, and skin flap compromise. These also typically manifest themselves with wound breakdown. If split thickness skin flap or full thickness skin flap was used to reconstruct the skin paddle donor site, these can manifest with poor take and blistering. Typically, these areas are full of granulation tissue, although if failure over paratenon occurs, exposure of the tendon is apparent and necrosis of the underlying tendon is sometimes observed. These wounds may require return to the operating room for debridement, negative pressure wound therapy, and eventual regrafting of the skin.

Many flap patients are seen at postoperative follow-up with speech and language pathologists. The patients are evaluated for swallow function when no concerns of flap healing are present. Most patients with uncomplicated course will have their swallow evaluation, and if no significant aspiration is present, they will be instructed in diet regimen, and the nasogastric feeding tube will be removed. If any concerns of per os tolerance or swallow efficiency are present, the nasogastric tube can be left in place, while the patient ramps up oral intake. Speech pathologists can also instruct the patient in maneuvers to help improve swallowing function. Furthermore, they continue to work with the patient to return speech function, especially when the flap is used for velum reconstruction or tongue reconstruction. Multiple studies verify higher quality of life scores and objective improvement of speech function, when speech therapist is involved in head and neck reconstruction [55, 56].

After adjunctive therapy such as radiation and chemotherapy is completed and the patient is stable from a functional and pathologic standpoint, patients may pursue functional or cosmetic rehabilitation. These are vast and based on patient's perceived importance. Common areas that require intervention include unwanted hair growth at the skin paddle, overly bulky flap, and acquired edentulism. For unwanted hair growth, laser can be utilized for hair removal [57] although some patients choose to trim the hair themselves. Debulking of the flap can be done prior or at the same time of implant placement but should be considered earlier if other surgical interventions are indicated, such as vestibuloplasty, and to aid in improvement of poor speech or impaired swallowing due to bulk and lip incompetence. Lastly, functional rehabilitation with endosseous implants will be determined by the patient's medical and surgical stability and after careful assessment of their flap.

Conclusion

Major reconstruction of the head and neck utilizing pedicled or microvascular tissue transfer is becoming a common duty of the oral and maxillofacial surgeon in the hospital care setting. Careful assessment of the patient and the flap allows prompt intervention and proactive rather than reactive care of the patient. Ultimately, these complex patients deserve equally methodical assessment that will give them the best chance of successful return to function.

References

1. Jarvis MA, Jarvis CL, Jones PR, Spyt TJ. Reliability of Allen's test in selection of patients for radial artery harvest. Ann Thorac Surg. 2000;70:1362–5.
2. Carli F, Scheede-Bergdahl C. Prehabilitation to enhance perioperative care. Anesthesiol Clin. 2015;33:17–33.
3. Dickinson KJ, Blackmon SH. Prehabilitation: prevention is better than cure. J Thorac Cardiovasc Surg. 2015;149(2):574–5. https://doi.org/10.1016/j.jtcvs.2014.10.078. Epub 2014 Oct 22.
4. Messmer K, Lewis DH, Sunder-Plassmann L, et al. Acute normovolemic hemodilution: changes of central hemodynamics and microcirculatory flow in skeletal muscle. Europ Surg Res. 1972;4:55–70.
5. Boldt J. New light on intravascular volume replacement regimens: what did we learn from the past three years? Anesth Analg. 2003;97:1595–604.
6. Pattani KM, Byrne P, Boahene K, Richmon J. What makes a good flap go bad? A critical analysis of the literature of intraoperative factors related to free flap failure. Laryngoscope. 2010;120:717–23. https://doi.org/10.1002/lary.20825.
7. Ettinger KS, Arce K, Lohse CM, Peck BW, Reiland MD, Bezak BJ, Moore EJ. Higher perioperative fluid administration is associated with increased rates of complications following head and neck microvascular reconstruction with fibular free flaps. Microsurgery. 2016. https://doi.org/10.1002/micr.30061.
8. Hoppe IC, Abernathie BL, Datiashvili RO. Examination of possible predictors of complications after free tissue transfer to the head and neck for oncologic defects. Ann Plast Surg. 2012;69:368–70.
9. Clark JR, McCluskey SA, Hall F, et al. Predictors of morbidity following free flap reconstruction for cancer of the head and neck. Head Neck. 2007;29:1090–101.
10. Szakmany T, Dodd M, Dempsey GA, et al. The influence of allogenic blood transfusion in patients having free-flap primary surgery for oral and oropharyngeal squamous cell carcinoma. Br J Cancer. 2006;94:647–53.
11. Taniguchi Y, Okura M. Prognostic significance of perioperative blood transfusion in oral cavity squamous cell carcinoma. Head Neck. 2003;25:931–6.
12. Fenner M, Vairaktaris E, Nkenke E, Weisbach V, Neukam FW, Radespiel-Tröger M. Prognostic impact of blood transfusion in patients undergoing primary surgery and free-flap reconstruction for oral squamous cell carcinoma. Cancer. 2009;115:1481–8. https://doi.org/10.1002/cncr.24132.
13. Hebert PC, Wells G, Blajchman MA, et al. A multicenter, randomized, controlled clinical trial of transfusion requirements in critical care. Transfusion Requirements in Critical Care Investigators, Canadian Critical Care Trials Group. N Engl J Med. 1999;340:409–17.
14. Rossmiller SR, Cannady SB, Ghanem TA, Wax MK. Transfusion criteria in free flap surgery. Otolaryngol Head Neck Surg. 2010;142:359–64.
15. Khouri RK, Sherman R, Buncke HJ Jr, et al. A phase II trial of intraluminal irrigation with recombinant human tissue factor pathway inhibitor to prevent thrombosis in free flap surgery. Plast Reconstr Surg. 2001;107:408–15. discussion 416–8
16. Lighthall JG, Cain R, Ghanem TA, et al. Effect of postoperative aspirin on outcomes in microvascular free tissue transfer surgery. Otolaryngol Head Neck Surg. 2013;148:40–6.
17. Bahl V, Shuman AG, Hu HM, Jackson CR, Pannucci CJ, Alaniz C, Chepeha DB, Bradford CR. Chemoprophylaxis for venous thromboembolism in otolaryngology. JAMA Otolaryngol Head Neck Surg. 2014;140(11):999–1005. https://doi.org/10.1001/jamaoto.2014.2254.
18. Caprini JA. Risk assessment as a guide for the prevention of the many faces of venous thromboembolism. Am J Surg. 2010;199(1 Suppl):S3–S10.
19. Drolet BC, et al. Evidence for safe tourniquet use in 500 consecutive upper extremity procedures. Hand (N Y). 2014;9(4):494–8.

20. Riot S, Herlin C, Mojallal A, Garrido I, Bertheuil N, Filleron T, et al. A systematic review and meta-analysis of double venous anastomosis in free flaps. Plast Reconstr Surg. 2015;136(6):1299–311.
21. Chen WF, Kung YP, Kang YC, Lawrence WT, Tsao CK. An old controversy revisited-one versus two venous anastomoses in microvascular head and neck reconstruction using anterolateral thigh flap. Microsurgery. 2014;34(5):377–83.
22. Fahmy HW, Moneim MS. The effect of prolonged blood stasis on a microarterial repair. J Reconstr Microsurg. 1988;4(2):139–43.
23. Fernandez EJ, Nadal RD, Gonzalez SM, Caffee HH. The effect of stasis on a microvascular anastomosis. Microsurgery. 1983;4(3):176–7.
24. Strecker WB, Wood MB, Schroeder AR. Stasis-induced thrombosis of rat microvascular anastomosis. J Reconstr Microsurg. 1987;4(1):69–73.
25. Heidekrueger PI, Ehrl D, Heine-Geldern A, et al. One versus two venous anastomoses in microvascular lower extremity reconstruction using gracilis muscle or anterolateral thigh flaps. Injury. 2016;47(12):2828–32.
26. Rozen WM, Chubb D, Whitaker IS, Acosta R. The efficacy of postoperative monitoring: a single surgeon comparison of clinical monitoring and the implantable Doppler probe in 547 consecutive free flaps. Microsurgery. 2010;30(2):105–10. https://doi.org/10.1002/micr.20706.
27. Um GT, Chang J, Louie O, Colohan SM, Said HK, Neligan PC, Mathes DW. Implantable Cook-Swartz Doppler probe versus Synovis Flow Coupler for the post-operative monitoring of free flap breast reconstruction. J Plast Reconstr Aesthet Surg. 2014;67(7):960–6. https://doi.org/10.1016/j.bjps.2014.03.034. Epub 2014 Apr 12.
28. Ho MW, Cassidy C, Brown JS, et al. Rationale for the use of the implantable Doppler probe based on 7 years' experience. Br J Oral Maxillofac Surg. 2014;52:530–4.
29. Kroll SS, Schusterman MA, Reece GP, et al. Timing of pedicle thrombosis and flap loss after free tissue transfer. Plast Reconstr Surg. 1996;98(7):1230–3.
30. Esclamado RM, Carroll WR. The pathogenesis of vascular thrombosis and its impact in microvascular surgery. Head Neck. 1999;21:355–62.
31. Kubo T, Yano K, Hosokawa K. Management of flaps with compromised venous outflow in head and neck microsurgical reconstruction. Microsurgery. 2002;22:391–5.
32. Goltz F. Ueber gefa¨ssserweiternde Nerven. Pflugers Arch Ges Physiol. 1874;9:174–97.
33. Genden EM, Rinaldo A, Suárez C, et al. Complications of free flap transfers for head and neck reconstruction following cancer resection. Oral Oncol. 2004;40(10):979–84.
34. Torre J, Hedden WH, Grant PM, et al. Retrospective review of the internal Doppler probe for intra- and postoperative microvascular surveillance. J Reconstr Microsurg. 2003;19:287–90.
35. Swartz WM, Izquierdo R, Miller MJ. Implantable venous Doppler microvascular monitoring: laboratory investigation and clinical results. Plast Reconstr Surg. 1994;93(1):152–63.
36. Neligan PC, Wei F-C. Microsurgical reconstruction of the head and neck. Microsurgery. 2010;30:507. https://doi.org/10.1002/micr.20783.
37. Elyassi AR, Terres J, Rowshan HH. Medicinal leech therapy on head and neck patients: a review of literature and proposed protocol. Oral Surg Oral Med Oral Pathol Oral Radiol. 2013;116(3):e167–72.
38. Koch CA, Olsen SM, Moore EJ. Use of the medicinal leech for salvage of venous congested microvascular free flaps of the head and neck. Am J Otolaryngol. 2012;33:26–30.
39. Jordan GH. Techniques of tissue handling and transfer. J Urol. 1999;162:1213–7.
40. Schreiber NTN, Mobley SR. Elegant solutions for complex paramedian forehead flap reconstruction. Facial Plast Surg Clin North Am. 2011;19(3):465–79. https://doi.org/10.1016/j.fsc.2011.06.003.
41. Davis RE, Wachholz JH, Jassir D, et al. Comparison of topical anti-ischemic agents in the salvage of failing random-pattern skin flaps in rats. Arch Facial Plast Surg. 1999;1:27–32.
42. Kutun S, Ay AA, Ulucanlar H, et al. Is transdermal nitroglycerin application effective in preventing and healing flap ischaemia after modified radical mastectomy? S Afr J Surg. 2010;48:119–21.
43. Bui DT, Cordeiro PG, Hu QY, et al. Free flap reexploration: indications, treatment, and outcomes in 1193 free flaps. Plast Reconstr Surg. 2007;119:2092–100.
44. Lin CM, Huang CC, Hsu H, Chiu CH, Chien SH. Advancements in free flap monitoring in the last decade: a critical review. Plast Reconstr Surg. 2010;126:679. author reply 679–80
45. Lohman RF, Langevin CJ, Bozkurt M, et al. A prospective analysis of free flap monitoring techniques: physical examination, external Doppler, implantable Doppler, and tissue oximetry. J Reconstr Microsurg. 2013;29(1):51–6. https://doi.org/10.1055/s-0032-1326741. Epub 2012 Nov 12
46. Steele MH. Three-year experience using near infrared spectroscopy tissue oximetry monitoring of free tissue transfers. Ann Plast Surg. 2011;66(5):540–5. https://doi.org/10.1097/SAP.0b013e31820909f9.
47. Khalid AN, Quraishi SA, Zang WA, et al. Color Doppler ultrasonography is a reliable predictor of free tissue transfer outcomes in head and neck reconstruction. Otolaryngol Head Neck Surg. 2006;134:635–8.
48. Few JW, Corral CJ, Fine NA, Dumanian GA. Monitoring buried head and neck free flaps with high-resolution color-duplex ultrasound. Plast Reconstr Surg. 2001;108:709–12.
49. Chao AH, Meyerson J, Povoski SP, et al. A review of devices used in the monitoring of microvascular free tissue transfers. Expert Rev Med Devices. 2013;10(5):649–60.
50. Hallock GG. Acoustic Doppler sonography, color duplex ultrasound, and laser Doppler flowmetry as

tools for successful autologous breast reconstruction. Clin Plast Surg. 2011;38:203–11.

51. Yetzer JG, Pirgousis P, Li Z, et al. Clinical pathway implementation improves efficacy of care in a maxillofacial head and neck surgery unit. J Oral Maxillofac Surg. 2016. pii: S0278-2391(16)30590-0. https://doi.org/10.1016/j.joms.2016.06.194.
52. O'Connell DA, Barber B, Klein MF, al e. Algorithm based patient care protocol to optimize patient care and inpatient stay in head and neck free flap patients. J Otolaryngol Head Neck Surg. 2015;44:45. https://doi.org/10.1186/s40463-015-0090-6.
53. Stoelting RK, Hines RL, Marschall KE. Cancer. In: Stoelting's anesthesia and co-existing disease. Philadelphia: Churchill Livingstone/Elsevier; 2012. p. 493–515. Print.
54. Spiro JD, Spiro RH, Strong EW. The management of chyle fistula. Laryngoscope. 1990;100:771.
55. Rieger JM, Tang JA, Harris J, et al. Survey of current functional outcomes assessment practices in patients with head and neck cancer: initial project of the head and neck research network. J Otolaryngol Head Neck Surg. 2010;39(5):523–31.
56. Beck-Broichsitter BE, Huck J, Küchler T, et al. J Cancer Res Clin Oncol. 2016. https://doi.org/10.1007/s00432-016-2287-0.
57. Shim TN, Abdullah A, Lanigan S, Avery C. Hairy intraoral flap—an unusual indication for laser epilation: a series of 5 cases and review of the literature. Br J Oral Maxillofac Surg. 2011;49:e50–2.

Part 4

Complications in Managing the Surgical Patient

38 Chest Pain as a Complication of Maxillofacial Surgery

Virginia Workman and Andre Ghantous

Abstract

Chest pain is a common occurrence in the perioperative patient. Although chest pain has many potential etiologies, a worrisome syndrome is cardiac angina, which may herald acute myocardial infarction. Angina occurs commonly in perioperative patients, even those who have not previously experienced angina in everyday life, due to increased stress on the heart in the perioperative period. In patients who do have a history of angina and myocardial infarction, cessation of chronic medications to minimize post-operative bleeding risk can also play a role in precipitating angina and cardiac complications. A familiarity with the initial steps in diagnosis and management of myocardial infarction is the responsibility of the oral and maxillofacial surgeon; consultation with a cardiologist should also be pursued for aid with management of acute coronary syndromes. The definitive management of myocardial infarction requires anticoagulation and often revascularization, but in the perioperative population, the risks and benefits of these therapies must be weighed carefully.

38.1 Complication—Chest Pain

38.1.1 Cause of the Complication

The differential diagnosis for chest pain is broad and includes musculoskeletal, gastrointestinal, and neurological etiologies among others. Most of these diagnoses are self-limited and benign. The most concerning etiology of chest pain is cardiac. Cardiac chest pain, or *angina pectoris*, is a manifestation of myocardial ischemia: an inadequate supply of oxygen to the *myocardium*, or heart muscle, to match metabolic demands. If left untreated, angina can progress rapidly to *myocardial infarction* or irreversible cell death and tissue necrosis. The resulting myocardial scar can lead to fatal arrhythmia, myocardial rupture, or heart failure. Therefore, the rapid diagnosis of chest pain as angina is of paramount importance to prevent potentially fatal complications of myocardial infarction.

V. Workman, M.D. • A. Ghantous, M.D. (✉)
Division of Cardiology, Department of Internal Medicine, Yale University School of Medicine, New Haven, CT, USA
e-mail: Andre.Ghantous@ynhh.org

© Springer International Publishing AG 2018

E.M. Ferneini, J.D. Bennett (eds.), *Perioperative Assessment of the Maxillofacial Surgery Patient*,
https://doi.org/10.1007/978-3-319-58868-1_38

In contrast to many other potential etiologies of chest pain, the physiologic stress of surgery and the perioperative state increases the likelihood that a patient may experience angina, even if the patient does not give a history of angina during a preoperative interview. This makes determining a patient's baseline level of metabolic demand, or exercise tolerance, a particularly important task in the preoperative evaluation, which is discussed in detail in Part 2.

38.1.2 Pathophysiology

The myocardium is supplied by three main arteries called *coronary arteries* that are contained within the outer endothelium of the myocardium, termed the *epicardium*. Normal epicardial coronary arteries deliver sufficient blood and oxygen to the myocardium to sustain the myocardial metabolic demands at rest and at a significant level of exertion. However, in a state of coronary disease, the blood flow and oxygen delivery to the myocardium become compromised at progressively lower workloads. The clinical syndrome of angina parallels this phenomenon, with symptoms initially occurring only with significant exertion. As coronary disease progresses, patients become increasingly symptomatic with diminishing exercise tolerance. In severe states, patients may have symptoms even in a resting state. The severity of angina is often described clinically by a patient's workload tolerance, as measured by scale developed by the Canadian Cardiovascular Society (Table 38.1) [1].

Table 38.1 The Canadian Cardiovascular Society angina grading scale

I	Occurs only with prolonged activity at a strenuous workload
II	Occurs with climbing more than one flight of stairs or walking more than two blocks on level ground
III	Occurs with climbing one flight of stairs or walking one—two blocks on level ground
IV	Occurs with any activity at all or at rest

Clinically, a distinction is made between *stable angina* and *unstable angina*. The latter syndrome encompasses angina occurring with progressively lower workloads and all angina occurring at rest. Unstable angina, non-ST elevation myocardial infarction (NSTEMI), and ST elevation myocardial infarction (STEMI) are known collectively as *acute coronary syndromes* and require urgent recognition and treatment.

Disease in the coronary arteries is caused by *atherosclerosis* or plaque buildup within the lumen of the artery that causes a narrowing that can progress to be hemodynamically significant and can in some cases progress to total occlusion of the lumen of the artery. In these cases, the myocardium distal to the diseased artery segment receives inadequate blood and oxygen supply. Atherosclerosis begins with an insult to the inner cell layer of the vascular wall or *endothelium* [2]. At the site of endothelial injury, platelets aggregate and smooth muscle proliferate, forming an atherosclerotic plaque. Mild atherosclerotic plaques are not hemodynamically significant, meaning that blood flow and perfusion are not impeded. Mildly diseased arteries are also responsive to vasodilatory stimuli in states of increased oxygen demand, which can improve blood flow in these arteries.

As disease progresses, small thrombi continually form and are incorporated into growing atherosclerotic plaques, which eventually result in significant narrowing of blood vessels and decreased myocardial perfusion. In severe stenosis, blood vessels are maximally dilated even in a resting state and therefore cannot respond to vasodilatory stimuli in the event of increased oxygen demand. In this setting, angina and myocardial ischemia may occur. Alternatively, plaques may fissure or rupture, causing an acute thrombus to form at the site and either partially or totally obstruct the lumen of the artery [3]. This process leads to acute myocardial infarction. In general, the acute coronary syndromes can be thought of as a spectrum from unstable angina (least malignant) to STEMI (highest mortality), where plaque damage increases along this spectrum. As plaque damage increases, thrombus becomes less labile and more fixed [4].

38.1.3 Prevalence

Globally, as the population ages, cardiac disease is among the most common morbidities. This is particularly true in more economically developed countries. The oromaxillofacial population is no different; in fact, given the strong link between gingival and cardiac disease, cardiac comorbidities are especially common in this population. A survey of 590 periodontal patients revealed that the most common chronic medical comorbidity in this population was cardiovascular disease, with 20% of participants affected [5]. (The only more common finding in the medical history was drug allergy, affecting 21.7% of participants).

Based on a survey of 1250 general dental practitioners, the incidence of angina during a dental visit was estimated to be approximately 1 case per practicing lifetime (assuming a 40-year career) [6]. The incidence of myocardial infarction was estimated to be 0.08 in a practicing lifetime or a complication occurring in 1 out of 13 practicing lifetimes (Table 38.2, adapted from Chapman [7]).

38.1.4 Manifestations/Presentation of Disease

38.1.4.1 Angina in the Absence of Acute Coronary Syndrome

In the absence of progression of symptoms to myocardial infarction, there are generally few manifestations of angina on clinical examination or routine laboratory or imaging studies. Therefore, the diagnosis of chest pain as angina mostly relies on a careful medical history aimed at assessing the quality and duration of symptoms along with triggers and relieving factors.

Table 38.2 Occurrence of chest pain and angina in dental practice

Country	Australia [6]	UK [8]	UK [9]
Number of practitioners surveyed	811	302	1093
Chest pain cases per dentist per year	0.03	0.2	0.03
Chest pain cases diagnosed as angina (%)	93	96	90

William Heberden is widely credited with the first description of angina, given in an address to the Royal College of Physicians in 1768 [10]. He noted that the pain occurs with exercise and relieves promptly with rest. Despite the myriad stress tests and angiography that are available in the modern era to definitively diagnose angina or a patient's risk of developing angina, the diagnosis of angina itself remains largely a clinical diagnosis. Diamond and Forrester's clinical classification of chest pain as "noncardiac," "atypical angina," or "typical angina," the most popular and well-validated iteration published in 1983 [11], is still widely used today. Typical angina fulfills three characteristics:

1. Pain is located substernally.
2. Symptoms are provoked by exertion or emotional stress.
3. Symptoms are relieved either with rest or following administration of nitroglycerin (discussed in detail in Management section).

Patients whose symptoms fulfill two of the three characteristics are said to have "atypical angina," and patients who only attest to zero or one of these characteristics are diagnosed with "non-anginal chest pain."

Other characteristics of chest pain have been described to increase or decrease the likelihood of angina. A recent systematic review of elements of chest pain history noted that characteristics that increase the likelihood of true angina include pain radiating to one or both arms/shoulders and associated nausea, vomiting, and/or diaphoresis [12]. The same review found that symptoms that were pleuritic, positional, or reproducible with palpation of the chest wall decreased the likelihood of true angina.

38.1.4.2 Acute Coronary Syndrome

Coronary chest pain may also signify an acute coronary event. In these instances, additional clues may be present on the clinical examination.

Electrocardiogram and laboratory findings are discussed in detail in the patient assessment section. While electrocardiogram changes may be present in angina in the absence of acute coronary syndrome if tested simultaneously with symptoms, electrocardiogram findings are more reliably and sustainably present in cases of NSTEMI and STEMI.

38.2 Patient Assessment

38.2.1 Monitoring

When first evaluating patients for potential surgery, it is important that the surgeon be familiar with medical comorbidities that put patients at increased risk of major adverse cardiovascular events during surgery. In general, adverse cardiovascular events occur in patients with some baseline degree of coronary artery disease. However, mild coronary artery disease that may be subclinical in a nonstress environment may become significant in a perioperative setting. An artery with a moderate burden of atherosclerotic plaque in general is able to supply sufficient oxygen to a myocardium with average metabolic demands. However, during surgery and physiologic stress, myocardial oxygen consumption increases, and in this setting ischemia may occur. Furthermore, nonocclusive atherosclerotic plaque is frequently a substrate for rupture, and thrombotic occlusion of the artery may occur. Therefore, the preoperative assessment of a patient's risk for coronary heart disease and adverse events during surgery is of particular importance, and referral to a cardiologist for consideration of ischemic heart disease testing is appropriate in select populations. This is discussed in detail in Part 2.

The most important clinical data to evaluate in a patient with chest pain are routine vital signs, including blood pressure, heart rate, and blood arterial oxygen saturation. Intra- and perioperative monitoring of these hemodynamic data are discussed in detail in Part 4.

38.2.1.1 Blood Pressure

An elevated blood pressure signifies an elevated vascular resistance or "afterload" against which the heart must contract to maintain adequate circulation and end-organ perfusion. When blood pressure is markedly elevated, myocardial oxygen consumption is increased, and oxygen demands may not be adequately met in patients with atherosclerotic coronary arteries. Furthermore, elevated blood pressure can cause increased shear stress in coronary arteries that can lead to endothelial and plaque disruption [2]. Therefore, one focus of the initial management of chest pain symptoms is targeted to lowering blood pressure, which is discussed in detail in the management section of this chapter.

38.2.1.2 Heart Rate and Rhythm

Heart rate monitoring is equally important, and patients with chest pain should be monitored with continuous cardiac telemetry when possible. Elevated heart rates may occur in patients with chest pain for several reasons. First, there is a catecholamine surge associated with pain that may cause increased sympathetic tone and resultant tachycardia. Similar to hypertension, tachycardia also increases myocardial oxygen consumption by increasing the number of cardiac cycles the heart must complete in a given time. Telemetry monitoring is important in patients with tachycardia to distinguish sinus tachycardia, which is usually benign, from more malignant arrhythmias. In the setting of myocardial ischemia, patients are predisposed to ventricular tachyarrhythmias, including mono- and polymorphic ventricular tachycardia and ventricular fibrillation, which can result in hemodynamic instability and even circulatory collapse and death.

Ventricular fibrillation is the most common cause of death in the acute stage of a myocardial infarction [13], with reported 4.7% incidence in acute myocardial infarction [14]. Though monomorphic ventricular tachycardia is not always an unstable (pulseless) rhythm on initial presentation, it can rapidly devolve into a hemodynamically unstable rhythm and ventricular fibrillation. Therefore, familiarity with waveform morphology for these unstable rhythms is necessary for proper monitoring of the chest pain patient, and urgent consultation of a cardiologist should be pursued if there is any concern for these arrhythmias.

38.2.1.3 Oxygenation

Arterial blood oxygen saturation can be estimated with noninvasive pulse oximetry. As the vasculature supplying the myocardium with oxygen is compromised in acute ischemia, optimizing the partial pressure of oxygen in arterial blood is an important aspect of therapy for myocardial ischemia. Many patients with acute ischemia have low oxygen saturations, often due to acute pulmonary edema in setting of acute systolic or diastolic heart failure.

38.2.2 Workup

There are two main pieces of information that are of great diagnostic value in a patient complaining of chest pain. They are:

1. The 12-lead surface electrocardiogram.
2. The serum troponin level. This is discussed in detail in the following section.

In general, all surgical facilities should have the equipment and properly trained staff necessary to perform a routine electrocardiogram within minutes of an initial complaint of chest pain. Additionally, rapid consultation with a cardiologist should be feasible if the results are not readily interpretable. Most vendors of electrocardiograph instruments include a software package that provides an automatic interpretation of electrocardiograms; however, it is unacceptable to rely solely on this interpretation to guide patient care.

STEMI is characterized by elevation of the ST segment of >1.5 mV in men and >0.2 mV in women in two or more leads in one of the following groups [15]:

- I, aVL
- II, III, aVF
- V1–V6

NSTEMI can be characterized by T-wave changes including peaking or inversion or ST-segment depression >0.05 mV in two leads. In patients with baseline ECG abnormalities, especially left ventricular hypertrophy, left bundle branch block, and ventricular pacing, the detection of ischemic ECG changes is more difficult. For any concerning ECG changes, consultation with a cardiologist should be considered.

Not only do ECG abnormalities signify myocardial injury or infarction but they lend important clues to assess the size, acuity, and location of an infarction. In fact, the most important distinction in myocardial infarction (NSTEMI vs. STEMI) is made solely based on ECG findings. A rapid diagnosis or exclusion of STEMI is of paramount importance, as this diagnosis is considered a medical emergency due to its high complication and mortality rates.

38.2.3 Laboratory Tests and Anticipated Results

The mainstay of biochemical assessment of chest pain is serial measurements of biomarkers of myocardial injury. Elevated levels of these biomarkers make the distinction between angina and true myocardial infarction. Both processes describe a condition in which myocardial tissue does not receive sufficient oxygen supply to meet metabolic demands, but only in myocardial infarction is there a sufficient mass of cell injury to produce detectable cardiac biomarkers. In angina, there is no consistent pattern of laboratory abnormalities. Therefore, carefully eliciting a detailed description of the presenting symptoms is of special importance in making this diagnosis (see Sect. 38.1.4).

In making the diagnosis of myocardial infarction, several biomarkers of myocardial ischemia may be used. These markers include CK-MB, myoglobin, and troponin. Whereas myoglobin is uniquely sensitive in the first 6 h following myocardial infarction, it is much less specific for cardiac muscle when compared to CK-MB and troponin [16]. Overall, troponin is the preferred diagnostic test as it remains sensitive for 72 h following an event, compared to 48 h for CK-MB. In fact, the ACC/AHA consensus guidelines for diagnosis of acute myocardial infarction state that CK-MB and myoglobin levels are of no benefit in making the diagnosis of acute coronary syndrome if modern troponin assays are available [17]. As none of these markers become reliable until 6 h following the onset of symptoms, maintaining a high clinical suspicion for patients with classic symptoms despite undetectable biomarkers remains important, as it is for patients presenting with angina in the absence of myocardial infarction.

There are many assays available to quantify serum troponin levels. Since these assays have varying sensitivity, it is important to maintain familiarity with the reference cutoff values for "normal" troponin levels for the specific assay used in each individual practice. In general, one of two isoforms of troponin (troponin I or troponin T) is detected with each assay. Troponin-I and troponin-T levels correlate in most instances and therefore are usually interchangeable; however, several case series have described instances of chronic elevation of troponin T with undetectable troponin I in patients with renal insufficiency [18].

A shared property of all of these markers that lends great clinical utility is the rapid rise and fall in serum levels over a matter of hours following the onset of symptoms. These changes in serum levels reflect the kinetics of accumulation and degradation of these proteins following myocardial injury. In fact, the definition of myocardial infarction requires a demonstrated rise and fall in serum troponin levels, as the rapid rise and fall of levels signifies an acute event (such as coronary thromboembolism), as opposed to other etiologies of myocardial injury, which tend to be more subacute or chronic in nature [19]. More recently, "point-of-care" troponin assays, in which a blood sample is collected and tested at the bedside, allowing results within minutes without sending samples to a central lab, have gained popularity.

Despite the excellent specificity of the troponin assays for myocardial tissue, troponin levels are detectable in many instances in which myocardial injury is present and are not specific to acute coronary syndrome as an etiology of myocardial injury. In the perioperative setting, there is a wide range of conditions that may cause myocardial injury that is not secondary to an acute coronary syndrome, and the management for these conditions is distinct from the management discussed for a primary coronary event in this chapter. Common alternate causes of troponin elevation in the perioperative population include sepsis (which may occur in the postoperative population due to disruption in barrier pathogen defense mechanisms) and distributive shock, such as in postoperative hemorrhage. Pulmonary embolism is also a common cause of both chest pain and troponin elevation and is common in the postoperative population due to venous stasis, disruptions in vascular integrity, and inflammatory milieu.

38.3 Management

38.3.1 Potential Problems

The symptoms of angina represent a state of myocardial ischemia; therefore, ongoing symptoms without proper treatment aimed at relieving these symptoms can lead to several complications. Angina can represent a vasospasm or unstable plaque that can lead to myocardial infarction with extensive myocardial necrosis. The cell death and resultant loss of function of part of the myocardium elevate a patient's risk for congestive heart failure, cardiogenic shock, and malignant arrhythmia. Initial management for all patients with angina and myocardial infarction has two main objectives:

1. Reducing myocardial metabolic demand to reduce the amount and duration of myocardial ischemia
2. Increasing "stability" of atherosclerotic plaque, thereby decreasing the likelihood of plaque rupture and thrombus formation

A third consideration in the setting of myocardial infarction is the need for urgent or emergent revascularization to restore coronary blood flow.

Revascularization is achieved either through the use of thrombolytic agents or, much more commonly, through percutaneous coronary intervention and coronary angioplasty. In general revascularization is deferred in the perioperative setting due primarily to increased bleeding risk, since anticoagulation agents are used intraprocedurally and antiplatelet medications are required continually for at least 1 month following the placement of a coronary stent to maintain stent patency and decrease risk of thrombus formation [20].

In the preoperative setting, pursuing revascularization generally requires a delay for pursuing surgery for at least 1 month. During coronary angioplasty procedures, coronary stents are placed in the majority of cases. "Drug-eluting" stents are the most commonly used in most centers; these stents carry a lower risk of late restenosis of a coronary lesion but in turn require a longer duration of antiplatelet therapy (at least 3 months vs. at least 1 month for "bare-metal" stents) [20]. Bare metal stents are used if the need for surgery in the next 3 months is expected. Patients are at significantly increased risk for major adverse cardiac events and mortality if surgery is pursued before the 3-month interval following a drug-eluting stent or before the 1-month interval following a bare-metal stent [21]. Most of this risk is attributable to cessation of antiplatelet therapy before the appropriate interval.

In the postoperative setting, pursuing revascularization with the appropriate anticoagulation and antiplatelet agents increases a patient's risk of postoperative bleeding and hemorrhage. The majority of postoperative bleeding events can be easily managed with local hemostasis; postoperative bleeding of clinical significance includes events continuing longer than 12 h, requiring a blood transfusion, requiring return to the emergency department or dental practice, and bleeding resulting in large hematoma or ecchymosis within the dental soft tissues [22]. The incidence of postoperative bleeding not controllable with local measures has been estimated to be between 0 and 3.5% in patients on anticoagulation therapy [23].

There are risks associated with thrombotic complications of coronary disease (in both angina and myocardial infarction and in patients with recent percutaneous coronary intervention), and there is a risk of bleeding in surgical patients on antiplatelet and anticoagulant medications. Therefore, the decision to pursue or delay revascularization with the requisite anticoagulation and antiplatelet therapy should be made in close collaboration between a cardiologist and a surgeon for both preoperative and postoperative patients.

38.3.2 Patient Management

The American Heart Association (AHA) and American College of Cardiology (ACC) publish joint recommendations for the management of acute coronary syndromes based on evidence from the medical literature, including observational studies and randomized controlled trials, and expert opinion. The recommendations presented here are representative of their consensus statements published in 2014 [17]. The recommendations outlined here represent only initial management during initial presentation of chest pain, prior to definitive diagnosis of myocardial infarction or other pathology. This management is aimed at improving myocardial oxygen supply and reducing myocardial oxygen demand, which can both improve symptoms and reduce the risk of progression from angina to myocardial ischemia to myocardial infarction.

38.3.2.1 Oxygen

As discussed in the monitoring section, arterial oxygen saturation should be measured noninvasively in chest pain patients. Supplemental oxygen should be available to every patient and should be especially administered to patients with oxygen saturations <90% or in patients with subjective dyspnea. Oxygen supplementation should not be administered indiscriminately to all patients, as there is some evidence that it may increase coronary arterial resistance and reduce coronary blood flow. Therefore oxygen saturation should be measured either continuously or at frequent intervals, and supplemental oxygen should be titrated to avoid unnecessary oxygen supplementation.

38.3.2.2 Nitrates

Nitroglycerin improves anginal symptoms and reduces myocardial oxygen consumption by reducing preload, afterload, and ventricular wall strain. Nitroglycerin also vasodilates coronary arteries and can in some instances improve coronary blood flow. Nitroglycerin is available in several formulations, including intravenous (typically administered as a continuous infusion), transdermal ointment or paste (applied to the sternum), and sublingual tablets and sprays. Sublingual nitroglycerin has a rapid onset and should be used in initial therapy. Patients with angina should be given 0.3–0.4 mg sublingual nitroglycerin every 5 min for up to three doses. If chest pain persists, a longer-acting formulation of nitroglycerin may be administered. Nitroglycerin is contraindicated in patients who have recently taken a phosphodiesterase inhibitor (such as sildenafil, tadalafil, or vardenafil) and in patients with hypotension.

38.3.2.3 Beta-Blockers

Beta-blockers are indicated in the setting of angina because they decrease heart rate and blood pressure, thereby decreasing myocardial oxygen consumption. They also decrease myocardial contractility, which also decreases demand, but for this reason are contraindicated in patients in whom acute heart failure is suspected. Furthermore, beta-blockers are used in preventing and controlling arrhythmia early following acute myocardial infarction [24]. In setting of bradycardia and hypotension, beta-blockers are contraindicated. In general, initial recommended dosing of beta-blockers is low-dose oral formulations for prevention of arrhythmias or low-dose intravenous formulations delivered as an intravenous bolus for treatment of acute arrhythmias.

38.3.2.4 Aspirin

Aspirin is the first-line antiplatelet therapy for acute coronary syndrome. Patients should be given a 162–325 mg "loading dose" of aspirin at the onset of suspicion for acute coronary syndrome. Non-enteric-coated formulations are preferred, and tablets (either enteric coated or non-enteric coated) may be crushed or chewed for more rapid absorption. For patients who are on a maintenance dose of aspirin and have received aspirin in the preceding 24 h, additional aspirin should be administered to total the recommended 162–325 mg loading dose. Aspirin has shown a mortality benefit among patients with acute coronary syndrome, stable angina, and high-risk patients [25].

Though aspirin and other antiplatelet medications inhibit platelet aggregation, there is increasing comfort among practitioners with continuing aspirin therapy uninterrupted during surgery. It has been commonly recommended for patients on aspirin therapy to continue taking aspirin uninterrupted through dental surgery in patients without coagulopathy [26]. A recent small single-center observational study found no significant increase in bleeding risk postoperatively in patients maintained on uninterrupted clopidogrel therapy or uninterrupted dual antiplatelet therapy with aspirin and clopidogrel, in patients receiving osteotomy [27]. All bleeding events were able to be treated with local measures and did not require hospitalization or transfusion. Therefore, if there is concern for a presentation of acute coronary syndrome in a perioperative patient, aspirin should be given without hesitation, or medical consultation may be pursued for careful risk-benefit analysis.

38.3.2.5 Morphine

In patients who continue to have chest pain despite nitroglycerin therapy, morphine 1–5 mg IV can be considered for additional pain control and may be given every 30 min under close monitoring of hemodynamics and respiratory status. Morphine increases venous dilation and decreases blood pressure and heart rate. The most common complications with morphine use are hypotension and respiratory depression. In perioperative patients who already received pharmacologic therapy for anxiolysis and analgesia, special care should be taken to avoid oversedation that may compromise respiratory status. Naloxone, an opioid reversal agent, should be readily available if morphine is used.

In contrast to the other recommendations for management above, morphine has not been studied in a randomized interventional study, and there are some observational studies that have suggested increased mortality with this approach [28]. Therefore, the other therapies described in this section should be prioritized, and morphine should only be added if blood pressure, heart rate, and respiratory rate remain acceptable.

38.4 Prevention

The most important tool in prevention is the preoperative evaluation, to determine a patient's risk of an adverse coronary event prior to surgery. A knowledge of the inherent cardiovascular risk associated with each surgery in a practitioner's repertoire is of equal importance. Patients at unacceptably high coronary risk should not be offered high-risk surgeries, especially in the elective setting. Carefully selecting surgical candidates is the best strategy for prevention. Preoperative medical and cardiology consultation may be considered for patients thought to be high risk.

In the preoperative setting, it is important to continue cardioprotective medications (both for secondary prevention and for primary prevention in high-risk individuals) to further minimize risk. Though patients may be instructed to take nothing by mouth prior to surgery to minimize aspiration risk with anesthesia, it should be stressed that certain medications must still be taken using small sips of water. As discussed in the management section, aspirin should be continued uninterrupted through surgery for patients who take the medication chronically, and consideration should be given to continuing dual antiplatelet therapy. Antihypertensive medications in general may also be continued through the morning of surgery, with a few exceptions. This is discussed in detail in Sect. 40.2.2.

In addition to the physiologic stress associated with surgery, there is also a component of psychological stress in many patients, which can cause catecholamine surge and tachycardia and hypertension similar to the response to physical pain. This alone can create a state of increased myocardial oxygen consumption that can place a patient at risk for angina or an acute coronary event. In fact, as discussed in the Manifestation/Presentation of Disease section, emotional stress as a trigger for pain is one criterion used to describe angina. It has been suggested that dental patients with cardiac comorbidities be scheduled for early morning procedures when possible to minimize anticipation and anxiety that may contribute to increased myocardial oxygen demand [29].

Conclusion

The oral and maxillofacial surgeon should maintain a high suspicion for cardiac or coronary etiology of symptoms in a patient with chest pain in the perioperative setting. Ideally, the surgeon should be well-informed regarding a patient's preoperative risk of a coronary event prior to the day of operation, which may influence initial workup and management. In patients in whom chest pain is suspicious for an acute coronary event, electrocardiogram and serum troponins should be used as the main diagnostic tools. Routine hemodynamic monitoring is equally necessary to stratify a patient's acuity and risk for complications. For patients meeting criteria for an acute coronary syndrome, consultation with a cardiologist should be pursued for individualized decision-making regarding need for revascularization, antiplatelet agents, and anticoagulation.

References

1. Campeau L. Letter: grading of angina pectoris. Circulation. 1976;54:522–3.
2. Von Dohlen TW, Rogers WB, Frank MJ. Pathophysiology and management of unstable angina. Clin Cardiol. 1989;12:363–9.
3. Davies MJ, Thomas AC. Plaque fissuring—the cause of acute myocardial infarction, sudden ischaemic death, and crescendo angina. Br Heart J. 1985;53:363–73.
4. Fuster V, Badimon L, Cohen M, Ambrose JA, Badimon JJ, Chesebro J. Insights into the pathogenesis of acute ischemic syndromes. Circulation. 1988;77:1213–20.
5. Peacock ME, Carson RE. Frequency of self-reported medical conditions in periodontal patients. J Periodontol. 1995;66:1004–7.
6. Chapman PJ. Medical emergencies in dental practice and choice of emergency drugs and equipment: a survey of Australian dentists. Aust Dent J. 1997;42:103–8.

7. Chapman PJ. Chest pain in the dental surgery: a brief review and practical points in diagnosis and management. Aust Dent J. 2002;47:259–61.
8. Girdler NM, Smith DG. Prevalence of emergency events in British dental practice and emergency management skills of British dentists. Resuscitation. 1999;41:159–67.
9. Atherton GJ, McCaul JA, Williams SA. Medical emergencies: medical emergencies in general dental practice in Great Britain Part 1: their prevalence over a 10-year period. Br Dent J. 1999;186:72–9.
10. Heberden W. Some account of a disorder of the breast. Med Transact. 1772;2:59–67.
11. Diamond GA. A clinically relevant classification of chest discomfort. J Am Coll Cardiol. 1983;1:574–5.
12. Swap CJ, Nagurney JT. Value and limitations of chest pain history in the evaluation of patients with suspected acute coronary syndromes. JAMA. 2005;294:2623–9.
13. Zipes DP, Wellens HJJ. Sudden cardiac death. Circulation. 1998;98:2334–51.
14. Benito B, Josephson ME. Ventricular tachycardia in coronary artery disease. Revista Española de Cardiología (English Edition). 2012;65:939–55.
15. Thygesen K, Alpert JS, White HD. Universal definition of myocardial infarction. J Am Coll Cardiol. 2007;50:2173–95.
16. Wu A, Feng Y, Contois J, Pervaiz S. Comparison of myoglobin, creatine kinase-MB, and cardiac troponin I for diagnosis of acute myocardial infarction. Ann Clin Lab Sci. 1996;26:291–300.
17. Amsterdam EA, Wenger NK, Brindis RG, Casey DE, Ganiats TG, Holmes DR, Jaffe AS, Jneid H, Kelly RF, Kontos MC, Levine GN, Liebson PR, Mukherjee D, Peterson ED, Sabatine MS, Smalling RW, Zieman SJ. 2014 AHA/ACC guideline for the management of patients with non-ST-elevation acute coronary syndromes: a report of the American College of Cardiology/American Heart Association Task Force on Practice Guidelines. Circulation. 2014;130:e344–426.
18. Bhayana V, Gougoulias T, Cohoe S, Henderson AR. Discordance between results for serum troponin T and troponin I in renal disease. Clin Chem. 1995;41:312–7.
19. Thygesen K, Alpert JS, Jaffe AS, Simoons ML, Chaitman BR, White HD. Third universal definition of myocardial infarction. Circulation. 2012;126:2020–35.
20. Levine GN, Bates ER, Bittl JA, Brindis RG, Fihn SD, Fleisher LA, Granger CB, Lange RA, Mack MJ, Mauri L, Mehran R, Mukherjee D, Newby LK, O'Gara PT, Sabatine MS, Smith PK, Smith SC. 2016 ACC/AHA guideline focused update on duration of dual antiplatelet therapy in patients with coronary artery disease: a report of the American College of Cardiology/American Heart Association Task Force on Clinical Practice Guidelines. J Am Coll Cardiol. 2016;68:1082–115.
21. Schouten O, van Domburg RT, Bax JJ, de Jaegere PJ, Dunkelgrun M, Feringa HHH, Hoeks SE, Poldermans D. Noncardiac surgery after coronary stenting: early surgery and interruption of antiplatelet therapy are associated with an increase in major adverse cardiac events. J Am Coll Cardiol. 2007;49:122–4.
22. Lockhart PB, Gibson J, Pond SH, Leitch J. Dental management considerations for the patient with an acquired coagulopathy. Part 1: coagulopathies from systemic disease. Br Dent J. 2003;195:439–45.
23. Pototski M, Amenábar JM. Dental management of patients receiving anticoagulation or antiplatelet treatment. J Oral Sci. 2007;49:253–8.
24. López-Sendó J, Swedberg K, McMurray J, Tamargo J, Maggioni AP, Dargie H, Tendera M, Waagstein F, Kjekshus J, Lechat P, Pedersen CT, Priori SG, Alonso García MA, Blanc J-J, Budaj A, Cowie M, Dean V, Deckers J, Fernandez Burgos E, Lekakis J, Lindahl B, Mazzotta G, McGregor K, Morais J, Oto A, Smiseth OA, Alonso García MA, Ardissino D, Avendano C, Lundqvist CB, ment DC, Drexler H, Ferrari R, Fox KA, Julian D, Kearney P, Klein W, ber LK, Mancia G, Nieminen M, Ruzyllo W, Simoons M, Thygesen K, Tognoni G, Tritto I, Wallentin L, Task Force on Beta-Blockers of the European Society of Cardiology. Expert consensus document on β-adrenergic receptor blockers. Eur Heart J. 2004;25:1341–62.
25. Collaboration AT. Collaborative meta-analysis of randomised trials of antiplatelet therapy for prevention of death, myocardial infarction, and stroke in high risk patients. BMJ. 2002;324:71–86.
26. Daniel NG, Goulet J, Bergeron M, Paquin P, Landry PE. Antiplatelet drugs: is there a surgical risk? J Can Dent Assoc. 2002;68:683–7.
27. Gröbe A, Fraederich M, Smeets R, Heiland M, Kluwe L, Zeuch J, Haase M, Wikner J, Hanken H, Semmusch J, Al-Dam A, Eichhorn W. Postoperative bleeding risk for oral surgery under continued clopidogrel antiplatelet therapy. Biomed Res Int. 2015;2015:823651.
28. Meine TJ, Roe MT, Chen AY, Patel MR, Washam JB, Ohman EM, Peacock WF, Pollack CV Jr, Gibler WB, Peterson ED. Association of intravenous morphine use and outcomes in acute coronary syndromes: results from the CRUSADE quality improvement initiative. Am Heart J. 2005;149:1043–9.
29. Jowett NI, Cabot LB. medical matters: Patients with cardiac disease: considerations for the dental practitioner. Br Dent J. 2000;189:297–302.

39

Respiratory Distress as a Complication of Maxillofacial Surgery

Carolyn McDonald and Rishal Ambaram

Abstract

Respiratory compromise is a serious panoperative complication that requires urgent and accurate diagnosis and treatment. This chapter will review differential diagnosis of respiratory distress. Appropriate diagnosis and early management will be emphasized.

39.1 Introduction

Vital organs need oxygen to survive. Oxygenation depends of ventilatory exchange, which requires both a patent airway and effective gas exchange of oxygen and carbon dioxide within the alveoli. This chapter will focus on respiratory compromise: the etiology, pathology, management, and potential adverse consequences of management.

Respiratory compromise can be separated into different categories: apnea/hypopnea, airway collapse/obstruction, inability/impaired ability to ventilate, and impaired diffusion. In order to predict and avoid states of respiratory compromise, one needs to be able to assess a patient's oropharyngeal airway and respiratory function to offer the safest and most predictable treatment options. Understanding airway anatomy helps in determining where an obstruction is and what rescue devices would work best in keeping an airway patent and a patient breathing.

Conditions that compromise an airway include body habitus (particularly obesity), neck immobility, incomplete frontal dentition, oral obstruction (tumor, mechanical), significant class II malocclusion (mandibular hypoplasia), short neck, enlarged tonsils, short thyromental distance, C-spine fusions, ankylosing spondylitis, medications, and other comorbidities. The structural features of the upper airway limit the airway caliber. The American Society of Anesthesiologists Task Force on the management of the difficult airway defines a difficult airway as the "clinical situation in which a conventionally trained anesthesiologist experiences problems with (a) face *mask ventilation* of the upper airway or (b) *tracheal intubation*, or both."

C. McDonald, C.R.N.A. (✉)
Department of Anesthesiology, Richard L. Roudebush VA Medical Center, Indianapolis, IN, USA
e-mail: carolyn.mcdonald@va.gov

R. Ambaram, D.D.S.
Division of Oral and Maxillofacial Surgery, School of Dental Medicine, University of Connecticut, Farmington, CT, USA

© Springer International Publishing AG 2018
E.M. Ferneini, J.D. Bennett (eds.), *Perioperative Assessment of the Maxillofacial Surgery Patient*,
https://doi.org/10.1007/978-3-319-58868-1_39

Qualitative clinical signs of ventilation include adequate chest rise and respiratory rate. The qualitative signs for oxygenation are not as reliable. Observing for signs of cyanosis and pallor before performing rescue measures not only increases a patient's morbidity but also could prove to be fatal. It is now standard of care to measure oxygenation with a pulse oximeter that measures the peripheral oxygen saturation of the arterial blood. However, understanding the limitations of using the pulse oximeter is important for anyone performing sedations. For example, in a case of a patient experiencing hypoventilation, hypoxia causes a reduction in the oxygen saturation obtained from the pulse oximeter; however, the time it takes for the SpO_2 to reflect the level of hypoxia can take up to 30 s, significantly affecting the risk profile for this patient. Assessing the waveform capnography would reflect the hypoventilation and subsequent respiratory acidosis much earlier. Peripheral vascular disease, vasoconstriction, and hypovolemia are factors that impact the limitations of fully relying on a pulse oximeter to assess oxygenation. Additionally, conventional pulse oximeters lack the ability to differentiate between carboxyhemoglobin and methemoglobin from oxyhemoglobin, decreasing the reliability to accurately assess peripheral oxygen saturation. Newer-generation pulse oximeters now use multiple wavelengths of light to detect carboxyhemoglobin from oxyhemoglobin, making readings more reliable [1].

In patients with acute respiratory distress, clinical findings that reflect an increase in work of breathing include retractions and the use of accessory muscles to breathe, inability to speak full sentences, inability to lie flat, extreme diaphoresis, and restlessness with declining level of consciousness. An important supplement in many patients experiencing respiratory distress is oxygen administration. Natural air has an O_2 concentration of about 20% (which is to say, the FiO_2, or the fraction of inspired O_2, is 20%). Oxygen supplementation provides air with a higher FiO_2. The PaO_2 is the partial pressure of the oxygen that is dissolved in the blood, measured in mmHg. Hypoxemia is defined as having a low PaO_2. A rule of thumb for a patient on supplemental O_2 is the PaO_2 should be $5 \times FiO_2$. So if a patient is breathing in 40% O_2, the PaO_2 should be $5 \times 40 = 200$ mmHg. A key differentiation is between the O_2 saturation and the PaO_2. The O_2 saturation, as mentioned earlier, is the percentage of hemoglobin binding sites in the blood that are bound to O_2. This measurement follows the HgB dissociation curve. The PaO_2 is a measure of the O_2 that is freely dissolved in the blood. The PaO_2 can be an additional index to assess if there is adequate ventilation and diffusion across the alveoli, with $5 \times FiO_2$ estimating appropriate oxygen supplementation [2].

In order to form a differential diagnosis of a patient experiencing respiratory distress in the outpatient setting, clinical symptoms and vitals are invaluable in leading your treatment plan. In patients experiencing wheezing and shortness of breath, typically an asthma or COPD exacerbation should be ruled out first. When patients display symptoms of coughing, increased work of breathing—like costal retractions and paradoxical chest wall and abdominal wall movement patterns—and stridor, one should think of an obstruction as a likely cause. Obstructions come in many different forms such as foreign body aspiration, laryngospasm causing partial or complete closure of the vocal cords, and even angioedema. Understanding the pathophysiology of each of these outcomes helps guide the management of these patients. Many of these topics will be covered in the remainder of the chapter, with the pathophysiology and treatment of each of these conditions. With that said, many of these respiratory complications should be addressed emergently, which also means that the treatment of many of these conditions in the emergency setting relies on a few major guiding principles. As stressful as it can be to be effective in responding to a patient declining precipitously, going back to the basics of (A) airway, (B) breathing, and (C) circulation can be a simple way of managing most emergencies. Maintaining a patent airway should always be the first response. Performing the chin lift/jaw thrust to open the airway and performing bag-valve-mask ventilation are lifesaving skills all medical professionals should have. Providing supplemental oxygen (FiO_2) and monitoring vitals are also simple ways that may stabilize a patient in respiratory distress and buy you time to call for help. The most important lesson to take away from this chapter, aside from how to manage patients in respiratory distress, is to always take a complete history and perform an adequate physical exam prior to performing any procedures. Obtaining such information not only helps in preventing these complications but also gives you an idea of what the problem is that incited the patient's adverse reaction.

39.2 Laryngospasm

Laryngospasm is an involuntary defense mechanism—from the entry of anything but air into the lungs—that involves muscle spasms of the vocal cords, creating a partial or complete airway closure, thereby making it difficult to breathe. A laryngospasm can be caused by allergies, anxiety, asthma exacerbation, cold air, and foreign bodies entering the upper airway and can quickly result in hypoxemia and hypercarbia [3]. A delayed reaction in a patient with this sort of response, especially in an outpatient setting, where there is fewer auxiliary staff to help in emergency situations, can result in significant morbidity and mortality. A strict management plan for a patient having a laryngospasm should routinely be reviewed to be able to respond expeditiously and regain a patent airway.

39.2.1 Pathophysiology

Closure of the glottis is produced by the recruitment of the laryngeal muscles that adduct the vocal cords. An afferent response from the thermal, chemical, and mechanical fibers travels along the sensory vagus nerve. This afferent limb carries a stimulatory response from areas that include the nasal mucosa, soft palate, pharynx, larynx, epiglottis, tracheobronchial tree, and even abdominal viscera. The subsequent motor response is performed by three intrinsic laryngeal muscles: the lateral cricoarytenoids, the thyroarytenoids, and the cricoarytenoids, all of which are innervated by the recurrent laryngeal nerve (the superior laryngeal nerve innervates only the cricothyroid muscle) [4]. The glottis closes either by adduction of just the true vocal cords or the combination of the true and false vocal cords. A collapse of the soft tissues may also occur from the translaryngeal inspiratory pressure gradient as it increases after closure of the true and false vocal cords. The supraglottic soft tissues become rounded and redundant and draw into the laryngeal inlet [5]. The soft tissue effect is known as the ball-valve effect.

39.2.2 Diagnosis

A laryngospasm is always an emergency, either stemming from a partial or complete airway obstruction. The patient is usually in noticeable respiratory distress, and identifying the problem is key to avoiding significant morbidity or, in some unfortunate cases, mortality. Inspiratory stridor is a hallmark sign. In cases seen by the oral and maxillofacial surgeon, many patients may cough to clear the foreign body obstruction or secretions that irritated the larynx. If the patient is unconscious, a bucking motion or abdominal rocking motion is seen as the patient attempts to breathe against a closed glottis [6]. Also noticeable are paradoxical chest wall and abdominal movements. In severe laryngospasm with complete airway obstruction, there are chest wall movements but a lack of breath sounds (sine qua non). In 77% of cases, a laryngospasm is clinically obvious and easily diagnosed [7].

39.2.3 Management

Initial assessment of the patient should begin with evaluation of the airway (A), breathing (B), and circulation (C). In an incomplete airway obstruction, the airway should be evaluated first, to note for any signs of obvious obstruction, removing the irritating surgical stimulus and debris. Next is perform the chin lift/jaw thrust and provide positive airway pressure with a well-sealed face mask. The jaw thrust lengthens the thyrohyoid muscle and unfolds any supraglottic tissue. Deepening the level of anesthesia/sedation can be also helpful. In a complete airway obstruction (after evaluating the airway and performing the jaw thrust), IV atropine and succinylcholine (4 mg/kg) are pushed [3]. The succinylcholine will relax the vocal chords within 1 min and provide adequate time to intubate the patient. In cases when a laryngospasm does not break and the patient continues to decline, an emergent cricothyrotomy or tracheostomy is performed to obtain a patent airway [7].

39.3 Hyperkalemia: Consequence of Succinylcholine

39.3.1 Pathophysiology

Severe, life-threatening hyperkalemia can occur when succinylcholine is given to patients with genetic skeletal muscle myopathies or with long-term immobility, extensive denervation of skeletal muscle, or upper motor neuron injuries.

There appear to be two pathways that contribute to the development of hyperkalemia. In the case of denervation, with upper motor neuron lesions due to stroke, brain or spinal cord pathology, closed head injury, or encephalitis and immobilization, the cause is likely upregulation of the receptors. In normal situations, junctional membrane depolarization results in a small leakage of potassium. However, after when the receptor is upregulated, very large amounts of K+ may leak—enough to produce severe hyperkalemia. The risk of this phenomenon increases with the severity and time from the denervation event, and it usually peaks at 7–14 days post event. This time frame corresponds to the time it takes for upregulation to reach its zenith. The second mechanism is a direct toxic effect of succinylcholine on the muscle cells of myopathy and dystrophy patients in whom succinylcholine greatly increases the permeability of muscle cell membranes, causing either rhabdomyolysis or massive leakage of potassium. Hyperkalemia resulting from rhabdomyolysis tends to be more severe than that from upregulation [8].

Myopathies are often occult at the time of surgery—especially among children—and that is one of the reasons why succinylcholine is prescribed for elective surgery in children though it remains an option for emergency intubation.

39.3.2 Management

Use the usual treatments for hyperkalemia using intravenous calcium to counteract the membrane effects of hyperkalemia and insulin glucose infusions to draw the potassium into the cells as well as ion exchange resins and/or dialysis as needed.

39.4 Atypical Pseudocholinesterase: Adverse Effect Associated with Succinylcholine

39.4.1 Pathophysiology

Pseudocholinesterase, also known as plasma cholinesterase and butyrylcholinesterase (BuChE), is a glycoprotein enzyme, serine hydrolase, that "catalyzes the hydrolysis of choline esters" (openanesthesia.org). It is produced in the liver and circulates in the blood (NIH.org-pseudocholinesterase). It should be distinguished from its close cousin erythrocyte cholinesterase that is found in red cells and neuromuscular junctions. Pseudocholinesterase rapidly breaks down succinylcholine, mivacurium, ester local anesthetics (e.g. procaine), and to a lesser extent cocaine [9]. However, in the face of pseudocholinesterase deficiency, succinylcholine is not broken down in the usual 3–15 min. It may take 20 min to 2 h, or much longer in rare cases, to metabolize a typical dose [9].

A variety of mutations of pseudocholinesterase are located on chromosome site 3q26 that result in reduction or loss of enzyme function [9]. These mutations prolong the effect of both succinylcholine and mivacurium, which can greatly prolong the duration of paralysis. Mivacurium is no longer available in the USA, so it is not a focus of this section, but it still is used in many countries. Pseudocholinesterase also breaks down ester-based *local* anesthetics. If a patient has inherited, an inactive or less active form of pseudocholinesterase, such ester local anesthetic agents will not be broken down as rapidly in the blood resulting in a higher plasma concentration, which may increase the chance for an adverse systemic effect. This is an important issue for maxillofacial surgery where large amounts of local anesthetic might be used either as primary or as a supplementary anesthetic. In such cases, use an amide-based, instead of an ester-based, local anesthetic to avoid any risk of an undiagnosed pseudocholinesterase deficiency.

39.4.2 Prevalence of the Genetic Defect

More than 64 variants of the pseudocholinesterase gene that reduce the activity of pseudocholinesterase by varying degrees have been reported [10]. Approximately 1:3000 people are homozygous for abnormal alleles [9]. Less than 1% of the population carries homozygous gene mutations that prolong succinylcholine paralysis for more than an hour. The most severe form only occurs in 1:100,000 people and can prolong paralysis for over 8 h.

39.4.3 Screening

Pseudocholinesterase deficiency is usually first identified by a delayed recovery of muscle strength at the end of a surgical case. Patients can be screened with genetic testing, but such screening is not recommended because of its high cost and the fact that the NMB will wear off after a few hours of observation when cholinestera+se deficiency is first discovered after a dose of succinylcholine or mivacurium.

Cholinesterase activity can also be diminished by nongenetic factors, and these effects can be strong (e.g., severe liver disease and exposure to organophosphates) [11]. More modest reductions in cholinesterase activity are associated with severe burns, chronic infections, and pregnancy—with reductions or activity up to 75% reported (https://www.openanesthesia.org/pseudocholinesterase_synthesis/ (openanesthesia.org)); but other authors claim lesser effects with no clinical significance in the absence of a pseudocholinesterase mutation. Other factors, such as renal failure and interactions with esmolol, metoclopramide, oral contraceptives, and monoamine oxidase inhibitors [12], may slow pseudocholinesterase metabolism and lead to increase dosing requirements.

39.4.4 Prevention

Use a paralyzing agent that is not metabolized by pseudocholinesterase, in which case the genetic changes discussed above have no relevance. Rocuronium is such an alternative. It has a rapid onset like succinylcholine but a longer duration of action. However, its NMB effects can be quickly reversed with sugammadex diminishing that disadvantage [13].

39.4.5 Patient Management

When prolonged paralysis occurs, maintain ventilation, which can be achieved with either a bag valve mask or ventilator until full muscle strength returns. The patient should be kept sedated so that patient is not awake and still paralyzed. Continue with ASA standard monitors including HR, RR, BP, SPO_2, Temp, and $ETCO_2$ [14] until full breathing capabilities return to baseline. Do not use neostigmine (or other cholinergic agents) to reverse succinylcholine's paralytic effect as this will only delay recovery because it contributes to depolarization and blocks cholinesterase which is needed to break down succinylcholine.

39.5 Bronchospasm

A bronchospasm is a reactionary constriction of muscles around the walls of the bronchioles due to the release of mediators from mast cells and basophils. In an oral and maxillofacial surgery practice, the triggers for such an event include secretions, blood, foreign body lodging into the bronchial tree, and asthma exacerbations. The histamine release causes inflammatory edema and mucus plugging that further impairs airflow. In a patient with a reactive airway, emergence from anesthesia increases the risk of laryngospasm and bronchospasm. To understand the management of bronchospasm, a big picture look at the tracheobronchial tree may help.

The trachea divides into the right and left primary bronchi at the level of the sternal angle. The bronchi branch lobar bronchi, then segmental bronchi, and then into bronchioles. The bronchioles are the smallest airways and do not contain any cartilage or mucus-secreting goblet cells. There is, however, an abundance of surfactant lipoprotein produced by club cells that prevent the walls of the small airways from sticking together. Bronchioles have conducting passages that eventually lead to respiratory bronchioles, which are involved in actual gas exchange. In a case of an acute asthma exacerbation, the trigger (cold air, allergens, exercise, viruses, pollution, aspirin) results in sudden contraction of the smooth muscles that surround the bronchioles (bronchospasm), causing the characteristic wheezing noise on expiration [15].

39.5.1 Management

In the oral and maxillofacial surgery office, most patients do not have a protective airway in place, such as an endotracheal tube or an LMA. Identifying the etiology of the patient's respiratory distress is vital in avoiding detrimental effects of surgical stress to the patient. In a nonsedated or minimally sedated patient, the most common treatment for bronchospasm is inhaled beta-2 agonist (albuterol 4–8 puffs) [16]. If the patient is too deeply sedated or unable to inhale the metered dose inhaler, 100% oxygen through a face mask is immediately provided. When the patient can be adequately ventilated, nebulized beta-2 agonist is administered [16].

In the case where a bronchospasm persists despite all of the above procedures, an IM dose of 0.3–0.5 mg of epinephrine 1:1000 is administered with continued 100% oxygen through the face mask. A last resort when the bronchospasm still persists is intubating the patient with an endotracheal tube. If the patient is intubated or has a LMA, deepening the anesthetic with sevoflurane or isoflurane, a potent bronchodilator, can break the bronchospasm, and traditionally IV steroid, dexamethasone 10 mg IV, can be given concurrently as well [17].

39.5.2 Prevention

"A large retrospective review revealed that the incidence of intraoperative bronchospasm and laryngospasm was surprisingly low, ~1.7%, although complications were more frequent in older patients and those with active asthma" [18]. In patients with well-controlled asthma, there appears to be no additional risk of bronchospasm in the perioperative setting. Before any sedation procedure, a good history and physical exam is vital. With patients who have a history of asthma, be certain to confirm how often they use their rescue inhaler (beta agonist) and what dose they use, and having them bring their inhaler with them to the appointment may be prudent. With patients who have had complications with anesthesia in the past, knowing the trigger and how it was managed is important to ascertain [18]. The α-2 agonist dexmedetomidine has long been used in the ICU setting because of its opioid-sparing analgesic, anxiolytic, and hypnotic effects. The lack of interaction with opioid receptors makes it valuable to use in patients with reactive airways or those with cardiopulmonary comorbidities. In a recent double-blind, randomized controlled trial looking at dexmedetomidine and its effect on hemodynamics after extubation, a dose of 0.75 mcg/kg administered 15 min before extubation reduced the incidence of MAP spikes, respiratory depression, laryngospasm, bronchospasm, and hypotension [19].

39.6 Foreign Object (Aspiration/Obstruction)

Foreign bodies that make their way into the airway can be life-threatening emergencies. The object can lodge into the larynx or trachea and cause a partial or complete obstruction. In this case, immediate respiratory distress and choking ensue, with the patient wretchedly coughing and gasping. If the object descends past the carina and into a main stem bronchus (usually the right bronchus because of its more acute angle of the trachea), the patient may be completely asymptomatic at first [20]. Commonly aspirated objects include food, dental appliances, toys, coins, etc. In an oral and maxillofacial surgery office, common aspirated items include loose or extracted teeth or tooth fragments and dental implant parts/screws [21].

39.6.1 Pathophysiology

When an object is aspirated, it might change position or move further distally. Local inflammation with edema, cellular infiltration, and ulceration can occur, making visualization with bronchoscopy more challenging. In severe inflammatory cases, tracheoesophageal fistulas and mediastinitis can occur. This may occur if a patient is sedated and is unaware that a tooth fragment or implant screw gets lodged into the airway and eventually settles into a main stem bronchus. Clinically, the patient may have asymmetric chest expansion on careful exam and possibly a wheeze on end expiration. In the acute setting, noticeable sternal retractions and paradoxical breathing are present. A chest X-ray may identify foreign body in a main stem bronchus and possibly show air trapping, indicating an inability to move air out of the obstructed lung. Distal to the obstruction, atelectasis, pneumonia, or bronchiectasis may be apparent if sufficient time has surpassed. Taking lateral X-rays in children may show that the dependent lung with the obstruction remains inflated, instead of collapsed [22].

In a recent case report, a 59-year-old male presented to the ED with right-sided chest discomfort with a cough productive of yellow phlegm and a tint of blood for 2 months. The physical exam was notable for wheezing and rhonchi over the right lung field. A chest X-ray revealed a radiopacity in the right main stem bronchus. An emergency bronchoscopy was done and revealed a mandibular partial denture [23].

39.6.2 Management

Initial treatment of airway obstruction/aspiration is to perform the head tilt, chin lift/jaw thrust maneuver. Next is to grab the tongue with gauze, tissue forceps, or with a suture. If the object is not visibly apparent and feasible to grasp with Magill forceps, then chest/abdominal thrusts should be performed [24]. This increases the airway pressure to help thrust the object up and into the pharynx. Common complications of this maneuver are rib fracture and abdominal or thoracic viscera lacerations. According to the American Heart Association, blind finger sweeps are no longer recommended. If none of the above techniques are successful, positive-pressure ventilation should be initiated.

39.7 Angioedema

Angioedema is swelling of the subcutaneous tissues as a result of mast cell degranulation, bradykinin, or complement deficiency. Drugs, trauma, dental work, tongue piercings, viral illnesses, pollen, animal dander, and venom can trigger the reaction. In some cases, chronic use of ACE inhibitors has been known to cause angioedema. The characteristic swelling in angioedema is due to the increased vascular permeability leading to increased fluid extravasation.

39.7.1 Pathophysiology

With mast cell degranulation, the release of histamine not only causes increased vascular permeability in the subcutaneous tissues but also in the dermal-epidermal junction—where histamine release can incite pruritus and urticaria [25]. In bradykinin-induced angioedema, pruritus and urticaria are not seen because the dermal-epidermal junction is not involved. In complement deficiency-induced angioedema, the problem lies in a deficiency or defect in C1 inhibitor, a protein involved with regulating the complement system. C1 inhibitor regulates the activation of C1, which causes vasodilation and increased vascular permeability. With a C1 inhibitor deficiency or defect, there is over activation of C1 that subsequently leads to uncontrolled fluid shifts into the extravascular space that lead to angioedema. In hereditary angioedema, there is either a C1 deficiency or a C1 defect that is inherited in an autosomal dominant fashion. In acquired C1 inhibitor deficiencies, B-cell lymphoma and other cancers consume excessive amounts of C1 inhibitor leading to C1 inhibitor deficiency [26].

In over 90% of cases, angioedema is due to IgE-mediated mast cell degranulation triggered by allergens. In some acute cases of angioedema, an allergen can interact with mast cells directly, without IgE mediation. In the oral and maxillofacial surgery patient, the most likely trigger in patients susceptible to angioedema is an antibiotic. This underscores the importance of obtaining a complete history [27].

39.7.2 Signs and Symptoms

In angioedema that is a result of mast cell degranulation, the usual signs are edema of the face, lips, tongue, and also the hands and feet. If the edema involves the upper respiratory tract, the patient may have wheezing and/or stridor. These characteristic signs are always accompanied by pruritus, urticaria, and sometimes bronchospasm and flushing. Typically, mast cell-induced angioedema can be noticed within minutes, whereas the bradykinin-induced pathway develops over hours to days [28].

39.7.3 Management

A patient displaying symptoms of angioedema should be treated emergently. First order of assessment is the airway and making certain the patient is not in respiratory distress. In most cases of mast cell-mediated angioedema, an IM dose 0.3 mg epinephrine in the deltoid muscle, followed by repeat doses every 5–15 min if needed, may resolve the airway edema. In severe cases, IV methylprednisolone 125 mg and diphenhydramine 50 mg should be administered [29]. Just like any anaphylactic reaction, it's important to remove the offending agent and to avoid it in the future. An integral part of this is educating the patient about angioedema and his or her triggers.

39.8 Croup

Croup is constellation of symptoms in young children commonly caused by viruses. It usually falls into two categories: laryngotracheitis and spasmodic croup. In laryngotracheitis, an inflammatory infiltrate swarms the lateral walls of the trachea below the vocal cords, causing erythema and edema. Onset of symptoms resembles those of a cold, with rhinitis, cough, nasal irritation, and fever that starts within 24 h. Symptoms usually progress quickly to hoarseness, barking cough, and minimal to severe respiratory stridor. In spasmodic croup, we see a noninflammatory edema in the subglottic region. Symptoms almost always present at night time, when the child goes to bed with little to no symptoms but suddenly awakens with inspiratory stridor and cough. Symptoms usually progress quickly, similarly to laryngotracheitis. Viruses that are often responsible for laryngotracheitis and spasmodic croup include parainfluenza virus 1, parainfluenza virus 3, influenza virus A, RSV, measles virus, adenovirus, and rhinovirus [30].

In bacterial croup, also termed laryngotracheobronchitis and laryngotracheobronchopneumonitis, thick pus fills the lumen of the trachea and the distal airway passages, and the tracheal wall is infiltrated with inflammatory cells.

Since croup develops in only small group of children exposed to the parainfluenza virus, an allergic factor is thought to be the reason for the recurrent croup. The initial parainfluenza virus 3 exposures go unnoticed with no clinical symptoms. The subsequent infection with parainfluenza virus 1 and 2 sensitizes the patient and creates the characteristic symptoms described above.

39.8.1 Incidence

Croup is an upper respiratory illness in children 6 years and younger. The most common age that croup occurs is between 3 months and 3 years. "In a 14-year study of hospitalizations for croup in Ontario, Canada, between 1988 and 2002, a biennial mid-autumn peak and an annual summer trough were observed." The severity of croup can be numerically assessed based on the level of consciousness, cyanosis, stridor, air entry, and retractions.

39.8.2 Differential Diagnosis

Assessing upper airway disease and the correct diagnosis is vital and can decrease the risk of mortality. In epiglottitis, the child would lack a barking, seallike cough. In cases of foreign body aspiration or angioedema, an obstruction may result and often doesn't accompany a fever and other symptoms of infection. In bacterial causes of croup, patients often decline further despite treatment with epinephrine and corticosteroids. On a lateral X-ray, evidence of pus may be apparent with signs of soft densities on imaging.

39.8.3 Treatment

The mainstay treatment for croup is corticosteroid therapy. Most regimens include a single dose of dexamethasone (0.6 mg/kg) orally, with nebulized budesonide (2 mg in 4 mL water). Other treatments including "steaming" haven't gained much traction. A Cochrane review from three other studies concluded that there was no evidence that inhalation of humidified air in children with mild-to-moderate croup resulted in a substantial improvement in the croup score. In severe croup, epinephrine has been shown to decrease the need for intubation. In cases with laryngotracheobronchitis and laryngotracheobronchopneumonitis, antibiotics need to be administered to cover the bacterial cause of croup. The antibiotic of choice should cover organisms including *Staphylococcus aureus*, *Streptococcus pyogenes*, *Streptococcus pneumoniae*, *Haemophilus influenzae*, and *Moraxella catarrhalis* [31].

39.9 Residual Neuromuscular Blockade

39.9.1 Pathophysiology

It has become increasingly apparent that residual neuromuscular blockade persists longer than had previously been thought and that this persistence has important physiologic and clinical consequences.

A recent study showed that, despite the use of intermediate-duration neuromuscular-blocking drugs (NMBDs) and the use of pharmacologic reversal agents, between 33 and 64% of patients had inadequate neuromuscular recovery upon arrival in the PACU as assessed by train-of-four (TOF) [32]. The TOF fade ratio is the ratio of the strength of T1 (the first simulation) to T4 (the fourth stimulation) in the train-of-four [33]. Until recently a TOF fade ratio >0.70 was considered evidence of reversal of neuromuscular blockade. However, in normal volunteers, loss of ventilatory drive can occur at TOF of 0.7, upper airway obstruction (due to pharyngeal muscle weakness) at a TOF of 0.8, and aspiration at a TOF of 0.9. In a randomized trial, the risk of respiratory complications was greater when the TOF was below 0.7. *Additionally*, Eikermann et al. detected upper airway obstruction in two-thirds of volunteers at a TOF radio of 0.5 and one-third of them at TOF ratio of 0.8. Other studies report significant pharyngeal muscle dysfunction in healthy volunteers at TOF fade ratios below 0.9 [34]. Such effects would likely be worse in postanesthesia patients who may have the added burden of residual anesthesia effects and postoperative narcotics. In one study residual paralysis was present in almost a third of the cases with low SPO_2 <90%. Airway obstruction was the second most common critical respiratory event (CRE) and occurs in 0.3% of PACU patients overall, and in a third of the CRE cases in one study, the NMB was the potentiating cause [32].

39.9.2 Assessment Monitoring

The use of simple clinical methods, such as the inability to hold the head up or maintain a sustained handgrip for 5 s, can be used to assess the persistence of a residual neuromuscular blockade (NMB) and is easy to implement. The tool has good specificity but very poor sensitivity for identifying residual NMB. TOF ratios are much better and are the standard methods of assessing the degree of residual NMB. They require the electrical stimulation of a nerve and observation of the strength of contraction of the enervated muscle. Multiple different nerves—muscle pairs are used but the ulnar nerve—and adductor pollicis muscle of the thumb correlate best with TOF of 4. TOF numbers are usually derived from subjective judgments. Objective measurements of muscle strength after nerve stimulation are much more accurate. The mechanomyogram and electromyogram are gold standards, and acceleromyograph is quite good [34]. These objective measures of strength recovery are more difficult to set up and more expensive than the subjective ones so are underutilized in clinical practice.

39.9.3 Management

The key decision after the use of a neuromuscular blocker is when to give a reversal agent to reach full recovery in the shortest time. Moi points out that there must be some recovery—a subjective train-of-four count (TOFC) of at least 2 before starting a reversal agent such as neostigmine—and to use the reversal agents at intervals until the subjective TOF reaches 4 with a 0.9 TOF fade ratio. He suggests different thresholds when using an objective TOF measure and when the patient has been exposed to certain anesthetic agents that potentiate weakness [34].

When rocuronium is the NMB agent, sugammadex can revise the NMB quickly in 2 min from the time when the TOFC reaches 2. It has none of the side effects of neostigmine and can also be used to reverse effects of vecuronium but not quite as quickly.

39.9.4 Prevention of Residual NMB

Avoid the use of any NMB when possible. Avoid large doses of NMB when feasible. Stay with the intermediate-duration NMBs, i.e., rocuronium and vecuronium, rather than long-acting agents. Use the lightest depth of paralysis possible; deep intraoperative paralysis, i.e., a TOFC of zero, will yield the most residual NMB.

Conclusion

This chapter provides an overview of managing the surgical patient with respiratory distress. Being able to correctly identify the physiology that is causing the symptoms not only reduces patient morbidity, it reduces the provider's anxiety in stressful times because understanding the reaction allows one to predict what happens with certain interventions. Nothing replaces a thorough history and physical examination. Using appropriate monitoring devices—CO_2 capnography, for example, as a primary means in conjunction with a pulse oximeter—can predict adverse outcomes much sooner, allowing intervention before the patient displays acute symptoms. In those facing respiratory distress, symptoms can point either to an obstruction in the tracheobronchial tree, a reaction of angioedema, or poor airflow. Becoming abreast with the symptoms and the first-line treatment of these conditions is essential in any surgical patient.

References

1. Langeron O, Birenbaum A, Le Saché F, Raux M. Airway management in obese patient. Minerva Anestesiol. 2014;80(3):382–92. Epub Oct 14, 2013
2. Strohl KP, Butler JP, Malhotra A. Mechanical properties of the upper airway. Compr Physiol. 2012;2(3): 1853–72.
3. Lawson NW, Johnson JO. Autonomic nervous system: physiology and pharmacology. In: Barash PG, Cullen BF, Stoelting RK, editors. Clinical anesthesia. 5th ed. Philadelphia, PA: Lippincott-Raven Publishers; 2006. p. 275–333.
4. Gavel G, Walker RWM. Laryngospasm in anaesthesia. Contin Educ Anaesth Crit Care Pain. 2014;14(2):47–51. https://doi.org/10.1093/bjaceaccp/mkt031.
5. Fink BR. The etiology and treatment of laryngospasm. Anesthesiology. 1956;17:569–77.
6. American Thoracic Society. Standards for the diagnosis and care of patients with chronic obstructive pulmonary disease (COPD). Am J Respir Crit Care Med. 1995;152:s77–s120.
7. Becker DE, Haas DA. Management of complications during moderate and deep sedation: respiratory and cardiovascular considerations. Anesth Prog. 2007;54(2): 59–69. doi: 10.2344/0003-3006(2007)54[59:MOCDMA]2.0.CO;2
8. Sugita H, Kaneki M, Sugita M, Yasukawa T, Yasuhara S, Martyn JAJ. Burn injury impairs insulin-stimulated Akt/PKB activation in skeletal muscle. Am J Physiol Endocrinol Metab. 2005;288(3):E585–91.
9. Wecksell M, Koutsospyros D. Pseudocholinesterase deficiency in a octogenarian undergoing total intravenous anesthesia; implications for neuromonitoring. Mid East J Anaesthesiol. 2015;23(2):157–62.
10. Soliday FK, Conley YP, Henker R. Pseudocholinesterase deficiency: a comprehensive review of genetic, acquired, and drug influences. AANA J. 2010;78(4):313–20.
11. Nelson TC, Burritt MF. Pesticide poisoning, succinylcholine-induced apnea, and pseudocholinesterase. Mayo CLin Proc. 1986;61(9):750–2.
12. https://www.openanesthesia.org/pseudocholinesterase_synthesis/openanesthesia.org
13. Sparr HJ, Vermeyen KM, Beaufort AM, et al. Early reversal of profound rocuronium-induced neuromuscular blockade by sugammadex in a randomized multicenter study: efficacy, safety, and pharmacokinetics. Anesth. 2007;106(5):953–43.
14. Geralemou S, Gan TJ. Assessing the value of risk indices of postoperative nausea and vomiting in ambulatory surgical patients. Curr Opin Anaesthesiol. 2016;29(6):668–73.
15. American Association for Respiratory Care. Aerosol consensus statement: 1991. Respir Care. 1991;36:916–21.
16. Simons FE, Sheikh A. Anaphylaxis: the acute episode and beyond. BMJ. 2013;346:f602. https://doi.org/10.1136/bmj.f602.
17. Worm M, Eckermann O, Dolle S, et al. Triggers and treatment of anaphylaxis: an analysis of 4,000 cases from Germany, Austria and Switzerland. Dtsch Arztebl Int. 2014;111(21):367–75.
18. Woods BD, Sladen RN. Perioperative considerations for the patient with asthma and bronchospasm. Br J Anaesth. 2009;103(Suppl 1):i57–65. https://doi.org/10.1093/bja/aep271.
19. Bindu B, Pasupuleti S, Gowd UP, Gorre V, Murthy RR, Laxmi MB. A double blind, randomized, controlled trial to study the effect of dexmedetomidine on hemodynamic and recovery responses during tracheal extubation. J Anaesthesiol Clin Pharmacol. 2013;29(2):162–7. https://doi.org/10.4103/0970-9185.111665.
20. Isaacs RS, Sykes JM. Anatomy and physiology of the upper airway. Anesthesiol Clin North Am. 2002;20:733–45.
21. National Safety Council, Research and Statistics Department. Injury facts 2008 edition. Itasca, Ill: National Safety Council, 2008;8:14–15.
22. Saki N, Nikakhlagh S, Heshmati SM. 25-Year review of the abundance and diversity of radiopaque airway foreign bodies in children. Indian J Otolaryngol Head Neck Surg. 2015;67(3):261–6.
23. Safdar SA, Shaaban H, Miller RA. Foreign body aspiration. Heart Lung Circ. 2015;10:1033–4.
24. Debeljak A, Sorli J, Music E, Kecelj P. Bronchoscopic removal of foreign bodies in adults: experience with 62 patients from 1974-1998. Eur Respir J. 1999;14(4): 792–5.
25. Kumar SA, Martin BL. Urticaria and angioedema: diagnostic and treatment considerations. J Am Osteopath Assoc. 1999;99(3 Suppl):S1–4.
26. Cicardi M, Bergamaschini L, Cugno M, et al. Pathogenic and clinical aspects of C1 inhibitor deficiency. Immunobiology. 1998;199(2):366–76.
27. Lin RY, Levine RJ, Lin H. Adverse drug effects and angioedema hospitalizations in the United States from 2000–2009. Allergy Asthma Proc. 2013;34(1):65–71.
28. Reed KL. Basic management of medical emergencies: recognizing a patient's distress. J Am Dent Assoc. 2010;141(Suppl 1):20S–4S.
29. Hepner DL, Castells MC. Anaphylaxis during the perioperative period. Anesth Analg. 2003;97(5):1381–95.
30. Cherry JD. Croup. N Engl J Med. 2008;358:384–91. https://doi.org/10.1056/NEJMcp072022.

31. Bjornson CL, Johnson D. Croup. Lancet. 2008; 371(9609):329–39.
32. Murphy GS, Szokol JW, Marymont JH, et al. Residual neuromuscular blockade and critical respiratory events in the postanesthesia care unit. Anesth Analg. 2008;107(1):130–7.
33. Staals LM, Driessen JJ, Van Egmond J, De Boer HD, Klimek M, Flockton EA, Snoeck MMJ. Train-of-four ratio recovery often precedes twitch recovery when neuromuscular block is reversed by sugammadex. Acta Anaesthesiologica Scandinavica. 2011;55(6): 700–7.
34. Moi D. Residual neuromuscular blockade. Anesthesia tutorial of the week. www.totwi.anesthesiologists.org. Accessed 30 Nov 2017.

40 Hemodynamic Instability as a Complication of Maxillofacial Surgery

Kyle J. Kramer

Abstract

A multitude of surgical, anesthetic, and patient-specific factors negatively impacting the cardiovascular system, specifically causing alterations in preload, afterload, and/or myocardial functionality, can precipitate hemodynamic instability leading to cardiovascular collapse. Transient mild-moderate perioperative hypertension and hypotension are rather common occurrences for oral surgical patients, especially while receiving sedation or general anesthesia. Profound intervention, such as the use of vasoactive drugs, remains a relatively rare complication. However, due to the potential for significant patient harm, hemodynamic instability continues to demand attention from the oral and maxillofacial surgeon, especially with respect to patient management and emergency preparedness. In addition to several preventive management strategies, there are various pharmacologic options available for initial management of perioperative hypotension and hypertension. Clinicians must be capable of rapidly assessing the likely causes leading to the development of the perioperative hemodynamic instability, while simultaneously quickly ascertaining the severity of the situation. Successful management and satisfactory patient outcomes require a prompt, efficient, and proper response.

40.1 Complication: Hemodynamic Instability

40.1.1 Cause of the Complication

The term hemodynamics refers to those physiologic processes involved with moving the blood throughout the body. Therefore, hemodynamic instability refers to a compromised ability to move the blood around, which if left untreated

K.J. Kramer, D.D.S., M.S.
Department of Oral Surgery and Hospital Dentistry, Indiana University School of Dentistry, Indianapolis, IN, USA
e-mail: kjkramer@iu.edu

© Springer International Publishing AG 2018
E.M. Ferneini, J.D. Bennett (eds.), *Perioperative Assessment of the Maxillofacial Surgery Patient*,
https://doi.org/10.1007/978-3-319-58868-1_40

can lead to inadequate tissue perfusion, organ failure, and possibly death. During the perioperative period, hemodynamic instability may manifest as profound hypotension or initially as hypertension ultimately leading to cardiovascular collapse. The key components of the cardiovascular system that may attribute to the development of hemodynamic instability include:

1. Preload or intravascular volume status
2. Afterload or systemic vascular resistance
3. Myocardial functionality (rate, rhythm, and contractility)

Failure of any of these components is likely to ultimately lead to compromised tissue perfusion and inadequate support of the aerobic metabolic processes, otherwise known as shock [1]. Hypotension is commonly defined as an absolute (Fig. 40.1) or relative reduction (<20% of baseline) in blood pressure [2]. Hypertension can be defined as an absolute (Fig. 40.2) or a relative elevation (>20% of baseline) in blood pressure [3]. Hemodynamic instability becomes especially problematic once the vital organs become inadequately perfused leading to tissue ischemia, hypoxia, and end-organ damage [4]. The central nervous system, kidneys, and heart are especially at risk once blood pressure alterations extend beyond the limits of autoregulation [5]. Regardless of the actual cause, the oral and maxillofacial surgeon must be able to proficiently identify and manage perioperative hemodynamic instability.

40.1.2 Pathophysiology

Perioperative hemodynamic instability manifesting as hyper- or hypotension is a rather common complication for the oral and maxillofacial patient. The most difficult aspect for the clinician is often simply determining the primary cause or causes, which can be quite numerous. This can make identifying the exact pathophysiologic defect rather onerous. Pathologies involving the basic components of the cardiovascular system discussed previously are all potential causes of hemodynamic instability and therefore should be assessed in order. However, astute clinicians must appreciate the interconnected nature of those components rather than conceptualize each as being completely independent.

40.1.2.1 Pathophysiology

Preload/Intravascular Volume Status

As mentioned previously, hemodynamics refers to the ability to move the blood around the body. If there is insufficient blood/fluid for the heart to

Absolute Hypotension	Blood Pressure (mmHg)
Systolic	< 90
Diastolic	< 60
Mean Arterial Pressure (MAP)	< 65

Fig. 40.1 Classification of absolute hypotension

Category	Systolic Blood Pressure (mmHg)	Diastolic Blood Pressure (mmHg)
Normal	< 120	< 80
Prehypertension	120–139	80–89
Stage 1	140–159	90–99
Stage 2	≥ 160	≥ 100

Fig. 40.2 Classification of hypertension

pump, the cardiovascular system will begin to collapse. This is conceptually no different than a well pump which begins to fail once the well runs dry of water. Patients may experience a significant reduction in preload for a variety of underlying reasons. Trauma patients may present with significant hypotension secondary to massive bleeding and extensive blood loss. It is common for patients to present preoperatively with mild hypovolemia secondary to NPO (nil per os) requirements. Profound venous vasodilation can promote pooling of the blood peripherally, which reduces return back to the heart. Additionally, movement or accumulation of fluids into the transcellular space can lead to a depletion of the intravascular volume, triggering significant hypotension. Pregnant patients can have impaired venous return secondary to supine hypotensive syndrome [6, 7]. The underlying issue with all of these clinical scenarios remains the same, a net decrease in the preload or intravascular volume available to be pumped around the body.

Afterload/Systemic Vascular Resistance

The afterload or systemic vascular resistance is defined as the pressure the heart must overcome in order to move the blood around the body. Extreme alterations in afterload are troublesome, especially if acute in nature as the body does not have sufficient time to compensate accordingly. If the systemic vascular resistance drops too low, peripheral blood flow simply stops. It is conceptually similar to the stagnation that occurs to flowing water as a riverbed begins to widen. Precipitous drops in blood pressure, as noted with severe sepsis, septic shock, or anaphylaxis, can all lead to inadequate systemic perfusion and cardiovascular collapse. Alternatively, significant acute increases in afterload can be particularly deleterious due to the increased workload on the myocardium. Extreme hypertension can cause injury to blood vessels leading to end-organ damage. Most patients have primary or essential hypertension, for which there is no known cause for the elevation in afterload. In contrast, secondary hypertension has an appreciable underlying cause, such as renal artery stenosis.

Myocardial Functionality (Rate, Rhythm, and Contractility)

In order for the cardiovascular system to function correctly, the pump, or heart, must be in working order. Alterations in its normal functionality often lead to impaired or inadequate perfusion. Conceptually, this is similar to a broken or malfunctioning impeller on a water pump being unable to mechanically move the water sufficiently. Profound bradycardia leads to cardiovascular collapse if unable to maintain adequate cardiac output. Profound tachycardia is problematic, not only for the additional stress put on the myocardium but also for the reduced time given for the chambers of the heart to adequately fill, especially the left ventricle. For otherwise healthy adults, a heart rate exceeding 160–170 beats/min is associated with a decrease in cardiac output [8]. The development of arrhythmias or dysrhythmias may be intermittent, benign, or potentially serious leading to cardiac compromise. The potential sequelae that may result depend on the specific rhythm abnormality as well as other factors such as the patient's medical and surgical comorbidities. Finally, the cardiac contractility, which refers to the intrinsic ability of the myocardium to generate force necessary to propel the blood, is the remaining factor responsible for ensuring adequacy of perfusion. There are multiple factors that impact the contractility of the myocardium; however, impairment of this ability easily leads to reductions in cardiac output and possibly cardiovascular collapse.

Perioperative State

The perioperative period presents many additional factors which alter the normal functionality of the cardiovascular system and can predispose patients to developing hemodynamic instability. As mentioned previously, nonemergent surgical patients often present with a modest degree of volume depletion secondary to a lack of nutritional and fluid intake in preparation for anesthesia. Emergency or trauma patients may present with additional factors such as massive blood loss, third-spacing, fluid wasting, and shock, all of which can negatively impact the stability of the patient's cardiovascular system.

Noxious stimulation (pain) caused by the surgical procedure itself leads to an increase in the overall sympathetic tone, possibly precipitating hypertension and tachycardia [9]. Concurrent administration of vasoconstrictors can cause similar cardiovascular alterations. Additionally, the vast majority of the agents (sedative or hypnotic drugs) that are used for sedation and general anesthesia act not only as central nervous system depressive agents but also to depress the cardiovascular system. This often manifests as hypotension triggered by one or both of the following mechanisms:

1. Direct myocardial depression (depression of myocardial contractility via negative inotropic effects, negative chronotropic effects)
2. Decreased systemic vascular resistance (vasodilation due to suppression of the sympathetic nervous system, sympatholysis via vasomotor centers in the medulla, or increased parasympathetic tone via vagal pathways) [10]

Successful management of the patient's hemodynamic status can become quite complex during the perioperative period, especially considering the interplay between all of these potential factors. In fact, it is quite common for patients to exhibit significant swings in blood pressure throughout the entire perioperative period in response to the interconnected nature of these various factors.

40.1.3 Prevalence

The true prevalence of hemodynamic instability during oral and maxillofacial surgical procedures is rather difficult to ascertain mainly due to a paucity of data on this particular topic within the literature. A rather dated article by D'Eramo in 1992 [11] evaluated morbidity and mortality data collected via survey from 147 active members of the Massachusetts Society of Oral and Maxillofacial Surgeons as they treated 416,561 patients during 1989. This survey specifically evaluated the incidence of perioperative hypotension requiring drug therapy, identifying the risk as 1:4404 for general anesthesia, 1:7863 for parenteral sedation with local anesthesia, and 1:16,587 for local anesthesia alone. The same study reported a significantly lower probability of hypertension requiring drug therapy as 1:37,436 for general anesthesia, 0:102,225 for parenteral sedation with local anesthesia, and 0:199,045 for local anesthesia alone [11]. This particular study failed to assign cutoff values for hypertension and hypotension, relying instead on the use of drug therapy, which was also rather vague. A follow-up study in 2004 reported data consistent with the aforementioned study [12]. In all actuality, the prevalence of perioperative hypotension requiring some type of intervention is likely much higher. It often resolves adequately secondary to simple means, such as reducing the depth of anesthesia or fluid bolus challenge, negating the need for vasoactive agents. Perioperative hypertension is also likely more common and tends to respond well to non-antihypertensive pharmacologic options, such as increasing anesthetic depth or judicious use of local anesthetics.

One aspect of the issue regarding the difficulty assessing the incidence of perioperative hemodynamic instability is the lack of a universal definition. Many studies have set arbitrary definitions such as alterations in MAP or systolic blood pressure above or below a certain percentage, for a specific duration of time, or even those requiring pharmacologic interventions. This has led to a multitude of varying results regarding the incidence of perioperative hemodynamic instability [13]. Bijker et al. estimated the incidence of intraoperative hypotension during anesthesia varies as much as 5–99%, depending on the particular definition or parameters used [14]. Clearly, hemodynamic instability manifesting as intraoperative hypertension or hypotension is a rather frequent occurrence, especially when general anesthesia is utilized. As such, the oral and maxillofacial surgeon must be ever vigilant and prepared to intervene accordingly based on the severity of the particular clinical situation.

40.1.4 Manifestations/Presentation of Disease

Patients who present with hemodynamic instability in the preoperative period may or may not have appreciable signs or symptoms. Quite often, mild-to-moderate hypertension or hypotension may be unnoticed until the application of noninvasive monitors. Instances of more severe hemodynamic instability may be accompanied by signs and symptoms expected during periods of abnormal end-organ perfusion. Common symptoms may include headache, dizziness, visual disturbances, feeling faint, or nausea and/or vomiting. Patients who begin to experience hemodynamic instability following initiation of sedation or general anesthesia are unlikely to report any symptoms due to altered consciousness or unconsciousness. Clinicians must be alert for signs suggestive of hypotension, such as pallor, diaphoresis, flattening of the pulse oximeter waveform, or delayed capillary refill rates. Patients may also experience oliguria or anuria, which would be noted perioperatively assuming a Foley catheter is in place [15]. Hypotension during the immediate postoperative period has a presentation similar to the preoperative and intraoperative periods and warrants similar approaches. Hypertension tends to be even more occult in nature and may not have any appreciable signs aside from elevated blood pressure measurements.

40.2 Patient Assessment

40.2.1 Monitoring

The primary means for assessing a patient for the initial signs of hemodynamic instability include the use of a noninvasive blood pressure cuff in combination with an electrocardiogram. Additional means of assessing blood pressure during the perioperative period include the use of invasive devices, such as intra-arterial or central venous pressure monitors [4]. Cannulation of an artery, typically the radial, is an easy and reliable means for providing direct measurements of the patient's blood pressure in real time. Arterial lines do require additional equipment, such as a transducer and special pressurized tubing and are not without some risk. The use must be accompanied by a risk/benefit analysis prior to deployment. Placement of a central venous line can provide the means to assess the central venous pressure, as the venous return enters back into the right atrium. While this is not a direct measurement of blood pressure, it can be used to assist with proper fluid management, especially in critically ill patients. It must be noted, however, that the vast majority of oral and maxillofacial surgery patients typically do not require these types of invasive monitors outside of the traditional operating room with rather few exceptions.

40.2.2 Work-Up

40.2.2.1 Preoperative

A preoperative cardiovascular assessment consisting of a measurement of the patient's blood pressure and heart rate is essential. This establishes a baseline against which the subsequent intraoperative and postoperative values can be compared. If the preoperative assessment of the patient's vital signs reveals significant changes (absolute or relative) to previous assessments, it is likely prudent to delay elective treatment, with referral for further evaluation or immediate transfer for acute emergent care as dictated. Additional monitors are likely to be of use to help identify potentially insidious cardiovascular events, such as an impending myocardial infarction or precipitous arrhythmia.

Evaluation of the patient's current medication list is a vital component of the preoperative assessment. Generally speaking, most patients who take antihypertensive mediations should be advised to continue taking their medications during the perioperative period with a few key exceptions [16]. Angiotensin-converting-enzyme (ACE) inhibitors and angiotensin II receptor antagonists (ARBs) can cause significant intraoperative hypotension that is often refractory to the typical pharmacologic interventions [17]. It is generally recommended that patients receiving sedation or general anesthesia hold their ACE inhibitor or ARB on the day of surgery. Patients taking other antihypertensive medications (beta-blockers, calcium channel blockers, diuretics, etc.) should generally continue taking their medications normally [4]. Other essential components to evaluate include assessment of the patient's functional capacity or exercise tolerance.

40.2.2.2 Intraoperative and Postoperative

It is commonly recommended that a patient's blood pressure and pulse remain consistently within 20–30% of their established baseline. If profound hemodynamic instability develops acutely, all aspects of the surgical and anesthetic plan should be taken into consideration while establishing a differential diagnosis, especially the most recent aspects. For example, a patient who presents to the dental clinic for outpatient sedation and surgery who promptly experiences profound hypotension and unconsciousness during placement of the IV line is most likely experiencing a syncopal event and should be managed accordingly. Quite often, there are a multitude of causal factors leading to the development of acute hemodynamic instability. In those cases, clinicians should start with the most likely causes and the associated management strategies while continually reassessing the clinical situation (refer to Fig. 40.1). Activation of emergency medical services (EMS/911) should remain an early consideration for patients failing to respond adequately to normal measures in the ambulatory care setting. Early activation of EMS is absolutely paramount to help avoid morbid patient outcomes should outside medical assistance become necessary.

40.2.3 Laboratory Tests and Anticipated Results

40.2.3.1 Hypovolemia

Direct measurement of the patient's intravascular volume is rather difficult to assess in the absence of more invasive monitors. Simple measurement of the patient's urine production can serve as a rough guide to assist the clinician for fluid replacement as well as adequacy of perfusion to the kidneys. Normally urine production should approximate 0.5–1 mL/kg/h. Urine production below this threshold may indicate decreased hypovolemia or hypoperfusion secondary to hypotension. Additional causes of impaired urine production may include intrinsic renal and post-renal issues as well, all of which may complication interpretation of the true clinical situation.

40.3 Management

40.3.1 Potential Problems

With regard to hemodynamic instability, the most concerning issue pertains to the adequacy of perfusion to the organs and peripheral tissues. Inadequate perfusion leads to the development of tissue hypoxia, acidosis, damage, and death of the various organ systems. Those systems most at risk include the brain, kidneys, and myocardium. The degree of damage is directly related to the extent of the abnormal perfusion, both in terms of magnitude and duration. A "normal, healthy" patient is likely to tolerate short periods of hypertension or hypotension without development of long-term sequelae. Significant hypotension is a rather common but brief observation, typically seen immediately following anesthetic induction before placement of the endotracheal tube. Patients rebound rather quickly due to the stimulation that accompanies instrumentation of the airway often becoming rather hypertensive and tachycardic.

Elective hypotensive anesthesia is often deployed during oral and maxillofacial surgery procedures to help minimize blood loss for particularly at-risk aspects of various surgical procedures such as the down fracture of the maxilla for orthognathic surgery. The elective hypotension is typically limited in terms of degree (MAP >50–65 mmHg) as well as duration (as needed, only for high-risk aspect of surgery) [18, 19]. Patients with significant medical comorbidities often lack the reserve necessary to tolerate such cardiovascular challenges without insult. Therefore, approaches that take fewer liberties with respect to stability of their cardiovascular system may be more ideal.

Perhaps the biggest problem for the oral and maxillofacial surgeon operating in the office-based or ambulatory care setting tasked with the unexpected or emergent management of a patient with hemodynamic instability is the isolated nature of that specific environment leading to inadequate response and significant patient morbidity or mortality. Most dental offices have a rather limited capability in terms of emergent resuscitation following cardiovascular collapse, especially when compared to the asset-rich environment of the traditional hospital setting. As such, prudent selection of the patient, surgical procedure, and anesthetic plan are critical. Regardless of ASA status, all patients must be carefully evaluated to determine the following:

1. Severity and degree of optimization of any medical comorbidities
2. Appropriateness of the surgical and anesthetic plan
3. Appropriateness of the surgical venue

ASA I and II patients are generally excellent candidates for the vast majority of oral and maxillofacial surgical procedures and can safely receive the whole spectrum of anesthesia services in the office-based environment with minimal alterations. Patients who are ASA III or above often require additional testing beyond otherwise "healthy adults." Patients who present with poorly controlled comorbidities or who are less than optimized should be rescheduled once a better degree of control is at hand. The surgeon must also ensure appropriate measures are readily available should untoward surgical events arise, such as extensive bleeding. If the surgery is likely to cause extensive blood loss requiring transfusions, the office-based setting may not be appropriate. Likewise, a patient with severe aortic stenosis, decompensated heart failure, or liver failure with ascites is likely to develop severe hemodynamic instability during the perioperative period which may not respond to the measures available in the traditional dental setting. Being cautious, selective, and adequately prepared are key concepts for oral and maxillofacial surgeons in order to maximize patient safety and prevent complications from occurring in the first place.

40.3.2 Patient Management

40.3.2.1 Preoperative Hemodynamic Instability

Patients who present with hemodynamic instability during the preoperative period should receive additional assessment prior to beginning the anesthetic or surgical procedure. Further inquiry should include the severity and likely causes of the notable hypotension or hypertension. While a catastrophic emergency such as an impending myocardial infarction remains rather rare, clinicians must be wary of patients who present with suspicious signs and symptoms.

Unusual hypertension or hypotension noted preoperatively should be confirmed by subsequent measurements prior to instituting other interventions and after ruling out common errors like inappropriately sized cuffs or malfunctioning equipment. Patients who appear to be extremely anxious or presyncopal may respond well initially to non-pharmacologic methods such as reassurance and verbal guidance. Placing the anxious or presyncopal patient into Trendelenburg position to promote adequate cerebral perfusion as well as utilizing sedatives for anxiolysis and possibly anticholinergics to manage bradycardia should be strongly considered. Patients may exhibit a degree of hemodynamic instability following vasovagal syncope and should be assessed accordingly prior to proceeding with treatment.

Patients with significant hypotension secondary to hypovolemia may be managed by volume replacement during the immediate preoperative period. The type of fluid replacement is primarily dictated by the underlying causal factors present. Trauma patients with significant blood loss may require use of blood products such as allogenic or recovered red blood cells, fresh frozen plasma, cryoprecipitate, and/or platelets. Depending on the stability of the patient, transfusions may be performed prior to surgery or more likely during the intraoperative period if emergent need occurs. Replacement is guided by the clinical presentation of the patient (stability of vital signs, appreciable bleeding, etc.) as well as by laboratory studies (hemoglobin, hematocrit, platelet count, coagulation studies, etc.). Patients who present with hypovolemia secondary to preoperative fasting can be managed with fluid replacement using crystalloid or colloid solutions, with the use of isotonic crystalloid options (0.9% normal saline or lacted Ringer's) predominating initial management. Simple calculation of the individual patient's normal fluid requirements per hour based on their body weight using the 4, 2, 1 rule serves as a guide, which can be multiplied by the total hours the patient has been without fluids to identify the total fluid deficit.

- 4 mL/kg for the first 10 kg
- 2 mL/kg for the second 10 kg
- 1 mL/kg for the remaining kg
- Hourly Fluid Requirements × # Hours NPO = Total Fluid Deficit

The traditional approach to replacing the total fluid deficit during the intraoperative period includes replacement of half the total fluid deficit over the course of the first hour, with the remaining two quarters broken up over the following 2 h. Additional fluids were recommended based on estimated blood loss, evaporation, and other non-sensible fluid losses. However, more recent guidelines have challenged these ideas moving toward goal-directed therapy, with data suggesting more modest fluid administration for longer, more complex cases, and more liberal fluids for shorter, ambulatory procedures. For the vast majority of dental/oral surgical procedures performed in the traditional dental office setting, patients often respond well to minimal fluid replacement rates during the intraoperative period, then shifting to more aggressive, higher fluid replacement rates during emergence and recovery. Despite this overall trend, patients suspected of hypovolemia may benefit from early fluid replacement prior to induction leading to a more hemodynamically stable anesthetic and surgical course.

40.3.2.2 Intraoperative Hemodynamic Instability

The development of hemodynamic instability during the intraoperative period demands immediate attention. There are a multitude of potential causes that can lead to the development of intraoperative hypertension or hypotension; however, there are several basic steps that should be done in order to likely increase the potential of a satisfactory outcome.

1. Rapidly assess/reassess the patient's general condition

   A rapid assessment of the patient's vital signs and general appearance should occur immediately once the oral and maxillofacial surgeon appreciates the possible development of hemodynamic instability. It is recommended that this include a recycling of the automated sphygmomanometer to rule out an inaccurate initial reading. During the time taken for the blood pressure cuff to cycle, the clinician should assess the patient for additional signs suggestive of cardiovascular collapse. Clinicians can rapidly palpate for the presence of peripheral pulses in addition to evaluating the capillary refill rate, color of mucous membranes, and overall respiratory effort (signs of obstruction, apnea, tachypnea, etc.). Other items that can quickly be assessed initially include other anesthesia monitors such as the EKG, capnography, and pulse oximeter waveforms and $etCO_2$. If no other abnormalities are noted and the subsequent assessment confirms the initial abnormal blood pressure reading, the clinician should move into the active management phase of treatment. Again, it must be stated that the degree of intervention depends heavily on the likely underlying causes in addition to the degree of hemodynamic instability noted. For example, it is quite common for patients to demonstrate profound hypotension immediately following induction [20]. This is most likely secondary to the liberal use of anesthetic medications which can cause varying degrees of myocardial depression as well as reductions in systemic vascular resistance. Thankfully, the vast majority of patients tend to rebound quickly once the larger induction doses begin to redistribute, be metabolized, or excreted. In fact, it is quite common for patients to "bottom out" temporarily and rebound so quickly that their blood pressure has normalized once the blood pressure cuff has recycled. This easily reflects the rapid action of many of the commonly used anesthetic medications used today, such as propofol, remifentanil, sevoflurane, and desflurane. If the patient's blood pressure normalizes quickly (2–3 min) following the reduction in drug dosages, usually no additional steps are needed. However, should the situation continue to deteriorate, additional interventions are needed.

2. Trendelenburg position
   Simply placing the patient in the Trendelenburg, or head down position, will promote increased venous return as well as increased perfusion to the brain, which can help buy the oral and maxillofacial surgeon additional time.
3. Alter the depth of anesthesia
4. Alter the IV fluid rate
   Turning off or reducing any continuously delivered anesthetic medications (propofol infusions, vaporizers, etc.) is crucial for rapidly correcting an overly deep anesthetic causing significant hypotension. Increasing the rate of fluid infusion will not only give the patient a modest fluid bolus (increasing their intravascular volume) but also increase speed of administration of any vasoactive intravenous agents used. Alternatively, patients with acute hypertension may be experiencing inadequate local anesthesia or be in an insufficiently light plane of anesthesia. Missed local anesthetic blocks are a common cause for intraoperative tachycardia and hypertension. The judicious use of local anesthesia is a crucial step to be considered prior to deepening the level of anesthesia.
5. Pharmacologic intervention
   Finally, the use of pharmacologic means to help normalize the patient's hemodynamic status should be considered if the patient continues to deteriorate. These agents can be used to further stabilize the patient, giving the oral and maxillofacial surgeon even more time to identify other complicating factors. There are several pharmacologic options available; however, the most common agents in the traditional dental/oral surgical office-type setting include anticholinergics (atropine, glycopyrrolate) and vasoactive agents (ephedrine, phenylephrine, epinephrine, and vasopressin) to manage hypotension and adrenergic antagonists (esmolol, metoprolol, and labetalol) and vasodilators (hydralazine) for hypertension. These pharmacologic agents will be discussed in greater detail shortly.
6. Activation of emergency medical services and termination of the procedure
   A key component to any emergency response is rapid activation of an emergency response team, which includes not only emergency medical services (911) to provide external assistance but also the internal response team (Code Team) to provide assistance immediately. This type of response is crucial when emergencies arise in the nontraditional hospital setting as resources and assistance may be scarce due to the rather isolated nature. Patients who fail to respond adequately should be transported as quickly as possible to a hospital for immediate assessment and care.

40.3.2.3 Intraoperative Hypotensive Pharmacologic Options: Anticholinergics

The two most common anticholinergic agents, or more specifically muscarinic receptor antagonists, are atropine and glycopyrrolate which cause parasympatholytic effects clinically. Atropine is a tertiary amine which also acts primarily outside of the central nervous system but is associated with CNS effects, especially with very low doses. The quaternary ammonium structure of glycopyrrolate prevents it from crossing the blood-brain barrier, rendering it essentially to the peripheral nervous system only [21]. Blockade of the parasympathetic innervation to the heart causes an appreciable increase in heart rate, conduction, and a variable increase in cardiac output. Adult dosing for atropine used to manage symptomatic intraoperative bradycardia is 0.5 mg via IV. Glycopyrrolate dosing is 0.1–0.2 mg via IV and can be titrated to the desired clinical effects. There is a significant difference between the onset speed of atropine (30–60 s) and glycopyrrolate (2–3 min), which makes atropine the preferred agent during emergencies. Aside from the onset speed, atropine causes a higher increase in heart rate, while glycopyrrolate produces stronger antisialogogue effects. Patients with hemodynamic instability and profound hypotension secondary to significant bradycardia, such as a vasovagal syncopal event, are likely to benefit from the vagolytic effects of atropine or glycopyrrolate.

40.3.2.4 Intraoperative Hypotensive Pharmacologic Options: Vasoactive Agents

There are several different vasoactive pharmacologic options readily available for intraoperative use such as temporary hemodynamic stabilizing agents. Their clinical profiles vary considerably, so the oral and maxillofacial surgeon must know reflexively which agent to select according to the specifics of the individual clinical scenario. The clinical effects all tend to be dose dependent, and as such clinicians are encouraged to titrate to the desired clinical endpoints.

Ephedrine

Ephedrine is another phenethylamine with direct and indirect agonistic activity involving both alpha (α1,2) and beta (β1,2) adrenergic receptors [22]. The main clinical effects observed following administration of ephedrine include vasoconstriction and increases in heart rate and contractility. It is the first-line agent to treat intraoperative hypotension [13]. Additional effects mimic those expected of nonselective adrenergic agonists such as epinephrine; however, ephedrine's effects tend to be more modest. Ephedrine is typically available in 50 mg/mL, 1 mL glass vials or ampules. For ease of administration, ephedrine can be diluted to a more useful 5 mg/mL concentration for IV administration. Ephedrine has recommended IV dosing for adults of 5–10 mg every 5–10 min as needed to manage significant intraoperative bradycardia and/or hypotension. Ephedrine is prone to tachyphylaxis due to the indirect action, triggering the release of stored norepinephrine from presynaptic adrenergic nerve terminals. Patients may begin to elicit impaired responses following repeated doses, necessitating either higher successive doses or alternative drug options.

Phenylephrine

Phenylephrine is phenethylamine selective alpha-1 (α1) direct-acting adrenergic agonist capable of causing potent vasoconstriction [23]. Typically phenylephrine is available in 10 mg/mL, 1 mL single dose vials, which can be double diluted to a more useable concentration of 0.1 mg/mL for IV use. Recommended IV dosing for adults is 0.1–0.2 mg IV boluses every 10–15 min to treat intraoperative hypotension [22]. Phenylephrine is noted to produce reflex bradycardia in response to profound vasoconstriction. As such, its use should be avoided in patients who are hypotensive and bradycardic.

Epinephrine

Epinephrine is a catecholamine that functions as a direct-acting nonselective alpha (α1,2) and beta (β1,2) directing-acting adrenergic agonist [22]. Clinically, epinephrine produces results typical of those anticipated following stimulation of adrenergic receptors. Cardiovascular effects include vasoconstriction and increased myocardial chronotropy, inotropy, and dromotropy all leading to increased cardiac output. However, these cardiovascular effects tend to be dose dependent. Higher plasma concentrations of epinephrine are associated with predominantly alpha-1 effects, while beta-1 and beta-2 effects predominate as plasma levels decline, respectively. Selection of epinephrine to manage intraoperative bradycardia and/or hypotension is typically reserved primarily for emergent use. Routine use is rather uncommon; however, epinephrine is the agent of choice when managing severe hypotension secondary to suspected anaphylaxis [24]. Epinephrine is readily available in a variety of concentrations and forms. Concentrated 1:1000 epinephrine (1 mg/mL) in 1 mL glass ampules or vials is reserved for IM/SQ administration only and should be diluted if IV administration is desired. Epinephrine 1:10,000 concentration (0.1 mg/mL) in prefilled syringes is available for IV use without the need for further dilution depending on the desired dose. Epinephrine can be administered as small boluses, or infusions at a rate of 2–10 mcg/min titrated to effect to manage modest bradycardia and/or hypotension. Severe hemodynamic instability or hypotension secondary to anaphylactic shock necessitates higher dosages such as 100–250 mcg IV every 3–5 min or 0.3–0.5 mg via IM injection for prolonged duration of action [25]. Epinephrine autoinjectors are also available, which use spring-loaded syringes to deliver fixed dosages of epinephrine and are designed to be used for intramuscular injections. The Epipen® and Epipen Jr® deliver 0.3 mg and 0.15 mg of epinephrine, respectively, and are the most well known; however, several generic alternatives are available in the market currently. For the oral and maxillofacial surgeon, the use of the prefilled 1:10,000 syringes or alternatively 1:1000 epinephrine vials or ampules is a more economical option with greater flexibility compared to the rather expensive IM autoinjectors. Regardless of the alternatives selected, clinicians must be competent and reflexively know how to utilize the epinephrine options at hand. Failure to do so is likely to lead to less than ideal patient outcomes should an emergency arise.

Vasopressin

Vasopressin, or antidiuretic hormone, is a synthetic version of the endogenous hormone produced by the posterior pituitary gland. In addition to increasing the reabsorption of water by the renal tubules via V_2 vasopressin receptor agonistic activity, vasopressin binds directly to V_1 vasopressor receptors on vascular smooth muscle causing vasoconstriction [23]. This mechanism of action is entirely different than the usual adrenergic agonists discussed previously. Vasopressin is typically supplied in 20 units/mL, 1 mL glass vials, which can be diluted to a concentration of 1 unit/mL for ease of administration. Recommended dosing for adults is 1–2 units administered intravenously every 10–20 min, titrated to desired clinical endpoint. Vasopressin is most useful for patients with intraoperative hypotension secondary to concomitant ACE inhibitor or ARB therapy who fails to respond adequately to other vasoactive therapy.

40.3.2.5 Intraoperative Hypertensive Pharmacologic Options: Adrenergic Antagonists

Esmolol

Esmolol hydrochloride is cardioselective beta-1 (β1) adrenergic antagonist that primarily acts to decrease myocardial chronotropy, inotropy, and dromotropy. It has a rapid onset of ~2 min and an ultrashort duration of action, with an elimination half-life of ~9 min [18]. This profile renders it extremely useful for management of intraoperative hypertension as it can be easily titrated to effect with no prolonged effects [26]. Esmolol is available for IV use as 10 mg/mL solution and can be administered as an infusion or more commonly as a bolus. A reduction in heart rate approximating 1 beat per 1 mg of esmolol administered can be expected.

Metoprolol

With a pharmacodynamic profile similar to esmolol, metoprolol is a selective β1 adrenergic antagonist that mainly differs with respect to its longer duration of action. Metoprolol tartrate is available as 1 mg/mL, 5 mL glass vials, for IV administration. IV metoprolol has a rapid onset approximating 2–3 min and has an elimination half-life approximating 3–4 h. It is primarily hepatically metabolized via CYP2D6. Patients exhibiting poor CYP2D6 metabolism may experience a prolonged elimination half-life up to 7–8 h [27]. Starting with a 1–2 mg initial bolus, metoprolol can be easily titrated to the desired clinical effect. Care must be taken when considering the use of metoprolol due to the prolonged duration of action.

Labetalol

Labetalol hydrochloride is a selective alpha-1 (α1), nonselective beta (β1,2) adrenergic antagonist available for IV administration as a 5 mg/mL solution. Its onset following IV administration is similar to metoprolol and approximates 2–3 min. The elimination half-life of labetalol is 5–8 h. The IV formulation has more appreciable beta antagonistic versus alpha antagonistic effects, reflecting the higher beta/alpha receptor blocking ratio (7:1) compared to oral formulations (3:1) [28]. It is packaged in a variety of different quantities, most commonly as 20 mL multidose vials and 4 mL single use syringes. Labetalol can be titrated slowly to the desired clinical endpoint using smaller, incremental 5–10 mg boluses [18]. Care should be taken in avoiding its use in patients with a history of significant reactive airway disease as it may negate the effects of any administered bronchodilators. Similar to metoprolol, clinicians must appreciate the prolonged duration of action compared to the ultrashort duration of esmolol.

40.3.2.6 Intraoperative Hypertensive Pharmacologic Options: Vasodilators

Hydralazine

Hydralazine is a potent direct-acting peripheral vasodilator that causes direct relaxation of vascular smooth muscle by interfering with the movement of calcium. Its actual mechanism of action remains poorly understood. Hydralazine is typically available in 20 mg, 1 mL single-dose glass vials for IV or IM administration. It has a fairly slow onset ~5 min, peak effect occurring in 10–80 min, and an elimination half-life approximating 3–7 h [13]. Hydralazine can be especially useful during the postoperative period for patients with persistent hypertension despite adequate pain control. It can be titrated to clinical effect using repeated 5 mg doses every 15–20 min, although its slower onset and delayed peak effect compared to other antihypertensives does require careful monitoring and a slower approach to minimize overdose and resultant hypotension.

Other Vasodilators

Several other vasodilating agents are available for management of hypertension during the perioperative period. Short-acting agents such as nitroglycerin, nitroprusside, and nicardipine, an ultrashort-acting dihydropyridine calcium channel blocker, typically require the use of continuous infusions to permit careful titration to the desired effect [13, 29]. Other alternatives that may be of interest include the non-dihydropyridine calcium channel blockers such as diltiazem and verapamil, although they are not commonly utilized in the typical oral surgery practice and are beyond the scope of this text.

40.3.2.7 Postoperative Hemodynamic Instability

Patients with persistent hemodynamic instability extending into the postoperative period should be evaluated in a similar fashion to those who exhibit signs and symptoms preoperatively or intraoperatively. Common potential causes of postoperative hypotension include excessive or lingering effects of anesthetic agents, potential overdose of local anesthetics, as well as total blood loss or stability of hemostasis postoperatively. The majority of anesthetic agents commonly utilized in the traditional dental/oral surgical ambulatory setting have durations of action that are relatively ideal for the shorter nature of most oral surgical procedures. However, prolonged durations of action extending beyond the stimulating intraoperative period may be of note for hyperresponsive patients as well as those with medical comorbidities likely to negatively impact normal drug pharmacokinetics. Additionally, selection of anesthetic agents with less than ideal or prolonged durations of action may be equally problematic leading to hypotension postoperatively. Excessive use of local anesthetic agents, specifically bupivacaine, can lead to the development of impaired cardiovascular function and even collapse. Bupivacaine is of particular note due to its high degree of protein binding and preference for myocardial tissues leading to cardiac toxicity.

Depending of the specifics of the surgical intervention, hemostasis or lack thereof may be an issue during the postoperative period. Particularly invasive procedures may have a higher risk of significant blood loss, which may lead to significant hypotension if uncontrolled.

Potential causes of hypertension in the immediate postoperative period include pain, excitement on emergence from anesthesia, anxiety, hypothermia, hypoxemia, hypercarbia, and bladder distention secondary to urine retention. These potential factors should be considered and ruled out prior to instituting any antihypertensive therapy. This will help prevent overcorrection errors and the patient becoming hypotensive as a result. Care must be taken to ensure the peak effect of any antihypertensives utilized has occurred. Discharge from the office should not occur until the patient's blood pressure approximates baseline and remains stable.

Regardless of the specific underlying cause, the oral and maxillofacial surgeon remains responsible for the patient throughout the entire postoperative period and should remain on hand to intervene if necessary. Under no circumstances should patients be "reversed" simply to facilitate a speedier recovery and discharge from the office. The surgeon should provide the final assessment regarding fitness for discharge to help prevent patients leaving the supervised setting prematurely. Finally, in regard to postoperative care following discharge from the office, it is absolutely crucial that the means to contact the oral and maxillofacial surgeon be provided should an emergency arise afterward.

40.4 Prevention

As with many emergency situations, the most important strategy in terms of the prevention of hemodynamic instability is ensuring a proper and thorough medical and physical assessment of the patient during the preoperative period. The old adage "an ounce of prevention is worth a pound of cure" rings true when discussing prevention of hemodynamic instability. Attention to detail during this phase of treatment is crucial to identifying potential causes likely to lead to significant hypertension or hypotension during the intraoperative and/or postoperative periods and taking the requisite steps to prevent the crisis from occurring in the first place. Patients who present during the consultation period with concerning medical comorbidities must be assessed properly prior to proceeding with the planned surgical and anesthetic interventions. For example, a patient who reports a history of severe aortic stenosis should be given proper consideration regarding the appropriateness in terms of the surgical/anesthetic plan and venue. Quite simply put, not all surgical patients are candidates for office-based or ambulatory care settings. Some patients should be managed instead in the traditional hospital OR setting due to the availability of abundant help and safety net systems that are in place should an emergency arise. Additionally this traditional OR setting provides the means for higher-risk patients to remain in a highly monitored care environment during an extended postoperative period, which can further reduce the risk should a complication arise.

Other prevention strategies include ensuring the office is adequately prepared should acute hemodynamic instability occur. This should include not only reviewing the indicated management protocols for hypertension and hypotension (differential diagnoses, various drug options, dosages, indications, contraindications, etc.) but also practicing the proper responses in advance. Inclusion of the various office-based team members (surgical assistants and front office staff) during regularly scheduled drills will help ensure a smooth, efficient response should an incident actually occur.

Conclusion

Hemodynamic instability is a common complication in our surgical patients. A multitude of surgical, anesthetic, and patient-specific factors can negatively impact the cardiovascular system causing alterations in preload, afterload, and/or myocardial functionality. This can precipitate hemodynamic instability leading to cardiovascular collapse. Early diagnosis and appropriate intervention is needed to treat and reverse this process. Surgeons must be capable of rapidly assessing and managing the likely causes leading to the development of the perioperative hemodynamic instability. Satisfactory patient outcomes require a prompt, efficient, and proper response.

References

1. Doyle CA, Rosenthal MH. Hypotension and shock states. In: Lobato EB, Gravenstein N, Kirby RR, editors. Complications in anesthesiology. Philadelphia: Lippincott Williams & Wilkins; 2008. p. 274–85.
2. Broussard D, Ural K. Cardiovascular problems in the post-anesthesia care unit (PACU). Philadelphia: Wolters Kluwer; 2016. https://www.uptodate.com/contents/cardiovascular-problems-in-the-post-anesthesia-care-unit-pacu?source=search_result&search=cardiovascular%20problems%20in%20the%20pacu&selectedTitle=1~150. Accessed 30 Aug 2016
3. Boysen PG. Perioperative hypertension. In: Lobato EB, Gravenstein N, Kirby RR, editors. Complications in anesthesiology. Philadelphia: Lippincott Williams & Wilkins; 2008. p. 286–94.
4. Matei VA, Haddadin AS. Systemic and pulmonary arterial hypertension. In: Hines RL, Marschall KE, editors. Stoelting's anesthesia and co-existing disease. 6th ed. Philadelphia, PA: Saunders/Elsevier; 2012. p. 104–19.
5. Erickson KM. Factors affecting cerebral blood flow. In: Murray MJ, Harrison BA, Mueller JT, Wass CT, Rose SH, Wedel DJ, editors. Faust's anesthesiology review. 4th ed. Philadelphia, PA: Elselvier/Saunders; 2015. p. 93–5.
6. Cengiz SB. The pregnant patient: considerations for dental management and drug use. Quintessence Int. 2007;38(3):e133–42.
7. Kurien S, Kattimani VS, Sriram RR, Sriram SK, Rao VKP, Bhupathi A, Bodduru RR, Patil NN. Management of pregnant patient in dentistry. J Int Oral Health. 2013;5(1):88–97.
8. Vijitpavan A. Physiologic determinants of cardiac output. In: Murray MJ, Harrison BA, Mueller JT, Wass CT, Rose SH, Wedel DJ, editors. Faust's anesthesiology review. 4th ed. Philadelphia, PA: Elselvier/Saunders; 2015. p. 74–6.
9. Varon J, Marik PE. Perioperative hypertension management. Vasc Health Risk Manag. 2008;4(3):615–27.
10. Morgan GE, Mikhail MS, Murray MJ. Clinical anesthesiology. 4th ed. New York: Lange Medical Books/McGraw Hill, Medical Pub. Division; 2006.
11. D'Eramo EM. Morbidity and mortality with outpatient anesthesia: the Massachusetts experience. J Oral Maxillofac Surg. 1992;50(7):700–4.
12. D'Eramo EM, Bontempi WJ, Howard JB. Anesthesia morbidity and mortality experience among Massachusetts oral and maxillofacial surgeons. J Oral Maxillofac Surg. 2008;66(12):2421–33. https://doi.org/10.1016/j.joms.2008.06.095.
13. Lonjaret L, Lairez O, Minville V, Geeraerts T. Optimal perioperative management of arterial blood pressure. Integr Blood Press Control. 2014;7:49–59. https://doi.org/10.2147/IBPC.S45292.
14. Bijker JB, van Klei WA, Kappen TH, van Wolfswinkel L, Moons KG, Kalkman CJ. Incidence of intraoperative hypotension as a function of the chosen definition: literature definitions applied to a retrospective cohort using automated data collection. Anesthesiology. 2007;107(2):213–20. https://doi.org/10.1097/01.anes.0000270724.40897.8e.
15. Lobato EB, Kirby RR. Oliguria. In: Lobato EB, Gravenstein N, Kirby RR, editors. Complications in anesthesiology. Philadelphia: Lippincott Williams & Wilkins; 2008. p. 429–42.
16. Fleisher LA, Fleischmann KE, Auerbach AD, Barnason SA, Beckman JA, Bozkurt B, Davila-Roman VG, Gerhard-Herman MD, Holly TA, Kane GC, Marine JE, Nelson MT, Spencer CC, Thompson A, Ting HH, Uretsky BF, Wijeysundera DN, American College of C, American Heart A. 2014 ACC/AHA guideline on perioperative cardiovascular evaluation and management of patients undergoing noncardiac surgery: a report of the American College of Cardiology/American Heart Association Task Force on practice guidelines. J Am Coll Cardiol. 2014;64(22):e77–137. https://doi.org/10.1016/j.jacc.2014.07.944.
17. Brabant SM, Bertrand M, Eyraud D, Darmon PL, Coriat P. The hemodynamic effects of anesthetic induction in vascular surgical patients chronically treated with angiotensin II receptor antagonists. Anesth Analg. 1999;89(6):1388–92.
18. Elliott BA. Deliberate hypotension. In: Faust RJ, Cucchiara RF, editors. Anesthesiology review. 3rd ed. New York: Churchill Livingstone; 2002. p. 158–60.
19. Posnick JC. Anesthesia techniques, blood loss/fluid replacement, airway management & convalescence in the treatment of dentofacial deformities. In: Posnick JC, editor. Orthognathic surgery: principles & practice, vol. 1. 1st ed. St. Louis, MO: Elselvier; 2014. p. 308–36.
20. Adlesic EC. Cardiovascular anesthetic complications and treatment in oral surgery. Oral Maxillofac Surg Clin North Am. 2013;25(3):487–506, vii. https://doi.org/10.1016/j.coms.2013.04.002.
21. Dietz NM. The pharmacology of atropine, scopolamine, and glycopyrrolate. In: Murray MJ, Harrison BA, Mueller JT, Wass CT, Rose SH, Wedel DJ, editors. Faust's anesthesiology review. 4th ed. Philadelphia, PA: Elselvier/Saunders; 2015. p. 187–8.
22. Jensen-Bundy P. Vasopressors and inotropes. In: Faust RJ, Cucchiara RF, editors. Anesthesiology review. 3rd ed. New York: Churchill Livingstone; 2002. p. 151–3.

23. Morozowich ST. Vasopressors. In: Murray MJ, Harrison BA, Mueller JT, Wass CT, Rose SH, Wedel DJ, editors. Faust's anesthesiology review. 4th ed. Philadelphia, PA: Elselvier/Saunders; 2015. p. 196–8.
24. Longrois D, Lejus C, Constant I, Bruyere M, Mertes PM. Treatment of hypersensitivity reactions and anaphylactic shock occurring during anaesthesia. Ann Fr Anesth Reanim. 2011;30(3):312–22. https://doi.org/10.1016/j.annfar.2010.12.010.
25. Selde W. Push dose epinephrine. A temporizing measure for drugs that have the side-effect of hypotension. JEMS. 2014;39(9):62–3.
26. Yu SK, Tait G, Karkouti K, Wijeysundera D, McCluskey S, Beattie WS. The safety of perioperative esmolol: a systematic review and meta-analysis of randomized controlled trials. Anesth Analg. 2011;112(2):267–81. https://doi.org/10.1213/ANE.0b013e3182025af7.
27. Borkar RM, Bhandi MM, Dubey AP, Ganga Reddy V, Komirishetty P, Nandekar PP, Sangamwar AT, Kamal A, Banerjee SK, Srinivas R. An evaluation of the CYP2D6 and CYP3A4 inhibition potential of metoprolol metabolites and their contribution to drug-drug and drug-herb interaction by LC-ESI/MS/MS. Biomed Chromatogr. 2016;30(10):1556–72. https://doi.org/10.1002/bmc.3721.
28. Kanto JH. Current status of labetalol, the first alpha- and beta-blocking agent. Int J Clin Pharmacol Ther Toxicol. 1985;23(11):617–28.
29. Cook DJ. Calcium channel blockers. In: Faust RJ, Cucchiara RF, editors. Anesthesiology review. 3rd ed. New York: Churchill Livingstone; 2002. p. 161–2.

41 Acute Renal Failure as a Complication of Maxillofacial Surgery

Marc Ciampi and George Sunny Pazhayattil

Abstract

Acute kidney injury continues to remain one of the most common yet serious complications of surgical patients. Despite having multiple definitions and criteria for diagnosing acute kidney injury along with introduction of new novel markers, acute kidney injury continues to be underdiagnosed, and the prevalence continues to rise. Patients who develop acute kidney injury or even small rises in serum creatinine have an increased risk of morbidity, mortality, and prolonged hospitalization. Medical therapies remain limited, and there are few advances in care and treatment. The cornerstone of therapy remains early recognition of preventable risk factors, early detection of renal pathology, and early consultative care with a nephrologist and targeted therapy to prevent further progression of kidney disease and promote renal recovery.

41.1 Complication: Acute Renal Failure (Acute Kidney Injury)

41.1.1 Definition of Acute Kidney Injury

Acute kidney injury (AKI) is defined by a sudden drop in kidney function or glomerular filtration rate (GFR) occurring over a short period of hours to days. With over 30 definitions of acute renal failure, the RIFLE criteria were adopted in 2004 to attempt to uniformly define acute kidney failure [1]. The term acute renal failure has now been replaced with acute kidney injury. This distinction attempts to identify various stages and progression of renal damage. The RIFLE acronym

M. Ciampi, M.D., F.A.C.P., F.A.S.N. (✉)
Yale University School of Medicine,
New Haven, CT, USA

Quinnipiac University Netter School of Medicine,
New Haven, CT, USA
e-mail: majciampi@me.com

G.S. Pazhayattil, M.D., F.A.C.P
Quinnipiac University Netter School of Medicine,
Hamden, CT, USA
e-mail: doclife@gmail.com

© Springer International Publishing AG 2018
E.M. Ferneini, J.D. Bennett (eds.), *Perioperative Assessment of the Maxillofacial Surgery Patient*,
https://doi.org/10.1007/978-3-319-58868-1_41

stands for risk, injury, failure, loss of function, and end-stage renal disease and uses serum creatinine and urine output and principal markers [2]. A simpler definition which is widely accepted is provided by Kidney Disease Improving Global Outcomes (KDIGO) clinical practice guidelines for AKI. According to KDIGO guidelines, definition of AKI is any of the following [3] (Table 41.1).

The development of AKI in patients undergoing surgery has several obvious and some silent consequences. The obvious complication is reduced urine output and eventual risk of volume overload and congestive heart failure. Patients who develop acute kidney injury will also begin to accumulate toxins (uremia) and can develop extreme electrolyte abnormalities such as elevated potassium and phosphorous levels and accumulation of acids. Less obvious is the development of impaired kidney filtration leading to increased drug metabolites and increased risk of adverse drug reactions. Additionally, the development of acute kidney injury postoperatively has importantly been associated with increased morbidity and mortality (see Chap. 18.1).

Table 41.1 KDIGO definition for diagnosing AKI

• Increase in SCr by ≥0.3 mg/dL within 48 h
• Increase in SCr to ≥1.5 times baseline, which is known or presumed to have occurred within the prior 7 days
• Urine volume ≤0.5 mL/kg/h for 6 h

41.1.2 Causes of Acute Kidney Injury

There are many causes of acute kidney injury; however, prerenal azotemia and acute tubular necrosis (ATN) account for more than half of the cases of renal failure in the hospital [4]. Hypotension or ischemia is the most common cause of acute kidney injury; however, it often goes unrecognized. Compared to detected hypotension, unobserved hypotension or a relative drop in blood pressure compared to the patient's baseline blood pressure may lead to modest reduction in renal perfusion and acute kidney injury. In surgical patients, anesthesia may lead to a lowering of systemic blood pressure and has direct effects on reduced renal perfusion leading to acute kidney injury. Common causes of acute kidney injury in the surgical patient are listed in Table 41.2.

41.1.3 Pathophysiology

AKI can be divided into three broad categories: prerenal, renal, or post-renal causes (Table 41.2). Prerenal causes of acute injury account for the majority (30–60%) of cases of postoperative renal failure [5]. Prerenal AKI traditionally involve a reduced effective circulating volume caused by volume loss, intense vasodilation, and low cardiac output. Volume loss is usually in the form of excessive bleeding or third spacing. Intense vasodilation could be in the form of sepsis or liver failure. Low cardiac output directly

Table 41.2 Common causes of AKI in surgical patients

Prerenal	Renal	Post-renal
Sepsis-hypotension	Ischemic injury—acute tubular necrosis (ATN)	Acute urinary retention-obstruction—hydronephrosis
Volume depletion	Nephrotoxic medications—nonsteroidal anti-inflammatory drugs (NSAIDs), antibiotics such as gentamycin and sulfamethoxazole/trimethoprim	
Low cardiac output	Contrast exposure	
Liver failure causing vasodilation	Acute interstitial nephritis	
Bilateral renal artery stenosis		

causes renal hypoperfusion. Patients with prerenal acute kidney injury have functionally preserved, normal-appearing kidneys without evidence of intrinsic damage and can correct rather quickly after restoring normal perfusion to the kidney.

Renal causes are intrinsic damage of the kidney microstructures such as the glomerulus, tubular, interstitium (matrix of kidney), or collecting system. While there are many causes of postoperative AKI, the most common cause of kidney damage postoperatively is ATN and accounts for 90% of intrinsic renal causes [6]. Briefly, ATN is caused by hypoxic damage to the medulla of the kidney leading to precipitous cellular death and sloughing of renal tubular epithelial cells that break off and lead to tubular obstruction. The duration of ATN may last days to weeks depending on the duration and degree of hypoperfusion or injury. Additional less common causes of "renal or intrinsic" acute kidney injury in the surgical patient include allergic interstitial nephritis (AIN) typically related to medications, direct nephrotoxicity from medications, rhabdomyolysis, and rarely renal infarct from atheroemboli [7].

Lastly, post-renal causes are any obstruction to urine flow leading to swelling of the kidney or hydronephrosis. Typically injury is caused by obstruction of the lower urinary tract, including urethra, prostate, or bladder outlet that is typically relieved by insertion of Foley catheter. During the perioperative period, exposure to anticholinergic agents and anesthetics can cause bladder dysfunction and obstructive uropathy, especially in patients with prostatic enlargement [7, 8]. Upper urinary tract disease, obstruction above the level of the bladder, is more occult and difficult to diagnose. Upper tract obstruction is not relieved with insertion of a Foley catheter and typically requires diagnosis with ultrasound. To develop worsening renal function, there needs to be involvement or obstruction of both kidneys. Although less common, obstruction of the ureter by an obstructing stone or urethral stricture in a patient with only a single functional kidney can present identically. Early relief of the obstruction with an internal stent or percutaneous nephrostomy with external drainage of the kidney typically corrects the urine flow and restores renal function. Obstructive nephropathy accounts for about 10% of cases of inpatient acute renal failure [9].

41.1.4 Risk Factors

Knowing that therapy options for acute kidney injury are somewhat limited, prevention or avoidance of acute kidney injury is essential. The greater the magnitude and duration of surgery coupled with the number of acute and chronic risk factors, there is a greater likelihood of perioperative acute kidney injury. The renal vasculature has the unique ability to adapt to changes in renal perfusion by vasoconstricting or vasodilating to ensure adequate renal blood flow and glomerular filtration rate. The kidneys, however, are very vulnerable to moderate hypoperfusion when autoregulation is impaired. Drugs like NSAIDs and renin-angiotensin-aldosterone (RAAS) blockade with angiotensin-converting enzyme inhibitors (ACEi) and angiotensin receptor blockers (ARBs) classically impair autoregulation and predispose patients to AKI [10]. AKI occurs more commonly in patients with advanced age or in people with atherosclerosis, hypertension, or chronic kidney disease who also have an acquired inability to adapt.

Understanding potential risk factors for the development of acute kidney injury can be helpful. If these patients have multiple or significant risk factors, more astute attention to the use of intravenous contrast, potential nephrotoxic medications, and appropriate fluid management is necessary. In noncardiac surgery, several independent risk factors for AKI have been identified by Kheterpal and colleagues. These risk factors include age, emergent surgery, liver disease, body mass index, high-risk surgery, peripheral vascular disease, and chronic obstructive pulmonary disease requiring chronic bronchodilator therapy [11, 12]. More recently, a clinical score to predict acute renal failure after cardiac surgery has been established and identified several additional risk factors for acute kidney injury [13]. All identified risk factors for AKI in surgical patient are listed under Table 41.3. Although there a multiple

Table 41.3 Risk factors for development of AKI in surgical patients

1. Advanced age over 65 years old
2. Preexisting chronic kidney disease (CKD)
3. Congestive heart failure
4. Recent exposure to nephrotoxic agents—aminoglycosides, NSAIDs, contrast, pigment nephropathy—bile, or rhabdomyolysis
5. Emergency surgery
6. Liver dysfunction
7. Diabetes mellitus type 2
8. Proteinuria
9. Volume depletion
10. Obesity

number of variables that increase the risk of postoperative renal damage, there remains unexplained variability in accurately predicting the outcome. While some of these risk factors are unavoidable, others are preventable yet sadly remain largely ignored in clinical practice [5].

41.1.5 Prevalence

Approximately 1 out of 20 hospitalized patients develop acute kidney injury, most often related to trauma or surgery [11]. Using general surgery statistics, 1% of all general surgery cases are complicated by acute kidney injury [14]. The prevalence is probably underestimated because a majority of surgeries occur as outpatients and inadequate follow-up bias occurs. The prevalence of acute kidney injury in patients undergoing dental or maxillofacial surgery is unknown. Despite recognizing the importance and high incidence of acute kidney injury, some studies have suggested that there continues to be a delay in involving nephrology. A delay in nephrology consultation was associated with a higher need for renal replacement therapy, worse renal outcome, and increased in hospital mortality [6, 15, 16].

The hospital and population-based reported incidences of AKI in North America and Europe are increasing. The incidence of AKI-requiring dialysis is also increasing [6]. The exact reasons for this growth are currently being investigated. Contributors to the growth of AKI include advancing age and increasing comorbidities of patients who suffer sepsis, major surgery, and congestive heart failure. There continues to be an increase in known precipitants of AKI such as patients with CKD, proteinuria, diabetes, obesity, and the exposure to several nephrotoxic medications that either are directly nephrotoxic or lower the threshold for sustaining acute injury [17].

41.2 Patient Assessment

41.2.1 Monitoring/Work-Up

Monitoring for complications of acute kidney injury is paramount. Guarding and protecting the body against progressive volume overload/congestive heart failure, hypertension, metabolic acidosis, and hyperkalemia are the essential cornerstone. In addition to blood urea nitrogen (BUN), serum creatinine (SCr), CBC, sodium, potassium, chloride, and bicarbonate levels, and possible arterial blood gas should be measured if impaired renal function is suspected. Monitoring intraoperative renal blood flow is currently limited, and there remains reliance on following urine output and hemodynamics. Measuring perioperative urine output however is also inaccurate and may not predict postoperative AKI in elective surgeries. A change in serum creatinine remains the most common metric to measure renal function, but this too can vary with age, body habits, sex, and ethnicity [10, 18]. Although elevations in BUN and SCr remain the hallmark features for worsening renal function, the rise in BUN and SCr is a late marker for renal dysfunction and may not begin to rise until several hours or days after the insult.

However, creatinine is a very poor predictor of kidney damage. Some of the delay in defining AKI is the concern that defining acute kidney injury based on the rise in creatinine alone has the potential for errors. There may a dilution of creatinine in patients who have received significant volume expansion with i.v. fluids. On the other hand, significant muscle injury or rhabdomyolysis can increase creatinine release and falsely raise SCr levels. SCr level alone is a relatively late and imprecise biomarker of kidney dysfunction, which may lead to delayed identification. Due to the delay in SCr, isolated serum creatinine level is an unreliable marker for glomerular filtration rate (GFR). Multiple factors may also interfere with the creatinine assay including cephalosporins, rhabdomyolysis, and impaired tubular secretion of creatinine caused by trimethoprim, cimetidine, probenecid, and even fenofibrates.

New biomarkers, most recently as many as 20, have been identified as potential new tests to detect acute kidney earlier that are more sensitive and specific than creatinine. Currently these remain experimental but are becoming more available [18].

Several lab tests are useful for assessing the cause of acute kidney injury. These include a fresh urinalysis and urine microscopy by a trained technician or physician. Examination of the urine and evidence of renal tubular epithelial cells, hyaline casts, muddy brown cast, protein, and or blood may help identify possible mechanisms of injury. In some cases, renal imaging with ultrasound may be useful. Unfortunately, there are very few prediction scores or tools to help highlight patients at higher risk of acute kidney injury. Most predictive scores have been validated in cardiac surgery or after exposure to contrast [12, 13].

41.2.2 Potential Complications

Even minor changes in postoperative serum creatinine are associated with adverse outcomes. Patients who develop AKI may develop a number of complex complications including the immediate risk of hyperkalemia, metabolic acidosis, and eventual volume overload and uremia. Additional common complications of acute kidney injury include increased risk of infections, arrhythmias and bleeding, and reduced red blood cell production from increased physiological stress. A study of both noncardiac surgery and cardiac surgical patients suggested that even minor changes in SCr (change Cr 25–49%) in noncardiac surgery, patients experienced a twofold risk of in hospital death and extended length of stay of 3 days [19].

41.3 Patient Management

Management of AKI is largely supportive, including preservation of existing renal function by avoiding further injury and management of potential complications of AKI. KDIGO guidelines for management of acute kidney injury include moderately aggressive glucose control and early nutritional support by providing 20–40 kcal/kg per day and avoiding protein-restricted diet [20]. Adequate nutritional support in surgical patients with AKI and increased catabolic state improves survival [3].

41.3.1 Intraoperative Fluid Management

An essential component of the treatment of acute kidney injury is hemodynamic monitoring and fluid resuscitation or replacement in the critically ill patient. Low perfusion states and risk factors for renal ischemia should be identified and adjusted promptly to prevent further renal damage, attempting to maintain MAP >60 mm Hg and >75 mm Hg in patients with chronic hypertension [21]. Intraoperative fluid requirements are important and vary according to the extent of the surgical insult (see Chap. 7 for a more detailed discussion). Rough estimates for a mild trauma is 4 mL/kg/h, moderate trauma 8 mL/kg/h, and severe trauma 15 mL/kg/h. There has been a significant shift and great deal of controversy in the choice of replacement fluid. Several studies have failed to show any benefit of colloids or plasma expanders such as hetastarch. Currently, the use of colloids or hetastarch solutions is not recommended for patients with or at risk for AKI. The current recommendation of using crystalloid with normal saline compared to more physiological solutions continues to be challenged [22]. Increased volumes of normal saline alone may cause hyperchloremic metabolic acidosis which may lead to reduced renal cortical perfusion [23]. Intravenous crystalloid—lactated ringers or ½ NS with 50–75 meq of bicarbonate—is becoming the replacement solution of choice.

Another new, important development in the management of acute kidney injury is the use of conservative fluid management compared to the traditional approach of aggressive fluid resuscitation. Beyond the initial aggressive management of hypotension with saline, there is increasing attention to avoid overzealous, continuous fluid resuscitation. Aggressive fluid resuscitation has been associated with lung injury—ARDS, prolonged mechanical ventilation, impaired wound healing, and delayed kidney recovery. A more conservative fluid management approach may lower morbidity and improve kidney recovery in patients with AKI [22–24]. Additional randomized trials will be needed to confirm these findings.

The use of loop diuretics such as furosemide has failed to show significant benefit in the treatment of acute kidney injury. Using a higher dose of a loop diuretic may convert oliguric renal failure into non-oliguric renal failure and help to prevent a positive fluid balance [25]. Although there was some initial interest in using dopamine and atrial natriuretic peptide to treat acute kidney injury, there is very little benefit and potential harm [26, 27].

41.3.2 Medications

Careful monitoring of medications is essential if perioperative acute kidney injury occurs. The presence of an abnormal GFR is associated with an increased incidence of adverse drug reactions. Avoidance of nephrotoxic agents including holding NSAIDs, diuretics, aminoglycosides, ACEi, ARBs, and intravenous contrast exposure is paramount. Dosing medications in patients with ensuing renal dysfunction can be challenging as the SCr continues to rise and steady state is not achieved. Conservative dose or frequency reduction of medications cleared by the kidney with the help of pharmacist or a nephrologist is recommended.

41.3.3 Use of Hemodialysis

Although largely deferred to the decision of the nephrologist, renal replacement or acute dialysis is occasionally required in patients with acute kidney injury. Renal replacement therapy in the acute setting may be required if there are no signs of meaningful renal recovery or the patient is developing complications of acute kidney injury. Traditionally, dialysis is performed for patients with specific indications. These indications are easily remembered using the mnemonic "AEIOU."

- Severe **a**cidosis or acidemia with low serum pH less than 7.0 or 7.1 that is not correctable with bicarbonate therapy.
- **E**lectrolyte abnormalities, marked by a potassium level traditionally greater than 6.0 and reduced urine output. **I**ntoxication, which is beyond the scope of this text, is used for the removal of specific poisons or intoxications.
- **O**verload or CHF, refractory to diuretics, may require hemodialysis to assist with fluid removal.
- Lastly, **u**remia which is marked by a rise in surrogate marker by the accumulation of high blood urea nitrogen.

Although there are many techniques to perform renal replacement therapy in the acute setting, the most common is hemodialysis which requires access to arterial and venous blood flow limbs. Blood cycles through a machine and a semipermeable membrane called a dialyzer which assist in removal of impurities and fluid. First used in 1944, dialysis techniques have continued to improve and evolve. Hemodialysis can be performed over a typical 3.5–5-h session. Additional modalities including slow efficient dialysis (SLED) over 6–8 h with slower blood flows. Continuous venovenous hemodiafiltration (CVVHD) that occurs continuously over 24 h is common in critical care settings. Much less common is acute peritoneal dialysis, performed through a catheter inserted into the abdominal peritoneal cavity. While all the modalities each have advantages and disadvantages, there does not appear to be any specific survival advantage, and the dialysis performed is largely hospital or nephrologist specific. Guidelines regarding the initiation of dialysis or threshold level of urea to commence dialysis remain controversial and remain outside the scope of this discussion.

41.4 Prevention

41.4.1 Background

There is currently limited data about preventing acute kidney injury. With the knowledge of hypoperfusion or hypotension as the leading cause of acute kidney injury, aggressive and early control of volume and blood pressure is essential. The most promising evidence for prevention of direct kidney injury is ensuring adequate volume resuscitation and providing maximal cardiac output. Greater attention to blood pressure and volume control and avoiding systemic vasodilation especially in patients with sepsis, liver disease, nephrotic syndrome (hypoalbuminemia), or congestive heart failure is crucial [21]. Being vigilant about patient's medications including over-the-counter medications that carry risk of renal injury and avoidance of these potential nephrotoxins remain paramount.

41.4.2 Loop Diuretics, Dopamine, Fenoldopam, and Others

Despite some earlier data, furosemide and other loop diuretics have no renal protective effects and may delay the detection of renal failure by increasing urine output [24]. Furthermore, looking at the medical folklore of "renal-dose dopamine," dopamine has no role in preventing acute renal failure. Despite the vasodilatory and diuretic effects of dopamine, dopamine has failed in multiple studies to show any sustained clinical advantage and is actually associated with greater risk of arrhythmias, tissue necrosis, worsening renal failure, and death [26, 27].

A few limited, positive studies using fenoldopam—specific agonist DA1—dopamine receptor to prevent acute kidney injury exist, yet controversy surrounds fenoldopam given its deleterious hypotensive effects. Fenoldopam has failed to have any true benefit of reducing the risk of significant renal failure and avoiding renal replacement therapy in high-risk patients. Pentoxifylline, a nonspecific phosphodiesterase (PDE) inhibitor with vasodilatory and anti-inflammatory properties produced conflicting results. Many other therapies have been investigated including atrial natriuretic peptide (ANP), adenosine, nitric oxide, and growth factors—insulin-like growth factor (IGF-1), epidermal growth factor (EGF), and hepatocyte growth factor (HGF) produced at the kidney with no clinical meaningful use presently [28, 29].

41.4.3 Contrast Exposure

The risk of contrast-induced acute kidney injury is quite high and carries significant morbidity. Although rare in patients with normal renal function, contrast-enhanced nephropathy is more common in patients with preexisting kidney disease, diabetes, volume depletion, and large or repeated exposure to contrast. Contrast-induced nephropathy has been reported to be responsible for up to 10% of all hospital-acquired cases of acute renal failure in the United States and Europe and is a common concern [30]. Currently, there is no established "safe level" of creatinine or estimated GFR value to allow the use of intravenous contrast.

Preventive measures to protect against contrast nephropathy have been established [31]. The most established strategy to protect from renal injury is optimal hydration and potentially holding diuretic therapy prior to contrast exposure. Another important strategy to limit contrast nephropathy is to reduce the dose of contrast or avoid contrast by asking if the use of intravenous contrast is absolutely neccessary. Most institutional guidelines for contrast exposure recommend volume expansion with normal saline 3 cc/kg 1 h prior to the contrast exposure, followed by 1 cc/kg for 6 h post-procedure or sodium bicarbonate infusion protocols, which may have slightly increased risk for congestive heart failure and volume overload. Despite being extensively studied, the use of *N*-acetyl cysteine (NAC) to prevent contrast nephropathy is controversial and is not universally recommended. Given the low risk of therapy, some protocols however continue to suggest to premedicate 24 h before contrast exposure with Mucomyst 600–1200 mg q 12 h for a total of four doses [32].

Similarly, the use of angiotensin-converting enzymes or angiotensin receptor blocker prior to use with contrast is controversial, but currently there is no evidence to discontinue this medication prior to intravenous contrast exposure [33]. Metformin should ideally be stopped 48 h before the administration of contrast due to the risk of lactic acidosis. Additionally, avoidance of diuretic therapy and NSAIDS for 24 h prior to contrast exposure is also recommended. Occasionally, intravenous contrast is required in the emergent setting and cannot be avoided in high-risk patients.

41.4.4 MRI with Gadolinium

The use of magnetic resonance imaging with gadolinium may serve as a better alternative in high-risk patients for contrast exposure. Unfortunately, in patients with impaired renal function with a known GFR below 30 cc/min, the use of MRI with gadolinium is currently contraindicated due to the significant growing concern for a rare, nonreversible systemic complication, nephrogenic systemic fibrosis (NSF). NSF was initially diagnosed in patients on dialysis and was limited to skin; has now been identified as a serious, untreatable disease mimicking systemic scleroderma with progressive, restrictive multiorgan involvement; and has been seen in patients with some reduction in renal function after exposure to gadolinium exposure. The current recommendations vary, but a discussion with your radiologist and or nephrologist is suggested. Some MRI studies can be performed "dry" without gadolinium or low-risk gadolinium agents that provide equal resolution [32].

41.5 Summary

Despite numerous small studies involving animal models and small populations that have suggested promise in preventing or treating acute tubular necrosis, large trials have been unsuccessful. Presently, supportive non-pharmacological care and avoidance of drugs that cause additional harm continue to be the principal therapy. Although this seems obvious, research has demonstrated that even simple preventive measures are not being followed [34]. At present the best strategy is to identify high-risk patients, optimize volume status and blood pressure, and ensure careful selection of perioperative medications. AKI continues to be a serious yet common complication that occurs in postsurgical patients. Perioperative AKI is a leading cause of morbidity and mortality and potentially progressive late stage chronic kidney disease. Given the absence of meaningful therapy, early identification of risk factors and prevention of AKI in the perioperative setting are essential.

References

1. Kellum JA, Levin N, Bouman C, Lameire N. Developing a consensus classification system for acute renal failure. Curr Opin Crit Care. 2002;8(6):509–14.
2. Lopes JA, Jorge S. The RIFLE and AKIN classifications for acute kidney injury: a critical and comprehensive review. Clin Kidney J. 2013;6(1):8–14.
3. Kellum JA, et al. Kidney disease: Improving Global Outcomes (KDIGO) Acute Kidney Injury Work Group: KDIGO clinical practice guideline for acute kidney injury. Kidney Int Suppl. 2012;2(1):1–138. https://doi.org/10.1038/kisup.2012.1.
4. Abuelo JG. Normotensive ischemic acute renal failure. N Engl J Med. 2007;357(8):797–805.
5. Calvert S, Shaw A. Perioperative acute kidney injury. Perioper Med. 2012;1:6.
6. Chertow GM, Burdick E, Honour M, Bonventre JV, Bates DW. Acute kidney injury, mortality, length of stay, and costs in hospitalized patients. J Am Soc Nephrol. 2005;16:3365–70.
7. Goren O, Matot I. Perioperative acute kidney injury. Br J Anaesth. 2015;115(Suppl 2):ii3–ii14.
8. Sear JW. Kidney dysfunction in the postoperative period. Br J Anaesth. 2005;95(1):20–32.
9. Hou SH, Bushinsky DA, Wish JB, Cohen JJ, Harrington JT. Hospital-acquired renal insufficiency: a prospective study. Am J Med. 1983;74(2):243–8.
10. Brenner BM, Rector FC. The kidney. Philadelphia: Saunders; 1991. Print
11. Kheterpal S, Tremper KK, et al. Predictors of postoperative acute renal failure after noncardiac surgery in patients with previously normal renal function. Anesthesiology. 2007;107(6):892–902.
12. Kheterpal S, Tremper K, et al. Development and validation of an acute kidney injury risk index for patients

undergoing general surgery: results from a National Data Set. Anesthesiology. 2009;10(3):505–15.
13. Khakar CV, Arrigain S, et al. A clinical score to predict acute renal failure after cardiac surgery has been established. J Am Soc Nephrol. 2005;16: 162–8.
14. Miller RD, Cohen NH. Miller's anesthesia. Philadelphia, PA: Elsevier/Saunders; 2015. Print
15. Meier P, et al. Referral patterns and outcomes in non critically ill patients with hospital-acquired acute kidney injury. Clin J Am Soc Nephrol. 2011;6(9): 2215–25.
16. Costa e Silva VT, Liaño F, Muriel A, Díez R, de Castro I, Yu L. Nephrology referral and outcomes in critically ill acute kidney injury patients. PLoS One. 2013;8(8):e70482. https://doi.org/10.1371/journal.pone.0070482.
17. Hobson C, et al. Cost and mortality associated with postoperative acute kidney injury. Ann Surg. 2015;261(6):1207–14.
18. Thomas ME, Blaine C, Dawnay A, et al. The definition of acute kidney injury and its use in practice. Kidney Int. 2015;87(1):62–73.
19. Kork F, Balzer F, Spies C, et al. Minor postoperative increases in creatinine are associated with higher mortality and longer hospital length of stay in surgical patients. Perioper Med. 2015;12:1301–11.
20. Chen J, Fang X, Jin X, Kang R, Liu K, Li J, Zhang S, et al. Expert consensus on the perioperative management of patients with sepsis. World J Emerg Med. 2015;6(4):245–60.
21. Joannidis M, Druml W, Forni LG, et al. Prevention of acute kidney injury and protection of renal function in the intensive care unit: expert opinion of the working group for nephrology, ESICM. Intensive Care Med. 2010;36:392–411.
22. Chowdhury AH, Cox EF, Francis ST, et al. A randomized, controlled, double-blind crossover study on the effects of 2-L infusions of 0.9% saline and plasmalyte® 148 on renal blood flow velocity and renal cortical tissue perfusion in healthy volunteers. Ann Surg. 2012;256:18–24.
23. Yunos NM, Bellomo R, Bailey M. Chloride-restrictive fluid administration and incidence of acute kidney injury—reply. JAMA. 2013;309:543–4.
24. Nadeau-Fredette AC, Bouchard J. Fluid management and use of diuretics in acute kidney injury. Adv Chronic Kidney Dis. 2013;20(1):45–55.
25. Grams ME, Estrella MM, Coresh J, et al. National Heart, Lung, and Blood Institute Acute Respiratory Distress Syndrome Network. Fluid balance, diuretic use, and mortality in acute kidney injury. Clin J Am Soc Nephrol. 2011;6:966–73.
26. Bellomo R, Chapman M, Finfer S, Hickling K, Myburgh J. Low-dose dopamine in patients with early renal dysfunction: a placebo-controlled randomised trial. Australian and New Zealand Intensive Care Society (ANZICS) Clinical Trials Group. Lancet. 2000;356(9248):2139–43.
27. Lauschke A, Teichgräber UK, Frei U, Eckardt KU. 'Low-dose' dopamine worsens renal perfusion in patients with acute renal failure. Kidney Int. 2006; 69(9):1669–74.
28. Bagshaw SM, Ghali WA. Theophylline for prevention of contrast-induced nephropathy: a systematic review and meta-analysis. Arch Intern Med. 2005;165(10): 1087–93.
29. Yilmaz MB, Yalta K, Yontar C, Karadas F, Erdem A, Turgut OO, Yilmaz A, Tandogan I. Levosimendan improves renal function in patients with acute decompensated heart failure: comparison with dobutamine. Cardiovasc Drugs Ther. 2007;21(6):431–5.
30. Briguori C, Tavano D, Colombo A. Contrast agent associated nephrotoxicity. Prog Cardiovasc Dis. 2003;45:493–503.
31. Barrett BJ, Parfrey PS. Preventing nephropathy induced by contrast medium. N Engl J Med. 2006;354: 379–86.
32. Rose TA, Choi J. Intravenous imaging contrast media complications: the basics that every clinician needs to know. Am J Med. 2015;128(9):943–9.
33. Arora P, Rajagopalam S, Ranjan R, Kolli H, Singh M, Venuto R, Lohr J, et al. Preoperative use of angiotensin-converting enzyme inhibitors/angiotensin receptor blockers is associated with increased risk for acute kidney injury after cardiovascular surgery. Clin J Am Soc Nephrol. 2008;3(5):1266–73.
34. Vanmassenhove J, Veys N, Van Biesen W. Prevention and conservative management of acute kidney injury. Minerva Urol Nefrol. 2016;68(1):58–71.

Check for updates

42 Altered Mental Status as a Complication of Maxillofacial Surgery

Roger S. Badwal

Abstract

The reversible and controlled alteration of the mental state by anesthesia is a hallmark of the clinical practice of oral and maxillofacial surgery. Polypharmacy and medical comorbidities can place patients at risk of uncontrolled changes in mental status with consequences. It is incumbent upon the oral and maxillofacial surgeon to be prepared to recognize, understand, and manage a multitude of adverse situations involving unintended alterations in mental status.

Altered mental status is a broad non-specific term referring to the change in the awareness and appropriate interaction within acceptable neuropsychiatric bounds. Altered mental status describes the whole spectrum of brain dysfunctions, such as dementia, delirium, and psychiatric disorders occurring in any age group, but is more frequently observed in the elderly, particularly with the onset of dementia. Altered mental status is a result of cerebral dysfunction with a very wide range of etiologies. It is estimated that 4–10% of non-traumatic emergency department patients present with altered mental status [1].

R.S. Badwal, D.M.D., M.D.
Division of Oral and Maxillofacial Surgery, Danbury Hospital, Danbury, CT, USA
e-mail: facedocb@yahoo.com

The pathophysiology of altered mental status is directly related to the underlying cause, which can be the result of trauma and physiological disturbances including psychiatric diseases. Altered mental status in the presence of psychiatric disease may complicate the evaluation of patients with head trauma.

In the typical office setting, a new patient is *not likely to present* with acute signs and symptoms of altered mental status. However, patients can develop changes in mental status while under care perioperatively. The office consultation for preoperative surgical and medical evaluation should alert the practitioner to possible complications that would make the patient susceptible to perioperative changes in the mental status.

Oral and maxillofacial surgeons (OMS) by nature of their training induce a controlled state of altered mental status on a routine basis during IV/GA (intravenous, general anesthesia) in the

© Springer International Publishing AG 2018
E.M. Ferneini, J.D. Bennett (eds.), *Perioperative Assessment of the Maxillofacial Surgery Patient*,
https://doi.org/10.1007/978-3-319-58868-1_42

office. This pharmacologically controlled state of depressed central nervous functioning is a continuum from lightly altered as with nitrous oxide to fully incapacitated under general anesthesia. One should develop the ability coupled with the knowledge of the medical history to understand the abnormalities of mental status changes not congruent with normal postanesthesia emergence. There are several entities, e.g., stroke and myocardial infarction, that can present intraoperatively which herald physiological problems that will affect the emergence and recovery of normal mental functioning. Patients affected by dementia or psychiatric disease present a significant management challenge when postanesthesia mental status does not return to baseline.

Kanich et al. [1] study involving emergency department patients with chief complaint of altered mental status revealed that the history of the present illness provided positive data leading to the diagnosis 51% of the time. The other six types of data in the study were (i) past medical history, 43%; (ii) physical exam, 41%; (iii) response to medications, 39%; (iv) imaging, 16%; (v) laboratory testing (11%); and (vi) the electrocardiogram (7%) in determining possible causes. Generally the etiology of altered mental status can fall into the broad categories listed in Table 42.1 [2].

Table 42.1 Categories of common etiologies of altered mental status

Metabolic: B_{12} or thiamine deficiency, serotonin syndrome
Hypoxemia: pulmonary, cardiac, anemia
Vascular: hypertensive emergency, ischemic/hemorrhagic, CVA, vasculitis, MI
Electrolytes and endocrine
Seizures: status epilepticus, postictal
Tumor, trauma, temperature, toxins: lead, mercury, CO, toxidromes
Uremia: renal or hepatic dysfunction with hepatic encephalopathy
Psychiatric, porphyria
Infection inflammatory
Drugs: including withdrawal, anticholinergics, tricyclic antidepressants, monoamine oxidase inhibitors (MAOIs), selective serotonin reuptake inhibitors (SSRIs), serotonin-norepinephrine reuptake inhibitors (SNRIs), benzodiazepines, barbiturates, alcohol

42.1 Manifestation of Altered Mental Status

Clinical features of patients who are described as having altered mental status include confusion, hyperalertness, obtundation, stupor, and frank coma. Altered mental status, diagnosed as delirium, carries the highest morbidity and mortality when missed [3]. Delirium has been described as "brain failure" and is a true medical emergency because the mortality is high if unrecognized and untreated. Studies have demonstrated that delirium is associated with cerebral hypoperfusion, particularly in the frontal, temporal, and parietal regions. This hypoxic state is associated with increased levels of oxidative markers, including higher levels of anticholinergic activity [4, 5]. The full description, manifestations, and treatment of delirium will not be addressed specifically in this chapter.

42.2 Mental Status Changes Encountered in the Outpatient Setting (Office)

Oral and maxillofacial surgeons routinely perform surgery in an outpatient clinic setting, as both operator and anesthetist. We will focus on this aspect and possible perioperative sequela. Unlike many patients who present with altered mental status to the hospital emergency department, your patient will have had an evaluation, including a full medical and surgical history on record. As discussed earlier, the medical history is the most important factor in determining possible causes of altered mental status affecting the patient [1]. Knowing the medical history will narrow the differential for managing the patient who experiences an adverse event. Regardless of the etiology of the altered mental status, the patient should be stabilized using the fundamentals of BLS (basic life support) and ACLS (advanced cardiac life support) measures.

The vast majority of patients who present for surgery can be quite apprehensive. Heightened anxiety makes patients prone to syncope or near syncope events, which may or may not be coupled with hyperventilation and panic attacks. Coupled with the NPO status in preparation for the IV/GA procedure, the susceptibility of an untoward event is higher. Patients with poorly controlled or marginal cardiovascular reserve are at increased risk for serious hemodynamic instability with consequences involving depressed cerebral functioning [6].

Acute changes in mental status may be associated with these events. The changes may spontaneously resolve in mild cases or with more severe pathology, be prolonged, and need hospitalization for treatment and management of the underlying etiology. Initial management consists of supportive therapy and treating the symptoms and signs according to established principles in BLS and ACLS. OMS should be trained and comfortable in the initial management and stabilization of any of these events until, if necessary, the patient can be transported for definitive care to a hospital.

42.3 Differential Diagnosis for Mental Status Change

Syncope is defined as a transient, self-limited loss of consciousness, with loss of motor tone that is followed by spontaneous recovery—"fainting." This results from temporary hypotension and loss of blood flow and oxygen to the brain. The etiology of syncope in most patients is benign, but can be the precipitating sentinel event with serious underlying pathology. The mental status changes accompanying this common form of syncope (loss of consciousness) are self-limited. The patient tends to recover their mental status readily after the episode terminates. This event is the most frequent emergency that is known to occur in dental offices [6]. In the OMS office, syncope could occur prior to or after procedures. Typically, pre-procedural syncope is related to anxiety and is usually vasovagal mediated. Common presyncopal vasovagal symptoms are related to parasympathetic stimulation—nausea, diaphoresis, blurry vision, and light-headedness. Uncomplicated post-procedural syncope may be related to orthostatic hypotension, hypovolemia, or lingering effects of IV/GA. Knowledge of the patient's medical history and the vital signs will guide the management. In general, Trendelenburg positioning (legs/feet higher than heart, supine), oxygen, and airway support are indicated. The use of smelling salts or a sharp stimulus may shorten the episode of uncomplicated syncope. In cases of persistent loss of consciousness (30–60 s) or an unresponsive patient, ACLS/BLS measures should be instituted, including the possible activation of the emergency management system (EMS) system.

42.4 Postural Hypotension (Orthostatic)

This condition occurs when the patient moves from either a sitting or supine position to a standing position, with an inadequate blood pressure response resulting in compromised cerebral blood flow. The decreased cerebral perfusion causes signs and symptoms of light-headedness, headache, blurred vision, warm or clammy sensation, weakness, fatigue, or syncope. Orthostatic hypotension is defined as a decrease in systolic blood pressure of 20 mmHg or a decrease in diastolic blood pressure of 10 mmHg within 3 min of standing compared with blood pressure from the sitting or supine position [7].

As most dental patients are recumbent for dental procedures, this is a fairly common finding in offices. In the Malamed study, there were almost 2500 such cases. This represents about 8% of the patients in the study. It is not uncommon for OMS patients to be both groggy and dizzy postanesthesia; however, orthostatic hypotension will cause these patients to behave erratically and be unable to respond appropriately. Hypotension that is purely postural could be related to anxiety (vasovagal) related to the dental procedure, hypovolemia, autonomic dysfunction, or iatrogenic from polypharmacy prescription medications, e.g., antihypertensive and antihistamines [8].

Management consists of bringing the patient into Trendelenburg position and incrementally bringing the patient upright. Repeated attempts that are unsuccessful with persistent unstable cardiac signs or symptoms should prompt reexamination of the patient's medical history and reevaluation of the differential diagnosis.

42.5 Seizures

Seizures are an uncontrolled discharge of cerebral electrical activity accompanied by altered mental status. The cerebral origin, frequency, and intensity determine the character of the seizure activity. Epilepsy is the chronic condition in which seizures require long-term medication control. It is present in 0.5–1% of the population, with a 10% lifetime risk of experiencing a single seizure. There are a multitude of different types of epilepsy and seizure types, which are beyond this scope of this discussion.

The symptoms of epilepsy can be as vague as a quiet transient inability to respond to normal verbal and tactile stimuli to full-fledged tonic-clonic activity, which may place the patient's life at immediate risk. Seizures are accompanied by alterations in alertness, communicability, confusion and amnesia, and inability to communicate during the episode. The post-seizure state is often referred to as postictal in which the patient continues to manifest signs of confusion, amnesia, drowsiness, hypertension, and headaches/migraine. The postictal state can last for several minutes to several hours. In general seizures must be terminated within a few minutes to prevent long-term brain damage. Seizure activity lasting more than 5 min is considered status epilepticus. This serious condition carries a short-term mortality of up to 22% and long-term mortality of 43% [9]. In general intravenous benzodiazepines (lorazepam, diazepam) are the first-line choice to terminate active seizure activity.

Understanding the patient's medical and seizure history (including type, prodrome, triggers, frequency, and therapeutic medications) will allow the practitioner to anticipate and manage perioperative complications. It is not uncommon for the patient to have routine serum concentrations evaluated for therapeutic drug levels, and this data should be part of the medical evaluation by the oral and maxillofacial surgeon. In addition there are common events and situations which predispose patients to seizures such as NPO status, sleep deprivation, fatigue, stress, surgical pain, adverse drug reactions, changes in drug regimens due to patient noncompliance, and interactions between anesthetics and anticonvulsants.

There is no published data studying the perioperative incidence of seizures in OMS either in the inpatient or outpatient setting.

The incidence of perioperative seizure has been reported as 3.1 per 10,000 patients by Akavipat. This study found that 30.19% were related to anesthesia, while 67.9% was related to the surgery, and 54.73% was related to patient factors [10]. The study by Niesen in 641 patients with pre-existing seizure disorder had a perioperative seizure incidence of 3.4% [11].

Multiple studies in patients with depression requiring electroconvulsive therapy (ECT) lean toward showing certain drug combinations used in anesthesia lowering seizure threshold or prolonging excitatory phase of the induced seizures. A Cochrane review concluded that many of the studies had high risk of bias, and quality of evidence was low. A list of the common anesthetic drugs used in OMS and their possible effect on seizure threshold is listed. The list of medications which were in the original final draft is now missing. If insufficient space does not allow the list of medications then this paragraph should be modified to reflect their absence. Many drugs have both pro- and anticonvulsant effects. The lowering of the seizure threshold or the promotion of seizure foci is dose/concentration dependent and can be ameliorated by the concomitant use of benzodiazepines [12, 13].

42.6 Hypoglycemia

This is defined as the condition in which the blood/plasma glucose drops below a threshold needed by the body to meet metabolic demands, causing cerebral and cardiovascular instability. The incidence of this in the dental office was reported by Malamed as about 3% of emergencies. The actual incidence of hypoglycemia in the general population with BG below 50 mg/dL is about 5–10% of those presenting with symptoms suggestive of hypoglycemia. The actual level at which a patient may become hypoglycemic is highly variable. The Whipple triad is documentation of low blood sugar, symptoms, and reversal of symptoms with normalization of blood sugar levels. The symptoms are sympathetically mediated with sweating, palpitations, anxiety, and tremulousness. The sympathetic symptoms and signs tend to precede the cerebral manifestations. The cerebral signs are confusion, difficulty with concentration, irritability, and hallucinations. Delay in recognition can lead to focal neurological symptoms, e.g., hemiplegia, and in fragile or medically compromised patients may result in coma or death [14].

Certain disease states make patients more susceptible to hypoglycemia. The most common cause is a diabetic patient using insulin who forgets to eat or administers excess insulin. Other common causes are suppression of the pituitary-hypothalamic-adrenal axis, thyrotoxicosis, fasting, and polypharmacy. Many patients whether or not they will receive GA/IV will have fasted, and, coupled with anxiety, may become hypoglycemic. Certain drugs known to increase the risk of hypoglycemia are ethanol, propranolol, haloperidol, pentamidine, quinine, salicylates, and sulfonamides (including the oral hypoglycemic sulfonylurea agents). Other commonly prescribed drugs known to increase patient's susceptibility to hypoglycemia include tramadol, stanozolol, isoniazid, methotrexate, tricyclic antidepressants, cytotoxic agents, chlorpromazine, fluoxetine, sertraline, fenfluramine, trimethoprim, 6-mercaptopurine, thiazide diuretics, angiotensin-converting enzyme (ACE) inhibitors, and lithium [15].

In two studies (Erikson, Gautier), patients with type 2 diabetes treated with the combination of metformin and sulfonylurea carry a greater risk for severe hypoglycemia, cardiovascular disease, and all-cause mortality than does the combination of metformin and dipeptidyl peptidase-4 inhibitors (gliptin class of medications, the first being sitagliptin (Januvia)) [16, 17].

Treatment is exogenous glucose either orally or intravenously. In the office this will likely take care of the vast majority of patients who have uncomplicated hypoglycemia. Patients who do not respond to glucose supplementation or continue to remain hypoglycemic (blood sugar via glucometer) should be transported to the hospital for management.

42.7 Hyperglycemia

Chronic untreated diabetes or acute episodes of hyperglycemia can lead to altered mental status, autonomic dysfunction, and cardiovascular instability. The symptoms of hyperglycemia are classically described as polydipsia, polyuria, and polyphagia. All of these symptoms are associated with diabetic ketoacidosis (DKA) or hyperosmolar hyperglycemia (HH). The distinguishing feature between these two entities is the presence of acidosis ($pH < 7.3$) in the former. The presentation of altered mental status associated with either entity is correlated to the level of serum hyperosmolarity in excess of 320 mOsm/L. Typical signs of mental status changes in DKA are lethargy, confusion, and possibly coma. In the HH state, more pronounced neurological signs are likely to present ranging from hemiparesis, seizures, to coma.

Management of hyperglycemia involving DKA or HHS requires correction by insulin and managing the associated electrolyte disturbances. A full discussion is beyond the scope of this chapter [15].

42.8 Adrenal Crisis

Adrenal crisis occurs when cortisol production cannot meet the physiological demands of the human body under stress. There can be a primary defect in cortisol production by the adrenal glands or as a secondary impairment from depressed hypothalamic-pituitary axis feedback. Cortisol is responsible for mediating a number of important physiological processes that involve both metabolism and immunity. Metabolically cortisol stimulates gluconeogenesis by the liver in the acute fasting state via proteolysis (consequently it inhibits protein synthesis). This results in hyperglycemia, forcing an increase in insulin release, but it also reduces the peripheral muscle sensitivity to insulin (by decreasing the translocation of glucose transporters). Cortisol influences the immune system by depressing B-cell humoral immunity, the inflammatory cascade via stabilization of lysosomes, reducing leukocyte activity, and inhibiting cytokine production as well as IgG and IgM (but not IgE) [18].

The OMS will likely encounter patients who may have chronic hypothalamic-pituitary-adrenal (HPA) suppression from exogenous steroids for a multitude of diseases like asthma, rheumatoid arthritis, and autoimmune diseases (Crohn's, ulcerative colitis, vasculopathies). There is a linear correlation with inhaled corticosteroids used (for control of asthmatic patients) and the level of HPA suppression. One meta-analysis study found that the daily dose of fluticasone at 500, 1000, 1500, and 2000 μg/day was correlated to HPA axis suppression in 6, 7, 10, and 13% of the study cohort of 732 children and adults [19].

In patients taking oral steroids, HPA is considered suppressed if 20 mg of prednisone or its equivalent is taken for more than 5 days in the preceding 12 months. In patients taking physiological doses (5 mg/day), suppression may be mild. The data on the quantity and length of time of exogenous steroid administration resulting in the inadequate production of cortisol by the adrenal glands is variable. Erring on the side of assuming suppression of the HPA is preferred [20, 21].

Suppression of the normal HPA axis renders the body's metabolic and endocrine responses to stress compromised. Symptoms of inadequate cortisol response lead to signs of autonomic instability, labile hemodynamics, and electrolyte disturbances. In the awake patient, this can present as nausea, vomiting, diarrhea, and altered mental status. The overall incidence of secondary adrenal insufficiency has been reported as 3.6 cases per 100 person-years [22]. Treatment is directed toward administering steroids in the form of hydrocortisone (has both mineralocorticoid and glucocorticoid functions) and fluid resuscitation. In the outpatient setting, management of the electrolyte disturbances is not truly possible; thus, the patient will need to be transported to a hospital setting for continued resuscitation measures.

Serotonin syndrome is a condition precipitated by the presence of excessive serotonin and the toxic side effects on the CNS. It is characterized by a triad of symptoms, which include altered mental status, neuromuscular hyperactivity, and autonomic instability or hyperactivity, which can lead to death. The increasing toxicity of serotonin manifests in the deterioration of autonomic function and impaired regulation of extrapyramidal neural circuitry [23].

There are a significant number of medications which have serotoninergic activity. These either block the reuptake of serotonin or augment serotonin release. The most commonly employed class of drugs which intentionally increase the intra-synaptic levels of serotonin are the SSRIs (selective serotonin reuptake inhibitors) and are used as antidepressants and mood stabilizers. The table shows all the common drugs which have serotonin-related activity [24, 25].

Serotonin reuptake inhibitors	Selective serotonin reuptake inhibitors: fluoxetine, fluvoxamine, paroxetine, citalopram, sertraline, escitalopram
Other antidepressants	
Serotonin-norepinephrine reuptake inhibitors	Venlafaxine, duloxetine, TCA, clomipramine, imipramine
Opioid analgesics	Tramadol, fentanyl, dextromethorphan
Herbal products	St. John's wort
Monoamine oxidase inhibitors	Irreversible monoamine oxidase A inhibitors: phenelzine, tranylcypromine
	Reversible monoamine oxidase A inhibitors: moclobemide
	Others: linezolid (antibiotic for gram-positive infections)
Serotonin-releasing agents	Fenfluramine
	Amphetamines
	Methylenedioxymethamphetamine (MDMA, ecstasy)
Miscellaneous	Lithium, tryptophan

The diagnosis is based on a clinical exam, and currently the Hunter Serotonin Toxicity Criteria show good specificity and sensitivity in narrowing the diagnosis. Serum levels of serotonin do not correlate with signs and symptoms; however, urinary levels of the breakdown product of serotonin (5-hydroxyindoleacetic acid, 5-HIAA) may be used to confirm serotonin syndrome. It has been reported that 60% of the cases will present within 6 h of drug administration, but the onset can be within minutes of administration of an offending drug or medication combination [24].

Hunter's criteria emphasize clonus (muscular spasm involving rhythmic contractions) as the most important sign of serotonin toxicity. These criteria have been shown to have 84% sensitivity and 97% specificity. These criteria are less sensitive in patients with very mild signs [24].

The criteria state that there must be use of a serotonergic drug, in addition to one or more of the following:

- Spontaneous clonus (involuntary rhythmic muscular contractions and relaxation)
- Inducible clonus with agitation or diaphoresis
- Ocular clonus with agitation or diaphoresis
- Tremor and hyperreflexia
- Hypertonia, temperature above 100.4 °F (38 °C) with ocular or inducible clonus

42.9 Moderate Symptoms

- Agitation
- Easily startled
- Hyperactive bowel sounds
- Hypervigilance
- Increased confusion
- Inducible clonus
- Myoclonus
- Ocular clonus
- Pressured speech
- Temperature of at least 40 °C

42.10 Severe Clinical Findings

- Acute respiratory distress syndrome
- Coma
- Delirium
- Diffuse intravascular clotting
- Disseminated intravascular coagulopathy
- Dramatic swings in pulse rate and blood pressure
- Elevation of serum aminotransaminases and creatinine
- Hypertension (can deteriorate to shock)
- Hypotonicity
- Metabolic acidosis
- Muscle rigidity
- Myoglobinuria
- Renal failure
- Respiratory failure
- Rhabdomyolysis
- Seizures
- Spontaneous clonus
- Tachycardia
- Temperature greater than 41.1 °C

Fentanyl is a very common drug found in the arsenal of anesthetic medications in the practice of outpatient OMS anesthesia. It has been implicated in multiple case reports of serotonin syndrome. Currently there is no predictable way to ascertain who is susceptible and what dosing is critical. When the clinical findings are mild, these may be missed or easily dismissed by the OMS during anesthesia or postanesthesia, e.g., mild hypertension, diaphoresis, tachycardia, and tremor or shivering. Such mild clinical findings can resolve over 24 h in many cases, but if severe may last several days, requiring hospitalization. Until the symptoms become clinically moderate and persistent, the patients' altered mentation may also be attributed to the lingering effects of the anesthesia.

Initial treatment should be supportive and directed to stabilizing vital signs with oxygen, IV fluids, cardiac monitoring, and temperature monitoring. Agitation may be managed with benzodiazepines. Postanesthesia emergence may be a muddled picture of clinical findings unless one is familiar with this entity. When recognized, appropriate referral to a hospital for continued monitoring and management is prudent.

42.11 Toxic CNS Effects of Local Anesthetics

Local anesthesia is an integral component to the practice of dentistry and surgery. Its routine administration with minimal side effects can lead one to downplay the serious side effects when inadvertent overdose or misplaced administration takes effect. One study revealed the incidence of aspiration-positive inferior alveolar nerve (IAN) blockade to be 15.3% [26].

There are two differing complications with the use of local anesthetics, which can contribute to a patient's change in mental status. The first aspect is of toxic overdose, and the second is the adverse biochemical effect, methemoglobinemia.

The progressively toxic side effects of local anesthetics on the central nervous system and cardiovascular system are biphasic in presentation with the excitatory preceding the inhibitory [27, 28].

The CNS is more sensitive to local anesthetic toxicity and typically affected before the CVS, but depending on the amount, route, and speed of administration, the signs and symptoms may overlap making the distinction academic. However, with patients who are under GA/IV, the toxic manifestations will be primarily of cardiovascular in origin.

The CNS is the sentinel organ affected first by the toxicity of the local anesthetics resulting in classic signs and symptoms, including altered mental status. The first phase of CNS effects is excitatory as the cortical inhibitory pathways are affected. Progressive toxicity associated during the secondary phase of inhibition will rapidly transform into global cerebral depression.

Phase 1 signs and symptoms	Phase 2 signs and symptoms
Circumoral and/or tongue numbness (local blockade may alter this symptom)	Muscle twitching
Metallic taste	Convulsions
Tinnitus	Coma
Light-headedness	Respiratory depression and arrest
Dizziness	
Confusion, disorientation, and drowsiness	

All commonly used local anesthetics can induce cardiac dysrhythmias and are myocardium depressants. There is a dose-dependent negative inotropic effect with decreasing cardiac output from the blockage of the sodium channels that affects impulse conduction throughout the myocardium.

The initial phase of blockade of the conduction pathways results in excitatory signs and symptoms (from prolonged PR interval to complete heart block, sinus arrest, and asystole). The secondary phase results from negative inotropic effect and global myocardial depression. The myocardium is frequently not responsive to traditional drug therapies (ACLS) for ameliorating the compromised cardiac status. If the index of suspicion for the change in mental status etiology is considered to be local anesthetic derived, then using lipid emulsion therapy has been shown to be relatively successful in reversing the cardiac toxicity of local anesthetic overdose [29].

The myocardial toxicity of the local anesthetics is shown below and is related to their protein binding and pKa.

Potency pot	Toxicity	LWPC	Onset	pKa	$t\frac{1}{2}$ (min)	%PB
Bupivacaine	8	2	27.5 slow	8.1	162	95.6
Articaine	3	3.3	17 fast	7.8	20	94
Lignocaine	2	2	2.9 fast	7.9	96	64.3
Mepivacaine	2	2.2	19.3 fast	7.8	114	78
Prilocaine	2	2.7	0.9 fast	7.7	93	55
Ropivacaine	4	2.25	2.9 mod	8.1	96	94

Patients under GA/IV may have arrhythmias which may not respond to typical ACLS protocols [29].

When the suspicion for local anesthetic toxicity is high, the patient should be transported to the nearest hospital facility where further management and support can be provided, including lipid therapy if required.

42.12 Stroke

Stroke is a medical emergency in which part of the brain has either obstructed blood flow (ischemic) or hemorrhage (hemorrhagic). It is characterized by a corresponding loss of neurologic function. Acute ischemic stroke is caused by thrombotic or embolic occlusion of a cerebral artery and is more common than hemorrhagic stroke. Depending on the severity and the cerebral territory involved, changes in mental status may accompany focal neurological deficits. Clinically it is not possible to ascertain the difference between ischemic and hemorrhagic strokes [30].

There is no data regarding perioperative stroke unique to dentistry or oral and maxillofacial surgery. However, there is data drawn from head and neck surgery. This data from the early 1990s had an incidence of 4.8% involving neck dissections and carotid endarterectomy. This was higher than the risk associated with general surgery (0.08–0.7%) and orthopedic surgery (0.2–0.9%). The incidence of stroke rises with age and comorbidities. The incidence increases with age: 0.1–0.2% for age up to 65 years, 0.5% for age 65–74 years, and 1.0% for age over 75 years. Perioperative mortality is very high at 18–26%. Other than age, other factors increasing the risk for perioperative stroke are female gender, prior stroke, hypertension, diabetes mellitus, renal insufficiency, dialysis, smoking, chronic obstructive pulmonary disease, peripheral vascular disease, atrial fibrillation, cardiac valvular disease, and *withholding antithrombotic therapy prior to surgery* [31].

42.13 Signs and Symptoms

Consider stroke in any patient presenting with acute neurologic deficit or any alteration in level of consciousness. Common stroke signs and symptoms include the following. The presentation is typically a combination of these signs and symptoms [32].

- Sudden decrease in level of consciousness
- Abrupt onset of hemiparesis, paresis, or (rarely) quadra-paresis
- Unilateral sensory deficits
- Monocular or binocular visual loss and visual field deficits
- Diplopia
- Dysarthria
- Facial droop
- Ataxia
- Vertigo (rarely in isolation)
- Nystagmus
- Aphasia

In younger patients, a history of recent trauma, coagulopathies, illicit drug use (especially cocaine), migraines, or use of oral contraceptives should be elicited. The increasing use of antithrombotics and the risks of holding them prior to surgery should be weighed heavily against the risk of stroke. Oral and maxillofacial surgeons should understand the risk factors for stroke. Consultation with the physician managing the antithrombotic is a prudent course prior to unilaterally deciding upon withholding antithrombotic therapy.

42.14 Chapter Summary

The increasing complexity of the aging population and the extensive polypharmacy management of medical conditions can frequently lead to drug interactions which can potentially compromise the stability of CNS. Perioperative management of the oral and maxillofacial patients requires the surgeon/anesthetist to remain vigilant of myriad side effects by understanding the medical history and potential drug interactions.

References

1. Kanich W, Brady WJ, Huff J, et al. Altered mental status: evaluation and etiology in the ED. Am J Emerg Med. 2002;20(7):613–7. https://doi.org/10.1053/ajem.2002.35464.
2. Odiari EA, Sekhon N, Han JY, David EH. Stabilizing and managing patients with altered mental status and delirium. Emerg Med Clin North Am. 2015;33(4):753–64. https://doi.org/10.1016/j.emc.2015.07.004.
3. Neufeld KJ, Thomas C. Delirium: definition, epidemiology, and diagnosis. J Clin Neurophysiol. 2013;30(5):438–42. https://doi.org/10.1097/wnp.0b013e3182a73e31.
4. Ely EW. Delirium as a predictor of mortality in mechanically ventilated patients in the intensive care unit. JAMA. 2004;291(14):1753. https://doi.org/10.1001/jama.291.14.1753.
5. Thomason JW, Shintani A, Peterson JF, Pun BT, Jackson JC, Ely EW. Intensive care unit delirium is an independent predictor of longer hospital stay: a prospective analysis of 261 non-ventilated patients. Crit Care. 2005;9(4):R375–81. https://doi.org/10.1186/cc3729.
6. Adlesic EC. Cardiovascular anesthetic complications and treatment in oral surgery. Anesthesia. 2013;25(3): 487–506. https://doi.org/10.1016/j.coms.2013.04.002.
7. Welker KL, Mycyk MB. Pharmacology in the geriatric patient. Emerg Med Clin North Am. 2016;34(3):469–81. https://doi.org/10.1016/j.emc.2016.04.003.
8. Hamid AA, Ghaleb M, Aljadhey H, Aslanpour Z. A systematic review of hospitalization resulting from medicine-related problems in adult patients. Br J Clin Pharmacol. 2014;78(2):202–17. https://doi.org/10.1111/bcp.12293.
9. Murdoch D. Mechanisms of status epilepticus: an evidence-based review. Curr Opin Neurol. 2007;20(2): 213–6. https://doi.org/10.1097/01.wco.0000263155.48598.41.
10. Akavipat P, Rungreungvanich M, Lekprasert V, Srisawasdi S. The Thai Anesthesia Incidents Study (THAI Study) of perioperative convulsion. J Med Assoc Thail. 2005;88:S106–12.
11. Niesen AD, Jacob AK, Aho LE, et al. Perioperative seizures in patients with a history of a seizure disorder. Anesth Analg. 2010;111(3):729–35. https://doi.org/10.1213/ane.0b013e3181e534a4.
12. Bajwa SJS, Jindal R. Epilepsy and nonepilepsy surgery: recent advancements in anesthesia management. Anesth Essays Res. 2013;7(1):10–7. https://doi.org/10.4103/0259-1162.113978.
13. Lihua P, Su M, Ke W, Ziemann-Gimmel P. Different regimens of intravenous sedatives or hypnotics for electroconvulsive therapy (ECT) in adult patients with depression. Cochrane Database Syst Rev. 2014. https://doi.org/10.1002/14651858.cd009763.pub2.
14. Park E, Abraham MK. Altered mental status and endocrine diseases. Emerg Med Clin North Am. 2014;32(2): 367–78. https://doi.org/10.1016/j.emc.2013.12.007.
15. Hamdy O. Hypoglycemia: practice essentials, background, pathophysiology. http://emedicine.medscape.com/article/122122-overview. 2016. Accessed 13 Nov 2016.
16. Eriksson JW, Bodegard J, Nathanson D, Thuresson M, Nyström T, Norhammar A. Sulphonylurea compared to DPP-4 inhibitors in combination with metformin carries increased risk of severe hypoglycemia, cardiovascular events, and all-cause mortality. Diabetes Res Clin Pract. 2016;117:39–47. https://doi.org/10.1016/j.diabres.2016.04.055.
17. Gautier J, Monguillon P, Verier-Mine O, et al. Which oral antidiabetic drug to combine with metformin to minimize the risk of hypoglycemia when initiating basal insulin? Diabetes Res Clin Pract. 2016;116:26–8. https://doi.org/10.1016/j.diabres.2016.04.008.
18. Kirkland L. Adrenal crisis: background, pathophysiology, epidemiology. http://emedicine.medscape.com/article/116716-overview. 2016. Accessed 13 Nov 2016.
19. Bondugulapati LNR, Rees DA. Inhaled corticosteroids and HPA axis suppression: how important is it and how should it be managed? Clin Endocrinol. 2016;85(2):165–9. https://doi.org/10.1111/cen.13073.
20. Liu D, Ahmet A, Ward L, et al. A practical guide to the monitoring and management of the complications of systemic corticosteroid therapy. Allergy Asthma Clin Immunol. 2013;9(1):30. https://doi.org/10.1186/1710-1492-9-30.
21. Raff H, Sharma ST, Nieman LK. Physiological basis for the etiology, diagnosis, and treatment of adrenal disorders: Cushing's syndrome, adrenal insufficiency, and congenital adrenal hyperplasia. Compr Physiol. 2014;4(2):739–69. https://doi.org/10.1002/cphy.c130035.
22. Hopkins RL, Leinung MC. Exogenous Cushing's syndrome and glucocorticoid withdrawal. Endocrinol Metab Clin N Am. 2005;34(2):371–84. https://doi.org/10.1016/j.ecl.2005.01.013.
23. Dunkley E, Isbister G, Sibbritt D, Dawson A, Whyte I. The hunter serotonin toxicity criteria: simple and accurate diagnostic decision rules for serotonin toxicity. QJM. 2003;96(9):635–42. https://doi.org/10.1093/qjmed/hcg109.
24. Greenier E, Lukyanova V, Reede L. Serotonin syndrome: fentanyl and selective serotonin reuptake inhibitor interactions. AANA J. 2014;82(5):340–5.
25. Sansone RA, Sansone LA. Serotonin norepinephrine reuptake inhibitors: a pharmacological comparison. Innov Clin Neurosci. 2014;11(3/4):37–42. http://innovationscns.com/serotonin-norepinephrine-reuptake-inhibitors-a-pharmacological-comparison/. Accessed 13 Nov 2016
26. Taghavi Zenouz A, Ebrahimi H, Mahdipour M, Pourshahidi S, Amini P, Vatankhah M. The incidence of intravascular needle entrance during inferior alveolar nerve block injection. J Dent Res Dent Clin Dent Prospects. 2008;2(1):38–41. https://doi.org/10.5681/joddd.2008.008.

27. Heavner J. Cardiac toxicity of local anesthetics in the intact isolated heart model: a review. Reg Anesth Pain Med. 2002;27(6):545–55. https://doi.org/10.1053/rapm.2002.36458.
28. Ciechanowicz S, Patil V. Lipid emulsion for local anesthetic systemic toxicity. Anesthesiol Res Pract. 2012;2012:131784. https://doi.org/10.1155/2012/131784.
29. Kapitanyan R. Local anesthetic toxicity: practice essentials, background, pathophysiology. http://emedicine.medscape.com/article/1844551-overview. 2016. Accessed 13 Nov 2016.
30. Jauch EC. Ischemic stroke: practice essentials, background, anatomy http://emedicine.medscape.com/article/1916852-overview. 2016. Accessed 13 Nov 2016.
31. Macellari F, Paciaroni M, Agnelli G, Caso V. Perioperative stroke risk in nonvascular surgery. Cerebrovasc Dis. 2012;34(3):175–81. https://doi.org/10.1159/000339982.
32. American Heart Association and American Stroke Association. http://www.strokeassociation.org/STROKEORG/WarningSigns/Stroke-Warning-Signs-and-Symptoms_UCM_308528_SubHomePage.jsp, http://www.strokeassociation.org/STROKEORG/WarningSigns/Learn-More-Stroke-Warning-Signs-and-Symptoms_UCM_451207_Article.jsp#.Wg43k7bMwUF. Accessed 8 Nov 2016.

43 Postoperative Cognitive Dysfunction as a Complication of Maxillofacial Surgery

Jagdev S. Heir

Abstract

It is often discovered beyond 30 days postoperatively; family and co-workers notice a lack of performance in everyday common tasks that the patient was able to do preoperatively. This decrease in cognitive ability is termed postoperative cognitive dysfunction (POCD). This is a diagnosis of exclusion. There is a lack of uniform criteria and guidelines for assessing, diagnosing, and treatment. The current literature is reviewed including animal studies along with the current science and theories of this condition.

43.1 Complication: Postoperative Cognitive Dysfunction

43.1.1 Cause of the Complication

Postoperative cognitive dysfunction (POCD) is a complication resulting from many causes. It involves patient factors such as gender and age, surgical trauma, inflammatory process, hemodynamic changes leading to ischemia, prolonged surgical and anesthetic times, and the natural progression of underlying disease [1].

POCD is defined as a decrease in cognitive performance based on a set of neuropsychological testing from before surgery to after surgery that is more than the expected norm and has been shown in certain patients to last greater than 30 days and in some cases beyond 6 years [2].

There have been numerous reports of traffic accidents on patients undergoing ambulatory surgery and then driving shortly thereafter. Initially it was thought that POCD was caused by general anesthesia (GA) and cardiac bypass; however, research over the years has found no specific direct cause despite animal studies showing a link between inflammation and the development of POCD. POCD has been studied in animal and human models where high-quality animal data shows one set of results, and human studies do not prove the hypothesis set out by the animal studies. Thus, the causes for POCD related to surgery and anesthesia are not completely clear.

POCD should be distinguished from delirium or dementia. Delirium describes an acute confusional state featuring disturbances in attention and decreased awareness of the environment.

J.S. Heir, M.D., D.M.D., F.A.C.S.
Sacramento Surgical Arts, PC, Sacramento, CA, USA
e-mail: drheir@sacramentosurgicalarts.com

© Springer International Publishing AG 2018
E.M. Ferneini, J.D. Bennett (eds.), *Perioperative Assessment of the Maxillofacial Surgery Patient*,
https://doi.org/10.1007/978-3-319-58868-1_43

Delirium symptoms fluctuate during the course of the day, and the patient often is disoriented along with hallucinations and inappropriate communication or behavior [1].

Some other risk factors that may lead to POCD can be increasing age, genetic predisposition, pre-existing cognitive impairment, use of neurotoxic drugs, low cerebral oxygenation leading to neuroinflammation, longer procedures, and hospital stays [3].

Other risk factors for developing POCD include larger and more invasive operations, duration of anesthesia, advanced age, history of alcohol abuse, use of anticholinergic medications, previous cerebral vascular accident, previous POCD, poor cognition, respiratory complications, infectious complications, and multiple surgeries [4].

Use of diazepam premedication nearly doubled the incidence of POCD at 7 days when compared to the general incidence of cognitive dysfunction after noncardiac surgery [5]. Patients kept at lower BIS levels during the majority of surgery performed better in testing for information processing speed compared to patients that were lightly anesthetized showing that the depth of anesthesia will affect cognitive performance [6].

Cardiac surgery and certain orthopedic procedures have a high incidence of POCD and have been attributed to microembolic events during the use of the bypass pump. The microembolic events may cause focal cerebral infarcts that lead to POCD. Fat emboli have also been linked to POCD [4].

43.1.2 Pathophysiology

The pathophysiology of postoperative cognitive dysfunction is poorly understood as are the risk factors that predispose patients to the development of POCD. Some of this is due to the lack of standardization of preoperative and postoperative testing methods along with the timing of administration of these tests [4].

The majority of the research has focused on cardiac surgery with the cardiopulmonary bypass pump being suggested as the major contributor to the POCD as the patient is warmed and taken off of the bypass pump due to the inflammatory process. In a rat model, slow rewarming and prolonged postoperative hypothermia decreased the incidence of POCD [4].

Predisposing factors to POCD include:

- Increasing age
- Lower levels of education
- Alcohol intake
- Patient's preoperative cognitive status
- Genetic predisposition (not well understood) [1]

Since the mechanisms leading to POCD are not fully clear, animal studies have been undertaken which suggest that a contributing factor to POCD is the immune response to surgery.

43.1.2.1 Animal Models

POCD may be caused by either excessive neuroinflammation after surgery, a failure to resolve this inflammation, blood-brain barrier and endothelial dysfunction, or pre-existing Alzheimer's disease pathology which can activate the innate immune system which is increasingly appreciated as an underlying factor in several neurodegenerative conditions.

Neuroinflammation in non-CNS surgery has been associated with behavioral dysfunction and memory deficits. Upregulation of systemic proinflammatory cytokines, including tumor necrosis factor-alpha (TNF-), interleukins (IL) 1 and 6, chemokines, and damage-associated molecular patterns (DAMPs) like high-mobility group box 1 (HMGB1), have been shown to activate bone-marrow-derived macrophages and contribute to the overall brain pathology after aseptic trauma [2].

HMGB1 is a chromatin protein that is secreted by immune cells mediating macrophage cytokine release. Several mechanisms including humoral, cellular, and neuronal pathways have been proposed in this bidirectional communication between the immune system and the brain following surgery. Clinical studies are uncovering potential roles for blood and CSF inflammatory markers involved with POCD; however, it remains unclear how the findings in animal models translate to human patients [2].

Through animal studies, it has been suggested that postoperative memory deficits may be due to anesthetic-induced upregulation of the alpha 5 subunit containing GABA-A receptors in the hippocampus. These receptors inhibit long-term potentiation (LTP) which is a cellular correlate of learning and memory. If these receptors became upregulated, then they would cause learning and memory deficits, which would play a role in contributing to human POCD. If this is blocked by an anti-inflammatory cholinergic signal cascade, then cognitive function remains unimpaired [2].

43.1.2.2 Human Models

Similar to animals, surgery has been associated with a central neuroinflammatory response in humans. Unlike in animal models, there has been no study that links this neuroinflammatory response to POCD. Pre-existing Alzheimer's disease pathology has been associated with increased perioperative decline in some cognitive tests but not in others. Patients with mild cognitive impairment (MCI) have larger cognitive deficits in some tests after perioperative care than surgical patients without MCI. Another cause could be pre-existing white matter damage causing postoperative executive function deficits in patients who underwent knee arthroplasty. Cardiac surgery has been shown to increase the incidents of "silent strokes" seen on magnetic resonance imaging (MRI), and this link has yet to be established as contributing to POCD [2].

Numerous human studies have failed to find plasma biomarkers associated with POCD. In one study, co-peptin which is a peptide co-released with arginine vasopressin from the hypothalamus was associated with increased risk of POCD [2].

Through observation, POCD arises after extensive surgery under general anesthesia as well as when there are postoperative complications. No definitive evidence has been found linking anesthesia or the type of anesthesia (general vs. regional) as a causative agent. In general, the shorter the duration of surgery and anesthesia, the shorter the duration of POCD [2]. Postoperative pain, a change from a familiar environment, and sleep deprivation after surgery are also possible reasons contributing to POCD [4].

43.1.3 Prevalence

The prevalence varies depending enormously due to the lack of formal criteria for the assessment, the standardization of timing for assessment, and the diagnosis of POCD. Further, it is usually not apparent until patients or family members complain about memory loss or difficulties with normal activities once the patient is home or returns to work to assess a diagnosis of POCD is considered [4].

The International Study of Post-Operative Cognitive Dysfunction 1 estimated that POCD incidence is 25.8% at 1 week and 9.9% after 3 months with age being a significant and independent risk factor for POCD. In the nonsurgical control patients, a 3% incidence of POCD was found at every time interval [4, 7].

In patients that had undergone noncardiac surgery, POCD documented occurrence at the time of discharge from the hospital occurred in 36.6% of the patients aged 18–39, 30.4% in patients aged 40–59, and 41.4% in patients over the age of 60. Higher prevalence occurred in patients that underwent cardiac surgery and tended to last longer than 5 years post-surgery [2].

Furthermore, the prevalence of POCD varies greatly depending on the age of the patient, the testing used to establish a diagnosis, the timing of the testing, and inclusion and exclusion criteria of both the group of patients and the control group. POCD can arise at any age but tends to affect everyday life and lasts longer in patients over the age of 60 [2].

43.1.4 Manifestations/Presentation of Disease

Cognitive decline is associated with a loss of independence, a reduction in the quality of life, and ultimately death. A lot of times, due to lack of knowledge and a definitive diagnostic process, POCD does not present itself until after the surgery when the patient's family or co-workers see a decrease in the ability to carry out normal tasks. Most of these patients experience mild problems after surgery such as:

- Inability to write a letter
- Concentrate
- Read a book
- Increased forgetfulness
- Unable to attend to regular life such as meetings, shopping, and traveling

43.2 Patient Assessment

43.2.1 Monitoring

There is no consensus of timing for assessment of cognitive dysfunction postoperatively. Based on information from other studies, POCD can be divided into acute, intermediate, and long-term changes based on information from previous studies. Acute POCD has been used to define cognitive decline detected within 1 week after surgery, intermediate POCD for changes within 3 months, and long-term POCD for changes 1–2 years following surgery [1].

Many studies have used composite measures of cognitive functioning to assess patients for the presence of POCD. The most commonly used composite measure was the Mini-Mental State Examination (MMSE). Unfortunately, composite testing does not differentiate which areas of neuropsychological functioning are affected by the surgical experience [1].

In a study done by Li et al., the development of POCD in patients undergoing laparoscopic pancreaticoduodenectomy is associated with alterations of rSO_2 (regional cerebral oxygen saturation) and A-beta (beta-amyloid protein); thus, monitoring of rSO_2 might be useful in the prediction of POCD, and A-beta might be used as a sensitive biochemical marker to predict the occurrence of POCD [7].

43.2.2 Work-Up

With proper preoperative levels of education and brain function assessment, patients at risk for POCD may be better identified. Cognitive performance testing is the main approach to diagnose POCD in patients after surgery; however, to date, there are no formal criteria to use in diagnosing POCD. This combined with the fact that preoperative testing is rarely done other than for research criteria makes the diagnosis more difficult. Also, there are no ideal tests accepted internationally to diagnose POCD. In order to make up for the lack of criteria and testing, it is advised to use a variety of tests to assess cognitive function [4].

Recent reviews of POCD after cardiac and noncardiac surgery reveal that the two most commonly assessed cognitive domains were:

- Learning and memory
- Attention and concentration

43.2.3 Laboratory Tests and Anticipated Results

The diagnosis of POCD is based on cognitive psychometric testing performed pre- and postoperatively. Mini-Mental State Examination (MMSE) cannot be utilized as there is a marked learning effect and can impair results in POCD. Neuropsychological testing provides the most reliable and sensitive indicator of postoperative cognitive impairment [4].

In general, various aspects of cognitive function should be assessed such as memory, concentration, orientation, mathematical functions, and executive functions. In the older patient or one that is female or the patient that does not have a high level of education, it may be beneficial to perform these tests preoperatively as well as postoperatively to determine the changes [4].

Comprehensive testing can take up to 2–3 h. The testing consists of:

- The Trail Making Test, Part A, where a patient is asked to connect numbers in and ascending order by drawing a line

- The Digit Span Test which measures how many digits are presented in a sequence that the patient can remember
- The Rey Auditory Verbal Learning Test
- The Trail Making Test, Part A and B, where combined tasks are measured
- The Grooved Pegboard Test to test manual dexterity
- The Digit Span Test which also measures the ability to remember a sequence of numbers [8]

Due to patients undergoing surgery and shortage of time preoperatively, shorter tests such as the Erzigkeit's Short Cognitive Performance Test (SKT) have been developed. Multiple other types of testing exist such as a driving simulator; however, there is a lack of uniformity in the various studies toward the type of testing used. Finally, an analysis of anxiety and depression should be performed as they affect cognitive performance [2].

A test that allows measurement of learning ability and memory retrieval is the visual verbal learning test which is a visual version of a test of secondary memory. Two consecutive trials are performed in which the patient has to memorize and reproduce a 15-word list. This test is done such that there is immediate recall at 5 min and then recall at 20 min [9].

Although a variety of test scoring methods for the detection of POCD have been used across studies, researchers generally agree that methods should consider:

- Baseline performance
- Practice effects
- Change on more than one neuropsychological test [1]

Due to POCD not being a formal psychiatric diagnosis, it is a diagnosis of exclusion. Once delirium, dementia, and amnestic disorder are ruled out and neuropsychological testing has been performed a diagnosis of POCD can be rendered.

43.3 Management

43.3.1 Potential Problems

Long-term cognitive decline is controversial, but several studies show that patients who underwent noncardiac surgery reported that acute POCD was associated with increased mortality after surgery. Unfortunately, there are no standards in diagnosing, and thus no standard treatment has been developed for the POCD patient [1].

43.3.2 Patient Management

The treatment for POCD is unclear, and the best treatment is prevention. Preoperative cognitive assessment should be performed, especially in the longer, more severe surgeries as POCD has higher rates of occurrence in this patient subgroup. There has been no study that shows less tissue trauma will cause less POCD due to decreasing the postoperative inflammatory response [2]. Studies with Xenon gas has shown that patients wake up quickly, but in randomized controlled studies, there is no difference in the occurrence of POCD when compared to other gases [10].

There is evidence that as time progresses, the incidence of POCD declines; however, in certain patients it can persist beyond 30 days; thus, it is important to assess the patient prior to 30 days [9].

Very few controlled studies have examined whether any intervention can treat or improve POCD once it has occurred. In one study acetylcholinesterase inhibitor donepezil was administered in patients who displayed cognitive decline 1 year after cardiac surgery. Donepezil improved some aspects of memory performance in these patients, which is consistent with the role of acetylcholinesterase inhibitors in improving memory in patients with early-stage Alzheimer's disease. In one report, selective serotonin reuptake inhibitor (SSRI) citalopram was used to treat POCD successfully [11].

43.4 Prevention

As there is no definitive cure for POCD, prevention is the best cure. Preoperative cognitive training can be used as a prophylactic intervention; the use of propofol instead of anesthetic agents such as sevoflurane, administration of lidocaine, ketamine, and magnesium sulfate helped reduce the incidence of POCD in some studies [12]. Additionally, making certain that the patient's day-night rhythm is physiologic and that the patient maintains social contacts, shorter periods of fasting before surgery and early discharge from hospital might be used to reduce POCD occurrence as well [4, 14].

Intraoperative lidocaine, magnesium, complement cascade suppression, and high-dose dexamethasone have all been shown to not prevent POCD in humans. Ketamine given at induction of anesthesia has been shown to be associated with a decrease in POCD occurrence after cardiac surgery due to a reduction in serum CRP levels. It is unclear as to how exactly ketamine prevents POCD [11].

Providing adequate intraoperative oxygen and maintaining appropriate perfusion of organs and glycemic balance are essential in order to avoid postoperative cerebral dysfunction. Since studies have shown that type of anesthesia, regional anesthesia (RA) versus general anesthesia (GA), found no causative relationship for decreased cognitive function, however, certain drugs such as benzodiazepines should be avoided. There is evidence that inhalational anesthetics may alter cognitive function due to amyloid beta accumulation in animals, but there has been no link of this in humans [9].

Patients and their families should be counseled to perform all cognitively challenging tasks before surgery and to have strong family support network to help with assistance, etc. A potential prevention of POCD was elicited in a study conducted by Chen et al. where they noticed in a retrospective study that IL-6 and TNF-alpha were decreased in patients that received intraoperative dexmedetomidine as a drip during the surgical procedure. This decrease led to lower rate of POCD measured which suggests an anti-inflammatory role of dexmedetomidine and its protective effects on POCD [13, 14].

Conclusion

Postoperative cognitive disorder is a multicausal life affecting diagnosis of exclusion. More clear-cut studies in humans with defined criteria must be undertaken with regard to timing of testing, type and kind of testing implemented, and follow-up care along with what is tested must be determined to achieve clear-cut answers. Without this, POCD will continue to be a diagnosis of exclusion affecting more and more people over time as people are living longer and therefore undergoing more surgical care.

References

1. Tsai TL, et al. An update on postoperative cognitive dysfunction. Adv Anesth. 2010;28(1):269–84.
2. Rundshagen I. Postoperative cognitive dysfunction. Dtsch Arztebl Int. 2014;111(8):119–25.
3. Kline RP, et al. Surgery and brain atrophy in cognitively normal elderly subjects and subjects diagnosed with mild cognitive impairment. Anesthesiology. 2012;116:603–12.
4. Wang W, et al. Postoperative cognitive dysfunction: current developments in mechanism and prevention. Med Sci Monit. 2014;20:1908–12.
5. Rasmussen LS, et al. Benzodiazepines and postoperative dysfunction in the elderly. Br J Anaesth. 1999;83:585–9.
6. Farg E, et al. Is depth of anesthesia, as assessed by the bispectral index, related to postoperative cognitive dysfunction and recovery? Anesth Analg. 2006;103:633–40.
7. Li XM, et al. Relationship between post-operative cognitive dysfunction and regional cerebral oxygen saturation and beta-amyloid protein. J Zhejiang Univ Sci B. 2014;15(10):870–8.
8. Murkin JM, et al. Statement of consensus on assessment of neurobehavioral outcomes after cardiac surgery. Ann Thorac Surg. 1995;59:1289–95.
9. Kotekar N, et al. Post-operative cognitive dysfunction in the elderly: a prospective clinical study. Indian J Anaesth. 2014;58(3):263–8.
10. Hoecker J, et al. Postoperative neurocognitive dysfunction in elderly patients after xenon versus propofol anesthesia for major noncardiac surgery. Anesthesiology. 2009;110:1068–76.
11. Berger M, et al. Postoperative cognitive dysfunction: minding the gaps in our knowledge of a common postoperative complication in the elderly. Anesthesiol Clin. 2015;33(3):517–50.

12. Bilotta F, et al. Pharmacological perioperative brain neuroprotection: a qualitative review of randomized clinical trials. Br J Anaesth. 2013;110:113–20.
13. Chen W, et al. The effects of dexmedetomidine on post-operative cognitive dysfunction and inflammatory factors in senile patients. Int J Clin Exp Med. 2015;8(3):4601–5.
14. Guay J. General anesthesia does not contribute to long-term post-operative cognitive dysfunction in adults: a meta-analysis. Indian J Anaesth. 2011;55(4):358–63.

Check for updates

44 Postoperative Delirium as a Complication of Maxillofacial Surgery

Michael P. Johnson

Abstract

Postoperative delirium (POD) is a temporary state of acute confusion that can occur immediately following surgery to several days postoperatively, frequently having an initial lucid state. POD is the most common postsurgical complication in older adults and if unrecognized can lead to other major postoperative complications, prolonged hospitalization, and possibly death. Various terms have been used to describe POD, such as "sundowning," "ICU psychosis," or "ICU syndrome," but delirium is the medically accepted term. There are many causes of POD, and the pathophysiology is uncertain and likely multifactorial. The best management is prevention through recognition of those patients who are high risk. Treatment consists of both non-pharmacologic and pharmacologic interventions. Prognosis is excellent if recognized early and managed effectively.

44.1 Complication: Postoperative Delirium (POD)

44.1.1 Cause of the Complication

Postoperative delirium (POD) was first described in the late 1950s and early 1960s as a postoperative "psychosis" in cardiac surgery patients [1] with an incidence of approximate 40%. Since then, many studies have confirmed that POD is one of the most common postsurgical complications, particularly in the elderly population and with those with preexisting neurodegenerative or psychiatric disease [2].

Delirium is an acute state of confusion and agitation and tends to have a fluctuating course. Delirium symptoms include impaired cognitive function, disorientation, inattentiveness, memory loss, and/or an inability to plan or organize thoughts. Additionally, delirium may cause a disturbance to the sleep—wake cycle, thought process, perception, and activity levels [3, 4].

Gleason et al. in 2015 [5] demonstrated that the presence of delirium substantially influenced adverse outcomes in a study of 566 older patients (mean age, 76) undergoing a variety of elective

M.P. Johnson, D.M.D., F.A.C.S.
Oral and Maxillofacial Surgery, Yale New Haven Hospital, Yale University, New Haven, CT, USA
e-mail: Michael.Johnson@YNHH.ORG

© Springer International Publishing AG 2018

E.M. Ferneini, J.D. Bennett (eds.), *Perioperative Assessment of the Maxillofacial Surgery Patient*,
https://doi.org/10.1007/978-3-319-58868-1_44

surgical procedures. 23.9% of the patients developed postoperative delirium (POD), and this was associated with increased risk for prolonged hospital length of stay, increased discharge to a facility other than home, and increased 30-day readmission. Additionally, Gleason et al. showed that POD increased the potential for undesirable postsurgical outcomes such as return to the operating room, wound infection, myocardial events, and sepsis.

Postoperative delirium (POD) should be viewed as a *postoperative complication* and an *emergent medical condition*.

The following is becoming standard for those patients identified as high risk for POD:

- Surgeon and nursing staff screening, both preoperative and postoperative
- Preventative interventions
- Thorough and systematic medical workup upon first signs of POD symptoms
- Swift management to avoid increased morbidity, prolonged hospital length of stay, and delayed recovery

44.1.1.1 "Sundowning," "ICU Psychosis," or "ICU Syndrome"

Various terms have been used to describe the clinical manifestations of postoperative delirium (POD) in the postsurgical period, such as "sundowning," "ICU psychosis," or "ICU syndrome." These are not considered acceptable terms to describe patients who develop acute postoperative onset confusion, agitation, or restlessness. "Delirium" is the accepted term by the American Psychiatric Association and experts in critical care medicine [6].

Postoperative delirium (POD) increases morbidity and delays recovery and discharge. POD has been shown to increase mortality rates in cardiac, orthopedic, and head and neck oncologic surgery. Early diagnosis and management are critical [7].

44.1.1.2 Causes

Various mnemonics have been used to determine the causes of postoperative delirium, but one of the more popular mnemonics used to systematically approach a determination of cause is:

I WATCH DEATH [8]

- Infections (encephalitis, meningitis, UTI, pneumonia)
- Withdrawal (alcohol, barbiturates, benzodiazepines)
- Acute metabolic disorder (electrolyte imbalance, hepatic or renal failure)
- Trauma (head injury, postoperative)
- CNS pathology (stroke, hemorrhage, tumor, seizure disorder, Parkinson's)
- Hypoxia (anemia, cardiac failure, pulmonary embolus)
- Deficiencies (vitamin B12, folic acid, thiamine)
- Endocrinopathies (thyroid, glucose, parathyroid, adrenal)
- Acute vascular (shock, vasculitis, hypertensive encephalopathy)
- Toxins, substance use, and medication (alcohol, anesthetics, anticholinergics, narcotics)
- Heavy metals (arsenic, lead, mercury)

44.1.2 Pathophysiology

The pathophysiology of postoperative delirium (POD) is multifactorial and complex. The multifactorial theories include:

- Cholinergic deficiency
- Dopamine excess
- Serotonin fluctuation
- Inflammation-induced ACH neurotransmission impairment

44.1.2.1 Cholinergic Deficiency

The cholinergic deficiency hypothesis originated from observations that delirium occurred with consumption of toxins and drugs that impair cholinergic function [9].

Acetylcholine plays a major role in attention and consciousness by acting as a modulator of signal-to-noise ratio in sensory and cognitive input. If there are irregularities in these brain functions, symptoms of delirium may precipitate [10].

Acetylcholine deficiency therefore appears to play a central role in the development of delirium. Additionally, an increase in age correlates with a decrease in ACH neurotransmission—reduced "cholinergic reserve," which would explain a higher incidence of POD in the geriatric population.

44.1.2.2 Dopamine Excess

The stress of surgery increases dopamine production. An increase in the production of toxic metabolites of dopamine has been associated with delirium, especially hallucinations and delusions. Dopamine increase may cause symptoms of the hyperactive type of delirium [11].

44.1.2.3 Serotonin Fluctuations

Serotonin is a major excitatory neurotransmitter in the brain and may fluctuate based on the production of its precursor, tryptophan. Some studies have shown a decrease in tryptophan production in postoperative patients [12].

44.1.2.4 Inflammation-Induced Acetylcholine Neurotransmission Impairment

Postsurgical perivascular edema may increase the diffusion time for oxygen to reach the nerve cells, decreasing metabolism of neurons. Metabolism of neurons cannot keep up with the requirements of their synthetic functions. Additionally, acetylcholine (ACH) synthesis and release are sensitive to hypoxia. Since ACH plays a major role in regulation of many brain functions, the lack of ACH (and excess of dopaminergic transmission) has been connected with the development of hallucinations and delusions [13]. This explains why many drugs with anticholinergic effect are known to cause memory and concentration impairment, whereas cholinomimetics can compensate for this.

44.1.2.5 Initial Lucid Period

Patients many times do not develop postoperative delirium (POD) immediately following surgery. Some patients will exhibit POD on subsequent postoperative days, having an initial "lucid period" where there are no symptoms. This delay in onset of symptoms may be explained by peak inflammation occurring 1–2 days postoperatively, increasing extravascular edema, increasing leukocyte adhesion, and decreasing perfusion of certain brain areas. This may explain why patients with stenosis of cerebral arteries and atherosclerotic arterial changes are prone to POD [13].

44.1.3 Prevalence

44.1.3.1 POD in the General Population

The incidence of postoperative delirium (POD) varies. In general, lengthy procedures common to the elderly will have a higher incidence of POD.

General surgery, orthopedic surgery, and heart surgery incidence have been reported between a range of 11 and 42%, with age over 70 being a predictor (Young). In an ICU setting, the incidence increases to 20–80% [14, 15]. POD has the potential to affect up to 50% of all elderly patients in the postoperative period. As such, POD is one of the most common postsurgical complications [15–17].

44.1.3.2 Risk Factors

Postoperative delirium (POD) is one of the most common postoperative complications and can increase postoperative morbidity and mortality. POD increases with advanced age (greater than 70 years) and prolonged length of the operation and presence of neurodegenerative disease [18]. Additionally, frailty, dementia, functional dependence, malnutrition, and medication and alcohol abuse are risk factors for POD [19].

Postoperative delirium (POD) incidence increases with those with preexisting dementia, decreased cognitive ability, polypharmacy, decreased ability to metabolize drugs, and visual and hearing impairment. Additionally, there is a higher incidence of POD seen in elderly with COPD, CAD, and cerebrovascular disease. POD increased in patients with depression, psychiatric illness, and underlying brain disease.

The presence of multiple medical comorbidities increases POD, in particular those who take multiple medications. High-risk medications include anticholinergics, tricyclic antidepressants (TCA), antihistamines, opioids, benzodiazepines, antiparkinsonians, and h2 blockers.

44.1.3.3 Oral and Maxillofacial Surgery

The overall incidence of postoperative delirium (POD) in oral and maxillofacial surgery has not been reported. With the exception of two case reports of POD in patients following orthognathic surgery [20–22] and a few retrospective reviews of POD in head and neck cancer surgery, there is little discussion of POD in the oral and maxillofacial surgery and head and neck literature.

44.1.4 Manifestations/Presentation of Disease

44.1.4.1 Clinical Presentation

There are three clinical subtypes of delirium:

1. Hyperactive (hyperaroused, hyperalert, or agitated)
2. Hypoactive (hypoaroused, hypoalert, or lethargic)
3. Mixed (alternating features of hyperactive and hypoactive types)

The hyperactive type of delirium represents about 25 percent of cases and is known as the "classic" presentation of delirium; patients who exhibit the classic form of delirium are generally wildly agitated, confused, uncooperative, and agitated.

The hypoactive type, also known as the "quiet" form of delirium, represents over half of all POD patients. The quiet form of delirium is more common in older patients than the other forms of delirium but can be frequently missed since these patients are easier to manage due to the drowsiness and quiet presentation.

The mixed type has alternating features of both and is managed according to the clinical symptoms.

The onset of postoperative delirium (POD) may be acute with a fluctuating course. Onset can be within hours of surgery or several days after surgery. POD may be diurnal, typically at night, referred to frequently as "sundowning."

The core features of delirium are as follows [11]:

- Disturbance of consciousness (reduced clarity and awareness of the environment) with reduced ability to focus, sustain, or shift attention
- Change in cognition (e.g., disorientation, memory impairment, reduced problem-solving capability, and language disturbance) or perceptual disturbance
- Onset of hours to days with fluctuation during the course of day
- Disturbance directly linked to physiological consequences of a general medical condition with evidence from the history, physical examination, or laboratory findings

Clinical features of delirium include [23]:

- Change in level of arousal:
  - Drowsiness or decreased arousal or increased arousal with hypervigilance
- Delayed awakening from anesthesia
- Abrupt change in cognitive function:
  - Worsening confusion over hours or days, including problems with attention, difficulty concentrating, new memory problems, and new disorientation
- Difficulty tracking conversations and following instructions
- Thinking and speech that is more disorganized, difficult to follow, slow, or rapid
- Quick-changing emotions:
  - Easy irritability, tearfulness, and uncharacteristic refusals to engage with postoperative care
- Expression of new paranoid thoughts or delusions (i.e., fixed false beliefs)
- New perceptual disturbances (e.g., illusions, hallucinations)
- Motor changes:
  - Slowed or decreased movements, purposeless fidgeting or restlessness, new difficulties in maintaining posture such as sitting or standing
- Sleep/wake cycle changes such as sleeping during the day and/or awake and active at night

- Decreased appetite
- New incontinence of urine or stool
- Fluctuating symptoms and/or level of arousal over the course of minutes to hours

44.2 Patient Assessment

44.2.1 Monitoring

Understanding the risk factors for delirium is critical in effectively monitoring for postoperative delirium.

Oral and maxillofacial surgeons should consider routinely performing a preoperative assessment of delirium risk factors when planning major surgery in patients with multiple risk factors.

These risk factors include [23]:

- Age greater than 65 years
- Chronic cognitive decline
- Dementia
- Poor vision
- Poor hearing
- Severe illness
- Presence of infection
- Polypharmacy
- Major surgery

A thorough presurgical assessment of geriatric patients is important in monitoring for POD in the postoperative period.

Patients identified as high risk should be considered for daily postoperative screening in order to initiate delirium treatment as early as possible.

Dworkin's prospective cohort study of older adults undergoing elective surgery identified a short and simple screening tool called the "Mini-Cog" as a means to stratify those patients at highest risk for POD. The "Mini-Cog" is a screening tool with a high sensitivity and specificity for cognitive impairment in those not diagnosed with dementia; low scores may identify an undiagnosed early dementia. Dementia being one of the highest risk factors for developing POD, the mini-cog served as a simple tool with adequate predictive power to identify risk for POD [24].

Several screening tools are available for use in the postoperative period, including:

- Confusion Assessment Method (CAM)
- Confusion Assessment Method for the Intensive Care Unit (CAM-ICU)
- Nursing Delirium Screening Scale (Nu-DESC)
- Delirium Detection Scale (DDS)
- Delirium Symptom Interview (DSI)

44.2.2 Workup

The American Geriatric Society Expert Panel on Postoperative Delirium [23] in Older Adults made the following recommendation with regard to diagnosis and workup of postoperative delirium (POD):

- Health-care professionals caring for postsurgical patients should be trained to recognize and document signs and symptoms of POD.
  - Understand both hyperactive and hypoactive forms: the hypoactive form can be easily missed and thus more dangerous.
- Health-care professionals should assess preoperative cognitive function in older adults undergoing major surgery.
  - Cognitive impair increases the risk for POD and thus necessitating the need to monitor for POD.
- Health-care professionals competent in diagnosing POD should perform a full clinical assessment in those suspected of having symptoms of POD.

44.2.2.1 Screening Tools

In an observation study, Radtke et al. [25] compared the Confusion Assessment Method (CAM), Nursing Delirium Screening Scale (Nu-DESC), and the Delirium Detection Scale (DDS) to screen for delirium. They found the Nu-DESC was the most sensitive and CAM the next most sensitive and the most specific, with 0.99 specificity. The DDS had lowest sensitivity with a high specificity [25].

44.2.2.2 Neelon and Champagne (NEECHAM) Confusion Scale

The NEECHAM was designed to assess acute confusion on the basis of criteria identified by nurses as representing acute confusion [26].

Subscale I level of responsiveness-information processing
• Attention and alertness (0–4 points)
• Verbal and motor response (0–5 points)
• Memory and orientation (0–5 points)
Subscale II level of behavior
• General behavior and posture (0–2 points)
• Sensory motor performance (0–4 points)
• Verbal responses (0–4 points)
Subscale III vital functions
• Vital signs (0–2 points)
• Oxygen saturation level (0–2 points)
• Urinary continence (0–2 points)
Scores: 0–19 points = moderate to severe confusion
20–24 points = mild or early development of delirium
25–30 points = not confused or normal function

44.2.2.3 Confusion Assessment Method (CAM)

The CAM is a standardized evidence-based tool that enables nonpsychiatrically trained clinicians to identify and recognize delirium quickly and accurately in both clinical and research settings [27]. The CAM includes four features found to have the greatest ability to distinguish delirium from other types of cognitive impairment. There is also a CAM-ICU version for use with nonverbal mechanically ventilated patients.

44.2.2.4 The Confusion Assessment Method (CAM) Diagnostic Algorithm

Feature 1: *Acute Onset or Fluctuating Course* This feature is usually obtained from a family member or nurse and is shown by positive responses to the following questions: Is there evidence of an acute change in mental status from the patient's baseline? Did the (abnormal) behavior fluctuate during the day, that is, tend to come and go, or increase and decrease in severity?

Feature 2: *Inattention* This feature is shown by a positive response to the following question: Did the patient have difficulty focusing attention, for example, being easily distractible, or having difficulty keeping track of what was being said?

Feature 3: *Disorganized thinking* This feature is shown by a positive response to the following question: Was the patient's thinking disorganized or incoherent, such as rambling or irrelevant conversation, unclear or illogical flow of ideas, or unpredictable switching from subject to subject?

Feature 4: *Altered Level of consciousness* This feature is shown by any answer other than "alert" to the following question: Overall, how would you rate this patient's level of consciousness (alert [normal], vigilant [hyperalert], lethargic [drowsy, easily aroused], stupor [difficult to arouse], or coma [unarousable])?

The *diagnosis of delirium* by CAM requires the presence of features 1 and 2 and either 3 or 4.

44.2.2.5 Confusion Assessment Method for the Intensive Care Unit (CAM-ICU)

The CAM-ICU is a validated assessment tool used to check for fluctuations in mental status, inattention, altered level of consciousness, and disorganized thinking [28]. This method evaluates the level of consciousness using the Richmond Agitation Sedation Score (RASS), which quantifies level of consciousness on a 10-point scale ranging from unarousable to combative [29].

44.2.2.6 Nursing Delirium Screening Scale (Nu-DESC)

The Nu-DESC is a fast screening (it takes about 1 min) used to evaluate delirium based on observation of the following five features, as defined by the instrument:

(i) Disorientation, (ii) inappropriate behavior, (iii) inappropriate communication, (iv) illusions/hallucinations, and (v) psychomotor retardation.

Each item is scored based on its severity (0 = absence, 1 = mild, and 2 = severe).

The cutoff for delirium is reported to be 2. It takes 1 min to complete the instrument. Nu-DESC has been shown to have a sensitivity of 85.7% and specificity of 86.8% [30–32].

44.3 Management

Management of postoperative delirium should be viewed as two phases:

1. Prevention with the use of prophylactic interventions
2. Accurate diagnosis of postoperative delirium and treatment once it has occurred

44.3.1 Prevention

There are non-pharmacologic and pharmacologic preventative interventions used for patients at risk for postoperative delirium.

Non-pharmacologic interventions include the use of multicomponent intervention strategies such as the use of a "Hospital Elder Life Program (HELP)" [33, 34] and "Proactive Geriatric Consultation" [18] or implementing a "Specialized Geriatric Ward" [14].

Pharmacologic intervention to prevent POD includes avoiding the use of narcotic pain control postoperatively, avoiding the prophylactic use of antipsychotic medications in older patients, and avoiding the use of cholinesterase inhibitors and anticholinergic medications.

44.3.1.1 Non-pharmacologic Interventions to Prevent POD

Non-pharmacologic interventions are important supportive elements of preventative intervention that may not be adequately utilized in the everyday management of elderly postoperative patients [35]. Nursing staff and the patient's environment are critical in preventing POD. For example, aids to orientation, protecting patients from stimuli, avoiding environmental changes, minimizing staff changes, and ensuring that a patient has adequate sensory aids can prevent delirium in hospitalized patients [35]. Aids to orientation include a clock, a calendar, or a familiar photo. Protecting patients from stimuli includes not changing the patient's room and having minimal staff changes. Sensory aids for the patient such as glasses or hearing aids should be used as well. Adequate lighting is important, so that a proper sleep-wake cycle is ensured [36]. In addition, personal attention and the involvement of friends or relatives have a positive effect [35].

Hospital Elder Life Program (HELP)

The Hospital Elder Life Program (HELP) was developed by Dr. Sharon K. Inouye [33, 34] and her colleagues at the Yale University School of Medicine for the prevention, diagnosis, and treatment of delirium in general hospitals. HELP is an innovative approach to improving the hospital care of older patients by maintaining cognitive and physical functioning of high-risk older adults throughout hospitalization, maximizing independence at discharge, assisting with the transition from hospital to home, and preventing unplanned hospital readmissions.

HELP uses a multicomponent strategy through the following interventions:

- Patients are activated and supported by trained volunteers.
- Relatives are involved.
- Patients are regularly screened for delirium.
- Specialist nurses advise ward staff and relatives.
- In-hospital training is provided for nursing and medical staff.

Implementation of the HELP has been shown to significantly reduce the development of delirium and functional decline in older patients [33, 34].

Proactive Geriatric Consultation Services

Proactive geriatric consultation model services involve a geriatrician making daily visits for the duration of the hospitalization and making targeted recommendations based on a structured protocol. Many hospitals have these services available. Orthopedic and trauma studies have shown that the use of proactive geriatrics consultations services can be successfully implemented after major surgery in high-risk patients. Compared to "usual care," geriatric consultation reduces delirium by over one-third and reduced severe delirium by over one-half [18].

Specialized Geriatric Wards or Units

Lundstrom et al. showed in 2007 [14] that postoperative delirium can be reduced and outcomes improved in elderly orthopedic trauma patients by using specialize geriatric wards or units. Additionally Chong et al. and Flaherty et al. [37–39] both described models of delirium care, where the important concepts of delirium prevention and management are integrated into geriatric specific units or wards. These concepts of consolidating specialized elderly care to units or wards have shown to improve delirium prevention and treatment outcomes.

44.3.1.2 Pharmacologic Interventions to Prevent POD

Several pharmacologic approaches to preventing postoperative delirium have been studied. These include the prophylactic perioperative use of:

- Antipsychotic medications
  - Haloperidol
  - Olanzapine
- Cholinesterase inhibitor medications
  - Rivastigmine
  - Donepezil

The antipsychotic medications commonly used to treat postoperative delirium (POD) can be used to prevent POD. These include haloperidol and olanzapine. Both have mixed results in showing reduced incidence of POD, but studies show that antipsychotics administered prophylactically during the perioperative period can reduce the severity and duration of POD when it occurred [40–43].

Cholinesterase inhibitors have been studied to prevent POD. This is based on the hypothesis that anticholinergic excess may be involved in the pathogenesis of delirium. Most studies have concluded that the use of these medications is not effective in preventing POD [44, 45].

44.3.2 Treatment

Postoperative delirium is considered a medical emergency and requires immediate attention.

Once postoperative delirium is confirmed, the treatment is based on the identification of the underlying disorder since delirium can be multifactorial.

A thorough history and physical exam should be performed, including:

- Review of current medications and adjust as needed
- Alcohol or drug withdrawal evaluation
- Vital signs monitoring
- Pulse oximetry monitor for hypoxia
- Consider arterial blood gas ABG
- EKG to rule out dysrhythmia
- Review of fluid status, to ensure adequate hydration
- Evaluation of the surgical site for infection, to monitor for surgical site infection
- Thorough neurological exam
- Sepsis workup if indicated
- Labs: CBC, electrolyte panel, urinalysis to rule out infection/sepsis, electrolyte imbalance, and/or UTI

If there is no identifiable cause, treatment is supportive through non-pharmacologic approaches:

- Adjust medications if determined to be a possible cause.
- Frequent reorientation and reassurance, both verbal and visual.
- Ask family and/or friends to stay with the patient.
- Keep hearing aids, eyeglasses, dentures, and other aids with the patient to help them stay oriented and alert to his or her surroundings.
- Make the hospital room more familiar by asking family to post some photos.
- Encourage physical activity, games, and conversation.

If the delirious patient fails to respond favorably to non-pharmacologic approaches or becomes agitated or threatening harm to self or others, pharmacologic approaches may be indicated to prevent injury to self or others and to allow further evaluation and treatment.

Neuroleptics, such as haloperidol, risperidone, and olanzapine, are the first line for non-withdrawal-related postoperative delirium. If alcohol or benzodiazepine withdrawal is suspected, benzodiazepines should be considered.

Haloperidol is considered the drug of choice, despite the lack of evidence that it is the better agent. Neuroleptics are preferred because they have fewer sedative, anticholinergic, hemodynamic, and respiratory side effects.

References

1. Kornfeld DS, Zimberg S, Malm JR. Psychiatric complications of open-heart surgery. N Engl J Med. 1965;273(6):287–92.
2. Shim JJ, Leung JM. An update on delirium in the postoperative setting: prevention, diagnosis and management. Best Pract Res Clin Anaesthesiol. 2012;26(3):327–43.
3. Robinson TN, Eiseman B. Postoperative delirium in the elderly: diagnosis and management. Clin Interv Aging. 2008;3(2):351–5.
4. Kawaguchi Y, Kanamori M, Ishihara H, Abe Y, Nobukiyo M, Sigeta T, Hori T, Kimura T. Postoperative delirium in spine surgery. Spine J. 2006;6(2):164–9.
5. Gleason LJ, Schmitt EM, Kosar CM, Tabloski P, Saczynski JS, Robinson T, Cooper Z, Rogers SO, Jones RN, Marcantonio ER, Inouye SK. Effect of delirium and other major complications on outcomes after elective surgery in older adults. JAMA Surg. 2015;150(12):1134–40.
6. Montes DM. Postoperative delirium in head and neck cancer patients: a survey of oncologic oral and maxillofacial surgeon practices. J Oral Maxillofac Surg. 2014;72(12):2591–600.
7. Yudofsky SC, Hales RE, editors. The American psychiatric press textbook of neuropsychiatry. 2nd ed. Washington, DC: American Psychiatric Publishing; 1992.
8. Smith DA, Seirafi J. Delirium and dementia. In: Textbook of family medicine. 8th ed. Saunders Elsevier: Philadelphia, PA; 2011.
9. Tune LE, Damlouji NF, Holland A, Gardner TJ, Folstein MF, Coyle JT. Association of postoperative delirium with raised serum levels of anticholinergic drugs. Lancet. 1981;2(8248):651–3.
10. Hshieh TT, Fong TG, Marcantonio ER, Inouye SK. Cholinergic deficiency hypothesis in delirium: a synthesis of current evidence. J Gerontol A Biol Sci Med Sci. 2008;63(7):764–72.
11. Ali S, Patel M, Jabeen S, Bailey RK, Patel T, Shahid M, Riley WJ, Arain A. Insight into delirium. Innov Clin Neurosci. 2011;8(10):25–34.
12. Robinson TN, Raeburn CD, Angles EM, Moss M. Low tryptophan levels are associated with post-operative delirium in the elderly. Am J Surg. 2008;196(5):670–4. https://doi.org/10.1016/j.amjsurg.2008.07.007.
13. Hála M. Pathophysiology of postoperative delirium: systemic inflammation as a response to surgical trauma causes diffuse microcirculatory impairment. Med Hypotheses. 2007;68(1):194–6.
14. Lundström M, et al. Postoperative delirium in old patients with femoral neck fracture: a randomized intervention study. Aging Clin Exp Res. 2007;19(3):178–86.
15. Ansaloni L, Catena F, Chattat R, et al. Risk factors and incidence of postoperative delirium in elderly patients after elective and emergency surgery. Br J Surg. 2010;97(2):273–80.
16. Young J, Inouye SK. Delirium in older people. BMJ. 2007;334:842–6.
17. Siddiqi N, House AO, Holmes JD. Occurrence and outcome of delirium in medical in-patients; a systematic literature review. Age Ageing. 2006;35:350–64.
18. Marcantonio ER, Flacker JM, Wright RJ, Resnick NM. Reducing delirium after hip fracture: a randomized trial. J Am Geriatr Soc. 2001;49(5):516–22.
19. Zenilman ME. Delirium: an important postoperative complication. JAMA. 2017;317(1):77–8.
20. Kunimatsu T, Misaki T, Hirose N, et al. Postoperative mental disorder following prolonged oral surgery. J Oral Sci. 2004;46:71.
21. da Costa FH, et al. Postoperative delirium following orthognathic surgery in a young patient. J Oral Maxillofac Surg. 2017;75(2):284.e1–4.
22. Galen DM, Beck M, Buchbinder D. Steroid psychosis after orthognathic surgery: a case report. J Oral Maxillofac Surg. 1997;55(3):294–7.
23. Panel, The American Geriatrics Society Expert. Postoperative delirium in older adults: best practice statement from the American Geriatrics Society. J Am Coll Surg. 2015;220(2):136–48.
24. Dworkin A, et al. A simple tool to predict development of delirium after elective surgery. J Am Geriatr Soc. 2016;64:11.
25. Radtke FM, et al. Comparison of three scores to screen for delirium in the recovery room. Br J Anaesth. 2008;101(3):338–43.
26. Neelon VJ, et al. The NEECHAM Confusion Scale: construction, validation, and clinical testing. Nurs Res. 1996;45(6):324–30.
27. Inouye S, van Dyck C, Alessi C, Balkin S, Siegal A, Horwitz R. Clarifying confusion: the confusion assessment method. Ann Intern Med. 1990;113(12):941–8.
28. Ely EW, Inouye SK, Bernard GR, Gordon S, Francis J, May L, Truman B, Speroff T, Gautam S, Margolin R, Hart RP, Dittus R. Delirium in mechanically ventilated patients: validity and reliability of the confusion assessment method for the intensive care unit (CAM-ICU). JAMA. 2001;286(21):2703–10. Table 1, p. 2705
29. Sessler CN, Gosnell MS, Grap MJ, Brophy GM, O'Neal PV, Keane KA, Tesoro EP, Elswick RK. The Richmond Agitation-Sedation Scale: validity and reliability in adult intensive care unit patients. Am J Respir Crit Care Med. 2002;166(10):1338–44.

30. Gaudreau JD, Gagnon P, Harel F, Tremblay A, Roy MA. J Pain Symptom Manag. 2005;29(4):368–75.
31. Neufeld KJ, Leoutsakos JS, Sieber FE, Joshi D, Wanamaker BL, Rios-Robles J, Needham DM. Evaluation of two delirium screening tools for detecting post-operative delirium in the elderly. Br J Anaesth. 2013;111(4):612–8.
32. Grover S, Kate N. Assessment scales for delirium: a review. World J Psychiatr. 2012;2(4):58–70. https://doi.org/10.5498/wjp.v2.i4.58.
33. Inouye SK, Bogardus ST, Charpentier PA, Leo-Summers L, Denise A, Holford TR, Cooney LM. A multicomponent intervention to prevent delirium in hospitalized older patients. N Engl J Med. 1999;340:669–76.
34. Inouye SK, Bogardus ST Jr, Baker DI, Leo-Summers L, Cooney LM Jr. The Hospital Elder Life Program: a model of care to prevent cognitive and functional decline in older hospitalized patients. Hospital Elder Life Program. J Am Geriatr Soc. 2000;48:1697–706.
35. Kratz T, Heinrich M, Schlauß E, Diefenbacher A. Preventing postoperative delirium: a prospective intervention with psychogeriatric liaison on surgical wards in a general hospital. Dtsch Arztebl Int. 2015;112(17):289–96. https://doi.org/10.3238/arztebl.2015.0289.
36. Zaubler TS, Murphy K, Rizzuto L, et al. Quality improvement and cost savings with multicomponent delirium interventions: replication of the hospital elder life program in a community hospital. Psychosomatics. 2013;54:219–26.
37. Chong MS, Chan MP, Kang J, Han HC, Ding YY, Tan TL. A new model of delirium care in the acute geriatric setting: geriatric monitoring unit. BMC Geriatr. 2011;11:41. https://doi.org/10.1186/1471-2318-11-41.
38. Chong MS, Chan M, Tay L, Ding YY. Outcomes of an innovative model of acute delirium care: the geriatric monitoring unit (GMU). Clin Interv Aging. 2014;9:603–12.
39. Flaherty JH, Tariq SH, Raghavan S, Bakshi S, Moinuddin A, Morley JE. A model for managing delirious older inpatients. J Am Geriatr Soc. 2003;51:1031–5.
40. Kalisvaart KJ, de Jonghe JF, Bogaards MJ, Vreeswijk R, Egberts TC, Burger BJ, Eikelenboom P, van Gool WA. Haloperidol prophylaxis for elderly hip-surgery patients at risk for delirium: a randomized placebo-controlled study. J Am Geriatr Soc. 2005;53(10):1658–66.
41. Vochteloo AJ, Moerman S, van der Burg BLB, de Boo M, de Vries MR, Niesten DD, Pilot P. Delirium risk screening and haloperidol prophylaxis program in hip fracture patients is a helpful tool in identifying high-risk patients, but does not reduce the incidence of delirium. BMC Geriatr. 2011;11(1):39.
42. Wang W, Li HL, Wang DX, Zhu X, Li SL, Yao GQ, Zhu SN. Haloperidol prophylaxis decreases delirium incidence in elderly patients after noncardiac surgery: a randomized controlled trial. Crit Care Med. 2012;40(3):731–9.
43. Larsen KA, Kelly SE, Stern TA, Bode RH, Price LL, Hunter DJ, Cotter JJ. Administration of olanzapine to prevent postoperative delirium in elderly joint-replacement patients: a randomized, controlled trial. Psychosomatics. 2010;51(5):409–18.
44. Overshott, R., Karim, S., & Burns, A. (2008). Cholinesterase inhibitors for delirium. Cochrane Database Syst Rev;(1):CD005317.
45. Demeure MJ, Fain MJ. The elderly surgical patient and postoperative delirium. J Am Coll Surg. 2006;203(5):752–7.

Fever as a Complication of Maxillofacial Surgery

45

H. Alexander Crisp and Martin B. Steed

Abstract

Fever is the presence of an elevated body temperature above normal and a manifestation of cytokine release in response to a variety of conditions. There is some evidence that IL-6 is the cytokine most closely correlated with postoperative fever. The emergence of fever, defined as a temperature greater than 38 °C (100.4 °F), within the perioperative course, presents a diagnostic and management challenge for the oral and maxillofacial surgeon. Symptoms of fever include sweating, shivering, headache, muscle aches, loss of appetite, dehydration, and generalized weakness. In severe instances, the symptoms may include hallucinations, confusion, irritability, convulsions, or severe dehydration. The body is normally able to maintain a fairly steady temperature via a balancing act between excess heat production and heat dissipation from the skin and lungs (Porat, http://www.uptodate.com, 2016; Weed, http://www.uptodate.com, 2016; Lee-Chiong and Stitt, Compr Ther 21:697, 1995). Throughout this chapter, we will explore the causes of fever development, the importance of identifying time of onset, the significance of fever, and its management in the perioperative oral and maxillofacial surgery patient.

45.1 Complication: Postoperative Fever

45.1.1 Cause of the Complication

As our conversation is going to center around the regulation of body temperature, or rather the deviation from its norm in the postoperative setting, it is only appropriate that we begin at the body's thermoregulatory center – the anterior hypothalamus. The anterior hypothalamus is able

H.A. Crisp, D.M.D. • M.B. Steed, D.D.S., F.A.C.S. (✉)
Department of Oral and Maxillofacial Surgery, Medical University of South Carolina College of Dental Medicine, Charleston, SC, USA
e-mail: steedma@musc.edu

© Springer International Publishing AG 2018

E.M. Ferneini, J.D. Bennett (eds.), *Perioperative Assessment of the Maxillofacial Surgery Patient*,
https://doi.org/10.1007/978-3-319-58868-1_45

Table 45.1 Causes of postoperative fever

Noninfectious	Infectious
Atelectasis	Abscess
Dehydration	Sinusitis
Drug fever	Clostridium difficile colitis
Thrombophlebitis	Bloodstream infections
Tissue trauma	Surgical site infections (SSI's)
Alcohol withdrawal	Intravascular device infections
Transfusion reaction	Parotitis
Adrenal insufficiency	Pneumonia
Factitious	Urinary tract infections
Malignant hyperthermia	Cholecystitis
Myocardial infarction	Endocarditis
Pancreatitis	Prostatitis
Pulmonary embolism	
Thyrotoxicosis	
Pheochromocytoma	
Pericarditis	

to maintain core temperature at a steady state despite excess heat production and heat dissipation. Normal daily body temperature fluctuates between 97 °F (36.1 °C) and 100 °F (37.8 °C), with the average body temperature being 98.6 °F (37 °C). Though the anterior hypothalamus is the thermoregulatory center, it is not the true source of fever development. In the febrile postoperative patient, the body's temperature has deviated from its norm because of an inciting stimulus. The etiology of postoperative fever can be multifaceted, and there are numerous patient-specific factors to consider [1–6]. A thorough differential diagnosis of postoperative fever includes noninfectious and infectious conditions that can occur following oral and maxillofacial surgery (Table 45.1).

45.1.2 Pathophysiology

Since the hypothalamus is the body's thermoregulatory center of temperature, it makes sense that the development of fever would also begin in this area. In response to infection, illness, or stress (e.g., in the postsurgical setting), and in conjunction with the initiation of the immune response, the hypothalamic thermoregulatory center takes an upward shift from normothermia. Elevated levels of prostaglandin E2 (PGE2) appear to be the trigger for the upward deviation from baseline in the anterior hypothalamus. Once the hypothalamic setting has risen, neurons in the vasomotor center are activated to commence vasoconstriction and warm-sensing neurons to slow their firing rate, thus increasing heat production in the periphery. Vasoconstriction leads to blood shunting away from the periphery, toward the internal organs, thus decreasing heat loss from the skin. This physiological response produces a noticeable cold sensation in the hands and feet, and this also leads to the patient reporting a sense of feeling cold [1–6].

45.1.3 Prevalence

Data regarding the prevalence of postoperative fever following oral and maxillofacial surgical procedures is difficult to ascertain. This is in part due to the fact that the topic has not been well studied. Numerous publications address the potential sources of postoperative fever and management strategies in the surgical patient. However, few literature sources define commonality, or lack thereof, when it comes to postoperative fever following oral and maxillofacial surgery.

45.1.4 Manifestations/Presentation of Disease

In an adult patient, fever is considered to be low-grade when the oral temperature is between 37.5 °C and 38 °C (99.5 °F and 100.4 °F). Furthermore, fever is considered to be high-grade when the oral temperature is above 38 °C (100.4 °F) or when the rectal or ear temperatures are above 38.3 °C (101 °F). In pediatric patients, a rectal temperature of at least 38 °C (100.4 °F) is considered a fever. Fever up to 38 °C is common in the first few days after major surgery, as early postoperative fever can commonly be a result of the inflammatory stimulus of surgery itself [2, 6–8]. More often than not, this low-grade fever resolves spontaneously and does not warrant intervention.

38 °C (100.4 °F) is not a hard and fast threshold by which to declare or exclude postoperative fever. Older adult patients may display only a modest increase in body temperature despite severe infections. A reduced temperature or absent fever may make the diagnosis more difficult in immunocompromised patients. Glucocorticoids, cancer chemotherapy, and post-transplant immunosuppression all attenuate fever development [9, 10].

45.2 Patient Assessment

45.2.1 Monitoring

When evaluating a patient for fever, consider whether the temperature measurement route is oral, rectal, tympanic, or axillary. Rectal and tympanic temperatures are about 1 °F higher, and axillary temperatures are about 1 °F lower than oral temperatures. Also consider whether the patient has smoked or consumed hot or cold liquids around the time of determination and whether the patient is taking antipyretics. Furthermore, remember that daily temperature varies by approximately 0.5 °C (0.9 °F), being lower in the morning (e.g., 4 a.m.) and higher in the evening (e.g., 8 p.m.) [4, 5, 9].

45.2.2 Work-Up

General fever work-up should be completed in a standard and stepwise fashion. Review the patient's medical health record, past medical history, medications, operative note, etc. prior to evaluation. Question and examine the patient to identify the obvious sources of fever. Questions pertaining to the ears, nose, throat, and sinuses are particularly helpful with children. Identification of neck pain upon flexion, adenopathy, pathologic heart and lungs sounds, erythema, edema, and inflammation will assist in determining the source of fever.

The etiology of postoperative fever can be multifaceted and with numerous factors determining the likely cause. Degree of elevation, timing of fever, cause of fever, and type of surgery all factor into properly diagnosing the source of the patient's postoperative fever [1, 2, 5]. As mentioned previously, a low-grade fever (a temperature up to 38 °C) is common in the first few days after major surgery. However, this does not make all fevers within the first 24 h dismissible.

Potential causes of fever in the operative and immediate postoperative period are mainly limited to medications, reactions to blood products, the surgery itself, and in rare cases malignant hyperthermia. Malignant hyperthermia in the postoperative setting is most unlikely because the symptoms have an onset that is within minutes of exposure to the inhalation anesthetic.

In the 24–72 h period after surgery, the likely source of fever shifts. The "5 W's" is an acronym used to describe five categories of common sources of postoperative fever. The five "W's" consist of wind, water, wound, walking, and wonder drugs, in that order. Surgeons should reflect on the acronym in this order as it reflects the timing and progression of the likely diagnosis: pneumonia ("wind"), urinary tract infection ("water"), surgical site infection ("wound"), venous thromboembolic event ("walking"), and reaction to medication ("wonder drugs") [1–3, 5, 10].

"Wind" represents postoperative fever associated with pulmonary function. Pneumonia, pulmonary embolism, aspiration, and atelectasis are sources of postoperative fever as they relate to pulmonary function. Pneumonia may be nosocomial or as a result of aspiration. If pulmonary function is the source of postoperative fever, the oxygen saturation will be diminished.

More recently, atelectasis has been a topic of controversy in medical literature. Historically, atelectasis has been used as an explanation for otherwise unexplained postoperative fever. However, their concurrence has come into question, and questions have been raised as to whether they are coincidental rather than causal. If pneumothorax has not been shown to cause fever, why would atelectasis cause fever? [1, 2, 5].

"Water" represents the next potential source of postoperative fever. Specifically, the sites of indwelling catheters such as the intravenous catheters and Foley catheters should be examined. The patient may have signs of erythema, edema, or calor at the site. Also, there may be visible phlebitis proximal to the site of the indwelling catheter. For intravenous catheters, a positive physical exam is diagnostic to determine if an indwelling line is the source of infection. To resolve the infection, removing the catheter, acquiring intravenous access at a different site, and administering antibiotics is often sufficient. When the urine catheter is the source of infection, physical exam in conjunction with urinalysis is diagnostic. White blood cells (leukocytes), red blood cells (erythrocytes), nitrites, and bacteria in the urinalysis may indicate a UTI, a frequent cause of postoperative fever in patients with indwelling urethral catheters. The risk of UTI increases with the duration of catheterization; indwelling catheters should be replaced every 72 h [1, 2, 5].

"Walking," or the lack thereof, may lead to the development of deep venous thrombosis (DVT), and subsequent pulmonary embolism (PE) in the postoperative patient. DVTs and PEs are most common following procedures resulting in direct or indirect venous stasis. Prolonged venous stasis may result from a patient's confinement to the hospital bed for several days or weeks, or as a result of multiple hours of surgery. A DVT may also develop status posttrauma. DVT may lead to the development of ischemia in the distal extremity, and mobilization of the DVT may lead to thrombus mobilization and subsequent PE. Symptoms of DVT include pain and edema in the affected leg; the pain often feels similar to cramping or soreness. Homan's sign was previously pathognomonic for DVT, but is no longer used because dorsiflexion of the foot is thought to lead to thrombus mobilization and subsequent PE.

Symptoms of PE include: sudden shortness of breath, acute chest pain which may worsen with deep inspiration or coughing, tachypnea and tachycardia, anxiety, diaphoresis, and heart palpitations. Oftentimes PE can be difficult to distinguish from other conditions with similar clinical presentations, such as a myocardial infarction (MI). Persistent high-grade fever and dyspnea are oftentimes the clinical signs that differentiate PE from MI [11–13].

"Wonder drugs" cause an increase in temperature in reaction to medication and represent the final "W." Other times this response is known as "drug fever." Drug fever is a transient postoperative fever that coincides with the administration of a medication and subsequently dissipates after discontinuation of the offending agent. Furthermore, drug fever is oftentimes diagnosed by process of exclusion. Though challenging, early diagnosis of drug fever can reduce the chance of future iatrogenic harm to the patient. Early diagnosis may also avoid unnecessary patient costs; diagnostic test and therapeutic interventions will be necessary if the patient has future adverse reactions to the offending medication. Some medical texts suggest that readministering the suspected offending medication will lead to a similar reaction and cause recurrence of fever within a few hours. Though this may confirm the diagnosis, readministering the medication is controversial because the patient may have a more severe reaction. If the decision has been made to readminister the suspected offending medications, it should be performed with extreme caution [1, 2, 5, 10, 13, 14].

45.2.3 Laboratory Tests and Anticipated Results

Laboratory studies such as CBC, CBC with differential, urinalysis, gram stains, and cultures assist with the identification of the source of infection. With a CBC, the normal range for leukocytes is 4000–11,000. An elevation in leukocytes is not commonly associated with an infectious process until the leukocyte count is greater than 11,000. A CBC with differential provides more detail information about the specific cellular changes. CBC with differential can present a left shift in neutrophil count. This is valuable information because it is indicative of an acute infection. Specifically, the left shift suggests an acute infection because there is a rapid release of immature neutrophils occurring in an effort to combat the inciting pathogen.

An elevation of white blood cells (leukocytes), red blood cells (erythrocytes), nitrites, and bacteria in the urinalysis are highly suggestive of a urinary tract infection (UTI). However, many medical professionals argue that a positive nitrate result alone is enough to diagnose a UTI. The justification behind this notion lies in the fact that the most common bacteria that lead to UTI release nitrates as a byproduct. Therefore, the elevation of nitrates must be indicative of the infectious bacteria's presence [5, 14–17].

Gram staining is essential for assistance in choosing an antibiotic for quick administration. Gram staining allows the surgeon to know whether the bacteria is gram positive or gram negative and can then lead the surgeon to choose the most appropriate antibiotic until culture sensitivities are available. Bacterial cultures allow multiple antibiotics to be tested against the infectious bacterial sample, and the most efficacious antibiotic to be selected based upon how each antibiotic prevents bacterial growth. Culture results assist in identifying the best antibiotic for patient care [17].

Radiographs should be used as an adjunct in identification of postoperative infection, especially when aspiration is the likely source of infection. A chest x-ray that reveals radiopacities within lung lobes will guide the clinician to (1) determine if aspiration is the likely source of infection and (2) locate the aspirate that has led to the infection. When chest x-ray is not conclusive, bronchoalveolar lavage is another adjunct to assist in determining if aspiration is the source of the infection. Lumbar puncture, thoracocentesis, and paracentesis are more aggressive procedures that are not commonly warranted to determine the source of postoperative infection. However, they may be necessary to identify the source of fever when other tests have failed [2, 17].

45.3 Management

45.3.1 Potential Problems

There is controversy over the need for clinician intervention when it comes to treatment of postoperative fever. There are pros and cons to fever and treatment of fever. Fever plays a role in the host's ability to resist infection. Increased body temperature creates an environment inhospitable to bacteria and viruses. Bacteria and viruses grow and multiply at normothermia, but fail to thrive at higher body temperatures. Au contraire, fever is noxious and can also leave a patient in a state of discomfort. Furthermore, dehydration may result from prolonged fever. Another reason commonly given to treating fever is that the metabolic cost of fever exceeds its clinical benefit. The metabolic cost of fever is most substantial when a patient shivers as a result of having chills. Shivering induces an increase in metabolic rate, increasing body temperature, but also consuming glucose [1–3, 18].

Wound infections, or surgical site infections (SSIs), are the most common type of nosocomial infection and are associated with substantial morbidity and mortality. SSIs are defined as infections related to the operative procedures that occur at or near the surgical incision within 30 days of an operative procedure or within 1 year of an implant. Whether a SSI occurs is dependent upon a complex interaction between numerous factors including the nature and number of organisms contaminating the surgical site, the health of the patient, and the skill and technique of the surgeon. Patient-related risk factors for SSI include diabetes, obesity, cigarette smoking, immunosuppression, malnutrition, colonization with microorganisms, the presence of pre-existing infection at a nonsurgical site, duration of preoperative hospitalization, and the severity of underlying illnesses.

In a SSI, clinical signs of infection include erythema, edema, crepitus upon palpation, and purulent discharge or abscess formation. Patient symptoms often include fever, tenderness to palpation, and constant pain at the surgical site. SSIs have different depths, which correlate with the type of surgery completed: superficial incisional SSI, deep incisional SSI, and organ or space SSI. Depending on the depth of SSI, the presentation of the infection will vary. Fever is often very high when the SSI is the source. Most SSIs can be treated with antibiotics. However, the treatment decision should be based upon clinician's interpretation of the infection. Return to the operating room may be warranted and is a clinical call the surgeon must make [1, 2, 11, 13, 19].

45.3.2 Patient Management

Reducing fever with antipyretics helps to attenuate the noxious state experienced by the patient. Antipyretics assist in reducing systemic symptoms of headache, myalgia, and arthralgia. Aspirin and NSAIDs are proven oral antipyretics, but they cause unwanted side effects on platelets, the gastrointestinal tract, and kidneys. Acetaminophen has no effect on platelets, the gastrointestinal tract, or the kidneys and is therefore generally the preferred antipyretic. A combination of acetaminophen and aspirin or acetaminophen and an NSAID is more effective than either alone, but the patient's present illness must be taken into consideration to avoid organ toxicity [1, 2, 20, 21].

45.4 Prevention

No matter what type of surgery, no matter what wound class, and no matter whether the surgery has been deemed sterile or non-sterile, postoperative complications are a known risk. The development of postoperative infections may not always be preventable and should therefore be explained to the patient at the time of acquiring consent. Although modern medicine has allowed antibiotic coverage to become specific for surgeries and surgical sites, all postoperative infections cannot be prevented. Yet and still, every effort must be made to prevent the development of postoperative infections.

Prevention of postoperative infections begins before the patient enters the operating room. Prior to the surgical date, the surgeon should make every effort to see that the patient is optimized for surgery. Whether this means consulting another service, acquiring labs or imaging, or delaying the surgery date because the patient has a common cold, the patient should be in their best health if at all possible prior to surgery.

On the day of surgery, additional steps can be taken to prevent postoperative infection. Prior to entering the OR, proper scrubbing is the first step the surgeon can take to prevent surgical site infection and subsequent postoperative infection. Furthermore, proper preparation of the patient, draping of the patient, antibiotic coverage, aseptic technique throughout the procedure, and closure of surgical site are a few of the perioperative steps every surgeon can take to prevent postoperative infections.

Assuring that all instruments have been properly sterilized will assist with prevention of a surgical site infection and postoperative infection. Also, as the surgeon, you are also the leader of the operation. The anesthesia team, the nursing team, the assistants, and the technicians are all important parts of the operation, but ultimately the patient's success rests upon your performance. Therefore, it is within reason that the surgeon also ensures that all other parties in the OR also adhere to the proper aseptic technique.

Postoperatively, along with continuing antibiotic coverage, preventing the development of fever follows the 5 "W's." We will discuss "wind" or aspiration and atelectasis first. Preventing aspiration begins prior to the operation. If the patient is not likely going to be able to independently maintain their airway, prolonged intubation with the patient in the intensive care unit (ICU) may be the best option for initial postoperative care. Conversely, if independently maintaining the airway is not of concern, having the patient ambulate and/or use an incentive spirometer (in the instance when they cannot ambulate) will assist in preventing postoperative atelectasis [1, 2, 5, 6, 15, 16].

Intravenous catheters and Foley catheters are the potential sources of postoperative infections that result from "water." As mentioned previously, clinical signs of erythema, edema, and calor at the site of intravenous catheters and Foley catheters are pathognomonic for infection. Ensuring that indwelling catheters are replaced every 72 h will help to prevent "water"-related postoperative infections [15].

Preventing postoperative surgical site infections, or "wound" infections, in the preoperative and intraoperative settings has been discussed above. There has been recent debate in the oral and maxillofacial surgery literature over whether or not antibiotics are always necessary postoperatively (see Chap. 10).

As mentioned previously, "walking," or the lack thereof, often leads to the development of deep venous thrombosis (DVT), with the potential for subsequent development of a pulmonary embolism (PE). Among several other clinical signs and symptoms, fever develops in the postoperative patient. DVTs and PEs are most common following procedures resulting in direct or indirect venous stasis; prolonged venous stasis most commonly results from a patient's confinement to the hospital bed for several days or weeks or as a result of multiple hours of surgery. Therefore, no matter the patient age or health status, DVT prophylaxis is necessary.

The form of DVT prophylaxis can vary depending on the patient's health and the length of the operation. If the patient is scheduled to undergo a short procedure, and he/she is considered healthy, sequential compression devices (SCDs) may suffice as an appropriate form of DVT prophylaxis. Conversely, if the patient has an ASA classification more consistent with a disease that is a constant threat to his/her well-being, and the length of the surgery is expected to last several hours, subcutaneous heparin or lovenox is the more appropriate DVT prophylaxis option [11–14].

If the patient is able to ambulate postoperatively, ambulation may provide sufficient DVT prophylaxis. However, if continued confinement to the hospital bed is anticipated, the patient should be continued on an anticoagulant in the postoperative setting to prevent the development of DVT.

Finally, "wonder drugs" are the fifth and last likely source of the development of postoperative fever. Preventing this nosocomial fever is best done through early diagnosis. Some medical texts suggest that readministering the suspected offending medication will lead to a similar reaction and cause recurrence of fever within a few hours. Though this may confirm the diagnosis, readministering the medication is controversial because the patient may have a more severe reaction. If the decision has been made to readminister the suspected offending medications, it should be performed with extreme caution. Or simple cessation of the suspected offending medication may resolve the fever and confirm the surgeon's suspicion [2, 5, 6, 18, 21].

References

1. Porat R. Pathophysiology and treatment of fever in adults. Uptodate.com. 2016. http://www.uptodate.com
2. Weed H. Postoperative fever. (2016). http://www.uptodate.com
3. Lee-Chiong TL Jr, Stitt JT. Disorders of temperature regulation. Compr Ther. 1995;21:697.
4. Niven DJ, Gaudet JE, Laupland KB, et al. Accuracy of peripheral thermometers for estimating temperature: a systematic review and meta-analysis. Ann Intern Med. 2015;163:768.
5. Sonnenberg EM. Wind, water, wound, walk—do the data deliver the dictum? (2015). https://www.ncbi.nlm.nih.gov/pubmed
6. Galicier C, Richet H. A prospective study of postoperative fever in a general surgery department. Infect Control. 1985;6:487.
7. Hobar PC, Masson JA, Herrera R, et al. Fever after craniofacial surgery in the infant under 24 months of age. Plast Reconstr Surg. 1998;102:32.
8. Bergman DA, Mayer ML, Pantell RH, et al. Does clinical presentation explain practice variability in the treatment of febrile infants? Pediatrics. 2006;117:787.
9. Advanced Trauma Life Support Manual; American College of Surgeons Committee on Trauma. Advanced trauma life support (ATLS®): the ninth edition. J Trauma Acute Care Surg. 2013;74(5):1363–6.
10. Garibaldi RA, Brodine S, Matsumiya S, Coleman M. Evidence for the non-infectious etiology of early postoperative fever. Infect Control. 1985;6:273.
11. Stein PD, Afzal A, Henry JW, Villareal CG. Fever in acute pulmonary embolism. Chest. 2000;117:39–42.
12. Murray HW, Ellis GC, Blumenthal DS, Sos TA. Fever and pulmonary thromboembolism. Am J Med. 1979;67:232–5.
13. Kokturk N, Demir N, Oguzulgen IK, Demirel K, Ekim N. Fever in pulmonary embolism. Blood Coagul Fibrinolysis. 2005;16:341–7.
14. Livelli FD Jr, Johnson RA, McEnany MT, et al. Unexplained in-hospital fever following cardiac surgery. Natural history, relationship to postpericardiotomy syndrome, and a prospective study of therapy with indomethacin versus placebo. Circulation. 1978;57:968.
15. Sedor J, Mulholland SG. Hospital-acquired urinary tract infections associated with the indwelling catheter. Urol Clin North Am. 1999;26:821.

16. Ghosh S, Charity RM, Haidar SG, Singh BK. Pyrexia following total knee replacement. Knee. 2006;13:324.
17. Kiragu AW, Zier J, Cornfield DN. Utility of blood cultures in postoperative pediatric intensive care unit patients. Pediatr Crit Care Med. 2009;10:364.
18. Gomez B, Mintegi S, Bressan S, et al. Validation of the "step-by-step" approach in the management of young febrile infants. Pediatrics. 2016;138:e20154381.
19. Garibaldi RA, Burke JP, Dickman ML, Smith CB. Factors predisposing to bacteriuria during indwelling urethral catheterization. N Engl J Med. 1974;291:215.
20. Garcia S, Mintegi S, Gomez B, et al. Is 15 days an appropriate cut-off age for considering serious bacterial infection in the management of febrile infants? Pediatr Infect Dis J. 2012;31:455.
21. Guinn S, Castro FP Jr, Garcia R, Barrack RL. Fever following total knee arthroplasty. Am J Knee Surg. 1999;12:161.

46 Drug–Drug Interactions as a Complication of Maxillofacial Surgery

James J. Omlie and Andrew Herlich

Abstract

All too often clinicians resort to a fixed regimen during the care of surgical patients in the perioperative period. The patient population is becoming increasingly ill, and it is commonplace for patients to be on several medications, which can potentially interact with those utilized in the perioperative period. Each drug that is used when managing these patients must be carefully evaluated for its potential interactions with anesthetic medications in the perioperative period. The goal for this chapter is to provide a framework to assist the clinician in understanding drug-drug interactions, which will be illustrated by examples of fatal to near-fatal reactions that have been documented in the literature.

46.1 Review of Pharmacology and How It Applies to Drug-Drug Interactions

46.1.1 Pharmacodynamics

The basic principles of pharmacodynamics relate to what a drug does to the body. The concentration of a drug at the receptor site and the degree of the resulting drug effect is studied to identify dose-response curves and the relative safety of the concentration of a drug.

An example of a dose-response curve is given in Fig. 46.1. This figure demonstrates the concentration of the drug and its efficacy, which can be therapeutic, subtherapeutic, or supratherapeutic (toxicity) [1]. Drugs act as ligands and they have specificity for their respective receptors. Certain medications have a specificity for several different receptors, such as diphenhydramine (histamine and muscarinic). Conversely, ondansetron has a high degree of specificity for the 5-HT3 receptor over other serotonin receptors [1]. However, the drug action at the receptor differs in that it can be an agonist, partial agonist, or antagonist. Non-depolarizing neuromuscular blocking drugs (NMBD) demonstrate competi-

J.J. Omlie, D.D.S., M.D.
Department of Oral and Maxillofacial Surgery, University of Pittsburgh Medical Center, Pittsburgh, PA, USA
e-mail: omliejj@upmc.edu

A. Herlich, D.M.D., M.D., F.A.A.P. (✉)
Department of Anesthesiology, University of Pittsburgh School of Medicine, Pittsburgh, PA, USA
e-mail: herlicha@upmc.edu

© Springer International Publishing AG 2018
E.M. Ferneini, J.D. Bennett (eds.), *Perioperative Assessment of the Maxillofacial Surgery Patient*,
https://doi.org/10.1007/978-3-319-58868-1_46

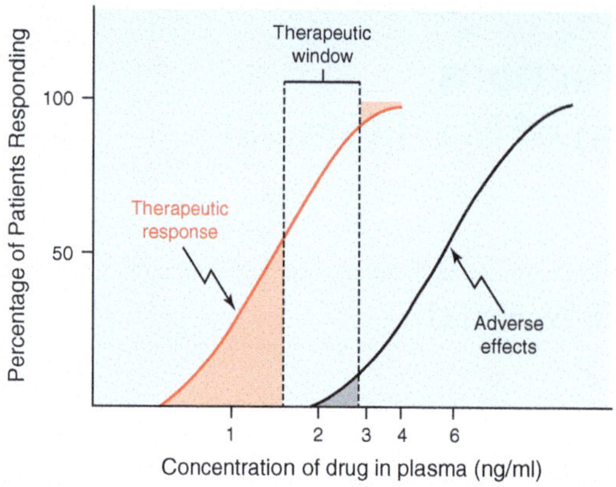

Fig. 46.1 Relationship of the therapeutic window of drug concentration to the subtherapeutic and adverse effects in the patient population [1] [Adapted from Wittwer ED and WT Nicholson. Pharmacodynamic Interactions: Core Concepts. In: Marcucci C et al., editor. A Case Approach to Perioperative Drug-Drug Interactions. New York: Springer; 2015. p. 9–14 with permission from Springer]

tive antagonism. There can be a "ceiling effect" as is seen with NMBD where all receptors are occupied and competitive reversal agents can become largely ineffective; however, a novel drug sugammadex may facilitate complete removal of the NMBD until quantitative evidence can demonstrate a partial return of neuromuscular function [1].

Not all antagonists work in the same manner. Competitive antagonists can be displaced from the receptors by increasing the concentration of agonists; however, this is not the case for noncompetitive antagonists which are bound irreversibly (aspirin) or the ligand slowly dissociates.

Over time patients develop tolerance to certain medications with upregulation or downregulation of receptors, requiring more of a single drug or drugs of a similar class which is known as cross-tolerance. Not necessarily all drugs demonstrate tolerance, but those that do, the degree of tolerance is not equal for all effects of that medication. For example, adequate analgesia from an opioid may require increased dosage; however, the increased dosage causes greater GI side effects and respiratory depression [1].

When two drugs are given simultaneously, pharmacodynamic interactions can cause additive or synergistic effects. Drug synergy is when the pharmacologic effect of both drugs together is greater than "the sum of their individual effects." Additive interactions occur when the combined effect of the medications equals the sum of their individual effects. These drug properties can be utilized to enhance the effect. This interaction may create a drug-drug interaction (DDI) causing dangerous effects, such as hypotension, apnea, or even death when one of these drugs on their own is less likely to cause this action. Drugs that act at the same receptor tend to act in an additive manner and conversely act in synergistic manner with those that act at different receptors [2].

46.1.2 Pharmacokinetics

Pharmacokinetics is what the body does to a drug (absorption, distribution, metabolism, and excretion). It is important to understand these concepts due to the many DDIs that involve pharmacokinetic properties. There are a variety of routes of administration with differing bioavailability of the medication. The different routes include IV, PO, PR, transdermal, sublingual, subcutaneous, and inhalational. Bioavailability is the fraction of drug that reaches systemic circulation. For example, intravenous administration is 100% bioavailable; however, there is greater variability for other routes. Additionally, the amount of drug reaching the systemic circulation may be reduced due to absorption in the GI tract or first pass effect (high hepatic extraction before entering systemic circulation) [3].

The GI tract has several routes of DDI interferences, of note are the two drug transporters P-glycoprotein and organic anion-transporting peptides (OATPs). Drug absorption and transport can be increased or decreased resulting in altered levels in systemic circulation. CYP3A is the major intestinal drug enzyme and can cause potentially serious increases in midazolam when taken orally with grapefruit juice [4].

Significant DDIs occur at the level of drug metabolism in the classically known phase I and phase II reactions. Phase I reactions are through the workhorse of drug metabolism, the CYP450 enzyme system. The CYP450 system performs oxidation, reduction, and hydrolysis of substrates that are both endogenous and exogenous. Phase II reactions revolve around the conjugation/addition of molecules to the drug substrate, such as glucuronidation, acetylation, methylation, and glutathione conjugation. The DDIs occur at this level when the medications are metabolized by the same enzyme system resulting in inhibition or induction of the respective enzymes. Inhibition causes a slower rate of drug metabolism and can either be competitive or noncompetitive. These drug interactions occur earlier than those observed with inducers, because inhibition can occur immediately whereas the induction of enzymes requires gene expression and synthesis [5, 6].

The CYP3A subfamily is responsible for 50% of oxidative reactions [3, 7]. These enzymes in the intestinal tract and liver undergo induction and inhibition with several common drugs. It is important to consider what the affected enzyme actually does to a drug. For example, whether it inactivates and creates an active metabolite or is a prodrug. If it is a prodrug or active metabolite, an inducer would increase the systemic concentration to potentially toxic levels [3].

An area of unrecognized clinical significance is the drug-gene interactions known as pharmacogenomics. Patients can be poor, intermediate, extensive, or ultra-rapid metabolizers depending on the allelic variations. This is similar to having an inducer or inhibitor co-administered, but this effect is primarily at the drug-gene level. The important example is the CYP2B6 polymorphisms and the potentially lethal reduced metabolism of methadone [8].

46.1.3 Clinically Relevant Cytochrome P450 Enzyme Systems, Substrates/Inhibitors/Inducers/Interactions (Table 46.1)

Table 46.1 Major cytochrome P450 system enzymes and the major enzyme systems and their respective substrates, inducers, inhibitors, and examples of DDIs [9–13]

Enzymes	Substrates	Inhibitors	Inducers	Interactions
CYP3A4	*Midazolam, ketamine, fentanyl, alfentanil, sufentanil, methadone, most local anesthetics (LA),* TCAs, antipsychotics, macrolide antibiotics, dihydropyridine calcium channel blockers, stains, carbamazepine, and steroid compounds	SSRIs, quinolone antibiotics, “azole” antifungals, and grapefruit juice	St. John’s wort, protease inhibitors (ritonavir), anticonvulsants, and rifampin	Midazolam levels can vary up to 800% depending on what medications are co-administered. Inhibitors (SSRIs, quinolone antibiotics, azole antifungals, and grapefruit juice) cause a significant increase in midazolam levels [14, 15]
CYP2D6	*Opioids (codeine, hydrocodone, dihydrocodone, and tramadol), ondansetron, β-blockers,* several SSRIs, TCAs, and metoclopramide	*Celecoxib, diphenhydramine, ropivacaine, cimetidine, methadone, and amiodarone*	No known biological inducers [16]	Paroxetine and tramadol resulted in development of central serotonin syndrome and seizures secondary to increased tramadol levels that lower the seizure threshold [17]

(continued)

Table 46.1 (continued)

Enzymes	Substrates	Inhibitors	Inducers	Interactions
CYP2E1	Ethanol, isoniazid, halogenated anesthetics *(enflurane, halothane, methoxyflurane, isoflurane, sevoflurane, and desflurane)* [18]	Disulfiram	Isoniazid, tobacco smoke, ethanol [19]	*Inducers (isoniazid, tobacco smoke, chronic alcohol, and uncontrolled diabetes)* resulting in increased rate of metabolism and increased halogenated anesthetic requirement
CYP2B6	*Propofol, ketamine, meperidine, methadone, bupropion*, antineoplastic agents (cyclophosphamide and ifosfamide), efavirenz [20, 21]	SSRIs (paroxetine and sertraline), estradiol, thiotepa, ticlopidine, and clopidogrel [21–23]	Phenobarbital, phenytoin, carbamazepine, rifampin, ritonavir, and dexamethasone [24]	Responsible for over 50% of the conversion of meperidine to the neurotoxic metabolite nor meperidine [25]. *Inducers (phenobarbital, phenytoin, carbamazepine, rifampin, ritonavir, dexamethasone)* should be noted on any drug history with co-administration of meperidine
CYP2C9	*Celecoxib, ibuprofen, indomethacin, diclofenac, hydromorphone, propofol, ketamine, phenobarbital, diazepam, halothane, warfarin,* phenytoin, carvedilol, clopidogrel, sulfonylureas, angiotensin II receptor blockers (ARBs), sertraline, and fluvastatin [26]	Amiodarone [27], fluconazole, sulfa drugs	Barbiturates	Amiodarone is an inhibitor with a long half-life. The long duration of inhibition results in significantly increased levels of warfarin and phenytoin [27]

46.1.4 The Fatal Forty and Its Application in Patient Care

The Fatal Forty drugs are a must to know when taking into consideration DDIs. This requires intimate knowledge of the CYP (P450) enzyme system and the transporter systems. There are several approaches to memorizing this list. The first is the card catalogue approach where one memorizes the 40 drugs and keeps a regular list with them when encountering cases. The second is the pharmacology approach which is endorsed by the authors of *A Case Approach to Perioperative DDIs* [28, 29].

1. *Drugs with a low therapeutic index:* Small changes in blood levels can have significant clinical effects often involving inhibitors.
   - Clozapine—seizures and oversedation
   - Cyclobenzaprine—common drug in pain clinic, 1A2 substrate
   - Digoxin—arrhythmias
   - Lamotrigine—toxic dermatologic syndromes (Stevens Johnson syndrome, toxic epidermal necrolysis, angioedema)
   - Lithium—nephrotoxicity
   - Methadone—arrhythmias and CNS/cardiopulmonary depression
   - Pimozide—malignant QT prolonger
   - Thioridazine—malignant QT prolonger

- Tricyclic antidepressants—QT prolongation
- Warfarin—hypocoagulable or non-therapeutic

2. *Drugs that are pan-inhibitors or pan-inducers:* The dangers with these drugs are that they inhibit or induce many enzymes and therefore have a high potential for DDIs.
   - Amiodarone—pan-inhibitor of cytochrome P450 enzymes (CYP450)
   - Cimetidine—pan-inhibitor of CYP450
   - Fluoxetine—pan-inhibitor of CYP450
   - Fluvoxamine—CYP450 pan-inhibitor
   - Ritonavir—pan-inhibitor and pan-inducer of CYP450
   - Phenobarbital—pan-inducer of CYP450
   - Carbamazepine—pan-inducer of CYP450, P-glycoprotein substrate and CYP3A4 substrate
   - Phenytoin—CYP2C9 greater than 2C19 substrate, P-glycoprotein substrate, CYP450 pan-inducer (except 1A2), and high plasma protein binding
   - Rifampin—pan-inducer of CYP450 and P-glycoprotein inducer
3. *Drugs that are CYP3A4 inhibitors:* 3A4 is the workhorse of the P450 enzyme system. The importance of CYP3A4 is illustrated by the fact that there is no poor metabolizer genotype as is seen with other P450 enzymes because such mutations may be lethal.
   - Ketoconazole—most potent 3A4 inhibitor. Fluconazole was developed due to the inhibition of 3A4 metabolism of endogenous cortisol by ketoconazole. Patients actually developed cushingoid symptoms.
   - Diltiazem and verapamil—potent 3A4 inhibitors.
   - Grapefruit juice—potent 3A4 inhibitor. Not allowed on hospital food trays.
   - Macrolides—common 3A4 inhibitors with the exception of azithromycin.
   - Note that the pan-inhibitors mentioned before also inhibit 3A4.
4. *Prodrugs:* Prodrugs must be converted to a biologically active form through CYP450 metabolism. The DDIs associated with these medications are under-recognized and poorly understood. Many of the DDIs act by preventing the pharmacological conversion step and commonly involve CPY2D6.
   - Codeine—prodrug at CYP2D6
   - Tamoxifen—prodrug at CYP2D6
   - Tramadol—prodrug at CYP2D6
   - Clopidogrel—prodrug at 3A4 and 2C19
5. *Common drugs:* Often mixed up with DDIs due to the relatively common use in the general population.
   - Calcium channel blockers (CCBs)—CYP3A4 substrates, diltiazem, and verapamil are also 3A4 and P-glycoprotein inhibitors.
   - Clopidogrel—prodrug at CYP3A4 and 2C19.
   - Omeprazole—CYP2C19 substrate and inhibitor; P-glycoprotein inhibitor.
   - Ethinylestradiol—CYP3A4 substrate, 2C19 and 1A2 inhibitor, and uridine 5′-diphosphoglucornoslytransferase 1A4 (UGT1A4) inducer.
   - Grapefruit juice—3A4 and 1A2 inhibitor.
   - Macrolides—3A4 and P-glycoprotein inhibitors with the exception of azithromycin.
   - Statins—lovastatin, simvastatin, and atorvastatin are CYPA4 substrates; simvastatin is also a 2D6 substrate; fluvastatin is a 2C9 substrate and inhibitor; all seem to be P-glycoprotein inhibitors.
   - Sulfonylureas—2C9 substrates.
   - Smoked tobacco—1A2 and 2E1 inducer.
6. *Drugs with rare but serious complications.*
   - Statins—excessively elevated blood levels associated with muscle cramping and possible rhabdomyolysis. Unpredictable time course. Complicated metabolic profile—atorvastatin, simvastatin, and lovastatin are CYP3A4 substrates. Simvastatin is a 2D6 substrate. Fluvastatin is a 2C9 substrate and inhibitor. Most statins are P-glycoprotein inhibitors with variable effects on warfarin.
   - Smoked tobacco—short time frame for inducer effects on 1A2 (1–3 days instead of 1–3 weeks).

46.1.5 Six Basic Patterns of Pharmacokinetic Drug-Drug Interactions

Pattern 1 is where an inhibitor is added to a substrate, which results in increased substrate levels secondary to decreased enzymatic activity. This can be potentially dangerous when a medication with a low therapeutic index is utilized. The example given by Sandson [30] is paroxetine being added to nortriptyline, which is metabolized by CYP2D6. Paroxetine is a 2D6 inhibitor which can result in toxic levels of nortriptyline.

Pattern 2 is essentially the same as pattern 1, but differs in that a substrate is added to an inhibitor increasing the bioavailability of the added substrate due to an already inhibited CYP450 enzyme. Sandson [30] noted fentanyl being given to a patient with HIV being treated with ritonavir which is a potent CYP3A4 inhibitor, which can result in respiratory depression, hypoxia, and death.

Pattern 3 is where an inducer is added to a substrate, which results in decreased substrate levels several weeks later because an inducer takes time to upregulate the respective enzyme system. An example is phenytoin being added to cyclosporine [30]. Phenytoin is a pan-inducer which requires increased substrate to reach therapeutic drug levels.

Pattern 4 is the opposite of pattern 3 where an inducer is already in use with the addition of a substrate. If the preset dosing guidelines are used, the effects would be subtherapeutic. The example given is midazolam added to carbamazepine with the recommendation to titrate to effect.

Pattern 5 is where a substrate and an inhibitor have been co-administered followed by the withdrawal of the inhibitor. The discontinuation of the inhibitor results in a return to normal enzymatic function causing decreased or subtherapeutic drug levels. An example of this is discontinuation of fluconazole in a patient taking prednisone [30]. The decreased levels of prednisone can result in an addisonian crisis.

Pattern 6 is similar to pattern 5, but involves the co-administration of a substrate and an inducer resulting in subtherapeutic drug levels. Several weeks after the withdrawal of the inducer, there are decreased levels of enzyme leading to increased levels of substrate. This must be recognized in substrates with a narrow therapeutic index which could result in substrate toxicity.

Exception: Prodrugs such as codeine, hydrocodone, tramadol, and cyclophosphamide must be considered in the opposite manner where addition of inhibitor causes loss of efficacy. The addition of an inducer would result in toxicity rather than loss of efficacy.

46.2 Fatal and Near-Fatal Drug-Drug Interactions

46.2.1 Meperidine and MAOIs and Other Medications Noted to Cause Serotonin Syndrome

Meperidine has widespread notoriety dating back to the Libby Zion case and its lethal DDIs. Meperidine was used in the perioperative period, specifically when encountering a shivering patient in the PACU. The critical issue pertaining to the Libby Zion case was that she was taking a monoamine oxidase inhibitor (MAOI), which precipitated a fatal DDI causing serotonin syndrome. Co-administration of these two medications is an example of a pharmacodynamic interaction resulting in both the inhibition of serotonin metabolism and reuptake of serotonin from the synaptic cleft. This ultimately results in increased intrasynaptic serotonin concentrations, which can result in central toxicity [31]. There are several different serotonin receptors, but agonism at the 5-HT2A has been identified as causing the most toxicity [32]. Serotonin syndrome is recognized by the triad of neuroexcitatory features (1) neuromuscular hyperactivity (tremor, clonus, myoclonus, hyperreflexia, and pyramidal rigidity), (2) autonomic hyperactivity (diaphoresis, fever, tachycardia, and tachypnea), and (3) altered mental status (agitation, excitement, and in more advanced cases confusion is observed) [31]. The rapid onset of these symptoms must be recognized immediately due to the fatal nature of these reactions. A case provided by Kenyon et al. noted a young woman's suicide attempt after beginning an MAOI, and in the PACU, she was subsequently given meperidine [33]. The signs of serotonin syndrome were promptly recognized, and the patient was given chlorpromazine and midazolam to counteract the effects of serotonin toxicity. The gold standard treatment involves use of 5-HT2A receptor antagonists (chlorprom-

Table 46.2 Medications associated with serotonin toxicity [31, 37, 39–41]

Drug class	Medications
MOAIs	Linezolid (weak), moclobemide, selegiline, hydrochloride, phenelzine sulfate, isoniazid, procarbazine hydrochloride, toloxatone, tranylcypromine
SSRIs	Paroxetine HCl, sertraline HCl, fluoxetine HCl, citalopram hydrobromide, venlafaxine HCl, fluvoxamine maleate, duloxetine HCl
SRIs	Clomipramine HCl, imipramine pamoate, chlorpheniramine maleate, brompheniramine maleate
Opioids	Meperidine HCl, tramadol HCl, methadone HCl, dextromethorphan hydrobromide
Illicit drugs	Methylenedioxymethamphetamine, amphetamine sulfate, cocaine HCl
Direct serotonin receptor agonists	Carbamazepine, buspirone HCl, lithium carbonate

azine (IV) and cyproheptadine hydrochloride (oral)) to reduce the signs and symptoms of toxicity, as well as benzodiazepines to decrease the hyperadrenergic response [31, 33]. It should be taken into consideration the genetic variability that can play a role in the different susceptibility to drug metabolism due to the inherently weak SRI actions of meperidine.

There are several drugs that when used concomitantly with meperidine or other noted medications can precipitate serotonin toxicity [34, 35]. Although linezolid is an antimicrobial used to treat enterococcus, pneumonia, and other infections, it has been associated with serotonin syndrome when given with SSRIs and meperidine [36, 37]. The mechanism of action for the linezolid and meperidine serotonin syndrome is due to the decreased metabolism of serotonin due to linezolid and the concomitant decreased reuptake of serotonin caused by meperidine. Successful treatment and ultimately survival is based on quick recognition of the syndrome, discontinuation of the drugs, and possible use of serotonin antagonists [38, 39]. There are several relatively common medications that have been associated with serotonin syndrome which are listed below (Table 46.2).

46.2.2 Bupropion and Pseudoephedrine: Cardiac Events in Young Patients

Antidepressants are increasingly encountered in the patient population. Certain classes, such as bupropion (a norepinephrine and dopamine reuptake inhibitor), have potentially lethal pharmacodynamic interactions with medications. The example reported in the literature is the combination with pseudoephedrine [42]. Pseudoephedrine is a common decongestant used by otolaryngologists and oral and maxillofacial surgeons in certain clinical scenarios. A case report was given for a healthy Jehovah's Witness that succumbed to a myocardial infarction intraoperatively due to the use of pseudoephedrine intranasally when the patient became hypotensive [42]. The pharmacodynamic interaction was secondary to sympathetic mediated coronary artery vasospasm resulting in myocardial ischemia and infarction [42–44]. These incidents have been reported mostly within a young, healthy population, and caution must be used when considering co-administration of sympathomimetics.

46.2.3 Phenytoin, Valproic Acid: CYP2C9 (Patient Death Secondary to Acute Liver Failure)

The maxillofacial patient encountered in the setting of traumatic head injuries may require antiepileptic medications. Although these patients are typically managed by a trauma/general surgery service at a tertiary care center, the potential for dangerous pharmacokinetic interactions must be avoided. The combination of phenytoin and valproic acid has a complex pharmacokinetic interaction. This interaction is at the level of metabolism and drug distribution, more specifically protein binding between phenytoin and albumin. Valproic acid is a moderate inhibitor of CYP2C9 and displaces phenytoin from albumin [45–48]. Consequently, there is a significant increase in free and total phenytoin concentrations due to the slowed metabolism and displacement of phenytoin from albumin. This can result in decreased seizure control and more significantly phenytoin toxicity [49–52]. Phenytoin toxicity is secondary to the production of a hepatotoxic metabolite with case reports showing death secondary to fulminant liver failure [53]. Metabolism of phenytoin is complex, and any other drug, changes in liver function, or protein binding (albumin level) can result in unpredictable drug levels. There are other antiepileptic medications available, but if these two are co-administered, free drug levels and LFTs should be monitored to screen for potential hepatic toxicity [51]. This typically occurs in the first 6 weeks when starting the drug [54]. Certain clinical correlations such as ataxia, confusion, nystagmus, and fever, rash, and confusion should prompt concern for possible increase in serum ammonia levels.

46.2.4 Summation Interactions with Local Anesthetics

Local anesthetic (LA) toxicity is an example of a synergistic or additive pharmacodynamic DDI. These drugs have identical mechanisms of action at the receptor sites, and consequently the total response is typically a summation of the individual effects [55, 56]. This concept is described by [57] with the doses of two interacting drugs plotted showing a linear diagonal function indicative of additive drug interactions. In this example, the median toxic dose of mepivacaine and tetracaine falls on this diagonal line; however, those LA combinations with median additive toxic doses above or below the line demonstrate less than additive or greater than additive (synergistic) interactions [55, 58]. Table 46.3 lists the dosages of LAs.

LA toxicity resulting in fatalities is well documented in the literature, especially when treating children. Understandably the combination of multiple LAs, specifically lidocaine and bupivacaine, was given a clinical significance rating of 1 [55]. In the perioperative period, notably in the operating room, it is relatively easy to overlook the amount of LA given to a child or adult. The use of lidocaine topical ointments for nasal tubes and the administration of lidocaine prior to induction with propofol or topical ointments are all additives. These additional doses are imperative to acknowledge in max dose calculations in children and the elderly to prevent the observation of LA toxicity reactions (CNS, convulsions, respiratory depression, cardiac arrest, and death) [61, 62].

Exparel is a relatively new local anesthetic utilizing bupivacaine encapsulated within multivesicular liposomes. This allows for slow release of bupivacaine for 72 h [63, 64]. However, the agent must be recognized for its potential interactions with other anesthetics, notably lidocaine. When lidocaine (or any other nonbupivacaine anesthetic) is administered within 20 min prior to Exparel, the bupivacaine is immediately released which can cause toxic levels of bupivacaine [63, 65]. The maximum dosage for an adult is 90 mg, and each vial of Exparel has 20 mL of solution containing 13.3 mg/mL, which can result in toxicity if all of the LA was released at once [64]. Additionally, Exparel looks very similar to propofol in an unmarked syringe, and heightened awareness of labeling the correct syringe is required.

Table 46.3 Recommended maximum LA dosages [59, 60]

Anesthetic agent	Max. dose with epinephrine (mg/kg)	Max. dose without epinephrine (mg/kg)	Maximum total dosage (mg)
2% lidocaine (1:100,000 epi)	7.7	4.4	500 with epi
3% mepivacaine	6.6	4.4	400
4% articaine	7.0		500
0.5% bupivacaine	1.3		90
4% prilocaine	8		400

46.2.5 Local Anesthetics with Opioid Sedation: Pediatric Disasters

The use of local anesthetics in combination with opioid sedation has resulted in pediatric disasters, most notably with the use of meperidine. LAs are readily absorbed and act as membrane depressants resulting in alteration of CNS and cardiovascular function [55]. These systemic manifestations when co-administered with CNS depressants are augmented and most evident in pediatric dental patients [55]. Always know the maximum recommended dose (MRD) when administering local anesthetic to a child and the difference when dosing a child and an adult. It is misconceiving in that the lower body mass is significantly less than an adult; however, the orofacial anatomy does not have such a disproportionate difference, therefore requiring similar amounts of local anesthetic. For example, a 50 lb. child does not require 1/3 the amount of anesthetic of a 150 lb. adult, which is how clinicians can easily exceed the MRD [55, 66]. Therefore, LA toxicity is more frequently seen in the pediatric population. Additionally, systemic drug interactions involving LA and CNS depressants become an even greater concern. Several studies have shown the interaction between local anesthetics and opioids, specifically meperidine [62, 67]. There is a clear association between opioid and LA co-administration with a decreased seizure threshold. Animal studies have shown the decrease in convulsant threshold when pretreated with opioids, mostly with meperidine [8, 68]. A respiratory acidosis ensues because of the respiratory depression caused by meperidine. The consequent acidosis and increased pCO_2 cause decreased protein binding of LA as well as greater cerebral perfusion resulting in increased delivery of free drug to the CNS [69–72]. The combination of increased free drug and increased CNS blood flow potentiates the sensitivity of the CNS to LA toxicity-related convulsions. These interactions are especially concerning due to the high potential to occur in an outpatient setting where it is more difficult to treat convulsions and respiratory depression.

46.2.6 Methadone and CYP2B6 Gene Mutations: An Example of a Drug-Gene Interaction

CYP2B6 polymorphisms cause interindividual variability in the metabolism of methadone. Of importance are slow metabolizers of methadone resulting in respiratory depression and death. This is a clinically significant drug-gene interaction that plays a role in the variability seen in toxic levels of methadone in overdose cases [73].

The number of patients being treated for opioid addiction and chronic pain has increased substantially. Methadone prescriptions have increased significantly between 2000 and 2009 with a fivefold increase (five million annually) [74]. In 2009, methadone accounted for 2% of prescriptions yet was attributed to 30% of prescription pain killer deaths. Methadone is a safe and effective drug when used properly; however, the relatively analgesic effect coupled with its long half-life increases the risk of toxic levels and drug interactions [75].

The mutation is most commonly seen in 33–50% of African Americans, 10–21% Asians, and 14–27% Caucasians [76, 77]. Those with the poor metabolizing polymorphism have a greater risk of methadone toxicity. Preoperative planning for pain management in the patient on methadone therapy is critical due to the risk for respiratory depression. The interindividual and intraindividual variability has confounded reliable dosing parameters predisposing those at risk to adverse events. In methadone-related deaths, blood levels can be in the therapeutic range for individuals with a normal rate of metabolism. Recommendations are given to monitor for symptoms of overdose closely as well as peak trough levels and serum methadone levels.

Most methadone-related deaths fall into three areas:

1. *Single overdose*: this is seen in opioid intolerant individuals or those with prior tolerance followed by a period of abstinence. Similar to other opioids, the primary effect is respiratory depression and hypoxia.

2. *Accumulated toxicity*: this is seen during the induction period when doses accumulate over several days and with SMLs increasing into toxic levels.
3. *Combining prescribed methadone with another drug*: combining other CNS depressants with methadone can result in toxic levels of the drug [75].

Most commonly associated with reported deaths is the use of a benzodiazepine. Caution must be used in patients taking psychiatric medications as well (fluoxetine, amitriptyline, quetiapine, and alprazolam). The largest proportion of methadone-associated deaths fall in category 2 during the induction phase (first 2 weeks). This is attributed to overestimation of the patient's tolerance to opioids [78–82]. The propensity for overestimation and the relatively recent discovery of CYP2B6 polymorphisms causing slower metabolism poses a greater risk for toxic methadone levels. Furthermore, it is not unreasonable to delay any elective procedures until after the induction period due to the risks posed with toxic drug levels secondary to the induction period and/or additional anesthetics utilized during the surgery.

46.3 Clinically Relevant DDIs

46.3.1 Nonsteroidal Anti-inflammatory Drugs (NSAIDs), Renal Disease, and DDIs

NSAIDs have a variety of effects involving both medical conditions and DDIs. They have adverse effects involving the gastrointestinal, cardiovascular (CV), and genitourinary systems (renal). Adverse CV effects involve both raising the blood pressure and increasing overall cardiovascular risk. NSAIDs utilized at doses to reduce inflammation and pain can increase blood pressure in normotensive and hypertensive patients, especially with patients taking selective cyclooxygenase-2 (COX-2) inhibitors [83].

NSAIDs can cause several different forms of kidney injury. These include hemodynamically mediated acute kidney injury (AKI), electrolyte and acid-base disorders, acute interstitial nephritis (AIN) with possible nephrotic syndrome, and papillary necrosis. Adverse renal events occur in 1–5% of patients taking NSAIDs [84]. Use of NSAIDs results in a decrease in the mean GFR due to its inhibition of prostaglandin synthesis, resulting in less dilation of the afferent arteriole to the glomerulus. Due to the effect on hemodynamic function, the combination with various antihypertensive medications with renal targets is associated with increased incidence of AKI. A case-control cohort study showed that the use of diuretics, ACE inhibitors, or ARBs increases the risk of NSAID-induced AKI [85]. Therefore, NSAID use should be limited and/or avoided in these patients. Additionally, the hemodynamic effects worsen GFR and understandably should be avoided in a patient with chronic kidney disease with a GFR less than 60 mL/min. This could result in an acute or long-term worsening of renal function. NSAID-induced AKI should be treated in a similar manner to other forms of AKI with the immediate cessation of the offending agent followed by volume resuscitation.

NSAID use as well as other medications effecting renal function should be used with caution in a bipolar patient treated with lithium. Lithium has a narrow therapeutic index and is excreted through the kidneys without being metabolized. NSAIDs along with diuretics and ACE inhibitors are associated with changes in renal function and salt balance which affects lithium excretion [86].

46.3.2 Anticoagulant DDIs (Warfarin, IIa Inhibitors, Xa Inhibitors)

Warfarin is a vitamin K antagonist that reduces production of factors II, VII, IX, and X as well as proteins C and S. This medication has a narrow therapeutic index and has several DDIs of note. There are three mechanisms of interaction: (1) prolonged PT/INR, (2) increased bleeding risk independent of PT/INR, and (3) reduced anticoagulation.

There are several ways that the INR can be prolonged. Several studies have noted altered intestinal flora which affects intestinal vitamin K synthesis. Antibiotics that have been documented to reduce vitamin K synthesis via this mechanism include co-trimoxazole (Bactrim), metronidazole, macrolides, and fluoroquinolones. Warfarin is metabolized by CYP2C9, which is inhibited by several medications. These agents include fluconazole, miconazole, fluoxetine (SSRI), amiodarone, gemfibrozil, simvastatin, atorvastatin, and Bactrim (trimethoprim/sulfamethoxazole) [87]. Acetaminophen has been associated with increased INR and is explained by the interruption of vitamin K recycling with inhibition at the vitamin K epoxide reductase and vitamin K-dependent carboxylase [87]. Any medication that displaces warfarin from albumin results in increased drug levels; however, this effect is usually minor.

There are several medications that cause increased bleeding risk without affecting the PT/INR. Aspirin and NSAIDs can cause increased bleeding risk due to injury to the gastrointestinal mucosa via reduced prostaglandin synthesis. This in combination with an impeded coagulation cascade due to warfarin and the antiplatelet effect of NSAIDs and ASA can result in a significant GI bleed. Clopidogrel and ticlopidine also have antiplatelet effects. There are several over-the-counter supplements that have incompletely characterized increased bleeding risk such as ginkgo biloba, dong quai, fenugreek, and chamomile [88].

Subtherapeutic levels result in reduced anticoagulation. This can occur with DDIs causing induction of CYP2C9 causing increased warfarin metabolism. This has been associated with rifampin, which is a pan-inducer of the CYP450 system. Additionally, the use of herbal medication St. John's wort has been associated with reduced anticoagulation, but the mechanism hasn't been characterized.

There are CYP2C9 variants resulting in a reduced rate of warfarin metabolism causing excessive anticoagulation and bleeding [89]. Additionally, 25% of Coumadin variability can be attributed to genetic variation at the vitamin K epoxide reductase gene, which plays a critical role in vitamin K recycling [90].

Dabigatran is a direct thrombin (IIa) inhibitor under the brand name Pradaxa. Dose modification and/or drug avoidance is recommended in certain clinical scenarios such as renal insufficiency, use of P-glycoprotein inhibitors or inducers, and obesity with a BMI > 40 kg/m^2. Dabigatran is not metabolized by the CYP450 system, but is a substrate for P-glycoprotein (P-Glp). Use of dabigatran with inducers of P-Glp, such as rifampin, reduces the anticoagulant effect. The anticoagulant effect is enhanced when used concomitantly with P-Glp inhibitors such as ketoconazole, cyclosporine, dronedarone, or verapamil, especially in patients with renal failure [91].

Rivaroxaban is a direct factor Xa inhibitor under the brand name Xarelto. This medication should be avoided in patients with renal failure (Cr clearance <30 mL/min). DDIs are noted in medications that are dual inhibitors of CYP-3A4 and P-Glp (ketoconazole, itraconazole, voriconazole, or ritonavir). However, those that inhibit one of the two pharmacokinetic systems do not have the same peak drug levels [91]. Strong inducers of CYP-3A4 have been shown to cause subtherapeutic levels of rivaroxaban in patients [92]. Strong inducers mentioned in the case report include rifampin, phenytoin, carbamazepine, and phenobarbital.

Apixaban is another factor Xa inhibitor under the brand name Eliquis. Apixaban has the least dependence on renal clearance, and it is recommended to avoid use or alter dosage in medications that inhibit both CYP-3A4 and P-Glp. Additionally, strong inducers of either pharmacokinetic system can cause subtherapeutic anticoagulation. The use of aspirin or NSAIDs in combination with direct oral anticoagulants carries a higher bleeding risk due to the additional antiplatelet effect [93].

46.3.3 Antiplatelet DDIs

Clopidogrel is often utilized in dual antiplatelet therapy following revascularization procedures, and several studies have demonstrated variability of the antiplatelet effect. Clopidogrel is a prodrug with several steps involved in its metabolism with several DDIs involving the CYP450 system. Earlier studies showed a relationship with CYP3A4-metabolized statins (atorvastatin and simvastatin) and decreased effect of clopidogrel. However, recent studies showed that patients receiving both CYP3A4-metabolized statin and clopidogrel had less major adverse cardiovascular events than those not taking statins [94].

Proton pump inhibitors (PPIs) have been associated with a decreased antiplatelet effect in patients taking clopidogrel, but a recent systemic review [95] showed little validity to prior conclusions with no adverse effects seen clinically. Calcium channel blockers inhibit CYP3A4 which can result in decreased metabolism of clopidogrel. Several studies have shown that CCB attenuates the platelet inhibition of clopidogrel [96]; however, not all studies show that this effect is clinically significant. A study involving 56,800 patients with 24,923 on clopidogrel of which 13,380 were taking CCBs showed no increase in adverse cardiovascular events [97], and it is recommended to continue CCBs in light of dual antiplatelet therapy. Additionally, if a patient is receiving DAPT, the necessity of an elective maxillofacial procedure is questionable. Other medications that inhibit CYP3A4 are erythromycin, troleandomycin, and ketoconazole. Upregulation/induction of CYP3A4 activity is caused by St. John's wort and rifampin. Therefore, patients receiving these medications concomitantly may have increased risk of bleeding and/or excessive bleeding.

Aspirin is an essential antiplatelet medication used in the DAPT following coronary revascularization procedures. Aspirin is unique in that it has relatively less DDIs than other antiplatelet agents due to its metabolism involving carboxylesterase rather than the CYP450 system. The antiplatelet effect occurs through irreversible inhibition of COX-1 and its production of thromboxane A2 with 99% inhibition over 7–10 days. Interestingly, when ibuprofen is administered prior to or concomitantly, the COX-1 effect was transient with only 50% following discontinuation of the NSAID. However, if given with rofecoxib, acetaminophen, or diclofenac prior to aspirin, or ibuprofen following aspirin, the thromboxane 2 serum levels at 24 h were similar to that of aspirin alone [98, 99]. An observational study involving 7000 patients on secondary prevention demonstrated a higher cardiovascular mortality in patients taking both aspirin and ibuprofen versus aspirin alone [100]. Therefore, the DDI between aspirin and some NSAIDS might increase cardiovascular risk in those taking both agents.

Aspirin and PPIs is an area of controversy with large retrospective study showing increased cardiovascular events in patients taking aspirin and a PPI [101]. A follow-up study in the UK showed the opposite in that there was no difference between the groups [102]. Theoretically the higher pH from PPI use could limit the absorption of aspirin from the stomach as shown in rat studies [103]. Largely the data shows that PPI blunting the antiplatelet effect of aspirin is unproven.

SSRIs alone inhibit platelet aggregation due to decreased intra-granule storage of serotonin [104]. SSRIs in combination with aspirin act synergistically with an inhibitory effect on platelets [99]. A large retrospective study involving 27,000 post-MI patients demonstrated a 42% difference in hospitalization due to bleeding in patients taking both SSRIs and aspirin vs. those taking aspirin alone [105]. Therefore, it is worth exploring other options for control of depression in patients at risk for bleeding or procedures that may have increased risk of perioperative bleeding.

Low-dose aspirin has relatively little effect on renal hemodynamics due to little inhibition of renal prostaglandin production. Patients receiving multiple medications to treat hypertension will have little to no effect on the blood pressure [106]. Multiple large studies such as the ACE Inhibitors Collaborative Group, OPTIMIZE-HF (Organized Program to Initiate Lifesaving Treatment in Hospitalized Patients with Heart Failure), and LIFE (Losartan Intervention for Endpoint Reduction in Hypertension) Trial showed no adverse effects in patients receiving both aspirins with either an ACE inhibitor or an ARB [107–110].

46.3.4 Heparin-Induced Thrombocytopenia, Drug Interaction, and Treatment

Heparin-induced thrombocytopenia (HIT) is different from other conditions affecting the number of platelets in that it is a paradoxical prothrombotic state [111]. This prothrombotic state must be recognized quickly and treated promptly. One in 5000 patients develops HIT and is more often seen in those receiving unfractionated heparin for 7–10 days with a history of recent major surgery. Studies have reported a 1–3% incidence following cardiac surgery [112]. HIT typically develops between 5 and 10 days following initiation of heparin therapy and those who have received heparin therapy within the past 90 days prior to restarting therapy [113, 114]. The latter example is due to circulating antiplatelet fact 4 (PF4)—heparin antibodies, which can cause an abrupt onset following reexposure. HIT is identified by decrease in platelet count of more than 50% from the highest platelet count prior to exposure, hypercoagulability, and presence of heparin-dependent, platelet-activating IgG antibodies. When HIT is recognized, the clinician must immediately stop heparin therapy and start one of two drugs approved for the treatment of HIT. These medications are the direct thrombin inhibitor argatroban and the antithrombin-dependent factor Xa inhibitor danaparoid [115]. An analysis of danaparoid-treated HIT outcomes showed a 90% success. Success was defined as a platelet count recovery without new thrombosis and no major adverse events requiring cessation of danaparoid [116]. A review of prospective cohort studies showed a significant reduction in risk of new thrombosis, amputation due to thrombosis, or death due to thrombosis in patients treated with argatroban [117]. Fondaparinux and bivalirudin have been used in this context with several studies showing good outcomes; however, its use has not been evaluated by the FDA [115, 118–120]. Additionally, vitamin K antagonists (VKA) should not be used in the setting of HIT until the condition has abated (platelets >150,000 per cubic millimeter) because of the decreased protein C levels, which can result in limb gangrene and limb loss [115]. A patient can eventually be switched to warfarin or another VKA when the platelet count has normalized. It is recommended to continue anticoagulation for at least 3 months following HIT associated with thrombosis, but evidence is lacking for duration of treatment for HIT without thrombosis [118]. HIT is an example of a drug interaction resulting in a prothrombotic state, and the immediate recognition and prompt treatment with the proper anticoagulants can significantly increase the chances of successful treatment.

Conclusion

A review of pharmacology, the enzyme systems, and patterns of interactions facilitate the use of the framework provided in this chapter to recognize potential DDIs. Computer-based systems do not have the capability to alert or flag these interactions, and the use of this framework will help circumvent avoidable complications. The clinical importance of recognizing drug-drug interactions cannot be overemphasized. The use of fixed drug regimens in the perioperative period can be lethal for the patient. The potential for serious morbidity and mortality is illustrated by examples of fatal to near-fatal DDIs documented in the literature.

References

1. Wittwer ED, Nicholson WT. Pharmacodynamic interactions: core concepts. In: Marcucci C, et al., editors. A case approach to perioperative drug-drug interactions. New York: Springer; 2015. p. 9–14.
2. Hendrickx JF, Eger EI 2nd, Sonner JM, et al. Is synergy the rule? A review of anesthetic interactions producing hypnosis and immobility. Anesth Analg. 2008;107:409–506.
3. Wittwer ED, Nicholson WT. Pharmacokinetic interactions: core concepts. In: Marcucci C, et al., editors. A case approach to perioperative drug-drug interactions. New York: Springer; 2015. p. 15–20.
4. Kupferschmidt HH, Ha HR, Ziegler WH, et al. Interaction between grapefruit juice and midazolam in humans. Clin Pharmacol Ther. 1995;58:20–8.
5. Badyal DK, Dadhich AP. Cytochrome P450 and drug interactions. Indian J Pharmacol. 2001;33:248–59.
6. Leucuta SE, Vlase L. Pharmacokinetics and metabolic drug interactions. Curr Clin Pharmacol. 2006;1:5–20.

7. Williams JA, Ring BJ, Cantrell VE, et al. Comparative metabolic capabilities of CYP3A4, CYP3A5, and CYP3A7. Drug Metab Dispos. 2002;30:883–91.
8. Moore PA, Burney RG. The interaction of morphine and meperidine with analgesic, convulsant and lethal properties of lidocaine in mice. Toxicol Appl Pharmacol. 1979;49:279–82.
9. DeCou J, Birgenheier N, RO DullCYP3A4: the workhorse. In: Marcucci C et al., editor. A case approach to perioperative drug-drug interactions. New York: Springer; 2015. p. 37–40.
10. Sanders JC, Koll R, Dull RO. CYP2D6: where it All Began. In: Marcucci C, et al., editors. A case approach to perioperative drug-drug interactions. New York: Springer; 2015. p. 29–32.
11. Gmelch BS, Dull RO. CYP2E1: the anesthesia enzyme. In: Marcucci C, et al., editors. A case approach to perioperative drug-drug interactions. New York: Springer; 2015. p. 33–6.
12. Coyle D, Dull RO. CYP2B: 2B or not 2B? In: Marcucci C, et al., editors. A case approach to perioperative drug-drug interactions. New York: Springer; 2015. p. 45–6.
13. Fergerson BD, Wallentine CB, Dull RO. CYP2C9: the support crew I. In: Marcucci C, et al., editors. A case approach to perioperative drug-drug interactions. New York: Springer; 2015. p. 49–51.
14. Dresser GK, Spence JD, et al. Pharmacokinetic-pharmacodynamic consequences and clinical relevance of cytochrome P-450 3A4 inhibition. Clin Pharmacokinet. 2000;38(1):41–57.
15. Pal D, Mitra AK. MDR- and CYP3A4-mediated drug-herbal interactions. Life Sci. 2006;78(18):2131–45.
16. Voronov P, Przybylo HJ, Jagannathan N. Apnea in a child after oral codeine: a genetic variant—an ultra-rapid metabolizer. Paediatr Anaseth. 2007;17(7):684.
17. Lantz MS, Buchalter EN, Giambanco V. Serotonin syndrome following the administration of tramadol with paroxetine. Int J Geriatr Psychiatry. 1998;13(5):343–5.
18. Kharasch ED, Thummel KE. Identification of cytochrome P450 2 E1 as the predominant enzyme catalyzing human liver microsomal defluorination of sevoflurane, isoflurane, and methoxyflurane. Anesthesiology. 1993;79:795–807.
19. Sandson NB. Drug-drug interaction primer: a compendium of case vignettes for the practicing clinician. Aerlington: American Psychiatric Publishing, Inc; 2007. p. 359–60.
20. Stresser D, Kupfer D. Monospecific antipeptide antibody to cytochrome P-450 2B6. Drug Metab Dispos. 1999;27(4):517–25.
21. Turpeinen M, Raunio H, Pelkonen O, et al. The functional role of CYP2B6 in human drug metabolism: substrates and inhibitors in vitro, in vivo, and in silico. Curr Drug Metab. 2006;7(7):705–14.
22. Palovaara S, Pelkonen O, Uusitalo J, et al. Inhibition of cytochrome P450 2B6 activity by hormone replacement therapy and oral contraceptive as measure by bupropion hydroxylation. Clin Pharmacol Ther. 2003;74(4):326–33.
23. Turnpeinen M, Tolonen A, Uusitalo J, et al. Effect of clopidogrel and ticlopidine on cytochrome P450 2B6 activity as measured by bupropion hydroxylation. Clin Pharmacol Ther. 2005;77(6):553–9.
24. Faucette SR, Wang H, Hamilton GA, et al. Regulation of CYP2B6 in primary human hepatocytes by prototypical inducers. Drug Metab Dispos. 2004;32(3):348–58.
25. Ramirez J, Innocenti F, Schuetz EG, et al. CYP2B6, CYP3A4, and CYP2C19 are responsible for the in vitro N-demethylation of meperidine in human liver microsomes. Drug Metab Dispos. 2004;32(9):930–6.
26. Zhou SF, Zhou ZW, Huang M. Polymorphisms of human cytochrome P450 2C9 and the functional relevance. Toxicology. 2010;278(2):165–88.
27. Miners JO, Birkett DJ. Cytochrome P4502C9: an enzyme of major importance in human drug metabolism. Br J Clin Pharmacol. 1998;45(6):525–38.
28. Sandson NB, Hutchens MP, Seagull FJ, Marucci C. The "Fatal Forty". In: Marcucci C, et al., editors. A case approach to perioperative drug-drug interactions. New York: Springer; 2015. p. 73–80.
29. Ketter TA, Flockhart DA, Post RM, et al. The emerging role of cytochrome P450 3A in psychopharmacology. J Clin Psychopharmacol. 1995;15(6):387–98.
30. Sandson NB, Marcucci C. The six patterns of pharmacokinetic drug-drug interactions. In: Marcucci C, et al., editors. A case approach to perioperative drug-drug interactions. New York: Springer; 2015. p. 81–5.
31. Gillman PK. Monoamine oxidase inhibitors, opioid analgesics, and serotonin toxicity. Br J Anaesth. 2005;95:434–41.
32. Boyer EW, Shannon M. The serotonin syndrome. N Engl J Med. 2005;352:1112–20.
33. Stack CG, Rogers P, Linter SP. Monoamine oxidase inhibitors and anesthesia: a review. Br J Anaesth. 1988;60:222–7.
34. Altman EM, Manos GH. Serotonin syndrome associated with citalopram and meperidine. Psychosomatics. 2007;48:361–3.
35. Guo SL, TJ W, Liu CC, et al. Meperidine-induced serotonin syndrome in a susceptible patient. Br J Aneasth. 2009;103:369–70.
36. Das PK, Warkentin DI, Hewko R, et al. Serotonin syndrome after concomitant treatment with linezolid and meperidine. Clin Infect Dis. 2008;46:264–5.
37. Taylor JJ, Wilson JW, Estes LL. Linezolid and serotonergic drug interactions: a retrospective survey. Clin Infect Dis. 2006;43:180–7.
38. Sporer KA. The serotonin syndrome: implicated drugs, pathophysiology and management. Drug Saf. 1995;13:94–104.

39. Isbister GK, Buckley NA, Whyte IM. Serotonin toxicity: a practical approach to diagnosis and treatment. Med J Aust. 2007;187:361–5.
40. Kenyon Laundre CA, Flick R, Sprung J. A shuddering interaction (Meperidine, phenelzine, serotonin syndrome). In: Marcucci C, et al., editors. A case approach to perioperative drug-drug interactions. New York: Springer; 2015. p. 275–9.
41. Wittwer ED, Weingarten TN, Sprung J. Linezolid (II) hyper and hot (linezolid, meperidine, serotonin syndrome). In: Marcucci C, et al., editors. A case approach to perioperative drug-drug interactions. New York: Springer; 2015. p. 509–12.
42. Pederson KJ, Kuntz DH, Gerbe GJ. Acute myocardial ischemia associated with ingestion of bupropion and pseudoephedrine in a 21-year-old man. Can J Cardiol. 2001;17(5):599–601.
43. Manini AF, Kabrhel C, Thomsen TW. Acute myocardial infarction after over-the-counter use of pseudoephedrine. Ann Emerg Med. 2005;45(2):213–6.
44. Wiener I, Tilkian AG, Palazzolo M. Coronary artery spasm and myocardial infarction in a patient with normal coronary arteries: temporal relationship to pseudoephedrine ingestion. Catheter Cardiovasc Diagn. 1990;20(1):51–3.
45. Yap KY, Chui WK, Chan A. Drug interactions between chemotherapeutic regimens and antiepileptics. Clin Ther. 2008;30:1385–407.
46. Mamiya K, Yukawa E, Matsumoto T, et al. Synergistic effect of valproate co-administration and hypoalbuminemia on the serum-free phenytoin concentration in patients with severe motor and intellectual disabilities. Clin Neuropharmacol. 2002;25:230–1.
47. Johnson GJ, Kilpatrick CJ, Bury RW, et al. Unbound phenytoin plasma concentrations in patients co-medicated with sodium valproate—the predictive value of plasma albumin concentration. Br J Clin Pharmacol. 1989;27:843–9.
48. Dahlqvist R, Borga O, Rane A, et al. Decreased plasma protein binding of phenytoin in patients on valproic acid. Br J Clin Pharmacol. 1979;8:547–52.
49. Palm R, Silseth C, Alvan G. Phenytoin intoxication as the first symptom of fatal liver damage induced by sodium valproate. Br J Clin Pharmacol. 1984;17:597–9.
50. Levy RH, Koch KM. Drug interactions with valproic acid. Drugs. 1982;24:543–56.
51. Von Winckelmann SL, Spriet I, Willems L. Therapeutic drug monitoring of phenytoin in critically ill patients. Pharmacotherapy. 2008;28:1391–400.
52. Nau H, Loscher W. Valproic acid and metabolites. Pharmacologic and toxicological studies. Epilepsia. 1984;25(Suppl 1):S14–22.
53. Bjornsson E. Hepatoxicity associated with antiepileptic drugs. Acta Neurol Scand. 2008;118:281–90.
54. Macri E, Brambrink AM, Sandson N. The funeral is on Monday (fatal forty DDI: phenytoin, valproic acid, CYP2C9). In: Marcucci C, et al., editors. A case approach to perioperative drug-drug interactions. New York: Springer; 2015. p. 757–61.
55. Moore PA. Adverse drug interactions in dental practice: interactions associated with local anesthetics, sedatives, and anxiolytics (part IV of a series). Clin Pharm. 1999;130:541–54.
56. Yagiela JA, Picozzi A. General mechanisms of drug interactions. In: Yagieal JA, Niede EA, Dowd FJ, editors. Pharmacology and therapeutics for dentistry. 4th ed. St. Louis: Mosby-Year Book; 1998. p. 61–8.
57. Loewe S. Antagonism and antagonists. Pharmacol Rev. 1957;9:237–42.
58. Daos FG, Lopez L, Virtue RW. Local anesthetic toxicity modified by oxygen and combination of agents. Anesthesiology. 1962;23:755–9.
59. Haas DA. An update on local anesthetics in dentistry. J Can Dent Assoc. 2002;68(9):546–51.
60. Council on Clinical Affairs, American Academy of Pediatric Dentistry. Guideline on use of local anesthesia for pediatric dental patients. Pediatr Dent. 2015;37:71–7.
61. Moore PA. Prevention of local anesthesia toxicity. JADA. 1983;123:60–4.
62. Goodson J, Moore PA. Life-threatening reactions following pedodontic sedation: an assessment of narcotic, local anesthetic and antiemetic drug interaction. JADA. 1983;107:239–45.
63. Burbridge M, Jaffe RA. Exparel®: a new local anesthetic with special safey concerns. Anesth Analg. 2015;121(4):1113–4.
64. Uskova A, O'Connor JE. LipΓsomal bupivacaine for regional anesthesia. Curr Opin Anesthesiol. 2015;28(5):593–7.
65. Exparel [Package Insert]. San Diego: Pacira Pharmaceuticals, Inc.; 2014.
66. Cianco SG, editor. ADA guide to dental therapeutics. Chicago: ADA Publishing Co.; 1998.
67. Moore PA, Goodson JM. Risk appraisal of narcotic sedation for children. Anesth Prog. 1985;32:129–39.
68. Smudski JW, Sprecher RL, Elliot HW. Convulsive interactions of promethazine, meperidine and lidocaine. Arch Oral Biol. 1964;9:595–600.
69. Burney RG, DiFazio CA, Foster JA. Effects of pH on protein binding of lidocaine. Anesth Analg. 1978;57:478–80.
70. Lambertsen CJ, Wendel H, Longenhagen JB. The separate and combine respiratory effects of chlorpromazine and meperidine in normal men controlled at 46 mmHg alveolar pCO_2. J Pharmacol Exp Ther. 1961;131:381–93.
71. deJong RH, Wagman IH, Prince DA. Effect of carbon dioxide on the cortical seizure threshold to lidocaine. Exp Neurol. 1967;17:221–32.
72. Sokoloff L. The effect of carbon dioxide on the cerebral circulation. Anesthesiology. 1960;21:664–73.
73. Kharasch ED, Regina KJ, Blood J, Friedel C. Methadone pharmacogenetics: CYP2B6 polymor-

phisms determine plasma concentrations, clearance, and metabolism. Anesthesiology. 2015;123:1142–53.
74. Paulozzi LJ, Mack KA, Jones CM. Vital signs: risk for overdose from methadone used for pain relief—United State, 1999–2010. Morb Mortal Wkly Rep. 2012;61:493–7.
75. Baxter LE Sr, Campbell A, Deshields M, Levounis P, Martin JA, McNicholas L, Payte JT, Salsitz EA, Taylor T, Wilford BB. Safe methadone induction and stabilization: report of an expert panel. J Addict Med. 2013;7:3777–86.
76. Zanger UM, Klein K. Pharmacogenetics of cytochrome P450 2B6 (CYP2B6): advances on polymorphisms, mechanisms, and clinical relevance. Front Genet. 2013;4:24.
77. Colic A, Alessandrini M, Pepper MS. Pharmacogenetics of CYP2B6, CYP2A6, and UGT2B7 in HIV treatment in African populations: focus on efavirenz and nevirapine. Drug Metab Rev. 2015;47:111–23.
78. Srivastava A, Kahan M. Methadone induction doses: are our current practices safe? J Addict Dis. 2006;25(3):5–13.
79. Shields LB, Hunsaker JC, Corey TS, et al. Methadone toxicity fatalities: a review of medical examiner cases in a large metropolitan area. J Forensic Sci. 2007;52(6):1389–95.
80. Center for Substance Abuse Treatment (CSAT). Medication-assisted treatment for opioid addiction in opioid treatment programs (Treatment improvement protocol [TIP] series 43). HHS publication no. (SMA) 08-4214. Rockville, MD: CSAT, Substance Abuse and Mental Health Services Administration; 2008.
81. Modesto-Lowe V, Brooks D, Petry N. Methadone deaths: risk factors in pain and addicted populations. J Gen Intern Med. 2010;9:898.
82. Webster LR, Cochella S, Dasgupta N, et al. An analysis of root causes for opioid-related overdose deaths in the United States. Pain Med. 2011;12:S26–35.
83. Warner TD, Mitchell JA. COX-2 selectivity alone does not define the cardiovascular risks associated with non-steroidal anti-inflammatory drugs. Lancet. 2008;371(9608):270–3.
84. Whelton A. Nephrotoxicity of nonsteroidal anti-inflammatory drugs: physiologic foundations and clinical implications. Am J Med. 1999;106:13S.
85. Lapi F, Azoulay L, Yin H, Nessim SJ, Suissa S. Concurrent use of diuretics, angiotensin converting enzyme inhibitors, and angiotensin receptor blockers with non-steroidal anti-inflammatory drugs and risk of acute kidney injury: nested case-control study. BMJ. 2013;346(8525):1–11.
86. Labbate LA, Fava M, Rosenbaum JF, et al. Drugs for treatment of bipolar disorders. In: Handbook of psychiatric drug therapy. 6th ed. Philadelphia: Lippincott Williams & Wilkins; 2010. p. 110.
87. Lopes RD, Horowitz JD, Garcia DA, Crowther MA, Hylek EM. Warfarin and acetaminophen interaction: a summary of the evidence and biologic plausibility. Blood. 2011;118(24):6269–73.
88. Bone KM. Potential interaction of *Ginkgo biloba* leaf with antiplatelet or anticoagulant drugs: what is the evidence? Mol Nutr Food Res. 2008;52:764–71.
89. Joffe HV, Xu R, Johnson FB, Longtine J, Kucher N, Goldhaver SZ. Warfarin dosing and cytochrome P450 2C9 polymorphisms. Thromb Haemost. 2004;91(6):1123–8.
90. Sconce EA, Khan TI, Wynne HA, et al. The impact of CYP2C9 and VKORC1 genetic polymorphism and patient characteristics upon warfarin dose requirements: proposal for a new dosing regimen. Blood. 2005;106:2329–33.
91. Nutesco E, Chuatrisorn I, Hellenbart E. Drug and dietary interactions of warfarin and novel oral anticoagulants: an update. J Thromb Thrombolysis. 2011;31:326–43.
92. Altena R, van Roon E, Folkeringa R, de Wit H, Hoogendoorn M. Clinical challenges related to novel oral anticoagulants: drug-drug interactions and monitoring. Haematologica. 2014;99(2):e26–7.
93. Walenga JM, Adiguzel C. Drug and dietary interactions of the new and emerging oral anticoagulants. Int J Clin Pract. 2010;64:835–8.
94. Schmidt M, Johansen MB, Maeng M, et al. Concomitant use of clopidogrel and statins and risk of major adverse cardiovascular events following coronary stent implantation. Br J Clin Pharmacol. 2012;74(1):161–70.
95. Focks J, Brouwer MA, van Oigen MGH, Lanas A, Bhatt DL, Verheugt FWA. Concomitant use of clopidogrel and proton pump inhibitors: impact on platelet function and clinical outcome—a systematic review. Heart. 2013;99:520–7.
96. Gremmel T, Steiner S, Seidinger D, Koppensteiner R, Panzer S, Kopp CW. Calcium-channel blockers decrease clopidogrel-mediated platelet inhibition. Heart. 2010;96:186–9.
97. Olesen JB, Gislason GH, Charlot MG, et al. Calcium-channel blockers do not alter clinical efficacy of clopidogrel after myocardial infarction. J Am Coll Cardiol. 2011;57(4):409–17.
98. Catella-Lawson F, Reilly MP, Kapoor SC, et al. Cyclooxygenase inhibitors and the antiplatelet effects of aspirin. N Engl J Med. 2001;345(25):1809–17.
99. Russo NW, Petrucci G, B Rocca. Aspirin, stroke, and drug-drug interactions. Vascul Pharmacol. 2016; 87:14-22. http://dx.doi.org/10.106/j.vph.2016.10.006. Accessed 17 Nov 2016.
100. MacDonald TM, Wei L. Effect of ibuprofen on cardioprotective effect of aspirin. Lancet. 2003;361:573–4.
101. Charlot M, Grove EL, Hansen PR, et al. Proton pump inhibitor use and risk of adverse cardiovascular events in aspirin treated patients with first time myocardial infarction: nationwide propensity score matched study. BMJ. 2011;342:2690.
102. Garcia Rodriguez LA, Johnsson S, Nagy P, Cea SL. Use of proton pump inhibitors and the risk of coronary events in new users of low-dose acetyl-

salicylic acid in UK primary care. Thromb Haemost. 2014;111:131–9.

103. Giraud MN, Sanduja SK, Felder TB, Illich PA, Dial EJ, Lichtenberger LM. Effect of omeprazole on the bioavailability of unmodified and phospholipid-complexed aspirin in rate. Aliment Pharmacol Ther. 1997;11:899–906.

104. Hoirisch-Clapauch S, Nardi AE, Gris JC, Brenner B. Are the antiplatelet and profibrinolytic properties of selective serotonin reuptake inhibitors relevant to their brain effects? Thromb Res. 2014;134:11–6.

105. Labos C, Dasgupta K, Nedjar H, Turecki G, Rahme E. Risk of bleeding associated with combined use of selective serotonin reuptake inhibitors and antiplatelet therapy following acute myocardial infarction. CMAJ. 2011;183:1835–43.

106. Hansson L, Zanchetti A, et al. Effects of intensive blood-pressure lowering and low-dose aspirin in patients with hypertension: principal results of the hypertension optimal treatment (HOT) randomized trial. HOT Study Group. Lancet. 1998;351:1755–62.

107. Zanchetti A, Hansson L, Leonetti G, Rahn KH, Ruilope L, Warnold I, Wedel H. Low-dose aspirin does not interfere with the blood pressure-lowering effects of antihypertensive therapy. J Hypertens. 2002;20:1015–22.

108. Teo KK, Yusuf S, Pfeffer M, Torp-Pedersen C, Kober L, Hall A, Pogue J, Latini R, Collins R. Effects of long-term treatment with angiotensin-converting-enzyme inhibitors in the presence or absence of aspirin: a systematic review. Lancet. 2002;360:1037–43.

109. Levy PD, Nandyal D, Welch RD, Sun JL, Pieper K, Ghali JK, Fonarow GC, Gheorghiade M, O'Connor CM. Does aspirin use adversely influence intermediate-term post-discharge outcomes for hospitalized patients who are treated with angiotensin-converting enzyme inhibitors or angiotensin receptor blockers? Findings from Organized Program to Facilitate Life-Saving Treatment in Hospitalized Patients with Heart Failure (OPTIMIZE-HF). Am Heart J. 2010;159:222–30.

110. Fossum E, Moan A, Kjeldsen SE, Devereux RB, et al. The effect of losartan versus atenolol on cardiovascular morbidity and mortality in patients with hypertension taking aspirin: the Losartan Intervention for End-point Reduction in hypertension (LIFE) study. J Am Coll Cardiol. 2005;46:770–5.

111. Greinacher A. Heparin-induced thrombocytopenia. N Engl J Med. 2015;373(3):253–61.

112. Warkentin TE, Levine MN, Hirsh J, et al. Heparin-induced thrombocytopenia in patients treated with low-molecular-weight heparin or unfractionated heparin. N Engl J Med. 1995;332:1330–5.

113. Warkentin TE, Kelton JG. Temporal aspects of heparin-induced thrombocytopenia. N Engl J Med. 2001;344:1286–92.

114. Warkentin TE, Greinacher A. Heparin-induced anaphylactic and anaphylactoid reactions: two distinct but overlapping syndromes. Expert Opin Drug Saf. 2009;8:129–44.

115. Warkentin TE, Greinacher A, Koster A, Lincoff AM. Treatment and prevention of heparin-induced thrombocytopenia: American College of Chest Physicians evidence- based clinical practice guidelines (8th edition). Chest. 2008;133(6 Suppl):340S–80S.

116. Chong BH, Magnani H. Danaparoid for the treatment of heparin-induced thrombocytopenia. In: Warkentin TE, Greinacher A, editors. Heparin-induced thrombocytopenia. 5th ed. New York: Informa Healthcare; 2013. p. 466–88.

117. Lewis BE, Wallis DE, Hursting MJ, Levine RL, Leya F. Effects of argatroban therapy, demographic variables, and platelet count on thrombotic risks in heparin- induced thrombocytopenia. Chest. 2006;129:1407–16.

118. Linkins LA, Dans AL, Moores LK, et al. Treatment and prevention of heparin-induced thrombocytopenia: antithrombotic therapy and prevention of thrombosis, 9th ed: American College of Chest Physicians evidence-based clinical practice guidelines. Chest. 2012;141(2 Suppl):e495S–530S.

119. Kang M, Alahmadi M, Sawh S, Kovacs MJ, Lazo-Langner A. Fondaparinux for the treatment of suspected heparin-induced thrombocytopenia: a propensity score-matched study. Blood. 2015;125: 924–9.

120. Bartholomew JR, Prats J. Bivalirudin for the treatment of heparin-induced thrombocytopenia. In: Warkentin TE, Greinacher A, editors. Heparin-induced thrombocytopenia. 5th ed. New York: Informa Healthcare; 2013. p. 429–65.

Postoperative Nausea and Vomiting as a Complication of Maxillofacial Surgery

47

Deepak G. Krishnan

Abstract

Postoperative and post-discharge nausea and vomiting are common complications following administration of general anesthesia or sedation for surgery. Postoperative nausea and vomiting (PONV) can severely impact postanesthetic recovery time and time to discharge and contribute to an overall patient dissatisfaction for the experience. The pathophysiology of PONV is clearly understood, and so are the risk factors associated with the complication. Management of the condition is done efficiently when all patients that present for surgery are assessed preoperatively and risk stratified for potential PONV. Consensus guidelines are available and updated frequently to help manage PONV. While management guidelines rely on pharmacologic agents, other strategies can also help prevent PONV and also help manage it effectively.

47.1 Complication

1. Cause of the complication: Postoperative and post-discharge nausea and vomiting are common complications following administration of general anesthesia or sedation for surgery. Postoperative nausea and vomiting (PONV) can severely impact postanesthetic recovery time and time to discharge and contribute to an overall patient dissatisfaction for the experience. PONV may be of greater concern for many patients than postoperative pain.

2. Pathophysiology: The terms used to describe symptoms of PONV may be confusing. The American Gastroenterological Association (AGA) has defined these entities separately [1]. Vomiting is defined as a forceful oral expulsion of gastric contents associated with contraction of the abdominal and chest wall musculature. Nausea on the other hand is an unpleasant sensation of the imminent need to vomit, usually referred to the throat or epigastrium, a sensation that may or may not ultimately lead to the act of vomiting. The AGA also has specific definitions of retching, regurgitation, and other terms associated with the conditions.

D.G. Krishnan, D.D.S., F.A.C.S.
Oral Maxillofacial Surgery, University of Cincinnati, Cincinnati, OH, USA
e-mail: deepak.krishnan@uc.edu

© Springer International Publishing AG 2018

E.M. Ferneini, J.D. Bennett (eds.), *Perioperative Assessment of the Maxillofacial Surgery Patient*, https://doi.org/10.1007/978-3-319-58868-1_47

While the pathways of the vomiting reflex are fairly well understood, the specific pathways related to PONV have not been studied in detail. It is assumed that the same pathways of initiation of the vomiting reflex in chemotherapy are in play following exposure to a multitude of stimuli in general anesthesia and the perioperative period. Certain kinds of surgery such as middle ear procedures, brain manipulation, and maxillofacial procedures have a propensity to cause PONV over an orthopedic procedure, for instance.

The vomiting center which is located within the medulla can initiate the vomiting reflex based on triggers it receives from trigger zones in the brain (area postrema, fourth ventricle) or the trigger zones in the GI tract. Vagal afferents are also present in the liver, in the vestibule-cochlear apparatus, and also in the higher cortical centers of the brain. These higher cortical centers of the brain are implicated in nausea or vomiting associated with sensory input such as pain, smell, or sight and emotions such as fear, anticipation, or memory. Chemotherapy can influence receptors both in the GI tract and the central trigger zones. The medications such as anesthetics and opioid analgesics primarily influence the chemoreceptor trigger zone in the area postrema which then triggers the vomiting reflex [2].

Regardless of the pathway of the triggering of the reflex, the vomiting center influences the muscles of the thoracic cavity, the abdomen, and the diaphragm causing a cascade of well-orchestrated movements that forcefully expel the gastric contents.

3. Prevalence: The prevalence of this complication is high. It is estimated that about 25–30% of all surgical patients experience nausea and/or vomiting postoperatively [3–5]. Of these, about 30% of patients experience vomiting and close to 50% of all patients experience nausea. A subset of high-risk patients may have 70–80% incidence of PONV. PONV can often be a reason for unanticipated post-discharge readmissions.
4. Manifestations/presentation of disease. As noted above, a larger number of patients may experience nausea in the postoperative period than vomiting. Several patient-related factors are related to an increased risk of PONV. Manifestations of PONV are higher in the following group of patients [6]:
    - Adults
    - Non-smokers
    - History of motion sickness, previous history of PONV
    - Predisposing gastric disorders
    - Preoperative anxiety

Anesthetic risk factors that can predispose presentation of PONV include the following factors [6]:
- Preanesthetic medications—opioids, atropine
- Volatile anesthetics
- Intraoperative use of opioids
- Duration of anesthesia >120 min

Surgical risk factors that can contribute to the presentation of PONV include the following [6]:
- Duration of surgery (each 30 min increases PONV risk by 60%)
- Type of surgery—craniotomy, head and neck procedures, major breast procedures, strabismus surgery, laparoscopy, laparotomy, etc.

47.2 Patient Assessment

1. Monitoring: Standard gamut of ASA recommended PACU monitoring is recommended for patients with PONV in the acute postoperative phase. These include blood pressure and heart rate monitoring, oxygenation and ventilation monitoring, as well as temperature monitoring. Depending on the kind of procedure the patient had undergone, some specific wound monitoring may be indicated. Microvascular anastomosis may be disrupted from heaving and neck extension in vomiting. It is prudent to have closer flap monitoring for ensuring blood supply. Intraocular procedures require specific monitoring of globe pressures or implant position following vomiting. Pressure from the vomiting can also cause

bleeding in previously hemostatic wounds, and hematomas may not be uncommon. These can be extensive and may necessitate a trip back to the operatory.

2. Work-up

   History: Paying attention to the history of PONV is important in the preoperative assessment of the patient. A clear differentiation between a pre-existing nausea/vomiting problem and an anticipated PONV should be made early on. Pre-existing conditions that can cause nausea/vomiting may be acute or chronic. Some of the conditions that can cause acute nausea and vomiting may be associated with gastroenteritis, cholecystitis, pancreatitis, or an allergic reaction to a drug administered presurgically. Metabolic disorders, eating disorders, and psychiatric illnesses should be suspected in more chronic nausea and vomiting. The symptoms are defined as chronic if their duration is over a month. Pregnancy should be in the list of possible causes of new-onset or persistent nausea with or without vomiting in the age- and gender-appropriate patient. The characteristic of the vomiting may also provide a clue to its etiology. Projectile vomiting, for instance, may suggest an increase in intracranial pressure. Vomiting that occurs after about an hour of eating may suggest gastroparesis or gastric outlet obstruction, whereas in eating disorders such as anorexia nervosa or bulimia, vomiting happens immediately following ingestion of food. Weight loss associated with chronic vomiting may be suggestive of an underlying malignancy.

3. Risk scoring: Anticipation of the risk of PONV begins with appropriate preoperative assessment. The American Society of Anesthesiology (ASA) and the Society for Ambulatory Anesthesia (SAMBA) have published consensus guidelines for assessing risks for PONV in adults and postoperative vomiting (POV) in children [7].

   These guidelines present a risk scoring mechanism for all patients. The risk score calculator is a simplified risk scoring grid from a previous study from Apfel et al. [8] that helps predict a patient's risk for PONV. The calculator provides a point each for the female gender, non-smokers, history of PONV, and postoperative opioid administration. When 0, 1, 2, 3, and 4 of the risk factors are present, the corresponding risk for PONV is about 10%, 20%, 40%, 60%, and 80%, respectively. A similar scoring scale was adapted for children as well.

4. Laboratory tests and anticipated results

If chronic nausea and vomiting is suspected from the patient's history, further investigations may be warranted. The preoperative investigations will be directed by the patient's history. Basic laboratory testing including blood counts and electrolyte measures may be useful in identifying anemia or blood dyscrasias as well as electrolyte imbalances.

In patients presenting PONV in the PACU, investigations will be directed by the severity of the disease and presentation. Severe loss of fluids from emesis may warrant checking electrolytes. Severe heaving can cause rebleeds of wounds as well as pneumothoraxes. Lab testing may also provide initial clues to other underlying disorders that may be contributing to the condition such as hyponatremia in Addison's disease.

47.3 Management

1. Potential problems

   As noted earlier, management of PONV has significant implications on the patient's postsurgical recovery as well as discharge or readmission.

   General management strategies depend on the preoperative risk assessment of the potential PONV for every patient.

2. Patient management

The consensus guidelines published in 2014 [7] distill the current evidence behind preventive strategies and steps to minimize PONV. These are outlined in the following section on Prevention. While PONV prevention is recommended in a subset of patients, current evidence does not support giving prophylactic antiemetics to all patients who undergo surgical procedures. However, they suggest the following for pharmacologic interventions in prophylaxis of PONV in *adults*.

5-Hydroxytryptamine (5-HT_3) receptor antagonists (ondansetron, dolasetron, granisetron, tropisetron, ramosetron, and palonosetron)

Neurokinin-1 (NK-1) receptor antagonists (aprepitant, casopitant, and rolapitant)

Corticosteroids (dexamethasone and methylprednisolone)

Butyrophenones (droperidol and haloperidol)

Antihistamines (dimenhydrinate and meclizine)

Anticholinergics (transdermal scopolamine [TDS])

In those patients who have been deemed high risk for PONV by risk stratification, the recommendation is to administer prophylactic therapy with combination ($\geq$2) interventions/multimodal therapy. These patients benefit from not only the prophylactic administration of antiemetics but also combination of drugs such as midazolam and dexamethasone at induction as well as intraoperative strategies such as:

- Dexamethasone 8 mg IV at induction plus ondansetron 4 mg IV at the end of surgery plus ondansetron 8 mg PO postoperatively
- Haloperidol 2.5 mg plus dexamethasone 5 mg IV after induction

In patients that did not receive prophylaxis, if PONV does occur, the following guidelines are suggested:

- Treatment should be administered with an antiemetic from a pharmacologic class that is different from the prophylactic drug initially given.
- Or if no prophylaxis was given, the recommended treatment is a low-dose 5-HT_3 antagonist.
- Repeating the medication given for PONV prophylaxis within the first 6 h after the initial dose conferred no additional benefit.
- An evaluation should be performed to exclude an inciting medication or mechanical factor for nausea and/or vomiting.

47.3.1 Specific Drugs Used in Clinical Practice

5-HT_3 Receptor Antagonists: Ondansetron—trade name Zofran—is the current "gold standard" drug among antiemetics. Its recommended dose is 4 mg IV in adults, and the effect of an 8 mg disintegrating tablet has been proven to be the same as an IV dose. It is most effective when given at the end of surgery.

NK-1 Receptor Antagonists: Aprepitant—trade name Emend—is an antiemetic with a half-life of 40 h. Aprepitant (40 and 80 mg) has been shown to be similar to ondansetron in achieving complete response for 24 h after surgery. It is significantly more effective than ondansetron for preventing vomiting at 24 and 48 h after surgery and in reducing nausea severity in the first 48 h after surgery and thus proven to have a greater antiemetic effect compared with ondansetron. Our current clinical experience with this drug is limited, and its role in routine prophylaxis is not established.

Corticosteroid: Dexamethasone—trade name Decadron—has shown that a prophylactic dose of 4–5 mg IV for patients at increased risk for PONV works well especially when given after anesthesia induction rather than at the end of surgery. It has also been shown that dexamethasone 4 mg IV is similar to ondansetron 4 mg IV and droperidol 1.25 mg IV, when compared. Further, recent studies increasingly use the higher dose of dexamethasone 8 mg IV rather than the minimum effective dose of 4–5 mg. It enhances the post-discharge quality of recovery in addition to reducing nausea, pain, and fatigue, and patients that received it required less opioid and reported less nausea, sore throat, muscle pain, and difficulty falling asleep.

Transdermal Scopolamine Patch: It has been shown to be as useful as an adjunct to other antiemetic therapies. The patch effectively prevented nausea and vomiting postoperatively up to 24 h and can be applied the evening before surgery or 2–4 h before the start of anesthesia (2–4-h onset of effect). Its adverse events are generally mild, the most common being visual disturbances, dry mouth, and dizziness.

Propofol as an antiemetic: Propofol used as part of TIVA is recommended to reduce baseline risk for PONV. The use of propofol for induction and maintenance of anesthesia decreases the incidence of early PONV (occurring within the first 6 h). Propofol, in small doses (20 mg as needed), can be used for rescue therapy for patients in the direct care environment, for example, PACU, and has been found as effective as ondansetron.

Butyrophenones: Droperidol—Prophylactic doses of droperidol 0.625–1.25 mg IV are effective for the prevention of PONV. The efficacy of droperidol is similar to ondansetron for PONV prophylaxis and is most effective when administered at the end of surgery. The droperidol doses used for the management of PONV are extremely low, and at these dosing levels, droperidol is unlikely to be associated with significant cardiovascular events. Several studies have documented the equal QT effects of droperidol versus ondansetron.

47.4 Prevention

Prevention of PONV refers to the strategies recommended by the ASA in reducing baseline risk of the complication [9]. These include:

- Avoidance of general anesthesia and using regional or local anesthesia whenever possible in patients with high risk of PONV
- Avoidance of volatile anesthetics including nitrous oxide
- Preferential use of propofol infusions
- Minimizing administration of intraoperative and postoperative opioids
- Maintaining adequate hydration

Conclusion

It is estimated that about 25–30% of all surgical patients experience nausea and/or vomiting postoperatively. Preoperative risk assessment helps prevent and manage this complication effectively. The consensus guidelines published by the ASA in 2014 present management strategies based on the current evidence. A multimodal approach including pharmacologic and non-pharmacologic approaches helps prevent and manage PONV. There are newer-generation medications being tested in chemotherapy-induced nausea and vomiting that are expected to be useful in the management of PONV currently being tested. These offer further hope for managing this unpleasant complication in our patients.

References

1. American Gastroenterological Association. American Gastroenterological Association medical position statement: Nausea and vomiting. Gastroenterology. 2001;120:261–2.
2. Naylor RJ, Inall FC. The physiology and pharmacology of postoperative nausea and vomiting. Anaesthesia. 1994;49(Suppl):2–5.
3. Quigley EMM, Hasler WL, Parkman HP. AGA technical review on nausea and vomiting. Gastroenterology. 2001;120:263–86.
4. Koivuranta M, Läärä E, Snåre L, Alahuhta S. A survey of postoperative nausea and vomiting. Anaesthesia. 1997;52:443–9.
5. Sinclair DR, Chung F, Mezei G. Can postoperative nausea and vomiting be predicted? Anesthesiology. 1999;91:109–18.
6. ASHP therapeutic guidelines on the pharmacologic management of nausea and vomiting in adult and pediatric patients receiving chemotherapy or radiation therapy or undergoing surgery. Am J Health Syst Pharm. 1999;56(8):729–64.
7. Gan TJ, Diemunsch P, Habib AS, Kovac A, Kranke P, Meyer TA, Watcha M, Chung F, Angus S, Apfel CC, Bergese SD, Candiotti KA, Chan MT, Davis PJ, Hooper VD, Lagoo-Deenadayalan S, Myles P, Nezat G, Philip BK, Tramèr MR. Consensus guidelines for the management of postoperative nausea and vomiting. Society for Ambulatory Anesthesia. Anesth Analg. 2014;118(1):85–113.
8. Apfel CC, Läärä E, Koivuranta M, Greim CA, Roewer N. A simplified risk score for predicting postoperative nausea and vomiting: conclusions from cross-validations between two centers. Anesthesiology. 1999;91:693–700.
9. Apfel CC, et al. A factorial trial of six interventions for the prevention of postoperative nausea and vomiting. N Engl J Med. 2004;350:2441–51.

48 Aspiration as a Complication of Maxillofacial Surgery

Frank Paletta, Tian Ran Zhu, and Douglas Johnson

Abstract

Aspiration is a complication, though infrequent, that can occur with maxillofacial surgical procedures. The goal of this chapter is to review definitions and discuss prevalence, preoperative patient risk factors, potential preventive measures, identification, treatment, and the most recent standard of care protocols.

48.1 Introduction

Aspiration in maxillofacial surgery, while rare, is a known serious complication that warrants urgent clinical recognition and timely surgical and medical intervention to minimize potentially fatal consequences. Pulmonary aspirations of oropharyngeal secretions, gastric contents, and foreign bodies are some of the most feared complications of oral surgical procedures and have life-threatening consequences. We recommend these key principles of preventing aspiration by identifying patients with increased risk for aspiration, keeping patients nil per os (NPO) at least 6 h prior to surgery with strict exclusion of solid foods and liquids, administering appropriate medications aimed at promoting gastric emptying and inhibiting acid production in those patients deemed at increased aspiration risk, and employing necessary perioperative maneuvers by the anesthesia team. In particular, we will consider the epidemiology, etiology, underlying risk factors, and pathophysiology of this condition and discuss the management and preventative strategies for treating the complications of and minimizing the risks for pulmonary aspiration.

48.2 Cause of the Complication

Aspirated materials include foreign bodies, gastric contents, and oropharyngeal secretions. Foreign body aspiration during oral surgery includes whole or fragmented tooth, sponges, dentures, coagulated blood, bite blocks, and sur-

F. Paletta, M.D., D.M.D., F.A.C.S. (✉)
MSL Facial and Oral Surgery, Warwick, RI, USA

Warren Alpert Medical School, Brown University, Providence, RI, USA
e-mail: docpaletta@cox.net

T.R. Zhu, M.D.
Warren Alpert Medical School, Brown University, Providence, RI, USA

D. Johnson, D.M.D.
Oral and Facial Surgical Center, St. Augustine, FL, USA

© Springer International Publishing AG 2018
E.M. Ferneini, J.D. Bennett (eds.), *Perioperative Assessment of the Maxillofacial Surgery Patient*, https://doi.org/10.1007/978-3-319-58868-1_48

gical instruments. Not uncommonly, maxillofacial trauma involves fractured maxilla and mandible and concomitant teeth fragments that become imminent aspiration hazards. Initial management must prioritize airway, breathing, and circulation and include evaluation of cervical spine stability as part of advanced trauma life support. While aspiration in both the left and right bronchial trees has been reported in literature, foreign bodies are most commonly found on the right side of the bronchial tree due to its vertical framework compared to the oblique angle that the left main stem bronchi takes after bifurcation from the trachea carina [1].

Aspiration pneumonitis is defined as an acute lung parenchyma injury that results from inhaling regurgitated gastric contents. As Marik and colleagues describe, this syndrome predominantly affects patients who have a marked impairment in consciousness secondary to cerebrovascular incident, drug overdose, seizure, or prolonged exposure to anesthesia [2]. Adnet and Baud further demonstrated that the risk of aspiration pneumonitis increases with the degree of unconsciousness as measured by the Glasgow Coma Scale (GCS) [3]. Patients with inadequately managed gastroesophageal reflux disease have increased proclivity for regurgitation of acidic gastric contents at time of surgery. Uncorrected hiatal hernia and diminished lower esophageal sphincter tone may exacerbate the frequency and severity of reflux. Other medical conditions that heighten the risk for aspiration pneumonitis include delayed gastric emptying or, more severely, gastroparesis secondary to diabetic autonomic neuropathy, atherosclerosis, vasculitis, or collagen vascular disease. Last, the recumbent position of the patient during surgery and length of anesthesia must also be acknowledged as contributing factors to the impairment of the normal protective mechanism against aspiration pneumonitis. In particular, in the recumbent position, the counteracting effect of gravity is lost; the physiologic kink that maintains the lower esophageal sphincter tone at the gastroesophageal junction weakens; and the intraabdominal pressure rises. These changes increase intrathoracic pressure, decrease lung compliance, and increase the likelihood of regurgitation of gastric contents.

On the contrary, aspiration pneumonia is an acute lung parenchyma infection that develops after inhaling colonized oropharyngeal secretions. Unlike aspiration pneumonitis, most cases of aspiration pneumonia are not witnessed. Thus, diagnosis hinges on radiographically evident pulmonary infiltrate in patients who are at increased risk for aspiration pneumonia. The most common causative pathogens in community-acquired aspiration pneumonia include *Streptococcus pneumoniae*, *Staphylococcus aureus*, and *Haemophilus influenzae*, whereas nosocomial aspiration pneumonia is caused by Gram-negative pathogens including *Pseudomonas aeruginosa* and *Klebsiella* [4]. As Marik and colleagues describe, any medical condition that increases the volume or bacterial burden of oropharyngeal secretions or impairs the natural respiratory defense mechanisms of patients increases the risk for aspiration pneumonia [2]. Additionally, certain patient populations are at increased risk of aspiration pneumonia including patients with neurologic disabilities and handicaps that preclude functioning gag reflex and normal swallowing mechanisms, the institutionalized patients, the elderly, and those with poor oral hygiene [5]. In fact, the most common cause of morbidity and mortality in patients afflicted with stroke is pulmonary complications from aspiration pneumonia. Conversely, factors that decrease the volume or bacterial burden of oropharyngeal secretions decrease the risk for aspiration pneumonia. Indeed, edentulous patients and elderly patients receiving aggressive oral care have reported lower incidence of aspiration events than their counter-peers [6].

48.3 Epidemiology

Ingestion or aspiration of foreign body has been reported in the literature to disproportionately affect pediatric population . Up to 80% of the reported aspiration events involve children below the age of 3 and food and inanimate objects constitute the majority of aspirated foreign bodies [7, 8]. On the contrary, in a review by Tiwana and colleagues, the ingestion and aspiration cases in adult stem primarily from loose dentures and broken orthodontic appliances to iatrogenic causes including implant components, fragmented teeth, and dental instruments [9]. As it pertains to dental and oral procedures, the incidences of aspiration and ingestion have been reported by many literature reviews. As early as 1971, Grossman and colleagues documented that up to 87% of foreign bodies were ingested into the gastrointestinal tract whereas 13% were aspirated into the respiratory tract [10]. Moreover, the occurrences per year was reported to be 0.018 in a survey of accidental ingestion and aspiration at Tokyo Dental College Hospital in 2010 [11]. The literature also demonstrated that while 90% of ingested foreign objects could pass through the gastrointestinal tract uneventfully, an approximate 10% of ingested foreign objects require endoscopic removal to minimize chemical and mechanical injury to the esophageal-gastric mucosa and subsequent perforation [10, 11]. Black and colleagues further determined that although bronchoscopy is effective in 99% of pediatric cases to retrieve aspirated foreign objects, the complication rate is between 2.4% and 5% [12].

The lack of sensitive and specific markers of aspiration pneumonia and pneumonitis complicates the reporting, diagnosis, and management of these two diseases. Nonetheless, Daniels and colleagues reported that aspiration pneumonia is the most common cause of morbidity and mortality in patients with dysphagia secondary to neurologic impairment, a condition that affects up to 600,000 patients each year in the United States [13]. Aspiration pneumonitis occurs more frequently in patients with altered level of consciousness. Olsson and colleagues in a query of 185,358 anesthetics cases, demonstrated that this condition is a recognized complication of general anesthesia, occurring at an annual rate of 1 per 3000 cases and accounting for approximately 10% to 30% of all deaths associated with anesthesia [14].

Last, Warner and colleagues in a retrospective study of nearly 120,000 elective procedures that require general anesthesia over a 6 year period at Mayo clinic found no serious morbidity or mortality from 42 pulmonary aspiration cases [15]. Both the incidence and severity of the pulmonary complications were largely attributed to the presence of comorbid conditions and emergent procedures [15].

48.4 Pathophysiology

Aspiration is defined by the inhalation of oropharyngeal or gastric contents into the tracheobronchial tree. Up to half of all healthy adults aspirate small amounts of oropharyngeal secretions during sleep but do not develop acute pulmonary injury [16]. Inherent defenses critical to preventing the complications of aspiration include active mucociliary transport, vigorous cough, and normal innate and adaptive immune response. In maxillofacial surgery that involves general anesthesia, these defenses are temporarily attenuated by induction and maintenance anesthesia drugs, which impede normal protective mechanisms to counter aspirated contents. During initial intubation and at time of extubation, direct mechanical friction and force of instruments against the larynx and trachea can instigate laryngeal spasm and render the normal cough, gag, and laryngeal reflexes nonfunctional. Additionally, anesthesia induces a transient lower esophageal sphincter relaxation, which diminishes the acute angle between the proximal stomach and the distal esophagus, a change that increases likelihood of gastroesophageal reflux.

With regards to tissue injury, aspiration pneumonitis causes direct chemical burn of tracheobronchial tree and lung parenchyma from acidic and gastric material. Following initial surface epithelial desquamation, a milieu of cytokines and arachidonic acid metabolites instigate a neutrophilic orchestrated inflammatory response to lung injury. The sloughing of respiratory mucosa can result in expectoration of frothy blood-tinged sputum while the inflammatory milieu results in low-grade fever, tachypnea, and malaise. The severity of lung injury increases as the aspirated gastric content volume increases and its pH decreases [17]. Traditionally, gastric contents are sterile environments, which can be perturbed in the setting of enteral feeding, gastroparesis, small bowel obstruction, ileus, or use of antacids, histamine H_2 receptor blockers, or proton-pump inhibitors [18]. Because of the increased bacterial colonization burden, aspiration of altered gastric content incites both chemical injury and also inflammatory response to bacterial infection. Moreover, organic factors such as diabetic autonomic neuropathy and systemic sclerosis and nonorganic factors such as anxiety and stress impair and delay gastric emptying. The pathophysiologic mechanism is an increase in gastric distension that weakens the lower esophageal sphincter tone, thereby increasing the likelihood for gastroesophageal reflux and aspiration of regurgitated gastric contents.

Aspiration of bacterial colonized nasopharyngeal and oropharyngeal secretions instigates an immune response to infection of pulmonary parenchyma. In surgical patients who are more likely to aspirate while in a recumbent position, the pulmonary infiltrate localizes to the posterior segments of upper lung lobes and apical segments of lower lung lobes [2]. On the contrary, patients who aspirate in an upright position, the infiltrate localizes to the basal segments of lower lobes. Not uncommonly, patients who have concurrent medical comorbidity that predispose to aspiration pneumonia are at higher risk of anesthesia and surgical-associated aspiration consequences. Examples include neurologic disability and dysphagia, in which impairment in function of one or more stages of swallowing, oral, pharyngeal, and esophageal, increases the risk of aspiration pneumonia. Individuals who have an increased proclivity to aspirate oropharyngeal secretions often have an impaired protective airway reflex secondary to muscle fatigue, lack of coordination when swallowing and breathing, or neurologic deficits that limit their ability to detect, organize, and control a bolus for swallowing.

48.5 Manifestations/Presentation of Disease

Initial signs and symptoms of foreign body aspiration include coughing, choking, gasping for air, inspiratory stridor, increased work of breathing, arterial hemoglobin oxygen desaturation, and acral and central cyanosis. Early complications of aspiration if left untreated can result in asphyxiation, atelectasis, pneumothorax, laryngeal edema, cardiac arrest, and death. In particular, aspiration of objects with sharp edges such as fragmented tooth roots, in addition to causing airway obstruction, may traumatize the lining of the respiratory tract and result in subsequent lung abscess, pneumonia, and/or reactive airway disease. Patients who aspirate gastric contents commonly are asymptomatic or present with symptoms ranging from a nonproductive cough to tachypnea, bloody sputum, broncho-laryngospasm, and respiratory distress 2–5 h after aspiration [2]. On the contrary, patients who aspirate colonized oropharyngeal contents present with fever, tachypnea, dyspnea, productive cough, and ruddy sputum. Left unrecognized and untreated, chronic aspiration can cause inflammation of lung tissue with subsequent development of fibrosis, bronchiectasis, infection, decreased functional lung capacity, respiratory failure, and death. In particular, without treatment, aspiration pneumonia can result in higher incidence of pulmonary cavitation, lung abscess formation, empyema, and pneumothorax [2]. Clinical signs and symptoms of chronic aspiration include dyspnea, hoarseness, halitosis, and dysphagia manifesting as coughing, choking, or gagging. Voice change is secondary to the chemical and mechanical trauma to the laryngeal apparatus critical to normal sound and speech production.

48.6 Potential Complications

For a witnessed aspiration event during oral surgery, we recommend immediate suctioning of the upper airway. If the aspiration occurred after extubation, reintubation is warranted unless the aspirated object is entrapped in the tracheal-bronchial tree that precludes endotracheal intubation. As Warner and colleagues advocated, those patients with clinically established aspiration events and do not develop symptoms such as cough, wheezing, or drop in baseline preoperative arterial oxygen saturation on room air within 1–2 h of observation are unlikely to have further respiration sequelae [15]. In their retrospective analysis, in all 42 patients in whom pulmonary aspiration occurred, none required additional intensive respiratory support or developed pulmonary complications [15]. Thus, we recommend disposition of these patients to home without further intervention or imaging. However, we advise immediate follow-up the evening of operation or the following morning to ensure these patients remain asymptomatic. For patients who develop any of the aforementioned symptoms, we recommend urgent admission to the hospital, preferably to an intensive care unit with supplemental oxygen, flexible bronchoscopy, and/or ventilatory support if necessary to maintain an $Sp_{O2} \geq 90\%$.

When radiographic imaging has confirmed ingestion past the distal esophagus, a trial period of observation can be performed for spontaneous foreign object self-expectoration through vigorous cough [19]. Unsuccessful extrusion of foreign object may warrant endoscopic retrieval. Radiographically confirmed aspiration requires urgent intervention with endoscopy. These modalities depend on whether the aspiration event occurred when the patient is awake or under general anesthesia. In an emergency, the awake patient with an airway obstruction should be placed in an upright or comfortable position and allowed to cough. If indicated the surgical sight should be packed off with a 4 in. by 4 in. gauze and the oropharynx suctioned. Digital traction of the tongue with gauze, tongue forceps, hemostat, or suture should be performed for visualization. Should coughing fail to alleviate the obstruction, then back slaps and Heimlich abdominal maneuver must be performed. If these measures are ineffective, then the patient must be transported to the nearest hospital immediately. Should the patient become unconscious, he or she should be placed in a supine position and BLS/ACLS initiated and 911 activated according to Advanced Protocols for Medical Emergencies (AAOMS). In a controlled surgical environment, illumination of the oral cavity and the use of forceps can reveal and remove entrapped objects within the supratonsillar recess, epiglottic vallecular, or piriform recess [7]. However, should the aspirated object travel further downstream of the respiratory tract, then endoscopy-guided removal is necessary.

As Zitzmann and colleagues advocate, bronchoscopy is the initial standard of care for removing inhaled foreign objects [20]. Indeed, initial orotracheal intubation followed by flexible bronchoscopy affords superb control of the airway while providing excellent visualization and allows distal airway access and immediate foreign body removal [1]. Moreover, in contrast to rigid bronchoscopy, flexible bronchoscopy through the tube allows better manipulation of the object with forceps while minimizing the chance of dropping the object in the oropharynx [21]. If left untreated, aspirated contents in the lung parenchyma can instigate chemical pneumonitis and lung abscess. While antibiotic therapy is the standard of care in patients with aspiration pneumonia, prophylactic use of antibiotic in patients in whom aspiration is suspected or witnessed is not recommended [2]. Even in the setting of fever, leukocytosis, and radiographically evident pulmonary infiltrate, antibiotics should not be given for aspiration pneumonitis. We discourage this approach because indiscriminate use of antibiotics for all aspiration events has not been shown to improve the clinical outcome but rather selects for resistant pathogens in patients with uncomplicated aspiration pneumonitis [2]. However, as Marik and colleagues demonstrated, antibiotics can be given to patients with aspiration pneumonitis associated with increased gastric colonization secondary to small bowel obstruction or delayed gastric emptying and in those patients whose aspiration pneumonitis fails to resolve within 48 h [2].

For patients with heightened risk for pulmonary aspiration especially those with dysphagia due to stroke, we strongly recommend initial swallow evaluation followed by additional behavioral, dietary, and medical strategies to reduce aspiration risk. For instance, patients are to be given a soft pureed diet and encouraged to eat with small bites and gradually advanced to more solid foods. The benefits of percutaneous endoscopic gastrostomy (PEG) tube, since its introduction in the mid-1800s, have been controversial. While it has the advantage over nasogastric tube for more effective delivery of daily nutrition, PEG tube has not been shown to be superior to nasogastric tube for preventing aspiration in these patients [22]. Moreover, feeding tubes offer no protection from colonized oropharyngeal secretions. Thus, for patients who are healthy and have minimal dysphagia but can control their oropharyngeal secretions, we recommend against feeding tubes in the postoperative convalescence. More effective measures at decreasing aspiration include elevating the patient's bed, encouraging regular deep inspiration exercises, having patient ambulate as early as tolerated, and efficacious patient education on healthy eating habits and maintaining adequate nutrition.

The majority of the pulmonary infections that follow oral surgery is caused by Gram-negative bacilli and anaerobes from aspiration of oropharyngeal secretions. Broad-spectrum antibiotic therapy and adequate pulmonary toiletry must be initiated urgently while waiting sputum culture and sensitivity results to better refine the antibiotic regimen. Generally, we advocate antibiotic agents with activity against Gram-negative organisms such as third-generation cephalosporin, fluoroquinolones, or piperacillin-tazobactam. In patients with severe periodontal disease, putrid sputum, or radiographically evident lung abscess, anaerobic coverage with clindamycin or metronidazole is warranted [2]. Of note, prior to administering fluoroquinolones in the elderly, the surgeon must inquire lower extremity musculoskeletal pathologies and onset of any new symptoms because of the associated risk of fluoroquinolone and tendon rupture. Incentive spirometry, early ambulation, suction clearance of expectorated secretions, and chest physical therapy are instrumental in alleviating postoperative aspiration pneumonia complications.

48.7 Prevention

Fundamental surgical technique principles must be espoused to minimize the risk of aspiration in oral surgery. Careful handling of soft tissue and bone reduces postoperative swelling, pain, bleeding, and aspiration risks. Of paramount importance is to achieve an adequate access to the surgical field. Great operative site visualization is accomplished through optimal patient positioning, excellent lighting, appropriate suctioning, and assiduous hemostasis. Central to visualization is appropriate placement of a pharyngeal protector to prevent aspiration. Options include placing a folded 4 in. by 4 in. gauze in the posterior oral pharynx. As an alternative for non-intubated patients, we recommend the use of a protective C-Sponge (Xemax Surgical Products) that acts to imbibe fluid and acts as a barrier to the oral pharyngeal complex. We caution against the use of 2 in. by 2 in. gauze as a pharyngeal barrier or as a tamponade to achieve hemostasis perioperatively. The small dimensions of the gauze increase the likelihood that it can become easily displaced and aspirated. It behooves the oral surgeon to establish an unimpeded path whether to extract an impacted tooth or create a plane to raise a flap or place an osteotomy cut. By removing the soft tissue and bone in a systematic fashion, the oral surgeon is better able to assess the anatomy of the teeth. For instance, malpositioned, impacted, or carious teeth are inherently more difficult to extract and may be obstructed by an adjacent tooth.

Initial panoramic radiograph and/or CT imaging can further assist the surgeon in determining whether to-be-extirpated tooth roots are curved or hindered by the bone. Tooth sectioning is a critical intervention to address these findings. The astute oral surgeon will employ such operative strategy to reduce the untoward consequences of excessive force such as fracture of the tooth, maxilla, or mandible that eject showers of fragments into the oral cavity. Last, controlled force must be employed to the protective surrounding bone and soft tissues. The oral surgeon must develop a feel for instrument engagement, amount of torque exerted, and force applied when using drills, osteotomes, rongeurs, and other surgical instruments.

Enhancements and advances in anesthesia care have tremendously reduced the rate of complications from perioperative pulmonary aspiration of oropharyngeal secretions and gastric contents. As promulgated by the American Society of Anesthesiologists (ASA), specific clinical practices for surgery that include general anesthesia include withholding solids and liquids for at least 6 h prior to surgery and prescribing pharmacologic agents that decrease gastric volume, reduce gastric acidity, enhance gastric emptying, and diminish postoperative nausea and vomiting [8, 23]. We strongly recommend effective and clear communication to patients the need for and rationale of perioperative fasting requirements. Verification of patient compliance with such stringent fasting requirements must be assessed and documented at the time of surgery [23].

Specifically, the ASA practice guidelines recommend for otherwise healthy infants (younger than 2 years), children (2–16 years), and adults fast from intake of clear liquids at least 2 h before procedures requiring general, regional, or sedation anesthesia [23]. The ASA members recommend that neonates younger than 44 gestational weeks and infants fast from intake of breast milk at least 4 h and infant formula at least 6 h before procedures requiring general, regional, or sedation anesthesia [23]. The ASA practice guidelines recommend children (2–16 years) and adults fast from solids and nonhuman milk 6 h before procedures requiring general, regional, or sedation anesthesia [23]. Intake of fried or fatty foods or meat may prolong gastric emptying time, thereby warranting additional fasting time of 8 h [23]. For patients who have no increased risk for pulmonary aspiration, ASA members recommend against the preoperative use of antacids (e.g., sodium citrate), gastrointestinal stimulants (e.g., metoclopramide), gastric acid blockers such as proton-pump inhibitors (e.g., omeprazole) and histamine-2 receptor antagonist (e.g., cimetidine), antiemetics (e.g., ondansetron), anticholinergics (e.g., glycopyrrolate), or combined multiple agents [23]. While these agents reduce gastric volume or acidity, enhance gastric emptying, or decrease incidence of emesis and reflux, they have not been shown to decrease perioperative pulmonary aspiration events [23].

Summary of fasting recommendations (*ASA 2010 Practice Guidelines for Preoperative Fasting and the Use of Pharmacologic Agents to Reduce the Risk of Pulmonary Aspiration: Application to Healthy Patients Undergoing Elective Procedures*)*, the following recommendations apply to healthy patients who are undergoing elective procedures. They are not intended for women in labor. Both the amount and type of food ingested must be considered when determining an appropriate fasting period.

Ingested material	Minimum fasting requirements (h)
Clear liquids	2
Breast milk	4
Infant formula	6
Nonhuman milk	6
Light meal	6

A thorough review of pertinent medical history and physical exam should be performed at the time of preoperative evaluation. Patient selection carries tremendous weight in minimizing aspiration risks in maxillofacial surgery. In particular, patients with pre-existing medical comorbidities that impair their natural protective airway mechanisms or gastrointestinal motility are at high risk for aspiration. These include patients with impaired upper airway reflexes and/or gastric emptying and fluid volume, e.g., cerebrovascular disease, neurologic disability such as Parkinson's disease, neuromuscular disorder such as myasthenia gravis, autoimmune disorder such as diabetes or systemic sclerosis, gastroesophageal reflux disease, patients who have tracheostomy, and patients who have reduced consciousness secondary to trauma and/or sedative medications and drugs. Anesthesia providers must recognize that these aforementioned conditions increase the likelihood of perioperative regurgitation and pulmonary aspiration. If the risk of aspiration is deemed high, antiemetic pharmacotherapy such as ondansetron in combination with promotility agents such as metoclopramide or gastric acid blockers such as cimetidine or omeprazole can be administered preoperatively to reduce gastric volume and acidity and minimize the risk of emesis, reflux, and pulmonary aspiration [23]. Thus it behooves the oral surgeon to be cognizant of both patient risk factors as well as anticipate complications of oral surgery and meticulously account for all teeth as part of initial diagnostic work-up. While aspiration or ingestion of foreign objects including surgical instruments is relatively uncommon risk during dental and oral procedures, it is reported as the second most common reason for aspiration in the lung [9]. Because of the serious morbidity and mortality associated with aspiration incidents, the importance of implementing precautions and adequate monitoring measures cannot be overlooked.

Conclusion

Complications are a part of oral and maxillofacial surgery. Aspiration, though rare, should be understood thoroughly by the practicing surgeon. Both medical and surgical causes are reviewed and the accompanying pathophysiology. The prevalence and epidemiology are discussed as well as medical and surgical preventive measures. Finally, appropriate work-up and management are reviewed for diagnosis and to enhance outcomes. The latest anesthesia guidelines are included for review and familiarization for best practice in care.

References

1. Debeljak A, Sorli J, Music E, Kecelj P. Bronchoscopic removal of foreign bodies in adults: experience with 62 patients from 1974–1998. Eur Respir J. 1999;14(4):792–5.
2. Marik PE. Aspiration pneumonitis and aspiration pneumonia. N Engl J Med. 2001;344(9):665–71.
3. Adnet F, Baud F. Relation between Glasgow Coma Scale and aspiration pneumonia. Lancet. 1996;348(9020):123–4.
4. Tuomanen EI, Austrian R, Masure HR. Pathogenesis of pneumococcal infection. N Engl J Med. 1995;332(19):1280–4.
5. Mann R, Srinivasan B, Baker A. Managing aspiration. Br Dent J. 2012;212(10):464–5.
6. Terpenning M, Bretz W, Lopatin D, Langmore S, Dominguez B, Loesche W. Bacterial colonization of saliva and plaque in the elderly. Clin Infect Dis. 1993;16(Suppl 4):S314–6.
7. Umesan UK, Chua KL, Balakrishnan P. Prevention and management of accidental foreign body ingestion and aspiration in orthodontic practice. Ther Clin Risk Manag. 2012;8:245–52.
8. Park JH, Owtad P, Milde B. Incident management guidelines for an ingested orthodontic object. Int J Orthod Milwaukee. 2013;24(3):45–9.
9. Tiwana KK, Morton T, Tiwana PS. Aspiration and ingestion in dental practice: a 10-year institutional review. J Am Dent Assoc. 2004;135(9):1287–91.
10. Grossman LI. Prevention in endodontic practice. J Am Dent Assoc. 1971;82(2):395–6.
11. Hisanaga R, Hagita K, Nojima K, et al. Survey of accidental ingestion and aspiration at Tokyo Dental College Chiba Hospital. Bull Tokyo Dent Coll. 2010;51(2):95–101.
12. Black RE, Johnson DG, Matlak ME. Bronchoscopic removal of aspirated foreign bodies in children. J Pediatr Surg. 1994;29(5):682–4.
13. Daniels SK, Brailey K, Priestly DH, Herrington LR, Weisberg LA, Foundas AL. Aspiration in patients with acute stroke. Arch Phys Med Rehabil. 1998;79(1):14–9.
14. Olsson GL, Hallen B, Hambraeus-Jonzon K. Aspiration during anaesthesia: a computer-aided study of 185,358 anaesthetics. Acta Anaesthesiol Scand. 1986;30(1):84–92.
15. Warner MA, Warner ME, Weber JG. Clinical significance of pulmonary aspiration during the perioperative period. Anesthesiology. 1993;78(1):56–62.
16. Huxley EJ, Viroslav J, Gray WR, Pierce AK. Pharyngeal aspiration in normal adults and patients with depressed consciousness. Am J Med. 1978;64(4):564–8.
17. Exarhos ND, Logan WD, Abbott OA, Hatcher CR. The importance of pH and volume in tracheobronchial aspiration. Dis Chest. 1965;47:167–9.
18. Bonten MJ, Gaillard CA, van der Geest S, et al. The role of intragastric acidity and stress ulcus prophylaxis on colonization and infection in mechanically ventilated ICU patients. A stratified, randomized, double-blind study of sucralfate versus antacids. Am J Respir Crit Care Med. 1995;152(6 Pt 1):1825–34.
19. Hou R, Zhou H, Hu K, et al. Thorough documentation of the accidental aspiration and ingestion of foreign objects during dental procedure is necessary: review and analysis of 617 cases. Head Face Med. 2016;12(1):23.
20. Zitzmann NU, Elsasser S, Fried R, Marinello CP. Foreign body ingestion and aspiration. Oral Surg Oral Med Oral Pathol Oral Radiol Endod. 1999;88(6):657–60.
21. Donado Uña JR, de Miguel PE, Casado López ME, Alfaro Abreu JJ. Fiber optic bronchoscopy in extraction of tracheo-bronchial foreign bodies in adults. Arch Bronconeumol. 1998;34(2):76–81.
22. Grant MD, Rudberg MA, Brody JA. Gastrostomy placement and mortality among hospitalized Medicare beneficiaries. JAMA. 1998;279(24):1973–6.
23. Practice guidelines for preoperative fasting and the use of pharmacologic agents to reduce the risk of pulmonary aspiration: application to healthy patients undergoing elective procedures: an updated report by the American Society of Anesthesiologists Committee on Standards and Practice Parameters. Anesthesiology. 2011;114(3):495–511.

Check for updates

Ophthalmologic Injuries as a Complication of Maxillofacial Surgery

49

Jeremy D. Clark and Hui Bae Harold Lee

Abstract

Managing traumatic injuries to the orbit and periorbital structures requires an individualized approach to these complex patients. The ideal surgical and medical plan is not always clear. The orbital specialist must use the most updated and appropriate recommendations from our own and other subspecialty studies to help guide this decision-making process.

49.1 Introduction

Trauma is the second leading cause of blindness in the United States, with 40,000 new cases of visual impairment occurring each year. The incidence of ocular injury associated with facial fractures, in retrospective reviews, varies from 2.7 to 67% [1]. In prospective studies, ocular injuries occurred in 25–29% of patients [2].

The risk of ocular injury is naturally greatest when orbital bones are involved. Fractures that decrease orbital bony volume, produce orbital soft-tissue hemorrhage, and extend to the optic canal have an added risk of secondary ocular or optic nerve injury. Ocular and extraocular injuries accompanying fracture-associated contusions may be minor and may not represent a serious threat to vision. On the other hand, serious ocular injuries can occur in association with those traumas of less apparent significance.

Awareness of the possibility and prompt recognition of the eye injury are critical to improved visual prognosis. Additionally, seriously injured patients may be obtunded or intoxicated, making communication difficult and unreliable. In this atmosphere, the diagnosis of serious eye injuries must not be delayed or overlooked.

The visual pathways perform the function of receiving, relaying, and processing visual information. The eye is responsible for collecting light, focusing it, and encoding the first neural signals of the visual pathway. The majority of blood supply to structures of the eye arrives via the ophthalmic artery, which is the first branch of

J.D. Clark, M.D.
Oculofacial Plastic and Orbital Surgery, Indianapolis, IN, USA

Department of Ophthalmology and Visual Sciences, University of Louisville, Louisville, KY, USA
e-mail: docclark83@gmail.com

H.B. Harold Lee, M.D., FACS (✉)
Oculofacial Plastic and Orbital Surgery, Indianapolis, IN, USA
e-mail: huibae@gmail.com

© Springer International Publishing AG 2018
E.M. Ferneini, J.D. Bennett (eds.), *Perioperative Assessment of the Maxillofacial Surgery Patient*, https://doi.org/10.1007/978-3-319-58868-1_49

the internal carotid artery. The ophthalmic artery enters the orbit through the optic canal, traveling beside the optic nerve. Once in the orbit, the ophthalmic artery branches into vessels supplying the globe (central retinal artery, the muscular artery, the anterior ciliary arteries, and the long and short posterior ciliary arteries) and vessels supplying other orbital structures (lacrimal artery, supraorbital artery, ethmoidal arteries, frontal artery, and nasal artery).

When light reaches the retina, energy is converted by retinal photoreceptors into an electrochemical signal relayed by neurons to the optic nerve, and the visual pathway travels posterior into the optic chiasm where there is a decussation of visual fibers from the nasal ganglion cells. The optic tracts, containing axons from the ipsilateral temporal retina and contralateral nasal retina, travel posterior through the cortex in multiple pathways to reach the primary visual cortex in the occipital lobe.

This chapter provides information essential to early diagnosis and insight into vision-threatening ocular injuries that commonly accompany facial fractures. It also provides a template for the ocular examination by the non-ophthalmologist to aid in recognizing serious ophthalmic injury that will require immediate ophthalmology consultation. Clearly, the detailed description of managing ophthalmic condition is beyond the scope of this chapter. The primary focus is upon pure ocular and optic nerve injury, and only minor attention will be given to ocular motility disturbances and adnexal injuries.

49.2 Assessment of Visual Function

49.2.1 Afferent Visual Function

49.2.1.1 Visual Acuity

Accurate assessment of initial visual acuity is of utmost importance to the diagnosis and treatment of ocular injuries in trauma. A brief history of pre-existing ocular conditions and vision will help the examiner understand the changes trauma may have caused to baseline acuity. Subjective measurements based on patient response in trauma are inadequate, and objective testing must be performed with near and distance vision being tested first.

The Snellen chart is a widespread tool, commonly used in the emergency department to screen for ocular injury [3]. The Snellen chart does, however, have its limitations. Patients must be conscious and compliant and should ideally be assessed wearing their usual visual aids, such as spectacle correction. A pocket-sized visual acuity assessment, the Rosenbaum near vision screener, can be transported by any examiner and used effectively for near vision screening in trauma where patient mobility is limited or spectacles are not accessible. The patient should be tested with the left eye occluded (to examine the right eye). The opposite side of the Rosenbaum card has Lea symbols for pediatric testing. The examiner should keep in mind that near testing of patients in the presbyopic age range can limit test accuracy and bifocals should be used when at all possible for this population. Several smartphone apps can perform similar testing and are readily available.

Often, initial evaluation of vision in trauma can be difficult for a patient, and frustration may lead to a patient response such as "I can't see at all" or "I can't focus on the letters." In such instances, the patient's ability to count fingers, and the maximum distance at which this can be accomplished, should be noted. If the patient can't count fingers, then the ability to recognize hand motion from the affected eye or the ability to perceive light in all four quadrants should be tested. It is imperative during testing of light perception that the fellow eye be totally occluded with an opaque object and a bright light (such as muscle light or direct ophthalmoscope) be used to ensure testing reliability.

49.2.1.2 Pupils

Pupil testing should follow visual acuity testing because bright light may transiently reduce the patient's ability to read the acuity chart accurately. Size, shape, and symmetry should be noted. To relax accommodation, gaze should be fixed on a distant target (20 ft away). To test the direct response, a bright light, such as a direct ophthalmoscope or otoscope (usually in ER rooms, hospital rooms) or muscle light, can be used. Room lighting should be kept dim so reactions can more easily be assessed. Once the direct response is noted, the pupil is retested directly so the contralateral consensual response can be observed. The contralateral pupil can then be tested in a similar fashion.

After direct response is noted, the alternating light test is performed. This examination is critical to the trauma evaluation as it discerns if optic nerve or massive retina disease is present. The basis for the swinging light test is to assess for a relative afferent pupillary defect, or RAPD. A positive RAPD indicates a difference between the two eyes in the afferent pathway due to retinal or optic nerve disease. The test can be performed properly by the following steps:

- Use a bright torch which can be focused to give a narrow, even beam of light. Perform the test in a semi-darkened room. If the room is too dark, it will be difficult to observe the pupil responses, particularly in heavily pigmented eyes.
- Ask the patient to look at a distant object, and to keep looking at it. This is to prevent the near-pupil response (a constriction in pupil size when moving focus from a distant to a near object).
- The test light is passed briskly between the two eyes several times with the examiner's attention focused on the direct responses. Normal pupils will dilate slightly in the absence of stimulation as the light is moved between the two eyes. Therefore, the first movement of each pupil should be constriction to direct stimulation. A lack of pupil reaction indicates an abnormal pupil and should direct the examiner to gross abnormalities of the affected eye such as traumatic mydriasis, glaucoma, iris incarceration in a corneoscleral laceration, efferent third nerve lesion, massive internal derangement of the eye, or optic nerve injury [4].
- After direct and consensual response is noted, next we check relative afferent function. Keep the beam of light steadily on the first eye for at least 3 seconds. This allows the pupil size to stabilize.
- Move the light quickly to shine in the other eye. Again, hold the light steady for 3 seconds. Note whether the pupil being illuminated stays the same size, or whether it dilates.
- As there is much to observe, repeat the test, observing what happens to the pupils of both eyes when one and then the other eye is illuminated.

When the test is performed on someone with unilateral or asymmetrical retinal or optic nerve disease, a RAPD should be present. In a positive RAPD test, the following happens:

- When the light is shone into the eye with the retinal or optic nerve disease, the pupils of both eyes will not constrict fully due to a problem with the afferent pathway.
- When the light is shone into the other, normal (less abnormal) eye, both pupils will constrict further. This is because the afferent pathway of this eye is intact, or less damaged than that of the other eye.
- When the light is shone back into the abnormal eye, both pupils will get larger, even the pupil in the normal eye (Fig. 49.1).
- It doesn't matter whether you start with the eye you think has the injury or the healthier eye: if the light is switched from one eye to the other and back again, the signs should become apparent.
- When an absolute afferent pupillary defect (amaurotic pupil) is present, there is no reaction to direct stimulation even though a brisk consensual response will be present.

Table 49.1 shows a common grading scale for measurement of the relative afferent pupillary defect.

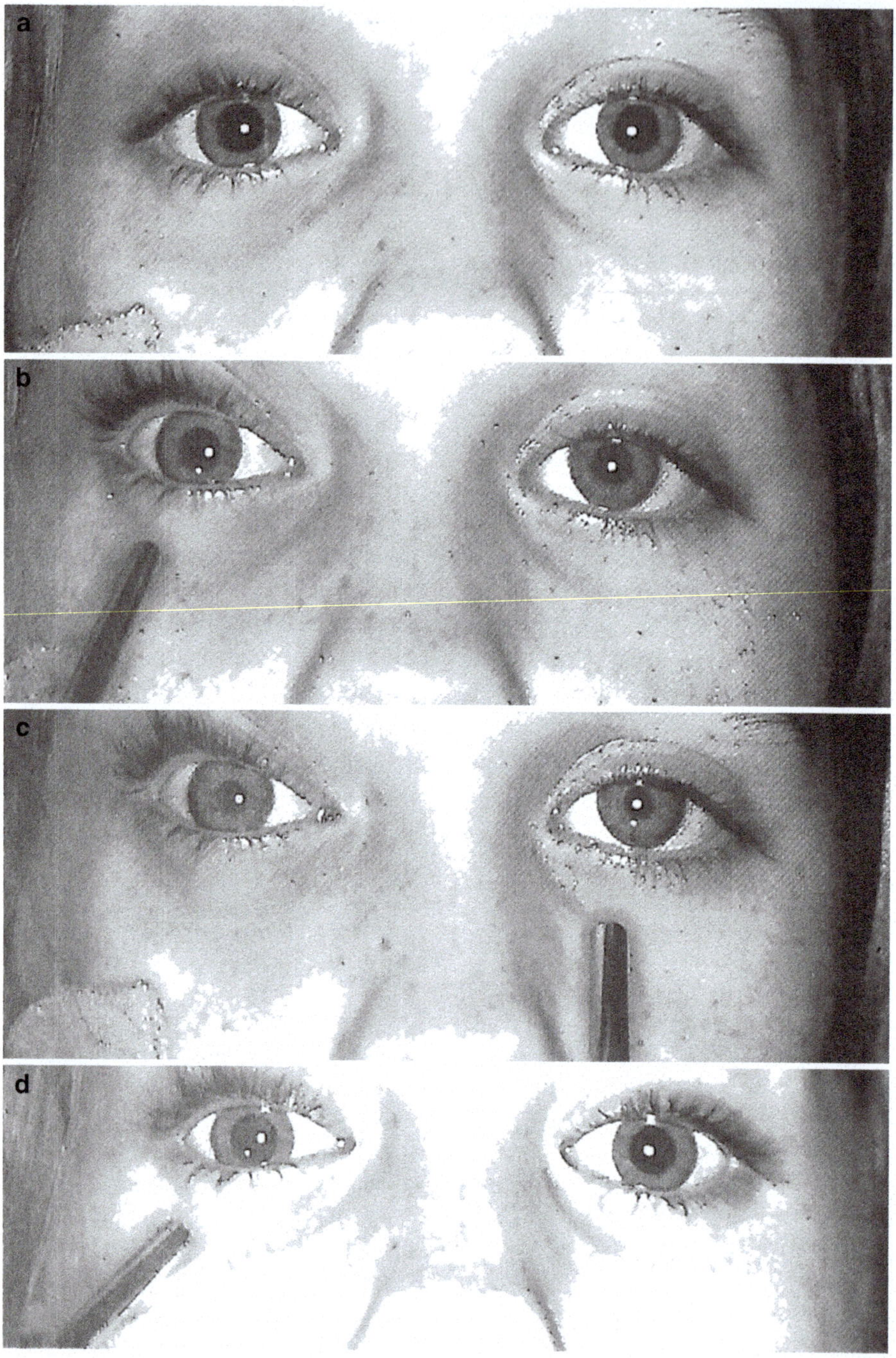

Fig. 49.1 The afferent pupillary defect: (**a**) Pupillary symmetry and size are observed in ambient room light. (**b**) The direct response is first tested with a bright light, and direct and consensual responses are observed. (**c**) The fellow eye is then tested. Comparing the reactions with those of figure (**b**) shows greater constriction of the left pupil and a more complete consensual response of the right pupil relative to the direct response. This pattern indicates an afferent pupil defect. (**d**) The alternating light test follows direct and consensual pupillary testing. The penlight is quickly moved between the eyes while the direct responses are observed. The first movement of the pupils should always be constriction; however, in this case the pupils dilate as the light is moved to the right eye. This is the typical pattern of an afferent pupillary defect as determined by the alternating light test. In the presence of a normal eye, this reaction indicates optic nerve injury

Table 49.1 The grading of a RAPD in the swinging light test

Amaurotic	This is seen when one eye has no perception of light. The pupil of this eye only constricts when light is shone into the other eye. When the light is shone back into the eye with no perception of light the pupil rapidly enlarges against the light
3–4+	The pupil enlarges as soon as the light is swung from the normal eye into the abnormal eye
1–2+	The pupil enlarges, but only after a short delay, after the light is swung from the normal eye into the abnormal eye
Subtle/trace	Sometimes the pupils of both eyes, can enlarge in the short time interval between shining the light in the normal eye and the abnormal eye. If this happens, the pupil of the abnormal eye may constrict a little bit before enlarging

The next section of the chapter will highlight specific conditions as it pertains to segmental evaluation of the globe.

49.3 Eyelid and Anterior Segment Evaluation

The anterior segment and ocular adnexa are examined following pupil evaluation. Without a slit lamp, only rudimentary evaluation of the anterior segment can be performed; however, vital information can be gleaned from subtle exam findings. Full-thickness eyelid lacerations should alert the examiner to possible globe rupture or conjunctival laceration. Medial canthal lacerations should raise suspicion to canalicular injury. Three hundred sixty-degree subconjunctival hemorrhage is a harbinger of posterior globe laceration and should be evaluated with this in mind. To examine the anterior segment, a penlight can be held temporally, slightly anterior and parallel to the plane of the iris, and perpendicular to the sagittal plane of the eye [4]. This will afford evaluation of corneal clarity, subconjunctival hemorrhage, and anterior chamber depth.

49.3.1 Eyelid Complications

49.3.1.1 Full-Thickness Eyelid Laceration

Periocular trauma can sometimes result in partial or full-thickness defects in the eyelid involving the skin and subcutaneous tissues (Fig. 49.2a). If the eyelid margin is involved, proper technique and repair are critical to secure a properly functioning eyelid. The most important step is to reapproximate the tarsus along its vertical axis with several sutures to allow for proper eyelid alignment and healing (Fig. 49.2b). Marginal repair alone will not provide structural integrity to the eyelid; the injured tarsus will splay apart, resulting in eyelid notching [5]. Care should be taken to avoid deeper, buried subcutaneous sutures that may incorporate the orbital septa, resulting in cicatricial eyelid tethering that can cause eyelid retraction and exposure keratopathy from lagophthalmos. Tarsal approximation should be lamellar, especially in the upper eyelid, to avoid penetration through conjunctiva and subsequent corneal abrasion.

49.3.1.2 Canalicular Laceration

A laceration medial to the upper or lower eyelid punctum, even without obvious canalicular involvement, should be probed and irrigated (Fig. 49.3). Repair can usually only be performed in the operating room as patient comfort, especially in the pediatric population, makes it difficult to perform bedside. Dog bites to the face and periocular region are notorious for causing canalicular lacerations. A recent review over an 11-year period found that 40% of dog bites to the ocular region resulted in canalicular injury [6]. If history elicits suspicion for a foreign body, then CT of the face should be obtained. For animal bites, if indicated, consider rabies vaccination and reporting of the animal to the local department of health. We typically perform bicanalicular stenting with Crawford-type stents for canalicular lacerations to promote structural integrity of the nasolacrimal system.

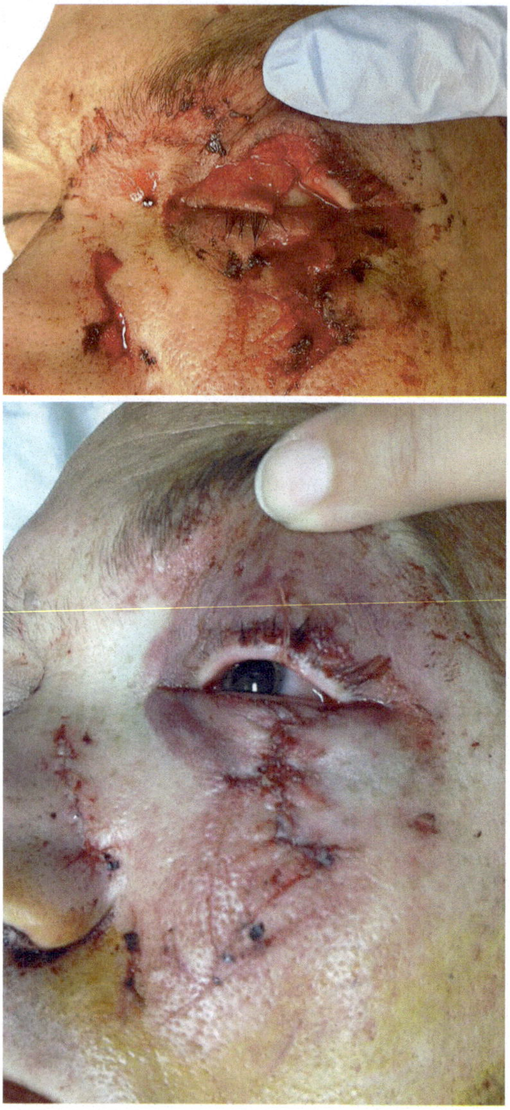

Fig. 49.2 (**a**) Clinical photograph demonstrating a left upper eyelid margin involving laceration. (**b**) Clinical photograph showing repair of the left upper eyelid margin laceration with proper grey line approximation

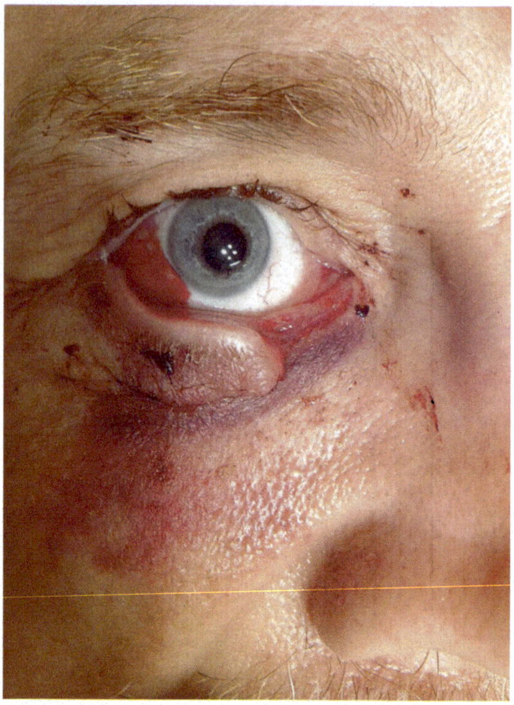

Fig. 49.3 Clinical photograph demonstrating a right medial canthal laceration with a dehiscence of lower eyelid showing the lacrimal punctum on the proximal side of the laceration. This loss of punctal approximation almost always indicates lacrimal outflow involvement

49.3.2 Anterior Segment Complications

49.3.2.1 Ruptured Globe

A ruptured globe must be excluded before repair of eyelid lacerations or orbital fractures. Careful inspection can easily diagnose a ruptured globe most of the time; however, sometimes it can be missed. Historical information that makes globe perforation more likely may include metal-on-metal strike, high-velocity projectile, sharp injuring object, and lack of eye protection [7].

Presentation

Signs that all facial trauma surgeons should look for when ruptured globe is suspected include 360-degree subconjunctival hemorrhage, shallow anterior chamber, peaked pupil (toward the open globe site), and exposed pigmented uvea through a globe wound. Anterior corneoscleral lacerations may present with an oblong pupil that points to the site of injury (Fig. 49.4a). Vision is usually severely reduced with hand motion and light perception vision common. Subconjunctival hemorrhage may obscure important signs of rupture such as uveal exposure and vitreous prolapse. Occult ruptures may develop beneath the rectus muscles at the time of impact causing deepening of the anterior chamber and dark red complete subconjunctival hemorrhage.

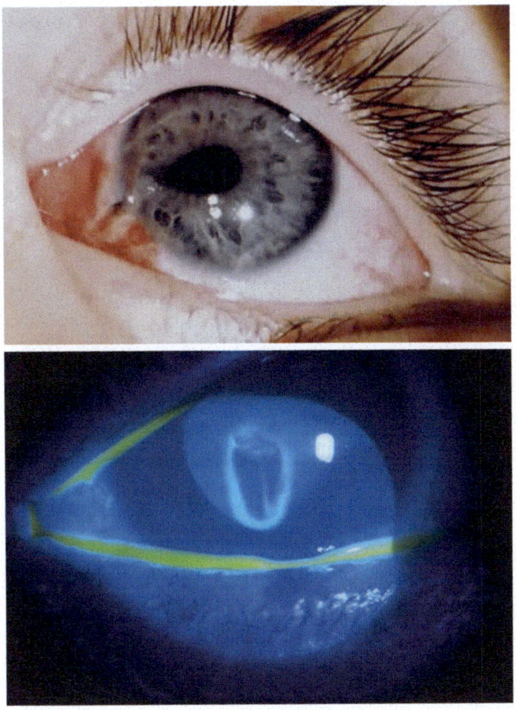

Fig. 49.4 (a) Clinical photograph showing a shallow anterior chamber with peaking of the nasal pupil toward a full thickness globe injury. Reprinted with permission from Duanes' Ophthalmology 2006. (b) The Seidel Test: A fluorescein strip containing 10% fluorescein is applied topically to the affected area and is examined with a cobalt blue filter. At this point, the fluorescein appears green, if the fluorescein pattern changes or enlarges from the corneal defect/abrasion this can indicate a full thickness globe laceration with aqueous egress through the wound

Monitoring/Workup

The eye should be protected at all times with a shield that vaults over the ocular surface (e.g., fox shield). A CT scan of the brain and orbits should be obtained to rule out an intraocular foreign body or intra-orbital foreign body. For corneal lacerations, the Seidel test can detect a corneal wound leak and can be performed by the non-ophthalmologist in the emergency setting. Concentrated fluorescein dye (drop or moistened strip) is applied directly over the potential site of perforation while observing the site at a slit lamp or under magnification (loupes). If a perforation and leak exist, the fluorescein dye is diluted by the aqueous and appears as a green (dilute) stream within the dark orange (concentrated) background. The stream of aqueous is best seen with a Wood's lamp or cobalt blue light of the slit lamp (Fig. 49.4b). Iris incarceration to the site of perforation is another presentation for corneal laceration.

Systemic antibiotics should be administered. Recommended agents for adults are cefazolin or vancomycin along with moxifloxacin which has better intraocular penetration. Preoperative visual acuity is the most reliable predictor of final visual outcome in traumatized eyes [8].

Patient Management

Once the diagnosis of ruptured globe is made urgent ophthalmologic evaluation is warranted, and further examination should be deferred until the time of surgical repair to avoid placing pressure on the globe that may extrude intraocular contents. Orbital and facial fracture repair is delayed in the setting of a ruptured globe until cleared by an ophthalmologist. This will prevent additional ocular complications.

49.3.2.2 Corneal Foreign Body

Presentation

Patients with a corneal or conjunctival foreign body often complain of foreign body sensation and pain with blink. A detailed history is important to identifying the type of foreign body that may be present. There is an increased infection risk associated with vegetable matter, and metallic foreign bodies are notorious in workers who use high-speed grinding tools and metal-on-metal hammering.

Monitoring/Workup

Foreign bodies can lodge in the inferior cul-de-sac or on the palpebral surface of the conjunctiva of the upper eyelid. Eversion of the lids can be performed to examine this area for a foreign body. Glass particles after a motor-vehicle accident can be difficult to locate with slit lamp magnification.

Patient Management

In cases of facial trauma when concerned for foreign body, it is always best to consult an ophthalmologist. Removal of an embedded corneal foreign body should be performed with minimal delay to ensure no central visual corneal scarring.

49.3.2.3 Hyphema

Presentation

Studies in the United States indicate that hyphemas occur in approximately 20 per 100,000 population per year [9]. Hyphemas result from injury to the vessels of the peripheral iris or anterior ciliary body. Anterior segment bleeding can be seen on penlight examination as a layering of blood inferiorly in the anterior chamber (Fig. 49.5). It most often will occur in young males. At presentation, more than 50% of hyphemas occupy less than one third of the height of the anterior chamber; fewer than 10% fill the whole chamber [10].

Monitoring/Workup

Hyphema is frequently associated with corneal abrasion, iritis, and mydriasis. The major concern is secondary hemorrhage (a rebleed) which may occur most frequently 3–5 days after the initial insult [11]. Secondary hemorrhage increases the likelihood of glaucoma, optic atrophy, and corneal blood staining [11]. Patients with sickle-cell hemoglobinopathies, and even those with sickle-cell trait, may require surgical intervention if intraocular pressure is not controlled within 24 hours [12].

Patient Management

Diagnosis of traumatic hyphema should alert the examiner that major blunt force has occurred to the eye and other posterior ocular injuries may have occurred. Urgent ophthalmologic consult should be obtained. The overall treatment plan for traumatic hyphema includes decreasing elevated intraocular pressure, decreasing inflammation, and preventing rebleed by maintaining a completely atraumatic environment for the patient. These measures may include a protective shield over the injured eye, restriction of physical activity, elevation of the head of the bed, and frequent ophthalmologic follow-up. Because there is a risk of rebleeding during fracture repair, the latter should be delayed at least until the period of greatest risk of rebleeding has passed—ideally, no sooner than 7 days. Intraocular surgery may sometimes be necessary to prevent irreversible corneal blood staining and optic atrophy from persistently elevated intraocular pressure [13].

49.3.2.4 Iridodialysis

Presentation

Blunt trauma may cause separation of the iris root from the ciliary body (Fig. 49.6). Usually this is associated with hyphema and not recognized until the hyphema clears.

Monitoring/Workup

Iridodialysis, if small, may be observed. Careful consideration should be given to rule out an intraocular foreign body that has traumatically caused the iridodialysis. If a hyphema is present, then monitoring should generally be aimed at treating

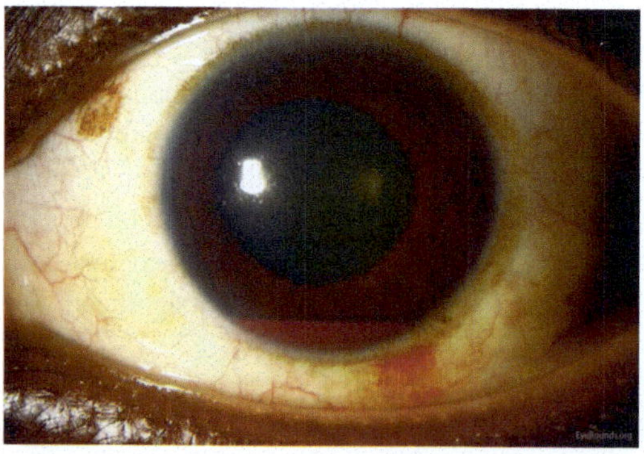

Fig. 49.5 Slit lamp photograph demonstrating a small traumatic hyphema with blood inferior in the anterior chamber angle. Reprinted with permission from Iowa Ophthalmology (webeye.ophth.uiowa.edu)

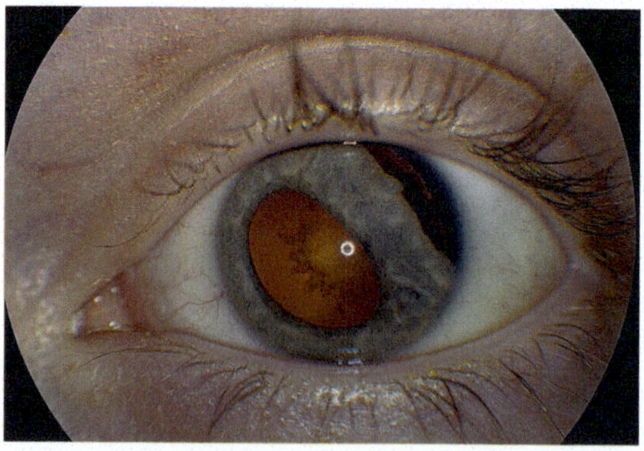

Fig. 49.6 Traumatic Iridodialysis: Slit lamp photograph of the left eye showing traumatic iridodialysis of the superotemporal iris from its insertion to the iris root. A traumatic stellate cataract can also be appreciated

the hyphema. Iridodialysis is frequently associated with other, more serious ocular injuries, which can preclude good vision.

Patient Management

Large iridodialysis may need surgical repair in the operating room; however, generally fracture repair can proceed if isolated iridodialysis is noted and ophthalmology has ruled out other causes of ocular damage.

49.3.2.5 Traumatic Iritis

Presentation

After blunt facial trauma, one of the most common ocular injuries seen is traumatic iritis. The patient will complain of photophobia, tearing, and ocular pain in the first 24 h after injury. Usually there is diminished vision and perilimbal conjunctival injection. It is not abnormal for a patient to have severe photophobia in the contralateral eye with direct illumination following traumatic iritis [14].

Monitoring/Workup

The pupil in traumatic iritis is usually stunned as a result of traumatic shockwaves that have traversed the globe. Therefore, it can be either smaller than the nontraumatized side (pupil dilates poorly) or potentially larger (caused by iris sphincter tears).

Patient Management

Treatment consists of a topical cycloplegic agent to relieve patient discomfort and often a topical steroid to decrease intraocular inflammation. Treatment agents should be given after ophthalmologic exam has ruled out corneal abrasions, angle closure glaucoma, and other ophthalmic conditions.

49.4 Posterior Segment Evaluation

The posterior segment of the eye encompasses the vitreous, retina, and optic nerve. In acute face trauma, surrounding periocular edema, ecchymosis, and patient discomfort can make examination of posterior ocular structures most challenging. It is not uncommon for eyelid edema to make it difficult for an examiner to accurately assess visual acuity, let alone try to assess retinal or optic nerve pathology. The posterior segment can adequately be examined only with an indirect ophthalmoscope or slit lamp dilated fundus exam. For initial screening, however, a direct ophthalmoscope is used. In this setting it is imperative for the physician to use subtle clues and techniques to help a patient obtain the best visual outcome.

A direct ophthalmoscope can help the facial trauma surgeon assess the clarity of the red reflex. The red reflex refers to the reddish-orange reflection of light from the eye's retina that is observed when using an ophthalmoscope or bright focused light. An asymmetric or absent red reflex should alert a physician that a serious problem with the retina could have occurred during the trauma. The red reflex can be appreciated best in a dimly lit room, but can often be challenging to examine when patients receive opioid analgesics which can cause pupillary miosis. In this setting, the reflection of light from the retina is minimized through a small pupil. Nonetheless, when evaluating ocular trauma in the setting of face trauma, red reflex testing can be a useful adjunct tool for the non-ophthalmologist.

Another test that can employed in most emergent settings is the bedside ocular ultrasound. This technique is simple and quick to perform and can diagnose a wide range of medical and traumatic conditions. It is free of ionizing radiation; can show the posterior chamber and retrobulbar structures when hyphema, cataract, or lid edema makes direct visualization impossible; and allows for dynamic evaluation of the eye [15–17]. Ocular point-of-care US has also proven useful in pediatric patients, who may be difficult to evaluate using traditional examination techniques [18]. The sonographer must be very careful to avoid any excess pressure so as not to extrude the vitreal contents. Thus, a ruptured globe is a relative contraindication to performing an ocular US [19]. Kilker et al. have designed a mnemonic for use of the ocular ultrasound in the setting of ocular trauma in an emergent setting

Table 49.2 Mnemonic for use of ocular ultrasound (FOVEA)

FOVEA: ocular ultrasound protocol	
Front of the eye	Foreign bodies, lens dislocations or subluxations, afferent pupillary defects, anterior chamber size changes
Optic nerve	Increased intracranial pressure in traumatic brain injury and idiopathic intracranial hypertension
Vitreous	Retinal hemorrhage, retinal detachment, vitreous hemorrhage, vitreous detachment, lens dislocation, endophthalmitis
Extraocular	Retrobulbar hemorrhage, globe disruption, foreign bodies
Artery/vascular	Central retinal artery occlusion, central retinal vein occlusion

Reprinted with permission from Kilker et al. European Journal of Emergency Medicine

(Table 49.2). Prompt consultation or referral to an ophthalmologist should still be made when the patient presents with a concerning history and exam [19].

49.4.1 Vitreous and Retinal Complications

49.4.1.1 Vitreous Hemorrhage

Presentation

Traumatic vitreous hemorrhage occurs as result of damage to blood vessels of the iris, ciliary body, retina, or choroid and can also be caused by retinal tears. A blunted red reflex in comparison to the nontraumatized eye is often seen. A patient will often have severely reduced acuity and may complain of a "reddish hue" or "black paint" in front of their vision. Pain is not a typical complaint of a patient with traumatic vitreous hemorrhage.

Monitoring/Workup

If vitreous hemorrhage is diagnosed and globe rupture has been ruled out, then ocular ultrasound examination can be performed to help view the retina and optic nerve. Sometimes bed rest with elevation of the patient's head causes the hemorrhage to settle sufficiently to allow ophthalmoscopic examination. Neuroimaging in some cases may be helpful to rule out a foreign body when a good ophthalmic examination is limited.

Patient Management

Traumatic vitreous hemorrhage without retinal detachment can be observed and allowed to clear. This will usually occur in 2–3 months, and, in some scenarios, surgical intervention may be needed to remove the hemorrhage from the eye. Treatment of facial fractures should be delayed, if possible, as vitreous hemorrhage from choroidal rupture may make the sclera weak and more prone to intraoperative globe rupture.

49.4.1.2 Commotio Retinae

Presentation

Commotio retinae appears as sheen-like retinal whitening hours following injury (Fig. 49.7). It occurs as a result of shock waves that traverse the eye and cause derangement of the outer retinal layers [20]. Visual acuity may decrease to as low as 20/200 but can also be normal.

Monitoring/Workup

Fortunately, commotio retinae will most often clear in 3–4 weeks and visual prognosis is good.

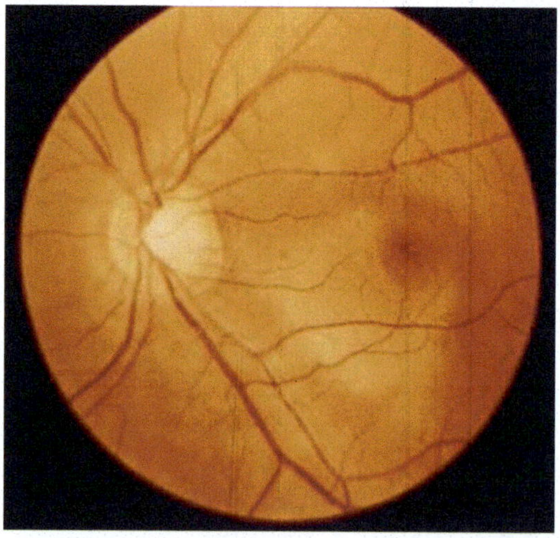

Fig. 49.7 Fundus Photograph of the left eye demonstrating retinal whitening in the fovea consistent with commotion retinae. This whitening occurs from degeneration of the layers of the retina secondary to shock waves caused by blunt trauma or blast injury. Reprinted with permission from Iowa Ophthalmology (webeye.ophth.uiowa.edu)

There is no acute treatment for the patient; however, an ophthalmology consult should be performed to rule out peripheral retinal tears or other retinal pathology that may predispose to retinal detachment.

Patient Management

Fracture repair may proceed without delay; however, long-term ophthalmologic follow-up is needed to detect possible late-developing retinal breaks in eyes with contusion retinopathy [21].

49.4.1.3 Retinal Detachment

Presentation

The incidence of retinal detachment in fractures of the orbital skeleton and midface has been cited between 2 and 6% [22, 23]. Traumatic retinal detachment is usually associated with severe vision loss, an afferent pupil defect, and vitreous hemorrhage. Blunt trauma compresses the eye along its anteroposterior diameter, and rapid compression seen in trauma can result in severe traction from vitreoretinal attachment sites and cause retinal breaks. Traumatic retinal breaks are often multiple and commonly found in the inferotemporal and superonasal quadrants.

Monitoring/Workup

Bedside ocular ultrasound can quickly and accurately diagnose and distinguish a retinal detachment. A retinal detachment will appear as hyperechoic or as a bright white membrane in the posterior chamber that is tethered to the optic nerve (Fig. 49.8). Traumatic retinal breaks that may lead to retinal detachment usually occur at the time of trauma [24], but their diagnosis is often delayed (and the opportunity for prophylactic treatment lost) for several reasons. For example, the patient may initially not complain of visual decline because a peripheral retinal tear is usually asymptomatic. Blood cells from a torn retina may take hours or a few days to permeate the vitreous and cause symptomatic floaters or a "veil"; however, sometimes patients disregard symptoms or may be conscious of them only much later [24].

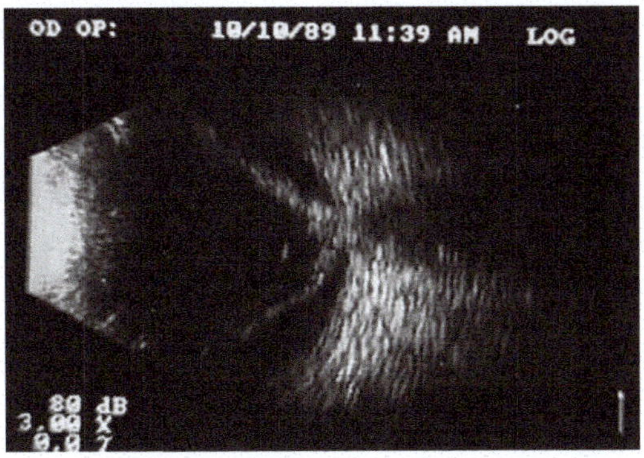

Fig. 49.8 Ocular ultrasound showing a retinal detachment. Demonstrated is the hyperechoic white membrane in the posterior chamber that is tethered to the optic nerve. Reprinted with permission from Duanes' Ophthalmology 2006

Patient Management

Retinal detachment is a relative ocular emergency and requires prompt ophthalmologic consultation. The patient is usually placed on bed rest until surgical repair can be performed urgently. All fracture repairs should be delayed until the patient can be cleared from an ophthalmic standpoint. Prompt recognition of this possible diagnosis will help the patient recover maximum vision, and delay in diagnosis can cause greater likelihood of irreversible vision loss.

49.4.2 Optic Nerve Complications

49.4.2.1 Traumatic Optic Neuropathy

Traumatic optic neuropathy (TON) can be classified as either direct or indirect. Direct TON arises from compression along the course of the optic nerve by bone fragments, hematoma, foreign body, or fractures involving the optic canal. Indirect TON is the most common form and will appear as severely reduced vision in the setting of trauma or facial fractures often without any evidence radiographically of injury to the orbital, intracanalicular, or intracranial optic nerve [25]. The exact etiology of indirect TON is speculative; however, secondary edema and vasospasm are thought to produce nerve ischemia and infarction [26]. Also, deformation of the optic canal during frontal impact with resultant nerve contusion and edema has also been suggested as a cause [27, 28].

Presentation

Traumatic optic neuropathy is a condition in which injury to the optic nerve can be clinically confirmed (i.e., patients demonstrate reduced visual acuity, color vision, and/or visual field, as well as a relatively afferent pupillary defect). Notably, this latter finding may not be present in bilateral cases. Direct ophthalmoscopy of the nerve is also expected to appear normal, though optic atrophy or pallor can develop in 4–8 weeks.

Monitoring/Workup

Suspected optic nerve injury requires neuroimaging to assess the extent of the injury and to detect any associated intracranial and facial injuries, infraorbital fragments, or hematoma [29]. Orbital or cranial surgery may be necessary but may not affect the prognosis for the optic nerve.

Patient Management

Therapy for indirect TON is controversial. It is known that some patients will experience spontaneous recovery, and the degree of recovery correlates inversely with the severity of initial visual loss [30, 31]. Most patients in the pediatric TON surveillance study improved or at least did not worsen from baseline acuity [32].

Treatment with high-dose corticosteroids is controversial. The rationale for their use is drawn from experience in the treatment of other optic neuropathies and experimental spinal cord trauma [33–35]. Optic canal decompression, either transcranial or transethmoidal, represents the primary surgical therapy attempted in treating indirect TON. The International Optic Nerve Trauma Study, a non-randomized, multicenter, comparative analysis of treatment outcomes, found no clear benefit for use of high-dose intravenous corticosteroids or optic canal decompression in the treatment of TON [36]. Moreover, Edwards in a study of over 10,000 head injury victims compared benefits of high-dose corticosteroids with placebo within an 8-h window following trauma. The study was terminated early when the group treated with corticosteroids had a statistically significant higher rate of mortality compared to the placebo group [37].

Dosage recommendations for indirect TON vary from 1 g/day up to megadosages (30 mg/kg loading dose). If visual function improves on corticosteroid therapy, the patient is generally converted to a tapering dose of oral therapy after 48 h. If no response, optic canal decompression may be considered. In the case of direct TON, surgical approaches have included early fracture reduction, orbital decompression, extracranial optic canal decompression, hematoma drainage, and optic nerve sheath fenestration [38, 39]. The technique chosen should be uniquely correlated to the individual patient, and there is no consensus to the efficacy of these approaches.

The authors advocate close observation in the setting of indirect TON as the current body of literature does not strongly support the use of high-dose steroids nor surgical decompression for indirect TON.

49.4.2.2 Optic Nerve Avulsion

Presentation

A forceful backward dislocation of the optic nerve from the scleral canal can occur in instances of extreme rotation of the globe or with penetrating orbital injury (Fig. 49.9).

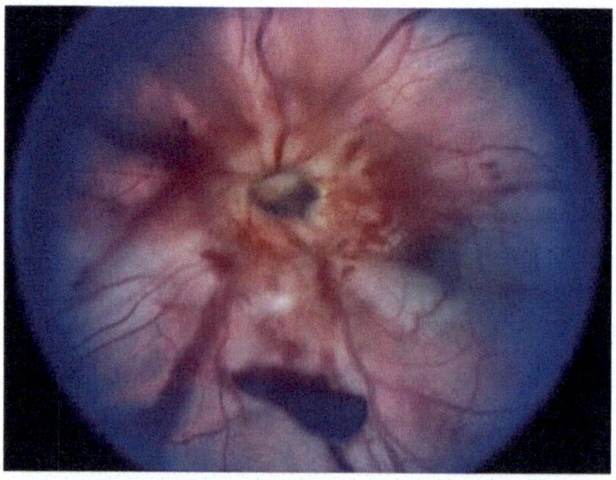

Fig. 49.9 Optic Nerve Avulsion: Fundus photograph demonstrating hemorrhage in all layers of the retina with loss of optic nerve architecture and a scleral ring at the site of previous optic nerve insertion

Patients usually present with no light perception vision if a complete avulsion has occurred, while partial avulsions cause variable degrees of visual loss.

Monitoring/Workup

The diagnosis may be suspected, but view of the fundus is usually obscured by a hyphema or vitreous hemorrhage. CT/MRI imaging is unlikely to demonstrate an optic nerve avulsion when present [40]. If the diagnosis is missed, the patient may receive unwarranted treatment with high-dose corticosteroids or optic canal decompression.

Patient Management

The visual prognosis in optic nerve avulsion depends on if the avulsion is complete or partial. Case reports have demonstrated late recovery of vision in partial avulsion and so delay of facial fracture repair that may further rotate the injured globe or orbit is warranted.

49.5 Extraocular Motility Examination

Vertical and horizontal positions should be tested after possibility of globe rupture has been eliminated [41]. The main objective in testing ocular ductions is to assess the likelihood of ocular muscle paresis or entrapment [42].

49.5.1 Corneal Light Reflex

In facial trauma, the initial examiner needs a quick and effective way to evaluate ocular alignment, and the corneal light reflection test can be a useful tool. The corneal light reflection test compares the position of the corneal light reflection in both eyes. In normally aligned eyes, the reflections should be symmetric on the cornea and in the same position relative to the pupil. The two most commonly used tests to measure corneal light reflection are the Hirschberg and Krimsky tests.

The Hirschberg test gives an estimation of ocular alignment by directly analyzing the angle of decentration of the corneal light reflection. Figure 49.10 illustrates estimated deviations. Every millimeter of decentration is equal to roughly 7°or 15 prism diopters (PD). Therefore, a light reflection at the pupillary margin (2 mm from the pupillary center) is equal to approximately 15° or 30PD of deviation; a reflection in the middle of the iris indicates a deviation of about 30° (60PD); and a reflection at the limbus is equivalent to a deviation of 45° (90PD).

The Krimsky test utilizes reflections from both corneas produced by an appropriately placed penlight that is fixated by the patient's better eye. The downside in this test is that prisms are needed and ocular prisms are rarely accessible in the emergency department or in the acute evaluation of midface trauma.

49.5.2 Forced Duction Testing

Also known as the traction test, forced duction testing helps to distinguish a paretic versus a restricted extraocular muscle. With the patient awake, a drop of topical anesthetic is instilled onto the globe. The eye is then moved with two-toothed forceps applied to the conjunctiva near the limbus in the direction opposite that in which mechanical restriction is suspected. For instance, to distinguish between lateral rectus paralysis and mechanical restriction involving the medial aspect of the globe (muscle entrapment in a medial wall fracture), we apply the forceps at the 6- and 12-o'clock positions and move the eye passively into abduction. If resistance is encountered, mechanical restrictions exist medially, and contracture of the medial rectus muscle or entrapment must be considered. It is important to not press the globe into the orbit during testing as this may artificially yield a positive test. In most cases, forced duction testing is not needed. Relying on versions and ductions is typically more than enough to assess the level of restriction in an orbit fracture. Extraocular muscle restriction is always a clinical diagnosis, not a radiologic one.

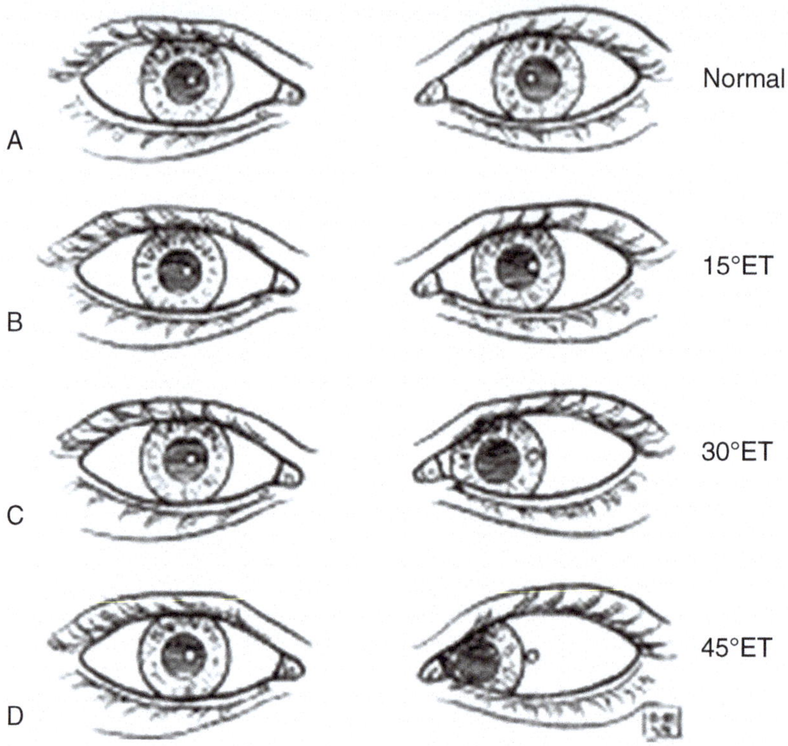

Fig. 49.10 Hirschberg ocular alignment test: (**a**) Pen Light showing corneal light centration bilaterally. (**b**) Left eye corneal light reflex displaced temporally 2 mm. Equivalent to 30 prism diopters of left eye esotropia. (**c**) Left eye corneal light reflex displaced temporally 4 mm. Equivalent to 60 prism diopters of left eye esotropia. (**d**) Left eye corneal light reflex displaced to the temporal limbus (6 mm). Equivalent to 90 prism diopters of left eye esotropia

49.6 Ocular Disorders Requiring Emergency Management

49.6.1 Orbital Compartment Syndrome

49.6.1.1 Presentation

The formation of retrobulbar hematomas is a known complication following facial trauma. Hislop reported an incidence of 0.6% in fractured zygomas involving the orbit and Gerbino identified an incidence of 0.45% after reviewing 1971 cases of blunt orbital trauma [43, 44]. Bleeding in the retrobulbar space, which quickly causes an increase in retrobulbar pressure due to the lack of distensibility of the surrounding structures, can cause orbital compartment syndrome. As orbital pressure rises, venous outflow is reduced and compression of nourishing arteries can lead to impairment of retinal and optic nerve perfusion, resulting in ischemic damage [45, 46]. The central retinal artery once occluded can lead to permanent, irreversible vision loss after as little 60–100 min of ischemia [47].

The patient usually presents with tight eyelids that are "rock hard" and resist retropulsion. Examination may also reveal proptosis, decreased visual acuity, afferent pupillary defect, and limited extraocular motility. Direct ophthalmoscope exam may show optic disc swelling or pulsations of retinal arterioles indicating impending occlusion.

49.6.1.2 Monitoring/Workup

Once identified, orbital compartment syndrome should be treated surgically without delay. Clinicians should not delay treatment to get imaging as this may affect visual outcome [48]. If imaging is available at the time of evaluation, "tenting" of the globe on axial imaging is usually noted and a harbinger of poor visual outcome [49]. The tenting sign indicates the optic nerve is at a maximum stretch and distorts (tents) the back of the globe into a teardrop shape.

49.6.1.3 Patient Management

The key to effective management of orbital compartment syndrome is timely and aggressive decompression. Lateral canthotomy and cantholysis of the inferior and superior crus of the lateral canthal tendon will allow the globe to displace anteriorly and inferiorly to relieve pressure in the orbital space and allow replenished blood flow to the retina and optic nerve [50]. After lateral canthotomy and cantholysis, patients will often feel a relief of orbital pressure. Reversal of the afferent pupillary defect and decrease in intraocular pressure can be immediate.

Patients should generally be watched closely for the next 24 h in an inpatient setting to ensure that continued bleeding or rebleeding does not occur and result in increased orbital pressure once again. If this occurs, more definitive orbital decompression may be needed [51].

Conclusion

Prompt recognition of ophthalmic injury is important in cases of facial fractures for several reasons. First, management of ocular injury often takes precedence over the treatment of midfacial and orbital fractures [22, 52]. Second, fracture repair in the setting of occult ocular injury (e.g., ruptured globe, retinal detachment) may result in exacerbation of the injury, resulting in devastating visual loss [53, 54]. Third, recognition of the extent and possible irreversibility of the ophthalmic injury is crucial preoperatively from a medicolegal standpoint, so that the fracture repair is not later claimed to be the etiology of permanent visual compromise [55]. The authors recommend ophthalmic consultation in all cases of facial fractures involving the orbit. Working together as a team optimizes patient outcomes. It is essential to have good consultation and communication with the ophthalmic and facial trauma services in the care of this patient population.

References

1. Ansari MH. Blindness after facial fractures: a 19-year retrospective study. J Oral Maxillofac Surg. 2005;63:229.
2. Al-Qurainy IA, Stassen LFA, Dutton GN, et al. The characteristics of midfacial fractures and the association with ocular injury: a prospective study. Br J Oral Maxillofac Surg. 1991;29:291.
3. Nagase DY, Courtemanche DJ, Peters DA. Facial fractures—Association with ocular injuries: a 13-year review of one practice in a tertiary care centre. Can J Plast Surg. 2006;14:167–71.
4. Gossman DM, Roberts DM, Barr CC. Ophthalmic aspects of orbital injury. Clin Plast Surg. 1992;19(1):71–85.
5. Ehlers JP, Shah CP. The Wills eye manual. Philadelphia: Lippincott Williams & Wilkins; 2008.
6. Prendes MA, Jian-Amadi A, Chang SH, Shaftel SS. Ocular trauma from dog bites: characterization, associations, and treatment patterns at a regional level I trauma center over 11 years. Ophthal Plast Reconstr Surg. 2016;32(4):279–83.
7. Spoor TC. An atlas of ophthalmic trauma. Mosby-Year Book: St Louis; 1997.
8. Barr CC. Prognostic factors in corneoscleral lacerations. Arch Ophthalmol. 1983;101:919–24.
9. Parver LM, Dannenberg AL, Blacklow B, et al. Characteristics and causes of penetrating eye injuries reported to the National Eye Trauma System Registry, 1985-91. Public Health Rep. 1993;108:625.
10. Reidy JJ. External disease and cornea: basic and clinical science course. San Francisco: American Academy of Ophthalmology; 2011.
11. Walton W, Von Hagen S, Grigorian R, et al. Management of traumatic hyphema. Surv Ophthalmol. 2002;47:297.
12. McCuen BW, Fung WE. The role of vitrectomy instrumentation in the treatment of severe traumatic hyphema. Am J Ophthalmol. 1979;88:930.
13. Nasrullah A, Kerr NC. Sickle cell trait as a risk factor for secondary hemorrhage in children with traumatic hyphema. Am J Ophthalmol. 1997;123:783.
14. Krachmer JH, Rapuano CJ, Luchs JI, et al. Anterior segment: the requisites of ophthalmology. St Louis: Mosby; 2000.
15. Ma OJ, Mateer JR, Blaivas M. Emergency ultrasound. 2nd ed. New York: McGraw-Hill; 2008. p. 449–62.
16. Blaivas M, Theodore D, Sierzenski P. A study of bedside ocular ultrasonography in the emergency department. Acad Emerg Med. 2002;9:791–9.
17. Blaivas M. Bedside emergency department ultrasonography in the evaluation of ocular pathology. Acad Emerg Med. 2000;7:947–50.
18. Tsung JW, Blaivas M, Cooper A, Levick NR. A rapid noninvasive method of detecting elevated intracranial pressure using bedside ocular ultrasound: application to 3 cases of head trauma in the pediatric emergency department. Pediatr Emerg Care. 2005;21:94–8.
19. Kilker BA, Holsta JM, Hoffman B. Bedside ocular ultrasound in the emergency department. Eur J Emerg Med. 2014;21:246–53.
20. Supperley JO, Quigley HA, Gass JDM. Traumatic retinopathy in primates. Arch Ophthalmol. 1978;96:2267–73.
21. Cox MS, Schepens CL, Freeman HM. Retinal detachment due to ocular contusion. Arch Ophthalmol (Chicago). 1966;76:678–85.

22. Guly CM, Guly HR, Bouamra O, Gray RH, Lecky FE. Ocular injuries in patients with major trauma. Emerg Med J. 2006;23:915–7.
23. Jamal BT, Pfahler SM, Lane KA, Bilyk JR, Pribitkin EA, Diecidue RJ, Taub DI. Ophthalmic injuries in patients with zygomaticomaxillary complex fractures requiring surgical repair. J Oral Maxillofac Surg. 2009;67:986–9.
24. Hoogewoud F, Chronopoulos A, Varga Z, Souteyrand G, Thumann G, Schutz JS. Traumatic retinal detachment—the difficulty and importance of correct diagnosis. Surv Ophthalmol. 2016;61:156–63.
25. Edmund J, Godtfredsen E. Unilateral optic atrophy following head injury. Acta Ophthalmol. 1963;41:693–7.
26. Walsh FB. Pathological-clinical correlations. I. Indirect trauma to the optic nerves and chiasm. II. Certain cerebral involvement associated with defective blood supply. Invest Ophthalmol. 1966;5:433–49.
27. Spetzler RF, Spetzler H. Holographic interferometry applied to the study of the human skull. J Neurosurg. 1980;52:825–8.
28. Panje WR, Gruss CE, Anderson RL. Sudden blindness following facial trauma. Otolaryngol Head Neck Surg. 1981;89:941–8.
29. BCSC Neuro Optic Neuropathy.
30. Feist RM, Kline LB, Morris RE. Recover of vision after presumed direct optic nerve injury. Ophthalmology. 1987;94:1567–9.
31. Hughes B. Indirect injury of the optic nerves and chiasm. Bull Johns Hopkins Hosp. 1962;111:90–126.
32. Ford RL, Lee V, Xing W, Bunce C. A 2-year prospective surveillance of pediatric traumatic optic neuropathy in the United Kingdom. J AAPOS. 2012;16:413–7.
33. Model AG. Reversal of blindness in temporal arteritis with methylprednisolone. Lancet. 1978;1:340.
34. Spoor TC, Rockwell DL. Treatment of optic neuritis with intravenous megadose corticosteroid. A consecutive series. Ophthalmology. 1988;95:131–4.
35. Young W, Flamm ES. Effect of high-dose corticosteroid therapy on blood flow, evoked potentials, and extracellular calcium in experimental spinal injury. J Neurosurg. 1982;57:667–73.
36. Levin LA, Beck RW, Joseph MP, Seiff S, Kraker R. The treatment of traumatic optic neuropathy: the International Optic Nerve Trauma Study. Ophthalmology. 1999;106:1268–77.
37. Edwards P, et al. Final results of MRC CRASH, a randomised placebo-controlled trial of intravenous corticosteroid in adults with head injury-outcomes at 6 months. Lancet. 2005;365(9475):1957–9.
38. Lipkin AF, Woodson GE, Miller RH. Visual loss due to orbital fracture: the role of early reduction. Arch Otolaryngol Head Neck Surg. 1987;113:81–3.
39. Walter JR. Subperiosteal hematomas of the orbit in young males: a serious complication of trauma or surgery in the eye region. Trans Am Ophthalmol Surg. 1979;77:104–15.
40. Foster BS, March GA, Lucarelli MJ, Samiy N, Lessel S. Optic nerve avulsion. Arch Ophthalmol. 1997;115:623–30.
41. Linz AM, Wennogle CP. Blow in fracture of the lateral wall of the orbit. Trans Congr Int Assoc Oral Surg. 1981;4:306–7.
42. Watson PG. The traumatic orbital apex syndrome: its differential diagnosis and treatment. Trans Ophthalmol Soc UK. 1969;88:361.
43. Hislop WS, Dutton GN, Duglas PS. Treatment of retrobulbar hematoma in accident and emergency departments. Br J Oral Maxillofac Surg. 1996;34:289–92.
44. Gerbino G, Ramieri GA, Nasi A. Diagnosis and treatment of retrobulbar hematomas following blunt orbital trauma: a description of eight cases. Int J Oral Maxillofac Surg. 2005;34:127–31.
45. Hartley JH Jr, Lester JC, Schatten WE. Acute retrobulbar hemorrhage during elective blepharoplasty. Plast Reconstr Surg. 1973;52:8–15.
46. Heinze JB, Hueston JT. Blindness after blepharoplasty: mechanism and early reveals. Plast Reconstr Surg. 1978;61:347–54.
47. Hayreh SS, Kolder HE, Weingeist TA. Central retinal artery occlusion and retinal tolerance. Ophthalmology. 1980;87:75–8.
48. Lima V, Bart B, Leibovitch I, Prabhakaran V, Goldberg RA, Selva D. Orbital compartment syndrome: the ophthalmic surgical emergency. Surv Ophthalmol. 2009;54:441–9.
49. Oester AE Jr, Sahu P, Fowler B, Fleming JC. Radiographic predictors of visual outcome in orbital compartment syndrome. Ophthal Plast Reconstr Surg. 2012;28(1):7–10.
50. Samples JR, Hedges JR. Ophthalmologic procedure. In: Roberts JR, Hedges JR, editors. Clinical procedures in emergency medicine. 3rd ed. Philadelphia: WB Saunders Co; 1998. p. 1089–119.
51. Chen YA, Singhal D, Chen YR, Chen CT. Management of acute traumatic retrobulbar haematomas: a 10 year retrospective review. J Plast Reconstr Aesthet Surg. 2012;65:1325–30.
52. Holt GR, Holt JE. Incidence of eye injuries in facial fractures: an analysis of 727 cases. Otolaryngol Head Neck Surg. 1983;91:276.
53. Ioannides C, Treffers W, Rutten M, et al. Ocular injuries associated with fractures involving the orbit. J Craniomaxillofac Surg. 1988;16:157.
54. Petro J, Tooze FM, Bales CR, et al. Ocular injuries associated with periorbital fractures. J Trauma. 1979;39:730.
55. Fonseca RJ. Oral and maxillofacial trauma. In: Weir CR, Dutton GN, Al-Qurainy IA, editors. Ophthalmic consequences of maxillofacial injuries. 3rd ed. Philadelphia: Elsevier Saunders; 2005. p. 693–719.

Check for updates

Vascular Injuries as a Complication of Maxillofacial Surgery

50

Dmitry Peysakhov and Antoine Ferneini

Abstract

This chapter discusses the etiology, diagnosis, and treatment of commonly encountered vascular injuries and complications related to the maxillofacial region. Basic topics discussed include vascular anatomy of the maxillofacial region, hemostatic mechanisms, and hemostatic agents. Adverse vascular events related to the specific surgical procedures and outside factors are also discussed. These include dentoalveolar procedures, implant surgery, epistaxis, maxillofacial infections, orthognathic surgery, TMJ surgery, and maxillofacial trauma. A review of advanced hemostatic procedures such as selective embolization and carotid artery ligation is also included.

50.1 Introduction

Vascular injuries associated with oral and maxillofacial surgery are rare but potentially serious complicating events. Vascular complications can be generally categorized as either bleeding and hemorrhage or a disruption in blood supply leading to ischemic tissue injury. Direct injury to a blood vessel can happen as a result of a surgical procedure, external traumatic event, arteriovenous malformation, or a pathologic condition that affects connective tissues. Patients who are on anticoagulation therapy are at increased risk for spontaneous bleeding [1] (Fig. 50.1).

Complete transection of a blood vessel wall usually leads to immediate bleeding or hemorrhage, whereas an incomplete tear can cause formation of pseudoaneurysm, which may expand and lead to a delayed hemorrhage. Hard and soft tissue ischemia and necrosis can be due to disruption of blood supply to the associated tissues, which can lead to a significant facial deformity and loss of function. One such example would be a LeFort I osteotomy for maxillary repositioning. Intraoperatively, accidental transection of descending palatine arteries can cause significant hemorrhage. Excessive tension on posterior pala-

D. Peysakhov, D.M.D.
Bothell Oral, Maxillofacial and Implant Surgery, Bothell, WA, USA

A. Ferneini, M.D., F.A.C.S. (✉)
Division of Vascular Surgery, Yale-New Haven Hospital/St. Raphael Campus, New Haven, CT, USA

Connecticut Vascular Center, PC, North Haven, CT, USA
e-mail: aferneini@ctvascularcenter.com

© Springer International Publishing AG 2018

E.M. Ferneini, J.D. Bennett (eds.), *Perioperative Assessment of the Maxillofacial Surgery Patient*,
https://doi.org/10.1007/978-3-319-58868-1_50

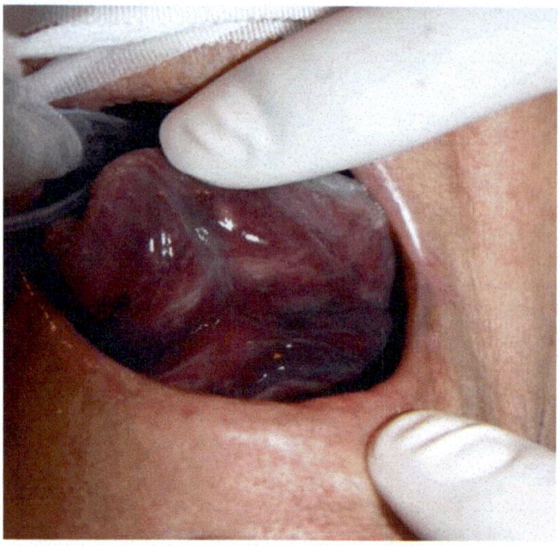

Fig. 50.1 Spontaneous sublingual hematoma as a result of anticoagulation therapy. With kind permission, Dr. Evgeni Brotfain

tal tissues can cause disruption of blood supply to the maxilla, causing necrosis and possible loss of premaxilla. Partial injury to the wall of descending palatine vessel can cause formation of pseudoaneurysm, which may lead to a significant delayed hemorrhage.

The objective of this chapter is to provide clinicians an overview of pertinent vascular anatomy applicable to the maxillofacial region, understanding of specific vascular complications related to common surgical procedures as well as traumatic injuries, and discussion of various treatment modalities including topical hemostatic agents, carotid artery ligation, and selective embolization.

50.2 Classification of Vascular Injury

In maxillofacial surgery, vascular injury occurs either from the external traumatic events or direct surgical trauma. In either case, there is a direct tissue trauma causing either indirect or direct endothelial injury [2]. Vascular complications can be generally divided into two broad categories: hemorrhagic and ischemic injuries. Bleeding and hemorrhage due to direct endothelial injury could lead to a significant blood loss and shock.

Table 50.1 Five types of vascular trauma

	Type of vascular injury	Etiology
Type I	Intimal injury	Blunt trauma
Type II	Complete endothelial defect	Penetrating trauma
Type III	Complete vessel transection	Penetrating trauma
Type IV	Arteriovenous fistula	Penetrating trauma
Type V	Arterial spasm	Blunt or penetrating trauma

Ischemia of the tissues in turn can be a result of either a direct injury to the supplying vessel or tissue pressure due to third spacing, hematoma formation, or excessive tissue stretching causing decrease in circulation and tissue necrosis. For example, following a LeFort I osteotomy, both the direct injury to the descending palatine vessels and excessive stretching of palatal tissues may increase the chance of maxillary necrosis. Detailed knowledge of the anatomy, anticipation of possible complicating events, and predisposing health conditions and meticulous surgical technique help minimize the chance of hemorrhage and loss of tissue due to vascular trauma.

When the injury to the blood vessel occurs, the degree of endothelial disruption can be categorized into five categories (Table 50.1) [3].

50.3 Topical Hemostatic Agents

In addition to standard suturing, and use of bone wax and vascular clips, topical hemostatic agents are routinely used as either adjunctive or alternative treatments to control bleeding in maxillofacial surgery [4]. These materials include gelatin, cellulose, hemostatic collagen, bone wax, topical thrombin, and fibrin sealant. Gelfoam is an absorbable gelatin compressed sponge that is prepared from purified porcine skin gelatin [4]. It can be placed into the tooth socket or any other bleeding site and acts as a scaffold for blood coagulation. Surgicel is an o-xidized regenerated methylcellulose dressing that like Gelfoam can be placed in the various bleeding sites. Due to its low pH, Surgicel binds platelets and chemically precipitates fibrin to form a blood clot. CollaTape and CollaPlug (Sulzer Denal, Carlsbad CA) are both made of highly cross-linked collagen that like gelfoam are compressed and are able to absorb large amounts of blood. They work by stimulating platelet adherence and clot stabilization. Unlike gelfoam, which liquefies within a week or less, cross-linked collagen products take 4–6 weeks to dissolve. Avitene is a powder made out of microfibrillar collagen, which can be mixed with saline and placed into bleeding cavities and wounds [5]. It acts similar to CollaTape and CollaPlug in stimulating the adherence of platelets and fibrin stabilization. Topical thrombin is a bovine-derived recombinant product, which is supplied in a fine powder that is mixed with $CaCl_2$ and can either be sprayed into the affected area or combined with gelfoam and applied directly. Topical thrombin cannot be used with Surgicel. Tisseel is a combination of bovine thrombin, human fibrin, $CaCl_2$, and aprotinin and works by its antifibrinolytic action. It requires a specialized mixing and heating delivery system and may be sprayed into the wounds and flaps.

Floseal is a human gelatin-thrombin matrix sealant that is commonly used as a topical surgical adjunct in regions where significant blood loss is expected such as rhytidectomy [6].

Tranexamic acid is a synthetic derivative of the amino acid lysine that exerts its antifibrinolytic effect through the reversible blockade of lysine-binding sites on plasminogen molecules [7]. It is supplied as a mouthwash solution and is used up to four times per day for several days to provide local antifibrinolytic treatment [8]. Aminocaproic acid (Amicar) is also an antifibrinolytic agent that can be given preoperatively to the patients at risk for bleeding such hemophiliacs [9].

50.4 Dentoalveolar Surgery

Life-threatening hemorrhage is seldom encountered in dentoalveolar surgery due to relatively small diameter vessel involvement and good access for direct control of bleeding. Like with any surgery, every effort should be made to identify patients with bleeding dyscrasias and to make sure that they are optimized for surgery [10–12].

Significant bleeding during mandibular dentoalveolar surgery is usually associated with injury to inferior alveolar artery and to a lesser degree lingual, sublingual, buccal, and submental arteries. Bleeding due to arteriovenous malformations has also been reported [13].

Bleeding encountered from the inferior alveolar artery after dental extractions can be troublesome due to difficulty in directly visualizing the vessel, and presence of inferior alveolar nerve, which prevents significant compression of the bleeding source due to the risk of injuring the nerve. In addition, often a pulsatile bleeding from a marrow channel can mimic the "arterial pulsation." When dealing with such bleeding, it is imperative to have good suction and light. In particular it is helpful to have very narrow suction tip to aid visualization in the apical portion of tooth socket. Unless the bleeding source is clearly visible, every effort should be made to conservatively pack the socket with either gelfoam or Surgicel. A topical thrombin mixed with gelfoam can provide an extremely successful treatment of extraction site bleeding. One should avoid using indiscriminate pressure, application of bone wax, and electrocautery, unless the source of bleeding is clearly visible and is away from neurovascular bundle.

Injury to the lingual artery may happen when a dental implant penetrates the lingual cortex, reflection of lingual flap for mylohyoid detachment, or direct injury to the floor of the mouth with a surgical drill.

Bleeding from lingual artery can be significant and can present a challenge due to possibility of significantly raising the floor of the mouth and obstructing airway, which is an emergency.

In cases where the lingual flap is reflected and the bleeding is directly visualized, clamping and ligation of the lingual artery can be attempted, being careful not to injure the lingual nerve or submandibular duct. If the bleeding source cannot be visualized, a prompt pressure on the floor of the mouth with a gauze and digital pressure should be made. In certain cases, the patient may need to be transferred to the hospital for a definite airway and exploratory surgery or selective embolization as this type of bleeding can be life-threatening. Similarly, bleeding from the submental artery can be encountered with mandibular symphyseal bone graft harvesting or after raising a lingual flap and is managed in a similar fashion as lingual artery bleeding.

Maxillary sources of bleeding during dentoalveolar surgery mainly involve the greater and lesser palatine arteries and infraorbital artery. Maxillary bleeding during dentoalveolar surgery is rarely serious and can usually be managed similarly to the bleeding in the mandible such as direct pressure, use of hemostatic agents, and direct electrocautery.

50.5 Dental Implant Surgery and Intraoral Bone Grafting

Significant bleeding associated with dental implant placement and intraoral bone grafting is uncommon [14]. Multiple case reports involving significant hemorrhage due to dental implant placement have been published [15–17, 36]. During the placement of dental implants in the mandible, either an inferior alveolar artery or lingual artery may be injured. Injury to the inferior alveolar nerve and artery are the most common complication during the posterior mandibular implant placement [14].

A careful preoperative planning with the aid of computer tomography allows localization of the inferior alveolar canal and location of mandibular lingual concavity and the lingual cortex in the interforaminal zone [18] (Fig. 50.2).The use of intraoperative X-rays to access the depth and direction of implant osteotomy, additionally, helps prevent accidental injury to the inferior alveolar neurovascular bundle [19]. Implant surgery in the anterior mandibular region in between the mental foramina may cause injury to either sublingual branch of lingual artery or submental artery [18, 20]. Such injury can cause severe floor of the mouth hemorrhage and airway compromise.

Sinus floor elevation is a common procedure used in cases where the alveolar bone resorption and increased sinus pneumatization led to insufficient bone height for placement of dental implants. Significant bleeding during the sinus lift surgery is rare [21]. The blood supply to the maxillary sinus is provided by an infraorbital, posterior superior alveolar (PSA), and greater palatine arteries.

Alveolar antral artery is a communicating branch between the PSA and infraorbital arteries. It travels either in the intrabony channel in the lateral antral wall or extrabony and can be injured during the sinus lift procedure [21, 22]. The use of Piezotome during the surgery can help isolate this vessel and prevent its transection. Significant

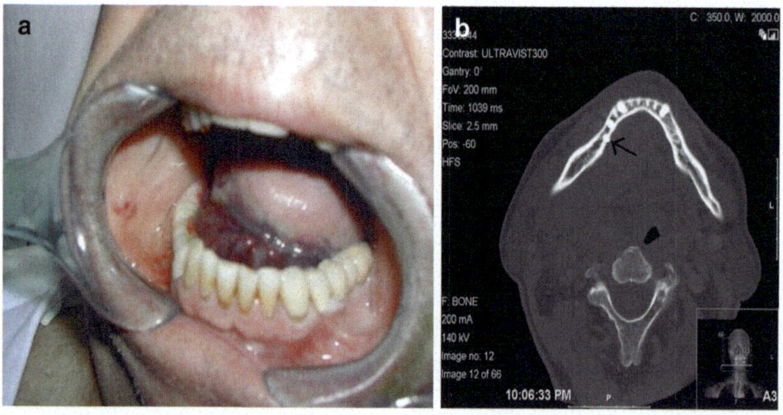

Fig. 50.2 (**a**) Floor of the mouth hematoma and tongue deviation following mandibular implant placement. (**b**) CT image of implant positioned in the mandibular right first molar site and perforation of lingual plate (arrow) (With kind permission. Dr. Elie Ferneini. *Ferneini et al. Floor of Mouth Hematoma. J Oral Maxillofac Surg 2009*)

bleeding during the sinus lift procedure can be managed by application of bone graft in combination with topical hemostatic agents to exert pressure on the wound, crushing the bleeding vessel within the antral bony channel, and use of electrocautery. Postoperative bleeding following this procedure may manifest as transient epistaxis, and patients should be instructed in sinus precautions for 5–7 days postoperatively.

Various intraoral sites for bone graft harvesting have been described and include mandibular symphysis, mandibular ramus, and maxillary tuberosity. Harvesting of autogenous bone graft from mandibular symphysis has a potential of injury to mental arteries, sublingual artery, and submental artery. The risk of bleeding complications with this procedure is rare, and most common sources of bleeding are from marrow or vascular bony channels which can be adequately controlled with topical hemostatic agents [23]. Bleeding risk depends on the surgical technique, degree of visualization of mental foramina, and the depth of osteotomy in the symphysis region. In most cases, harvesting of unicortical symphysis graft can provide adequate volume of bone for intraoral grafting. Bicortical mandibular symphysis bone graft harvesting which includes buccal and lingual cortices carries the risk of accidental transection of submental artery and severe hemorrhage.

Ascending ramus and mandibular body are common sources for autogenous intraoral graft harvesting. The ease of access and limited morbidity, when compared to the symphysis graft harvesting, make this site a popular choice for reconstruction of small- to medium-sized alveolar defects [23]. The pertinent vascular anatomy in the region includes inferior alveolar neurovascular bundle, buccal artery and vein, and facial artery. Although the risk of bleeding is small, several studies have reported bleeding as a complication [24, 25]. Careful subperiosteal dissection and the use of retractors during the osteotomy allow adequate soft tissue reflection and protection against accidental injury to the facial and buccal arteries. Preoperative CT assessment of the ramus allows clinician an opportunity to locate the position of the inferior alveolar canal in relation to the planned osteotomies, thus further reducing the risk of bleeding and nerve injury.

50.6 Epistaxis

Mild to life-threatening nasal bleeding is one of the most common emergencies encountered by head and neck surgical specialists and accounts for about 1 in 200 emergency department visits in the United States [26]. Epistaxis can be a result of direct trauma; physiologic changes such as hypertension, medications (anticoagulants), abnormal anatomy, and postsurgical trauma; and vascular changes.

The essential part of managing any epistaxis is early primary control with nasal packs, assessment of patient's hemodynamic status, adequate fluid or blood replacement, and a quick thorough patient assessment to identify possibly contributing local or systemic factors (Table 50.2).

The sources of intranasal bleeding usually involve Kiesselbach's plexus in the anterior septal region and Woodruff's plexus in the posteroinferior region.

Kiesselbach's plexus is one the most common sources of epistaxis [27, 28]. Also called Little's area, it is located 15 mm posterior to the anterior mucocutaneous junction. It is composed of anastomosis of posterior nasal artery, nasolabial artery, and anterior and posterior ethmoid arteries. Due to its more anterior location, isolated anterior nasal bleeding can usually be success-

Table 50.2 Local and systemic factors involved in epistaxis

Local factors	Systemic factors
Trauma	Hypertension
Topical medications (nasal sprays)	Vascular disorders
Foreign body	Allergies
Chemical irritants	Medications
Nasal pathology	Drugs
Anatomic abnormalities	Alcohol
Barometric changes	Infections
	Malnutrition
	Clotting disorders

fully managed by local means due to good visualization and good access.

Posterior nasal bleeding is most commonly located in Woodruff's region, which is located in the posterior aspect of inferior turbinate. It is composed of sphenopalatine artery, posterior nasal artery, and pharyngeal artery.

Initial patient presentation with epistaxis can vary between minor bleeding from one or both nostrils to severe bleeding with patient having trouble with maintaining airway. A good light and suction are the two most important tools for initial patient management. The patient should be placed in a semi-reclined position. The blood clots should be suctioned out from both nasal passages. All efforts should be made to identify the location of bleeding in order to choose the appropriate course of action. The direct examination usually involves visualization of nares, nasal roof, nasal floor, and anterior and posterior septal regions.

If not contraindicated, a topical anesthetic, with a vasoconstrictor can be applied via aerosolizing spray or cotton pledgets inside the nose for 7–10 min. This initial treatment may decrease or stop the bleeding allowing for a better exam and assessment. If available, a rigid or flexible endoscope can be used bedside to visualize the nasal cavity in order to determine the origin of bleeding [29]. In some instances, especially with brisk bleeding, it may not be possible to initially determine the location of bleeding. In these cases, the anterior and posterior intranasal regions should be packed to allow for bleeding stabilization and time for assessment and definitive treatment plan.

In cases of observed isolated anterior nasal bleeding, the nasal cavity can be packed with either petroleum jelly gauze, Merocel® sponges, Rapid Rhino® device, or a urinary catheter inflated to stop the bleeding (Fig. 50.3). These conservative procedures are often successful enough to stop the epistaxis and usually can be kept in place for up to several days. If posterior bleeding is encountered, then the initial line of treatment would be to use a Foley catheter to tamponade the nasopharynx. Although this treatment is usually used as a first-line therapy for posterior nasal bleeding, it is associated with a 26–50% failure rate [30]. For this reason, some investigators are advocating for endoscopic nasal cauterization as a first-line treatment in managing the posterior nasal bleeding [31, 32] (Fig. 50.1).

Once it is determined that the conservative measures are not adequate for management of epistaxis, the decision has to be made to either take the patient to the operating room in order to secure the airway and surgically stop the bleeding or to send the patient to interventional radiology for selective embolization.

The decision to operate versus the use of interventional radiology should be based upon the surgeon's experience with management of intranasal bleeding, experience in endoscopy, and availability of interventional radiology. Operative option allows a thorough assessment of hemorrhage with a secured airway and a controlled environment. Intraoperatively, isolated anterior nasal hemorrhage can be managed by a careful coagulation with either electrocautery or silver nitrate. Posterior nasal bleeding that is not responsive to electrocautery or is difficult to visualize can be addressed with sphenopalatine artery ligation (Fig. 50.4). If either of the above treatment modalities are unsuccessful in controlling the hemorrhage, then the surgeon must make a choice between carotid artery ligation or, if available, sending the patient for selective embolization.

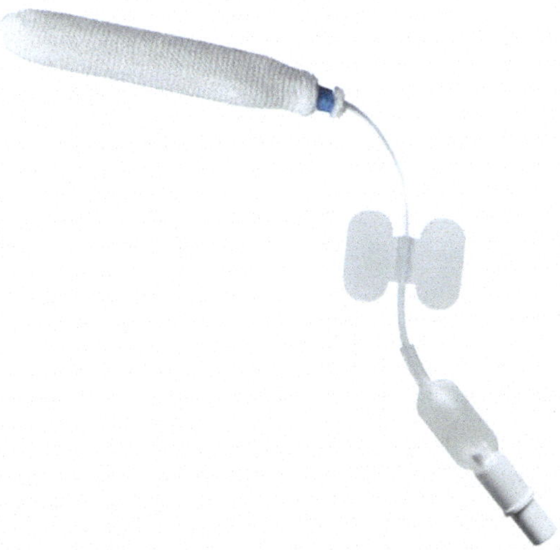

Fig. 50.3 Rapid Rhino epistaxis device. Reproduced with permission from Smith and Nephew

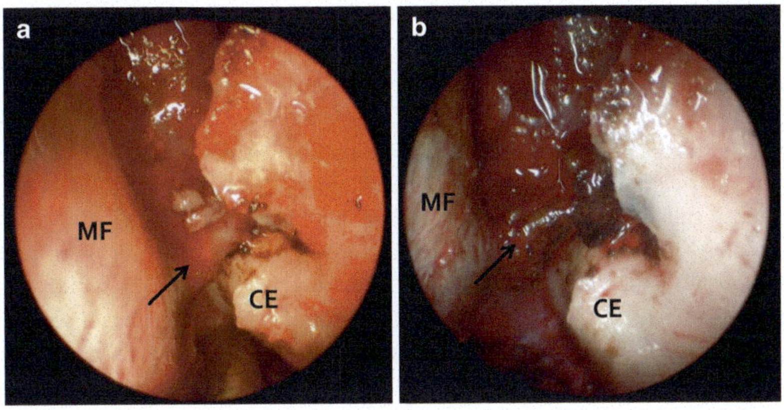

Fig. 50.4 An intra-operative endoscopic photo showing the left sphenopalatine artery (black arrow) before bipolar diathermy (**a**) and after bipolar diathermy (**b**). *CE* Crista Ethmoidalis, *ME* elevated mucosal flap. With kind permission from Dr. Hossam Thabet

50.7 TMJ Surgery

Temporomandibular joint (TMJ) region consists of mandibular condyle, squamous portion of glenoid bone, articular disk, fibrous capsule that is lined inside with synovial membrane, and accessory ligaments. The blood supply to the TMJ region is mainly derived from the branches of internal maxillary artery, superficial temporal artery, and maxillary artery.

The retrodiscal tissue is supplied by posterior auricular, anterior tympanic, and middle meningeal arteries, which are all branches of internal maxillary artery [33].

Temporomandibular surgery can be divided into three categories: arthrocentesis and arthroscopy, direct open arthroplasty, and total joint replacement.

Vascular complications of TMJ surgery can either involve the superficial vessels, which can be encountered during the entry into the joint, internal joint bleeding, or injury to the internal maxillary artery during the open surgical approaches.

The incidence of vascular injuries during TMJ arthroscopy is low. Carter et al. reported the incidence rate of 2% [34]. The initial entry into the TMJ with a trocar as it passes through the superficial temporal fascia can cause injury to the superficial vessels in the region. These include superficial temporal artery and vein, transverse facial artery and vein, and masseteric artery. Superficial temporal artery is located at a mean distance of 12.8 mm from the posterior aspect of the tragus [34]. This vessel is in particular vulnerable to puncture injuries during the initial entry into the TMJ with a trocar [35].

If the initial bleeding is encountered, it is rarely serious and can most of the time be treated with direct pressure using a gauze dressing. Ligation of the bleeding vessel, or selective embolization, is rarely required except in cases where the bleeding is due to arteriovenous (AV) malformations or vascular lesions [36].

Once the TMJ is entered, the most common cause of bleeding is during accidental medial wall puncture and bleeding in the retrodiscal tissue. In most cases, interarticular bleeding can be managed conservatively by increasing the hydraulic pressure in the joint during arthroscopy, injection of vasoconstrictors, electrocautery, or lateral compression with gauze.

During the open TMJ surgery, the most commonly used approach is either preauricular incision with or without Blair modification or endaural approach.

Once the superficial temporal fascia is reached, the location of superficial temporal vein is directly behind the superficial temporal artery. These vessels are usually well visualized and can be either protected or ligated. During inadvertent direct injury to the superficial temporal vessels, either electrocautery or ligation is usually enough to stop the bleeding due to good visualization.

Patients presenting with TMJ ankylosis are most commonly treated by gap arthroplasty, resection of proximal condylar segment, and a reconstruction with either costochondral graft or

TMJ prosthesis. Significant amount of bone removal is usually required in the glenoid fossa in order to remove the ankylosed tissue and prepare the space for TMJ reconstruction. There is a risk of direct injury to the internal maxillary artery during medial osteotomy [37]. Such injury could result in a significant hemorrhage, which could be difficult to manage intraoperatively due to poor visualization and poor access. Unless there is a clear visualization, blind clamping of the bleeding vessels should not be routinely performed in this location due to abundance of other anatomic structures that are passing medial to the condyle and ramus such as middle meningeal artery and mandibular branch (V3) of trigeminal nerve. In cases of injury to the internal maxillary artery or middle meningeal artery, the bleeding could be managed with gauze packing, injection of local anesthetic with vasoconstrictor, electrocautery, placement of hemostatic agents, arterial clipping, external carotid artery ligation, and selective embolization [38]. Cillo et al. reported successfully using gelatin-based hemostatic agents for superficial temporal and middle meningeal artery bleeding during the TMJ replacement surgery [39].

50.8 Orthognathic Surgery

Significant bleeding during or after orthognathic surgery is uncommon, but potentially serious complications as result of intraoperative direct vessel injury have been reported [40]. Most of the reported cases of hemorrhage associated with orthognathic surgery involve LeFort I osteotomy [40].

Bleeding encountered during or after LeFort I osteotomy is the most common vascular complication in orthognathic surgery and can be due to either arterial or venous injury [41]. The maxilla receives its blood supply mainly from the branches of maxillary artery with some contribution from ascending palatine and ascending pharyngeal arteries. Maxillary artery posteriorly gives off the descending palatine branch, which travels in intrabony channel in in the posterior lateral nasal wall [41]. It then courses inferiorly through the greater palatine canal on each side to give rise to greater and lesser palatine nerves.

Intraoperative bleeding during LeFort I osteotomy commonly occurs following the downfracture of the maxilla. The bleeding, which is usually transient, either emanates from the pterygoid plexus or descending palatine arteries which are located posteriorly in the lateral nasal wall. Injury to the descending palatine arteries is more likely to happen during significant forward advancement, posterior maxillary retrusion, posterior maxillary intrusion, and horseshoe palatal osteotomy [41].

When separating the lateral nasal walls, care should be taken not to advance the single guarded osteotome more than 25–30 mm posteriorly from the pyriform rim. The average distance of the descending palatine canal to the pyriform rim is 34 mm (Cheung LK et al. posterior maxillary anatomy).

During the pterygomaxillary disjunction, the curved osteotome should be angled anteroinferiorly because the maxillary artery is located 10 mm superior to the superior edge of the osteotome. The oozing encountered intraoperatively can be successfully treated with topical hemostatic agents and gauze packing in the posterior maxilla. The use of hypotensive anesthesia, especially right prior to downfracture of the maxilla can be helpful in decreasing the overall blood loss from this procedure [42–44]. If significant bleeding from the descending palatine arteries is encountered, then the arteries should be ligated with vascular clips. Clipping of the vessel is superior to electrocautery as the latter can destroy the visible part of the vessel and cause the proximal portion to retract superiorly inside the bony canal. In such an event, the area should be packed with a hemostatic material and situation reassessed.

Even in cases with relatively minimal intraoperative bleeding, prior to the final fixation of the maxillary segments, it is imperative to inspect the descending palatine arteries for minor bleeding or any tears. If any injury to the vessel is suspected, it is better to air on the side of caution and ligate the vessel to prevent the formation of pseudoaneurysm and delayed hemorrhage. Pseudoaneurysm, or false aneurysm, is a rare complication of orthognathic surgery and is caused by an incomplete arterial tear, causing bleeding into the surrounding soft tissues [45]. The continuity of the blood flow in the vessel is maintained, and bleeding occurs into the soft tissues surrounding the vessel. The perivascular hematoma increases in size until its pressure is greater than the arterial pressure. The resultant sac will form an endothelial lining that is continuous with the artery and be influenced by the arterial pressure [46]. The pseudoaneurysm can then expand and rupture.

Postoperative hemorrhage following the LeFort I osteotomy usually initially presents as an epistaxis two weeks postoperatively [45]. It is usually severe enough that the patient is brought into the emergency room. First line of treatment normally constitutes packing both nasal cavities with anterior and posterior nasal packs. If this treatment is ineffective then, opening of the incisions and packing the maxillary sinuses and pterygomaxillary regions with either a gauze or hemostatic agents can be performed [45–48]. In cases of severe hemorrhage, the surgeon may attempt either unilateral or bilateral external carotid artery ligation, reoperation to visualize the bleeding vessel, or selective embolization. If available, selective embolization should be the treatment of choice for delayed hemorrhage following the LeFort I surgery [49].

In addition to hemorrhage, avascular necrosis of the maxilla is a rare but serious complication that can lead to significant morbidity. This complication is usually due to disruption of maxillary blood supply through the posterior palatal pedicle and palatal soft tissues. Postoperatively, initial blanching and cyanosis of the attached gingiva can progress to sloughing off of soft tissues and maxillary necrosis [50]. Prevention is the best treatment and includes careful handling of soft tissues, making sure that the palatal soft tissue pedicle is not overstretched and cared to reduce the chance of palatal lacerations. In cases of initial suspicion of compromised blood supply, treatment steps include placement of maxilla into the original position, prevention of secondary infection with oral antiseptic rinses and antibiotics, use of nitroglycerin paste on the intraoral tissues, and hyperbaric oxygen (HBO) treatment. HBO does not stop or reverse avascular necrosis, but it can delineate the area of necrosis [50].

Hemorrhage associated with mandibular orthognathic surgical procedures is rare when compared to maxillary LeFort I osteotomy. Most common sources of arterial bleeding in the mandible may occur from damage to the inferior alveolar neurovascular bundle during bilateral sagittal split osteotomy (BSSO) and injury to the masseteric artery during intraoral vertical ramus osteotomy IVRO). Injury to the inferior alveolar neurovascular bundle most often occurs proximally near the lingula or during the actual split in the body of the mandible [51]. Such injuries can be prevented, by obtaining a preoperative CT scan to locate the mandibular canal and the position of lingula. Intraoperatively, attention should be directed to careful medial soft tissue reflection, adequate visualization of neurovascular bundle at the lingula, and careful use of medial retractor. During the actual sagittal split, the osteotome should be kept just beneath the cortical plate to prevent damage to the inferior alveolar nerve. In the event of witnessed transection of inferior alveolar neurovascular bundle, bleeding should be managed with topical hemostatic agents. Coagulation, clipping, or clamping of the bundle is contraindicated due to potentially serious damage to inferior alveolar nerve. After the cessation of bleeding, the bundle should be repaired prior to mandibular fixation.

Damage to the facial artery can occur during BSSO at the time of subperiosteal dissection near the inferior border of the mandible. The periosteal elevator could penetrate the periosteum and directly injure the facial artery causing significant hemorrhage. If the injured vessel can be clearly visualized intraorally, then it can be clamped and ligated or clipped, keeping in mind the close location of marginal mandibular branch of facial nerve. In rare cases where it is not possible to visualize the bleeding, it may be necessary to access the facial artery via an extraoral approach. Pseudoaneurysm formation following

BSSO has also been reported [52]. Masseteric artery passes through the sigmoid notch to the deep surface of masseter muscle. Injury to the masseteric artery during IVRO can be prevented with careful lateral soft tissue stripping, visualization of sigmoid notch, and use of Bauer retractors for good access [51].

Sliding genioplasty is the procedure that is commonly performed for the correction of chin positioning. Branches of the submental and sublingual arteries are the most common source of significant postoperative bleeding associated with this procedure. Postoperative hemorrhage can cause a significant floor of the mouth hematoma formation that could lead to airway embarrassment [53].

50.9 Trauma

The head, neck, and face injuries account for 12% of total body injuries [54].

Vascular complications related to maxillofacial trauma range from minor bleeding from superficial soft tissue injuries to late post-traumatic aneurysms associated with significant facial fractures [55–58]. Treatment of post-traumatic bleeding depends on the mode and degree of injury, as well as the anatomic regions involved.

When assessing a trauma patient, it is important to perform a systematic and thorough head and neck examination starting with the scalp and finishing in the subclavicular region. Any laceration, abrasion, and ecchymosis should be noted and documented. Superficial soft tissue trauma of the head and neck can present with significant hemorrhage, especially in the scalp region where there is a very rich vascular network [59–61]. Provided that the primary survey has been completed, any profuse head and neck bleeding should be managed immediately to prevent significant blood volume loss and shock. This can often be accomplished in the trauma bay using pressure dressings, coagulation, vascular clips, topical hemostatic agents, sutures. or staples. In rare cases, where it is not possible to find the source of significant bleeding, the patient may require an emergency exploratory surgery, carotid artery ligation, or selective embolization.

Thorough ophthalmologic, otoscopic, intranasal, and intraoral examinations should be performed because bleeding in these regions could indicate more serious injuries.

A finding of proptosis, severe pain, ophthalmoplegia, decrease in visual acuity, diplopia, chemosis, mydriasis, loss of direct pupillary reflex, and subconjunctival hemorrhage could indicate a retrobulbar hematoma and orbital compartment syndrome with increased intraocular pressure [62]. This is a rapidly progressing hemorrhage in the retrobulbar space and can lead to blindness if not treated. The conservative treatment ranges from bedrest and globe massage to mannitol infusion [62]. Emergent treatment usually requires a lateral canthotomy and inferior cantholysis to allow the accumulated blood to exit through the wound and relieve the pressure on the globe.

Bloody otorrhea could be a consequence of multiple conditions including internal ear injuries, subcondylar mandibular fractures, zygomatic fractures, and basilar skull fractures [63, 64]. Basilar skull fractures occur in 3.5–20% of all head injuries and correlate positively with orbital wall, rim, and ZMC fractures [64]. Some of the positive vascular clinical findings of basilar skull fractures include periorbital ecchymosis and edema, subconjunctival hemorrhage, bloody rhinorrhea, Battle sign, and otorrhea. These findings are important and can lead the medical team to perform additional tests in a timely fashion since vascular damage from skull fractures can occur in up to 50% of patients as delayed ischemic brain damage.

Traumatic epistaxis is a common finding in patients with maxillofacial trauma. It can be due to direct injury to Kiesselbach's or Woodruff's plexuses, maxillary fractures with injuries to maxillary artery and its branches, zygomatic fractures, and basilar skull fractures. Severe epistaxis that is associated with facial trauma often necessitates anterior and posterior nasal packs. Some of the nasal packs involve either dedicated balloon systems or urinary catheters. In patients with basilar skull fractures, placement of such devices poses a significant risk and can cause violation of cranial vault and intracranial placement of these devices that could lead to significant neurologic injury [65–69].

Significant hemorrhage as a result of facial fractures is not common [70]. Injuries to internal maxillary, infraorbital, posterior superior alveolar, and other branches of external and internal carotid arteries can happen as a result of vessel disruption from bony displacement. A thorough clinical and radiographic assessment is crucial in identifying the extent of injury to determine the possible source of bleeding.

Due to its facial prominence, nasal fractures account for 50% of all facial fractures in adults [71]. Hemorrhage related to isolated nasal fractures is almost always due to injuries to Kiesselbach's and Woodruff's plexuses, and its treatment has been described in the earlier section.

LeFort and zygomatic fractures almost always involve fractures in the maxillary sinus walls, which cause a steady bleeding in the antral and nasal cavities. Injury to the descending palatine artery during traumatic LeFort or zygomaticomaxillary complex fractures can cause significant hemorrhage and epistaxis requiring emergent treatment. The treatment for this type of injury is similar to the treatment of post-orthognathic LeFort I osteotomy bleeding, although in the midst of other facial fractures and injuries, the bleeding source may at first not be apparent. In such event, interventional radiology can prove invaluable in identifying the bleeding vessel and embolizing it.

Patients presenting with mandibular fractures are also at risk for significant hemorrhage, depending on the level of fracture.

Condylar process fractures account for 25–35% of all mandibular fractures [72]. Intracapsular fractures and subsequent bleeding into the TMJ can cause intra-articular hemarthrosis and progression to eventual TMJ ankylosis [73]. Significant posterior extracapsular displacement of the mandibular condyle may lacerate eternal auditory canal and cause tympanic membrane and internal ear injury and otorrhea [74]. Superior condylar displacement into middle cranial fossa is a rare complication but can cause vascular complications such as hemorrhage from middle meningeal artery and dural tears causing subdural and epidural hematoma formation [75]. Eao and colleagues described a case of maxillary artery hemorrhage as a result of bilateral subcondylar fractures causing progressive expansile preauricular edema [76]. In addition to direct airway compromise from bilateral mandibular body fractures, potential sublingual and submental hemorrhage can be caused by direct trauma to the floor of the mouth, submental and submandibular regions. In such cases, prior to any bony fixation, all vascular injuries have to be controlled with either direct examination and ligation of bleeding vessels or selective embolization.

The neck can be divided into three anatomic zones, which historically has been used for evaluation of injuries [77] (Table 50.3). Zone-driven selective surgical approach allowed surgeons systematic exploration of a particular zone and was successful based on the relative ease with which surgeons could access Zone II injuries compared with the more technically demanding Zones I and III. Exploration of all neck wounds deep to the platysma lead to a significant number of high negative exploration rates, increased patient mortality and increased costs [78]. Recently, however, advances in sensitive medical technology including CT angiography (CTA) are widely available. This modality, along with clinical examination, allows safe and noninvasive evaluation of trajectory of traumatic force, loca-

Table 50.3 Neck zones and vascular structures at risk

	Anatomic borders	Vascular structures at risk
Zone 1	From clavicle to cricoid cartilage	– Aortic arch – Subclavian arteries – Brachiocephalic veins – Common carotid arteries – Jugular veins
Zone 2	From cricoid cartilage to angle of the mandible	– Carotid arteries – Vertebral arteries – Jugular veins
Zone 3	From angle of the mandible to the base of the skull	– Carotid arteries – Jugular veins

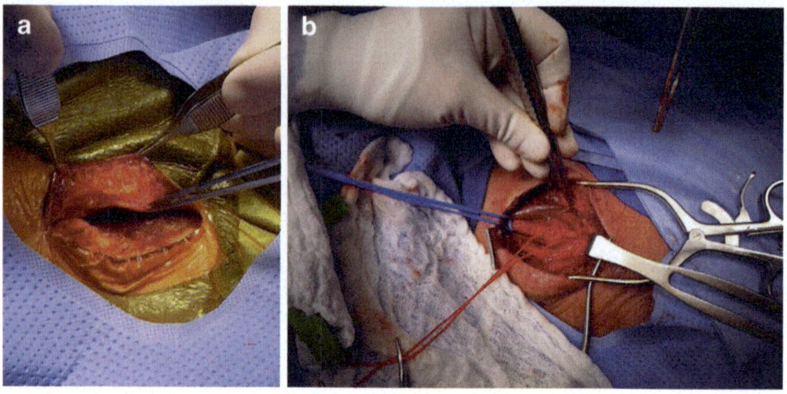

Fig. 50.5 (**a**) Neck dissection to expose carotid artery. (**b**) Common carotid bifurcation

tion, and degree of injury and is referred to as "no zone" approach [79].

Superficial soft tissue injuries make up the majority of traumatic injuries to the neck. Such injuries, which include lacerations, abrasions, and avulsions, can be treated directly with soft tissue closure, local and free flaps. Blunt neck trauma may at first not be as identifiable as direct injuries but has potential for serious vascular injuries. Direct blunt trauma to the anterior neck, especially in the Zone II, can compress and rupture the carotid arteries causing a rapidly expanding hematoma and airway occlusion [80]. Direct blows to the side of the head can cause rotational injury, resulting in hyperextension of the carotid artery across the cervical spine, causing a dissection, formation of pseudoaneurysm, and thrombosis [80, 81]. Penetrating neck injuries (PNIs) can cause a serious concern due to the proximity of vital structures such as blood vessels, nerves, and the airway. Management of neck trauma includes stabilization of airway and c-spine, use of Foley catheters and balloon inflation to stabilize bleeding, identification and ligation of bleeding vessels, electrocautery, use of hemostatic agents, and selective embolization [81].

50.10 External Carotid Artery Ligation

In maxillofacial surgery, significant bleeding can usually be at least temporarily controlled with conservative measures including the use of topical hemostatic agents and wound packing with gauze. If permanent bleeding arrest is not possible, then the external carotid artery (ECA) ligation and selective embolization can be used to achieve definitive control [82].

Although not commonly performed due to availability of interventional radiology and embolization, external carotid artery ligation has important implications in patients with severe and uncontrolled hemorrhage [82–85]. This is especially true in circumstances where selective embolization is not available, and ECA ligation is the only procedure that can prevent shock [85–87]. Complications of ECA ligation include bleeding, aneurysm formation, facial paresis, pain in muscles of mastication, diplopia, and gait disturbance [85, 87] (Fig. 50.5).

50.11 Angiography and Selective Embolization

In comparison to carotid ligation, the use of angiography and selective embolization (SE) in arresting severe hemorrhage has gained a wide popularity due to its low morbidity, minimally invasive nature, and its ability to highly selectively embolize the vessel very close to the site of bleeding, thus limiting the impact of collateral circulation [85, 88, 89]. This treatment modality was first used for management of head and neck bleeding in 1973 and has since become the standard of care in most major medical centers [89]. It is now routinely used for management of hemorrhage due to epistaxis, traumatic injuries, orthognathic surgery, TMJ surgery, and vascular lesions.

Depending on the source of bleeding, angiography with or without embolization can be performed either preoperatively to assess the arterial anatomy, intraoperatively to find the bleeding vessel and embolize it, or postoperatively to confirm the success of embolization. It is an extremely useful treatment modality in cases of arteriovenous malformations (Fig. 50.6a, b). These lesions, which are either high or low flow, contain enlarged arteries and veins soiled around each other. The high flow lesions have a high risk of spontaneous rupture and hemorrhage. They often have multiple sources of feeding vessels especially in cases of previous attempted therapy to sclerose the lesion. Preoperative angiography allows clear visualization of vascular anatomy and feeding vessels, which can be used as an intraoperative guide (Fig. 50.6c, d). The procedure involves insertion of catheter through either a femoral or radial vein. The catheter is then advanced to the site of suspected bleeding, and a contrast material is injected to visualize the anatomy. Once the decision is made to embolize the vessel, various particular or liquid agents can be used. Coils, acrylic microspheres, gelfoam, microfibrillar collagen, autologous clots, and detachable balloons can be used to embolize the vessel. Following embolization, angiography is then performed once again to assess the success of the procedure. Risk and complications of angiography and

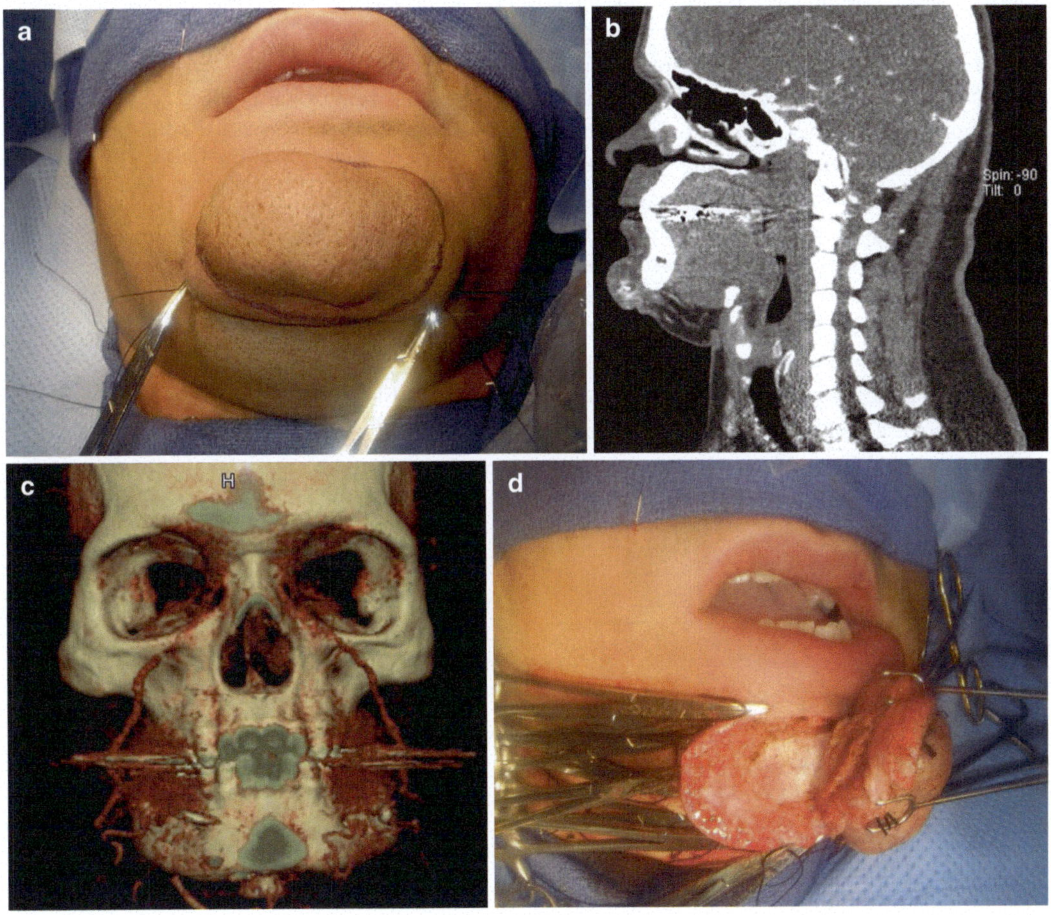

Fig. 50.6 (**a**) Vascular malformation of the chin. Although this lesion was previously treated with injection of sclerosing material, it did not change its behavior, and it continued to increase in size. (**b**) CT with contrast demonstrating vascularity of the lesion. (**c**) CT angiogram demonstrating feeding arteries from the left. (**d**) Excision of the vascular lesion by careful dissection toward the feeding vessels

embolization are rare and include hematoma formation at the site of percutaneous access, facial numbness, tissue necrosis, pulmonary embolism, stroke blindness, and distal tissue injury [85, 90].

Conclusion

Vascular injuries and complications of the maxillofacial region can be a result of traumatic injuries, pathologic processes, or direct surgical trauma. Detailed knowledge of head and neck vascular anatomy and hemostatic mechanisms is important in order to be able to quickly assess the source and severity of bleeding and plan on appropriate treatment. In particular, the location of internal maxillary artery and its terminal branches including their variations is integral in many procedures that are commonly performed including dentoalveolar surgery, dental implant surgery, TMJ surgery, orthognathic surgery, maxillofacial infections, and maxillofacial trauma. Pathologic processes and traumatic injuries to the head and neck and in particular penetrating neck injuries can cause a significant hemorrhage from the carotid and jugular systems. These injuries have to be recognized very early in the course of patient assessment, and their timely management is critical to patient survival. Finally, in the event of significant bleeding, a clinician has to be able to make a quick decision in regard to whether to perform a surgical exploration and treatment such as coagulation and ligation or to refer the patient for selective embolization if the resources are available.

References

1. Brotfain E, Koyfman L, Schwartz A, Rusabrov E, Frenkel A, Zlotnik A, Klein M. Spontaneous sublingual hematoma: surgical or non-surgical management? Int J Case Rep Images. 2012;3(1):1–4.
2. Feliciano DV. Management of peripheral arterial injuries. Curr Opin Crit Care. 2010;16(6):602–8.
3. Feliciano DV, Moore FA, Moore EE, West MA, Davis JW, Cocanour CS, Kozar RA, McIntyre RC Jr. Evaluation and management of peripheral vascular injury. Part 1. Western Trauma Association/critical decisions in trauma. J Trauma. 2011;70:1551–6.
4. Schonauer C, Tessitore E, Barbagallo G, Albanese V, Moraci A. The use of local agents: bone wax, gelatin, collagen, oxidized cellulose. Eur Spine J. 2004;13(Suppl 1):S89–96.
5. Sundaram CP, Keenan AC. Evolution of hemostatic agents in surgical practice. Indian J Urol. 2010;26(3):374–8.
6. Giordano S, Koskivuo I, Suominen E, Verejankorva E. Tissue sealants may reduce haematoma and complications in face-lifts: a meta-analysis of comparative studies. J Plast Reconstr Aesthet Surg. 2016;70(3):297–306.
7. Dunn CJ, Goa KL. Tranexamic acid: a review of its use in surgery and other indications. Drugs. 1999;57(6):1005–32.
8. Ramström G, Sindet-Pedersen S, Hall G, Blombäck M, Alander U. Prevention of postsurgical bleeding in oral surgery using tranexamic acid without dose modification of oral anticoagulants. J Oral Maxillofac Surg. 1993;51(11):1211–6.
9. Cooksey MW, Perry CB, Raper AB. Epsilon-aminocaproic acid therapy for dental extractions in haemophiliacs. Br Med J. 1966;2(5530):1633–4.
10. Olmos-Carrasco O, Pastor-Ramos V, Espinilla-Blanco R, Ortiz-Zárate A, García-Avila I, Rodríguez-Alonso E, Herrero-Sanjuán R, Ruiz-García MM, Gallego-Beuter P, Sánchez-Delgado MP, Terán-Agustín AI, Fernández-Behar M, Peña-Sainz I. Hemorrhagic complications of dental extractions in 181 patients undergoing double antiplatelet therapy. J Oral Maxillofac Surg. 2015;73(2):203–10.
11. Bajkin BV, Urosevic IM, Stankov KM, Petrovic BB, Bajkin IA. Dental extractions and risk of bleeding in patients taking single and dual antiplatelet treatment. Br J Oral Maxillofac Surg. 2015;53(1):39–43.
12. Nath D, Kumath M, Tandon S, Panwar M. Case report fatal hemorrhage following extraction of first molar. J Indian Acad Forensic Med. 2011;33(4):370–1.
13. Kriwalsky MS, Papadimas D, Maurer P, Brinkmann M, Jackowski J, Kunkel M. Life-threatening bleeding after tooth extraction due to vascular malformation: a case report and literature review. Oral Maxillofac Surg. 2014;18(3):279–82.
14. Shelley AM, Ferrero A, Brunton P, Goodwin M, Horner K. The impact of CBCT imaging when placing dental implants in the anterior edentulous mandible: a before–after study. Dentomaxillofac Radiol. 2015;44(4):20140316.
15. Kalpidis CDR, Setayesh RM. Hemorrhaging associated with endosseous implant placement in the anterior mandible: a review of the literature. J Periodontol. 2004;75(5):631–45.
16. Ten Bruggenkate CM, Krekeler G, Kraaijenhagen HA, Foitzik C, Oosterbeek HS. Hemorrhage of the floor of the mouth resulting from lingual perforation during implant placement: a clinical report. Int J Oral Maxillofac Implants. 1993;8(3):48–57.
17. Darriba MA, Mendonca-Caridad JJ. Profuse bleeding and life-threatening airway obstruction after

placement of mandibular dental implants. J Oral Maxillofac Surg. 1997;55(11):1328–30.
18. Burstein J, Mastin C, Le B. Avoiding injury to the inferior alveolar nerve by routing use of intraoperative radiographs during implant placement. J Oral Implantol. 2008;34(1):34–8.
19. Kusum KK, Mody PV, et al. Interforaminal hemorrhage during anterior mandibular implant placement: an overview. Dent Res. 2015;12(4): 291–300.
20. Valente NA, Harogiannis K, Andreana S. Alveolar antral artery management during sinus elevation: a case report of a novel approach with review of the literature. Int J Contemp Dent Med Rev. 2015;2015, Article ID: 100215.
21. Boyne PJ, James RA. Grafting of the maxillary sinus floor with autogenous marrow and bone. J Oral Surg. 1980;38(8):613–6.
22. Maridati P, Stoffella E, Speroni S, Cicciu M, Maiorana C. Alveolar antral artery isolation during sinus lift procedure with the double window technique. Open Dent J. 2014;8:95–103.
23. Pikos M. Mandibular block autografts for alveolar ridge augmentation. Atlas Oral Maxillofacial Surg Clin N Am. 2005;13:91–107.
24. Silva FM, Cortez AL, Moreira RW, Mazzonetto R. Complications of intraoral donor site for bone grafting prior to implant placement. Implant Dent. 2006;15(4):420–6.
25. Cordaro L, Torsello F, Tindara Miuccio M, Mirisola di Torresanto V, Eliopoulos D. Mandibular bone harvesting for alveolar reconstruction and implant placement: Subjective and objective cross-sectional evaluation of donor and recipient site up to 4 years. Clin Oral Implants Res. 2011;22:1320.
26. Newton E, Lasso A, Petrcich W, Kilty SJ. An outcomes analysis of anterior epistaxis management in the emergency department. J Otolaryngol Head Neck Surg. 2016;45:24. https://doi.org/10.1186/s40463-016-0138-2.
27. Paul J, Kanotra SP, Kanotra S. Endoscopic management of posterior epistaxis. Indian J Otolaryngol Head Neck Surg. 2011;63(2):141–4.
28. McCLURG SW, CARRAU R. Endoscopic management of posterior epistaxis: a review. Acta Otorhinolaryngol Ital. 2014;34(1):1–8.
29. Kumar MV, Prasad KUR, Gowda PRB. Rigid nasal endoscopy in the diagnosis and treatment of epistaxis. J Clin Diagn Res. 2013;7(5):831–3.
30. Pritikin JB, Caldarelli DD, Panje WR. Endoscopic ligation of the internal maxillary artery for treatment of intractable posterior epistaxis. Ann Otol Rhinol Laryngol. 1998;107:85–91.
31. Paul J, Kanotra SP, Kanotra S. Endoscopic management of posterior epistaxis. Indian J Otolaryngol Head Neck Surg. 2011;63(2):141–4. https://doi.org/10.1007/s12070-010-0054-0.
32. Traboulsi H, Alam E, Hadi U. Changing trends in the management of epistaxis. Int J Otolaryngol. 2015;2015:263987.
33. Hatcher DC, Blom RJ, Baker CG. Temporomandibular joint spatial relationships: osseous and soft tissues. J Prosthet Dent. 1986;56(3):344–53.
34. Carter JB, Testa L. Complications of TMJ arthroscopy: a review of 2225 cases: review of the 1988 scientific session abstracts. J Oral Maxillofac Surg. 1988;46:M14.
35. Greene MW, Hacknewy FL, JE VS. Arthroscopy of the temporomandibular joint: an anatomic perspective. J Oral Maxillofac Surg. 1989;47:386.
36. Manning MP, Marshall JH. Aneurysm after arthroscopy. J Bone Joint Surg Br. 1987;69:151.
37. Cuccia AM, Caradonna C, Caradonna D, et al. The arterial blood supply of the temporomandibular joint: an anatomical study and clinical implications. Imaging Sci Dent. 2013;43(1):37–44.
38. Peoples JR, Herbosa EG, Dion J. Management of internal maxillary artery hemorrhage from temporomandibular joint surgery via selective embolization. J Oral Maxillofac Surg. 1988;46(11): 1005–7.
39. Cillo J. Management of middle meningeal and superficial temporal artery hemorrhage from total temporomandibular joint replacement surgery with a gelatin-based hemostatic agent. J Craniofac Surg. 2005;16(2):309–12.
40. Madani M, Veznedaroglu E, Pazoki A, Danesh J, Matson S. Pseudoaneurysm of the facial artery as a late complication of bilateral sagittal split osteotomy and facial trauma. Oral Surg Oral Med Oral Pathol Oral Radiol Endo. 2010;110:579–84.
41. Lanigan DT, Hey JH, West RA. Major vascular complications of orthognathic surgery: hemorrhage associated with Le Fort I osteotomies. Oral Maxillofac Surg. 1990;48(6):561–73.
42. Fromme GA, MacKenzie RA, Gould AB Jr, Lund BA, Offord KP. Controlled hypotension for orthognathic surgery. Anesth Analg. 1986;65(6):683–6.
43. Praveen K, Narayanan V, Muthusekhar MR, Baig MF. Hypotensive anaesthesia reduces blood loss in orthognathic surgery: a clinical study. Br J Oral Maxillofac Surg. 2001;39:138–40.
44. Ettinger KS, et al. Hypotensive anesthesia is associated with shortened length of hospital stay following orthognathic surgery. J Oral Maxillofac Surg. 2016;74(1):130–8.
45. Lanigan DT, Hey JH, West RA. Major vascular complications of orthognathic surgery: false aneurysms and arteriovenous fistulas following orthognathic surgery. J Oral Maxillofac Surg. 1991;49(6):571–7.
46. Krempl GA, Noorily AD. Pseudoaneurysm of the descending palatine artery presenting as epistaxis. Otolaryngol Head Neck Surg. 1996;114:453–6.
47. Bradley JP, Elahi M, Kawamoto HK. Delayed presentation of pseudoaneurysm after Le Fort I osteotomy. J Craniofac Surg. 2002;13(6):746–50.
48. Manafi A, Ghenaati H, Dezham F, Arshad M. Massive repeated nose bleeding after bimaxillary osteotomy. J Craniofac Surg. 2007;18(6):1491–3.

49. Avelar RL, Goelzer JG, Becker OE, de Oliveira RB, Raupp EF, de Magalhães PS. Embolization of pseudoaneurysm of the internal maxillary artery after orthognathic surgery. J Craniofac Surg. 2010;21(6):1764–8.
50. Shanker M, Hamilton FMR. Critical ischemia of the maxilla treated with hyperbaric oxygen. Br J Oral Maxillofac Surg. 2003;41:346.
51. Balcioglu HA, Kilic C, Varol A, Ozan H, Kocabiyik N, Yildirim M. A morphometric study of the maxillary artery and lingula in relation to mandibular ramus osteotomies and TMJ surgery. Eur J Dent. 2010;4(2):166–70.
52. Silva AC, O'Ryan F, Beckley ML, Young HY, Poor D. Pseudoaneurysm of a branch of the maxillary artery following mandibular sagittal split ramus osteotomy: case report and review of the literature. J Oral Maxillofac Surg. 2007;65(9):1807–16.
53. Lindquist CC, Beid G. Complications of genioplasty done alone or in combination with sagittal split-ramus osteotomy. Oral Surg Oral Med Oral Pathol. 1998;66(1):13–6.
54. Mackenzie EJ, Rivara FP, Jurkovich GJ, et al. The national study on costs and outcomes of trauma. J Trauma. 2007;63(6 Suppl):S54–67; discussion S81–6.
55. Newman F, Cillo J. Late vascular complication associated with panfacial fractures. J Oral Maxillofac Surg. 2008;66(11):2374–7.
56. Mauldin FW, Cornay WJ 3rd, Mahaley MS Jr, Hicks JN. Severe epistaxis from a false aneurysm of the external carotid artery. Otolaryngol Head Neck Surg. 1989;101:588–90.
57. Suzuki S, Kimura Y, Kanaji M, Sudo M, Igarashi M, Yamamoto H. Traumatic maxillary artery aneurysm with rupture into the maxillary sinus. Pract Otol (Kyoto). 1999;92:1107–10.
58. Bozkurt M, Kapi E, Karakol P, Yorgancilar E. Sudden rupture of the internal maxillary artery causing pseudoaneurysm (mandibular part) secondary to subcondylar mandible fracture. J Craniofac Surg. 2009;20:1430–2.
59. Hamilton JR. Fatal hemorrhage from simple lacerations of the scalp. Forensic Sci Med Pathol. 2005;1(4):267–72.
60. Turnage B, Maull KI. Scalp laceration: an obvious "occult" cause of shock. South Med J. 2000;93(3):265–6.
61. Lemos MJ, Clark DE. Scalp lacerations resulting in haemorrhagic shock: case reports and recommended management. J Emerg Med. 1998;6(5):377–9.
62. Bailey W, Kud PC, Evans LS. Diagnosis and treatment of retrobulbar hemorrhage. J Oral Maxillofac Surg. 1993;51:780-782.
63. Vasconcelos BC, et al. Posterior dislocation in intact mandibular condyle: an unusual case. Int J Oral Maxillofac Surg. 2010;39(1):89–91.
64. Slupchynskyj OS, Berkower AS, Byrne DW, Cayten CG. Association of skull base and facial fractures. The Laryngoscope. 1992;102:1247–50.
65. Veeravagu A, Joseph R, Jiang B, et al. Traumatic epistaxis: skull base defects, intracranial complications and neurosurgical considerations. Int J Surg Case Rep. 2013;4(8):656–61.
66. Porras LF, Cabezudo JM, Lorenzana L, Garcia-Yague LM, Rodriguez-Sanchez JA. Inadvertent intraspinal placement of a Foley catheter in severe craniofacial injury with associated atlanto-occipital dislocation: case report. Neurosurgery. 1993;33:310–1; discussion 311–313.
67. Huang HM, Wei ST, Chen DC, Lin HL. Preventing iatrogenic injury from inadvertent intracranial migration of a urinary Foley catheter while controlling profuse epistaxis after severe craniofacial trauma. J Craniofac Surg. 2011;22:748–9.
68. Pawar SJ, Sharma RR, Lad SD. Intracranial migration of Foley catheter—an unusual complication. J Clin Neurosci. 2003;10:248–9.
69. Woo HJ, Bai CH, Song SY, Kim YD. Intracranial placement of a Foley catheter: a rare complication. Otolaryngol Head Neck Surg. 2008;138:115–6.
70. Siritongtaworn P. Management of life threatening hemorrhage from facial fracture. J Med Assoc Thai. 2005;3:88.
71. Kelley BP, Downey CR, Stal S. Evaluation and reduction of nasal trauma. Semin Plastic Surg. 2010;24(4):339–47.
72. Barron RP, et al. Management of traumatic dislocation of the mandibular condyle into the middle cranial fossa. J Can Dent Assoc. 2002;68(11):676–80.
73. Yan Y-B, Liang S-X, Shen J, Zhang J-C, Zhang Y. Current concepts in the pathogenesis of traumatic temporomandibular joint ankylosis. Head Face Med. 2014;10:35.
74. Psimopoulou M, Antoniades K, Magoudi D, Karakasis D. Tympanic plate fracture following mandibular trauma. Dentomaxillofac Radiol. 1997;26:344–6.
75. Yeo MS, Goh TLH, Nallathamby V, Cheong EC, Lim TC. Maxillary artery injury associated with subcondylar mandible fractures: a novel treatment algorithm. Craniomaxillofac Trauma Reconstr. 2012;5(2):83–8.
76. Thal ER, Meyer DM. Penetrating neck trauma. Curr Probl Surg. 1992;29(1):1–56.
77. Apffelstaedt JP, Müller R. Results of mandatory exploration for penetrating neck trauma. World J Surg. 1994;18:917.
78. Shiroff AM, Gale SC, Martin ND, et al. Penetrating neck trauma: a review of management strategies and discussion of the 'No Zone' approach. Am Surg. 2013;79:23.
79. Phrampus P, Walker L. Danger zone: the prehospital assessment and treatment of blunt and penetrating neck trauma. JEMS. 2002;27(11):26–38.
80. Brysczynski J, Barrett T, Lyon J, et al. Management of penetrating neck injury in the emergency department: a structured literature review. Emerg Med J. 2008;25(11):711–5.
81. Weppner J. Improved mortality from penetrating neck and maxillofacial trauma using Foley catheter balloon tamponade in combat. J Trauma Acute Care Surg. 2013;75(2):220–4.
82. Humaidi GA. Carotid system ligation in surgical management of some maxillofacial hemorrhagic lesions and ich njuries. Thi-Qar Med J. 2010;4(3):11–23.

83. Fanning NF, Kahn A, Corbally MT. External carotid artery ligation for life-threatening hemorrhage in exsanguinating orbital facial congenital hemangiopericytoma. J Pediatr Surg. 1997;32(8):1252–4.
84. Faverani LP, Gaetti-Jardim EC, Ramalho-Fereirra G, Gulinelli JL, Queiroz TP, IR GJ. Ligature of external carotid artery as an Optional Technique in a Patient with von Willebrand disease. Braz Dent J. 2011;22(5):435–8.
85. Bouloux GF, Perciaccante VJ. Massive hemorrhage during oral and maxillofacial surgery: ligation of the external carotid artery or embolization? J Oral Maxillofac Surg. 2009;67(7):1547–51.
86. Nasr MM. Bilateral external carotid artery ligation: a lifesaving procedure in severe maxillofacial trauma. Int J Surg Case Rep. 2015;8:81–3.
87. Liston SL, Siegel LG. Claudication on mastication following bilateral external carotid ligation. Head Neck. 1990;12:269–71.
88. Singam P, Thanabalan J, Mohammed Z. Superselective embolisation for control of intractable epistaxis from maxillary artery injury. Biomed Imaging Interv J. 2011;7(1):e3.
89. Dubel GJ, Ahn SH, Soares GM. Transcatheter embolization in the management of epistaxis. Semin Intervent Radiol. 2013;30(3):249–62.
90. Nishimoto K, Minoda R, Yoshida R, Hirai T, Yumoto Y. A case of periodontal necrosis following embolization of maxillary artery for epistaxis. Case Rep Otolaryngol. 2016;2016, Article ID: 6467974.

51 Malignant Hyperthermia as a Complication of Maxillofacial Surgery

Adriana D. Oprea

Abstract

Malignant hyperthermia (MH) is a rare anesthetic complication. This chapter will discuss the prevalence, pathophysiology, and manifestations of the condition. The surgeon must be familiar as to how to work up and manage a patient who is at risk or has a diagnosis or family history of malignant hyperthermia. Offices in which agents associated with malignant hyperthermia are used must be appropriately equipped and supplied to monitor and intervene as the patient can rapidly deteriorate once the process begins.

51.1 Medical Disease

51.1.1 Pathophysiology

Malignant hyperthermia (MH) is a genetic and pharmacologic disorder characterized by development of a hypermetabolic state in susceptible patients exposed to "triggers" such as succinylcholine or inhalational anesthetics (with the exception of nitrous oxide) [1]. Susceptible individuals have genetic mutations resulting in skeletal muscle receptor abnormalities. In the presence of triggering factors (halogenated inhalational anesthetics or succinylcholine), excessive amounts of calcium are released from the sarcoplasmic reticulum in the cytoplasm leading to a hypermetabolic crisis. It is unclear what the interaction between anesthetics and the muscle receptor is.

51.1.2 Prevalence

While the exact prevalence of MH is unknown, the latest data show an MH episode can complicate 1:100,000 surgeries in adults and 1:30,000 in children. The genetic susceptibility for MH is more prevalent, being as high as 1:2000 patients in the general population, recent data reporting up to 1:400 prevalence in certain family cohorts [2, 3]. The prevalence varies by geographic location with Nebraska, Michigan, West Virginia, and Wisconsin having a higher incidence in the USA [2].

A.D. Oprea, M.D.
Department of Anesthesiology, Yale School of Medicine, New Haven, CT, USA
e-mail: adriana.oprea@yale.edu

© Springer International Publishing AG 2018

E.M. Ferneini, J.D. Bennett (eds.), *Perioperative Assessment of the Maxillofacial Surgery Patient*,
https://doi.org/10.1007/978-3-319-58868-1_51

51.1.3 Manifestations of Disease

Susceptible individuals do not manifest any clinical features unless exposed to triggering anesthetics.

In susceptible patients, exposure to triggering anesthetics can lead to a malignant hyperthermia crisis—characterized by a severe hypermetabolic state. Not all susceptible patients develop a crisis in response to a triggering anesthetic during the first exposure. It is believed that it may take up to three exposures before a crisis ensues.

In the presence of a triggering anesthetic (or sometimes due to excessive heat and stress), there is uncontrolled release of calcium from the sarcoplasmic reticulum mediating excessive excitation-contraction coupling cycles. This results in excessive muscle contraction, eventually leading to rhabdomyolysis.

The MH crisis manifests as a hypermetabolic state characterized by sinus tachycardia, hypercarbia (the first sign is a rising $EtCO_2$ in the absence of a decrease in minute ventilation), hyperthermia (with an increase in temperature of 1–2 degrees every 5 min), muscle rigidity, and metabolic acidosis.

The profound hypermetabolic states are further complicated by rhabdomyolysis leading to hyperkalemia and myoglobinuria resulting in acute renal failure. Further complications include congestive heart failure, bowel ischemia, compartment syndrome due to marked swelling, and DIC (which is the most usual cause of death when the hyperthermia exceeds 41 °F).

51.1.4 Anesthetic Risk

Susceptible individuals are those with mutations to the ryanodine receptor gene (RYR1) and the dihydropyridine receptor gene (DHP), either inherited in an autosomal dominant fashion or as new mutations. Also patients with a proven or suspected prior episode of malignant hyperthermia and patients with a family history of malignant hyperthermia should be considered susceptible and treated accordingly.

51.2 Preoperative Assessment

51.2.1 Preoperative Evaluation

Patients known to be susceptible to MH and those with a known causative RYR1 mutation do not require further testing, and a nontriggering anesthetic should be planned.

Patients with a personal or family history of an episode during anesthesia suspicious for MH should have the anesthetic record reviewed. Nonetheless, most patients susceptible to MH do not develop an acute MH episode with their first anesthetic. Most patients have a history of 2–3 episodes of uneventful anesthetics even with the use of triggering agents (succinylcholine or volatile anesthetics).

If the anesthetic records of a suspicious episode are available, a grading system can be used to determine whether a certain episode is likely to represent a true MH event.

This clinical grading system takes into account several clinical and laboratory values and based on the total score gives a probability of an episode representing an MH crisis [4] (Table 51.1).

Patients with a prior personal or familial episode graded at a score >20 should be tested for susceptibility to MH.

51.3 Laboratory Testing

The gold standard diagnostic method is the caffeine/halothane contracture test (CHCT). This consists in taking a fresh muscle biopsy from the thigh (3–4 in.) and testing the strength of muscle contracture to caffeine and halothane. The test can be done in special MH muscle biopsy centers in the USA (Winston-Salem, NC; Bethesda, MD; Davis, CA; Minneapolis, MN), and an unusually strong contracture indicates susceptibility to MH. The biopsy is collected under general anesthesia, using agents other than succinylcholine or volatile anesthetics, and can be performed in a patient with an episode concerning for MH crisis after 3–6 months since the event. Cost of muscle biopsy is ~ 2500 $ and most insurances cover the costs at least partially.

Table 51.1 Clinical grading for MH probability (Adapted with permission from Larach MG et al. Anesthesiology. 1994;80(4):771–9)

Process	Indicator (points)
Rigidity	Generalized muscular rigidity without shivering during or immediately following emergence from inhalational anesthesia (15 points) Masseter muscle spasm shortly following succinylcholine administration (15 points)
Rhabdomyolysis	CK >20,000 IU after anesthesia with succinylcholine (15 points) CK >10,000 IU after anesthesia without succinylcholine (15 points) Cola-colored urine in perioperative period (10 points) Urine myoglobin >60 mcg/L (5 points) Serum myoglobin >170 mcg/L (5 points) Serum K >6 mEq/L (without renal failure) (3 points)
Respiratory acidosis	Controlled ventilation $PETCO_2$ >55 (15 points) Controlled ventilation $PaCO_2$ >60 (15 points) Spontaneous ventilation $PETCO_2$ >60 (15 points) Spontaneous ventilation $PaCO_2$ >65 (15 points) Inappropriate hypercarbia (judgment) (15 points) Inappropriate tachypnea (judgment) (10 points)
Fever	Inappropriate rapid increase in temperature (judgment) (15 points) Inappropriate perioperative temperature >38.8 °C (judgment) (10 points)
Tachycardia	Inappropriate sinus tachycardia (3 points) Ventricular tachycardia or ventricular fibrillation (3 points)
Others	Base excess below −8 mEq/L (10 points) Arterial pH <7.25 (10 points) Rapid reversal of MH signs with dantrolene (5 points) Positive family history together with positive personal anesthetic history (not including elevated resting CK) (10 points) Resting elevated serum CK (in patient with positive family history) (10 points)

0 points MH rank = 1 and MH likelihood is almost never
3–9 points MH rank = 2 and MH likelihood is unlikely
10–19 points MH rank = 3 and MH likelihood is somewhat less than likely
20–34 points MH rank = 4 and MH likelihood is somewhat greater than likely
35–49 points MH rank = 5 and MH likelihood is very likely
50–108 points MH rank = 6 and MH likelihood is almost certain

Indications for the CHCT include:

- Patient with known MHS relative (as determined by positive muscle contracture test)
- Patient with MHS family member (as determined by past suspicious MH episode, but without a known RYR1 causative genetic mutation)
- Patient with past suspected MH event (wait 3–6 months post event, depending upon the degree of rhabdomyolysis)
- Patient with severe masseter muscle rigidity (MMR) during anesthesia with a triggering agent
- Patient with moderate to mild MMR with evidence of rhabdomyolysis

In addition, other patients are referred for CHCT, even without a history of anesthetic reaction. These include patients with a history of heat stroke, exercise-induced rhabdomyolysis, statin-induced myopathy, or myopathy of unknown etiology [5–9].

The test has a sensitivity of 97–99%, and a negative result practically rules out MH susceptibility [10]. Patients with a positive result should be considered MH susceptible, and a non-triggering anesthetic should be planned. There are reports of false positive results to the CHCT, but since not all mutations responsible for MH susceptibility have been identified, genetic testing would not change management.

Genetic testing should be offered to:

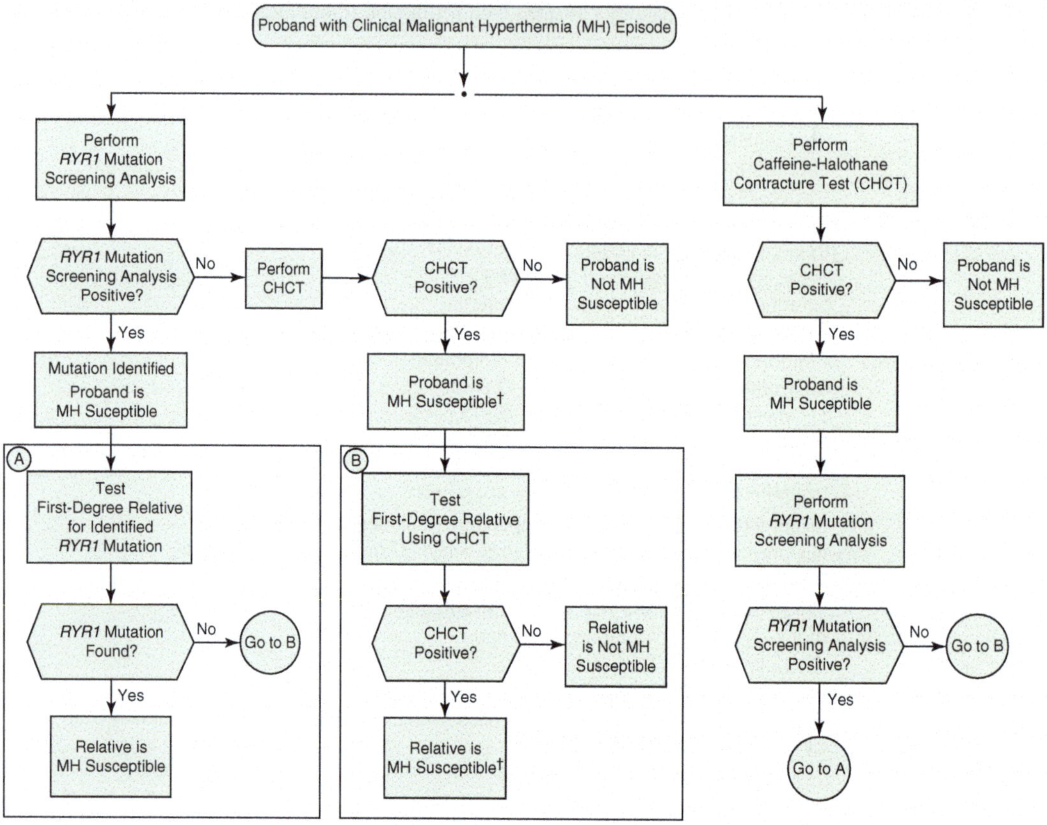

Fig. 51.1 Algorithm for testing family members of patients diagnosed with MH (adapted with permission from Litman RS. JAMA. 2005 Jun 15;293(23):2918–24)

- Patients with a positive CHCT (to assess for a specific mutation)
- Patient with a confirmed or highly suspicious clinical episode of MH
- Patients who have relatives with positive CHCT or genetic tests
- Patients who refuse to undergo CHCT despite having an episode suspicious for MH
- Patients with relatives with known causal RYR1 mutation

The advantage of the genetic testing is that it is noninvasive and less expensive; the disadvantage is that it only tests for specific known RYR1 mutations that represent only a percentage of the mutations responsible for MH susceptibility. However, in families where a causative mutation is identified, genetic testing obviates the need to undergo the CHCT in order to identify susceptibility to MH for family members of the affected individual [11].

A patient with a positive test is considered susceptible for MH, but a negative genetic test does not rule out MH, and the patient should be considered susceptible if the clinical scenario suggests it. Therefore, an MH negative diagnosis cannot be made using DNA testing.

Family members of patients diagnosed with malignant hyperthermia should be counseled and tested according to the following algorithm (Fig. 51.1).

51.4 Intraoperative Management

51.4.1 Anesthesia for the Malignant Hyperthermia-Susceptible Patient

Patients susceptible to MH can safely tolerate anesthesia as long as the anesthetic plan does not involve the use of succinylcholine or volatile anesthetics.

Patients should be monitored according to American Society of Anesthesiologists standards, including pulse oximeter, capnogram, ECG leads, blood pressure cuff, and temperature probe. Additional monitoring (i.e., arterial catheter) should be dictated by the patient's underlying medical conditions and the procedure planned, rather than the MH susceptibility status.

As per the Malignant Hyperthermia Association of the United States (MHAUS), the anesthesia machine should be prepared specifically for MH-susceptible cases. The preparation aims at removing any trace of volatile anesthetics from the machine. This preparation involves removal of anesthetic vaporizers from the machine, changing the soda lime to a new canister, flushing the machine with high flow (>10 L) oxygen for at least 20 min, and attaching a new circuit and a new bag [2]. The recommendation of 20-min flushing of the machine with high flow oxygen is based on older machines; therefore, for newer machines, manufacturer guideline recommendations should be followed to ensure lack of volatile anesthetics, until new recommendations from the MHAUS are formulated [12]. Also, placing a charcoal filter in the inspiratory limb of the circuit rapidly decreases the amount of volatile anesthetic [13].

In addition, an MH cart should be available outside the OR where an MH-susceptible patient is anesthetized. The contents of the MH cart are summarized below, according to recommendations from MHAUS [2] (Table 51.2).

Safe anesthetic options for MH-susceptible patients include monitored anesthesia care, neur-

Table 51.2 MH cart content

Medications	**Dantrium®/Revonto®** (36 vials) or **Ryanodex®** (3 vials) **Sterile water for injection (non-bacteriostatic)** (36 vials of 100 mL or 3 vials of 5 mL) **Sodium bicarbonate** 8.4%, 50 mL (5 prefilled syringes or vials) **Dextrose** 50%, 50 mL (2 prefilled syringes or vials) **Calcium chloride** 10%, 10 mL (2 vials) **Lidocaine** 2%, 100 mg/5 mL or 1% 100 mg/10 mL (4 prefilled syringes or vials)
Refrigerated drugs and solutions	**Insulin regular** 100 units/mL, 10 mL (1 vial) **0.9% normal saline** 1000 mL for IV cooling (4 bags and sterile pour bottles) **Cold packs** (8)
General equipment	**Syringes** 60 mL to dilute dantrolene (5 syringes) **IV catheters** (for IV access and arterial line) (4 each) **Nasogastric tubes** (various sizes) 60 cc **irrigation syringe** (2)
Monitoring equipment	**Esophageal or other core temperature probes** (e.g., for nasopharyngeal, tympanic membrane, rectal or bladder sites, or a pulmonary artery catheter) **Central venous pressure kits** (sizes appropriate to your patient population) **Transducer kits** for arterial and central venous cannulation
Nursing supplies	**Large sterile plastic drape** (e.g., Steri-Drape, for rapid drape of wound) (1) **Urine meter** (1) **Irrigation tray with piston** (60 cc irrigation) syringe (1) **Small and large clear plastic bags for ice** (4 each) **Bucket for ice** (1) **Test strips**: urine analysis for hemoglobin and finger-stick glucose (1 vial)
Laboratory testing supplies	**Syringes** (3 mL) for blood gas analysis or **ABG kits** × 6 or point-of-care monitors; **ISTAT** with TB syringes **Blood specimen tubes** for CPK, myoglobin, LDH, electrolytes, thyroid studies, PT/PTT, fibrinogen, fibrin split products, lactate, CBC **Urine collection container** for myoglobin level

axial or regional anesthetics, and general anesthetics as long as they don't involve triggering agents.

Anesthetic agents that are imperative to be avoided in patients with susceptibility to MH are:

- Succinylcholine (fastest onset of MH, regardless of other anesthetics used).
- Volatile anesthetics (sevoflurane, desflurane, halothane, enflurane, isoflurane)—onset of MH is faster with halothane and sevoflurane than with desflurane and isoflurane.

Safe anesthetics include:

- Nitrous oxide and xenon (as the only volatile anesthetics)
- Local anesthetics (e.g., bupivacaine, ropivacaine, mevacaine, lidocaine)
- Intravenous anesthetics (e.g., propofol, etomidate, thiopental, methohexital, ketamine, dexmedetomidine)
- Anxiolytics (midazolam)
- Narcotics (e.g., morphine, hydromorphone, fentanyl, remifentanil, alfentanil, sufentanil, demerol, methadone)
- Nondepolarizing muscle relaxants (e.g., rocuronium, vecuronium, cisatracurium, pancuronium)

Ambulatory/outpatient/office surgery is appropriate for MH-susceptible patients. A nontriggering anesthetic technique should be used. The same precautions should be observed when treating an MH-susceptible patient in the outpatient setting as far as machine preparation (charcoal filter, removal of the vaporizers, flushing the machine for >20 min) and avoidance of succinylcholine. The MHAUS recommends that an MH cart should be present in any facility (ambulatory center/office) where triggering anesthetics are present on site (succinylcholine, volatile anesthetics). Patients should be observed in the PACU postoperatively for ~2 h (concordant with standard recommendations) since an MH episode can be apparent up to 2 h postoperatively [14]. The ambulatory centers should have a plan in place in case of an MH crisis, which includes transferring the patient to the hospital for further management [15].

51.4.2 The Malignant Hyperthermia Crisis

The clinical manifestations of the MH crisis are nonspecific and usually include sinus tachycardia, hypercarbia, a rapid rise in temperature, and generalized muscle contracture. These signs appear most of the time during general anesthesia but can also develop in the early postoperative period (first 1–2 h). Temperature can rise abruptly by more than 1–2 °C per minute. Extreme temperature of >44 °C put the patient at risk for widespread organ failure and disseminated intravascular coagulation (DIC).

The rise in end-tidal CO_2 uncorrected by hyperventilation is the earliest sign, but since the decrease in the use of succinylcholine, the rise in CO_2 seen is less prominent than previously observed [1]. Due to the increased production of CO_2, the CO_2 absorbent rapidly changes color, and the canister becomes warm to touch due to the exothermic reaction of CO_2 neutralization.

Severe masseter muscle rigidity to the administration of succinylcholine is a concerning sign for development of MH (mild rigidity is a normal response and is of no concern).

Going unrecognized, the crisis progresses to generalized muscle contracture (pathognomonic for MH), hypermetabolism, depletion of intracellular ATP store, and rhabdomyolysis.

Later signs include metabolic acidosis, hyperkalemia with EKG changes, acute kidney failure due to myoglobinuria, ventricular arrhythmias due to hyperkalemia, and DIC.

51.4.2.1 Diagnosis of MH Crisis

The diagnosis of MH relies on a high index of suspicion, clinical features as described above, and laboratory tests. A suspicious episode should be considered MH if under general anesthesia when triggering agents have been used since most patients presenting with a crisis have a negative personal and family history of MH.

As detailed above, clinical signs include tachycardia, rise in end-tidal CO_2 uncorrected by ventilation, hyperthermia, and generalized muscle contracture especially in the presence of neuromuscular blockade.

Supporting laboratory values include a mixed respiratory and metabolic acidosis, hyperkalemia, increased CPK (>10,000 without succinylcholine and >20,000 with succinylcholine), increased serum, and urine myoglobin.

As the definitive diagnosis is done only by susceptibility testing with the use of the CHCT, a high index of suspicion should lead to initiation of treatment for MH (unless an alternate diagnosis is more likely).

51.4.3 Treatment of MH Crisis

Treatment of the MH crisis includes calling for additional personnel to help mix the dantrolene and declaring an emergency [16]. The MH cart should be brought to the OR where the MH case occurs and additional information is available from MHAUS Hotline at 1-800-644-9737. The surgeon should be informed and surgery should be postponed or aborted.

Treatment includes:

1. Optimization of ventilation: The respiratory rate and tidal volumes should be increased in order to increase minute ventilation and decrease the end-tidal CO_2. The patient should be placed on 100% O_2, and if not intubated, an endotracheal tube should be used to secure the airway (helped by the use of nondepolarizing muscle relaxants only)—change the system if a volatile agent was being used or is attached to the machine in a patient who was not known to be MH.
2. All triggering agents should be discontinued (volatile anesthetics should be stopped and replaced by total intravenous anesthetics) and all the vaporizers removed. There is no need to change the machine/circuit as it may take up valuable time in this emergent setting [16].
3. Administration of dantrolene: Dantrolene is the antidote for MH that abates the crisis within minutes of administration. The dose of dantrolene is 2.5 mg/kg and is administered as an intravenous bolus, followed by additional 1 mg/kg boluses given until the crisis resolves. The initial dose leads to resolution of the crisis in most cases, except for muscular patients who may require up to 10 mg/kg total dose or cases where the diagnosis is wrong.
   Dantrolene is available in the USA in two preparations:
   - Dantrium and Revonto are older preparations of 20 mg of lyophilized dantrolene, mixed with mannitol to maintain a certain pH. The vials are reconstituted with 60 mL sterile water. This preparation requires warming in order to help dissolve the drug and to hasten reconstitutions. Mixing nine vials gives the appropriate dose for a 70 kg man. Mixing dantrolene in these preparations requires additional personnel to be present and help.
   - Ryanodex is a more recent lyophilized preparation, the vials containing 250 mg of dantrolene each. The reconstitution is done with 5 mL sterile water vials and warming is not necessary. Therefore using Ryanodex is much easier, and this preparation may be more appropriate for the ambulatory center/office where limited resources may be available. The convenience of use should be balanced against the increase in cost (~7000 $ for Ryanodex versus ~ 3500–3600 $ for the older preparations) and by the shorter shelf life of Ryanodex (2 years versus 3 years for the older preparations).

   Dantrolene use can lead to muscle weakness, dizziness, dysphagia, and dyspnea and decrease inspiratory capacity. It should not be extravasated into the surrounding tissue, which can lead to tissue necrosis.

4. Treatment of hyperthermia: All patients with MH should have their core temperature monitored, and cooling should be initiated for patients with core temperatures of >39 °C. These measures should be continued until the core temperature drops below 38.5 °C. Options include infusing 2000–3000 mL of chilled (4 °C) saline solution intravenously, surface cooling with wet sheets, fans and axillary placed ice packs, and other cooling devices [16].

5. Treatment of acidosis: Hypercapnia should be addressed with hyperventilation, and bicarbonate solutions should be used if the pH is <7.2 [16].
6. Treatment of hyperkalemia: In patients where rhabdomyolysis is prominent, hyperkalemia needs to be monitored and treated with insulin/dextrose (50% dextrose, 50 mL and 50 IU of insulin), bicarbonate solution, or calcium chloride 0.1 mmol/kg (if EKG peaked T waves are present) [16]. These modalities lead to intracellular potassium transport but do not help eliminate potassium from the body. Definitive treatment for hyperkalemia entails administration of loop diuretics (furosemide, bumetanide) or exchange resins (Kayexalate).
7. Treatment of arrhythmias: Amiodarone 300 mg IV and beta blockers should be administered to treat the ventricular arrhythmias, and ACLS protocols should be followed.
8. Monitoring and treatment of metabolic acidosis: While the metabolic disturbances usually start as a respiratory acidosis, MH leads to a combined respiratory and metabolic acidosis. Bicarbonate boluses or infusion should be used to control the metabolic acidosis [16].
9. Monitoring of rhabdomyolysis: The patient should be clinically monitored for the development of compartment syndrome, and serum CPK, serum, and urine myoglobin should be measured. Compartment syndrome may require fasciotomy.
10. Monitoring the renal function: A Foley catheter should be inserted, and the urine output measured. Presence of red-/tea-colored urine, testing negative for RBCs but positive for blood, is indicative of myoglobinuria. Measures should be instituted to reduce the risk of acute tubular necrosis due to pigment nephropathy—these include hydration and maintenance of a urine output of >2 mL/kg/h and urine alkalinization with sodium bicarbonate. In addition, mannitol 1 g/kg or furosemide 0.5–1 mg/kg can be used to maintain the urine output as long as aggressive hydration is also undertaken [16].
11. Monitoring for DIC: Patients that reach high temperatures (>40 °C) are at higher risk of developing DIC and should be monitored with measurement of standard coagulation tests (PT/INR, PTT, fibrinogen, fibrin split products).

51.5 Postoperative Management

Postoperative monitoring should be done for at least the first 24 h after the episode of MH. Stable patients whose crises have been aborted early can be safely observed in a step down unit [16].

Patients with full-blown crises should be admitted to the intensive care unit until fever decreases to <38 °C, muscle rigidity resolves, metabolic stability is ensured, CPK levels decrease, and myoglobinuria resolves.

There can be recurrence of symptoms in a fourth of cases up to 24 h after the initial episode. Therefore, the patient with a full-blown crisis should be maintained on dantrolene 1 mg/kg every 4–6 h or an intravenous infusion of 0.25 mg/kg/h for the first 24 h.

Following recovery from the MH episode, the patient should be counseled appropriately, including being referred to a muscle biopsy center for definitive diagnosis and avoiding strenuous exercise which can result in excessive rhabdomyolysis. Family members should be also counseled given the disease's genetic component.

Conclusion

Malignant hyperthermia can rapidly result in significant morbidity and mortality. The first step in management is to recognize the at-risk patient and modify the anesthetic appropriately. Patients who are at risk can be managed safely if the appropriate modifications are taken. All facilities that administer anesthetics associated with malignant hyperthermia must be equipped to intervene immediately.

References

1. Rosenberg H, Pollock N, Schiemann A, Bulger T, Stowell K. Malignant hyperthermia: a review. Orphanet J Rare Dis. 2015;10:93.
2. Malignant Hyperthermia Association of the United States; 2016.
3. Gonsalves SG, Ng D, Johnston JJ, Teer JK, Stenson PD, Cooper DN, Mullikin JC, Biesecker LG, Program NCS. Using exome data to identify malignant hyperthermia susceptibility mutations. Anesthesiology. 2013;119:1043–53.
4. Larach MG, Localio AR, Allen GC, Denborough MA, Ellis FR, Gronert GA, Kaplan RF, Muldoon SM, Nelson TE, Ording H. A clinical grading scale to predict malignant hyperthermia susceptibility. Anesthesiology. 1994;80:771–9.
5. Tobin JR, Jason DR, Challa VR, Nelson TE, Sambuughin N. Malignant hyperthermia and apparent heat stroke. JAMA. 2001;286:168–9.
6. Köchling A, Wappler F, Winkler G, Schulte am Esch JS. Rhabdomyolysis following severe physical exercise in a patient with predisposition to malignant hyperthermia. Anaesth Intensive Care. 1998;26:315–8.
7. Wappler F, Fiege M, Steinfath M, Agarwal K, Scholz J, Singh S, Matschke J, Schulte Am Esch J. Evidence for susceptibility to malignant hyperthermia in patients with exercise-induced rhabdomyolysis. Anesthesiology. 2001;94:95–100.
8. Vladutiu GD, Isackson PJ, Kaufman K, Harley JB, Cobb B, Christopher-Stine L, Wortmann RL. Genetic risk for malignant hyperthermia in non-anesthesia-induced myopathies. Mol Genet Metab. 2011;104:167–73.
9. Krivosic-Horber R, Dépret T, Wagner JM, Maurage CA. Malignant hyperthermia susceptibility revealed by increased serum creatine kinase concentrations during statin treatment. Eur J Anaesthesiol. 2004;21:572–4.
10. Allen GC, Larach MG, Kunselman AR. The sensitivity and specificity of the caffeine-halothane contracture test: a report from the North American Malignant Hyperthermia Registry. The North American Malignant Hyperthermia Registry of MHAUS. Anesthesiology. 1998;88:579–88.
11. Stowell KM. DNA testing for malignant hyperthermia: the reality and the dream. Anesth Analg. 2014;118:397–406.
12. Kim TW, Nemergut ME. Preparation of modern anesthesia workstations for malignant hyperthermia-susceptible patients: a review of past and present practice. Anesthesiology. 2011;114:205–12.
13. Wappler F. Anesthesia for patients with a history of malignant hyperthermia. Curr Opin Anaesthesiol. 2010;23:417–22.
14. Barnes C, Stowell KM, Bulger T, Langton E, Pollock N. Safe duration of postoperative monitoring for malignant hyperthermia patients administered non-triggering anaesthesia: an update. Anaesth Intensive Care. 2015;43:98–104.
15. Brandom BW. Ambulatory surgery and malignant hyperthermia. Curr Opin Anaesthesiol. 2009;22:744–7.
16. Glahn KP, Ellis FR, Halsall PJ, Müller CR, Snoeck MM, Urwyler A, Wappler F. Recognizing and managing a malignant hyperthermia crisis: guidelines from the European Malignant Hyperthermia Group. Br J Anaesth. 2010;105:417–20.

The manufacturer's authorised representative in the EU is Springer Nature Customer Service Centre GmbH, Europaplatz 3, 69115 Heidelberg, Germany. If you have any concerns regarding our products, please contact ProductSafety@springernature.com

Printed and bound by CPI Group (UK) Ltd, Croydon, CR0 4YY
05/10/2026
02228134-0006